Differential Dia nary Disease

Charles V. Pollack, Jr.
Editor

Differential Diagnosis of Cardiopulmonary Disease

A Handbook

Springer

Editor
Charles V. Pollack, Jr.
Department of Emergency Medicine
Thomas Jefferson University
Philadelphia, PA, USA

ISBN 978-3-319-63894-2   ISBN 978-3-319-63895-9 (eBook)
https://doi.org/10.1007/978-3-319-63895-9

Library of Congress Control Number: 2019935819

This Springer imprint is published by the registered company Springer Nature Switzerland AG
The registered company address is: Gewerbestrasse 11, 6330 Cham, Switzerland

Preface

This book is intended to be a ready resource and guide for the evaluation of common symptoms and syndromes that originate in the primary cardiopulmonary system. It should prove particularly useful in the generation of a working differential diagnosis, consideration of diagnostic approach, and initial management decisions. It is not intended to be a comprehensive resource; rather, it follows the classic "emergency medicine approach" of considering first the worst-case scenario, and then exploring other possibilities quickly and efficiently. The image, video, and audio links embedded in the text should help the learner correlate bedside findings with reference material.

It is our hope that this guide will streamline the diagnostic approach to patients with "thoracic" complaints and make the learner more confident in his or her skills. The focus of this book is on differential diagnosis, confirmation of diagnosis, and essential steps towards initiating treatment. Therapeutic modalities change more rapidly that diagnostic approach and may have evolved since a specific chapter was completed. Treatment should always be guided by the latest literature, but is founded upon solid diagnostic acumen.

Philadelphia, PA, USA

Charles V. Pollack, Jr.

Contents

Contributors

Jaime Friel Blanck, MLIS, MPA Welch Medical Library, Johns Hopkins University, Baltimore, MD, USA

Richard M. Cantor, MD, FAAP, FACEP Department of Emergency Medicine and Pediatrics, State University of New York Upstate Medical University, Syracuse, NY, USA

Melissa Platt, MD, FACEP Department of Emergency Medicine, University of Louisville, Louisville, KY, USA

Charles V. Pollack, Jr. MA, MD, FACEP, FAAEM, FAHA, FESC, FCPP Department of Emergency Medicine, Thomas Jefferson University, Philadelphia, PA, USA

Christopher J. Rees, MD Emergency Department, Pennsylvania Hospital, Philadelphia, PA, USA

Victoria G. Riese, MLIS, AHIP Librarian Consultant, Eldersburg, MD, USA

Chapter 1
Achalasia

Christopher J. Rees, Victoria G. Riese, and Charles V. Pollack, Jr.

Name and Synonyms

Achalasia

Incidence/Epidemiology

- Achalasia is a rare disease with an annual incidence of 1–2/100,000 persons.
- It affects men and women with equal frequency.
- It usually presents between the ages of 20 and 40, but may occur at any adult age.
- Onset before adolescence is rare.

Differential Diagnosis

- Achalasia is the most common motility disorder of the esophagus.
- It most often causes dysphagia (difficulty swallowing, as opposed to odynophagia—painful swallowing), so the differential is the differential for dysphagia.

C. J. Rees
Emergency Department, Pennsylvania Hospital, Philadelphia, PA, USA

V. G. Riese
Librarian Consultant, Eldersburg, MD, USA

C. V. Pollack, Jr. (✉)
Department of Emergency Medicine, Thomas Jefferson University,
Philadelphia, PA, USA

C. V. Pollack, Jr. (ed.), *Differential Diagnosis of Cardiopulmonary Disease*,
https://doi.org/10.1007/978-3-319-63895-9_1

- Other diseases that may present with dysphagia and associated esophageal dilatation (secondary achalasia) include gastric cancer; infiltrative diseases such as amyloidosis, sarcoidosis, eosinophilic gastritis, and neurofibromatosis; and infections such as Chagas disease in South America.

Pathophysiology and Etiology

- Achalasia is a motility disorder of the esophagus; the cause is unknown.
- Histopathologically, achalasia is associated with degeneration of neurons in the myenteric plexus of the esophageal wall near the lower esophageal sphincter (LES). There is also an associated inflammatory response with an influx of inflammatory cells.
- The degeneration is most marked within the inhibitory neurons that allow for relaxation of the LES. This leads to a sustained contraction/increase in tone of the LES, resulting in an increase in LES pressure.
- Degeneration of the inhibitory neurons within the myenteric plexus in the lower two thirds of the esophagus affects the smooth muscle and causes aperistalsis.
- The cause of the degeneration is unknown. It has been ascribed to autoimmune phenomenon and sometimes to chronic viral infections from herpes simplex virus, measles virus, and HSV-1, but there is no conclusive evidence for any of these putative mechanisms.

Presentation

Typical/"Classic"

- Dysphagia (difficulty with swallowing) is the most common presenting symptom of achalasia, occurring in about 90 % of patients. Typically, the dysphagia is to solids and liquids equally.
- Most patients (about 75 %) also report regurgitation of undigested food. The regurgitated food remains in the esophagus, so usually there is no "acid taste" as in reflux. This has been described as a "bland reflux."
- Many patients describe an epigastric or retrosternal fullness after eating that may be severe enough to provoke attempts to induce vomiting, leading to confusion with eating disorders.
- Other commonly reported symptoms include difficulty belching, substernal chest pain associated with reflux, and frequent hiccups.
- Symptoms usually progress gradually. The mean time from symptom onset until diagnosis is about 5 years. This reflects the insidious nature of the symptoms, more than any particular difficulty in diagnosis.

- Some patients are noted to perform mechanical maneuvers (raising the arms above the head, standing erect and hyperextending the back) to help clear the esophagus. These actions may be noticed more by family members.

Atypical

- In retrospect, most patients will have years of somewhat typical symptoms before presentation.
- Most patients will have been treated for gastroesophageal reflux (GERD) before consideration of the diagnosis.
- Patients may present with chest pain, especially with eating. This may have been considered esophageal spasm and not responded to treatment.

Primary Differential Considerations

- Other causes of dysphagia should be considered, including
  - Esophageal tumors
  - Reflux /GERD
  - Connective tissue disorders, such as systemic sclerosis
  - Esophageal perforation
  - Esophageal spasm or stricture
  - Gastric cancer that involves the lower esophagus
  - Much rarer considerations:
    - Chagas disease
    - Plummer–Vinson syndrome

History and Physical Exam

Findings That Confirm Diagnosis

- The history usually is very suggestive of the diagnosis, although there are no absolutely confirmatory findings on history and physical exam. Physical exam usually is normal, although patients may have unintended weight loss.
- Confirmation is with esophageal manometry.

Factors That Suggest Diagnosis

- The historical features as described above suggest the diagnosis.
- An especially suggestive historical feature is dysphagia to solids and liquids equally.

Factors That Exclude Diagnosis

- Early in the course of illness, esophageal manometry may be nondiagnostic, so a high index of suspicion needs to be maintained if the symptoms continue or progress.

Ancillary Studies

Laboratory

- Lab tests generally are not helpful in the diagnosis.

Imaging

- Chest x-ray may demonstrate widening of the esophagus or mediastinum, but more commonly is normal, especially early in the disease course.
- Barium swallowing studies may be helpful in suggesting the diagnosis, especially later in the course of illness.
- Classically, the barium esophagram demonstrates a proximally dilated esophagus that narrows to a contracted gastroesophageal junction, giving the classic "bird-beak" appearance of the esophagus.

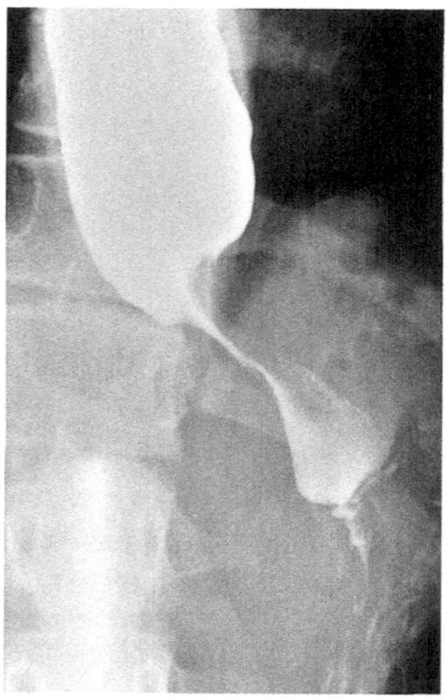

Classic "bird-beak" appearance of the esophagus on barium esophagram in achalasia. [Mittal R. Esophageal motor disorders. In: Orlando RC, editor. Atlas of esophageal diseases. 2nd ed. Philadelphia: Current Medicine; 2002. p 163–78.]

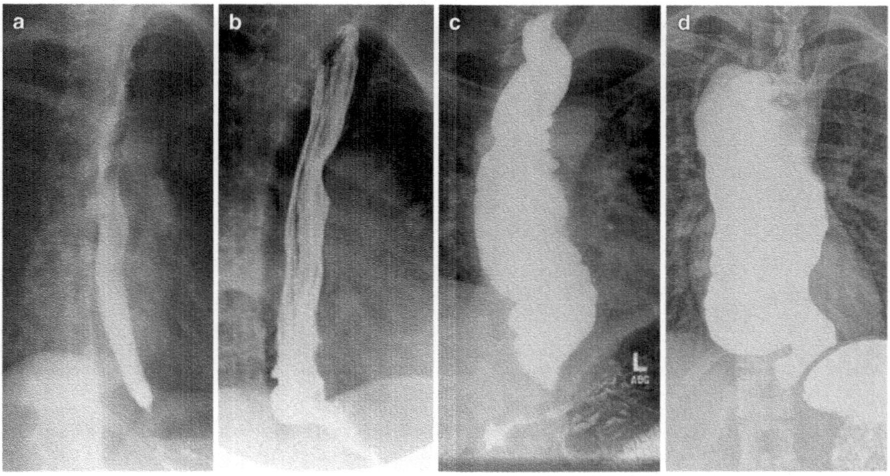

Examples of progressive dilation of the esophagus in different patients with achalasia. a Normal diameter esophagus leading to a bird's beak at the LES. b Minimal esophageal dilation (from 4 to 7 cm). c Progressive esophageal dilation (from 7 to 10 cm) with preserved esophageal axis. d Greater dilation (>10 cm) and initial sigmoidal course of the distal esophagus. [From article: A controversy that has been tough to swallow: is the treatment of achalasia now digested? J Gastrointest Surg. 2010 Feb;14 Suppl 1:S33-45. https://doi.org/10.1007/s11605-009-1013-5, at http://link.springer.com/article/10.1007%2Fs11605-009-1013-5; by Garrett R. Roll, Charlotte Rabl, Ruxandra Ciovica, Sofia Peeva, Guilherme M. Campos, © The Author(s) 2009; licensed under Creative Commons Attribution Noncommercial License https://creativecommons.org/licenses/by-nc/2.0/] *Caption from original*

- Other suggestive findings on barium study include a dilated esophagus, aperistalsis of the esophagus, and poor/delayed emptying of the barium into the stomach.
- Barium studies may be falsely negative in up to one third of cases.
- The diagnosis usually is confirmed by esophageal manometry, which is usually performed at specialized, experienced centers.
- Currently, the procedure of choice is high-resolution manometry (HRM) with or without esophageal pressure topography (HRMEPT).
- The classic finding on manometry is aperistalsis of the distal two thirds of the esophagus with incomplete relaxation of the LES. Increased pressure within the LES is a supportive finding but is not diagnostic.
- HRMEPT allows subtyping of achalasia, which may help in deciding treatment.
- Endoscopy (usually done when considering esophagitis, peptic ulcer disease, or gastritis in the diagnosis) usually is normal, though itmay demonstrate a dilated esophagus with retained products.

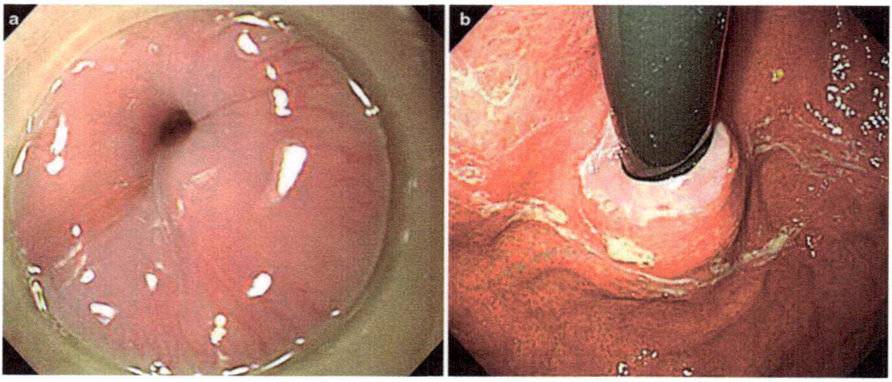

Endoscopic appearance of achalasia. (**a**) Sustained contraction of the lower esophageal sphincter as viewed from the proximal esophagus. (**b**) Retroflexed view of the LES from the stomach. [Park JM. Miscellaneous esophageal diseases. In: Chun HJ, Yang S-K, Choi M-G, editors. Clinical gastrointestinal endoscopy: a comprehensive atlas. Heidelberg: Springer. 2014. p. 87–98.] *Caption adapted from original*

Special Populations

Age

- Achalasia usually presents between the ages of 20 and 40 but may occur at any adult age.
- May be seen in adolescence, but is rare.

Pitfalls in Diagnosis

Critical Steps Not to Miss

- Consideration of the diagnosis is the first step.
- It is critical to consider malignancy in the differential diagnosis.

Mimics

- Any disease process that presents predominately with dysphagia can mimic achalasia.

- It is important to consider malignancy and other mechanical causes of dysphagia.
- Gastric cancer close to the gastroesophageal junction is a mimic of achalasia that must be considered.
- Space-occupying lesions (such as cancer) usually present with dysphagia that is greater with solids than liquids, but as they enlarge, they may produce dysphagia to both.
- Another diagnosis that may be confused with achalasia when evaluating a patient for dysphagia is myasthenia gravis. Myasthenia usually produces both dysphagia and dysphonia (decrease in tone/quality of voice).

Time-Dependent Interventions

- There are no particular time-dependent interventions in the evaluation of achalasia other than consideration of and evaluation for malignancy.

Overall Principles of Treatment

- Treatment is aimed at reducing the resting pressure of the LES.
- The first step usually is progressive, endoscopy-guided dilatation of the LES.
- If symptoms persist after three attempts at dilatation, or patients cannot tolerate dilatation, surgical myotomy often is performed.
- Patients who are not surgical candidates, or those who decline surgery, may be offered a trial of endoscopically guided direct injection of botulinum toxin into the LES.
- If all other treatments are unsuccessful, or the patient is not a candidate for surgery or endoscopy, a trial of oral nitrates or calcium channel blockers may be attempted.

Disease Course

- Achalasia is a chronically progressive disease; without treatment, esophageal dilatation will continue.
- Ten to fifteen percent of patients will develop end-stage disease even with treatment.
- Up to 5 % eventually may require complete esophagectomy, especially when the esophageal diameter exceeds 6 cm (megaesophagus).
- Patients with achalasia are at increased risk for squamous cell carcinoma of the esophagus. The absolute risk is low, however, so endoscopic surveillance is not recommended.

Related Evidence

Papers of particular interest have been highlighted as:
*** Of key importance*

Practice Guideline

Vaezi MF, Pandolfino JE, Vela MF. ACG clinical guideline: diagnosis and management of achalasia. Am J Gastroenterol. 2013 Aug;108(8):1238–49; quiz 1250. https://doi.org/10.1038/ajg.2013.196. PMID: 23877351. http://www.ncbi.nlm.nih.gov/pubmed/23877351 **

Stefanidis D, Richardson W, Farrell TM, Kohn GP, Augenstein V, Fanelli RD; Society of American Gastrointestinal and Endoscopic Surgeons. SAGES guidelines for the surgical treatment of esophageal achalasia. Surg Endosc. 2012 Feb;26(2):296–311. https://doi.org/10.1007/s00464-011-2017-2. PMID: 22044977. http://www.ncbi.nlm.nih.gov/pubmed/22044977 **

Review

Dobrowolsky A, Fisichella PM. The management of esophageal achalasia: from diagnosis to surgical treatment. Updates Surg. 2014 Mar;66(1):23–9. https://doi.org/10.1007/s13304-013-0224-1. PMID: 23817763. http://www.ncbi.nlm.nih.gov/pubmed/23817763 **

Boeckxstaens GE, Zaninotto G, Richter JE. Achalasia. Lancet. 2014 Jan 4;383(9911):83–93. https://doi.org/10.1016/S0140-6736(13)60651-0. PMID: 23871090. http://www.ncbi.nlm.nih.gov/pubmed/23871090 **

Allaix ME, Patti MG. What is the best primary therapy for achalasia: medical or surgical treatment? Who owns achalasia? J Gastrointest Surg. 2013 Sep;17(9):1547–9. https://doi.org/10.1007/s11605-013-2252-z. PMID: 23780637. http://www.ncbi.nlm.nih.gov/pubmed/23780637

O'Neill OM, Johnston BT, Coleman HG. Achalasia: a review of clinical diagnosis, epidemiology, treatment and outcomes. World J Gastroenterol. 2013 Sep 21;19(35):5806–12. https://doi.org/10.3748/wjg.v19.i35.5806. PMID: 24124325. http://www.ncbi.nlm.nih.gov/pubmed/24124325 **

Pandolfino JE, Kahrilas PJ. Presentation, diagnosis, and management of achalasia. Clin Gastroenterol Hepatol. 2013 Aug;11(8):887–97. https://doi.org/10.1016/j.cgh.2013.01.032. PMID: 23395699. http://www.ncbi.nlm.nih.gov/pubmed/23395699 **

Cohort Study

Sadowski DC, Ackah F, Jiang B, Svenson LW. Achalasia: incidence, prevalence and survival. A population-based study. Neurogastroenterol Motil. 2010 Sep;22(9):e256–61. https://doi.org/10.1111/j.1365-2982.2010.01511.x. PMID: 20465592. http://www.ncbi.nlm.nih.gov/pubmed/20465592

Use PubMed Clinical Queries to find the most recent evidence. Use this search strategy:
"Esophageal Achalasia"[Mesh] OR "Achalasia"

Chapter 2
Acute Coronary Syndrome: Non–ST-Segment Elevation Myocardial Infarction

Charles V. Pollack, Jr. and Victoria G. Riese

Name and Synonyms

Non–ST-Segment Elevation Myocardial Infarction

- NSTEMI, subendocardial MI, non-Q-wave MI (NQMI), troponin-positive ACS

Incidence/Epidemiology

- In the middle of the continuum of diagnoses collectively called acute coronary syndrome (ACS)—between unstable angina (UA) and ST-segment elevation MI (STEMI).
- More common than STEMI.

C. V. Pollack, Jr. (✉)
Department of Emergency Medicine, Thomas Jefferson University, Philadelphia, PA, USA

V. G. Riese
Librarian Consultant, Eldersburg, MD, USA

C. V. Pollack, Jr. (ed.), *Differential Diagnosis of Cardiopulmonary Disease*,
https://doi.org/10.1007/978-3-319-63895-9_2

	STEMI	NSTEMI/UA
Pathogenesis	Fully occlusive thrombus	Less than fully occlusive thrombus
Incidence		Higher than that of STEMI
Patient profile		Older; higher co-morbidity (diabetes, renal failure) than STEMI patients
Time course	Minutes to hours	Up to a few days
Clinical manifestations		Similar to STEMI
Imaging studies		Similar to STEMI
EKG	ST elevations	No ST elevations[a]
Biomarkers	Elevated	Elevated
Therapy	See Table 2.54	See Table 2.54
Rehabilitation		Similar to STEMI
Complications		Similar to STEMI
Prognosis		Mortality lower in-hospital, higher at 6 months and 4 years than with STEMI

[a]ST elevations may be seen in Prinzmetal's angina

STEMI and NSTEMI/UA: a comparison. [Adelmann GA. Coronary artery disease. In: Adelmann GA, editor. Cardiology essentials in clinical practice. London: Springer; 2011. p. 23–95. Book https://doi.org/10.1007/978-1-84996-305-3] *Caption from original*

- Incidence varies widely by demographics and risk profiles; patients with NSTEMI tend to be older and have more co-morbidities than STEMI patients.
- Of the more than 1.2 million MIs in United States each year; most are NSTEMI, and as troponin assays become increasingly sensitive, there are fewer cases diagnosed as UA and more as NSTEMI.

Differential Diagnosis

- Includes all other causes of chest pain.
- Includes other causes of "anginal equivalents" in susceptible populations, e.g.:
  - Dyspnea
  - Back pain
  - Jaw pain
  - Shoulder pain
  - Epigastric pain
  - Palpitations
  - Dizziness
  - Weakness
  - Nausea
  - Syncope

Pathophysiology and Etiology

- ACS is the result of ischemia (diminished blood flow / oxygen delivery) to myocardium.
- If ischemia persists, frank infarction (muscle death) may occur.
- Infarction results in breakdown of cell membranes, allowing release of intracellular proteins (such as myoglobin, troponins, and CPK-MB) into the circulation, where they may be detected in peripheral blood.
- NSTEMI is defined by this protein (enzyme) "leak," and it is that lab finding that differentiates it from UA.
  - Other causes of elevated troponin include:
    - Renal insufficiency
    - Heart failure
    - Pulmonary embolism
    - Septic shock
    - Nonthrombotic causes

Demand ischemia: a mismatch between myocardial oxygen demand and supply in the absence of flow-limiting stenosis (i.e., systemic inflammatory response, hypotension, tachyarrthmias)
Myocardial ischemia in the absence of fixed obstructive coronary disease: an imbalance of the autonomic nervous system and increased catecholamine effect on the myocardial cells (i.e., vasospastic angina, acute stroke or intracranial hemorrhage and subarachnoid hemorrhage)
Direct myocardial damage: cell injury by traumatic or inflammatory process (i.e., pericarditis and myocarditis)
Myocardial strain: volume and pressure overload of both ventricles (i.e., congestive heart failure, pulmonary embolism)

Nonthrombotic mechanisms of troponin elevation in ICU setting. [Lazzeri C, Bonizzoli M, Cianchi G, Gensini GF, Peris A. Troponin I in the intensive care unit setting: from the heart to the heart. Intern Emerg Med. 2008 Mar;3(1):9-16. https://doi.org/10.1007/s11739-008-0089-3] *Caption from original*

- Most NSTEMI occurs as a result of fracture or frank rupture of atherosclerotic plaque in an epicardial artery, but often the artery that is fully occluded is downstream from the plaque and is actually occluded by a platelet aggregate embolism from upstream. It also may occur from incomplete obstruction at the site of plaque and poor collateral circulation upstream.

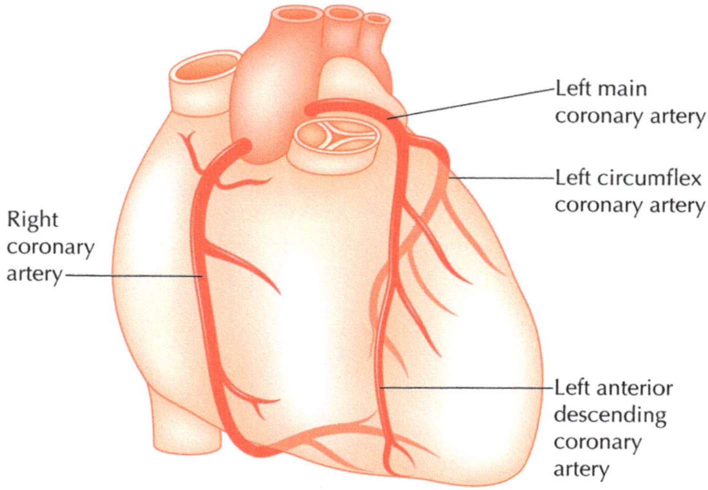

Normal coronary anatomy. [Achenbach S. Normal coronary anatomy. In: Budoff MJ, Narula J, Achenbach SS, editors. Atlas of cardiovascular computed tomography. Philadelphia: Current Medicine; 2007] *Caption from original*

- Atherosclerosis is a product of diverse inherited and acquired conditions, including:
  - Family history
  - Hyperlipidemia
  - Hypertension
  - Diabetes mellitus
  - Tobacco abuse

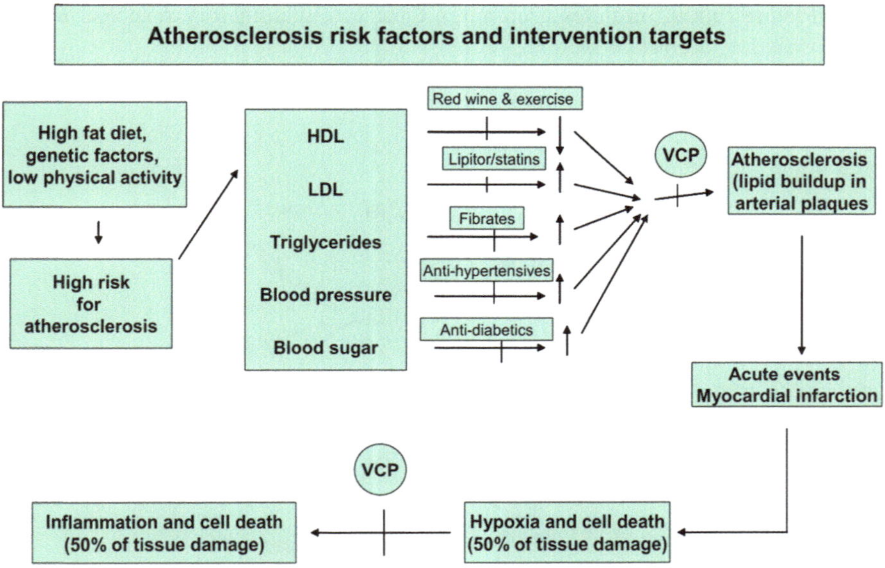

Atherosclerosis risk factors and intervention targets. [Thorbjornsdottir P, Thorgeirsson G, Kotwal GJ, Arason GJ. Control of inflammation with complement control agents to prevent atherosclerosis. In: Suri JS, Kathuria C, Molinari F, editors. Atherosclerosis disease management. New York: Springer; 2011. p. 633-75. Book https://doi.org/10.1007/978-1-4419-7222-4] *Caption adapted from original*

Risk factors	No. of patients
Individual	
Smoking	6
Hypertension	11
Hypercholesterolemia	9
Diabetes mellitus	4
Clusters	
Smoking and hypercholesterolemia	1
Hypertension and hypercholesterolemia[a]	4
Hypertension and diabetes	2
Smoking, hypertension and hypercholesterolemia	1
Smoking, hypertension, hypercholesterolemia and diabetes	2

[a] Hypertension was defined as a diastolic arterial pressure >95 mm Hg and hypercholesterolemia >6 mmol/l

Main known risk factors for atherosclerosis in 16 patients studied. [Watt S, Aesch B, Lanotte P, Tranquart F, Quentin R. Viral and bacterial DNA in carotid atherosclerotic lesions. Eur J Clin Microbiol Infect Dis. 2003 Feb;22(2):99-105. https://doi.org/10.1007/s10096-002-0867-1] *Caption adapted from original*

- Plaque rupture initiates a complex thrombo-inflammatory response locally including activation of:
  - Coagulation

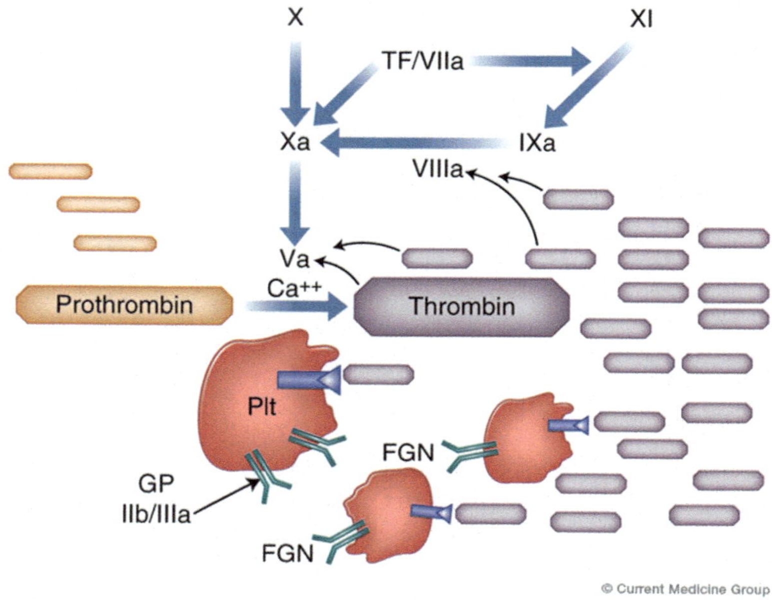

Networking of coagulation cascade and aggregation of platelets (Plt). The extrinsic limb triggers activation of the coagulation cascade when tissue factor (TF) is exposed in a disrupted plaque. Coagulation factor VII is activated (VIIa) and can activate factor X to Xa and promote perpetuation of the coagulation process via the intrinsic limb that results in formation of IXa and VIIIa. The prothrombinase complex of Xa, Va, Ca^{++} forms on a phospholipid surface (*eg*, membrane of a platelet) and converts prothrombin to thrombin. The thrombin that is formed binds to the thrombin receptor on platelets promoting activation and aggregation of platelets, as well as amplifying the coagulation cascade by promoting formation of VIIIa and Va. This diagram depicts the amplification nature of the coagulation process because one molecule of Xa leads to the downstream production of a large number of thrombin molecules (stoichiometric relationship not completely depicted to prevent obscuring the diagram with thrombin molecules). Activated platelets express numerous copies of the active form of the fibrinogen receptor GP IIb/IIIa on their surface. GP IIb/IIIa recognizes specific amino acid sequences on circulating ligands. One such ligand is fibrinogen (FGN), which has multiple copies of the RGD amino acid sequence and serves to bridge platelets together, promoting formation of aggregates. The more aggregates formed, the greater the surface area for the prothrombinase complex and amplification of the reactions of the coagulation cascade. [Antman E. Acute coronary syndromes. In: Libby P, editor. Essential atlas of cardiovascular disease. Philadelphia: Current Medicine; 2009. ISBN: 978-1-57340-309-2] *Caption from original*

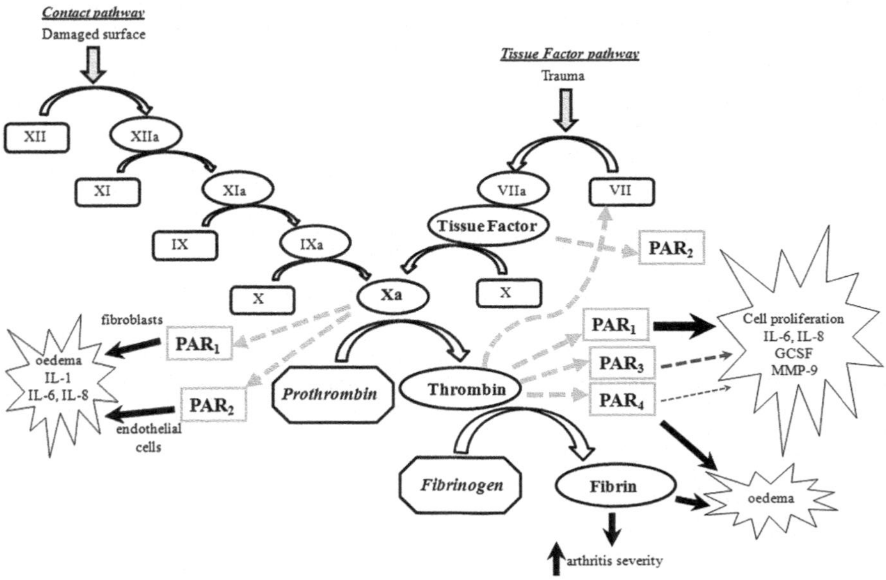

A simplified diagram of the coagulation cascade and its links with PARs and inflammation. Two pathways are involved in coagulation, with the major one being the tissue factor pathway. Most of the coagulation factors are serine proteinases that are present as inactive zymogens (rectangles) that when activated (ovals; lowercase 'a' indicates an active form) can catalyze the next reaction in the cascade. The two pathways converge to activate factor X, thrombin and fibrin. [Russell FA, McDougall JJ. Proteinase-activated receptors and arthritis. In: Vergnolle N, Chignard M, editors. Proteases and their receptors in inflammation. Basel: Springer; 2011. p. 217-42. Book https://doi.org/10.1007/978-3-0348-0157-7] *Caption adapted from original*

- Platelets

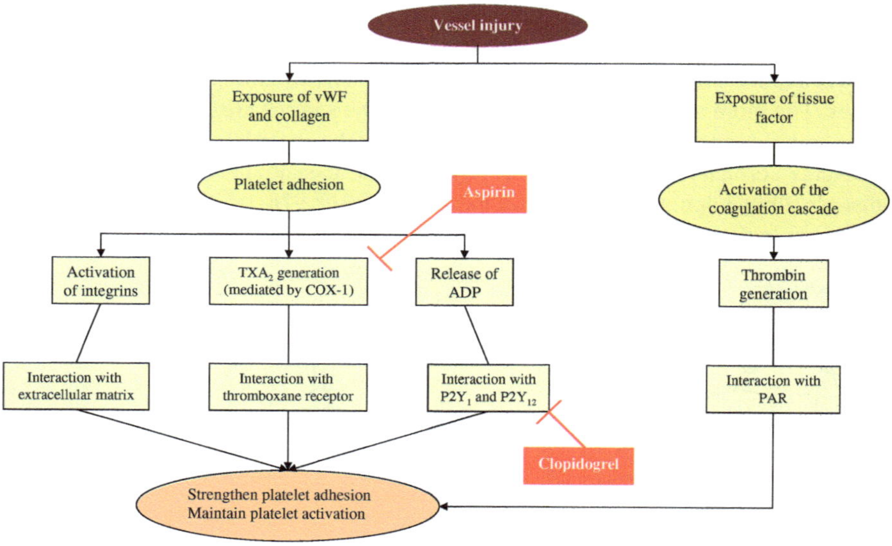

Mechanisms of platelet activation. [Ajjan R, Storey RF, Grant PJ. Aspirin resistance and diabetes mellitus. Diabetologia. 2008 Mar;51(3):385-90. https://doi.org/10.1007/s00125-007-0898-3] *Caption adapted from original*

- Complement

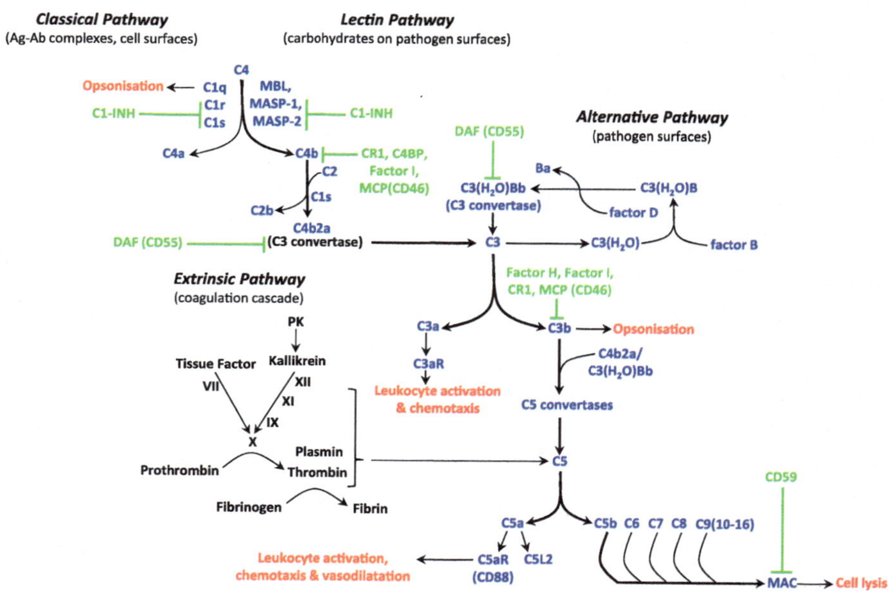

Common pathways for complement activation. [From article: Complement activation in the injured central nervous system: another dual-edged sword? J Neuroinflammation. 2012 Jun 21;9:137. https://doi.org/10.1186/1742-2094-9-137

at http://link.springer.com/article/10.1186/1742-2094-9-137 by Faith H Brennan, Aileen J Anderson, Stephen M Taylor, Trent M Woodruff, Marc J Ruitenberg, © 2012 Brennan et al.; licensee BioMed Central Ltd.; licensed under Creative Commons Attribution License BY 2.0 http://creativecommons.org/licenses/by/2.0] *Caption adapted from original*

- This response results in local aggregation of activated platelets that are subsequently linked via strands of fibrinogen connecting the platelets' glycoprotein IIb/IIIa membrane receptors.

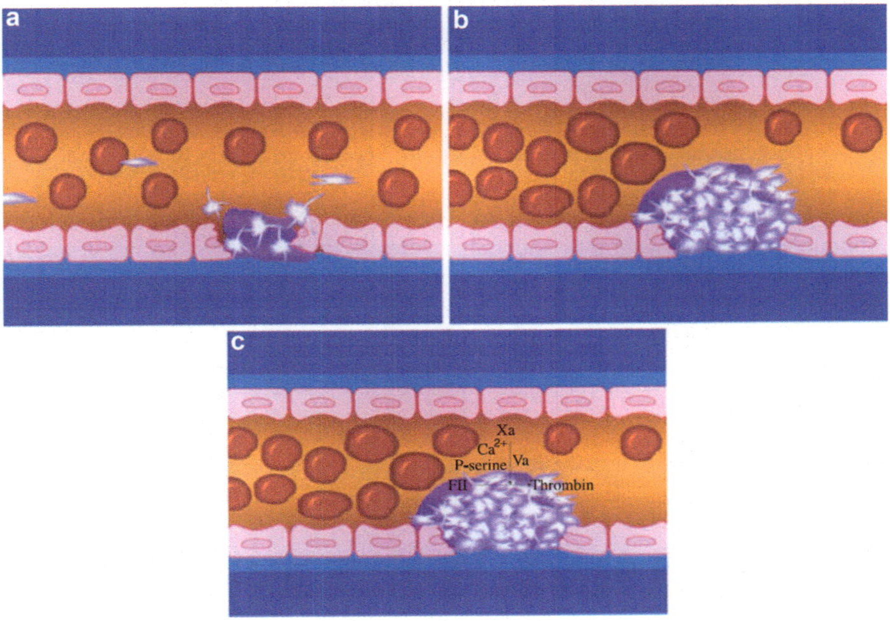

Platelet adhesion at the site of injury and aggregation with one another (a). Platelet plug consolidation (b) and platelets expressing procoagulant activity on their surface with subsequent thrombin generation (c). Procoagulant factors are represented by roman numbers. P-serine, phosphatidylserine. [Tripodi A. Haemostasis abnormalities in chronic liver failure. In: Ginès P, Kamath PS, Arroyo V, editors. Chronic liver failure. New York: Springer; 2011. p. 289-303. Book https://doi.org/10.1007/978-1-60761-866-9] *Caption from original*

- Alternative and much rarer etiologic considerations:
  - Pure arterial spasm without plaque rupture
  - Arteritis
  - Lupus

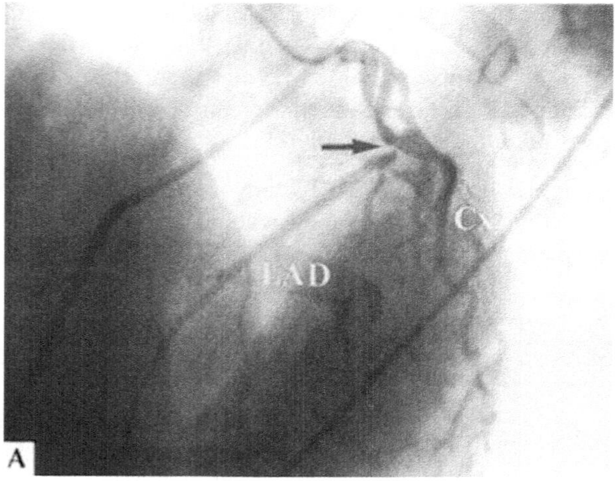

Anteroapical myocardial infarction in a patient with SLE. A, Cranial left anterior oblique view on arteriography showing severe proximal stenosis (arrow) of the left anterior descending (LAD) coronary artery that led into an anteroapical infarction in a 41-year-old woman with flaring SLE. [Roldan CA. Rheumatic and connective tissue diseases and the heart. In: Braunwald E, Crawford MH, editors. Atlas of heart diseases; vol. 6. Philadelphia: Current Medicine; 1996. ISBN: 1-878132-28-8] *Caption adapted from original*

- Takayasu's disease
- Kawasaki's disease

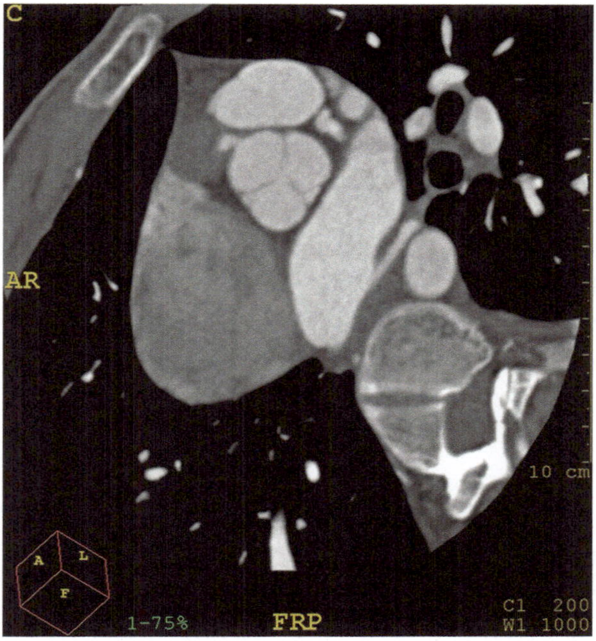

Image obtained from a patient with an acute myocardial infarction caused by thrombosis of a right coronary artery Kawasaki aneurysm (*arrow*). Kawasaki disease results from a mucocutaneous viral infection acquired during childhood. Typically, multiple aneurysms may develop in the coronaries and in other systemic vessels. Thrombosis of these aneurysms may occur later in life. [Garcia MJ. Intracardiac, myocardial and extracardiac abnormalities. In: Budoff MJ, Achenbach S, Narula J, editors. Atlas of cardiovascular computed tomography. Philadelphia: Current Medicine; 2007] *Caption from original*

- Cocaine- or methamphetamine-induced vasospasm

Presentation

Typical/"Classic"

- Pressure-like chest pain starting substernally and radiating toward left shoulder or left jaw.
- Pain is classically associated with diaphoresis, dyspnea, and nausea.
- Pain often accompanied by tachycardia; blood pressure is variable, with very high and very low presenting blood pressures associated with poorer prognosis.

- Pain often starts with exertion; may be improved with rest or with use of nitroglycerin. May also start at rest and often persists >20 minutes before presentation.
- Pain unchanged with movement, positioning, or deep breathing.
- In describing pain, patient may hold clenched fist over chest ("Levine sign").
- Notable for absence of specific, diagnostic ECG findings:
  - Persistent ST-segment elevation is ABSENT
  - ST-segment depression confers higher risk of poor outcomes but IS NOT diagnostic of NSTEMI
    - Particularly high risk when depression is "dynamic"—that is, present when patient is experiencing pain and resolved when that pain is relieved.

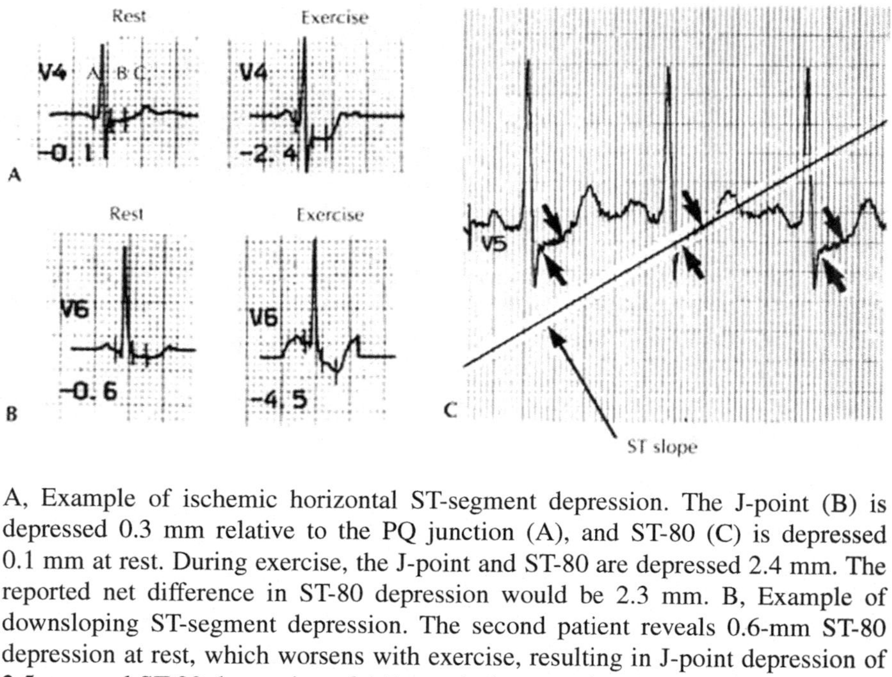

A, Example of ischemic horizontal ST-segment depression. The J-point (B) is depressed 0.3 mm relative to the PQ junction (A), and ST-80 (C) is depressed 0.1 mm at rest. During exercise, the J-point and ST-80 are depressed 2.4 mm. The reported net difference in ST-80 depression would be 2.3 mm. B, Example of downsloping ST-segment depression. The second patient reveals 0.6-mm ST-80 depression at rest, which worsens with exercise, resulting in J-point depression of 2.5 mm and ST-80 depression of 4.5 mm during exercise. The reported net difference in ST-80 depression would be 3.9 mm. [Chaitman B. Chapter 2. In: Beller GA. Chronic ischemic heart disease. Philadelphia: Current Medicine; 1995 (Braunwald E, editor. Atlas of heart diseases; vol. 5). ISBN: 1-878132-29-6, 2002-01-23; Chaitman, Bernard; Beller, George; Braunwald, Eugene] *Caption adapted from original*

- T-wave inversion confers higher risk in patients with symptoms of ACS but IS NOT diagnostic of NSTEMI.

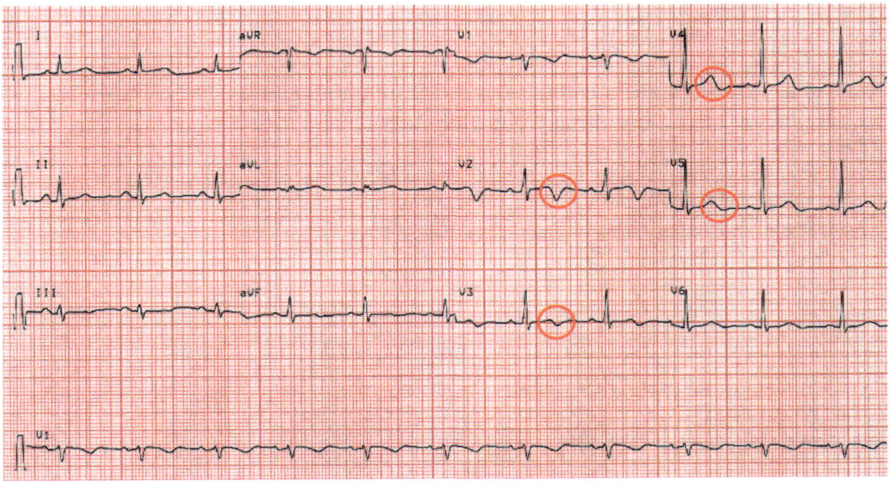

Electrocardiogram with T-wave inversions in leads V1 to V4. [From article: Triptans and troponin: a case report. Orphanet J Rare Dis. 2009 Jun 18;4:15. https://doi.org/10.1186/1750-1172-4-15, at http://link.springer.com/article/10.1186/1750-1172-4-15; by Claudia R Weder, Markus Schneemann, © Weder and Schneemann. 2009; licensee BioMed Central Ltd.; licensed under Creative Commons Attribution License BY 2.0 http://creativecommons.org/licenses/by/2.0] *Caption from original*

Atypical

- NSTEMI has been discovered in patients with virtually any complaint localized above the umbilicus.
- "Anginal equivalents" listed above include different distributions of pain (e.g. epigastric, jaw, neck, back) and some presentations that are not painful at all (e.g. palpitations, nausea, syncope).
  - Patients with NSTEMI who present without chest pain as their chief complaint frequently experience delays in diagnosis and therefore delays in treatment.
  - Atypical presentations more common in women, in elderly, and in diabetics.
- Elevated troponin levels are the defining and unifying feature of all NSTEMI presentations. Because of the time required for troponin to leak out of dying myocardial cells, the first troponin assay is often not elevated in patients who present soon after onset of symptoms.

Primary Differential Considerations

- Primary differential considerations include pain mimics to NSTEMI and are diverse, including life-threatening and more benign causes:
    - Aortic dissection
    - Pulmonary embolism
    - Peptic and esophageal disease, hiatal hernia
    - Costochondritis
    - Pneumonia
    - Pneumothorax
    - Pleurisy
    - Anxiety and panic disorders
    - Biliary colic
    - Herpes zoster

	Helpful clinical features
Cardiovascular	
Angina	Retrosternal chest pressure, squeezing, heaviness. Associated with exertion or emotional stress, relieved by rest or nitroglycerin. Usually between 2 and 20 min in duration.
Aortic stenosis	Similar features as for angina, but with late-peaking systolic murmur radiating to carotids. May be associated with syncope or signs of left heart failure.
Pericarditis	Sharp, retrosternal, pleuritic chest pain lasting hours to days. May be associated with friction rub and may be alleviated by leaning forward.
Aortic dissection	Sudden onset of tearing, ripping chest pain radiating to back. Associated with underlying hypertension.
Pulmonary embolism	Ipsilateral pleuritic pain associated with dyspnea, tachycardia, possible cor pulmonale. May have irritative cough or hemoptysis or present with syncope. Usually sudden onset.
Pulmonary	
Pneumonia/pleuritis/pleural effusion	Pleuritic pain, lateralizing to side of infection/inflammation. May be associated with fevers, dyspnea, cough. Exam with pleural rub, consolidation, or dullness to percussion.
Asthma/COPD exacerbation	Chest "tightness" associated with more prominent findings of dyspnea, tachypnea and diffuse wheezing.
Spontaneous pneumothorax	Sudden onset of pleuritic pain. Unilateral and associated with dyspnea. More common in thin, young males or patients with emphysematous disease. Decreased breath sounds and hyperresonance on side of pneumothorax.
Chest wall	
Muscle spasm/strain	Associated with prior increased physical activity/weight lifting. Pain variable in character but usually reproducible with palpation.

	Helpful clinical features
Costochondritis	Sharp, sudden onset pain that is short in duration. May be reproducible with palpation.
Herpes zoster	Sharp, burning, superficial neuropathic pain. May have allodynia, vesicular rash on exam. Unilateral dermatomal distribution.
Rib fracture	Prior trauma or known metastatic disease of bone. Point tenderness over affected rib(s). Pain is usually pleuritic.
Cervical/thoracic nerve root compression	Intermittent neuropathic pain often associated with neck movement or position. Usually unilateral.
Gastrointestinal	
Mediastinitis/ esophageal rupture	Often preceded by esophageal procedure or forceful vomiting. Pt. may have fever, associated septic shock. Symptoms vary from burning chest discomfort to severe dyspnea.
Esophageal reflux	Burning pain, often associated with nausea, belching. Usually worse at night and after large meals. Alleviated by antacids.
Esophageal spasm	Sudden onset, sharp, retrosternal pain. May be relieved by nitroglycerine and exacerbated by cold liquids. Sometimes associated with dysphagia.
Pancreatitis	Sharp epigastric pain, usually constant and prolonged. Exacerbated by food and often associated with nausea/vomiting. Alcohol and gallstones are risk factors.
Peptic ulcer	Sharp or burning epigastric pain. Often relieved by food or antacids. May be associated with occult GI bleeding or massive acute blood loss.
Psychogenic	
Anxiety/panic disorder	May be unable to distinguish from anginal pain, but usually has atypical features such as prolonged duration and no exertional component. Should be a diagnosis of exclusion at initial workup.

Differential diagnosis of acute chest pain. [McClintic BR, Rosenblatt RL. Approach to the patient with chest pain. In: Bisognano JD, Beck R, Connell R, editors. Manual of outpatient cardiology. London: Springer; 2012. p. 349-71. Book https://doi.org/10.1007/978-0-85729-944-4] *Caption from original*

History and Physical Exam

Findings That Confirm Diagnosis

- None

Factors That Suggest Diagnosis

- Nature and history of pain with presence of risk factors

Factors That Exclude Diagnosis

- None

Ancillary Studies

Laboratory

- CBC: no diagnostic findings.
- Electrolytes: no diagnostic findings.
- Renal function: no diagnostic findings, but renal insufficiency/failure is a risk factor for ACS and may complicate treatment.
- Coagulation studies: no diagnostic findings but should be performed before initiation of therapy.
- Cardiac enzymes: Elevation in troponin (I or T) levels is a required part of universal diagnosis of myocardial infarction.
  - Elevated enzyme levels differentiate NSTEMI from UA
  - Time course is critical
    - Depending on specific troponin assay and volume of muscle infarcted, generally takes about 6 hours after onset of symptoms for troponin levels to rise
    - A negative troponin within 6 hours of reliable onset time of symptoms is not particularly helpful
      - If onset time unclear, start at time of presentation
      - Negative troponin does NOT exclude angina

    - Positive troponin is *always* helpful, but use caution in interpreting levels in patients with renal insufficiency
- Levels of MB band of CPK enzyme still sometimes used to identify NSTEMI
    - Can sometimes be specifically helpful, e.g., in repeated chest pain presentations within 2-3 days, when troponin levels from first infarct will remain elevated, but CPK-MB may have returned to normal in interim

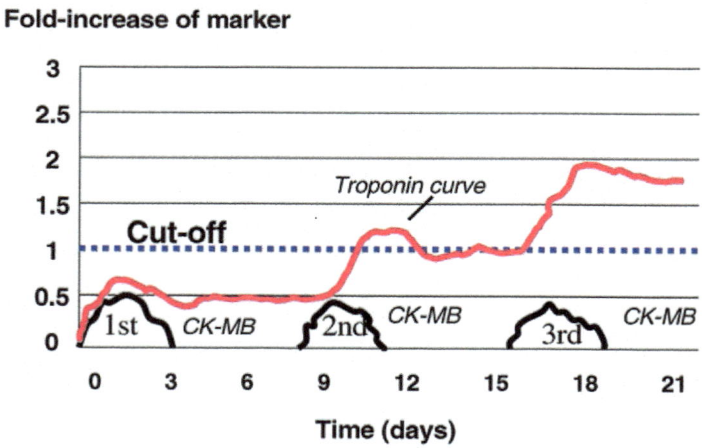

Summation model. Temporal release of cardiac markers CK-MB and troponins during repetitive episodes of ischaemia causing myocardial necroses in the setting of an acute coronary syndrome. Compared with the release and clearance of CK-MB 48-72 h after each episode (indicated as 1st, 2nd and 3rd), troponin release is cumulative. [From article: Implications of troponin testing in clinical medicine. Curr Control Trials Cardiovasc Med. 2001; 2(2): 75–84. https://doi.org/10.1186/cvm-2-2-075, at http://link.springer.com/article/10.1186/cvm-2-2-075; by Britta U Goldmann, Robert H Christenson, Christian W Hamm, Thomas Meinertz, E Magnus Ohman, © BioMed Central Ltd 2001; Available under Open Access, licensed under Creative Commons Attribution License https://creativecommons.org/licenses/by/2.0/] *Caption from original*

- BNP levels may offer some prognostic significance.

Electrocardiography

- No diagnostic findings.
- Per national quality standards in the United States, ECG should be obtained within 10 minutes of arrival in an emergency department.

Imaging

- No diagnostic findings for NSTEMI on chest x-ray (CXR).
- Findings of heart failure (cardiomegaly, pulmonary congestion) on CXR portend a poorer prognosis for NSTEMI.

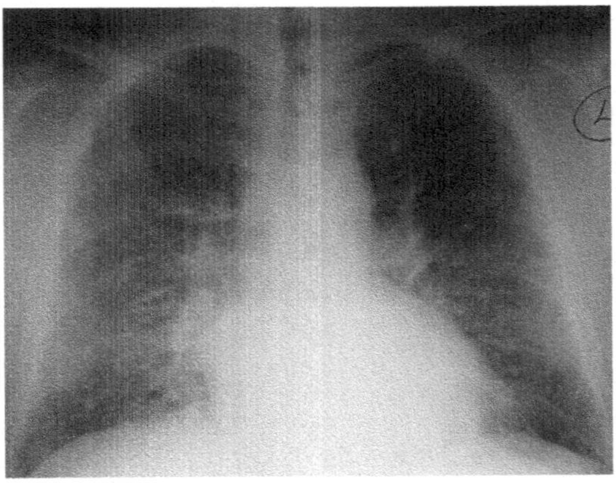

Frontal chest radiograph reveals typical features of pulmonary interstitial edema in a patient with congestive heart failure, manifested by peribronchial cuffing, indistinctness of the pulmonary vessels, and Kerley B lines. Note the cephalization or redistribution of the pulmonary vasculature and mild cardiomegaly. [Boiselle PM, Dass C, Steiner RM. Radiologic imaging in the critically ill patient. In: Criner GF, Barnette RE, D'Alonzo GE, editors. Critical care study guide. 2e, New York: Springer; 2010. p. 181-207. Book https://doi.org/10.1007/978-0-387-77452-7] *Caption from original*

- Findings of a widened mediastinum suggest consideration of aortic dissection but do not exclude NSTEMI. Check differential blood pressures in the upper extremities.

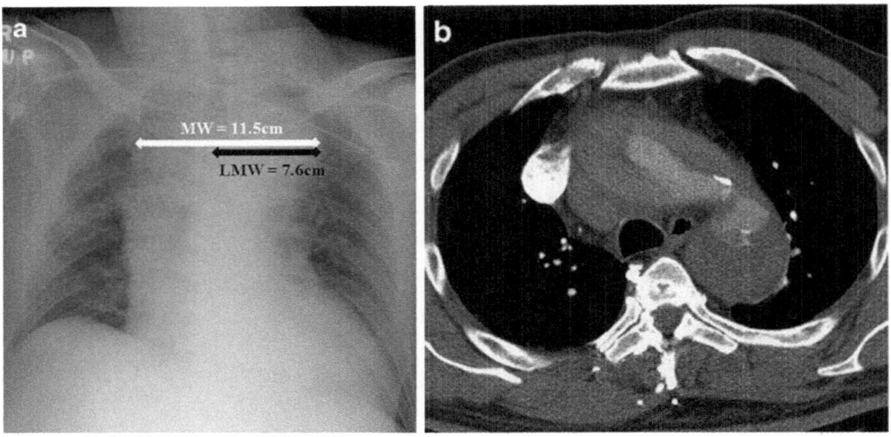

Acute type A aortic dissection in a 46-year-old man. A) AP chest radiograph showing marked widening of the mediastinum with MW and LMW measuring 11.5 and 7.6 cm, respectively. B) Corresponding selected image of CT aortogram confirms type A aortic dissection. [From article: Diagnostic accuracy of mediastinal width measurement on posteroanterior and anteroposterior chest radiographs in the depiction of acute nontraumatic thoracic aortic dissection. Emerg Radiol. 2012 Aug;19(4):309-15. https://doi.org/10.1007/s10140-012-1034-3 at http://link.springer.com/article/10.1007/s10140-012-1034-3 by Vincent Lai, Wai Kan Tsang, Wan Chi Chan, Tsz Wai Yeung, licensed under Creative Commons Attribution License, https://creativecommons.org/licenses/by/2.0/] *Caption from original*

- Findings of pneumonia suggest consideration of that differential but do not exclude NSTEMI. Check for signs of infection. Frank septic shock may result in elevated troponin levels.

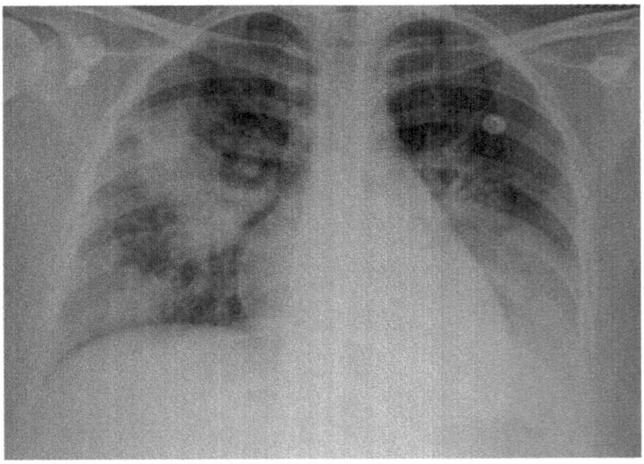

Chest radiograph showing right upper/lower lung field opacities and left lower lung field opacity consistent with pneumonia. [Tsigrelis C, Mohammad M, Fraimow HS, Dellinger RP, Marchesani D, Reboli AC. Secondary bacterial pneumonia due to Staphylococcus aureus complicating 2009 influenza A (H1N1) viral infection. Infection. 2010 Jun;38(3):237-9. https://doi.org/10.1007/s15010-010-0009-0, 2010-06-01] *Caption adapted from original*

- Findings of pneumothorax suggest consideration of that differential but do not exclude NSTEMI. Evaluate oxygenation status.

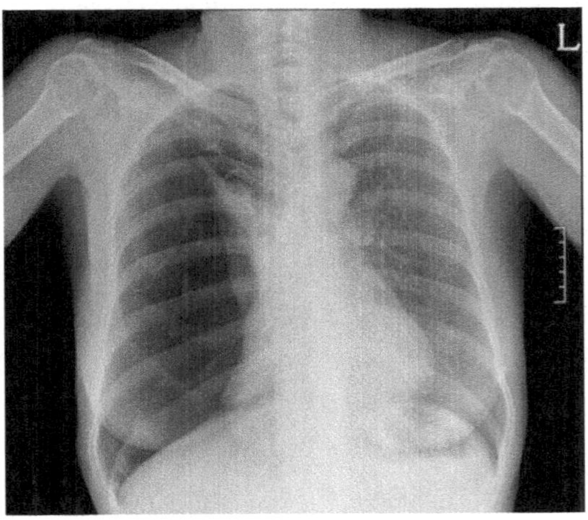

Posteroanterior upright chest X-ray shows large pneumothorax of the right lung. [Kim SH, Yoo WH. Recurrent pneumothorax associated with pulmonary nodules after leflunomide therapy in rheumatoid arthritis: a case report and review of the literature. Rheumatol Int. 2011 Jul;31(7):919-22. https://doi.org/10.1007/s00296-009-1240-9] *Caption adapted from original*

- Findings of hiatal hernia suggest consideration of that differential but do not exclude NSTEMI.

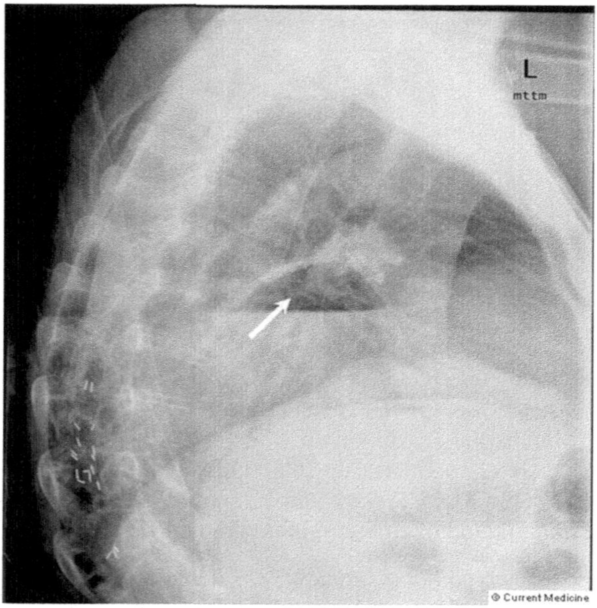

Radiograph of large hiatal hernia. [Aurigemma G, Tighe D, Oh J, Espinoza R. Pericardial disease and cardiac masses. In: Solomon S, editor. Atlas of echocardiography. Philadelphia: Current Medicine; 2008. ISBN: 1-57340-217-6] *Caption from original*

Risk Scoring

- TIMI Risk Score may be helpful in establishing short-term prognosis, which helps drive intensity of therapy.

- Age ≥65 years
- History of known CAD (documented prior coronary artery stenosis >50%)
- ≥3 conventional cardiac risk factors (age, male sex, family history, hyperlipidemia, diabetes mellitus, smoking, obesity)
- Use of aspirin in the past 7 days
- ST-segment deviation (persistent depression or transient elevation)
- Increased cardiac biomarkers (troponins)
- ≥2 anginal events in the preceding 24 h

TIMI = Thrombosis in Myocardial Infarction; CAD = coronary artery disease

Score = sum of number of above characteristics

TIMI = Thrombosis in Myocardial Infarction; CAD = coronary artery disease

Score = sum of number of above characteristics

TIMI risk score for unstable angina and NSTEMI. [Stillman AE, Oudkerk M, Ackerman M, Becker CR, Buszman PE, Feyter PJ, Hoffmann U, Keadey MT, Marano R, Lipton MJ, Raff GL, Reddy GP, Rees MR, Rubin GD, Schoepf UJ, Tarulli G, Beek EJR, Wexler L, White CS. Use of multidetector computed tomography for the assessment of acute chest pain: a consensus statement of the North American Society of Cardiac Imaging and the European Society of Cardiac Radiology. Int J Cardiovasc Imaging. 2007 Aug;23(4):415-27. https://doi.org/10.1007/s10554-007-9226-8] *Caption from original*

Value	TIMI risk score[a] (95% CI)	Modified TIMI risk score[b] (95% CI)
Sensitivity	53.7 (44.9–62.3)	58.1 (49.8–66.4)
Specificity	75.2 (72.1–78.2)	82.6 (80.0–85.2)
Negative predictive value	90.6 (88.2–927)	92.2 (90.2–94.1)
Positive predictive value	26.6 (21.5–32.3)	35.9 (29.6–42.2)

[a] Using a cut point of 3 (less than 3 vs. 3 or greater)

[b] Using a cut point of 2 (less than 2 vs. 2 or greater)

A summary of the TIMI risk score and modified TIMI risk scores as predictors of 30-day myocardial infarction/revascularization/death. [Jaffery Z, Hudson MP, Jacobsen G, Nowak R, McCord J. Modified Thrombolysis in Myocardial Infarction (TIMI) risk score to risk stratify patients in the emergency department with possible acute coronary syndrome. J Thromb Thrombolysis. 2007 Oct;24(2):137-44. DOI: https://doi.org/10.1007/s11239-007-0013-0] *Caption from original*

Special Populations

Age

- Risk for NSTEMI increases with age, starting at age 40 in men and at menopause in women.
  - Age is a risk factor for mortality from NSTEMI.
  - Likelihood of atypical presentation with NSTEMI increases with age.

Co-morbidities

- Hypertension, diabetes, and renal failure are important co-morbidities in NSTEMI risk and prognosis.
- Obesity is a weaker predictor of NSTEMI risk.

Pitfalls in Diagnosis

Critical Steps Not to Miss

- ECG must be performed as soon as the diagnosis of ACS is even considered.

Mimics

- All differential considerations listed under Primary Differential Considerations.
  - Of these, only aortic dissection and pulmonary embolism are also life-threatening.

Time-Dependent Interventions

- Stabilization of the NSTEMI patient is time sensitive; unlike in STEMI, restoration of perfusion is not extremely time sensitive.
  - Current guidelines call for diagnostic angiography in 24–48 hours to establish preferred course of management.

- Unless contraindicated (allergy, active bleeding), 324–325 mg aspirin should be administered immediately upon suspicion of an acute coronary syndrome.
- Anticoagulation therapy should be initiated upon confirmation of ACS diagnosis or with high suspicion in high-risk patients.
- Extremes of blood pressure should be promptly treated to avert shock (hypotension) or undue myocardial oxygen demand (hypertension).
- Airway and oxygenation should be monitored and supported as necessary.
- Patients with NSTEMI should be on continuous cardiac monitoring to evaluate for dangerous arrhythmias.
- Consider early initiation of dual antiplatelet therapy (aspirin plus an ADP receptor antagonist—ticagrelor or clopidogrel).

Overall Principles of Treatment

- Immediate stabilization of the patient with control of blood pressure, pulse rate, and pain is critical. The patient may require resuscitation, intubation, and intensive support.
- Medical management with anticoagulation and antiplatelet therapy is important.
  - Bleeding risk should also be assessed so that the risk of treatment-related hemorrhage can be minimized
- The higher the patient's risk, the more disproportionately s/he benefits from aggressive therapy.

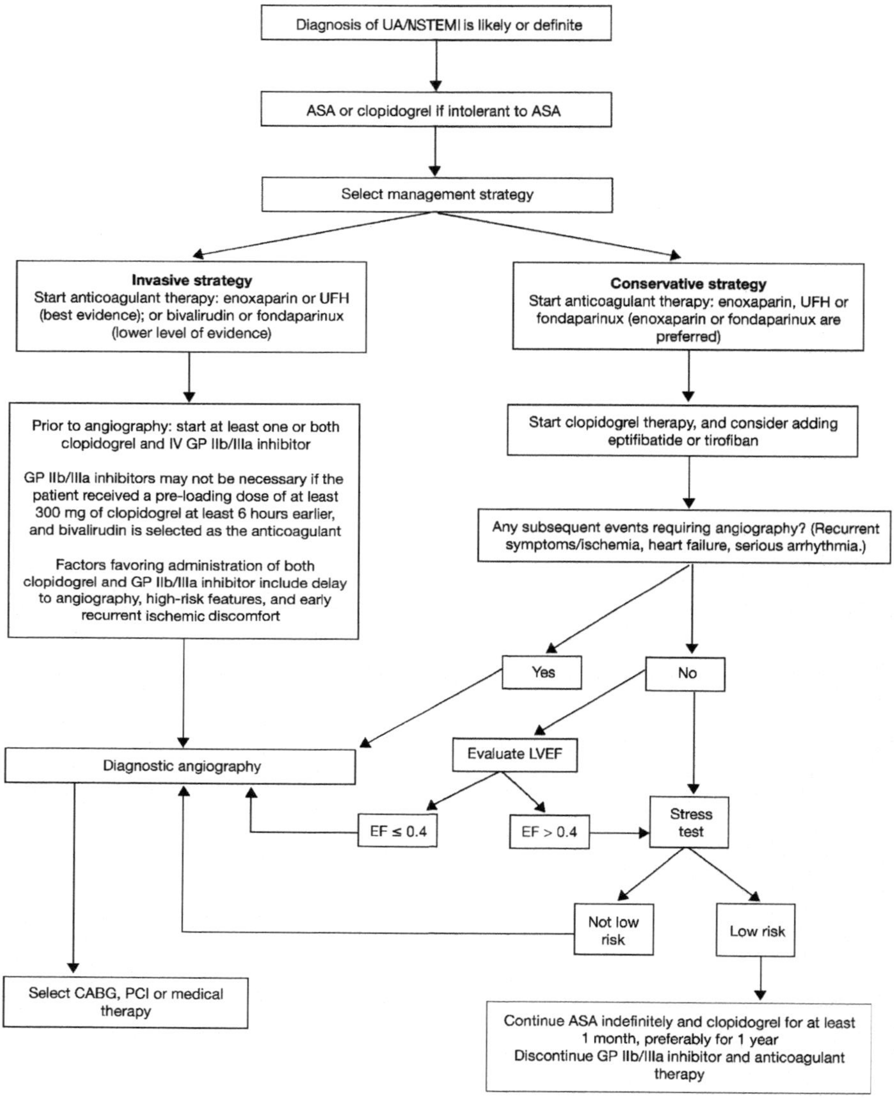

Algorithm for the initial management of patients with UA/NSTEMI with an invasive or conservative treatment strategy [1] Abbreviations: ASA, aspirin; CABG, coronary artery-bypass grafting; EF, ejection fraction; GP, glycoprotein; IV, intravenous; LVEF, left ventricular ejection fraction; PCI, percutaneous coronary intervention; UA/NSTEMI, unstable angina/non-ST-elevation myocardial infarction; UFH, unfractionated heparin. [Cohen M. High-risk acute coronary syndrome patients with non-ST-elevation myocardial infarction: definition and treatment. Cardiovasc Drugs Ther. 2008 Oct;22(5):407-18. https://doi.org/10.1007/s10557-008-6120-0] *Caption from original*

Disease Course

- NSTEMI mortality is 6–10 %, depending on the population studied, over 6 months.

Related Evidence

Papers of particular interest have been highlighted as:
*** Of key importance*

Practice Guideline

Anderson JL, Adams CD, Antman EM, Bridges CR, Califf RM, Casey DE Jr, Chavey WE 2nd, Fesmire FM, Hochman JS, Levin TN, Lincoff AM, Peterson ED, Theroux P, Wenger NK, Wright RS, Jneid H, Ettinger SM, Ganiats TG, Lincoff AM, Philippides GJ, Zidar JP; American College of Cardiology Foundation/American Heart Association Task Force on Practice Guidelines. 2012 ACCF/AHA focused update incorporated into the ACCF/AHA 2007 guidelines for the management of patients with unstable angina/non-ST-elevation myocardial infarction: a report of the American College of Cardiology Foundation/American Heart Association Task Force on Practice Guidelines. Circulation. 2013 Jun 11;127(23):e663-828. https://doi.org/10.1161/CIR.0b013e31828478ac. Erratum in: Circulation. 2013 Jun 18;127(24):e863-4. PMID: 23630129. http://www.ncbi.nlm.nih.gov/pubmed/23630129 **

2012 Writing Committee Members, Jneid H, Anderson JL, Wright RS, Adams CD, Bridges CR, Casey DE Jr, Ettinger SM, Fesmire FM, Ganiats TG, Lincoff AM, Peterson ED, Philippides GJ, Theroux P, Wenger NK, Zidar JP, Anderson JL; American College of Cardiology Foundation; American Heart Association Task Force on Practice Guidelines. 2012 ACCF/AHA focused update of the guideline for the management of patients with unstable angina/Non-ST-elevation myocardial infarction (updating the 2007 guideline and replacing the 2011 focused update): a report of the American College of Cardiology Foundation/American Heart Association Task Force on practice guidelines. Circulation. 2012 Aug 14;126(7):875-910. https://doi.org/10.1161/CIR.0b013e318256f1e0. PMID: 22800849. http://www.ncbi.nlm.nih.gov/pubmed/22800849

Task Force for Diagnosis and Treatment of Non-ST-Segment Elevation Acute Coronary Syndromes of European Society of Cardiology, Bassand JP, Hamm CW, Ardissino D, Boersma E, Budaj A, Fernández-Avilés F, Fox KA, Hasdai D, Ohman EM, Wallentin L, Wijns W. Guidelines for the diagnosis and treatment of non-ST-segment elevation acute coronary syndromes. Eur Heart J. 2007 Jul;28(13):1598-660. PMID: 17569677. http://www.ncbi.nlm.nih.gov/pubmed/17569677 **

Review

Tricoci P, Leonardi S, White J, White HD, Armstrong PW, Montalescot G, Giugliano RP, Gibson CM, Van de Werf F, Califf RM, Harrington RA, Braunwald E, Mahaffey KW, Newby LK. Cardiac troponin after percutaneous coronary intervention and 1-year mortality in non-ST-segment elevation acute coronary syndrome using systematic evaluation of biomarker trends. J Am Coll Cardiol. 2013 Jul 16;62(3):242-51. https://doi.org/10.1016/j.jacc.2013.04.043. PMID: 23684676. http://www.ncbi.nlm.nih.gov/pubmed/23684676

Lippi G, Franchini M, Cervellin G. Diagnosis and management of ischemic heart disease. Semin Thromb Hemost. 2013 Mar;39(2):202-13. https://doi.org/10.1055/s-0032-1333543. PMID: 23378254. http://www.ncbi.nlm.nih.gov/pubmed/23378254 **

Giugliano RP, Braunwald E. The year in non-ST-segment elevation acute coronary syndrome. J Am Coll Cardiol. 2012 Nov 20;60(21):2127-39. https://doi.org/10.1016/j.jacc.2012.08.972. PMID: 23103037. http://www.ncbi.nlm.nih.gov/pubmed/23103037 **

Trost JC, Lange RA. Treatment of acute coronary syndrome: Part 1: Non-ST-segment acute coronary syndrome. Crit Care Med. 2011 Oct;39(10):2346-53. https://doi.org/10.1097/CCM.0b013e31821e855f. PMID: 21602671. http://www.ncbi.nlm.nih.gov/pubmed/21602671 **

Sami S, Willerson JT. Contemporary treatment of unstable angina and non-ST-segment-elevation myocardial infarction (part 1). Tex Heart Inst J. 2010;37(2):141-8. PMID: 20401284. http://www.ncbi.nlm.nih.gov/pubmed/20401284

Sami S, Willerson JT. Contemporary treatment of unstable angina and non-ST-segment-elevation myocardial infarction (part 2). Tex Heart Inst J. 2010;37(3):262-75. PMID: 20548800. http://www.ncbi.nlm.nih.gov/pubmed/20548800

Thomas D, Giugliano RP. Day 1 care in patients with non-ST-segment elevation myocardial infarction. Cardiovasc Revasc Med. 2010 Jan-Mar;11(1):41-51. https://doi.org/10.1016/j.carrev.2009.07.005. PMID: 20129360. http://www.ncbi.nlm.nih.gov/pubmed/20129360

Kalra S, Duggal S, Valdez G, Smalligan RD. Review of acute coronary syndrome diagnosis and management. Postgrad Med. 2008 Apr;120(1):18-27. https://doi.org/10.3810/pgm.2008.04.1756. PMID: 18467805. http://www.ncbi.nlm.nih.gov/pubmed/18467805

Mauric AT, Oreto G. STEMI or NSTEMI, i.e. ST-evaluation or non-ST-evaluation myocardial infarction? J Cardiovasc Med (Hagerstown). 2008 Jan;9(1):81-2. https://doi.org/10.2459/JCM.0b013e328013d630. PMID: 18268425 http://www.ncbi.nlm.nih.gov/pubmed/18268425

Clinical Trial

Berry C, Layland J, Sood A, Curzen NP, Balachandran KP, Das R, Junejo S, Henderson RA, Briggs AH, Ford I, Oldroyd KG. Fractional flow reserve versus angiography in guiding management to optimize outcomes in non-ST-elevation myocardial infarction (FAMOUS-NSTEMI): rationale and design of a randomized controlled clinical trial. Am Heart J. 2013 Oct;166(4):662-668.e3. https://doi.org/10.1016/j.ahj.2013.07.011. PMID: 24093845. http://www.ncbi.nlm.nih.gov/pubmed/24093845

Chenevier-Gobeaux C, Meune C, Freund Y, Wahbi K, Claessens YE, Doumenc B, Zuily S, Riou B, Ray P. Influence of age and renal function on high-sensitivity cardiac troponin T diagnostic accuracy for the diagnosis of acute myocardial infarction. Am J Cardiol. 2013 Jun 15;111(12):1701-7. https://doi.org/10.1016/j.amjcard.2013.02.024. PMID: 23540652. http://www.ncbi.nlm.nih.gov/pubmed/23540652

Di Stefano R, Di Bello V, Barsotti MC, Grigoratos C, Armani C, Dell'Omodarme M, Carpi A, Balbarini A. Inflammatory markers and cardiac function in acute coronary syndrome: difference in ST-segment elevation myocardial infarction (STEMI) and in non-STEMI models. Biomed Pharmacother. 2009 Dec;63(10):773-80. https://doi.org/10.1016/j.biopha.2009.06.004. PMID: 19906505. http://www.ncbi.nlm.nih.gov/pubmed/19906505

Cohort Study

Khan NA, Daskalopoulou SS, Karp I, Eisenberg MJ, Pelletier R, Tsadok MA, Dasgupta K, Norris CM, Pilote L; GENESIS PRAXY Team. Sex differences in acute coronary syndrome symptom presentation in young patients. JAMA Intern Med. 2013 Nov 11;173(20):1863-71. https://doi.org/10.1001/jamainternmed.2013.10149. PMID: 24043208. http://www.ncbi.nlm.nih.gov/pubmed/24043208

Acharjee S, Roe MT, Amsterdam EA, Holmes DN, Boden WE. Relation of admission high-density lipoprotein cholesterol level and in-hospital mortality in patients with acute non-ST segment elevation myocardial infarction (from the National Cardiovascular Data Registry). Am J Cardiol. 2013 Oct 15;112(8):1057-62. https://doi.org/10.1016/j.amjcard.2013.05.050. PMID: 23891245. http://www.ncbi.nlm.nih.gov/pubmed/23891245

Ferrara LA, Russo BF, Gente R, Esposito G, Rapacciuolo A, de Simone G. STEMI and NSTEMI: a mono versus a multivessel disease? Int J Cardiol. 2013 Oct 3;168(3):2905-6. https://doi.org/10.1016/j.ijcard.2013.03.154. PMID: 23643429. http://www.ncbi.nlm.nih.gov/pubmed/23643429

Patel JH, Gupta R, Roe MT, Peng SA, Wiviott SD, Saucedo JF. Influence of Presenting Electrocardiographic Findings on the Treatment and Outcomes of Patients With Non-ST-Segment Elevation Myocardial Infarction. Am J Cardiol. 2013 Oct 2. doi:pii: S0002-9149(13)01926-7. https://doi.org/10.1016/j.amjcard.2013.09.009. PMID: 24290492. http://www.ncbi.nlm.nih.gov/pubmed/24290492

Bahrmann P, Christ M, Bahrmann A, Rittger H, Heppner HJ, Achenbach S, Bertsch T, Sieber CC. A 3-hour diagnostic algorithm for non-ST-elevation myocardial infarction using high-sensitivity cardiac troponin T in unselected older patients presenting to the emergency department. J Am Med Dir Assoc. 2013 Jun;14(6):409-16. https://doi.org/10.1016/j.jamda.2012.12.005. PMID: 23375478. http://www.ncbi.nlm.nih.gov/pubmed/23375478

Antonsen L, Jensen LO, Thayssen P, Christiansen EH, Junker A, Tilsted HH, Terkelsen CJ, Kaltoft A, Maeng M, Hansen KN, Ravkilde J, Lassen JF, Madsen M, Sørensen HT, Thuesen L. Comparison of outcomes of patients ≥ 80 years of age having percutaneous coronary intervention according to presentation (stable vs unstable angina pectoris/non-ST-segment elevation myocardial infarction vs ST-segment elevation myocardial infarction). Am J Cardiol. 2011 Nov 15;108(10):1395-400. https://doi.org/10.1016/j.amjcard.2011.06.062. PMID: 21890087. http://www.ncbi.nlm.nih.gov/pubmed/21890087

Movahed MR, John J, Hashemzadeh M, Hashemzadeh M. Mortality trends for non-ST-segment elevation myocardial infarction (NSTEMI) in the United States from 1988 to 2004. Clin Cardiol. 2011 Nov;34(11):689-92. https://doi.org/10.1002/clc.20968. PMID: 22095658. http://www.ncbi.nlm.nih.gov/pubmed/22095658

García-García C, Subirana I, Sala J, Bruguera J, Sanz G, Valle V, Arós F, Fiol M, Molina L, Serra J, Marrugat J, Elosua R. Long-term prognosis of first myocardial infarction according to the electrocardiographic pattern (ST elevation myocardial infarction, non-ST elevation myocardial infarction and non-classified myocardial infarction) and revascularization procedures. Am J Cardiol. 2011 Oct 15;108(8):1061-7. https://doi.org/10.1016/j.amjcard.2011.06.003. PMID: 21791326. http://www.ncbi.nlm.nih.gov/pubmed/21791326

Case Study

McManus DD, Gore J, Yarzebski J, Spencer F, Lessard D, Goldberg RJ. Recent trends in the incidence, treatment, and outcomes of patients with STEMI and NSTEMI. Am J Med. 2011 Jan;124(1):40-7. https://doi.org/10.1016/j.amjmed.2010.07.023. PMID: 21187184. http://www.ncbi.nlm.nih.gov/pubmed/21187184 **

Yeh RW, Sidney S, Chandra M, Sorel M, Selby JV, Go AS. Population trends in the incidence and outcomes of acute myocardial infarction. N Engl J Med. 2010 Jun

10;362(23):2155-65. https://doi.org/10.1056/NEJMoa0908610. PMID: 20558366. http://www.ncbi.nlm.nih.gov/pubmed/20558366 **

Use PubMed Clinical Queries to find the most recent evidence. Use this search strategy:

"non ST segment elevation myocardial infarction" OR "NSTEMI"

Chapter 3
Acute Coronary Syndrome: ST-Segment Elevation Myocardial Infarction

Charles V. Pollack, Jr., Richard M. Cantor, and Victoria G. Riese

Name and Synonyms

ST-Segment Elevation Myocardial Infarction

- STEMI, ST-elevation MI, acute MI, transmural MI, Q-wave MI

Incidence/Epidemiology

- At the highest-acuity end of the continuum of diagnoses collectively called acute coronary syndrome (ACS)
- Highest pre- and in-hospital 30-day mortality of ACS spectrum
- Incidence varies widely by demographics and risk profiles
- More than 1.2 million MIs in US each year; about 20 % are STEMI

Differential Diagnosis

- Includes all other causes of chest pain

C. V. Pollack, Jr. (✉)
Department of Emergency Medicine, Thomas Jefferson University, Philadelphia, PA, USA

R. M. Cantor
Department of Emergency Medicine and Pediatrics, State University of New York Upstate Medical University, Syracuse, NY, USA

V. G. Riese
Librarian Consultant, Eldersburg, MD, USA

C. V. Pollack, Jr. (ed.), *Differential Diagnosis of Cardiopulmonary Disease*,
https://doi.org/10.1007/978-3-319-63895-9_3

- Includes other causes of “anginal equivalents” in susceptible populations, e.g.:
- Dyspnea
- Back pain
- Jaw pain
- Shoulder pain
- Epigastric pain
- Palpitations
- Dizziness
- Weakness
- Nausea
- Syncope

Pathophysiology and Etiology

- ACS is the result of ischemia (diminished blood flow / oxygen delivery) to myocardium
- If ischemia persists, frank infarction (muscle death) may occur
- Infarction results in breakdown of cell membranes, allowing release of intracellular proteins (such as myoglobin, troponins, and CPK-MB) into the circulation, where they may be detected in peripheral blood draw
- STEMI is most extreme and acute form of ACS, with “transmural” ischemia that results in characteristic acute findings on ECG (see below)
- Most STEMI occurs as a result of fracture or frank rupture of atherosclerotic plaque in an epicardial artery

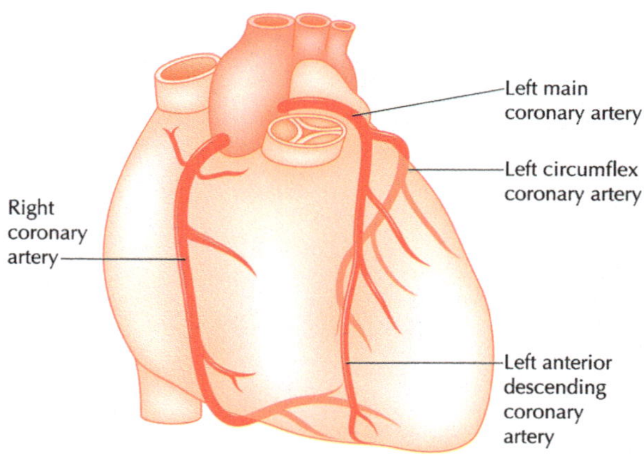

Normal coronary anatomy. [Achenbach S. Normal coronary anatomy. In: Budoff MJ, Achenbach S, Narula J, editors. Atlas of cardiovascular computed tomography. Philadelphia: Current Medicine; 2007 (Braunwald E, editor. Atlas of heart diseases; vol. 1)] *Caption from original*

- Atherosclerosis is a product of diverse inherited and acquired conditions, including:
  - Family history
  - Hyperlipidemia
  - Hypertension
  - Diabetes mellitus
  - Tobacco abuse

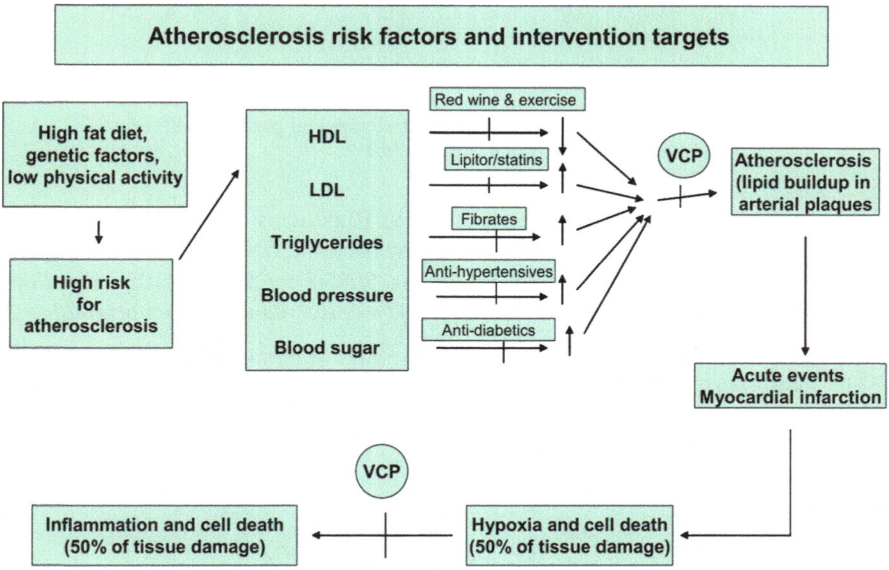

Atherosclerosis risk factors and intervention targets. [Thorbjornsdottir P, Thorgeirsson G, Kotwal GJ, Arason GJ. Control of inflammation with complement control agents to prevent atherosclerosis. In: Suri JS, Kathuria C, Molinari F, editors: Atherosclerosis disease management. New York: Springer. p. 633-75. Book https://doi.org/10.1007/978-1-4419-7222-4; Chapter: 20; Chapter https://doi.org/10.1007/978-1-4419-7222-4_20, 2011-01-01] *Caption adapted from original*

Risk factors	No. of patients
Individual	
Smoking	6
Hypertension	11
Hypercholesterolemia	9
Diabetes mellitus	4
Clusters	
Smoking and hypercholesterolemia	1
Hypertension and hypercholesterolemia[a]	4
Hypertension and diabetes	2
Smoking, hypertension and hypercholesterolemia	1
Smoking, hypertension, hypercholesterolemia and diabetes	2

[a] Hypertension was defined as a diastolic arterial pressure >95 mm Hg and hypercholesterolemia >6 mmol/l

Main known risk factors for atherosclerosis in 16 patients studied. [Watt S, Aesch B, Lanotte P, Tranquart F, Quentin R. Viral and bacterial DNA in carotid atherosclerotic lesions. Eur J Clin Microbiol Infect Dis. 2003 Feb;22(2):99-105. https://doi.org/10.1007/s10096-002-0867-1, 2003-02-01] *Caption adapted from original*

- Plaque rupture initiates a complex thrombo-inflammatory response locally, including activation of:
  - Coagulation

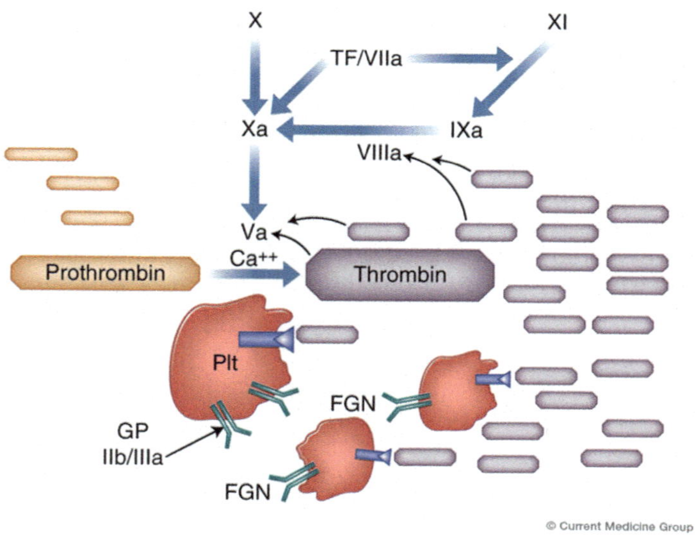

Networking of coagulation cascade and aggregation of platelets (Plt). The extrinsic limb triggers activation of the coagulation cascade when tissue factor (TF) is exposed in a disrupted plaque. Coagulation factor VII is activated (VIIa) and can activate factor X to Xa and promote perpetuation of the coagulation process via the intrinsic limb that results in formation of IXa and VIIIa. The prothrombinase complex of Xa, Va, Ca^{++} forms on a phospholipid surface (*eg*, membrane of a platelet) and converts prothrombin to thrombin. The thrombin that is formed binds to the thrombin receptor on platelets promoting activation and aggregation of platelets, as well as amplifying the coagulation cascade by promoting formation of VIIIa and Va. This diagram depicts the amplification nature of the coagulation process because one molecule of Xa leads to the downstream production of a large number of thrombin molecules (stoichiometric relationship not completely depicted to prevent obscuring the diagram with thrombin molecules). Activated platelets express numerous copies of the active form of the fibrinogen receptor GP IIb/IIIa on their surface. GP IIb/IIIa recognizes specific amino acid sequences on circulating ligands. One such ligand is fibrinogen (FGN), which has multiple copies of the RGD amino acid sequence and serves to bridge platelets together, promoting formation of aggregates. The more aggregates formed, the greater the surface area for the prothrombinase complex and amplification of the reactions of the coagulation cascade. [Antman E. Acute coronary syndromes. In: Libby P, editor. Essential atlas of cardiovascular disease. Philadelphia: Current Medicine; 2009. ISBN: 978-1-57340-309-2, 2009-05-21; Antman, Elliott] *Caption from original*

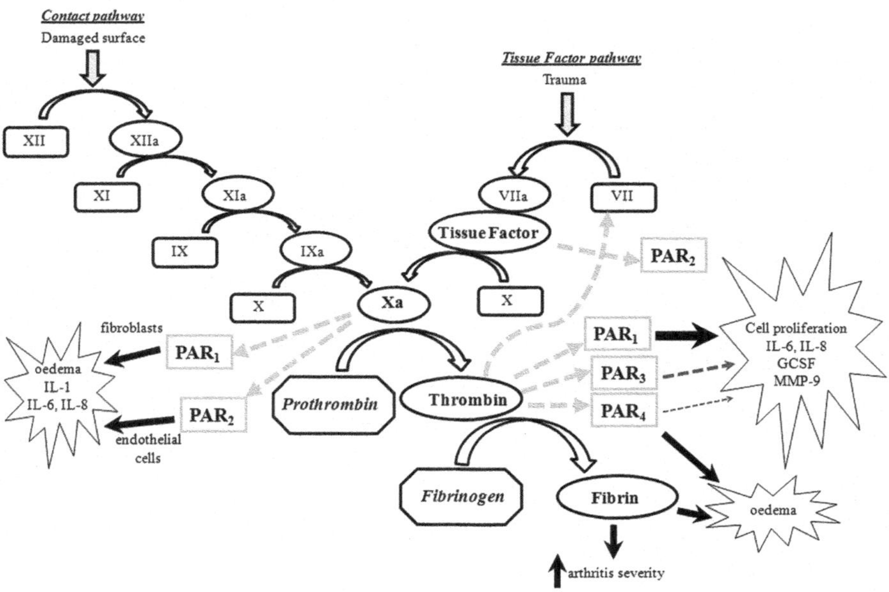

A simplified diagram of the coagulation cascade and its links with PARs and inflammation. Two pathways are involved in coagulation, with the major one being the tissue factor pathway. Most of the coagulation factors are serine proteinases that are present as inactive zymogens (rectangles) that when activated (ovals; lowercase 'a' indicates an active form) can catalyze the next reaction in the cascade. The two pathways converge to activate factor X, thrombin and fibrin. [Russell FA, McDougall JJ. Proteinase-activated receptors and arthritis. In: Vergnolle N, Chignard M, editors. Proteases and their receptors in inflammation. Basel: Springer; 2011. p. 217-42. Book https://doi.org/10.1007/978-3-0348-0157-7; Chapter: 9; Chapter https://doi.org/10.1007/978-3-0348-0157-7_9, 2011-01-01] *Caption adapted from original*

- Platelets

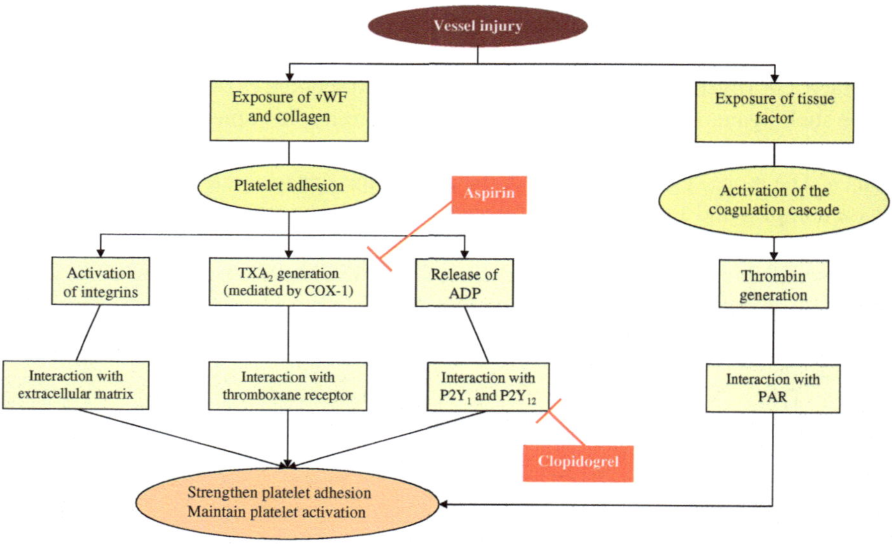

Mechanisms of platelet activation. [Ajjan R, Storey RF, Grant PJ. Aspirin resistance and diabetes mellitus. Diabetologia. 2008 Mar;51(3):385-90. https://doi.org/10.1007/s00125-007-0898-3, 2008-02-01] *Caption adapted from original*

- Complement

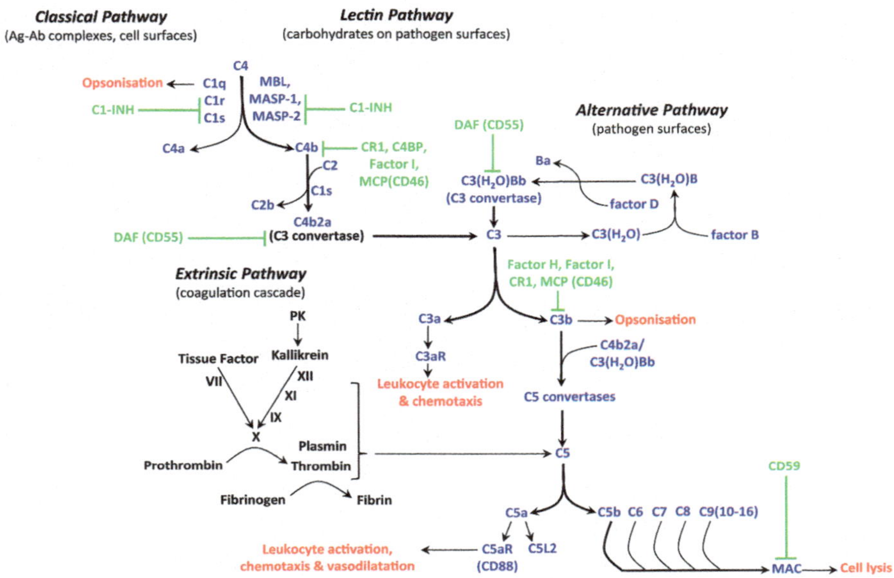

Common pathways for complement activation. [From article: Complement activation in the injured central nervous system: another dual-edged sword? J Neuroinflammation. 2012 Jun 21;9:137. https://doi.org/10.1186/1742-2094-9-137, at http://link.springer.com/article/10.1186%2F1742-2094-9-137; by Faith H Brennan, Aileen J Anderson, Stephen M Taylor, Trent M Woodruff, Marc J Ruitenberg, © Brennan et al.; licensee BioMed Central Ltd. 2012; licensed under Creative Commons Attribution License http://creativecommons.org/licenses/by/2.0] *Caption adapted from original*

- This response results in local aggregation of activated platelets that decreases and ultimately occludes downstream blood flow, leaving muscle distal to lesion ischemic and subject to infarction unless there is sufficient downstream collateral perfusion.

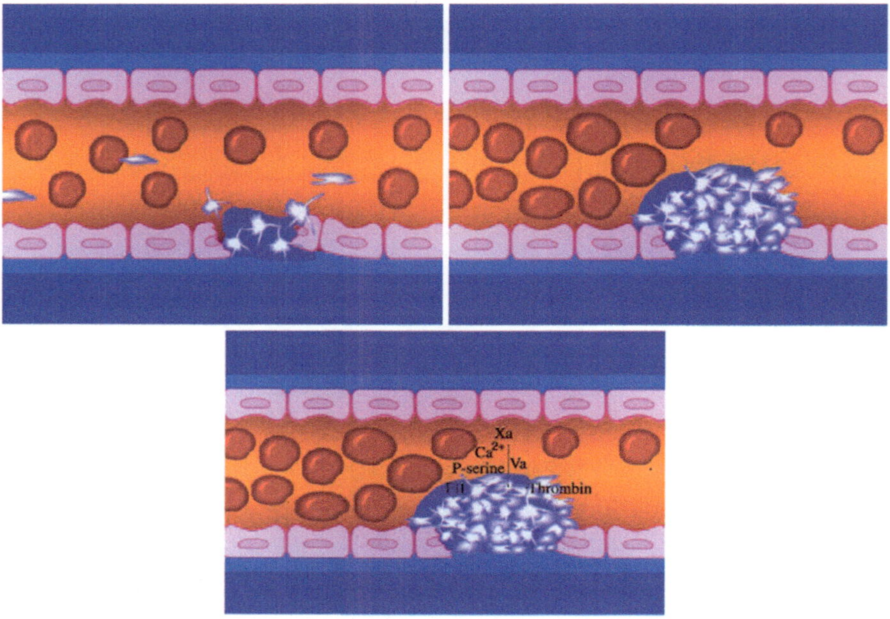

Platelet adhesion at the site of injury and aggregation with one another (a). Platelet plug consolidation (b) and platelets expressing procoagulant activity on their surface with subsequent thrombin generation (c). Procoagulant factors are represented by roman numbers. P-serine, phosphatidylserine. [Tripodi A. Haemostasis abnormalities in chronic liver failure. In: Ginès P, Kamath PS, Arroyo V, editors. Chronic liver failure. New York: Springer; 2011. p. 289-303. Book https://doi.org/10.1007/978-1-60761-866-9; Chapter: 14; Chapter https://doi.org/10.1007/978-1-60761-866-9_14, 2011-01-01] *Caption from original*

- Sudden acute ischemia from complete upstream artery occlusion results in characteristic ECG findings (see below).
- Alternative and much rarer etiologic considerations

- Pure arterial spasm without plaque rupture
- Arteritis
    - Lupus

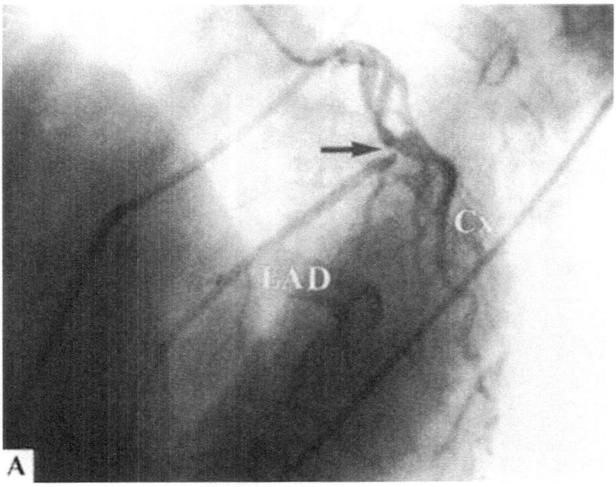

Anteroapical myocardial infarction in a patient with SLE. A, Cranial left anterior oblique view on arteriography showing severe proximal stenosis (arrow) of the left anterior descending (LAD) coronary artery that led into an anteroapical infarction in a 41-year-old woman with flaring SLE. [Roldan CA. Rheumatic and connective tissue diseases and the heart. In: Crawford MH, editor. Heart disease in the presence of disorders of other organ systems. Philadelphia: Current Medicine; 1996 (Braunwald E, editor. Atlas of heart diseases; vol. 6). ISBN: 1-878132-28-8, 2002-01-23] *Caption adapted from original*

- Takayasu's disease
- Kawasaki's disease

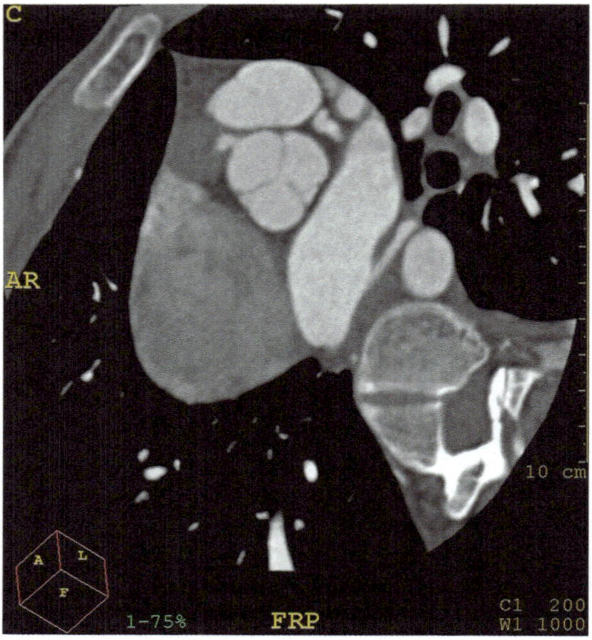

Image obtained from a patient with an acute myocardial infarction caused by thrombosis of a right coronary artery Kawasaki aneurysm (*arrow*). Kawasaki disease results from a mucocutaneous viral infection acquired during childhood. Typically, multiple aneurysms may develop in the coronaries and in other systemic vessels. Thrombosis of these aneurysms may occur later in life. [Garcia MJ. Intracardiac, myocardial and extracardiac abnormalities. In: Budoff MJ, Achenbach S, Narula J, editors. Atlas of cardiovascular computed tomography. Philadelphia: Current Medicine; 2007] *Caption from original*

- Cocaine- or methamphetamine-induced vasospasm

Presentation

Typical/"Classic"

- Pressure-like chest pain starting substernally and radiating toward left shoulder or left jaw
- Pain is classically associated with diaphoresis, dyspnea, and nausea
- Pain often accompanied by tachycardia; blood pressure is variable with very high and very low presenting blood pressures associated with poorer prognosis
- Pain often starts with exertion; may be improved with rest or with use of nitroglycerin. May also start at rest and often persists >20 minutes before presentation
- Pain unchanged with movement, positioning, or deep breathing

- In describing pain, patient may hold clenched fist over chest ("Levine sign")
- Defined (as name implies) by specific ECG findings:
    - ST-segment elevation in two or more contiguous leads OR

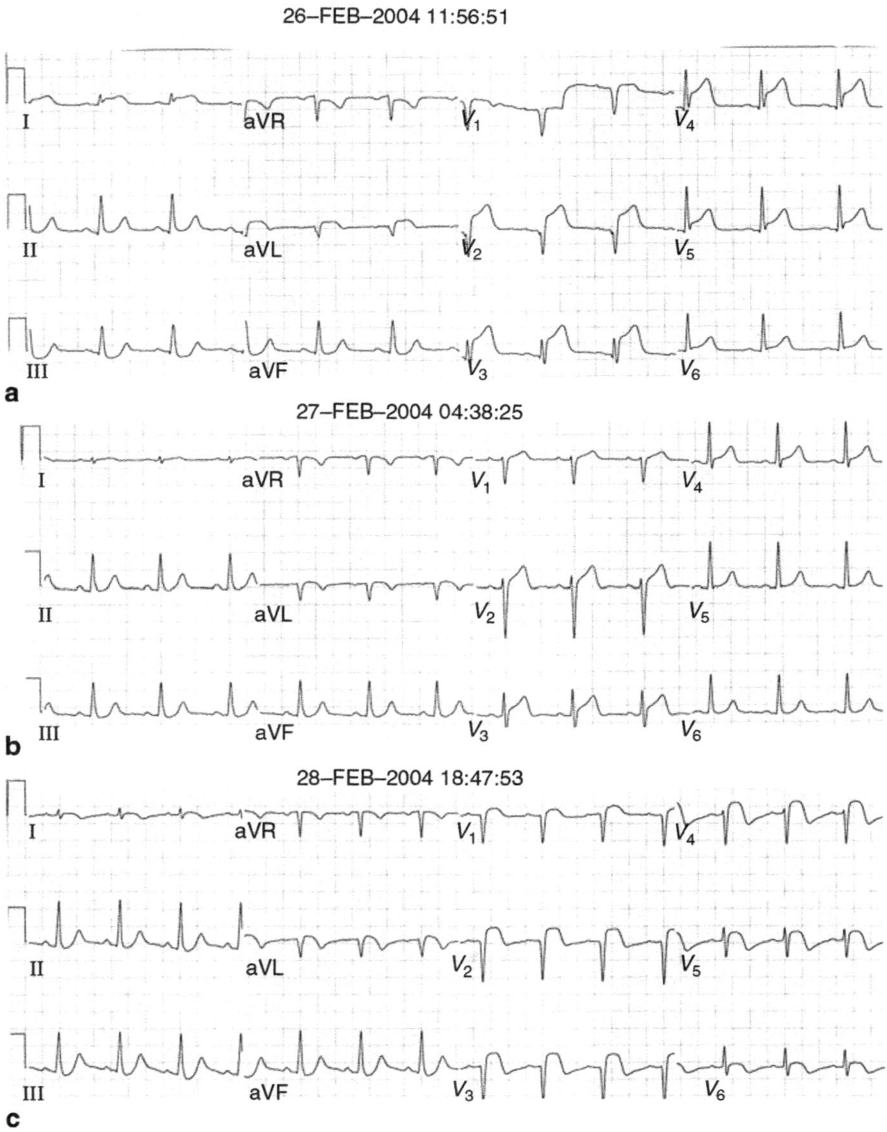

Electrocardiogram of a 51-year-old man with acute anterior-superior myocardial infarction caused by total occlusion of left anterior descending coronary artery proximal to the first septal perforator and the first diagonal branch; there was also

40% occlusion of the first obtuse marginal branch of the left circumflex artery and 70% occlusion of the right coronary artery. Kinesis involved large portion of the anterior wall and the apex. with an estimated left ventricular ejection fraction of 15%. In (a): ST elevation in leads aVL and V1–6, with reciprocal ST depression in leads III and aVR. In (b): one day later "pseudonormalization" with slight ST elevation in the leads V 2–3 and T wave inversion in lead aVL as the only abnormalities. In (c): on the following day when chest pain resolved. ST elevation and T wave inversion in leads I, aVL and V 1–6 with reciprocal ST depression in the leads III, aVF compatible with the evolution of the infarction pattern. Incipient T wave inversion in leads a VL, V 2–6. [Surawicz B. Ventricular repolarization in myocardial ischemia and myocardial infarction: theory and practice. In: Macfarlane PW, van Oosterom A, Pahlm O, Kligfield P, Janse M, Camm J, editors. Comprehensive electrocardiology. London: Springer; 2011. p. 803-31. Book https://doi.org/10.1007/978-1-84882-046-3; Chapter: 18; Chapter https://doi.org/10.1007/978-1-84882-046-3_18, 2010-01-01] *Caption from original*

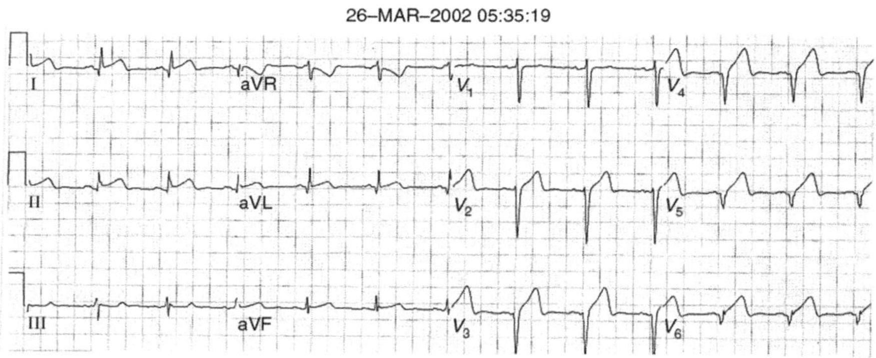

a

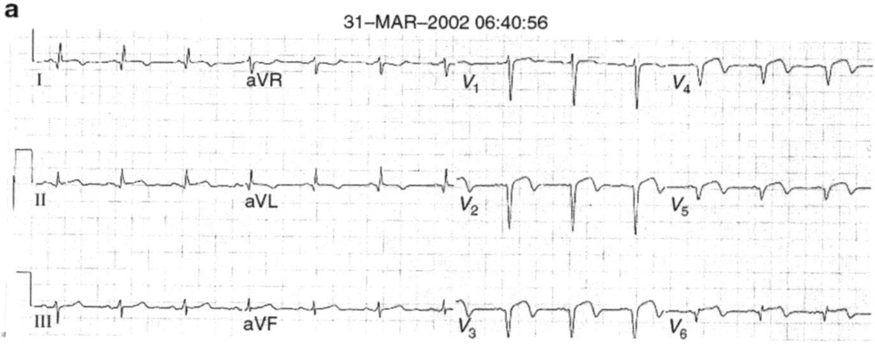

b

Electrocardiogram of a 47-year-old woman with anterolateral myocardial infarction (MI) caused by total occlusion of left anterior descending coronary artery in mid-portion associated with 50–70% occlusion of the co-dominant left anterior circumflex artery. Anterior wall and apex were akinetic with an estimated left ventricular ejection fraction of 30%. In (a): Q waves with ST elevation in leads I, aVL, V 3–6 and reciprocal ST depression in aVR. In (b) 5 days later after an emergent percutaneous intervention evolution of ECG pattern of anterior MI with T wave inversion in leads I, aVL and V 2–6. Residual ST elevation is present in the above leads. [Surawicz B. Ventricular repolarization in myocardial ischemia and myocardial infarction: theory and practice. In: Macfarlane PW, van Oosterom A, Pahlm O, Kligfield P, Janse M, Camm J, editors. Comprehensive electrocardiology. London: Springer; 2011. p. 803-31. Book https://doi.org/10.1007/978-1-84882-046-3; Chapter: 18; Chapter https://doi.org/10.1007/978-1-84882-046-3_18, 2010-01-01] *Caption from original*

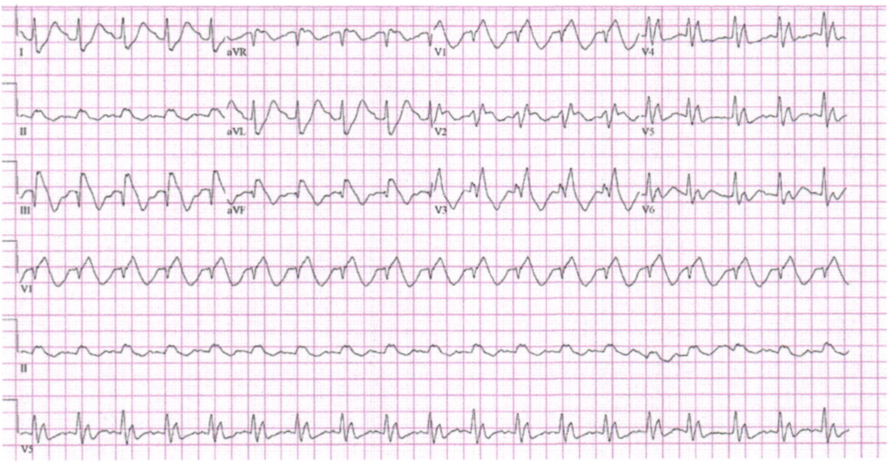

Electrocardiogram on presentation showing coved ST-segment elevation in precordial leads with simultaneous ST-segment elevation in leads II, III, and aVF. [Sheikh M, Kanjwal K, Kasmani R, Chutani S, Maloney JD. Simultaneous ST-segment elevation in inferior and precordial leads following ingestion of a lethal dose of desipramine: a novel Brugada-like EKG pattern. J Interv Card Electrophysiol. 2010 Jun;28(1):35-8. https://doi.org/10.1007/s10840-009-9412-9, 2010-04-13] *Caption from original*

- Known-to-be-new left bundle branch block in presence of anginal symptoms

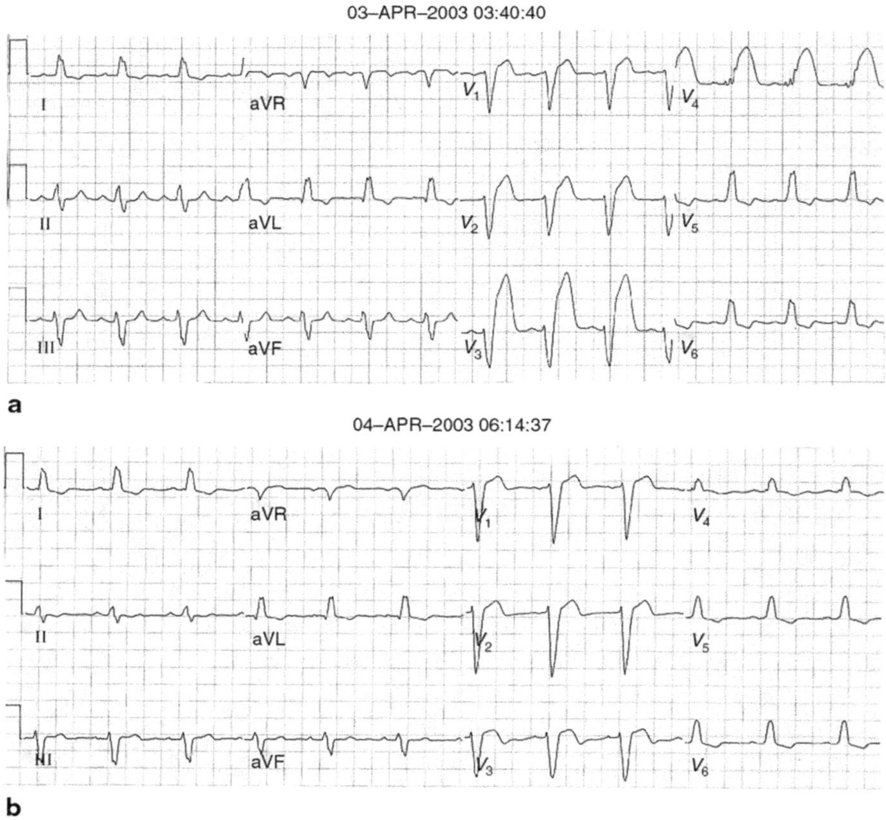

Electrocardiogram of a 58-year-old man with left bundle branch block (LBBB) and acute anterior myocardial infarction (MI). In (a), in addition to secondary ST and T changes of LBBB, there is primary ST elevation in leads V_{2-4}-indicative of acute injury pattern. No reciprocal ST depression is discernible. In (b), after percutaneous intervention, primary ST elevation subsided, but primary T-wave inversion in leads V_{2-3} is compatible with evolution of anterior MI pattern. [Surawicz B. Ventricular repolarization in myocardial ischemia and myocardial infarction: theory and practice. In: Macfarlane PW, van Oosterom A, Pahlm O, Kligfield P, Janse M, Camm J, editors. Comprehensive electrocardiology. London: Springer; 2011. p. 803-31. Book https://doi.org/10.1007/978-1-84882-046-3; Chapter: 18; Chapter https://doi.org/10.1007/978-1-84882-046-3_18, 2010-01-01] *Caption from original*

Atypical

- STEMI has been discovered in patients with virtually any complaint localized above the umbilicus.
- "Anginal equivalents" listed above include different distributions of pain (e.g., epigastric, jaw, neck, back) and some presentations that are not painful at all (e.g., palpitations, nausea, syncope).
  - Patients with STEMI who present without chest pain frequently experience delays in diagnosis and therefore delays in treatment.
  - Atypical presentations more common in women, in elderly, and in diabetics.
- Diagnostic ECG findings are the defining and unifying feature of all STEMI presentations.

Primary Differential Considerations

- Primary differential considerations include pain mimics to STEMI and are diverse, including life-threatening and more benign causes:
  - Aortic dissection
  - Pulmonary embolism
  - Peptic and esophageal disease, hiatal hernia
  - Costochondritis
  - Pneumonia
  - Pneumothorax
  - Pleurisy
  - Anxiety and panic disorders
  - Biliary colic
  - Herpes zoster

	Helpful clinical features
Cardiovascular	
Angina	Retrosternal chest pressure, squeezing, heaviness. Associated with exertion or emotional stress, relieved by rest or nitroglycerin. Usually between 2 and 20 min in duration.
Aortic stenosis	Similar features as for angina, but with late-peaking systolic murmur radiating to carotids. May be associated with syncope or signs of left heart failure.
Pericarditis	Sharp, retrosternal, pleuritic chest pain lasting hours to days. May be associated with friction rub and may be alleviated by leaning forward.
Aortic dissection	Sudden onset of tearing, ripping chest pain radiating to back. Associated with underlying hypertension.
Pulmonary embolism	Ipsilateral pleuritic pain associated with dyspnea, tachycardia, possible cor pulmonale. May have irritative cough or hemoptysis or present with syncope. Usually sudden onset.
Pulmonary	
Pneumonia/pleuritis/pleural effusion	Pleuritic pain, lateralizing to side of infection/inflammation. May be associated with fevers, dyspnea, cough. Exam with pleural rub, consolidation, or dullness to percussion.
Asthma/COPD exacerbation	Chest “tightness” associated with more prominent findings of dyspnea, tachypnea and diffuse wheezing.
Spontaneous pneumothorax	Sudden onset of pleuritic pain. Unilateral and associated with dyspnea. More common in thin, young males or patients with emphysematous disease. Decreased breath sounds and hyperresonance on side of pneumothorax.
Chest wall	
Muscle spasm/strain	Associated with prior increased physical activity/weight lifting. Pain variable in character but usually reproducible with palpation.

	Helpful clinical features
Costochondritis	Sharp, sudden onset pain that is short in duration. May be reproducible with palpation.
Herpes zoster	Sharp, burning, superficial neuropathic pain. May have allodynia, vesicular rash on exam. Unilateral dermatomal distribution.
Rib fracture	Prior trauma or known metastatic disease of bone. Point tenderness over affected rib(s). Pain is usually pleuritic.
Cervical/thoracic nerve root compression	Intermittent neuropathic pain often associated with neck movement or position. Usually unilateral.
Gastrointestinal	
Mediastinitis/ esophageal rupture	Often preceded by esophageal procedure or forceful vomiting. Pt. may have fever, associated septic shock. Symptoms vary from burning chest discomfort to severe dyspnea.
Esophageal reflux	Burning pain, often associated with nausea, belching. Usually worse at night and after large meals. Alleviated by antacids.
Esophageal spasm	Sudden onset, sharp, retrosternal pain. May be relieved by nitroglycerine and exacerbated by cold liquids. Sometimes associated with dysphagia.
Pancreatitis	Sharp epigastric pain, usually constant and prolonged. Exacerbated by food and often associated with nausea/vomiting. Alcohol and gallstones are risk factors.
Peptic ulcer	Sharp or burning epigastric pain. Often relieved by food or antacids. May be associated with occult GI bleeding or massive acute blood loss.
Psychogenic	
Anxiety/panic disorder	May be unable to distinguish from anginal pain, but usually has atypical features such as prolonged duration and no exertional component. Should be a diagnosis of exclusion at initial workup.

Differential diagnosis of acute chest pain. [McClintic BR, Rosenblatt RL. Approach to the patient with chest pain. In: Bisognano JD, Beck R, Connell R, editors. Manual of outpatient cardiology. London: Springer. p. 349-71. Book https://doi.org/10.1007/978-0-85729-944-4; Chapter: 13; Chapter https://doi.org/10.1007/978-0-85729-944-4_13, 2012-01-01] *Caption from original*

History and Physical Exam

Findings That Confirm Diagnosis

- None

Factors That Suggest Diagnosis

- Nature and history of pain with presence of risk factors.

Factors That Exclude Diagnosis

- None

Ancillary Studies

Laboratory

- CBC: no diagnostic findings
- Electrolytes: no diagnostic findings
- Renal function: no diagnostic findings, but renal insufficiency/failure is a risk factor for ACS and may complicate treatment
- Coagulation studies: no diagnostic findings but should be performed before initiation of anticoagulation therapy
- Cardiac enzymes: will be elevated in STEMI, but presentation often precedes abnormal test values. Elevation of enzymes is NOT required for diagnosis of STEMI.
  - Elevation in troponin (I or T) levels is part of universal diagnosis of myocardial infarction

Electrocardiography

- As above, STEMI is defined by the ECG
- Per national quality standards in the United States, ECG should be obtained within 10 minutes of arrival in an emergency department

Imaging

- No diagnostic findings for STEMI on chest x-ray (CXR)
- Findings of heart failure (cardiomegaly, pulmonary congestion) on CXR portend a poorer prognosis on STEMI

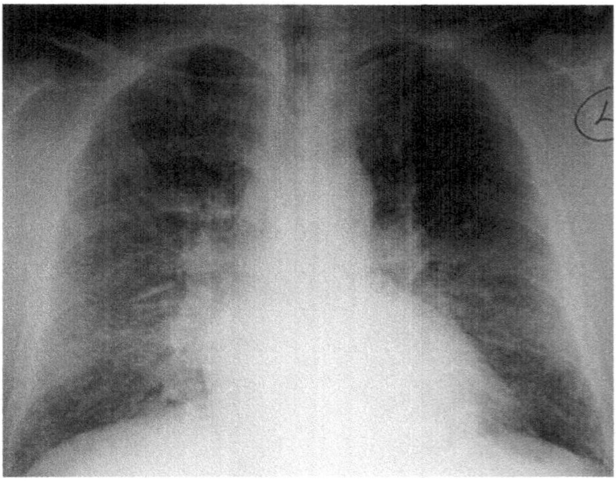

Frontal chest radiograph reveals typical features of pulmonary interstitial edema in a patient with congestive heart failure, manifested by peribronchial cuffing, indistinctness of the pulmonary vessels, and Kerley B lines. Note the cephalization or redistribution of the pulmonary vasculature and mild cardiomegaly. [Boiselle PM, Dass C, Steiner RM. Radiologic imaging in the critically ill patient. In: Criner GJ, Barnette RE, D'Alonzo GE, editors. Critical care study guide. New York: Springer; 2010. p. 181-207. Book https://doi.org/10.1007/978-0-387-77452-7; Chapter: 11; Chapter https://doi.org/10.1007/978-0-387-77452-7_11, 2010-01-01] *Caption from original*

- Findings of a widened mediastinum suggest consideration of aortic dissection but do not exclude STEMI. Check differential blood pressures in the upper extremities.

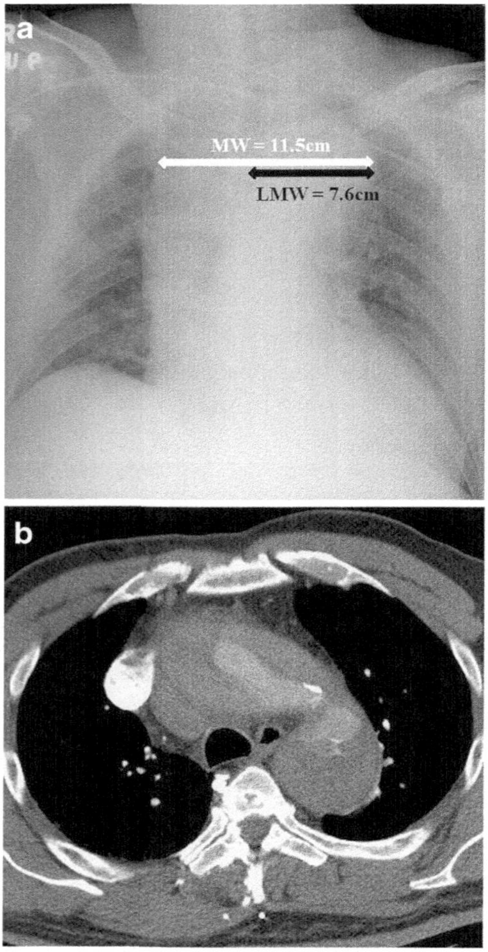

Acute type A aortic dissection in a 46-year-old man. A) AP chest radiograph showing marked widening of the mediastinum with MW and LMW measuring 11.5 and 7.6 cm, respectively. B) Corresponding selected image of CT aortogram confirms type A aortic dissection. [From article: Diagnostic accuracy of mediastinal width measurement on posteroanterior and anteroposterior chest radiographs in the depiction of acute nontraumatic thoracic aortic dissection. Emerg Radiol. 2012 Aug;19(4):309-15. https://doi.org/10.1007/s10140-012-1034-3, at http://link.springer.com/article/10.1007%2Fs10140-012-1034-3; by Vincent Lai, Wai Kan Tsang, Wan Chi Chan, Tsz Wai Yeung, © The Author(s) 2012; licensed under Creative Commons Attribution License https://creativecommons.org/licenses/by/2.0/] *Caption from original*

- Findings of pneumonia suggest consideration of that differential but do not exclude STEMI. Check for signs of infection.

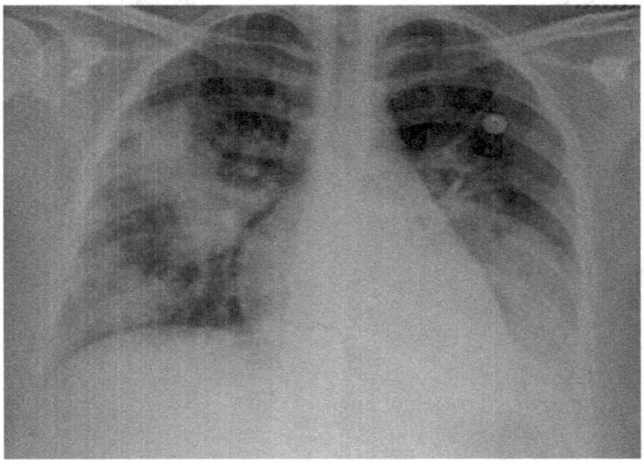

Chest radiograph showing right upper/lower lung field opacities and left lower lung field opacity consistent with pneumonia. [Tsigrelis C, Mohammad M, Fraimow HS, Dellinger RP, Marchesani D, Reboli AC. Secondary bacterial pneumonia due to Staphylococcus aureus complicating 2009 influenza A (H1N1) viral infection. Infection. 2010 Jun;38(3):237-9. https://doi.org/10.1007/s15010-010-0009-0, 2010-06-01] *Caption adapted from original*

- Findings of pneumothorax suggest consideration of that differential but do not exclude STEMI. Evaluate oxygenation status.

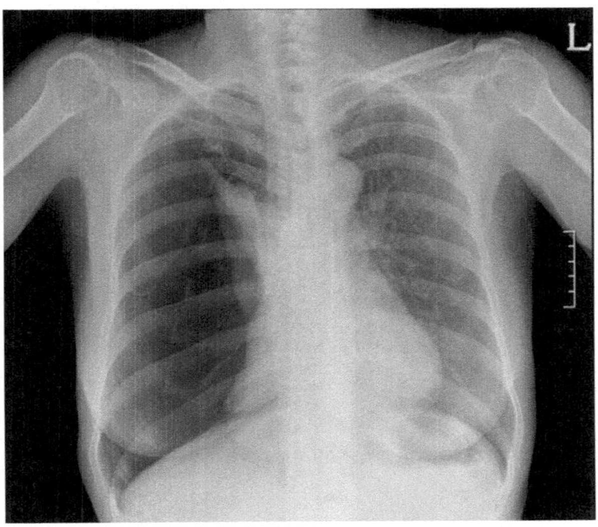

Posteroanterior upright chest X-ray shows large pneumothorax of the right lung. [Kim SH, Yoo WH. Recurrent pneumothorax associated with pulmonary nodules after leflunomide therapy in rheumatoid arthritis: a case report and review of the literature. Rheumatol Int. 2011 Jul;31(7):919-22. https://doi.org/10.1007/s00296-009-1240-9, 2011-06-21] *Caption adapted from original*

- Findings of hiatal hernia suggest consideration of that differential but do not exclude STEMI

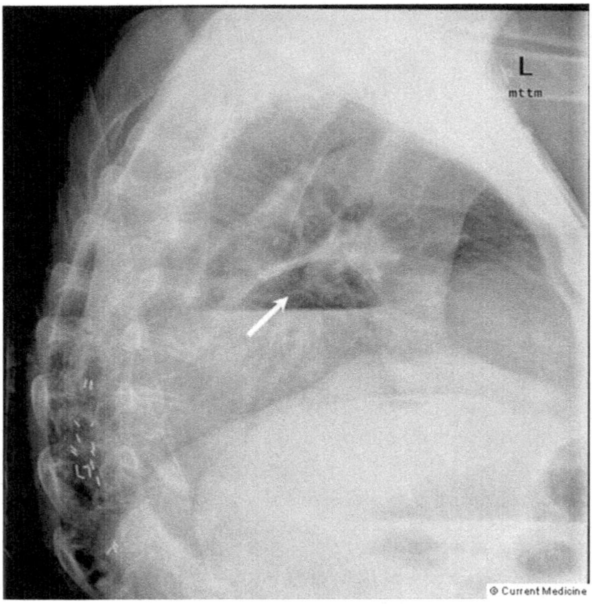

Radiograph of large hiatal hernia. [Aurigemma G, Tighe D, Oh J, Espinoza R. Pericardial disease and cardiac masses. In: Solomon S, editor. Atlas of echocardiography. Philadelphia: Current Medicine; 2008.] *Caption from original*

Special Populations

Age

- Risk for STEMI increases with age, starting at age 40 in men and at menopause in women.
  - Age is a risk factor for mortality from STEMI.
  - Likelihood of atypical presentation with STEMI increases with age.

Pediatric Considerations

- A congenital abnormality of the coronary vasculature, in which there is an anomalous origin of the left coronary artery arising from the pulmonary artery (ALCAPA), may occur in infancy. It presents with various symptoms of cardiac ischemia (diaphoresis when feeding) and if not recognized and corrected surgically, may cause irreversible myocardial damage.

Co-morbidities

- Hypertension, diabetes, and renal failure are important comorbidities in STEMI risk and prognosis.
- Obesity is a weaker predictor of STEMI risk.

Pitfalls in Diagnosis

Critical Steps Not to Miss

- ECG must be performed as soon as the diagnosis of STEMI is even considered.

Mimics

- All differential considerations listed above.
  - Of these, only aortic dissection and pulmonary embolism are also life-threatening.

Time-Dependent Interventions

- Restoration of myocardial perfusion is time sensitive.
  - If possible, STEMI should be managed in the cardiac cath laboratory within 90 minutes of initial evaluation.
  - Outcomes worsen with each 30–60-minute delay in restoration of flow.
  - If interventional management is not possible, evaluation for fibrinolytic therapy should be performed immediately, with a goal of delivering lytic therapy to appropriate STEMI patients within 30 minutes of initial evaluation.

- Unless contraindicated (allergy, active bleeding), 324-325 mg aspirin should be administered immediately upon suspicion of an acute coronary syndrome.
- Extremes of blood pressure should be promptly treated to avert shock (hypotension) or undue myocardial oxygen demand (hypertension).
- Airway and oxygenation should be monitored and supported as necessary.
- Patients with STEMI should be on continuous cardiac monitoring to evaluate for dangerous arrhythmias.

Overall Principles of Treatment

- Immediate stabilization of the patient with control of blood pressure, pulse rate, and pain is critical. The patient may require resuscitation, intubation, and intensive support.
- Measures to reperfuse infarcting myocardium are essential and are time sensitive.

Disease Course

- STEMI mortality is highest in the prehospital setting.
- Once at the emergency department, in-hospital STEMI mortality among patients receiving reperfusion therapy is around 6 %.

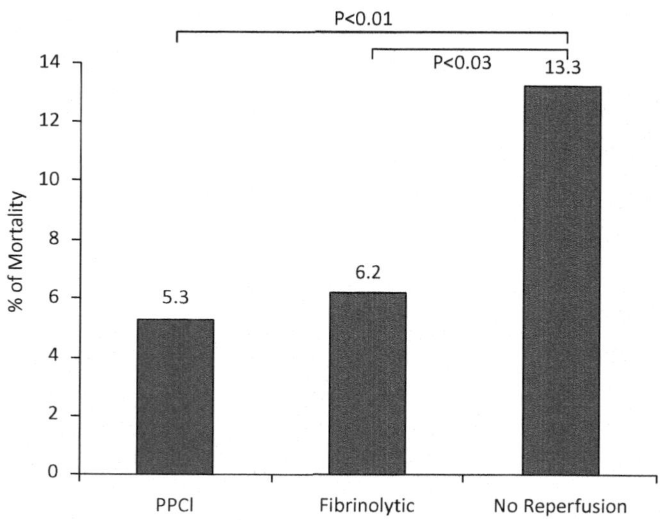

In-hospital mortality of STEMI patients. [Dharma S, Juzar DA, Firdaus I, Soerianata S, Wardeh AJ, Jukema JW. Acute myocardial infarction system of care in the third world. Neth Heart J. 2012 Jun;20(6):254-9. https://doi.org/10.1007/s12471-012-0259-9, 2012-06-01] *Caption from original*

Related Evidence

Papers of particular interest have been highlighted as:
*** Of key importance*

Practice Guideline

O'Gara PT, Kushner FG, Ascheim DD, Casey DE Jr, Chung MK, de Lemos JA, Ettinger SM, Fang JC, Fesmire FM, Franklin BA, Granger CB, Krumholz HM, Linderbaum JA, Morrow DA, Newby LK, Ornato JP, Ou N, Radford MJ, Tamis-Holland JE, Tommaso CL, Tracy CM, Woo YJ, Zhao DX, Anderson JL, Jacobs AK, Halperin JL, Albert NM, Brindis RG, Creager MA, DeMets D, Guyton RA, Hochman JS, Kovacs RJ, Kushner FG, Ohman EM, Stevenson WG, Yancy CW; American College of Cardiology Foundation/American Heart Association Task Force on Practice Guidelines. 2013 ACCF/AHA guideline for the management of ST-elevation myocardial infarction: a report of the American College of Cardiology Foundation/American Heart Association Task Force on Practice Guidelines. Circulation. 2013 Jan 29;127(4):e362-425. https://doi.org/10.1161/CIR.0b013e3182742cf6. PMID: 23247304. http://www.ncbi.nlm.nih.gov/pubmed/23247304 **

Tubaro M, Danchin N, Goldstein P, Filippatos G, Hasin Y, Heras M, Jansky P, Norekval TM, Swahn E, Thygesen K, Vrints C, Zahger D, Arntz HR, Bellou A, De La Coussaye JE, De Luca L, Huber K, Lambert Y, Lettino M, Lindahl B, McLean S, Nibbe L, Peacock WF, Price S, Quinn T, Spaulding C, Tatu-Chitoiu G, Van De Werf F. Pre-hospital treatment of STEMI patients. A scientific statement of the Working Group Acute Cardiac Care of the European Society of Cardiology. Acute Card Care. 2011 Jun;13(2):56-67. https://doi.org/10.3109/17482941.2011.581292. PMID: 21627394. http://www.ncbi.nlm.nih.gov/pubmed/21627394 **

Review

Uysal F, Bostan OM, Semizel E, Signak IS, Asut E, Cil E. Congenital anomalies of coronary arteries in children: the evaluation of 22 patients. Pediatr Cardiol. 2014 Jun;35(5):778-84. https://doi.org/10.1007/s00246-013-0852-8. PMID: 24337706. http://www.ncbi.nlm.nih.gov/pubmed/24337706

Lippi G, Franchini M, Cervellin G. Diagnosis and management of ischemic heart disease. Semin Thromb Hemost. 2013 Mar;39(2):202-13. https://doi.org/10.1055/s-0032-1333543. PMID: 23378254. http://www.ncbi.nlm.nih.gov/pubmed/23378254 **

Hartman SM, Barros AJ, Brady WJ. The use of a 4-step algorithm in the electrocardiographic diagnosis of ST-segment elevation myocardial infarction by novice interpreters. Am J Emerg Med. 2012 Sep;30(7):1282-95. https://doi.org/10.1016/j.ajem.2011.11.009. PMID: 22244224. http://www.ncbi.nlm.nih.gov/pubmed/22244224

Welch TD, Yang EH, Reeder GS, Gersh BJ. Modern management of acute myocardial infarction. Curr Probl Cardiol. 2012 Jul;37(7):237-310. https://doi.org/10.1016/j.cpcardiol.2012.03.002. PMID: 22664306. http://www.ncbi.nlm.nih.gov/pubmed/22664306 **

Wallace EL, Abdel-Latif A, Charnigo R, Moliterno DJ, Brodie B, Matnani R, Ziada KM. Meta-analysis of long-term outcomes for drug-eluting stents versus bare-metal stents in primary percutaneous coronary interventions for ST-segment elevation myocardial infarction. Am J Cardiol. 2012 Apr 1;109(7):932-40. https://doi.org/10.1016/j.amjcard.2011.11.021. PMID: 22221949. http://www.ncbi.nlm.nih.gov/pubmed/22221949

Huang HD, Birnbaum Y. ST elevation: differentiation between ST elevation myocardial infarction and nonischemic ST elevation. J Electrocardiol. 2011 Sep-Oct;44(5):494.e1-494.e12. https://doi.org/10.1016/j.jelectrocard.2011.06.002. PMID: 21871995. http://www.ncbi.nlm.nih.gov/pubmed/21871995

Perazzolo Marra M, Lima JA, Iliceto S. MRI in acute myocardial infarction. Eur Heart J. 2011 Feb;32(3):284-93. https://doi.org/10.1093/eurheartj/ehq409. PMID: 21112897. http://www.ncbi.nlm.nih.gov/pubmed/21112897

Nable JV, Brady W. The evolution of electrocardiographic changes in ST-segment elevation myocardial infarction. Am J Emerg Med. 2009 Jul;27(6):734-46. https://doi.org/10.1016/j.ajem.2008.05.025. PMID: 19751632. http://www.ncbi.nlm.nih.gov/pubmed/19751632

Peña E, Nguyen ET, Merchant N, Dennie G. ALCAPA syndrome: not just a pediatric disease. Radiographics. 2009 Mar-Apr;29(2):553-65. https://doi.org/10.1148/rg.292085059. PMID: 19325065. http://www.ncbi.nlm.nih.gov/pubmed/19325065

Mauric AT, Oreto G. STEMI or NSTEMI, i.e. ST-evaluation or non-ST-evaluation myocardial infarction? J Cardiovasc Med (Hagerstown). 2008 Jan;9(1):81-2. https://doi.org/10.2459/JCM.0b013e328013d630. PMID: 18268425 http://www.ncbi.nlm.nih.gov/pubmed/18268425

Kalra S, Duggal S, Valdez G, Smalligan RD. Review of acute coronary syndrome diagnosis and management. Postgrad Med. 2008 Apr;120(1):18-27. https://doi.org/10.3810/pgm.2008.04.1756. PMID: 18467805. http://www.ncbi.nlm.nih.gov/pubmed/18467805

Cohen M, Roubin G, Kuepper F. The challenge of ST-segment elevation myocardial infarction. Int J Clin Pract. 2007 Dec;61(12):2079-92. PMID: 17941831. http://www.ncbi.nlm.nih.gov/pubmed/17941831

Clinical Trial

Lopes RD, Siha H, Fu Y, Mehta RH, Patel MR, Armstrong PW, Granger CB. Diagnosing acute myocardial infarction in patients with left bundle branch block. Am J Cardiol. 2011 Sep 15;108(6):782-8. https://doi.org/10.1016/j.amjcard.2011.05.006. PMID: 21726838. http://www.ncbi.nlm.nih.gov/pubmed/21726838

Saltzman AJ, Stone GW, Claessen BE, Narula A, Leon-Reyes S, Weisz G, Brodie B, Witzenbichler B, Guagliumi G, Kornowski R, Dudek D, Metzger DC, Lansky AJ, Nikolsky E, Dangas GD, Mehran R. Long-term impact of chronic kidney disease in patients with ST-segment elevation myocardial infarction treated with primary percutaneous coronary intervention: the HORIZONS-AMI (Harmonizing Outcomes With Revascularization and Stents in Acute Myocardial Infarction) trial. JACC Cardiovasc Interv. 2011 Sep;4(9):1011-9. https://doi.org/10.1016/j.jcin.2011.06.012. PMID: 21939942. http://www.ncbi.nlm.nih.gov/pubmed/21939942

Cohort Study

Gregg RE, Helfenbein ED, Babaeizadeh S. New ST-segment elevation myocardial infarction criteria for left bundle branch block based on QRS area. J Electrocardiol. 2013 Nov-Dec;46(6):528-34. https://doi.org/10.1016/j.jelectrocard.2013.07.001. PMID: 23948522. http://www.ncbi.nlm.nih.gov/pubmed/23948522

Khan NA, Daskalopoulou SS, Karp I, Eisenberg MJ, Pelletier R, Tsadok MA, Dasgupta K, Norris CM, Pilote L; GENESIS PRAXY Team. Sex differences in acute coronary syndrome symptom presentation in young patients. JAMA Intern Med. 2013 Nov 11;173(20):1863-71. https://doi.org/10.1001/jamainternmed.2013.10149. PMID: 24043208. http://www.ncbi.nlm.nih.gov/pubmed/24043208

Ferraro S, Biganzoli E, Marano G, Santagostino M, Boracchi P, Panteghini M, Bongo AS. New insights in the pathophysiology of acute myocardial infarction detectable by a contemporary troponin assay. Clin Biochem. 2013

Aug;46(12):999-1006. https://doi.org/10.1016/j.clinbiochem.2013.03.026. PMID: 23578744. http://www.ncbi.nlm.nih.gov/pubmed/23578744

Bagai A, Jollis JG, Dauerman HL, Peng SA, Rokos IC, Bates ER, French WJ, Granger CB, Roe MT. Emergency department bypass for ST-Segment-elevation myocardial infarction patients identified with a prehospital electrocardiogram: a report from the American Heart Association Mission: Lifeline program. Circulation. 2013 Jul 23;128(4):352-9. https://doi.org/10.1161/CIRCULATIONAHA.113.002339. PMID: 23788525. http://www.ncbi.nlm.nih.gov/pubmed/23788525

Dündar C, Oduncu V, Erkol A, Tanalp AC, Sırma D, Karagöz A, Karabay CY, Kılıçgedik A, Pala S, Tigen K, Izgi A, Kırma C. In-hospital prognostic value of hemoglobin levels on admission in patients with acute ST segment elevation myocardial infarction undergoing primary angioplasty. Clin Res Cardiol. 2012 Jan;101(1):37-44. https://doi.org/10.1007/s00392-011-0361-9. PMID: 21931965. http://www.ncbi.nlm.nih.gov/pubmed/21931965

Rasoul S, Ottervanger JP, de Boer MJ, Dambrink JH, Hoorntje JC, Marcel Gosselink AT, Zijlstra F, Suryapranata H, van 't Hof AW; Zwolle Myocardial Infarction Study Group. Predictors of 30-day and 1-year mortality after primary percutaneous coronary intervention for ST-elevation myocardial infarction. Coron Artery Dis. 2009 Sep;20(6):415-21. https://doi.org/10.1097/MCA.0b013e32832e5c4c. PMID: 19641460. http://www.ncbi.nlm.nih.gov/pubmed/19641460

Comparative Study

McCabe JM, Armstrong EJ, Ku I, Kulkarni A, Hoffmayer KS, Bhave PD, Waldo SW, Hsue P, Stein JC, Marcus GM, Kinlay S, Ganz P. Physician accuracy in interpreting potential ST-segment elevation myocardial infarction electrocardiograms. J Am Heart Assoc. 2013 Oct 4;2(5):e000268. https://doi.org/10.1161/JAHA.113.000268. PMID: 24096575. http://www.ncbi.nlm.nih.gov/pubmed/24096575

Oduncu V, Erkol A, Kurt M, Tanboğa IH, Karabay CY, Şengül C, Bulut M, Özveren O, Fotbolcu H, Akgün T, Türkyilmaz E, Kırma C. The prognostic value of very low admission LDL-cholesterol levels in ST-segment elevation myocardial infarction compared in statin-pretreated and statin-naive patients undergoing primary percutaneous coronary intervention. Int J Cardiol. 2013 Jul 31;167(2):458-63. https://doi.org/10.1016/j.ijcard.2012.01.009. PMID: 22305817. http://www.ncbi.nlm.nih.gov/pubmed/22305817

Juliard JM, Golmard JL, Himbert D, Feldman LJ, Delorme L, Ducrocq G, Descoutures F, Sorbets E, Garbarz E, Boudvillain O, Aubry P, Vahanian A, Steg PG. Comparison of hospital mortality during ST-segment elevation myocardial infarction in the era of reperfusion therapy in women versus men and in older versus younger patients. Am J Cardiol. 2013 Jun 15;111(12):1708-13. https://

doi.org/10.1016/j.amjcard.2013.02.023. Epub 2013 Mar 20. PMID: 23523063. http://www.ncbi.nlm.nih.gov/pubmed/23523063

Jain S, Ting HT, Bell M, Bjerke CM, Lennon RJ, Gersh BJ, Rihal CS, Prasad A. Utility of left bundle branch block as a diagnostic criterion for acute myocardial infarction. Am J Cardiol. 2011 Apr 15;107(8):1111-6. https://doi.org/10.1016/j.amjcard.2010.12.007. PMID: 21296327. http://www.ncbi.nlm.nih.gov/pubmed/21296327 **

Case Study

Sadowski M, Janion-Sadowska A, Gąsior M, Gierlotka M, Janion M, Poloński L. Higher mortality in women after ST-segment elevation myocardial infarction in very young patients. Arch Med Sci. 2013 Jun 20;9(3):427-33. https://doi.org/10.5114/aoms.2013.35324. PMID: 23847662. http://www.ncbi.nlm.nih.gov/pubmed/23847662

McManus DD, Gore J, Yarzebski J, Spencer F, Lessard D, Goldberg RJ. Recent trends in the incidence, treatment, and outcomes of patients with STEMI and NSTEMI. Am J Med. 2011 Jan;124(1):40-7. https://doi.org/10.1016/j.amjmed.2010.07.023. PMID: 21187184. http://www.ncbi.nlm.nih.gov/pubmed/21187184

Yeh RW, Sidney S, Chandra M, Sorel M, Selby JV, Go AS. Population trends in the incidence and outcomes of acute myocardial infarction. N Engl J Med. 2010 Jun 10;362(23):2155-65. https://doi.org/10.1056/NEJMoa0908610. PMID: 20558366. http://www.ncbi.nlm.nih.gov/pubmed/20558366 **

Use PubMed Clinical Queries to find the most recent evidence. Use this search strategy:

"ST segment elevation myocardial infarction" OR "STEMI"

Chapter 4
Acute Coronary Syndrome: Unstable Angina

Charles V. Pollack, Jr. and Victoria G. Riese

Name and Synonyms

Unstable angina

- Troponin-negative acute coronary syndrome (ACS)

Incidence/Epidemiology

- Because unstable angina is a clinical diagnosis with inconsistent defining criteria, the true incidence is unknown.

C. V. Pollack, Jr. (✉)
Department of Emergency Medicine, Thomas Jefferson University, Philadelphia, PA, USA

V. G. Riese
Librarian Consultant, Eldersburg, MD, USA

C. V. Pollack, Jr. (ed.), *Differential Diagnosis of Cardiopulmonary Disease*,
https://doi.org/10.1007/978-3-319-63895-9_4

Progressive angina (grade IB)
Characterized by either new-onset angina pectoris or chronic angina with an increase in frequency or severity of episodes
Angina at rest (grades IIB and IIIB)
Recurrent angina with transient ST- or T-wave changes
Early postinfarction angina (grades IIC and IIIC)
Recurrent angina within 30 d following MI; angina either at rest or related to minimal exercise

Classification of unstable angina [Prasad A, Holmes D, Kleiman N. Use of percutaneous coronary intervention in unstable angina and acute myocardial infarction. In: Califf RM, editor. Acute myocardial infarction and other acute ischemic syndromes. 2nd ed. Philadelphia: Current Medicine; 2001. Chapter 7. (Braunwald E, editor. Atlas of heart diseases; vol. 8.)]

- Unstable angina is considered a "non-ST-segment-elevation" (NSTE) ACS. NSTE-ACS (which also includes NSTE myocardial infarction [NSTEMI]) is much more common than STEMI.

	STEMI	NSTEMI/UA
Pathogenesis	Fully occlusive thrombus	Less than fully occlusive thrombus
Incidence		Higher than that of STEMI
Patient profile		Older; higher co-morbidity (diabetes, renal failure) than STEMI patients
Time course	Minutes to hours	Up to a few days
Clinical manifestations		Similar to STEMI
Imaging studies		Similar to STEMI
EKG	ST elevations	No ST elevations[a]
Biomarkers	Elevated	Elevated
Therapy	See Table 2.54	See Table 2.54
Rehabilitation		Similar to STEMI
Complications		Similar to STEMI
Prognosis		Mortality lower in-hospital, higher at 6 months and 4 years than with STEMI

[a]ST elevations may be seen in Prinzmetal's angina

STEMI and NSTEMI/UA: a comparison. [Adelmann GA. Cardiology essentials in clinical practice. London: Springer; 2011. Chapter 2, Coronary artery disease; p. 23-95. Book https://doi.org/10.1007/978-1-84996-305-3; Chapter: 2; Chapter https://doi.org/10.1007/978-1-84996-305-3_2, 2010-01-01] Caption from original

- Incidence varies widely by demographics and risk profiles; patients with NSTE-ACS tend to be older and to have more comorbidities than STEMI patients.

- About 1 million patients are hospitalized with a diagnosis of unstable angina in the US each year, but in the absence of a consistent definition, it is likely that this is an overestimation, with some patients going on to complete MI and others more properly diagnosed as having either stable angina or noncoronary chest pain.

Differential Diagnosis

- Includes all other causes of chest pain
- Includes other causes of "anginal equivalents" in susceptible populations, e.g.:
  - Dyspnea
  - Back pain
  - Jaw pain
  - Shoulder pain
  - Epigastric pain
  - Palpitations
  - Dizziness
  - Weakness
  - Nausea
  - Syncope

Pathophysiology and Etiology

- ACS is the result of ischemia (diminished blood flow / oxygen delivery) to myocardium.
- If ischemia persists, frank infarction (muscle death) may occur.
- Infarction results in breakdown of cell membranes, allowing release of intracellular proteins (such as myoglobin, troponins, and CPK-MB) into the circulation, where they can be detected in peripheral blood draw.
- Unstable angina, as currently defined, is the clinical picture of ACS in the absence of both (1) ST-segment elevation on ECG and (2) elevated biomarker levels. These factors clearly differentiate unstable angina from NSTEMI and STEMI.
- The greatest consensus on the factors that make angina "unstable" include:
  - Anginal onset at rest (especially in patients who previously had only exertional angina)
  - Anginal symptoms do not resolve after

    - rest, if onset was with exertion
    - abortive therapy, such as sublingual nitroglycerin
    - 20 minutes
  - "crescendo" pattern of symptoms or change in usual anginal pattern
  - Multiple episodes within 24 hours
  - Association with signs of heart failure

- Most cases of ACS occur as a result of fracture or frank rupture of atherosclerotic plaque in an epicardial artery, but unstable angina also may result from "demand" ischemia, in which blood flow through a stenotic coronary artery is insufficient to meet increased myocardial oxygen demands (such as in exercise or physiologic stress). In the latter case, the plaque causing the stenosis need not be fractured or ruptured.

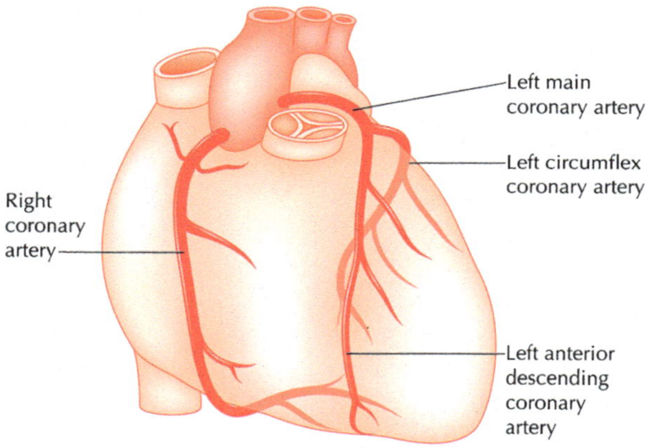

Normal coronary anatomy. [Achenbach S. Normal coronary anatomy. In: Budoff MJ, Achenbach S, Narula J, Braunwald E, editors. Atlas of cardiovascular computed tomography. Philadelphia: Current Medicine; 2007.] *Caption from original*

- Atherosclerosis, which is most often at the foundation of unstable angina, is a product of diverse inherited and acquired conditions, including:
  - Family history
  - Hyperlipidemia
  - Hypertension
  - Diabetes mellitus
  - Tobacco abuse

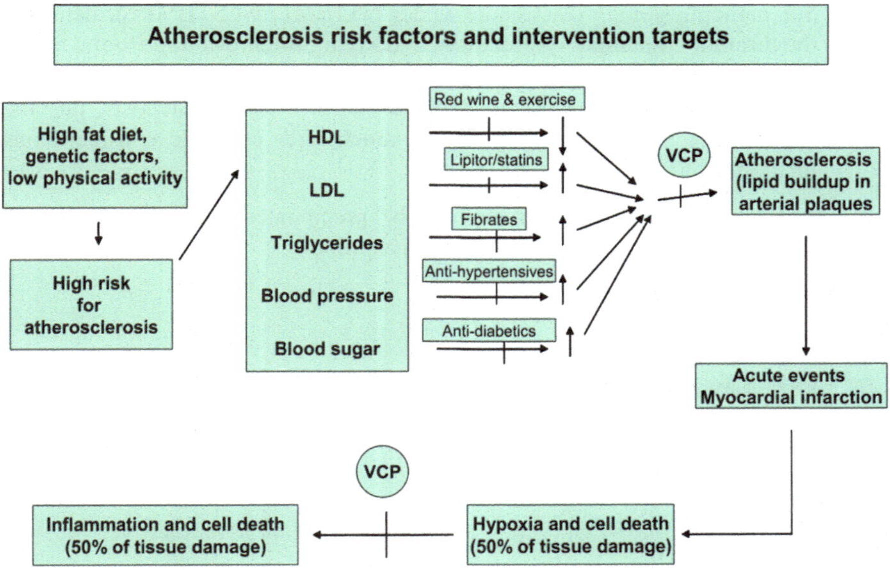

Atherosclerosis risk factors and intervention targets. [Thorbjornsdottir P, Thorgeirsson G, Kotwal GJ, Arason GJ. Control of inflammation with complement control agents to prevent atherosclerosis. In: Suri JS, Kathuria C, Molinari F, editors. Atherosclerosis disease management. New York: Springer; 2011. p. 633-75. Book https://doi.org/10.1007/978-1-4419-7222-4; Chapter: 20; Chapter https://doi.org/10.1007/978-1-4419-7222-4_20, 2011-01-01] *Caption adapted from original*

Risk factors	No. of patients
Individual	
Smoking	6
Hypertension	11
Hypercholesterolemia	9
Diabetes mellitus	4
Clusters	
Smoking and hypercholesterolemia	1
Hypertension and hypercholesterolemia[a]	4
Hypertension and diabetes	2
Smoking, hypertension and hypercholesterolemia	1
Smoking, hypertension, hypercholesterolemia and diabetes	2

[a] Hypertension was defined as a diastolic arterial pressure >95 mm Hg and hypercholesterolemia >6 mmol/l

Main known risk factors for atherosclerosis in 16 patients studied. [Watt S, Aesch B, Lanotte P, Tranquart F, Quentin R. Viral and bacterial DNA in carotid atherosclerotic lesions. Eur J Clin Microbiol Infect Dis. 2003 Feb;22(2):99-105. https://doi.org/10.1007/s10096-002-0867-1, 2003-02-01] *Caption adapted from original*

- See pathophysiology discussions under NSTEMI and STEMI for details of the thromboinflammatory processes underlying ACS resulting from a breach of an atherosclerotic plaque.
- Besides atherothrombosis and demand across a critical stenosis, unstable angina may result from a variety of much rarer etiologic considerations, including
    - Pure arterial spasm (which may be precipitated by sympathomimetic agents such as cocaine or methamphetamine)
    - Arteritis
        - Lupus
        - Takayasu disease
        - Kawasaki disease

Presentation

Typical/"Classic"

- Pressure-like chest pain starting substernally and radiating toward the left shoulder or left jaw.
- Pain is classically associated with diaphoresis, dyspnea, and nausea.
- Pain often accompanied by tachycardia; blood pressure is variable, with very high and very low presenting blood pressures associated with poorer prognosis.
- Pain often starts with exertion; may be improved with rest or with use of nitroglycerin. May also start at rest and often persists > 20 minutes prior to presentation.
- Pain unchanged with movement, positioning, or deep breathing.
- In describing pain, patient may hold clenched fist over chest ("Levine sign").
- Notable for absence of specific, diagnostic ECG findings:
    - Persistent ST-segment elevation is ABSENT
    - ST-segment depression confers a higher risk for poor outcomes but IS NOT diagnostic of NSTEMI.
        - Particularly high risk when depression is "dynamic"—that is, present when patient is experiencing pain and resolved when that pain is relieved

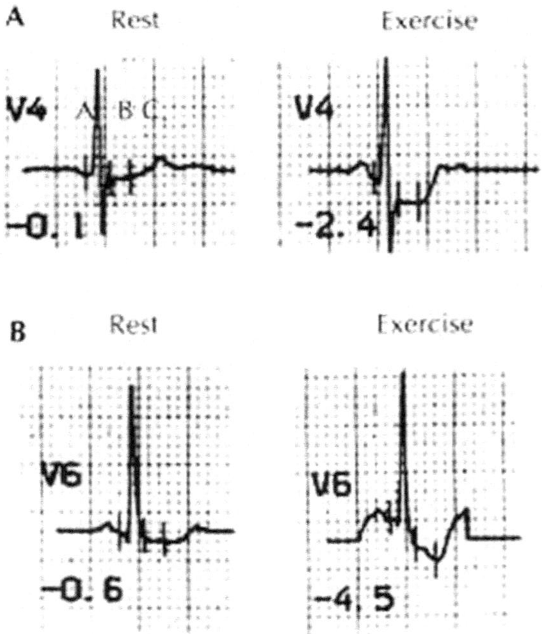

A, Example of ischemic horizontal ST-segment depression. The J-point (B) is depressed 0.3 mm relative to the PQ junction (A), and ST-80 (C) is depressed 0.1 mm at rest. During exercise, the J-point and ST-80 are depressed 2.4 mm. The reported net difference in ST-80 depression would be 2.3 mm. B, Example of downsloping ST-segment depression. The second patient reveals 0.6-mm ST-80 depression at rest, which worsens with exercise, resulting in J-point depression of 2.5 mm and ST-80 depression of 4.5 mm during exercise. The reported net difference in ST-80 depression would be 3.9 mm. [Chaitman B. Exercise electrocardiographic stress testing. In: Beller G, editor. Chronic ischemic heart disease. Philadelphia: Current Medicine; 1995. Chapter 2. (Braunwald E, editor. Atlas of heart diseases; vol. 5.) ISBN: 1-878132-29-6, 2002-01-23] *Caption adapted from original*

- T-wave inversion confers a higher risk in patients with symptoms of ACS but IS NOT diagnostic of unstable angina or NSTEMI.

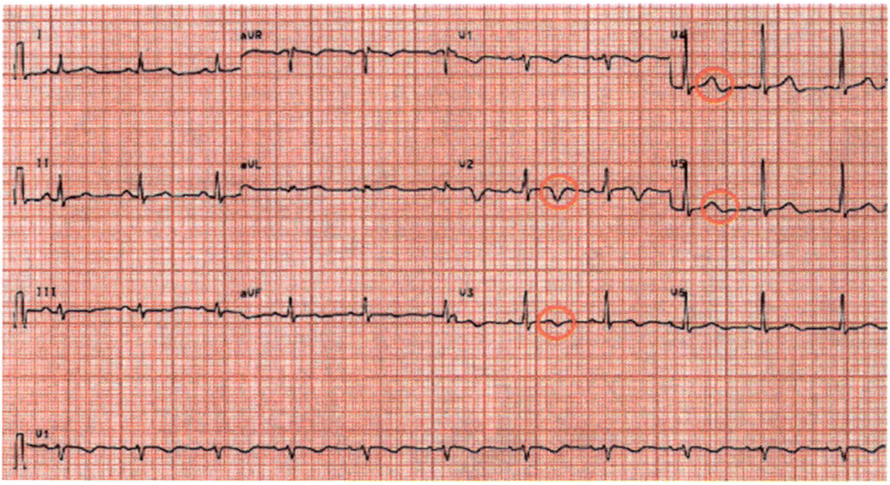

Electrocardiogram with T-wave inversions in leads V1 to V4. [From article: Triptans and troponin: a case report. Orphanet J Rare Dis. 2009 Jun 18;4: 15. https://doi.org/10.1186/1750-1172-4-15, at http://link.springer.com/article/10.1186/1750-1172-4-15; by Claudia R Weder, Markus Schneemann, © Weder and Schneemann. 2009; licensee BioMed Central Ltd.; licensed under Creative Commons Attribution License BY 2.0 http://creativecommons.org/licenses/by/2.0] *Caption from original*

Atypical

- Unstable angina has been diagnosed in patients with virtually any complaint localized above the umbilicus.
- "Anginal equivalents" listed above include different distributions of pain (e.g., epigastric, jaw, neck, back) and some presentations that are not painful at all (e.g., palpitations, nausea, syncope).
  - Patients with ACS who present without chest pain as their chief complaint frequently experience delays in diagnosis and therefore delays in treatment.
  - Atypical presentations are more common in women, in elderly people, and in diabetics.
- The absence of an elevated troponin level is required for the diagnosis of unstable angina, by current definitions.

Primary Differential Considerations

- Primary differential considerations include pain mimics to angina and are diverse, including life-threatening and more benign causes:
  - Aortic dissection
  - Pulmonary embolism
  - Peptic and esophageal disease, hiatal hernia
  - Costochondritis
  - Pneumonia
  - Pneumothorax
  - Pleurisy
  - Anxiety and panic disorders
  - Biliary colic
  - Herpes zoster

	Helpful clinical features
Cardiovascular	
Angina	Retrosternal chest pressure, squeezing, heaviness. Associated with exertion or emotional stress, relieved by rest or nitroglycerin. Usually between 2 and 20 min in duration.
Aortic stenosis	Similar features as for angina, but with late-peaking systolic murmur radiating to carotids. May be associated with syncope or signs of left heart failure.
Pericarditis	Sharp, retrosternal, pleuritic chest pain lasting hours to days. May be associated with friction rub and may be alleviated by leaning forward.
Aortic dissection	Sudden onset of tearing, ripping chest pain radiating to back. Associated with underlying hypertension.
Pulmonary embolism	Ipsilateral pleuritic pain associated with dyspnea, tachycardia, possible cor pulmonale. May have irritative cough or hemoptysis or present with syncope. Usually sudden onset.
Pulmonary	
Pneumonia/pleuritis/pleural effusion	Pleuritic pain, lateralizing to side of infection/inflammation. May be associated with fevers, dyspnea, cough. Exam with pleural rub, consolidation, or dullness to percussion.
Asthma/COPD exacerbation	Chest "tightness" associated with more prominent findings of dyspnea, tachypnea and diffuse wheezing.
Spontaneous pneumothorax	Sudden onset of pleuritic pain. Unilateral and associated with dyspnea. More common in thin, young males or patients with emphysematous disease. Decreased breath sounds and hyperresonance on side of pneumothorax.
Chest wall	
Muscle spasm/strain	Associated with prior increased physical activity/weight lifting. Pain variable in character but usually reproducible with palpation.

	Helpful clinical features
Costochondritis	Sharp, sudden onset pain that is short in duration. May be reproducible with palpation.
Herpes zoster	Sharp, burning, superficial neuropathic pain. May have allodynia, vesicular rash on exam. Unilateral dermatomal distribution.
Rib fracture	Prior trauma or known metastatic disease of bone. Point tenderness over affected rib(s). Pain is usually pleuritic.
Cervical/thoracic nerve root compression	Intermittent neuropathic pain often associated with neck movement or position. Usually unilateral.
Gastrointestinal	
Mediastinitis/ esophageal rupture	Often preceded by esophageal procedure or forceful vomiting. Pt. may have fever, associated septic shock. Symptoms vary from burning chest discomfort to severe dyspnea.
Esophageal reflux	Burning pain, often associated with nausea, belching. Usually worse at night and after large meals. Alleviated by antacids.
Esophageal spasm	Sudden onset, sharp, retrosternal pain. May be relieved by nitroglycerine and exacerbated by cold liquids. Sometimes associated with dysphagia.
Pancreatitis	Sharp epigastric pain, usually constant and prolonged. Exacerbated by food and often associated with nausea/vomiting. Alcohol and gallstones are risk factors.
Peptic ulcer	Sharp or burning epigastric pain. Often relieved by food or antacids. May be associated with occult GI bleeding or massive acute blood loss.
Psychogenic	
Anxiety/panic disorder	May be unable to distinguish from anginal pain, but usually has atypical features such as prolonged duration and no exertional component. Should be a diagnosis of exclusion at initial workup.

Differential diagnosis of acute chest pain. [McClintic BR, Rosenblatt RL. Approach to the patient with chest pain. In: Bisognano JD, Beck R, Connell R, editors. Manual of outpatient cardiology. London: Springer; 2012. p. 349-71. Book https://doi.org/10.1007/978-0-85729-944-4; Chapter: 13; Chapter https://doi.org/10.1007/978-0-85729-944-4_13, 2012-01-01] *Caption from original*

History and Physical Exam

Findings That Confirm Diagnosis

- None

Factors That Suggest Diagnosis

- Nature and history of symptoms with presence of risk factors

Factors That Exclude Diagnosis

- An elevated troponin level is inconsistent with the diagnosis of unstable angina.

Ancillary Studies

Laboratory

- CBC: no diagnostic findings.
- Electrolytes: no diagnostic findings.
- Renal function: no diagnostic findings, but renal insufficiency/failure is a risk factor for ACS and may complicate treatment.
- Coagulation studies: no diagnostic findings but should be performed before initiation of therapy.
- Cardiac enzymes: lack of elevation in troponin (I or T) levels is required to differentiate unstable angina from myocardial infarction.
  - Time course is critical.
    - Depending on specific troponin assay and volume of muscle infarcted, generally takes about 6 hours after onset of symptoms for troponin levels to rise.

- A negative troponin within 6 hours of reliable onset time of symptoms is not particularly helpful.
    - If onset time unclear, start at time of presentation.
    - Patients may be given the *clinical* diagnosis of unstable angina and then be "upgraded" to NSTEMI if a subsequent troponin assay shows an elevated level.
- Positive troponin is *always* helpful, but use caution in interpreting levels in patients with renal insufficiency.
- BNP levels may offer some prognostic significance.

Electrocardiography

- No diagnostic findings, although both ST-segment depression and T-wave inversion confer a poorer prognosis in the setting of unstable angina.

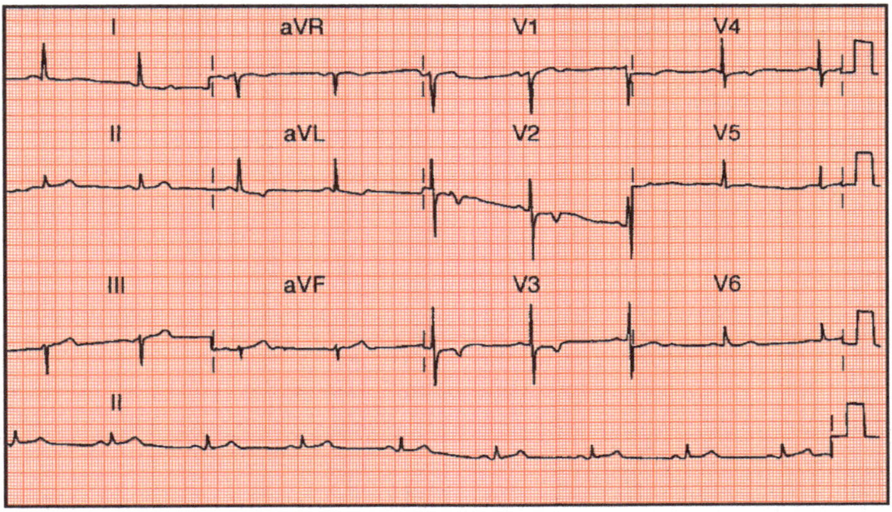

This 57-year-old patient presented with unstable angina, ischemic changes (T wave inversions) are noted in the anteroseptal leads (aVL, V2, V3, V4) (SM; 13/3/93). [Peters N, Gatzoulis MA, Vecht R. ECG diagnosis in clinical practice. London: Springer; 2009. Chapter 2, Ischaemic (coronary) heart disease; p. 11-66.] *Caption from original*

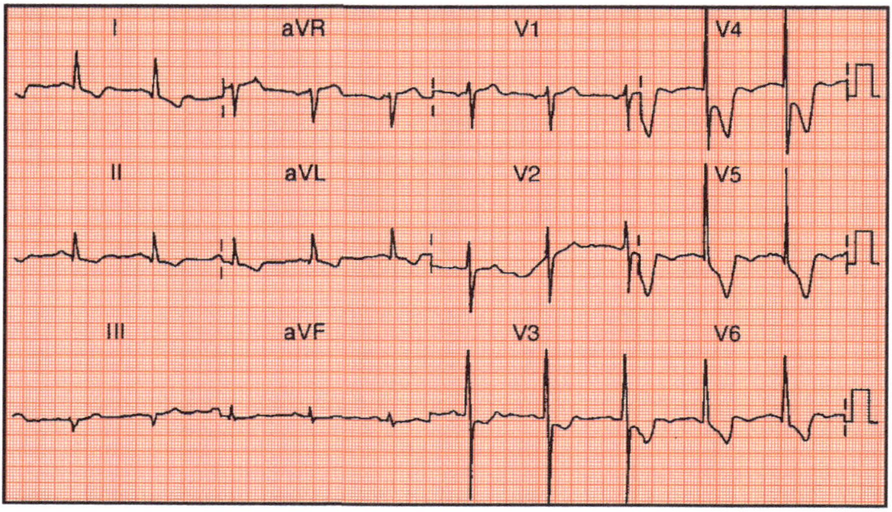

Unstable angina with marked anterolateral ischemic changes. Cardiac catheterization showed critical mainstem stenosis. The patient underwent surgery on the same day (MK; 5/12/95). [Peters N, Gatzoulis MA, Vecht R. ECG diagnosis in clinical practice. London: Springer; 2009. Chapter 2, Ischaemic (coronary) heart disease; p. 11-66.] *Caption from original*

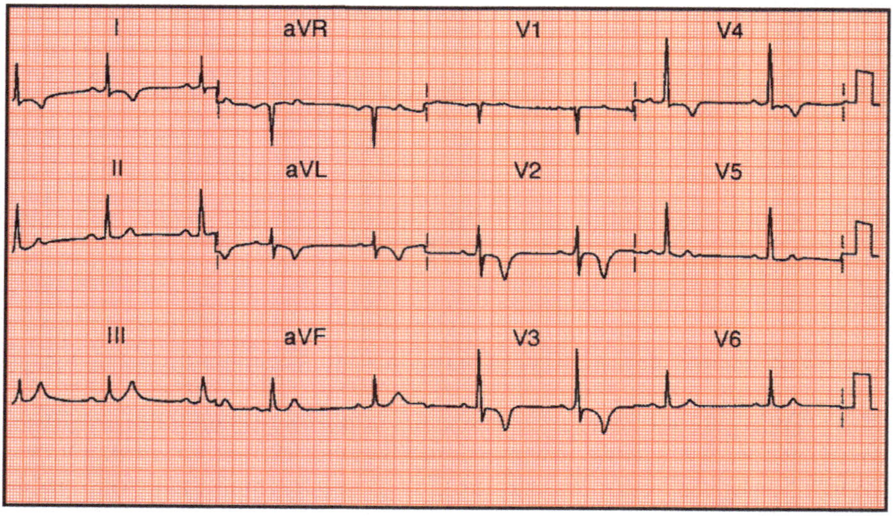

This 86-year-old man presented with severe unstable angina. His cardiac enzyme levels were not elevated. He was treated medically (PR; 16/4/95) [Peters N, Gatzoulis MA, Vecht R. ECG diagnosis in clinical practice. London: Springer; 2009. Chapter 2, Ischaemic (coronary) heart disease; p. 11-66.] *Caption from original*

- According to national quality standards in the United States, ECG should be obtained within 10 minutes of arrival at an emergency department.

Imaging

- No diagnostic findings for ACS on chest x-ray (CXR).
- Findings of heart failure (cardiomegaly, pulmonary congestion) on CXR portend a poorer prognosis in unstable angina.

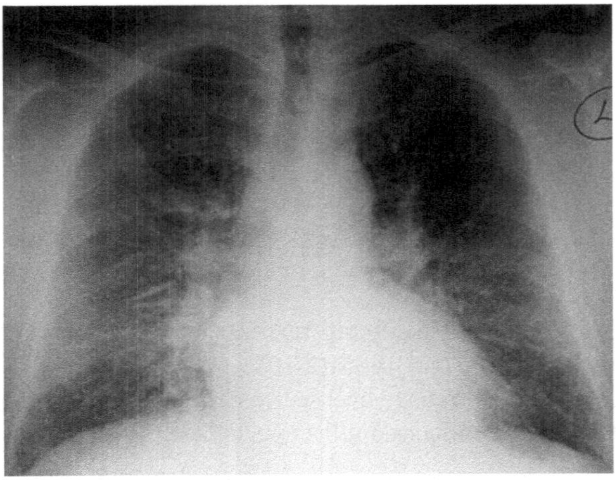

Frontal chest radiograph reveals typical features of pulmonary interstitial edema in a patient with congestive heart failure, manifested by peribronchial cuffing, indistinctness of the pulmonary vessels, and Kerley B lines. Note the cephalization or redistribution of the pulmonary vasculature and mild cardiomegaly. [Boiselle PM, Dass C, Steiner RM. Radiologic imaging in the critically ill patient. In: Criner GJ, Barnette RE, D'Alonzo GE, editors. Critical care study guide. 2nd ed. New York: Springer; 2010. p. 181-207. Book https://doi.org/10.1007/978-0-387-77452-7; Chapter: 11; Chapter https://doi.org/10.1007/978-0-387-77452-7_11, 2010-01-01] *Caption from original*

- Findings of a widened mediastinum suggest consideration of aortic dissection but do not exclude angina. Check differential blood pressures in the upper extremities.

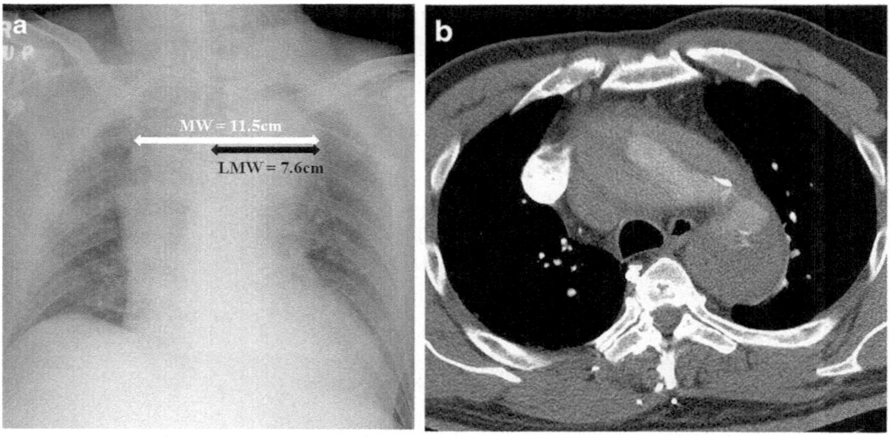

Acute type A aortic dissection in a 46-year-old man. A) AP chest radiograph showing marked widening of the mediastinum with MW and LMW measuring 11.5 and 7.6 cm, respectively. B) Corresponding selected image of CT aortogram confirms type A aortic dissection. [From article: Diagnostic accuracy of mediastinal width measurement on posteroanterior and anteroposterior chest radiographs in the depiction of acute nontraumatic thoracic aortic dissection. Emerg Radiol. 2012 Aug;19(4):309-15. https://doi.org/10.1007/s10140-012-1034-3 at http://link.springer.com/article/10.1007/s10140-012-1034-3 by Vincent Lai, Wai Kan Tsang, Wan Chi Chan, Tsz Wai Yeung, licensed under Creative Commons Attribution License, https://creativecommons.org/licenses/by/2.0/] *Caption from original*

- Findings of pneumonia suggest consideration of that differential but do not exclude angina. Check for signs of infection. Frank septic shock may result in elevated troponin levels.

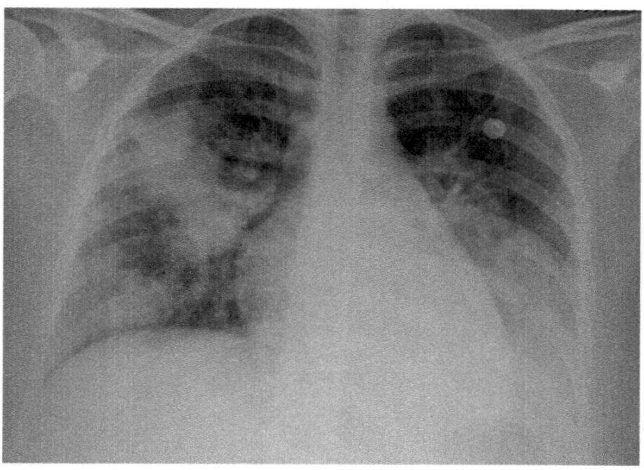

Chest radiograph showing right upper/lower lung field opacities and left lower lung field opacity consistent with pneumonia. [Tsigrelis C, Mohammad M, Fraimow HS,

Dellinger RP, Marchesani D, Reboli AC. Secondary bacterial pneumonia due to Staphylococcus aureus complicating 2009 influenza A (H1N1) viral infection. Infection. 2010 Jun;38(3):237-9. https://doi.org/10.1007/s15010-010-0009-0, 2010-06-01] *Caption adapted from original*

- Findings of pneumothorax suggest consideration of that differential but do not exclude angina. Evaluate oxygenation status.

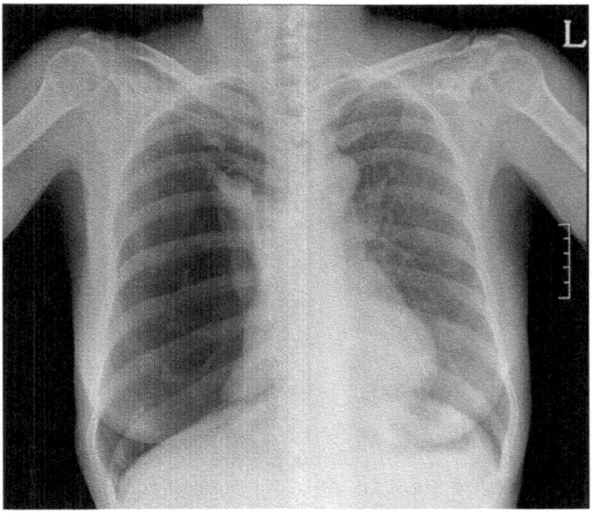

Posteroanterior upright chest X-ray showing large pneumothorax of the right lung. [Kim SH, Yoo WH. Recurrent pneumothorax associated with pulmonary nodules after leflunomide therapy in rheumatoid arthritis: a case report and review of the literature. Rheumatol Int. 2011 Jul;31(7):919-22. https://doi.org/10.1007/s00296-009-1240-9, 2011-06-21] *Caption adapted from original*

- Findings of hiatal hernia suggest consideration of that differential but do not exclude angina.

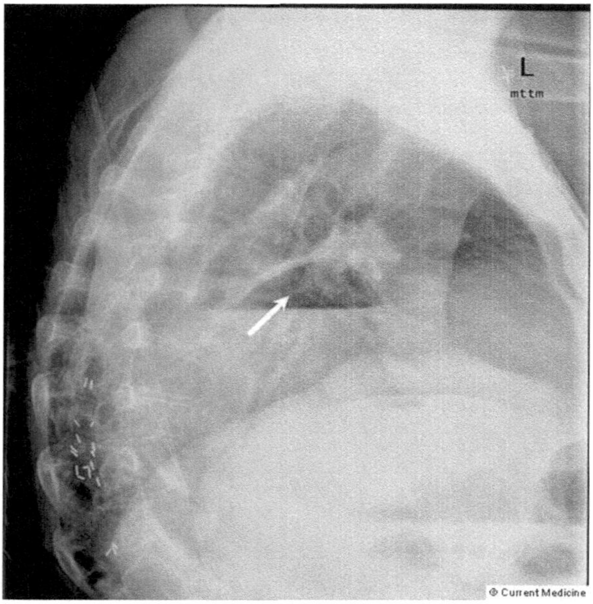

Radiograph of large hiatal hernia. [Aurigemma G, Tighe D, Oh Jae, Espinoza R. Pericardial disease and cardiac masses. In: Solomon SD, Braunwald E, editors. Atlas of echocardiography. 2nd ed. Philadelphia: Current Medicine; 2008. Chapter 16. ISBN: 1-57340-217-6, 2008-10-22;] *Caption from original*

Risk Scoring

TIMI risk score may be helpful in establishing short-term prognosis, which helps drive intensity of therapy.

- Age ≥65 years
- History of known CAD (documented prior coronary artery stenosis >50%)
- ≥3 conventional cardiac risk factors (age, male sex, family history, hyperlipidemia, diabetes mellitus, smoking, obesity)
- Use of aspirin in the past 7 days
- ST-segment deviation (persistent depression or transient elevation)
- Increased cardiac biomarkers (troponins)
- ≥2 anginal events in the preceding 24 h

TIMI = Thrombosis in Myocardial Infarction; CAD = coronary artery disease

Score = sum of number of above characteristics

TIMI = Thrombosis in Myocardial Infarction; CAD = coronary artery disease

Score = sum of number of above characteristics

TIMI risk score for unstable angina and NSTEMI. [Stillman AE, Oudkerk M, Ackerman M, Becker CR, Buszman PE, Feyter PJ, Hoffmann U, Keadey MT, Marano R, Lipton MJ, Raff GL, Reddy GP, Rees MR, Rubin GD, Schoepf UJ, Tarulli G, Beek EJR, Wexler L, White CS. Use of multidetector computed tomography for the assessment of acute chest pain: a consensus statement of the North American Society of Cardiac Imaging and the European Society of Cardiac Radiology. Int J Cardiovasc Imaging. 2007 Aug;23(4):415-27. https://doi.org/10.1007/s10554-007-9226-8, 2007-07-12] *Caption adapted from original*

Value	TIMI risk score[a] (95% CI)	Modified TIMI risk score[b] (95% CI)
Sensitivity	53.7 (44.9–62.3)	58.1 (49.8–66.4)
Specificity	75.2 (72.1–78.2)	82.6 (80.0–85.2)
Negative predictive value	90.6 (88.2–927)	92.2 (90.2–94.1)
Positive predictive value	26.6 (21.5–32.3)	35.9 (29.6–42.2)

[a] Using a cut point of 3 (less than 3 vs. 3 or greater)

[b] Using a cut point of 2 (less than 2 vs. 2 or greater)

A summary of the TIMI risk score and modified TIMI risk scores as predictors of 30-day myocardial infarction/revascularization/death. [Jaffery Z, Hudson MP, Jacobsen G, Nowak R, McCord J. Modified Thrombolysis in Myocardial Infarction (TIMI) risk score to risk stratify patients in the emergency department with possible acute coronary syndrome. J Thromb Thrombolysis. 2007 Oct;24(2):137-44. https://doi.org/10.1007/s11239-007-0013-0, 2007-08-02] *Caption adapted from original*

Special Populations

Age

- Risk for coronary artery disease that causes angina increases with age, starting at age 40 in men and at menopause in women.
  - Age is a risk factor for mortality from all types of ACS.
  - Likelihood of atypical presentation with unstable angina increases with age.

Comorbidities

- Hypertension, diabetes, and renal failure are important comorbidities in ACS risk and prognosis.
- Diabetes is associated with the likelihood of atypical presentation with unstable angina.
- Obesity is a weaker predictor of unstable angina risk.

Pitfalls in Diagnosis

Critical Steps Not to Miss

- ECG must be performed as soon as the diagnosis of ACS is even considered. By definition, in unstable angina, there will not be persistent ST-segment elevation.

Mimics

- All differential considerations are listed under Primary Differential Considerations.
  - Of these, only aortic dissection and pulmonary embolism are also life threatening.

Time-Dependent Interventions

- Stabilization of the unstable angina patient is time-sensitive.
- Derangements in blood pressure should be addressed immediately: hypertension results in increased myocardial oxygen demand, and hypotension reduces blood supply to the myocardium.

- Current guidelines call for diagnostic angiography in 24–48 hours to establish preferred course of management.
- Unless contraindicated (allergy, active bleeding), 324–325 mg aspirin should be administered immediately upon suspicion of an ACS.
- Anticoagulation therapy should be initiated upon determination of the diagnosis of unstable angina or when there is high suspicion in high-risk patients.
- Airway and oxygenation should be monitored and supported as necessary.
- Patients with a diagnosis of unstable angina should be on continuous cardiac monitoring to evaluate for dangerous arrhythmias.
- Consider early initiation of dual antiplatelet therapy (aspirin plus an ADP receptor antagonist—ticagrelor or clopidogrel).

Overall Principles of Treatment

- Immediate stabilization of the patient with control of blood pressure, pulse rate, and pain is critical. The patient with unstable angina only rarely requires resuscitation, intubation, and intensive support.
- Medical management with anticoagulation and antiplatelet therapy is important.
  - Bleeding risk should also be assessed so that the risk of treatment-related hemorrhage can be minimized.
- The higher the patient's risk, the more disproportionately s/he benefits from aggressive therapy.

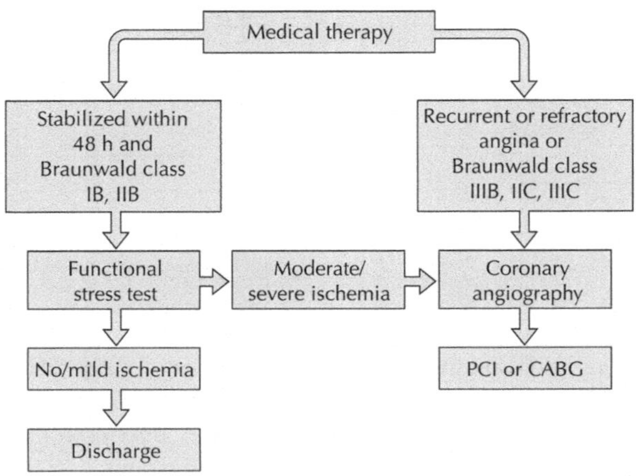

Treatment for unstable angina [Prasad A, Holmes D, Kleiman N. Use of percutaneous coronary intervention in unstable angina and acute myocardial infarction. In: Califf RM, editor. Acute myocardial infarction and other acute ischemic syndromes. 2nd ed. Philadelphia: Current Medicine; 2001. Chapter 7. (Braunwald E, editor. Atlas of heart diseases; vol. 8.)]

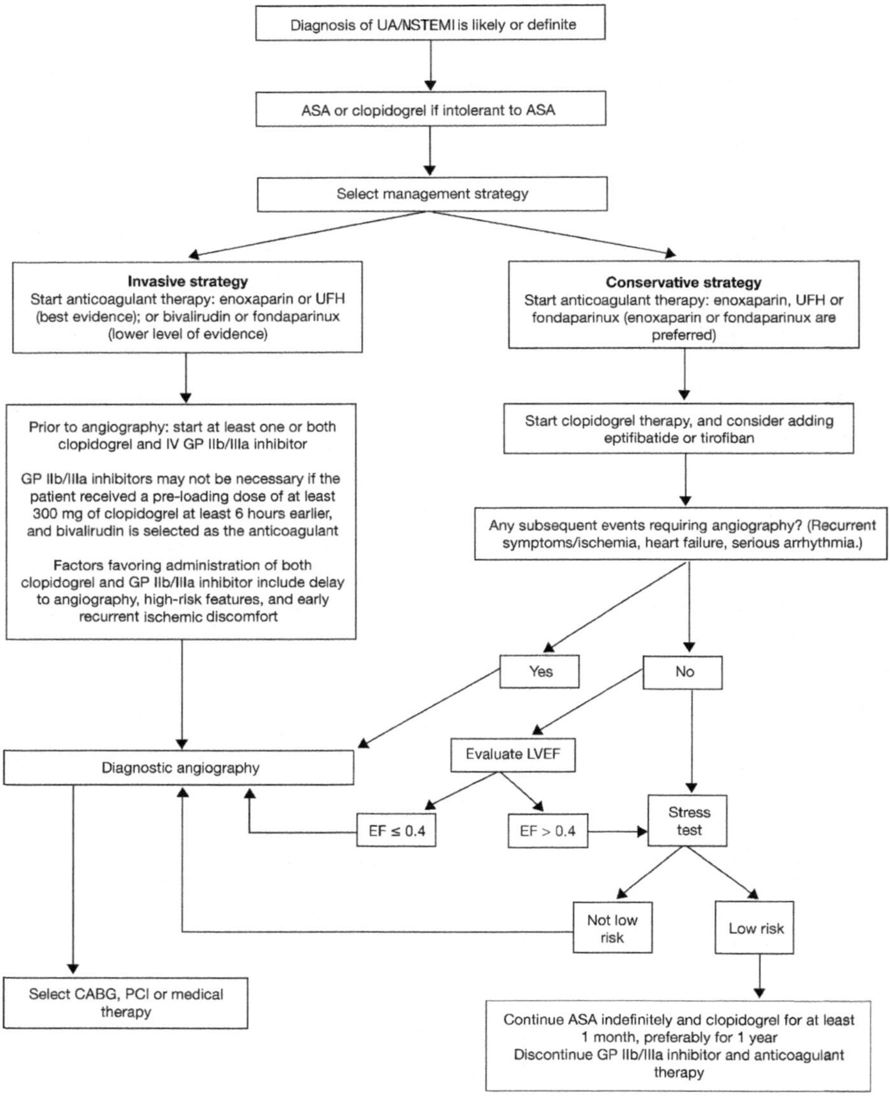

Algorithm for the initial management of patients with UA/NSTEMI with an invasive or conservative treatment strategy. Abbreviations: ASA, aspirin; CABG, coronary artery-bypass grafting; EF, ejection fraction; GP, glycoprotein; IV, intravenous; LVEF, left ventricular ejection fraction; PCI, percutaneous coronary intervention; UA/NSTEMI, unstable angina/non-ST-elevation myocardial infarction; UFH, unfractionated heparin. [Cohen M. High-risk acute coronary syndrome patients with non-ST-elevation myocardial infarction: definition and treatment. Cardiovasc Drugs Ther. 2008 Oct;22(5):407-18. https://doi.org/10.1007/s10557-008-6120-0, 2008-09-04] *Caption adapted from original*

Disease Course

- The expected mortality rate associated with unstable angina alone is not clear, owing to differences in the definition of the disease. Mortality in NSTEMI—the other component of NSTE-ACS—is 6–10 %, depending on the population studied, over 6 months.

Related Evidence

Papers of particular interest have been highlighted as:
*** Of key importance*

Practice Guideline

Anderson JL, Adams CD, Antman EM, Bridges CR, Califf RM, Casey DE Jr, Chavey WE 2nd, Fesmire FM, Hochman JS, Levin TN, Lincoff AM, Peterson ED, Theroux P, Wenger NK, Wright RS, Jneid H, Ettinger SM, Ganiats TG, Lincoff AM, Philippides GJ, Zidar JP; American College of Cardiology Foundation/American Heart Association Task Force on Practice Guidelines. 2012 ACCF/AHA focused update incorporated into the ACCF/AHA 2007 guidelines for the management of patients with unstable angina/non-ST-elevation myocardial infarction: a report of the American College of Cardiology Foundation/American Heart Association Task Force on Practice Guidelines. Circulation. 2013 Jun 11;127(23):e663-828. https://doi.org/10.1161/CIR.0b013e31828478ac. Erratum in: Circulation. 2013 Jun 18;127(24):e863-4. PMID: 23630129. http://www.ncbi.nlm.nih.gov/pubmed/23630129 **

Task Force for Diagnosis and Treatment of Non-ST-Segment Elevation Acute Coronary Syndromes of European Society of Cardiology, Bassand JP, Hamm CW, Ardissino D, Boersma E, Budaj A, Fernández-Avilés F, Fox KA, Hasdai D, Ohman EM, Wallentin L, Wijns W. Guidelines for the diagnosis and treatment of non-ST-segment elevation acute coronary syndromes. Eur Heart J. 2007 Jul;28(13): 1598-660. PMID: 17569677. http://www.ncbi.nlm.nih.gov/pubmed/17569677 **

Review

Meier P, Lansky AJ, Baumbach A. Almanac 2013: acute coronary syndromes. Heart. 2013 Oct;99(20):1488-93. https://doi.org/10.1136/heartjnl-2013-304649. PMID: 23945172. http://www.ncbi.nlm.nih.gov/pubmed/23945172

Tricoci P, Leonardi S, White J, White HD, Armstrong PW, Montalescot G, Giugliano RP, Gibson CM, Van de Werf F, Califf RM, Harrington RA, Braunwald E,

Mahaffey KW, Newby LK. Cardiac troponin after percutaneous coronary intervention and 1-year mortality in non-ST-segment elevation acute coronary syndrome using systematic evaluation of biomarker trends. J Am Coll Cardiol. 2013 Jul 16;62(3):242-51. https://doi.org/10.1016/j.jacc.2013.04.043. PMID: 23684676. http://www.ncbi.nlm.nih.gov/pubmed/23684676

Giugliano RP, Braunwald E. The year in non-ST-segment elevation acute coronary syndrome. J Am Coll Cardiol. 2012 Nov 20;60(21):2127-39. https://doi.org/10.1016/j.jacc.2012.08.972. PMID: 23103037. http://www.ncbi.nlm.nih.gov/pubmed/23103037 **

Trost JC, Lange RA. Treatment of acute coronary syndrome: Part 1: Non-ST-segment acute coronary syndrome. Crit Care Med. 2011 Oct;39(10):2346-53. https://doi.org/10.1097/CCM.0b013e31821e855f. PMID: 21602671. http://www.ncbi.nlm.nih.gov/pubmed/21602671 **

Sami S, Willerson JT. Contemporary treatment of unstable angina and non-ST-segment-elevation myocardial infarction (part 1). Tex Heart Inst J. 2010;37(2):141-8. PMID: 20401284. http://www.ncbi.nlm.nih.gov/pubmed/20401284 **

Cohort Study

Antonsen L, Jensen LO, Thayssen P, Christiansen EH, Junker A, Tilsted HH, Terkelsen CJ, Kaltoft A, Maeng M, Hansen KN, Ravkilde J, Lassen JF, Madsen M, Sørensen HT, Thuesen L. Comparison of outcomes of patients ≥ 80 years of age having percutaneous coronary intervention according to presentation (stable vs unstable angina pectoris/non-ST-segment elevation myocardial infarction vs ST-segment elevation myocardial infarction). Am J Cardiol. 2011 Nov 15;108(10):1395-400. https://doi.org/10.1016/j.amjcard.2011.06.062. PMID: 21890087. http://www.ncbi.nlm.nih.gov/pubmed/21890087

Use PubMed Clinical Queries to find the most recent evidence. Use this search strategy:

"Angina, Unstable"[Mesh] OR "unstable angina"

Chapter 5
Acute Pericarditis

Charles V. Pollack, Jr., Richard M. Cantor, and Victoria G. Riese

Name and Synonyms

Acute pericarditis

Incidence/Epidemiology

- Acute pericarditis is the admitting diagnosis in 0.1 % of hospital admissions. Acute pericarditis accounts for 1 % of cases of ST-segment elevation seen in the emergency department.
- Acute pericarditis occurs more commonly in men than in women. There are no known geographic predilections. There is a very rare familial form (Mulibrey nanism)

C. V. Pollack, Jr. (✉)
Department of Emergency Medicine, Thomas Jefferson University, Philadelphia, PA, USA

R. M. Cantor
Department of Emergency Medicine and Pediatrics, State University of New York Upstate Medical University, Syracuse, NY, USA

V. G. Riese
Librarian Consultant, Eldersburg, MD, USA

C. V. Pollack, Jr. (ed.), *Differential Diagnosis of Cardiopulmonary Disease*,
https://doi.org/10.1007/978-3-319-63895-9_5

Differential Diagnosis

- Acute pericarditis has many causes (see Pathophysiology and Etiology below), and often the differential exploration focuses on determining an etiology for the disease. This involves a search for co-morbidities as diverse as malignancy, renal failure, recent myocardial infarction, adverse effects of certain drugs, and collagen vascular diseases. Because the primary clinical manifestation of acute pericarditis is chest pain, the differential is broad.

Pathophysiology and Etiology

- The pathophysiology of acute pericarditis, regardless of etiology, is inflammation of the pericardium, a double (serous and parietal) membrane separated normally by 15-50 mL of fluid that is an ultrafiltrate of plasma.
- The function of the pericardium is to prevent sudden overdistention of the cardiac chambers and to help maintain the anatomic position of the heart and great vessels. By definition, acute pericarditis is present and symptomatic for less than 6 weeks; pericarditis for 6 weeks to 6 months is termed subacute, and beyond 6 months, chronic.
  - This inflammation may result from a myriad of potential causes:
    - Infectious:
      - Viral (Coxsackie, echovirus, adenovirus, HIV)
      - Tuberculous
      - Pyogenic (pneumococcal, streptococcal, staphylococcal)
      - Fungal (histoplasmosis, coccidioidomycosis, blastomycosis, *Candida*)
    - Noninfectious:
      - Post–myocardial infarction (Dressler's syndrome)
      - Uremia/renal failure
      - Neoplastic (primary or metastatic [lung, breast, lymphoma, Hodgkins])
      - Myxedema
      - Trauma (penetrating or nonpenetrating)
      - Aortic dissection into pericardium
      - Post–radiation therapy
      - Rheumatic fever
      - Collagen vascular disease (lupus, rheumatoid arthritis, scleroderma, Wegener's granulomatosis)
      - Drug-induced (procainamide, hydralazine, INH, phenytoin, doxorubicin, rifampin, methyldopa)
      - Idiopathic (most common)

Presentation

Typical/"Classic"

- Chest pain and a pericardial friction rub are most the common findings.

http://www.easyauscultation.com/acute-pericarditis
[Acute Pericarditis Page; Easy Auscultation; copyright 2015, MedEdu LLC]

- On electrocardiography, there are electrical changes suggesting acute pericarditis, and if there is also an effusion there is generalized low voltage.

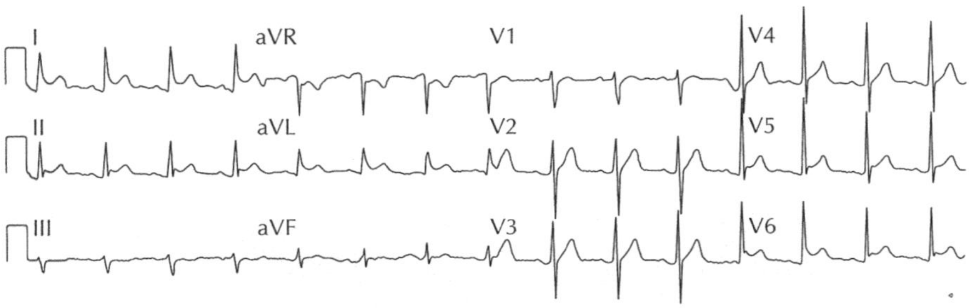

ECG finding in acute pericarditis [Oh J, Espinosa R. Pericardial disease. In: Vannan MA, Lang RM, Rakowski H, Tajik AJ, editors. Atlas of echocardiography. Philadelphia: Current Medicine; 2005 (Braunwald E, editor. Atlas of heart diseases; vol. 16).] *Caption from original*

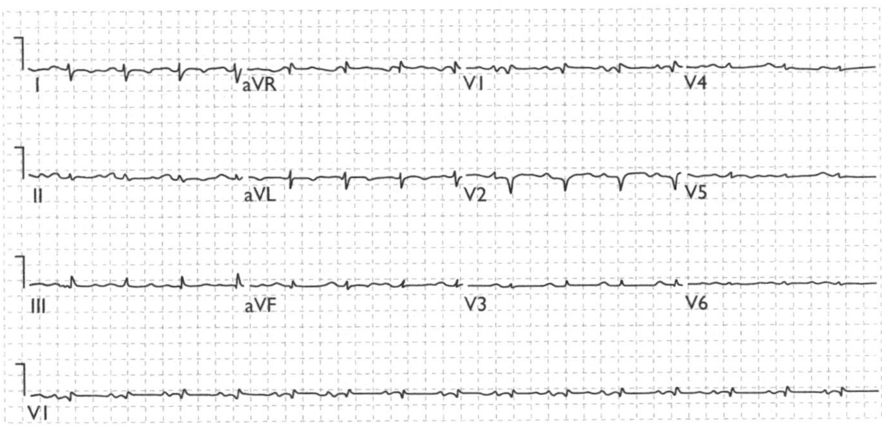

Typical amyloid ECG with diffuse low voltage [Wellens H, Subramaniam K. The electrocardiogram in heart failure. In: Shivkumar K, Weiss JN, Fonarow GC, Narula J, editors. Atlas of electrophysiology in heart failure. Philadelphia: Current

Medicine; 2005 (Braunwald E, editor. Atlas of heart diseases; vol. 15).] *Caption from original*

- On echocardiogram, an effusion may be visible but is not required for a diagnosis of acute pericarditis.

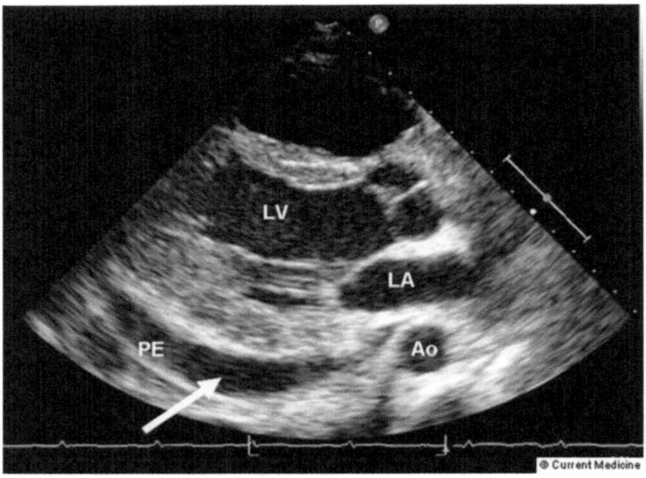

Echocardiogram of pericardial effusion. Arrow indicates descending thoracic aorta. [Aurigemma G, Tighe D, Oh J, Espinoza R. Pericardial disease and cardiac masses. In: Solomon SD, editor. Atlas of echocardiography. 2nd ed. Philadelphia: Current Medicine; 2008.] *Caption adapted from original*

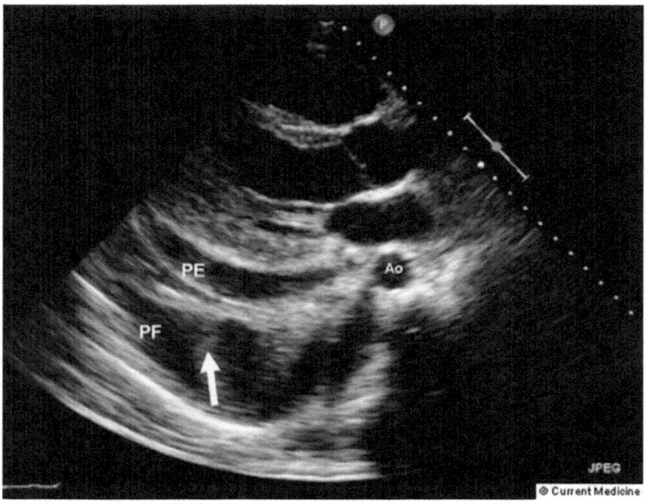

Echocardiogram of pericardial effusion. Arrow indicates lung parenchyma. [Aurigemma G, Tighe D, Oh J, Espinoza R. Pericardial disease and cardiac masses.

In: Solomon SD, editor. Atlas of echocardiography. 2nd ed. Philadelphia: Current Medicine; 2008.] *Caption adapted from original*

- If the effusion is large (>250 mL), the heart takes on a "water bottle" appearance on plain chest x-ray.

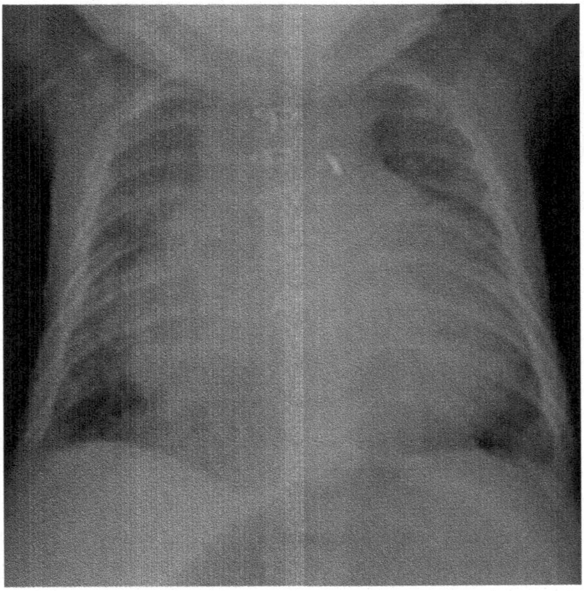

Chest X-ray in pericardial effusion: water bottle shaped heart. [Tissot C, Phelps CM, Cruz EM, Miyamoto SD. Pericardial diseases. In: Munoz R, Morell V, Cruz E, Vetterly C, editors. Critical care of children with heart disease. London: Springer; 2010. p. 521-41. https://doi.org/10.1007/978-1-84882-262-7_47; 2009-01-01] *Caption from original*

- Cardiac tamponade may develop, and the patient may have pulsus paradoxus.

http://www.youtube.com/watch?feature=player_embedded&v=jTsjCZ9QxW8
Stanford 25 video on pulsus paradoxus. Provides definition, guidance on testing, sound clip.

- The pain is often severe. It is most often substernal and left-sided. It often radiates to the back and to the trapezius ridge.

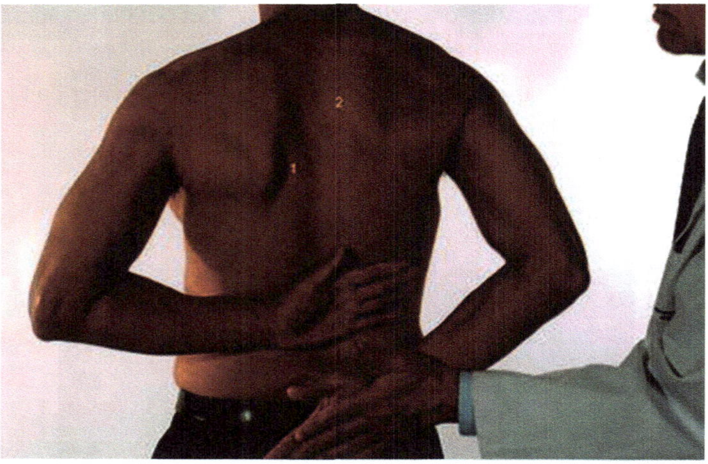

Trapezius ridge: the lower border of trapezius, 1; the rhomboids, 2. [Birch R. Surgical disorders of the peripheral nerves. London: Springer; 2010. Chapter 5, Clinical aspects of nerve injury; p. 145-90] *Caption adapted from original*

- The pain is often pleuritic in nature, so it is aggravated by deep inspiration, cough, and lying down as opposed to sitting up.
- The friction rub is the most important physical sign of acute pericarditis. It is often described as "scratching" or "grating," and it may be evanescent. It is best heard with the diaphragm of the stethoscope along the lower left sternal border, with the patient sitting up, during exhalation.
- The classic ECG findings of acute pericarditis are diffuse, mild ST-segment elevation across the precordium. Depression of the PQ segment is common. With large effusions, the overall voltage on the ECG is reduced. Occasionally, atrial fibrillation occurs with acute pericarditis. The ST-segment elevation associated with acute pericarditis can be differentiated from simple early repolarization, and from left ventricular hypertrophy with strain, by considering the ratio of the amplitude of ST segment to the amplitude of the T wave in leads I, V4, V5, and V6.

Atypical

- The most common form of pericarditis is idiopathic, and the diagnosis is one of exclusion. Patients with acute pericarditis and no effusion may present with chest pain and no audible friction rub, with limited to no ECG changes. In this case, acute pericarditis is just one of many differential considerations in the chest pain syndrome presentation. As in other etiologies of chest pain syndrome, the pain may occur in non-substernal locations.

- Pain may be mostly absent in slowly developing pericarditis (neoplastic, uremic, postradiation). Worsening exercise intolerance may be a clue to the diagnosis in these patients.

Primary Differential Considerations

- The initial differential elements to be considered in a patient with a presentation consistent with acute pericarditis are angina, aortic dissection, pulmonary embolism, and distal esophageal pain.

History and Physical Exam

Findings That Confirm Diagnosis

- A full classic presentation (substernal and/or left-sided pleuritic chest pain, a friction rub, and diffuse mild ST-segment elevation on ECG) should be considered confirmatory and should prompt a search for an etiology other than idiopathic.

Factors That Suggest Diagnosis

- Any of the classic findings in isolation should elevate acute pericarditis in the differential diagnosis of the chest pain patient.
- Onset of pain within 2–4 days of acute myocardial infarction (Dressler's syndrome) or after thoracic surgery should elevate acute pericarditis in the differential diagnosis of the chest pain patient.
- A presentation consistent with both acute pericarditis and an apparent cause of pericarditis (such as uremia, myxedema, acute infection, immunocompromise, collagen vascular disease, post chest irradiation) should elevate acute pericarditis in the differential diagnosis of the chest pain patient.
- Uremic pericarditis is most often seen in patients on hemodialysis (HD). A history of HD therefore is suggestive of the diagnosis. It should be noted that chest pain is often minimal or absent in uremic pericarditis, but a friction rub is common.

Factors That Exclude Diagnosis

- A normal echocardiogram excludes pericardial effusion and tamponade but not acute pericarditis.

Ancillary Studies

Laboratory

- Lab tests should include CBC; serum electrolyte, blood urea nitrogen (BUN), and creatinine levels; and erythrocyte sedimentation rate (ESR) and/or C-reactive protein (CRP) levels. In the evaluation of chest pain syndrome, cardiac biomarker measurements are often indicated.
- The ESR and CRP levels are elevated in acute pericarditis, consistent with the underlying inflammation. These tests also are abnormal in patients with collagen vascular diseases, which may be an etiology of acute pericarditis.
- Other laboratory tests may be pertinent to the evaluation of the etiology of the pericarditis:
  - Assessment of renal function in possible uremic pericarditis
  - Assessment of thyroid function in possible myxedema
  - An antistreptolysin O (ASO) titer is indicated if rheumatic fever is suspected.
  - If a pericardial effusion is sampled via pericardiocentesis, the fluid should be tested for cell count, glucose and protein, and culture growth. Other specialized tests may be needed, and fluid should be retained for "unusual" requests by consultants.

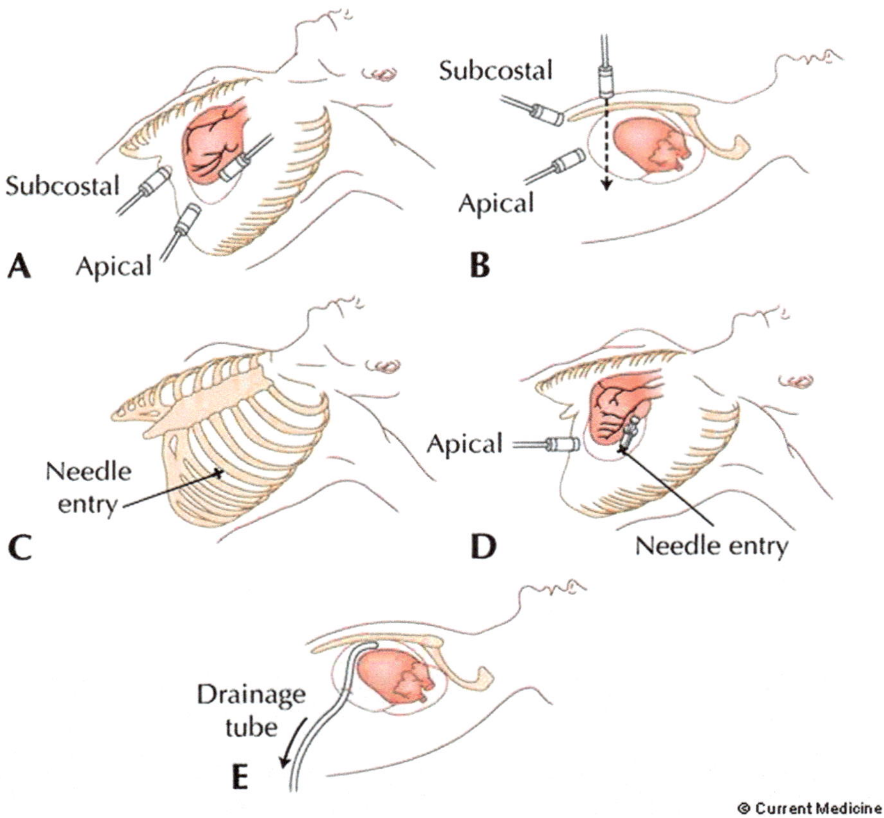

Echocardiographically guided pericardiocentesis procedure [Aurigemma G, Tighe D, Oh J, Espinoza R. Pericardial disease and cardiac masses. In: Solomon SD, editor. Atlas of echocardiography. 2nd ed. Philadelphia: Current Medicine; 2008.] *Caption from original*

https://www.youtube.com/watch?feature=player_embedded&v=BQTVqUPimdk
Video from The New England Journal of Medicine on pericardiocentesis. Covers indications, risk factors, contraindications, equipment, preparation, procedure (ultrasound-guided, electrocardiographic monitoring, and blind approaches), aftercare, and complications.

https://www.youtube.com/watch?v=y0-K2RcThi0
Video from MD Anderson Cancer Center explaining the anterior chest approach to pericardiocentesis.

Imaging

- There are no diagnostic imaging findings of acute pericarditis. When a pericardial effusion is present, transthoracic echocardiography will demonstrate an echo-free space between the visceral and parietal layers of the pericardium.
- Echocardiography should be performed in all cases of pericarditis, because any form of pericardial inflammation may induce pericardial effusion. It is important to note that in the absence of effusion, the pericardium may have a normal appearance in pericarditis.
- With large effusions, a "swinging heart" may be seen on echocardiography, as the heart "floats" in the effusion fluid.

https://www.youtube.com/watch?feature=player_embedded&v=huXuWp_eOKQ Brief clip of cardiac tamponade with swinging heart echocardiogram.

- Plain chest radiographs are usually normal in acute pericarditis. If there is an effusion of 250 mL or more fluid, the cardiac silhouette will take on an enlarged, "water bottle" appearance.
- Smaller effusions may be detected by MRI, which can also assess the thickness of the pericardium (normal, 4 mm). In acute pericarditis, the pericardium may be globally or locally thickened.

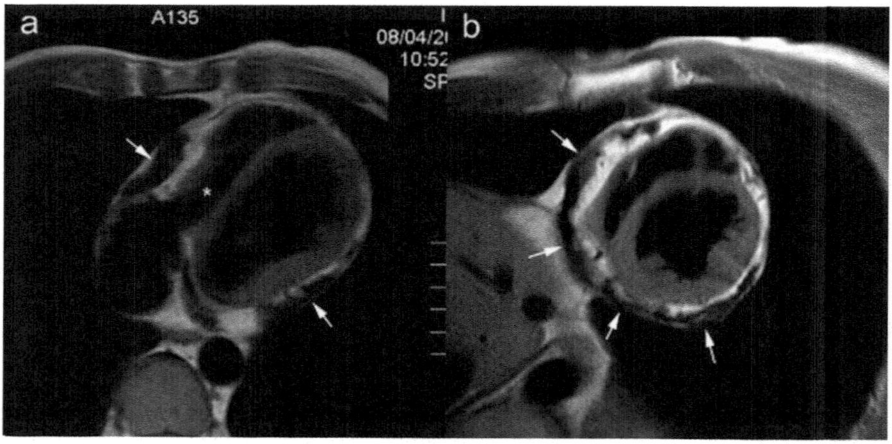

Classic presentation of constrictive pericarditis on T1-weighted fast spin-echo CMR, axial view (a), and short-axis view (b) [From article: Cardiovascular magnetic resonance in pericardial diseases. J Cardiovasc Magn Reson. 2009; 11(1):14. https://doi.org/10.1186/1532-429X-11-14, at http://link.springer.com/article/10.1186%2F1532-429X-11-14; by Jan Bogaert, Marco Francone, © Bogaert and Francone; licensee BioMed Central Ltd. 2009; licensed under Creative Commons Attribution License BY 2.0 http://creativecommons.org/licenses/by/2.0] *Caption from original*

Special Populations

Age

- Acute pericarditis is more common in adults than in children, but adolescents are more commonly affected than young adults
- The most common presenting complaint in children with pericarditis is chest pain, accompanied by the typical findings seen in patients of any age.
- In children, the clear majority of cases are viral in etiology, since autoimmune diseases usually present no earlier than late adolescence.

Co-morbidities

- Review of the etiologies of acute pericarditis will indicate co-morbidities of interest. Uremia, malignancy, and immunocompromise are the most worrisome of these.

Pitfalls in Diagnosis

Critical Steps Not to Miss

- Consideration of the diagnosis is the first critical step. In patients with hemodynamic compromise, an echocardiogram should be performed early to assess for effusion, or even tamponade, and to measure the pumping ability of the heart.
- Acute pericarditis is one of the few diagnoses in which an ESR and CRP are actually very helpful.

Mimics

- The entire constellation of diagnoses that underlies chest pain syndrome can mimic the pain and overall presentation of acute pericarditis.
- Because acute pericarditis is often associated with diffuse ST-segment elevation on ECG, acute coronary syndrome must be always considered as an alternative diagnosis. PR-segment depression usually is also seen in patients with acute pericarditis who have ST-segment elevation.

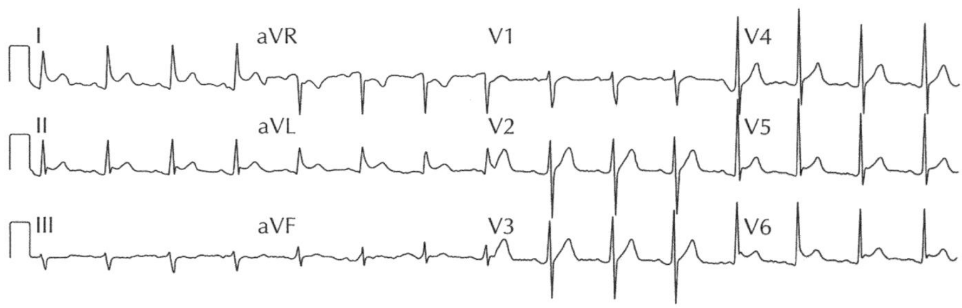

ECG finding in acute pericarditis [Oh J, Espinosa R. Pericardial disease. In: Vannan MA, Lang RM, Rakowski H, Tajik AJ, editors. Atlas of echocardiography. Philadelphia: Current Medicine; 2005 (Braunwald E, editor. Atlas of heart diseases; vol. 16).] *Caption from original*

Time-Dependent Interventions

- Time-dependent interventions in acute pericarditis are necessary only when cardiac function is compromised, which is usually the case only when there is a large pericardial effusion. In such patients, pericardiocentesis may be a lifesaving procedure.

Overall Principles of Treatment

- Because acute pericarditis is an inflammatory disease, the primary treatment in idiopathic pericarditis comprises anti-inflammatory agents (such as corticosteroids [e.g., prednisone] and nonsteroidal anti-inflammatory drugs [NSAIDs]). Resistant cases may require a surgical pericardiectomy, pericardiotomy, or pericardial window.
- Patients with an identified underlying cause of their pericarditis generally benefit from better control/specific treatment of the disease.

Disease Course

- Idiopathic pericarditis generally resolves within 1-2 weeks with anti-inflammatory therapy. The recurrence rate may reach 33 %.
- The course of secondary pericarditis typically follows control of the underlying disease.

Related Evidence

Papers of particular interest have been highlighted as:
*** Of key importance*

Practice Guideline

Maisch B, Seferović PM, Ristić AD, Erbel R, Rienmüller R, Adler Y, Tomkowski WZ, Thiene G, Yacoub MH; Task Force on the Diagnosis and Management of Pricardial Diseases of the European Society of Cardiology. Guidelines on the diagnosis and management of pericardial diseases executive summary; The Task force on the diagnosis and management of pericardial diseases of the European society of cardiology. Eur Heart J. 2004 Apr;25(7):587-610. PMID: 15120056. http://www.ncbi.nlm.nih.gov/pubmed/15120056**

Review

Imazio M, Adler Y. Treatment with aspirin, NSAID, corticosteroids, and colchicine in acute and recurrent pericarditis. Heart Fail Rev. 2013 May;18(3):355-60. https://doi.org/10.1007/s10741-012-9328-9. PMID: 22661042. http://www.ncbi.nlm.nih.gov/pubmed/22661042

Seferović PM, Ristić AD, Maksimović R, Simeunović DS, Milinković I, Seferović Mitrović JP, Kanjuh V, Pankuweit S, Maisch B. Pericardial syndromes: an update after the ESC guidelines 2004. Heart Fail Rev. 2013 May;18(3):255-66. https://doi.org/10.1007/s10741-012-9335-x. PMID: 22855353. http://www.ncbi.nlm.nih.gov/pubmed/22855353**

Shammas NW, Padaria RF, Coyne EP. Pericarditis, myocarditis, and other cardiomyopathies. Prim Care. 2013 Mar;40(1):213-36. https://doi.org/10.1016/j.pop.2012.11.009. Epub 2012 Dec 6. PMID: 23402470. http://www.ncbi.nlm.nih.gov/pubmed/23402470**

Imazio M. Treatment of recurrent pericarditis. Expert Rev Cardiovasc Ther. 2012 Sep;10(9):1165-72. https://doi.org/10.1586/erc.12.101. PMID: 23098152. http://www.ncbi.nlm.nih.gov/pubmed/23098152**

Dudzinski DM, Mak GS, Hung JW. Pericardial diseases. Curr Probl Cardiol. 2012 Mar;37(3):75-118. https://doi.org/10.1016/j.cpcardiol.2011.10.002. PMID: 22289657. http://www.ncbi.nlm.nih.gov/pubmed/22289657**

Sheth S, Wang DD, Kasapis C. Current and emerging strategies for the treatment of acute pericarditis: a systematic review. J Inflamm Res. 2010;3:135-42. https://doi.org/10.2147/JIR.S10268. Epub 2010 Nov 25. PMID: 22096363; PMCID: PMC3218740. http://www.ncbi.nlm.nih.gov/pubmed/22096363

Lotrionte M, Biondi-Zoccai G, Imazio M, Castagno D, Moretti C, Abbate A, Agostoni P, Brucato AL, Di Pasquale P, Raatikka M, Sangiorgi G, Laudito A, Sheiban I, Gaita F. International collaborative systematic review of controlled clinical trials on pharmacologic treatments for acute pericarditis and its recurrences. Am Heart J. 2010 Oct;160(4):662-70. https://doi.org/10.1016/j.ahj.2010.06.015. PMID: 20934560. http://www.ncbi.nlm.nih.gov/pubmed/20934560

Khandaker MH, Espinosa RE, Nishimura RA, Sinak LJ, Hayes SN, Melduni RM, Oh JK. Pericardial disease: diagnosis and management. Mayo Clin Proc. 2010 Jun;85(6):572-93. https://doi.org/10.4065/mcp.2010.0046. PMID: 20511488; PMCID: PMC2878263. http://www.ncbi.nlm.nih.gov/pubmed/20511488**

Imazio M, Spodick DH, Brucato A, Trinchero R, Adler Y. Controversial issues in the management of pericardial diseases. Circulation. 2010 Feb 23;121(7):916-28. https://doi.org/10.1161/CIRCULATIONAHA.108.844753. PMID: 20177006. http://www.ncbi.nlm.nih.gov/pubmed/20177006**

Imazio M, Brucato A, Derosa FG, Lestuzzi C, Bombana E, Scipione F, Leuzzi S, Cecchi E, Trinchero R, Adler Y. Aetiological diagnosis in acute and recurrent pericarditis: when and how. J Cardiovasc Med (Hagerstown). 2009 Mar;10(3):217-30. https://doi.org/10.2459/JCM.0b013e328322f9b1. PMID: 19262208. http://www.ncbi.nlm.nih.gov/pubmed/19262208

Syed FF, Mayosi BM. A modern approach to tuberculous pericarditis. Prog Cardiovasc Dis. 2007 Nov-Dec;50(3):218-36. Review. PubMed PMID: 17976506. http://www.ncbi.nlm.nih.gov/pubmed/17976506

Tingle LE, Molina D, Calvert CW. Acute pericarditis. Am Fam Physician. 2007 Nov 15;76(10):1509-14. PMID: 18052017. http://www.ncbi.nlm.nih.gov/pubmed/18052017**

Ariyarajah V, Spodick DH. Acute pericarditis: diagnostic cues and common electrocardiographic manifestations. Cardiol Rev. 2007 Jan-Feb;15(1):24-30. PMID: 17172880. http://www.ncbi.nlm.nih.gov/pubmed/17172880**

Permanyer-Miralda G. Acute pericardial disease: approach to the aetiologic diagnosis. Heart. 2004 Mar;90(3):252-4. PMID: 14966036; PMCID: PMC1768141. http://www.ncbi.nlm.nih.gov/pubmed/14966036

Ross AM, Grauer SE. Acute pericarditis. Evaluation and treatment of infectious and other causes. Postgrad Med. 2004 Mar;115(3):67-70, 73-5. PMID: 15038256. http://www.ncbi.nlm.nih.gov/pubmed/15038256**

Troughton RW, Asher CR, Klein AL. Pericarditis. Lancet. 2004 Feb 28;363(9410):717-27. PMID: 15001332. http://www.ncbi.nlm.nih.gov/pubmed/15001332**

Spodick DH. Acute pericarditis: current concepts and practice. JAMA. 2003 Mar 5;289(9):1150-3. PubMed PMID: 12622586. http://www.ncbi.nlm.nih.gov/pubmed/12622586**

Aikat S, Ghaffari S. A review of pericardial diseases: clinical, ECG and hemodynamic features and management. Cleve Clin J Med. 2000 Dec;67(12):903-14. PMID: 11127986. http://www.ncbi.nlm.nih.gov/pubmed/11127986

Goodman LJ. Purulent Pericarditis. Curr Treat Options Cardiovasc Med. 2000 Aug;2(4):343-350. PMID: 11096539. http://www.ncbi.nlm.nih.gov/pubmed/11096539

Clinical Trial

Imazio M, Brucato A, Barbieri A, Ferroni F, Maestroni S, Ligabue G, Chinaglia A, Cumetti D, Casa GD, Bonomi F, Mantovani F, Di Corato P, Lugli R, Faletti R, Leuzzi S, Bonamini R, Modena MG, Belli R. Good prognosis for pericarditis with and without myocardial involvement: results from a multicenter, prospective cohort study. Circulation. 2013 Jul 2;128(1):42-9. https://doi.org/10.1161/CIRCULATIONAHA.113.001531. PMID: 23709669. http://www.ncbi.nlm.nih.gov/pubmed/23709669

Cohort Study

Cakir O, Gurkan F, Balci AE, Eren N, Dikici B. Purulent pericarditis in childhood: ten years of experience. J Pediatr Surg. 2002 Oct;37(10):1404-8. PMID: 12378443. http://www.ncbi.nlm.nih.gov/pubmed/12378443

Roodpeyma S, Sadeghian N. Acute pericarditis in childhood: a 10-year experience. Pediatr Cardiol. 2000 Jul-Aug;21(4):363-7. PMID: 10865014. http://www.ncbi.nlm.nih.gov/pubmed/10865014

Case Study

Lilly LS. Treatment of acute and recurrent idiopathic pericarditis. Circulation. 2013 Apr 23;127(16):1723-6. https://doi.org/10.1161/CIRCULATIONAHA.111.066365. PMID: 23609551. http://www.ncbi.nlm.nih.gov/pubmed/23609551**

Spodick DH. Acute pericarditis: classic electrocardiogram. Am J Geriatr Cardiol. 2003 Jul-Aug;12(4):266. PMID: 12888710. http://www.ncbi.nlm.nih.gov/pubmed/12888710

Editorial/Comment

Mascitelli L, Pezzetta F. Electrocardiography in acute pericarditis. Cleve Clin J Med. 2006 Aug;73(8):705. PMID: 16917996. http://www.ncbi.nlm.nih.gov/pubmed/16917996

Use PubMed Clinical Queries to find the most recent evidence. Use this search strategy:"acute pericarditis" OR ("acute" AND ("Pericarditis"[Mesh] OR "pericarditis")

Chapter 6
Anomalous Coronary Arteries

Richard M. Cantor, Charles V. Pollack, Jr., and Victoria G. Riese

Name and Synonyms

- Anomalous Left Coronary Artery from the Pulmonary Artery (ALCAPA)
- Also known as Bland-White-Garland Syndrome

Incidence/Epidemiology

- A rare but serious congenital anomaly.
- Usually an isolated cardiac anomaly.
- If unaddressed, mortality rates reach 90 % in the first year of life.

Differential Diagnosis

- Dilated cardiomyopathy
- Myocarditis

R. M. Cantor
Department of Emergency Medicine and Pediatrics, State University of New York Upstate Medical University, Syracuse, NY, USA

C. V. Pollack, Jr. (✉)
Department of Emergency Medicine, Thomas Jefferson University, Philadelphia, PA, USA

V. G. Riese
Librarian Consultant, Eldersburg, MD, USA

C. V. Pollack, Jr. (ed.), *Differential Diagnosis of Cardiopulmonary Disease*,
https://doi.org/10.1007/978-3-319-63895-9_6

- Coronary artery fistula
- Severe mitral regurgitation

Pathophysiology and Etiology

- After birth, pulmonary pressures decrease, as does pulmonary arterial oxygen content.
- As a result of this, the left ventricular musculature is underperfused and underoxygenated.
- This is often accompanied by varying degrees of mitral insufficiency.

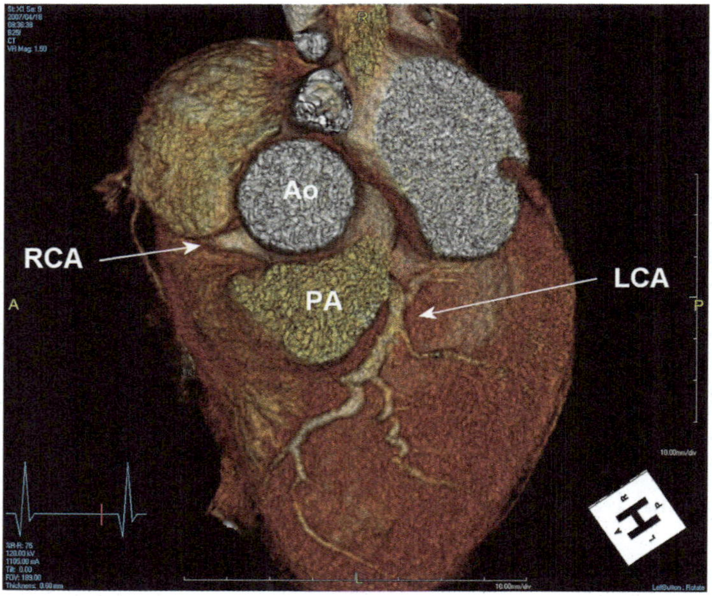

Three-dimensional image of patient. In this cranial view of the heart, the left coronary artery (LCA) can be seen to originate from the pulmonary artery (PA), a condition known as ALCAPA. The right coronary artery (RCA) has a normal origin from the right coronary cusp of the aorta (Ao) [de Jonge GJ, van Ooijen PMA, Piers LH, Dikkers R, Tio RA, Willems TP, van den Heuvel AFM, Zijlstra F, Oudkerk M. Visualization of anomalous coronary arteries on dual-source computed tomography. European Radiology. 2008 Nov;18(11):2425–32.] *Caption adapted from original*

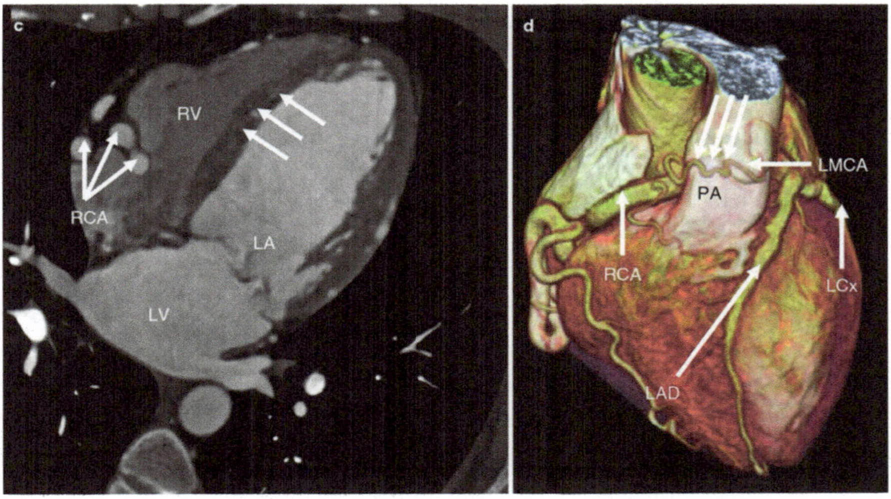

Anomalous pulmonary origin of left main coronary artery (LMCA) from the main pulmonary artery (MPA) also known as ALCAPA or Bland–White–Garland syndrome. Panels (a) and (b) are multiplanar reformats demonstrating the takeoff of the LMCA from the MPA. Panels (c) and (d) illustrate the very large and tortuous right coronary artery (RCA), which provides oxygenated myocardial blood supply for the whole myocardium via an extensive collateral circulation to the branches of the left coronary circulation, and seen best in panel (c and d) and shown by the arrows. Note the flow of blood from the left coronary artery to the MPA. Aoasc ascending aorta, LA left atrium, LAA left atrial appendage, LAD left anterior descending artery, LCx left circumflex artery, LV left ventricle, RA right atrium, RV right ventricle, SVC superior vena cava [Mazur W, Siegel MJ, Miszalski-Jamka T, Pelberg R. Coronary Artery Anomalies. CT Atlas of Adult Congenital Heart Disease [Internet]. London: Springer London; 2013 [cited 2016 May 31]. p. 183–202. Available from: http://link.springer.com/10.1007/978-1-4471-5088-6_16] *Caption from original*

Presentation

Typical/"Classic"

Typical signs and symptoms of ALCAPA appear in the first two months of life and include:

- Abnormal heart rhythm
- Enlarged heart
- Heart murmur (rare)

- Rapid pulse
- Crying or sweating during feeding ("splanchnic steal")
- Pale skin
- Poor feeding, poor weight gain
- Rapid breathing
- Sweating
- Symptoms of pain or distress in the baby (often mistaken for colic)

Atypical

- Poor feeding and fussiness in infant, at first attributed to colic.
- Occasionally ALCAPA does not present until adolescence or early adulthood.

Primary Differential Considerations

- Dilated cardiomyopathy due to other causes, such as myocarditis, should be considered.

History and Physical Exam

Findings That Confirm Diagnosis

- The combination of respiratory distress, diaphoresis, and pallor, accompanied by ECG findings consistent with myocardial ischemia, will point the clinician toward making the diagnosis.
- Auscultation may demonstrate a systolic murmur consistent with mitral valve regurgitation.

http://www.easyauscultation.com/mitral-regurgitation

Mitral regurgitation audio. [Mitral Regurgitation Page; Easy Auscultation; www.easyauscultation.com/mitral-regurgitation; copyright 2015, MedEdu LLC]

- In severe cases, signs of congestive heart failure (CHF) will be present, including tachycardia, tachypnea, gallop, poor perfusion, and signs of right sided failure (late).

Factors That Suggest Diagnosis

- ANY infant or child who presents with diaphoresis during feedings should be considered a candidate for a full cardiac workup.

Factors That Exclude Diagnosis

- ALCAPA cannot be excluded in symptomatic patients based on history and physical alone. Coronary angiography is required.

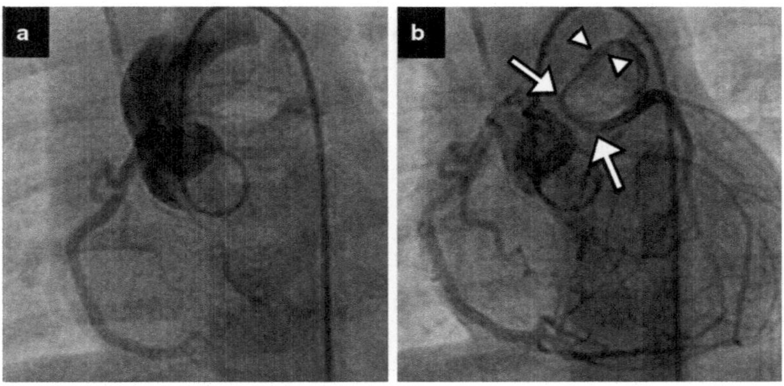

Still images (a, b) from the patient's digital subtraction angiogram (DSA). Injection of the aortic root demonstrates an enlarged and tortuous RCA with several epicardial collateral vessels; no sign of the LCA during early phase of injection (a). There is retrograde filling of the ALCAPA (arrows) (b) via multiple small collaterals from the right coronary system. There is retrograde flow of contrast through the ALCAPA and into the PA (arrowheads) [Day K, Avery R, Oliva I, Jokerst C. Coronary CTA appearance of anomalous left coronary artery arising from the pulmonary artery with Intramural Aortic Route. The International Journal of Cardiovascular Imaging. 2014 Feb;30(2):241–3.] Available from http://springerimages.com/Images/MedicineAndPublicHealth/1-10.1007_s10554-013-0334-3-1. *Caption from original*

Ancillary Studies

Electrocardiography

- In most cases, a pattern consistent with an anterolateral infarct with abnormal deep (>3 mm) and wide (>30 msec) q waves is observed in leads I, aVL, V_5, and V_6.

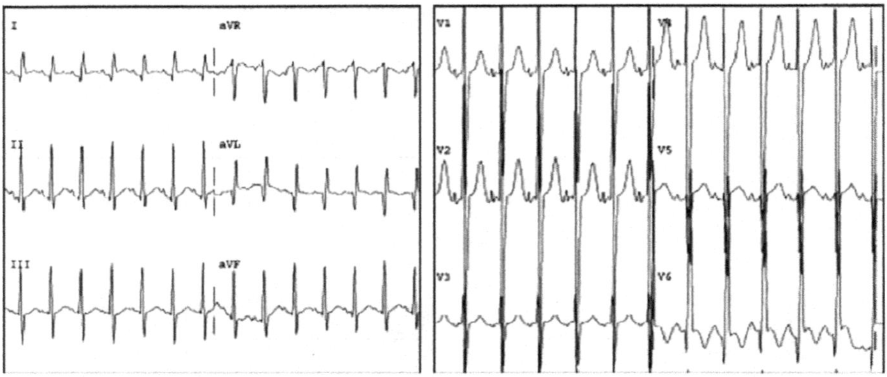

Typical electrocardiogram in anomalous left coronary artery arising from the pulmonary artery (ALCAPA) syndrome: Q waves in I and avL with prominent Q waves in V6 [Tissot C, da Cruz EM, Miyamoto S. Cardiac Failure. In: Munoz R, Morell V, Cruz E, Vetterly C, editors. Critical Care of Children with Heart Disease [Internet]. London: Springer London; 2009 [cited 2016 Jul 28]. p. 557–72. Available from: http://link.springer.com/10.1007/978-1-84882-262-7_49] *Caption from original*

Cardiac Enzymes

- Unfortunately, laboratory tests are not definitive.

Special Populations

Age

- ALCAPA is almost exclusively a pediatric disease, with only very rare presentations in adolescence or early adulthood.

Co-morbidities

- ALCAPA may occur with other congenital malformations.
- When ALCAPA coexists with other congenital malformations, particularly those associated with pulmonary hypertension, the initial presentation can be quite confusing and is often misinterpreted.

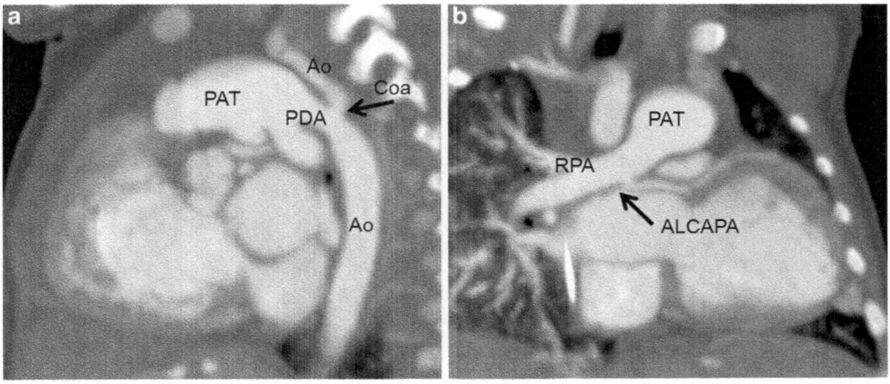

Computer tomographic (CT) images of aortic coarctation and anomalous left coronary artery connected to the pulmonary artery (ALCAPA). a Sagittal CT image showing an aortic coarctation (CoA, black arrow) bypassed by a large persistent arterial duct (PDA). The horizontal aortic arch is hypoplastic. b Coronal CT image with the anomalous left coronary artery (ALCAPA, black arrow) connected to the right pulmonary artery (RPA), a rather rare anatomic variant. PAT pulmonary artery trunk [Laux D, Bertail C, Bajolle F, Houyel L, Boudjemline Y, Bonnet D. Anomalous Left Coronary Artery Connected to the Pulmonary Artery Associated With Other Cardiac Defects: A Difficult Joint Diagnosis. Pediatric Cardiology. 2014 Oct;35(7):1198–205.] Available from http://springerimages.com/Images/MedicineAndPublicHealth/1-10.1007_s00246-014-0916-4-0. *Caption adapted from original*

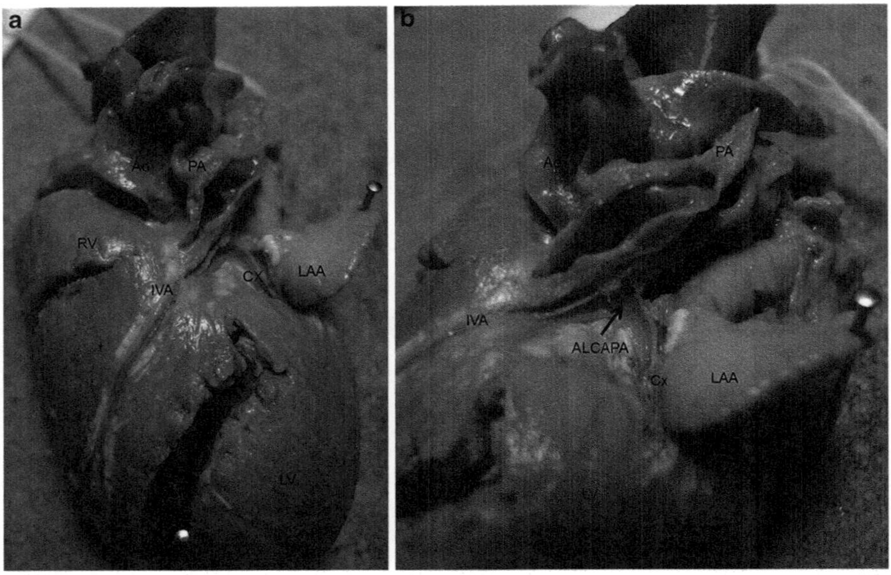

Macroscopic views of a heart with tetralogy of Fallot and pulmonary atresia associated with anomalous left coronary artery connected to the pulmonary artery (ALCAPA). **a** Frontal view of the heart in anatomic position with the apex to the left: The right (RV) and left (LV) ventricles have been opened, but the interior cannot be seen. The trunk of the pulmonary artery (PA) has been opened to confirm valvular atresia (not shown). The left coronary artery with its division in the infundibular anterior descending artery (IVA) and the circumflex (Cx) artery can be seen connecting to the PA. **b** A lateral, close-up view of the same heart with the opened ALCAPA and its two branches. LAA left atrial appendage, Ao aorta [Laux D, Bertail C, Bajolle F, Houyel L, Boudjemline Y, Bonnet D. Anomalous Left Coronary Artery Connected to the Pulmonary Artery Associated With Other Cardiac Defects: A Difficult Joint Diagnosis. Pediatric Cardiology. 2014 Oct;35(7):1198–205.] Available from http://springerimages.com/Images/MedicineAndPublicHealth/1-10.1007_s00246-014-0916-4-1. *Caption adapted from original*

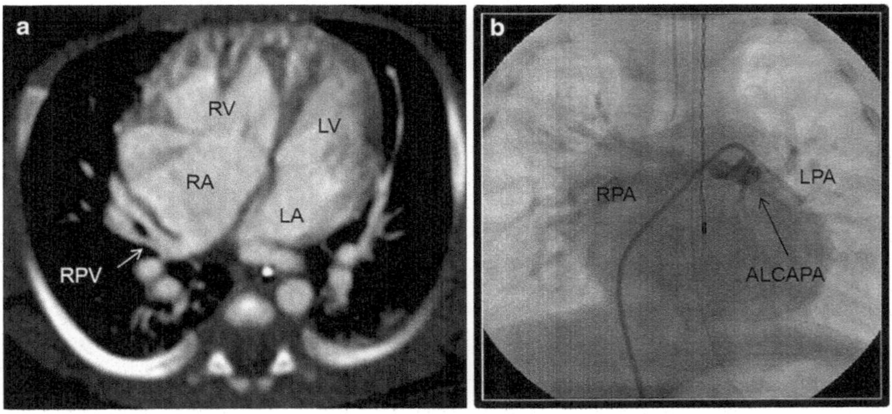

Computed tomography (CT) scan and cardiac catheter image of patient 9 with divided left atrium, partial anomalous pulmonary venous connection, and anomalous left coronary artery connecting to the pulmonary artery (ALCAPA).**a** Four-chamber view of the patient's heart on an axial CT image: The right pulmonary veins (RPVs) connect to the right atrium (RA). **b** Left coronary artery abnormally connecting to the pulmonary trunk (ALCAPA, black arrow) in the same patient shown by anterograde injection of contrast agent into the pulmonary trunk during cardiac catheterization (frontal view). RV right ventricle, LA left atrium, LV left ventricle, RPA right pulmonary artery, LPA left pulmonary artery [Laux D, Bertail C, Bajolle F, Houyel L, Boudjemline Y, Bonnet D. Anomalous Left Coronary Artery Connected to the Pulmonary Artery Associated With Other Cardiac Defects: A Difficult Joint Diagnosis. Pediatric Cardiology. 2014 Oct;35(7):1198–205.] Available from http://springerimages.com/Images/MedicineAndPublicHealth/1-10.1007_s00246-014-0916-4-2. *Caption from original*

Pitfalls in Diagnosis

Critical Steps Not to Miss

- The most important step in making the diagnosis of ALCAPA is to accept the fact that there is a congenital anomaly that will present *exactly* like the adult form of ischemic heart disease.

Mimics

- As previously mentioned, the feeding difficulties in these infants will often be misinterpreted as colic or some form of dietary intolerance.

Time-Dependent Interventions

- Immediate consultation with a Pediatric Cardiologist is recommended
- Focus is on diagnosis, not treatment; time-dependent interventions are limited.

Overall Principles of Treatment

- In cases that present with CHF, supplemental oxygen is indicated.
- The use of diuretics may be beneficial, but should be applied *only* after consultation with a Pediatric Cardiologist.

Disease Course

- The prognosis is excellent if surgical correction is carried out.

Related Evidence

Papers of particular interest have been highlighted as:
*** Of key importance*

Cohort Study

Weigand J, Marshall CD, Bacha EA, Chen JM, Richmond ME. Repair of Anomalous Left Coronary Artery From the Pulmonary Artery in the Modern Era: Preoperative Predictors of Immediate Postoperative Outcomes and Long Term Cardiac Follow-up. Pediatr Cardiol. 2014 Oct 10. PMID: 25301273. http://www.ncbi.nlm.nih.gov/pubmed/25301273 **

Uysal F, Bostan OM, Semizel E, Signak IS, Asut E, Cil E. Congenital anomalies of coronary arteries in children: the evaluation of 22 patients. Pediatr Cardiol.

2014 Jun;35(5):778-84. https://doi.org/10.1007/s00246-013-0852-8. PMID: 24337706. http://www.ncbi.nlm.nih.gov/pubmed/24337706 **

Latus H, Gummel K, Rupp S, Mueller M, Jux C, Kerst G, Akintuerk H, Bauer J, Schranz D, Apitz C. Cardiovascular magnetic resonance assessment of ventricular function and myocardial scarring before and early after repair of anomalous left coronary artery from the pulmonary artery. J Cardiovasc Magn Reson. 2014 Jan 5;16:3. https://doi.org/10.1186/1532-429X-16-3. PMID: 24387660. http://www.ncbi.nlm.nih.gov/pubmed/24387660 **

Kazmierczak PA, Ostrowska K, Dryzek P, Moll JA, Moll JJ. Repair of anomalous origin of the left coronary artery from the pulmonary artery in infants. Interact Cardiovasc Thorac Surg. 2013 Jun;16(6):797-801. https://doi.org/10.1093/icvts/ivt061. PMID: 23442939. http://www.ncbi.nlm.nih.gov/pubmed/23442939 **

Alexi-Meskishvili V, Nasseri BA, Nordmeyer S, Schmitt B, Weng YG, Böttcher W, Hübler M, Berger F, Hetzer R. Repair of anomalous origin of the left coronary artery from the pulmonary artery in infants and children. J Thorac Cardiovasc Surg. 2011 Oct;142(4):868-74. https://doi.org/10.1016/j.jtcvs.2011.04.006. PMID: 21665229. http://www.ncbi.nlm.nih.gov/pubmed/21665229

Browne LP, Kearney D, Taylor MD, Chung T, Slesnick TC, Nutting AC, Krishnamurthy R. ALCAPA: the role of myocardial viability studies in determining prognosis. Pediatr Radiol. 2010 Feb;40(2):163-7. https://doi.org/10.1007/s00247-009-1412-5. PMID: 19795113. http://www.ncbi.nlm.nih.gov/pubmed/19795113 **

Case Study

Lam JC, Giuffre M, Myers KA. Late intervention in an asymptomatic pediatric patient with anomalous left coronary artery. World J Cardiol. 2014 Aug 26;6(8):874-7. https://doi.org/10.4330/wjc.v6.i8.874. PMID: 25228967. http://www.ncbi.nlm.nih.gov/pubmed/25228967 **

Szmigielska A, Roszkowska-Blaim M, Gołąbek-Dylewska M, Tomik A, Brzewski M, Werner B. Bland-White-Garland syndrome - a rare and serious cause of failure to thrive. Am J Case Rep. 2013 Sep 16;14:370-2. https://doi.org/10.12659/AJCR.889112. PMID: 2408679. http://www.ncbi.nlm.nih.gov/pubmed/24086793 **

Varghese M, Kothari S. The caveats in the diagnosis of anomalous origin of left coronary artery from pulmonary artery (ALCAPA). Images Paediatr Cardiol. 2010 Jul;12(3):3-8. PMID: 22368564. http://www.ncbi.nlm.nih.gov/pubmed/22368564 **

Kurup RP, Daniel R, Kumar RK. Anomalous origin of the left coronary artery from the pulmonary artery in infancy with preserved left ventricular function: Potential pitfalls and clues to diagnosis. Ann Pediatr Cardiol. 2008 Jan;1(1):65-7. https://doi.org/10.4103/0974-2069.41061. PMID: 20300243. http://www.ncbi.nlm.nih.gov/pubmed/20300243 **

Brotherton H, Philip RK. Anomalous left coronary artery from pulmonary artery (ALCAPA) in infants: a 5-year review in a defined birth cohort. Eur J Pediatr. 2008 Jan;167(1):43-6. PMID: 18038147. http://www.ncbi.nlm.nih.gov/pubmed/18038147 **

Use PubMed Clinical Queries to find the most recent evidence. Use this search strategy:

"Bland White Garland Syndrome"[Mesh] OR "ALCAPA" OR "Bland White Garland"

Chapter 7
Anxiety

Charles V. Pollack, Jr., Richard M. Cantor, and Victoria G. Riese

Name and Synonyms

Anxiety, anxiety disorder, panic disorder, panic attacks

Incidence/Epidemiology

- Anxiety disorder is a very common psychiatric condition. It often manifests through physical symptoms; chest pain +/- dyspnea/hyperventilation +/- palpitations is a common presentation of anxiety disorder.
- There is no good estimate of the incidence of anxiety as a cause of chest pain that prompts medical evaluation.
- Around 25 % of individuals are thought to experience at least one panic attack in their lifetimes.

C. V. Pollack, Jr. (✉)
Department of Emergency Medicine, Thomas Jefferson University, Philadelphia, PA, USA

R. M. Cantor
Department of Emergency Medicine and Pediatrics, State University of New York Upstate Medical University, Syracuse, NY, USA

V. G. Riese
Librarian Consultant, Eldersburg, MD, USA

C. V. Pollack, Jr. (ed.), *Differential Diagnosis of Cardiopulmonary Disease*,
https://doi.org/10.1007/978-3-319-63895-9_7

Differential Diagnosis

- Presentation can be quite dramatic. The differential considerations for chest pain due to anxiety therefore include immediate life threats such as pulmonary embolism, acute coronary syndrome, and aortic dissection. Less severe differential considerations include pneumonia and pneumothorax, which can cause pleuritic pain; and chest wall pain.

Pathophysiology and Etiology

- Current thinking is that anxiety and panic result from an imbalance in CNS neurotransmitters.
- The diagnosis of anxiety as an etiology for chest pain that prompts medical evaluation should be made only after more serious causes have been evaluated and reasonably excluded.

Presentation

Typical/"Classic"

- The classic presentation of anxiety- or panic-related chest pain is:
  - Acute onset
  - Associated with dyspnea (the patient may confuse hyperventilation with dyspnea)
  - Associated with diaphoresis
  - Trembling or shaking
  - Fear of dying
  - Sense of loss of control
  - Nausea

Atypical

- Patients with anxiety or panic disorder may present with myriad complaints. Chest pain is common among these, but many other features may be present.

Primary Differential Considerations

- The differential diagnosis of acute anxiety is broad and includes both medical and psychiatric considerations.
- Medical:
  - Because acute anxiety may mimic acute somatic disease, one must consider such immediate life threats as acute myocardial infarction, aortic dissection, arrhythmias, pulmonary embolism, pneumothorax, or stroke.
  - Other concerns include hypo- and hyperglycemia, poisoning and drug abuse, delirium tremens, and encephalopathy.
- Psychiatric:
  - Acute anxiety may be confused with acute psychosis, conversion disorders, dissociative disorders, schizoaffective disorder, and Tourette's syndrome.

History and Physical Exam

Findings That Confirm Diagnosis

- History and physical examination are not diagnostic for anxiety.

Factors That Suggest Diagnosis

- Symptoms are out of proportion with physical findings.
- Patient-reported dyspnea is found on exam to be hyperventilation.

Video overview of the causes and treatment of hyperventilation
https://www.youtube.com/watch?v=p97HeXx0vN0

- History of anxiety or panic disorder.
- Young age and/or lack of risk factors for more serious conditions.
- Choking sensation accompanying chest pain.
- Current substance abuse.

Factors That Exclude Diagnosis

- There are no history or physical findings that conclusively exclude anxiety as a cause of chest pain.

Ancillary Studies

Laboratory

- There are no diagnostic laboratory studies for anxiety.
- Laboratory tests target suspected underlying disease.

Imaging

- There are no diagnostic imaging studies for anxiety.

Special Populations

Age and Gender

- The epidemiology of anxiety and panic disorder does not indicate any consistent patterns by age or gender. It may begin at a young age.
- Anxiety disorders are the most common psychiatric disturbances in childhood, usually representing negative outcomes of naturally occurring fears associated with childhood development.
- The literature describes multiple forms of anxiety disorders in children, including social anxiety, agoraphobia, panic attacks, separation anxiety, and specific phobias.

Co-morbidities

- It is important to consider and evaluate for the presence of serious underlying disease or psychiatric stress that could prompt situation anxiety, such as:
  - Recent death of a loved one
  - Recent relationship stress
  - Recent diagnosis of serious disease
- Other psychiatric issues may be discovered upon questioning.
- Substance abuse issues may be discovered upon questioning.

Pitfalls in Diagnosis

Critical Steps Not to Miss

- Because there are differential considerations that are immediate life threats, evaluation for acute coronary syndrome, pulmonary embolism, and pneumonia should be considered early.

Mimics

- The entire constellation of diagnoses that underlies chest pain syndrome can mimic or cause the pain and overall presentation of anxiety.

Time-Dependent Interventions

- Other than excluding life threats, there are no time-dependent interventions for chest pain deemed due to anxiety or panic disorder.
- Patients who also express suicidal or homicidal ideation should be promptly evaluated in an emergency care setting.

Overall Principles of Treatment

- Treatment of the acute symptoms of chest pain caused by panic or anxiety disorder may include:
  - Reassurance and support
  - Benzodiazepines
  - Monitoring while the effects of acute substance abuse diminish

Disease Course

- The course of patients with anxiety or panic disorder may vary widely, from no further episodes to debilitating psychiatric illness that limits or precludes productive engagement with society.

Related Evidence

Papers of particular interest have been highlighted as:
*** Of key importance*

Practice Guideline

Bandelow B, Sher L, Bunevicius R, Hollander E, Kasper S, Zohar J, Möller HJ; WFSBP Task Force on Mental Disorders in Primary Care; WFSBP Task Force on Anxiety Disorders, OCD and PTSD. Guidelines for the pharmacological treatment of anxiety disorders, obsessive-compulsive disorder and posttraumatic stress disorder in primary care. Int J Psychiatry Clin Pract. 2012 Jun;16(2):77–84. https://doi.org/10.3109/13651501.2012.667114. PMID: 22540422. http://www.ncbi.nlm.nih.gov/pubmed/22540422 **

Schaffer A, McIntosh D, Goldstein BI, Rector NA, McIntyre RS, Beaulieu S, Swinson R, Yatham LN; Canadian Network for Mood and Anxiety Treatments (CANMAT) Task Force. The CANMAT task force recommendations for the management of patients with mood disorders and comorbid anxiety disorders. Ann Clin Psychiatry. 2012 Feb;24(1):6–22.. PMID: 22303519. http://www.ncbi.nlm.nih.gov/pubmed/22303519 **

Review

Combs H, Markman J. Anxiety Disorders in Primary Care. Med Clin North Am. 2014 Sep;98(5):1007–1023. https://doi.org/10.1016/j.mcna.2014.06.003. PMID: 25134870. http://www.ncbi.nlm.nih.gov/pubmed/25134870 **

Stein DJ, Craske MA, Friedman MJ, Phillips KA. Anxiety disorders, obsessive-compulsive and related disorders, trauma- and stressor-related disorders, and dissociative disorders in DSM-5. Am J Psychiatry. 2014 Jun 1;171(6):611–3. https://doi.org/10.1176/appi.ajp.2014.14010003. PMID: 24880507. http://www.ncbi.nlm.nih.gov/pubmed/24880507 **

McConaghy JR, Oza RS. Outpatient diagnosis of acute chest pain in adults. Am Fam Physician. 2013 Feb 1;87(3):177–82. PMID: 23418761. http://www.ncbi.nlm.nih.gov/pubmed/23418761 **

Bystritsky A, Khalsa SS, Cameron ME, Schiffman J. Current diagnosis and treatment of anxiety disorders. P T. 2013 Jan;38(1):30–57. PMID: 23599668. http://www.ncbi.nlm.nih.gov/pubmed/23599668 **

Hoge EA, Ivkovic A, Fricchione GL. Generalized anxiety disorder: diagnosis and treatment. BMJ. 2012 Nov 27;345:e7500. https://doi.org/10.1136/bmj.e7500. PMID: 23187094. http://www.ncbi.nlm.nih.gov/pubmed/23187094 **

Kessler RC, Ruscio AM, Shear K, Wittchen HU. Epidemiology of anxiety disorders. Curr Top Behav Neurosci. 2010;2:21–35. PMID 21309104. http://www.ncbi.nlm.nih.gov/pubmed/21309104 **

Weisberg RB. Overview of generalized anxiety disorder: epidemiology, presentation, and course. J Clin Psychiatry. 2009;70 Suppl 2:4–9. PMID: 19371500. http://www.ncbi.nlm.nih.gov/pubmed/19371500

Case Study

Wolf L. Anxiety is the last diagnosis on the list. J Emerg Nurs. 2010 May;36(3):287–9. https://doi.org/10.1016/j.jen.2010.01.001. PMID: 20457335. http://www.ncbi.nlm.nih.gov/pubmed/20457335

Use PubMed Clinical Queries to find the most recent evidence. Use this search strategy:

“Anxiety”[Mesh] OR “Anxiety”

Chapter 8
Aortic Regurgitation

Christopher J. Rees, Charles V. Pollack, Jr., and Victoria G. Riese

Name and Synonyms

Aortic Regurgitation

- Aortic Insufficiency

Incidence/Epidemiology

- The most common causes of aortic regurgitation (AR) in the developed world are congenital bicuspid aortic valve and aortic root enlargement from diseases such as Marfan's syndrome.
- In the developing world, the most common cause of aortic regurgitation is rheumatic heart disease.
- The prevalence of aortic regurgitation increases with age, with about a 2 % prevalence of moderate to severe AR in men over 70, and about a 2.5 % prevalence of moderate to severe AR in women over 70.

C. J. Rees
Emergency Department, Pennsylvania Hospital, Philadelphia, PA, USA

C. V. Pollack, Jr. (✉)
Department of Emergency Medicine, Thomas Jefferson University, Philadelphia, PA, USA

V. G. Riese
Librarian Consultant, Eldersburg, MD, USA

C. V. Pollack, Jr. (ed.), *Differential Diagnosis of Cardiopulmonary Disease*,
https://doi.org/10.1007/978-3-319-63895-9_8

Differential Diagnosis

- The differential diagnosis of AR is broad, and includes all the pulmonary and cardiac causes of exertional dyspnea, such as myocardial ischemia, pulmonary edema/CHF, pulmonary embolism, and pneumonia.

Pathophysiology and Etiology

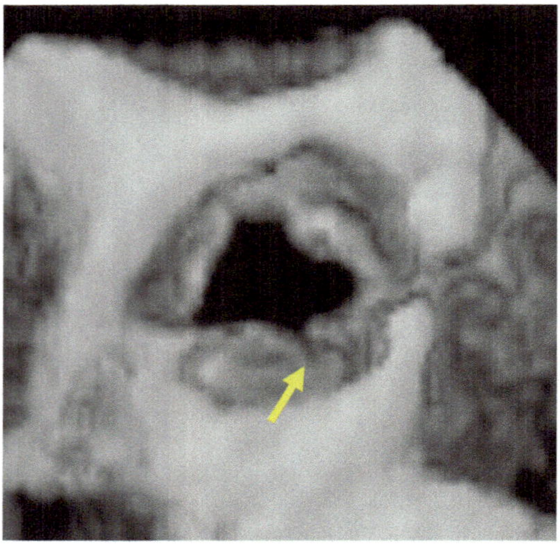

Aortic valve from a patient with aortic insufficiency. The three-dimensional transesophageal echocardiogram demonstrates a tear in the right cusp (arrow). [Garcia M, Liu Z, Rakowski H. Chapter 4. In: Vannan M, Lang RM, Rakowski H, Tajik AJ. Atlas of echocardiography. Philadelphia: Current Medicine; 2005. (Braunwald E, editor. Atlas of heart diseases; vol. 16). ISBN: 1-57340-217-6, 2005-12-05] *Caption from original*

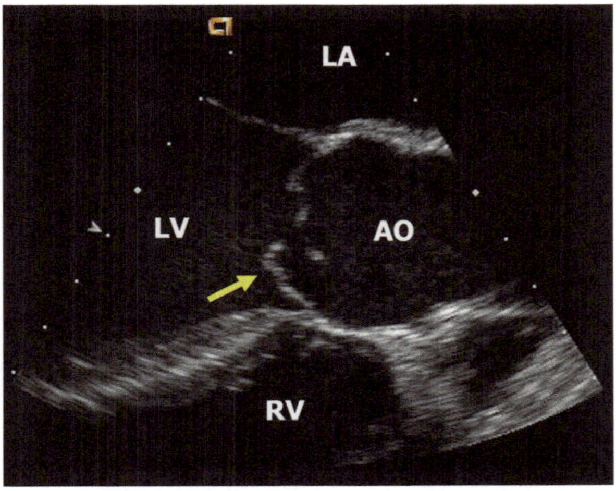

Aortic valve from a patient with aortic insufficiency. This transesophageal echocardiography image demonstrates a bicuspid valve with severe anterior cusp prolapse (arrow). Ao—aorta; LA—left atrium; LV—left ventricle; RV—right ventricle. [Garcia M, Liu Z, Rakowski H. Chapter 4. In: Vannan M, Lang RM, Rakowski H, Tajik AJ. Atlas of echocardiography. Philadelphia: Current Medicine; 2005. (Braunwald E, editor. Atlas of heart diseases; vol. 16). ISBN: 1-57340-217-6, 2005-12-05] *Caption from original*

- Aortic regurgitation may result from either primary aortic valvular disease or aortic root disease.
- Primary valve disease. There are multiple causes of primary valve disease that may result in aortic regurgitation. The final common pathophysiologic pathway involves some deformity/disease of the valve leaflets that prevents normal systolic opening and/or diastolic closure. Usually these processes cause fibrosis, scarring, and hypertrophy of the valve leaflets. The causes of primary valve disease include:
    - Rheumatic valve disease, which is usually associated with concomitant mitral valve disease.
    - Congenital bicuspid aortic valve, which more commonly results in aortic stenosis, but may also develop into aortic regurgitation.

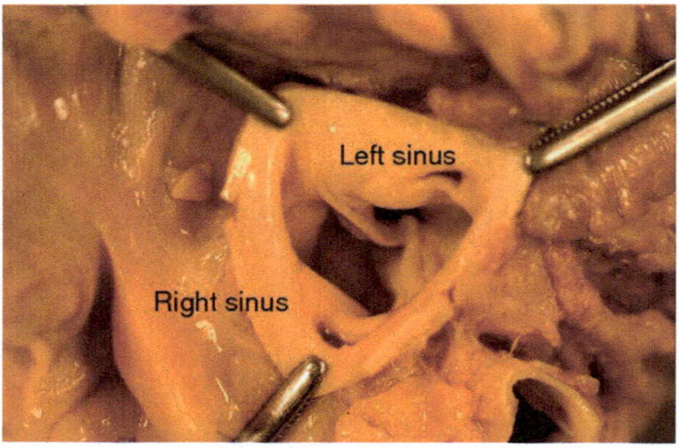

Bicuspid aortic valve. The origin of the coronary arteries can be appreciated in each of the sinuses. BAV was found during autopsy of a 41-year-old male who died from ischaemic heart disease [Suárez-Mier MP, Morentin B, Cobo M, Castedo E, García-Pavía P. Pathology of the Heart Valves. In: Lucena JS, García-Pavía P, Suarez-Mier MP, Alonso-Pulpon LA, editors. Clinico-Pathological Atlas of Cardiovascular Diseases [Internet]. Cham: Springer International Publishing; 2015 [cited 2016 Apr 4]. p. 171–200. Available from: http://link.springer.com/10.1007/978-3-319-11146-9_7] *Caption from original*

- Membranous, subaortic stenosis
- Infective endocarditis
- Syphilis
- Ankylosing spondylitis
- Ventricular septal defect
- Non-penetrating chest trauma
- Prior use of fenfluramine-phentermine

- Primary aortic root disease. Aortic root disease occurs with any process that causes widening and dilatation of the aortic root. This causes separation of the aortic valve leaflets and prevents normal opening and closing of the valve. Aortic root disease may result from:

  - Marfan's disease
  - Idiopathic
  - Annuloaortic ectasia
  - Osteogenesis imperfecta
  - Severe hypertension
  - Retrograde dissection of the aorta to the aortic root
  - Syphilitic aortitis
  - Ankylosing spondylitis

- Hemodynamic consequences. When the aortic valve does not close completely during diastole, regurgitant blood will flow back from the aorta into the left ventricle. This increases the total stroke volume of the left ventricle because in addition to normal blood flow from the left atrium, regurgitant blood flow from the aorta also fills the left ventricle during diastole. This results in an increased left ventricular end diastolic volume (LVEDV), or increased preload. Initially, the heart compensates for the volume increase with left ventricular (LV) dilatation and subsequent hypertrophy, maintaining a near-normal cardiac output and blood pressure. Eventually, however, the left ventricle can no longer dilate or hypertrophy any further, and the end-diastolic volume continues to increase, leading then to a decrease in stroke volume and forward flow. Initially, these changes manifest as exertional dyspnea and fatigue, as the cardiac output can be maintained during rest but not with exertion. These processes may take many years to develop, and there is generally a long asymptomatic period. It may take 15–20 years for symptoms to develop. This is typical, chronic aortic regurgitation.
- In some cases (especially with endocarditis, dissection, trauma) significant aortic regurgitation may develop acutely. In this situation, the left ventricle cannot handle the massive increase in LVEDV to sufficiently maintain stroke volume, and pulmonary edema or cardiogenic shock develops quickly.

Presentation

Typical/"Classic"

- Aortic regurgitation is generally a chronic, slowly progressive disease and may be asymptomatic for many (typically 15–20) years.
- Early complaints are somewhat nonspecific but may include:
- An unusual awareness of the heart beating, especially when lying down and on the left side. In these positions, the left ventricle becomes closer to the chest wall.
  - Persistent sinus tachycardia.
  - Palpitations with frequent ectopy. Ectopic beats may become even more uncomfortable than usual, as there is even more LV filling during the compensatory pause, so the eventual beat feels even "stronger" than usual.
  - Noticing that the head "bobs" with the heart beat when sitting quietly.
  - Chest pain, either exertional or nocturnal, often accompanied by severe diaphoresis and not significantly alleviated by sublingual nitroglycerin.
- The typical presentation is one of slowly worsening exertional dyspnea, associated with the typical diastolic murmur of aortic regurgitation. Often, the diastolic murmur is the first manifestation appreciated on routine examination, which then leads to the diagnosis.

Atypical

- The atypical presentation of aortic regurgitation is the acute presentation of pulmonary edema or cardiogenic shock.

Primary Differential Considerations

- The differential diagnosis of AR is basically limited to other valve disorders, acute coronary syndrome, very proximal aortic dissection, and infective endocarditis.

History and Physical Exam

Findings That Confirm Diagnosis

- A consistent history and physical examination should be confirmed with a transthoracic echocardiogram.

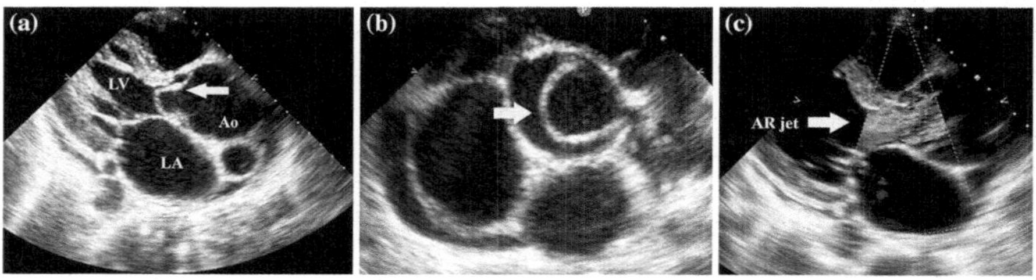

Transthoracic echocardiogram a parasternal long-axis view showing the dissection flap prolapsing into the LVOT (arrow), b parasternal short axis view showing a circular dissection flap (arrow) and c colour Doppler image showing severe aortic regurgitation (arrow). LVOT left ventricular outflow tract, LV left ventricle, LA left atria, Ao aorta, AR aortic regurgitation [Rajesh GN, Sajeer K, Anishkumar N, Sajeev CG, Krishnan MN. Intimo-intimal intussusception–circumferential aortic dissection: a rare mechanism of severe acute aortic regurgitation. Journal of Echocardiography. 2014 Sep;12(3):118–9.] *Caption from original*

Factors That Suggest Diagnosis

- Auscultatory findings.
  - Typical auscultatory findings can strongly suggest the diagnosis of aortic regurgitation.
  - The aortic closure sound (A2) may be soft or absent.
  - The classic murmur of chronic aortic regurgitation is a blowing, high-pitched, decrescendo, diastolic murmur, heard best in the third intercostal space along the left sternal border with the patient sitting up, leaning forward, at end expiration. There is little correlation between the intensity of the murmur and the degree of regurgitation. However, as the degree of regurgitation becomes greater, the duration of the murmur will increase and eventually become holosystolic. The murmur is usually accentuated by maneuvers that increase systemic vascular resistance, such as sustained handgrip, and squatting. The murmur decreases with Valsalva maneuver.

http://www.easyauscultation.com/cases-listing-details?caseID=124
The classic murmur of chronic aortic regurgitation. [Aortic Regurgitation (Decrescendo Diastolic Murmur); Easy Auscultation; www.easyauscultation.com; copyright 2014, MedEdu LLC]

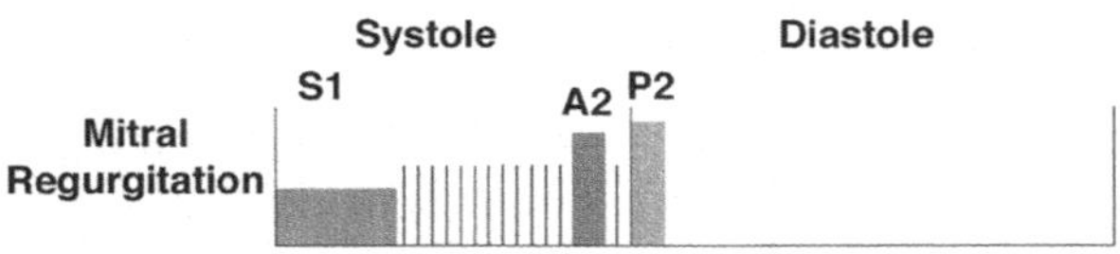

Caused by an insufficiency of the mitral valve, the mitral regurgitation murmur is a systolic murmur best heard over the mitral auscultation area. A2 = aortic valve closure; P2 = pulmonic valve closure; S1 = first heart sound [Bojanov G. Blood Pressure, Heart Tones, and Diagnoses. In: Iaizzo PA, editor. Handbook of Cardiac Anatomy, Physiology, and Devices [Internet]. Totowa, NJ: Humana Press; 2009 [cited 2016 Apr 4]. p. 243–55. Available from: http://link.springer.com/10.1007/978-1-60327-372-5_16] *Caption from original*

- There is often an associated midsystolic ejection murmur, heard best at the base of the heart, that radiates into the carotids.
- The Austin Flint murmur is sometimes heard in severe, chronic AR. It is a soft-pitched, rumbling, mid- to late diastolic murmur, heard best at the apex. It is caused by turbulence from the interaction of the usual antegrade blood flow from the left atrium and the retrograde flow from the aorta. This turbulence may result in displacement of the mitral valve leaflets.

https://www.youtube.com/watch?v=y5CcncRHl38
Video of the Austin Flint murmur.

  - Acute AR is associated with a softening of S1 due to the early closure of the mitral valve from the acutely increased LV end-diastolic volume. Often a soft, short, early diastolic murmur also is present.
- Many physical examination findings are associated with chronic, severe AR:
  - Widened pulse pressure. AR is often associated with systolic hypertension and a low diastolic pressure. A clue to disease progression is diastolic blood pressure that seems to increase over time, a result of the worsening regurgitant flow leading to increased end-diastolic volume. As the diastolic pressure approaches the LVEDV, they will eventually become equal and then rise, as the diastolic pressure cannot be below the LVEDV.
  - de Musset's sign: head bobbing with the heartbeat.
  - Corrigan (water hammer) pulse. The pulse is palpated with a forceful, rapid rise, and then quickly dissipates.

https://www.youtube.com/watch?v=OR19BOodAVI
Video demonstrating Corrigan's pulse in aortic regurgitation.

  - Quincke's pulse (capillary pulsations). While holding pressure at the tip of the nail, one can see pulsations of the skin at the nail bed; may also be seen at the lips.

https://www.youtube.com/watch?v=9m_0RAQDFHM
Video demonstrating Quincke's pulse

  - Traube's sign. A "pistol-shot" sound heard over the femoral artery.
  - Duroziez's sign. A back-and-forth bruit heard over the femoral artery after light compression with the head of the stethoscope.

Factors That Exclude Diagnosis

- A normal echocardiogram excludes aortic regurgitation.

Ancillary Studies

Laboratory

- Lab tests for patients with these nonspecific but questionably cardiac complaints should include a CBC, complete metabolic panel, cardiac biomarkers, and a B-type natriuretic peptide.

Electrocardiography

- The ECG in chronic, severe aortic regurgitation often shows LV hypertrophy with an associated strain pattern. This is usually seen as large-voltage QRS complexes with ST depression and T-wave inversions in the inferolateral leads.

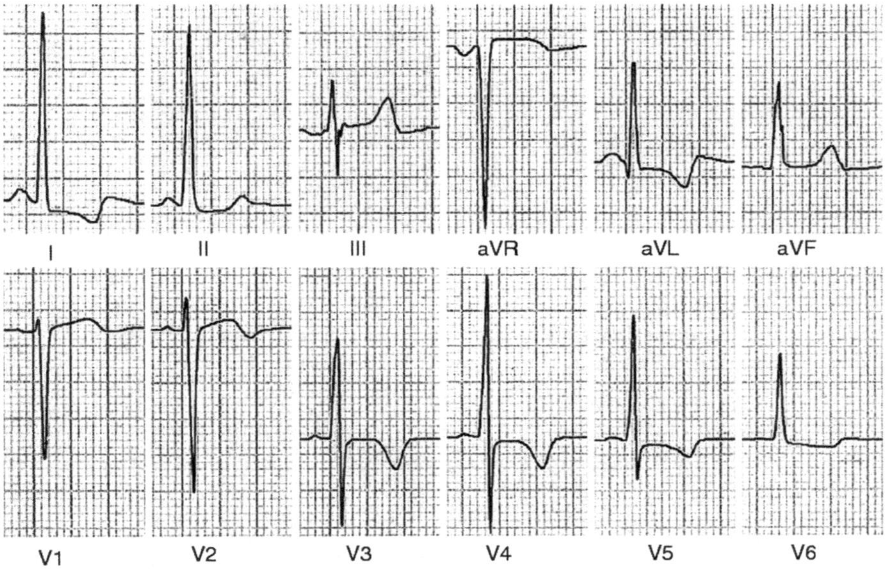

Electrocardiograph (ECG) in a patient with hypertrophic cardiomyopathy (HCM) showing left ventricular (LV) hypertrophy and T-wave inversion [Merlo M, Cocciolo A, Brun F, Sinagra G. Hypertrophic Cardiomyopathy: Clinical Assessment and Differential Diagnosis. In: Pinamonti B, Sinagra G, editors. Clinical Echocardiography and Other Imaging Techniques in Cardiomyopathies [Internet]. Cham: Springer International Publishing; 2014 [cited 2016 Apr 4]. p. 85–94. Available from: http://link.springer.com/10.1007/978-3-319-06019-4_9] *Caption from original*

Imaging

- A transthoracic echocardiogram is the diagnostic study of choice in the diagnosis and evaluation of aortic regurgitation. It can document the presence of aortic regurgitation, quantify the regurgitant flow, and define the cause of aortic regurgitation.
- A chest x-ray may be normal, but also may show cardiomegaly associated with LV hypertrophy. In acute aortic regurgitation, the chest x-ray may be consistent with pulmonary edema.

- Cardiac catheterization and angiography may be useful if all other imaging modalities (echo, cardiac MRI) are inconclusive, as well as for preoperative evaluation of aortic regurgitation. Before valve replacement surgery, coronary angiography is often performed to evaluate for concurrent coronary artery disease.

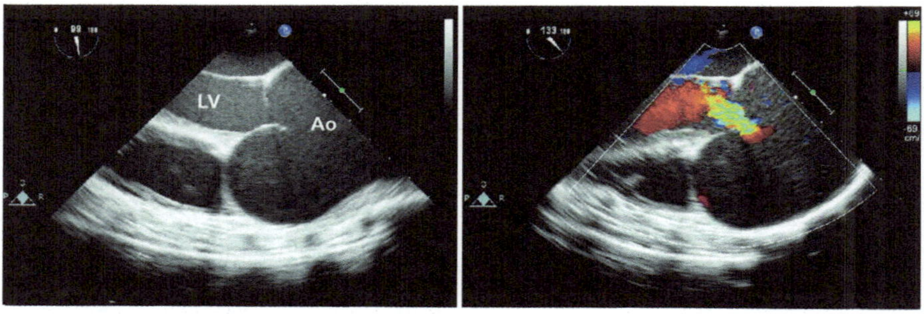

Markedly dilated aortic root as seen from the mid esophageal aortic valve long axis view without color mapping (left panel) and with color mapping, showing central aortic regurgitation (right panel). Ao aorta, LV left ventricle [Lopez L, Ventura R, Choueiter NF. Outflow Tract Anomalies. In: Wong PC, Miller-Hance WC, editors. Transesophageal Echocardiography for Congenital Heart Disease. London: Springer-Verlag London; 2014. p. 283-305. https://doi.org/10.1007/978-1-84800-064-3_11] *Caption from original*

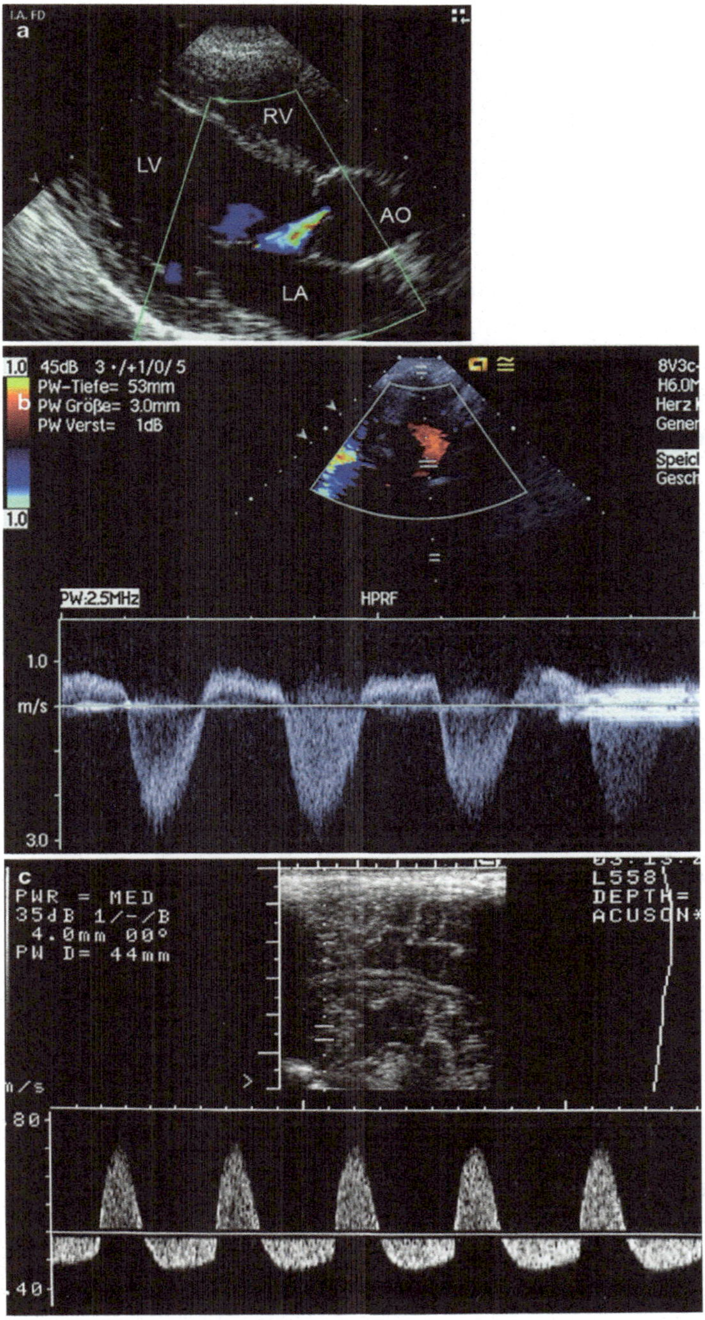

(a) Colour flow imaging of aortic insufficiency. Diastolic flow in the left ventricular outflow tract shown in the parasternal long axis view. The picture shows mild diastolic backflow from the aorta into the left ventricular outflow tract. AO aorta, LA left atrium, LV left ventricle, RV right ventricle. (b) Flow measurement in the aortic arch in severe aortic regurgitation. Colour Doppler shows retrograde flow in the aortic arch which is displayed red. Pulsed Doppler shows diastolic backflow displayed above the baseline. (c) Flow measurement in the anterior cerebral artery in a patient with severe aortic regurgitation. Diastolic backflow caused by severe aortic regurgitation [Deeg K-H. Cardiovascular Diseases Which Influence the Flow in the Extracardial Arteries. In: Deeg K-H, Rupprecht T, Hofbeck M, authors. Doppler Sonography in Infancy and Childhood [Internet]. Cham: Springer International Publishing; 2015 [cited 2016 Apr 4]. p. 679–730. Available from: http://link.springer.com/10.1007/978-3-319-03506-2_15] *Caption from original*

Special Populations

Age

- Aortic regurgitation is more common in middle-aged and older adults, especially because the latent period before the appearance of symptoms may be two decades.
- Aortic regurgitation may be seen in children, in whom it is usually associated with either severe aortic stenosis or a ventricular septal defect. Most cases in children are mild and asymptomatic, and need only be followed with serial exams and echocardiography.

Co-morbidities

- Aortic regurgitation may be diagnosed in relatively healthy patients but also may present in the setting of numerous other cardiovascular diseases and risks.

Pitfalls in Diagnosis

Critical Steps Not to Miss

- Consideration of the diagnosis is the first critical step. In patients with hemodynamic compromise, an echocardiogram should be performed early to assess all hemodynamic parameters and determine the need for urgent operative intervention.

Mimics

- The entire constellation of diagnoses that underlies dyspnea, chest pain, and other valvular diseases can mimic the presentation of aortic regurgitation.

Time-Dependent Interventions

- Time-dependent interventions in aortic regurgitation are necessary only when acute aortic regurgitation is considered and cardiac and pulmonary function is compromised. In such patients, urgent valve replacement may be a lifesaving procedure.
- For chronic aortic regurgitation, there must be a well-planned and considered approach to operative intervention.

Overall Principles of Treatment

- Acute aortic regurgitation.
  - In acute aortic regurgitation, urgent valve replacement is indicated. Intravenous diuretics and vasodilators (such as sodium nitroprusside) may be helpful as a bridge to surgery.
  - In acute aortic regurgitation, intra-aortic balloon counterpulsation (IABP) is contraindicated, as it may worsen the regurgitation. Intravenous beta-blockers are relatively contraindicated, as they may decrease cardiac output even further.
- Chronic aortic regurgitation.
  - All patients diagnosed with aortic regurgitation, even those who are asymptomatic, must have their systolic blood pressure controlled. Aortic regurgitation is often associated with difficult-to-control systolic hypertension due to increased stroke volume. The goal should be less than 140 mm Hg. Most patients may benefit from vasodilator therapy with ACE inhibitors, dihydropyridine calcium channel blockers, or hydralazine.
  - Patients with early symptoms and mild dyspnea often also benefit from the addition of a diuretic.
  - Surgery with aortic valve replacement is indicated for all symptomatic patients with chronic aortic regurgitation.
  - The optimal time for surgery seems to be after the onset of LV dysfunction but before the development of symptoms. It is important to remember that patients with chronic AR do not become symptomatic until after LV dysfunction develops.

- Appropriately timed surgery often may restore normal LV function. However, surgery delayed for more than 1 year after the onset of LV dysfunction or symptoms often fails to restore normal LV function.
- If there are no indications for surgery, it is generally recommended that the patient be followed up with exams and echocardiograms every 3–6 months.
- Indications for operation in the asymptomatic patient include:
    - An LV ejection fraction <50 %
    - An LV end-systolic dimension < 55 mm or an end-diastolic dimension <75 mm
    - A regurgitant fraction ≥50 %
    - A regurgitant volume ≥ 60 mL

Disease Course

- Patients with AR may remain asymptomatic for decades, but many patients eventually require valve replacement surgery.
- Overall operative mortality is 3 %, but in the presence of prolonged LV dysfunction, mortality approaches 10 % and is then also associated with a late mortality approaching 5 % per year from LV failure.

Related Evidence

Papers of particular interest have been highlighted as:
** *Of key importance*

Practice Guideline

Nishimura RA, Otto CM, Bonow RO, Carabello BA, Erwin JP 3rd, Guyton RA, O'Gara PT, Ruiz CE, Skubas NJ, Sorajja P, Sundt TM 3rd, Thomas JD; ACC/AHA Task Force Members. 2014 AHA/ACC Guideline for the Management of Patients With Valvular Heart Disease: a report of the American College of Cardiology/American Heart Association Task Force on Practice Guidelines. Circulation. 2014 Jun 10;129(23):e521-643. https://doi.org/10.1161/CIR.0000000000000031. PMID: 24589853. http://www.ncbi.nlm.nih.gov/pubmed/24589853 **

Lancellotti P, Tribouilloy C, Hagendorff A, Moura L, Popescu BA, Agricola E, Monin JL, Pierard LA, Badano L, Zamorano JL; European Association of Echocardiography. European Association of Echocardiography recommendations for the assessment of valvular regurgitation. Part 1: aortic and pulmonary regurgitation (native valve disease). Eur J Echocardiogr. 2010 Apr;11(3):223-44. https://doi.org/10.1093/ejechocard/jeq030. PMID: 20375260. http://www.ncbi.nlm.nih.gov/pubmed/20375260 **

Review

Iung B, Vahanian A. Epidemiology of acquired valvular heart disease. Can J Cardiol. 2014 Sep;30(9):962-70. https://doi.org/10.1016/j.cjca.2014.03.022. PMID: 24986049. http://www.ncbi.nlm.nih.gov/pubmed/24986049 **

Prodromo J, D'Ancona G, Amaducci A, Pilato M. Aortic valve repair for aortic insufficiency: a review. J Cardiothorac Vasc Anesth. 2012 Oct;26(5):923-32. https://doi.org/10.1053/j.jvca.2011.07.014. PMID: 22703946. http://www.ncbi.nlm.nih.gov/pubmed/22703946 **

Hamirani YS, Dietl CA, Voyles W, Peralta M, Begay D, Raizada V. Acute aortic regurgitation. Circulation. 2012 Aug 28;126(9):1121-6. https://doi.org/10.1161/CIRCULATIONAHA.112.113993. PMID: 22927474. http://www.ncbi.nlm.nih.gov/pubmed/22927474 **

Goldbarg SH, Halperin JL. Aortic regurgitation: disease progression and management. Nat Clin Pract Cardiovasc Med. 2008 May;5(5):269-79. https://doi.org/10.1038/ncpcardio1179. PMID: 18364707 http://www.ncbi.nlm.nih.gov/pubmed/18364707 **

Bekeredjian R, Grayburn PA. Valvular heart disease: aortic regurgitation. Circulation. 2005 Jul 5;112(1):125-34. PMID: 15998697. http://www.ncbi.nlm.nih.gov/pubmed/15998697 **

Enriquez-Sarano M, Tajik AJ. Clinical practice. Aortic regurgitation. N Engl J Med. 2004 Oct 7;351(15):1539-46. PMID: 15470217. http://www.ncbi.nlm.nih.gov/pubmed/15470217 **

Use PubMed Clinical Queries to find the most recent evidence. Use this search strategy:

"Aortic Valve Insufficiency"[Mesh] OR "Aortic Regurgitation"

Chapter 9
Aortic Stenosis

Charles V. Pollack, Jr., Melissa Platt, Richard M. Cantor, and Victoria G. Riese

Name and Synonyms

Aortic stenosis

Incidence/Epidemiology

The frequency of the causes of aortic valve disease varies geographically:

- Worldwide, rheumatic valve disease is the most common cause of aortic stenosis
- In North America, calcified disease is the primary cause of aortic stenosis

C. V. Pollack, Jr. (✉)
Department of Emergency Medicine, Thomas Jefferson University, Philadelphia, PA, USA

M. Platt
Department of Emergency, University of Louisville, Louisville, KY, USA

R. M. Cantor
Department of Emergency Medicine and Pediatrics, State University of New York Upstate Medical University, Syracuse, NY, USA

V. G. Riese
Librarian Consultant, Eldersberg, MD, USA

C. V. Pollack, Jr. (ed.), *Differential Diagnosis of Cardiopulmonary Disease*,
https://doi.org/10.1007/978-3-319-63895-9_9

Differential Diagnosis

- The main issue to recognize is that the symptoms may be attributed to other disease processes, and aortic stenosis can be missed in the acute setting
- Other diagnostic considerations include supravalvular aortic stenosis, congenital subvalvular aortic stenosis, and hypertrophic obstructive cardiomyopathy.

Pathophysiology and Etiology

- Three primary causes of aortic stenosis:
  - Congenital (unicuspid/bicuspid valve) with superimposed calcification
  - Calcified disease of a trileaflet aortic valve
  - Rheumatic valve

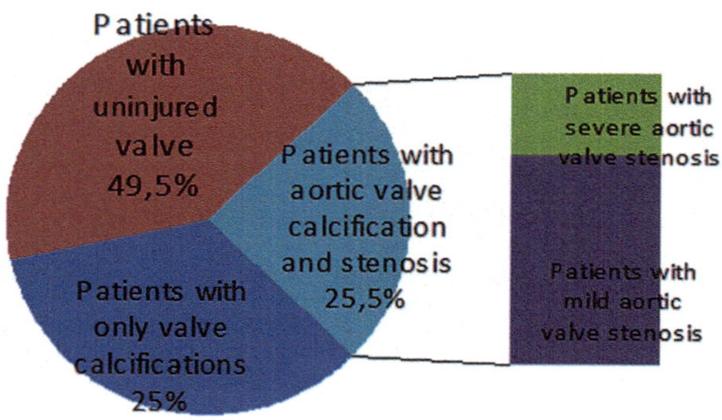

Distribution of population according to aortic valve degeneration. Patients with uninjured valve 49.5 %. Patients with aortic valve calcification and stenosis 25.5 %. Patients with only valve calcifications 25 %. [Fazio G, Caracciolo C, Barone R, D'angelo L, Di Maggio R, Vernuccio F, Siragusa S. An unknown cause of aortic valve stenosis: polycythemia vera. Journal of Thrombosis and Thrombolysis. 2013 Feb;35(2):282–5.] *Caption from original*

- Pathophysiology differs depending on the cause:
  - Calcified disease occurs when lipid accumulation triggers an inflammatory response by various mediators. There is local production of protein that promotes tissue calcification. Aortic stenosis occurs when the antegrade velocity across an abnormal valve is at least 2.6 m/sec.
  - Rheumatic valve disease causes fusion of the commissures between the leaflets leaving a small central opening.

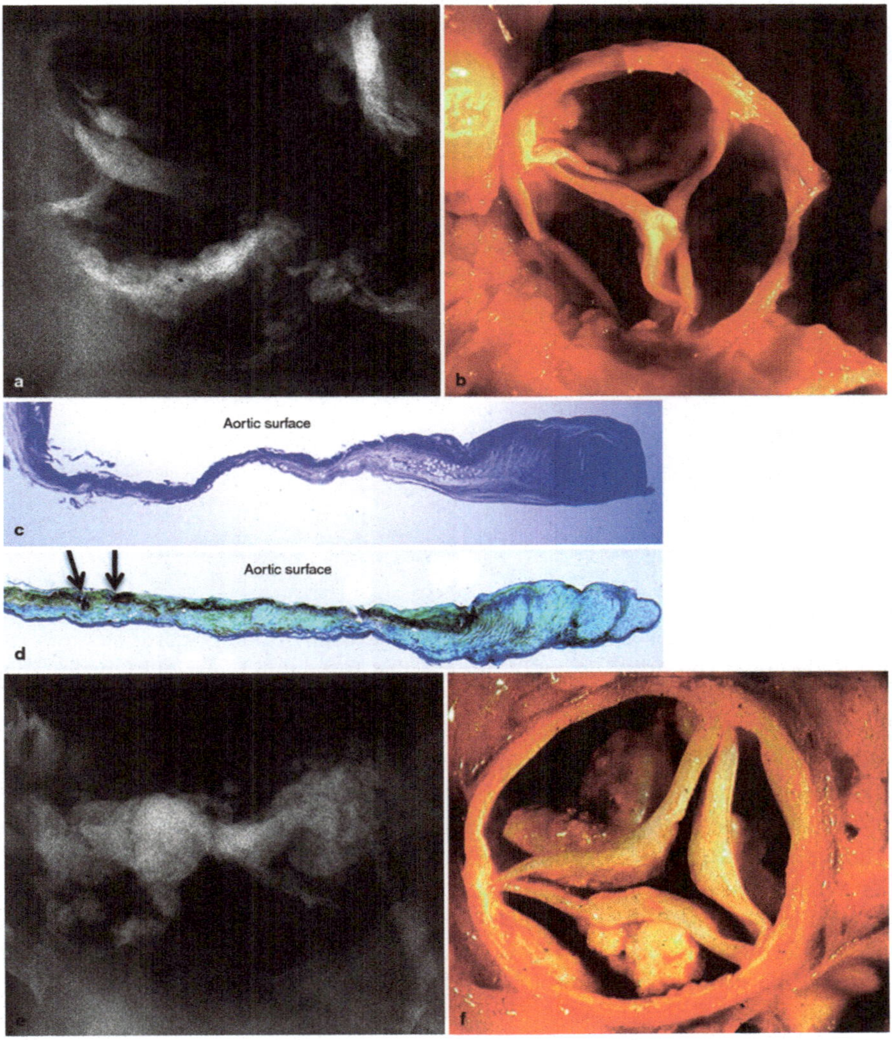

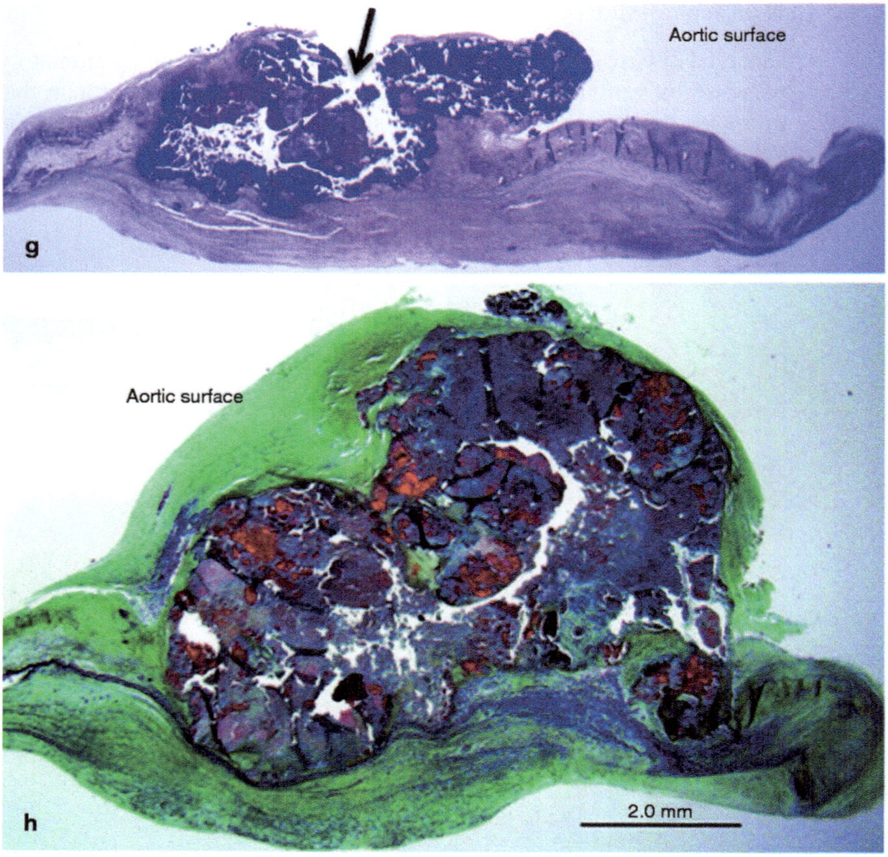

Two aortic valves seen at autopsy showing progression of calcific aortic stenosis. (a, b) Radiograph and gross image of aortic valve from an 83-year-old female. This valve shows mild calcification with small calcific deposits on aortic surface of cusps and sparing of the free edge. (c, d) Histologic sections of cusps showing fibrotic thickening and microscopic calcific deposits in the zona fibrosa (arrows). (e, f). Radiograph and gross image of stenotic aortic valve from an 82-year-old female. There is marked nodular calcification of the cusps with bulky deposits on the aortic surface. (g, h) Histologic sections of the cusps show calcific nodules superimposed on a fibrotic cusp with ulceration of the aortic surface (arrow). Note fibrotic thickening of the ventricular surface [Ladich E, Nakano M, Virmani R. Pathologic Findings in Aortic Stenosis. In: Min JK, Berman DS, Leipsic J, editors. Multimodality Imaging for Transcatheter Aortic Valve Replacement [Internet]. London: Springer London; 2014 [cited 2015 Aug 27]. p. 145–56. Available from: http://link.springer.com/10.1007/978-1-4471-2798-7_11] *Caption from original*

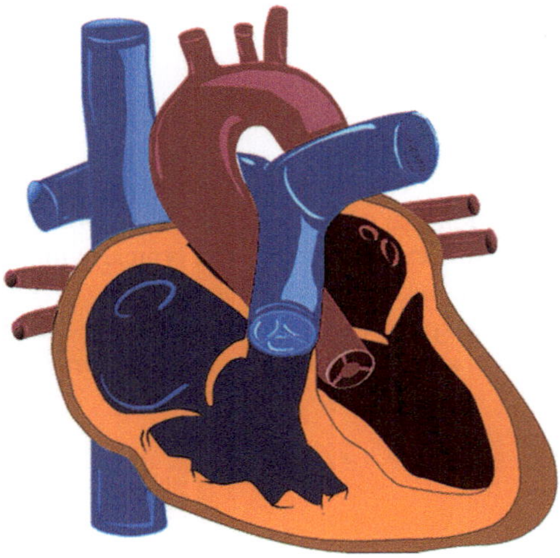

Aortic stenosis (AS). The aortic valve orifice is small; this may be a result of thickening of valve cusps, adhesion of cusp edges rendering separation between cusps during systole limited and/or due to small valve annulus [Holmes KW, McCarville MA. Aortic Stenosis. In: Abdulla R, editor. Heart Diseases in Children [Internet]. Boston, MA: Springer US; 2011 [cited 2015 Aug 27]. p. 149–58. Available from: http://link.springer.com/10.1007/978-1-4419-7994-0_11] *Caption from original*

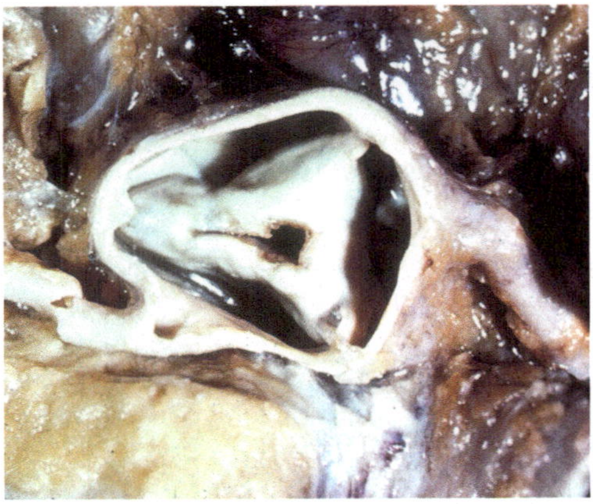

Rheumatic heart disease: aortic stenosis. In this aortic valve, there is diffuse fibrosis of the three cusps and fusion of the three commissures, producing a narrow central orifice [Buja LM, Cheong B. Cardiovascular Pathology. In: Krueger GRF, Buja LM, editors. Atlas of Anatomic Pathology with Imaging [Internet]. London: Springer London; 2013 [cited 2015 Aug 27]. p. 43–104. Available from: http://link.springer.com/10.1007/978-1-4471-2846-5_2] *Caption from original*

Presentation

Typical/"Classic"

- Typically asymptomatic for a prolonged period of time. There is a wide degree of outflow obstruction that causes symptoms. On average, symptoms develop once the aortic valve area is < 1.0 cm^2. The typical symptoms are heart failure, syncope, and angina, but they reflect late disease.
- In earlier disease dyspnea on exertion, decreased exercise tolerance, dizziness, and exertional angina are more common findings.

Atypical

- Aortic stenosis can manifest as sudden cardiac death, atrial fibrillation, or endocarditis.

Primary Differential Considerations

History and Physical Exam

Findings that Confirm Diagnosis

- There is no single or combination of findings that is sensitive or specific enough to confirm the diagnosis of aortic stenosis.

Factors that Suggest Diagnosis

- The quality of the arterial pulse reflects degrees of obstruction. This is often described as "parvus and tardus," meaning the pulse is weak and increases slowly.
- There is a harsh systolic ejection murmur heard best at the second intercostal space on the right. The murmur can be transmitted to the carotid arteries.

http://www.easyauscultation.com/cases?coursecaseorder=11&courseid=31

Aortic Stenosis (Diamond Shaped Systolic Murmur). [Aortic Stenosis (Diamond Shaped Systolic Murmur); Easy Auscultation; www.easyauscultation.com; copyright 2015, MedEdu LLC]

- The S2 heart sound can be paradoxically split with severe stenosis, and the S2 heart sound is soft.

http://www.easyauscultation.com/cases?coursecaseorder=3&courseid=31
Second Heart Sound – Splitting. [Second Heart Sound – Splitting; Easy Auscultation; www.easyauscultation.com; copyright 2015, MedEdu LLC]

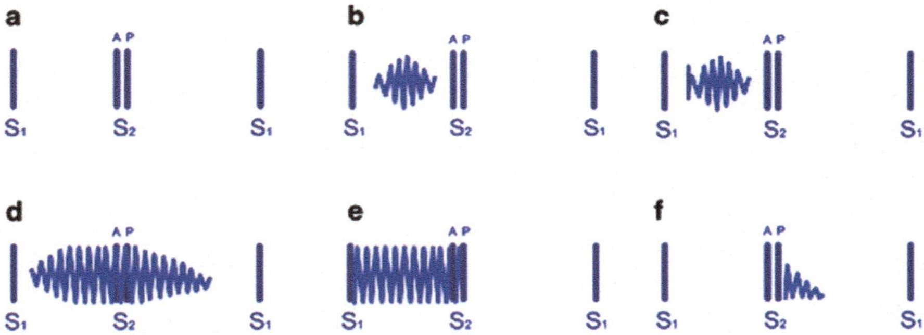

Heart sounds and murmurs. (a) Normal heart sounds: once the ventricles start to contract at the onset of systole, the tricuspid and mitral valves close. Closure of the atrioventricular valves contributes to the first heart sound which tends to be single. Aortic and pulmonary valves open soon after S1; however, this is usually inaudible in the normal heart. Flow across the aortic and pulmonary valves follows, which is again usually inaudible in the normal heart. The aortic valve closes first, followed by the pulmonary valve; the delay in closure of the pulmonary valve gives the "splitting" character of the second heart sound. Diastole, similar to systole is quiet; during diastole, blood flows through the tricuspid and mitral valves into the right and left ventricles. (b) Systolic flow murmur: increased blood flow across the pulmonary or aortic valve causes turbulence of blood flow which produces a systolic flow murmur heard over the left or right upper sternal border, respectively. In atrial septal defect, increased blood flow across the pulmonary valve causes a systolic ejection murmur along the left upper sternal border. Severe anemia with increase in blood volume to compensate for decreased oxygen-carrying capacity causes turbulence of blood flow and consequently a murmur across both aortic and pulmonary valves. These murmurs are distinguished from those caused by stenosis of the pulmonary or aortic valves by lack of a systolic ejection click heard just before the systolic murmurs. (c) Pulmonary or aortic valve stenosis: flow across the pulmonary and aortic valves occurs during midsystole; therefore, pulmonary or aortic stenosis produces a systolic ejection murmur preceded by a systolic ejection click. These murmurs are loudest over the right upper sternal borders in aortic stenosis and the left upper sternal border in pulmonary stenosis. The systolic ejection click is caused by the snap sound of opening of abnormal pulmonary or aortic valves. (d) Continuous murmur: a murmur heard over systole and most of diastole reflects abnormal shunting across a vascular structure connecting the systemic to pulmonary circulations, such as with patent ductus arteriosus. Murmur caused by PDA may be restricted to systole in children due to the soft and inaudible flow during diastole. (e) Early diastolic murmur: during early diastole, blood in the proximal portions of the pulmonary artery and aorta eject to the pulmonary and systemic circulations, respectively. Backward flow of blood into the right or left ventricles due to valve regurgitation will cause an early diastolic murmur. Aortic regurgitation is best heard over the mid or left sternal region. Pulmonary regurgitation is typically inaudible due to low pressures in the right heart and if heard may indicate pulmonary hypertension. (f) Mid-diastolic murmur: during mid-diastole blood flows from the atria to the respective ventricles. Excessive blood flow across the tricuspid valve, such as with atrial septal defect, or across the mitral valve such as with patent ductus arteriosus will cause a mid-diastolic murmur heard over the left lower sternal border in patients with atrial septal defect and at the apex in patients with patent ductus arteriosus [Thompson WR, Mehrotra SM. Cardiac History and Physical Examination. In: Abdulla R, editor. Heart Diseases in Children [Internet]. Boston, MA: Springer US; 2011 [cited 2015 Aug 27]. p. 3–16. Available from: http://link.springer.com/10.1007/978-1-4419-7994-0_1] *Caption from original*

	Severity of AS		
	Mild	Moderate	Severe
Arterial pulse	Normal	Slowly rising	Parvus et tardus
Jugular venous pulse	Normal	Normal	Usually normal
Carotid thrill	±	±	±
Cardiac impulse	Normal	Heaving	Heaving, sustained
Precordial thrill	±	±	Palpable *a* wave
			Usually ++
Auscultation			
S_4	–	±	++
ESC	+	±	–
Peak of ESM	Early systole	Mid systole	Late systole
S_2	Normal	Normal or single	Single or paradoxic

Physical examination for aortic stenosis. The findings on physical examination in patients with mild aortic stenosis (AS) are an ejection systolic click (ESC) and ejection systolic murmur (ESM) that peak in early systole. The ESC may be absent if the valve is calcified or is rigid. These patients may have a carotid or precordial thrill. Patients with severe AS display characteristic physical findings. The arterial pulse, which is best felt over the carotid or the suprasternal notch, shows a slowly rising pulse that takes longer to reach peak (parvus et tardus) (see). The jugular venous pulse is normal and a carotid thrill may be present. The cardiac impulse is left ventricular (LV) in type; it is heaving and sustained. Often a powerful presystolic wave (a wave) is felt. A precordial systolic thrill is often present. On auscultation, there is an S4gallop, the ESC is absent, the ESM peaks in late systole, and the S2 is single. S2 is at times paradoxic, but this usually occurs in the presence of associated left bundle branch block or LV failure. In addition, there is usually a faint diastolic murmur of minimal aortic regurgitation. In the presence of congestive heart failure, the jugular venous pressure is often increased, the LV is dilated, there is an S3, and the ESM may be very soft or absent. Frequently, a holosystolic murmur of mitral regurgitation is present. The findings on physical examination resemble those of heart failure from a variety of causes, eg, a cardiomyopathy, rather than AS. The physical findings in moderate AS are between those seen in mild and severe AS. [Rahimtoola S. Chapter 06. In: Braunwald E, editor. Atlas of Heart Disease: Valvular Heart Disease, Volume 11, 1e. St. Louis, Mo.: Current Medicine; 1997. ISBN: 1-878132-30-X] *Caption from original*

Factors that Exclude Diagnosis

- The presence of a normal split S2 heart sound most reliably excludes **severe** aortic stenosis in adults.

Ancillary Studies

Electrocardiography

- May see left ventricular hypertrophy, increased QRS voltage, ST-T wave changes that reflect subendocardial ischemia and left atrial hypertrophy. Atrial fibrillation is common in adults with aortic stenosis.

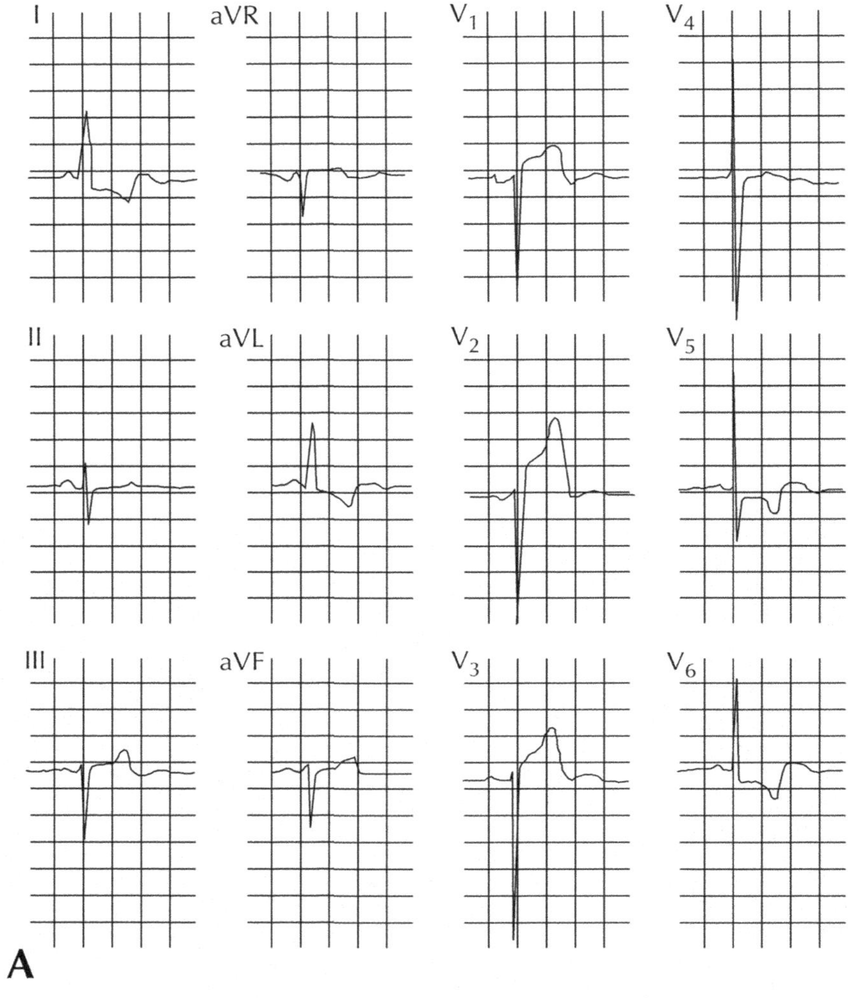

Electrocardiographic data in aortic stenosis. Electrocardiograph (ECG), chest radiographic, left ventricular (LV) and ascending aorta pressure pulses, LV diastolic pulmonary artery wedge (PAW) pressure pulses, and hemodynamic-LV function data. This 61-year-old man had recent onset of symptoms of mild shortness of breath on exertion. A, The ECG shows voltage criteria for LV hypertrophy and ST depression with T-wave inversion in leads I, aVL, V5, and V6. ECG standardization is 1 mV=10 mm. [Rahimtoola S. Chapter 06. In: Braunwald E, editor. Atlas of Heart Disease: Valvular Heart Disease, Volume 11, 1e. St. Louis, Mo.: Current Medicine; 1997. ISBN: 1-878132-30-X] *Caption adapted from original*

Imaging

- Chest radiography is usually normal.However, a rounding of the left ventricular apex may be seen, suggesting left ventricular hypertrophy or the calcification of the aortic leaflets and aortic root, but this is a rare finding

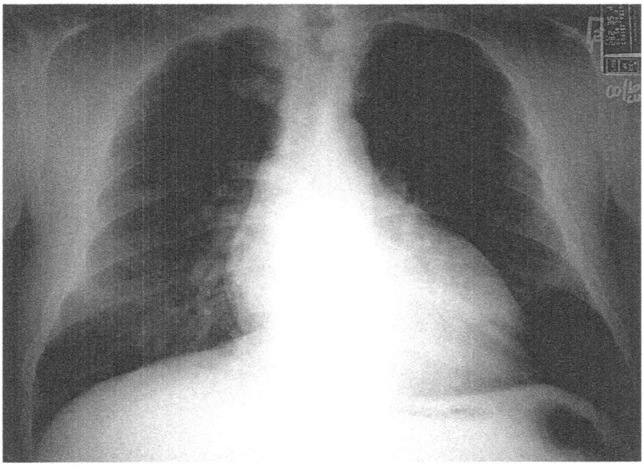

Chest radiographic diagnosis of aortic stenosis. Chest radiography (posteroanterior view) shows an increased heart size (cardiothoracic ratio, 0.53) and normal pulmonary vasculature. The cardiac silhouette is typical for LV hypertrophy associated with severe AS. Calcification of the aortic valve would be best appreciated in the lateral view of the chest. [Rahimtoola S. Chapter 06. In: Braunwald E, editor. Atlas of Heart Disease: Valvular Heart Disease, Volume 11, 1e. St. Louis, Mo.: Current Medicine; 1997. ISBN: 1-878132-30-X] *Caption adapted from original*

- Echocardiography is the most reliable way to evaluate aortic stenosis.
- Some findings include the finding of a bicuspid valve, thickened and calcified aortic leaflets, possible left ventricular hypertrophy, and probable concurrent aortic regurgitation.
- Echocardiography has reduced the need for cardiac catheterization with hemodynamic measurements.

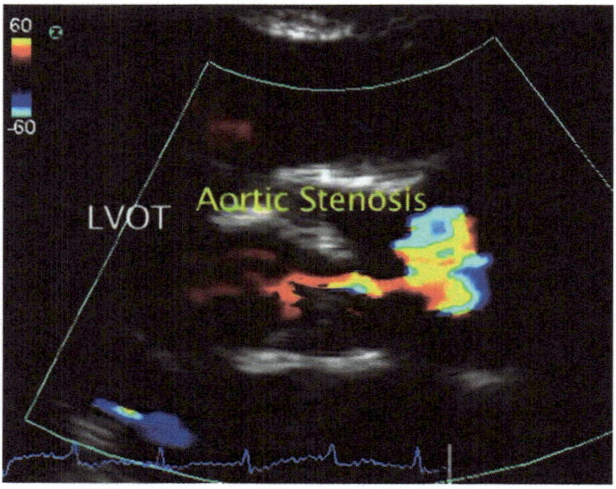

Critical aortic stenosis color Doppler LVOT view [Riley DC, Glassman G, Hodges K. Emergency department diagnosis of critical aortic stenosis using bedside ultrasonography. Critical Ultrasound Journal. 2010 Nov;2(2):87–9.] *Caption from original*

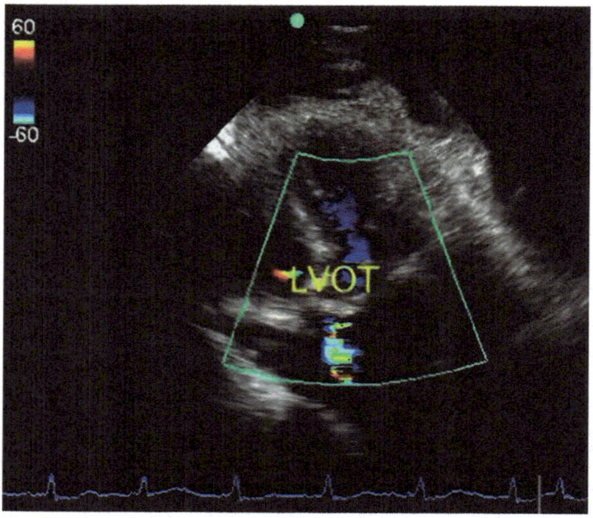

Critical aortic stenosis color Doppler apical 5-chamber view [Riley DC, Glassman G, Hodges K. Emergency department diagnosis of critical aortic stenosis using bedside ultrasonography. Critical Ultrasound Journal. 2010 Nov;2(2):87–9.] *Caption from original*

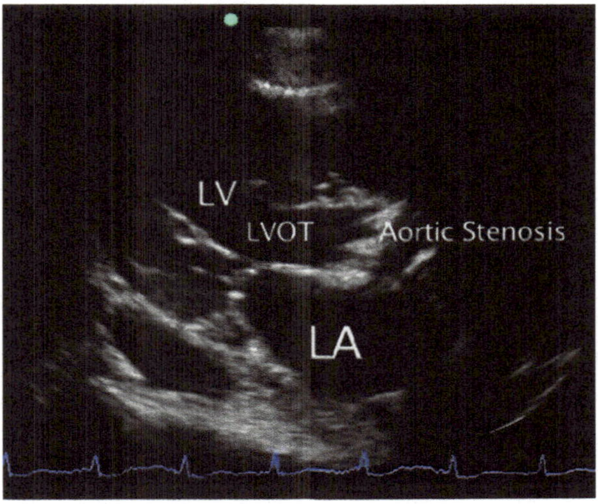

Critical aortic stenosis parasternal long-axis view [Riley DC, Glassman G, Hodges K. Emergency department diagnosis of critical aortic stenosis using bedside ultrasonography. Critical Ultrasound Journal. 2010 Nov;2(2):87–9.] *Caption from original*

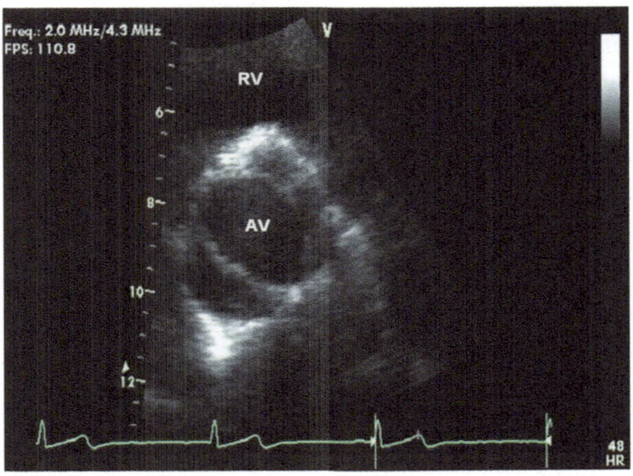

Bicuspid aortic stenosis. Parasternal short-axis view of a bicuspid aortic valve (AV) showing the typical bowing aortic cusps. [Sorajja P, Nishimura RA. Aortic Stenosis. In: Wang A, Bashore TM, editors. Valvular Heart Disease [Internet]. Totowa, NJ: Humana Press; 2009 [cited 2015 Aug 27]. p. 165–86. Available from: http://link.springer.com/10.1007/978-1-59745-411-7_7] *Caption adapted from original*

Special Populations

Age

- Severe isolated aortic stenosis is primarily a disease of older patients
- Aortic stenosis in infancy will often present with signs of CHF, with accompanying growth failure.
- AS in older children is usually asymptomatic.

Co-Morbidities

- Patients with aortic stenosis have an increased risk of bleeding. The increased risk appears to be due to an acquired Von Willebrand syndrome.

Pitfalls in Diagnosis

Critical Steps Not to Miss

- Once symptoms develop, prompt surgical intervention is needed to increase survival owing to the high risk of sudden death.

Mimics

- Symptoms may be attributed to other diseases, such as coronary artery disease or congestive heart failure, with the diagnosis of aortic stenosis being made only later in the work-up.

Time Dependent Interventions

- Once symptoms develop, even mild symptos, surgery is needed because without a valve replacement the survival rate is only 2 to 3 years.

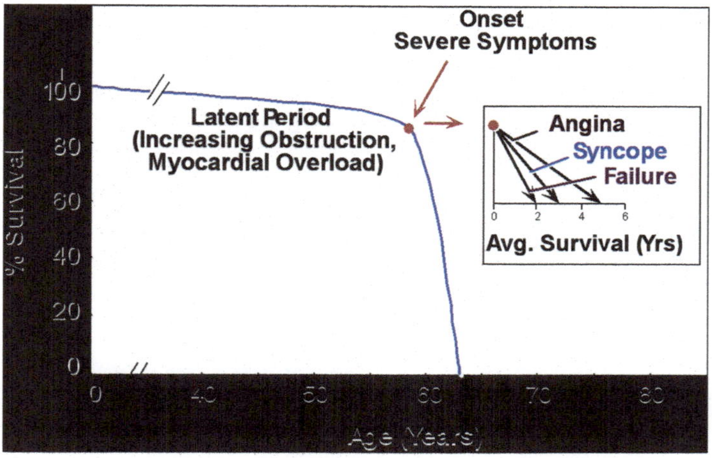

Classic survival curve aortic stenosis. [Ross J, Braunwald E. Aortic Stenosis. Circulation. 1968 Jul 1;38(1S5):V-61-V-67. Reprinted with permission.]

- Symptomatic patients with severe aortic stenosis alone or
  - Undergoing coronary artery bypass surgery
  - Undergoing surgery on the aorta or other heart valves
- Patients with moderate aortic stenosis and
  - Undergoing coronary artery bypass surgery
  - Undergoing surgery on the aorta
  - Undergoing surgery on other heart valves
- Asymptomatic patients with severe aortic stenosis and left ventricular systolic dysfunction typified by
  - Abnormal response to exercise (e.g., hypotension)
  - Ventricular tachycardia
  - Marked or excessive left ventricular hypertrophy (> 15 mm)
  - Valve area < 0.6 cm^2
  - Prevention of sudden death without the findings listed

Aortic valve replacement in aortic stenosis (Bonow RO, Carabello BA, Kanu C, et al. ACC/AHA guidelines for the management of patients with valvular heart disease. A report of the American College of Cardiology/American Heart Association Task Force on Practice Guidelines. Circulation 2006;114:e84–231.) [John R, Liao KK. Heart Valve Disease. In: Iaizzo PA, editor. Handbook of Cardiac Anatomy, Physiology, and Devices [Internet]. Totowa, NJ: Humana Press; 2009 [cited 2015 Aug 28]. p. 527–49. Available from: http://link.springer.com/10.1007/978-1-60327-372-5_31] *Caption from original*

Overall Principles of Treatment

- After repair of aortic stenosis, quality of life and survival generally return to those expected for age and comorbidity burden.

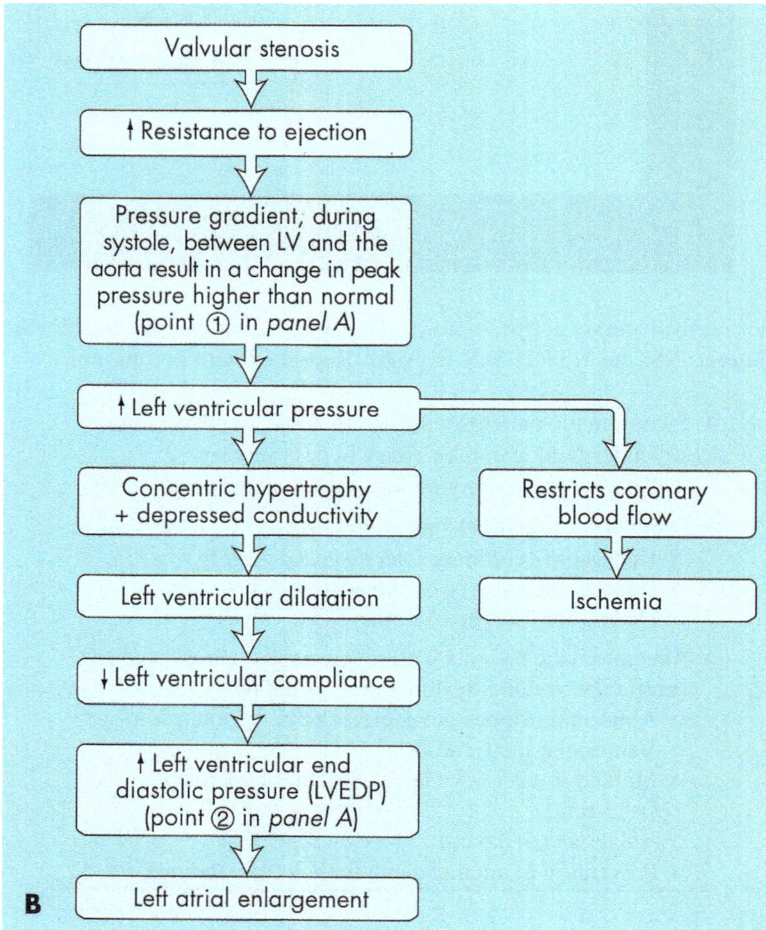

Aortic stenosis. The primary hemodynamic abnormality in aortic stenosis is obstruction to left ventricular outflow, which results in a pressure gradient (B) (which can be estimated by Doppler echocardiography) between the left ventricle (LV) and the aorta, leading to left ventricular hypertrophy. Loss of atrial contraction and contribution to ventricular filling may result in clinical deterioration. The increased left ventricular size necessitates an increase in myocardial oxygen demand, and intraventricular wall pressure may exceed coronary artery perfusion pressure, causing myocardial ischemia even in the absence of coronary artery disease. Cardinal signs are exertional dyspnea (inability to increase cardiac output and elevated pulmonary capillary pressure), angina pectoris, and exertional syncope (caused by decreased arterial pressure associated with vasodilatation in the exercising muscles or arrhythmias). Care must be taken to avoid intravascular volume depletion [Mulligan M, Cousins M. Chapter 4. In: Lichtor JL, editor. Preoperative preparation and intraoperative monitoring. Philadelphia: Current Medicine; 1997. (Miller RD, editor. Atlas of anesthesia; vol. 3)] *Caption adapted from original*

Disease Course

- After the onset of symptoms, patients with severe aortic stenosis have a survival rate as low as 50% at two years and 20% at five years without aortic valve replacement.

Related Evidence

Papers of particular interest have been highlighted as:
*** Of key importance*

Practice Guideline

Nishimura RA, Otto CM, Bonow RO, Carabello BA, Erwin JP 3rd, Guyton RA, O'Gara PT, Ruiz CE, Skubas NJ, Sorajja P, Sundt TM 3rd, Thomas JD, Anderson JL, Halperin JL, Albert NM, Bozkurt B, Brindis RG, Creager MA, Curtis LH, DeMets D, Guyton RA, Hochman JS, Kovacs RJ, Ohman EM, Pressler SJ, Sellke FW, Shen WK, Stevenson WG, Yancy CW; American College of Cardiology; American College of Cardiology/American Heart Association; American Heart Association. 2014 AHA/ACC guideline for the management of patients with valvular heart disease: a report of the American College of Cardiology/American Heart Association Task Force on Practice Guidelines. J Thorac Cardiovasc Surg. 2014 Jul;148(1):e1-e132. https://doi.org/10.1016/j.jtcvs.2014.05.014. PMID: 24939033. http://www.ncbi.nlm.nih.gov/pubmed/24939033 **

Vahanian A, Alfieri O, Andreotti F, Antunes MJ, Barón-Esquivias G, Baumgartner H, Borger MA, Carrel TP, De Bonis M, Evangelista A, Falk V, Lung B, Lancellotti P, Pierard L, Price S, Schäfers HJ, Schuler G, Stepinska J, Swedberg K, Takkenberg J, Von Oppell UO, Windecker S, Zamorano JL, Zembala M; ESC Committee for Practice Guidelines (CPG); Joint Task Force on the Management of Valvular Heart Disease of the European Society of Cardiology (ESC); European Association for Cardio-Thoracic Surgery (EACTS). Guidelines on the management of valvular heart disease (version 2012): the Joint Task Force on the Management of Valvular Heart Disease of the European Society of Cardiology (ESC) and the European Association for Cardio-Thoracic Surgery (EACTS). Eur J Cardiothorac Surg. 2012 Oct;42(4):S1–44. https://doi.org/10.1093/ejcts/ezs455. PMID: 22922698. http://www.ncbi.nlm.nih.gov/pubmed/22922698 **

Holmes DR Jr, Mack MJ, Kaul S, Agnihotri A, Alexander KP, Bailey SR, Calhoon JH, Carabello BA, Desai MY, Edwards FH, Francis GS, Gardner TJ, Kappetein AP, Linderbaum JA, Mukherjee C, Mukherjee D, Otto CM, Ruiz CE, Sacco RL, Smith D, Thomas JD; American College of Cardiology Foundation; American Association for Thoracic Surgery; Society for Cardiovascular Angiography and Interventions; Society for Thoracic Surgeons; American Heart Association; American Society of Echocardiography; European Association for Cardio-Thoracic Surgery; Heart Failure Society of America; Mended Hearts; Society of Cardiovascular Anesthesiologists; Society of Cardiovascular Computed Tomography; Society for Cardiovascular Magnetic Resonance. 2012 ACCF/AATS/SCAI/STS expert consensus document on transcatheter aortic valve replacement: developed in collaboration with the American Heart Association, American Society of Echocardiography, European Association for Cardio-Thoracic Surgery, Heart Failure Society of America, Mended Hearts, Society of Cardiovascular Anesthesiologists, Society of Cardiovascular Computed Tomography, and Society for Cardiovascular Magnetic Resonance. Ann Thorac Surg. 2012 Apr;93(4):1340–95. https://doi.org/10.1016/j.athoracsur.2012.01.084. PMID: 22300625. http://www.ncbi.nlm.nih.gov/pubmed/22300625 **

Meta-Analysis

Giordana F, D'Ascenzo F, Nijhoff F, Moretti C, D'Amico M, Biondi Zoccai G, Sinning JM, Nickenig G, Van Mieghem NM, Chieffo A, Dumonteil N, Tchetche D, Barbash IM, Waksman R, D'Onofrio A, Lefevre T, Pilgrim T, Amabile N, Codner P, Kornowski R, Yong ZY, Baan J, Colombo A, Latib A, Salizzoni S, Omedè P, Conrotto F, La Torre M, Marra S, Rinaldi M, Gaita F. Meta-Analysis of Predictors of All-Cause Mortality After Transcatheter Aortic Valve Implantation. Am J Cardiol. 2014 Nov 1;114(9):1447-1455. https://doi.org/10.1016/j.amjcard.2014.07.081. PMID: 25217456. http://www.ncbi.nlm.nih.gov/pubmed/25217456

Sannino A, Losi MA, Schiattarella GG, Gargiulo G, Perrino C, Stabile E, Toscano E, Giugliano G, Brevetti L, Franzone A, Cirillo P, Imbriaco M, Trimarco B, Esposito G. Meta-analysis of mortality outcomes and mitral regurgitation evolution in 4,839 patients having transcatheter aortic valve implantation for severe aortic stenosis. Am J Cardiol. 2014 Sep 15;114(6):875–82. https://doi.org/10.1016/j.amjcard.2014.06.022. PMID: 25092192. http://www.ncbi.nlm.nih.gov/pubmed/25092192

Coffey S, Cox B, Williams MJ. The prevalence, incidence, progression, and risks of aortic valve sclerosis: a systematic review and meta-analysis. J Am Coll Cardiol.

2014 Jul 1;63(25 Pt A):2852–61. https://doi.org/10.1016/j.jacc.2014.04.018. PMID: 24814496. http://www.ncbi.nlm.nih.gov/pubmed/24814496 **

Review

Singh A, Steadman CD, McCann GP. Advances in the understanding of the pathophysiology and management of aortic stenosis: role of novel imaging techniques. Can J Cardiol. 2014 Sep;30(9):994–1003. https://doi.org/10.1016/j.cjca.2014.03.008. PMID: 2501569. http://www.ncbi.nlm.nih.gov/pubmed/2501569 **

Iung B, Vahanian A. Epidemiology of acquired valvular heart disease. Can J Cardiol. 2014 Sep;30(9):962–70. https://doi.org/10.1016/j.cjca.2014.03.022. PMID: 24986049. http://www.ncbi.nlm.nih.gov/pubmed/24986049 **

Pandian NG, Ramamurthi A, Applebaum S. Role of echocardiography in aortic stenosis. Prog Cardiovasc Dis. 2014 Jul-Aug;57(1):47–54. https://doi.org/10.1016/j.pcad.2014.05.006. PMID: 25081401. http://www.ncbi.nlm.nih.gov/pubmed/25081401

Thaden JJ, Nkomo VT, Enriquez-Sarano M. The global burden of aortic stenosis. Prog Cardiovasc Dis. 2014 May-Jun;56(6):565–71. https://doi.org/10.1016/j.pcad.2014.02.006. PMID: 24838132. http://www.ncbi.nlm.nih.gov/pubmed/24838132 **

Saikrishnan N, Kumar G, Sawaya FJ, Lerakis S, Yoganathan AP. Accurate assessment of aortic stenosis: a review of diagnostic modalities and hemodynamics. Circulation. 2014 Jan 14;129(2):244–53. https://doi.org/10.1161/CIRCULATIONAHA.113.002310. PMID: 24421359. http://www.ncbi.nlm.nih.gov/pubmed/24421359 **

Dill KE, George E, Abbara S, Cummings K, Francois CJ, Gerhard-Herman MD, Gornik HL, Hanley M, Kalva SP, Kirsch J, Kramer CM, Majdalany BS, Moriarty JM, Oliva IB, Schenker MP, Strax R, Rybicki FJ. ACR appropriateness criteria imaging for transcatheter aortic valve replacement. J Am Coll Radiol. 2013 Dec;10(12):957–65. https://doi.org/10.1016/j.jacr.2013.09.002. PMID: 24183748. http://www.ncbi.nlm.nih.gov/pubmed/24183748 **

Akerström F, Barderas MG, Rodríguez-Padial L. Aortic stenosis: a general overview of clinical, pathophysiological and therapeutic aspects. Expert Rev Cardiovasc Ther. 2013 Feb;11(2):239–50. https://doi.org/10.1586/erc.12.171. PMID: 23405844. http://www.ncbi.nlm.nih.gov/pubmed/23405844 **

McLean KM, Lorts A, Pearl JM. Current treatments for congenital aortic stenosis. Curr Opin Cardiol. 2006 May;21(3):200–4. PMID: 16601457. http://www.ncbi.nlm.nih.gov/pubmed/16601457

Use PubMed Clinical Queries to find the most recent evidence. Use this search strategy:

"Aortic Valve Stenosis"[Mesh] OR "Aortic Stenosis"

Chapter 10
Aspiration

Christopher J. Rees, Richard M. Cantor, Charles V. Pollack, Jr., and Victoria G. Riese

Name and Synonyms

Aspiration; Aspiration Pneumonia; Aspiration Pneumonitis; Chemical Pneumonitis

Incidence/Epidemiology

- About half of all healthy adults aspirate to some degree during sleep, but this is usually not clinically significant. Healthy people have physiologic defenses (such as cough and glottic closure) against aspiration that helps to limit the damage that can be caused.
- Aspiration becomes clinically significant when the patient has some underlying condition that compromises the usual defenses.
- Up to 15 % of cases of typical community-acquired pneumonia (CAP) are due to aspiration of pathogenic bacteria from the oro-pharyngeal cavity and the stomach. The incidence increases with age, and up to 20 % of CAP in the elderly is from aspiration.

C. J. Rees
Emergency Department, Pennsylvania Hospital, Philadelphia, PA, USA

R. M. Cantor
Department of Emergency Medicine and Pediatrics, State University of New York Upstate Medical University, Syracuse, NY, USA

C. V. Pollack, Jr. (✉)
Department of Emergency Medicine, Thomas Jefferson University, Philadelphia, PA, USA

V. G. Riese
Librarian Consultant, Eldersburg, MD, USA

C. V. Pollack, Jr. (ed.), *Differential Diagnosis of Cardiopulmonary Disease*,
https://doi.org/10.1007/978-3-319-63895-9_10

- It is felt that the majority of hospital- and nursing home-acquired pneumonias are due to aspiration.
- Factors that can increase the risk of aspiration include: decreased level of consciousness; neurologic disorders that affect swallowing; mechanical disruption of the oro-pharynx, epiglottis, trachea, and esophagus, such as endotracheal intubation; nasogastric feeding tubes; tracheostomy, etc.

Differential Diagnosis

- Aspiration, especially aspiration of gastric contents causing aspiration pneumonitis, can present as acute shortness of breath with both tachypnea and hypoxia. As such, the differential is broad, and contains all the usual causes of acute dyspnea and respiratory compromise, such as ACS, pulmonary embolism, and pulmonary edema/CHF, among others.
- Aspiration pneumonia may present as typical CAP or HAP, with fever and cough with purulent sputum, but can also present sub-acutely when caused predominately by anaerobes.

Pathophysiology and Etiology

- Aspiration results in three broad clinical syndromes, often presenting with overlapping features:
  - Aspiration pneumonitis (chemical pneumonitis)
  - Bacterial Infection causing pneumonia, empyema, and/or pulmonary abscess
  - Airway obstruction from larger, solid matter
- The pathophysiology starts similarly in all syndromes. They are caused by the abnormal entry of endogenous secretions, fluids, and/or particulate matter into the lower airway.
- Aspiration/Chemical Pneumonitis. In this syndrome, there is aspiration of materials that have a direct, toxic effect on the lower airways and lung tissue. The best-known and studied substance is gastric acid, and serves as the pathophysiologic model for all other substances.
  - The airways and lungs are relatively resistant to injury. For clinically significant issues to result, there needs to be a large amount of aspirate (generally more than 25 ml in an adult), and the pH must be below 2.5.
  - When this condition is met, rapid physiologic changes occur (within 3 minutes), including atelectasis, peribronchial hemorrhage, pulmonary edema, and rapid death of bronchial epithelial cells.
  - After 4 hours, the alveolar spaces will become filled with an inflammatory exudate composed of inflammatory cells, fibrin, and desquamated tissue.

- Within 2 days there will be hyaline membrane formation, and the lungs will be edematous and hemorrhagic with consolidation of the alveolar spaces.
- Lungs that have been injured by acid or other directly toxic materials are more susceptible to subsequent bacterial infection.

- Bacterial Infection/Aspiration Pneumonia. The bacteria that cause aspiration pneumonia generally originate in the upper airways or stomach.
  - Classically, oral anaerobes (*Peptostreptococcus*, *Fusobacterium nucleatum*, *Prevotells*, and *Bacteroides* spp.) and streptococci caused aspiration pneumonia.
  - More recently, hospital- and healthcare-acquired aspiration pneumonia has been associated with more virulent organisms, such as Staphylococcus aureus, Pseudomonas aeruginosa, and gram-negative bacilli.
- Airway obstruction. Airway obstruction may result from either fluids or solid material aspiration.
  - The ingestion of fluids that are not directly toxic to lung tissue (saline, barium, etc.) can initiate a reflex airway closure, such as in drowning.
  - Solid objects cause differing levels of obstruction based upon their size relative to the airways.
  - Most foreign body aspirations occur in children between the ages of one and three.
  - Large objects can obstruct at the larynx, proximal trachea, tracheal bifurcation, or main stem bronchus. They cause nearly immediate respiratory distress, inability to talk, and cyanosis. Unless removed quickly, they can rapidly lead to death.
  - Smaller objects cause local atelectasis, and the patient will have a cough or focal wheezing.

Presentation

Typical/"Classic"

- Aspiration/Chemical Pneumonitis:
  - Acute onset of symptoms with profound dyspnea, and associated hypoxemia.
  - Often seen in the setting of known risk-factors for aspiration.
- Bacterial Infection. Presentation is variable, and depends upon the causative organisms and the overall health status of the affected patient.
  - Most patients present somewhat acutely with the typical symptoms of pneumonia, fever, productive cough, and dyspnea, especially when the infection is due to organisms other than anaerobes (such as Staph, Strep, Pseudomonas, etc.).

    - Infections from anaerobic organisms often present more slowly, over days and weeks. There is often necrotic-smelling sputum, and a notable lack of rigors. Most patients with anaerobic aspiration pneumonia will have an easily recognized risk factor for aspiration, and poor dental health.
- Airway Obstruction.
    - Large particle airway obstruction causes acute respiratory compromise and failure, with severe dyspnea, inability to talk, hypoxia/cyanosis, and rapid cardiovascular collapse if not removed.
    - Small particle airway obstruction can present in a more subtle fashion, with an indolent, irritative cough, associated with dyspnea that is sometimes present only with exertion.

Atypical

- There is a wide-spectrum of clinical presentations and syndromes for aspiration. As above, aspiration syndromes typically present acutely, but depending upon many factors, may be sub-acute or indolent. Also, as noted above, atypical presentations occur especially with aspiration pneumonia caused by anaerobic organisms, airway obstruction caused by small particles, or aspiration pneumonitis caused by small volume, higher pH substances.

Primary Differential Considerations

- Differential considerations for aspiration include:
    - Respiratory Distress Syndrome
    - Other respiratory failure
    - Status asthmaticus
    - Circulatory shock
    - RSV infection in children

History and Physical Exam

Findings That Confirm Diagnosis

- A witnessed aspiration event, followed by the typical clinical syndrome of aspiration pneumonitis, confirms the diagnosis.

Factors That Suggest Diagnosis

- A patient who presents with community- or hospital-acquired pneumonia, has risk factors for aspiration, and/or has infiltrates in the dependent lung zones (lower lobes if aspiration occurred in the upright position, or superior segments of the lower lobes and/or posterior segment of the upper lobes if aspiration occurred in the supine position) should be further evaluated for aspiration and swallowing difficulties.

Factors That Exclude Diagnosis

- Finding another cause for the dyspnea/respiratory distress makes aspiration unlikely.

Ancillary Studies

Laboratory

- Laboratory abnormalities in aspiration pneumonitis are usually non-specific. There may be a moderately elevated white blood cell count. Patients may be hypoxic with a respiratory acidosis on blood gas analysis, especially in the acute setting when they are tachypneic.
- Patients with bacterial pneumonia caused by aspiration will usually have laboratory findings of acute infection with a leukocytosis with bandemia and/or a leftward shift. These patients may also be hypoxic.
  - Sputum culture has a limited role in aspiration pneumonia. Most infections are polymicrobial, and many of the causative organisms are difficult to culture. Coughed sputum samples are not useful for culture, as the normal flora of the mouth and upper airway contaminates them.
- Laboratory studies are not helpful in the diagnosis of airway obstruction from particulate matter.

Imaging

- CXR findings in aspiration pneumonitis typically appear about 2 hours after an aspiration event. Typically, there are infiltrates in the dependent lung zones. These are the lower lobes when the patient was in an upright position during the aspiration event, and the superior segments of the lower lobes and posterior segments of the upper lobes if the patient was in the supine position during the aspiration event. Over time, if the disease progresses, the CXR may show evidence of ARDS with diffuse, fluffy infiltrates.

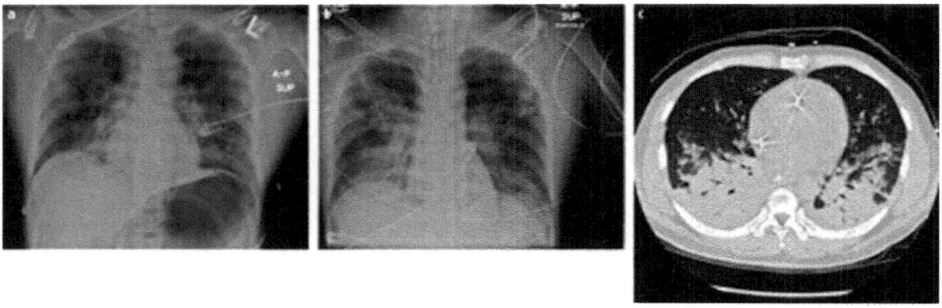

Aspiration pneumonia with infection: image progression. **a** Several hours after aspiration of gastric content, there are patchy infiltrates at both lung bases medially. **b** Three days after aspiration, the consolidation has increased in density and extent. At this phase, aspiration pneumonitis should be improving. This suggests secondary infection. **c** Four days after aspiration, computed tomography reveals dense consolidation in the posterior and lateral basal segments of both lower lobes. This degree of consolidation is more than one usually sees with uncomplicated aspiration pneumonitis. [Goodman LR. Imaging the Intensive Care Patient. In: Hodler J, von Schulthess GK, Zollikofer CL, editors. Diseases of the Heart and Chest, Including Breast 2011–2014 [Internet]. Milano: Springer Milan; 2011 [cited 2015 May 22]. p. 66–9. Available from: http://link.springer.com/10.1007/978-88-470-1938-6_10] *Caption adapted from original*

- The CXR in aspiration pneumonia caused by bacteria will also typically reveal an infiltrate in one or more of the dependent lung zones.
- Patients with pneumonia caused by anaerobic bacteria can have more indolent presentation and may develop either lung abscess or empyema that can be revealed on the CXR.

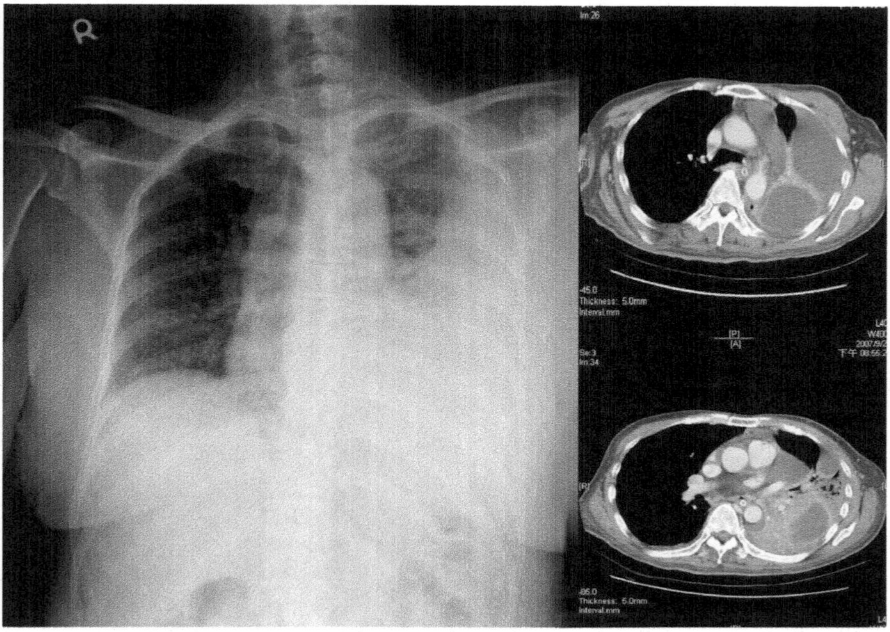

The chest radiograph and computed tomography scan showed pleural empyema without lung abscess. [From article: Lung abscess predicts the surgical outcome in patients with pleural empyema. Journal of Cardiothoracic Surgery. 2010;5(1):88. https://doi.org/10.1186/1749-8090-5-88, at http://link.springer.com/article/10.1186%2F1749-8090-5-88; by Hung-Che Huang, Heng-Chung Chen, Hsin-Yuan Fang, Yi-Chieh Lin, Chin-Yen Wu, Ching-Yuan Cheng, © Huang et al; licensee BioMed Central Ltd. 2010; licensed under Creative Commons Attribution License BY 2.0 http://creativecommons.org/licenses/by/2.0] *Caption from original*

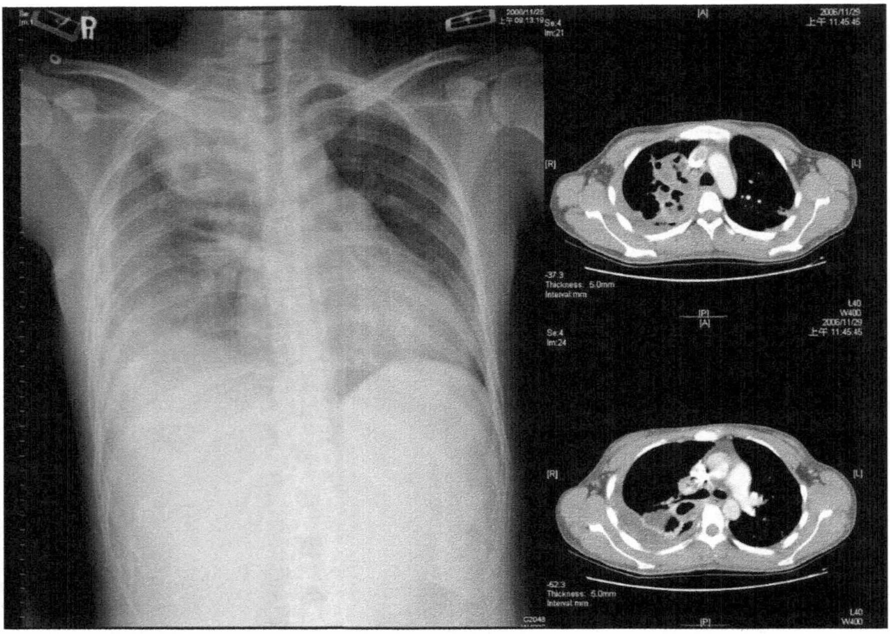

The chest radiograph and computed tomography showed pleural empyema with lung abscess. [From article: Lung abscess predicts the surgical outcome in patients with pleural empyema. Journal of Cardiothoracic Surgery. 2010;5(1):88. https://doi.org/10.1186/1749-8090-5-88, at http://link.springer.com/article/10.1186%2F1749-8090-5-88; by Hung-Che Huang, Heng-Chung Chen, Hsin-Yuan Fang, Yi-Chieh Lin, Chin-Yen Wu, Ching-Yuan Cheng, © Huang et al; licensee BioMed Central Ltd. 2010; licensed under Creative Commons Attribution License BY 2.0 http://creativecommons.org/licenses/by/2.0] *Caption from original*

- Airway obstruction from aspirated, large objects must be diagnosed prior to CXR, as the patients are in extremis and need rapid treatment. When the object is smaller, and the presentation not as severe or obvious, a CXR may be helpful. Many objects that are aspirated are biologic and radiolucent (peanuts, vegetables, other food objects), and some are radiodense (teeth, buttons, batteries, etc.). If the object itself is not visualized on the x-ray, there may be atelectasis with an elevated hemidiaphragm, and other signs of lung-volume loss.

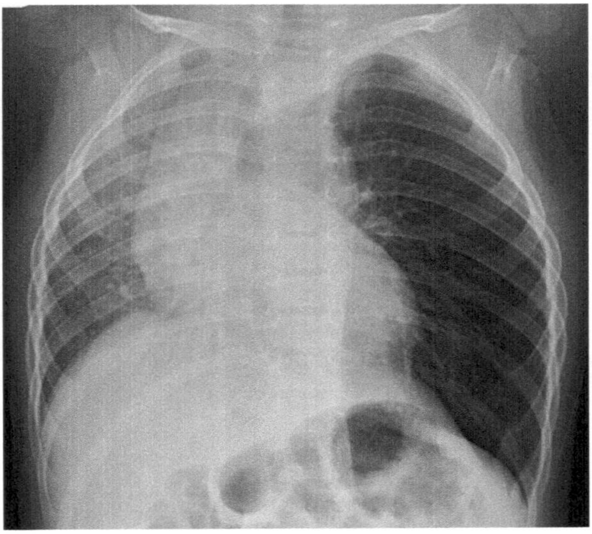

Frontal chest radiograph of a child with foreign body aspiration. The left lung is large and hyperlucent with less vessels due to air trapping caused by partial obstruction of the left main bronchus. Note the mediastinal shift to the right. [Soto G, Moënne K. Classic Chest Radiology Findings, Pearls and Pitfalls. In: Garcia-Peña P, Guillerman RP, editors. Pediatric Chest Imaging [Internet]. Berlin, Heidelberg: Springer Berlin Heidelberg; 2013 [cited 2015 May 22]. p. 13–30. Available from: http://link.springer.com/10.1007/174_2013_905] *Caption from original*

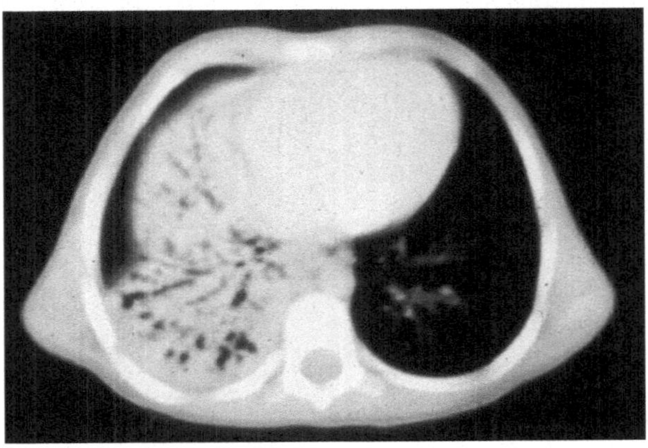

Axial CT of the lower chest in a case of chronic foreign body aspiration into the right intermediate bronchus, causing collapse and bronchiectasis in the right middle lobe and right lower lobe. [Koplewitz BZ, Bar-Ziv J. Foreign Body Aspiration: Imaging Aspects. In: Garcia-Peña P, Guillerman RP, editors. Pediatric Chest Imaging [Internet]. Berlin, Heidelberg: Springer Berlin Heidelberg; 2014 [cited 2015 May 22]. p. 305–26. Available from: http://link.springer.com/10.1007/174_2013_952] *Caption from original*

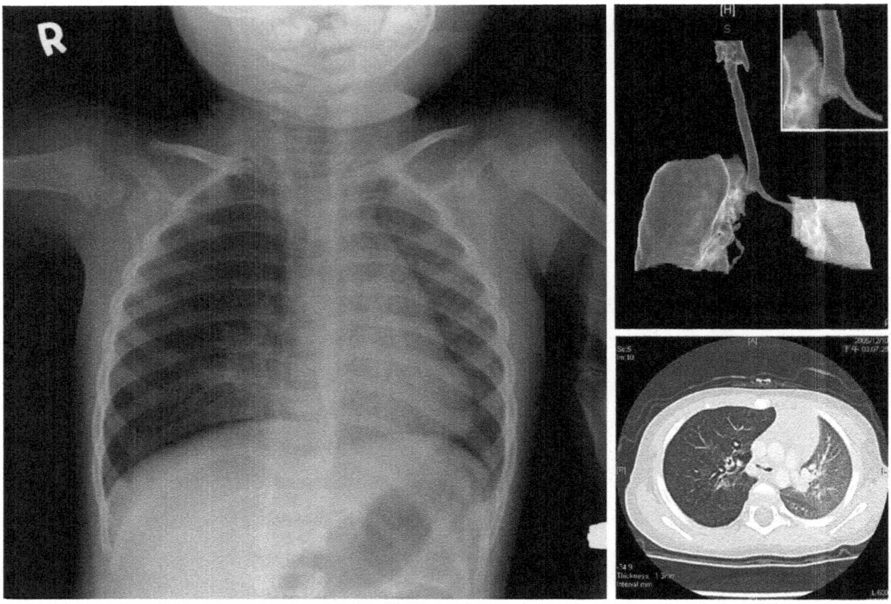

Plain chest radiograph showing a nearly left total opacity with ipsilateral mediastinal shift caused by foreign body aspiration. Three-dimensional chest computed tomography showing a nearly total occlusion in the right main bronchus [Huang H-J, Fang H-Y, Chen H-C, Wu C-Y, Cheng C-Y, Chang C-L. Three-dimensional computed tomography for detection of tracheobronchial foreign body aspiration in children. Pediatric Surgery International. 2008 Feb;24(2):157–60.] *Caption from original*

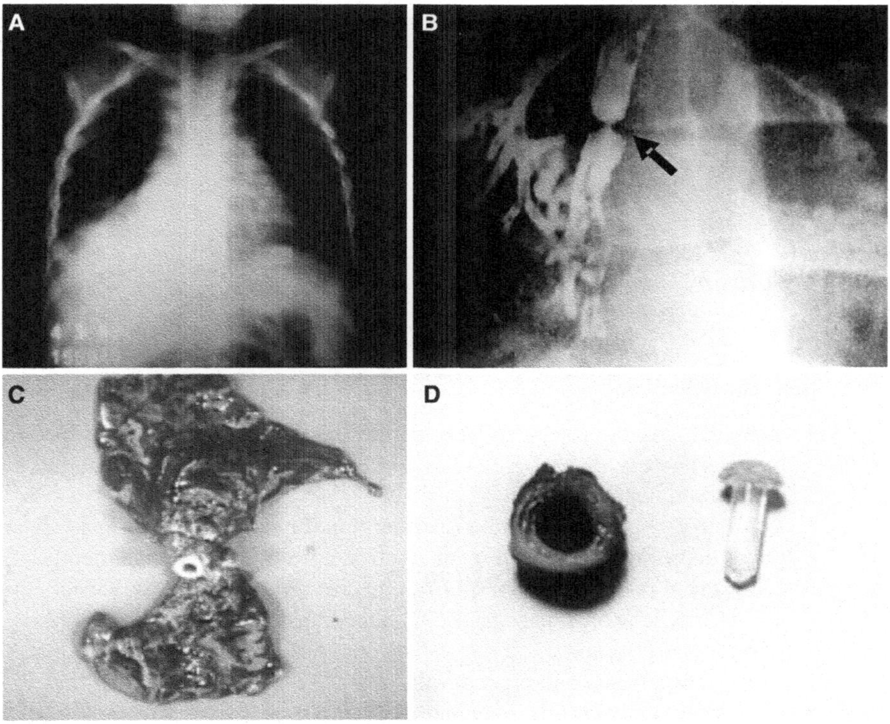

a Thorax X-ray showing atelectasis of the inferior and middle lobe of the right lung in a child with recurrent pneumonia for 2 years. b Bronchography showing stenosis of the intermediate segment, the foreign body cannot be seen. c Removed inferior and middle destroyed lobes. d Foreign body and blocked bronchus. When saw the foreign body, the mother said that it was part of a toy that had disappeared 2 years earlier [Cataneo AJM, Cataneo DC, Ruiz RL. Management of tracheobronchial foreign body in children. Pediatric Surgery International. 2008 Feb;24(2):151–6.] *Caption from original*

Special Populations

Age

- Aspiration pneumonitis is more common in the elderly, especially those with neurologic and other swallowing difficulties.
- Aspiration of objects is more common among children between the ages of one and three.
- Gastroesophogeal reflux (GER) is common in infancy, resulting in vomiting, albeit without complications.

- The diagnosis of gastroesophogeal reflux disease (GERD) applies when reflux events are associated with pathologic outcomes or debilitating symptoms.
- Concomitant aspiration events are rarely seen in infants with GERD, except in patients with swallowing disorders, e.g., neurological impairment scenarios.

Co-morbidities

- There are multiple co-morbidities that increase the risk of all types of aspiration. These include:
    - Reduced consciousness, which depresses the gag and glottic closure reflexes and can be brought on by causes such as alcohol and drug intoxication, and hepatic failure.
    - Prior stroke or neuromuscular disorder that impairs the ability to swallow.
    - Other neurologic conditions such as stroke, head injury, and dementia.
    - Mechanical instrumentation of the upper airway, such as endotracheal intubation, tracheostomy, nasogastric tube feedings, and upper endoscopy.
    - Periodontal disease.
    - General anesthesia and procedural sedation.
    - Gastroesophageal reflux, esophageal dysmotility.

Pitfalls in Diagnosis

Critical Steps Not to Miss

- Consideration of the diagnosis is the first critical step. Patients presenting with respiratory compromise need all appropriate supportive care until a diagnosis can be established.
- CXR should be performed early, but findings may be delayed by several hours.
- Patients who are felt to have a syndrome-consistent aspiration should have their swallowing function evaluated.

Mimics

- Many conditions can cause acute dyspnea and respiratory compromise, including ACS, pulmonary embolism, pneumothorax, pulmonary edema/CHF, among others.

Time-Dependent Interventions

- Airway obstruction with a large object causing complete airway obstruction is a medical emergency and can be fatal within minutes if not recognized and treated appropriately.
- Aspiration pneumonia from bacterial infection can present with acute respiratory compromise, so the rapid support of ventilatory function and administration of empiric antibiotics for likely pathogens is necessary.
- A witnessed aspiration event should be treated urgently with airway suctioning to remove as much fluid and solid matter as possible, and ventilatory and respiratory function should be supported.

Overall Principles of Treatment

- Aspiration pneumonitis.
  - As noted above, a patient with a witnessed or presumed acute aspiration event should have tracheal suctioning, administration of supplemental oxygen, and all respiratory and ventilator necessary.
  - The use of glucocorticoids is controversial. There are no good data supporting their use in aspiration pneumonitis.
  - Empiric or prophylactic antibiotics are commonly given in aspiration pneumonitis. Chemically injured lungs are at an increased risk for developing bacterial superinfection in the coming days, but there is no good evidence that prophylactic antibiotics administration prevents these infections. It is appropriate to administer antibiotics if the diagnosis is in doubt and bacterial pneumonia remains on the differential.
- Bacterial Aspiration Pneumonia.
  - Antibiotics are necessary in the treatment of aspiration pneumonia due to bacteria.
  - Most of these infections are polymicrobial, and include anaerobes. As such, most patients will be treated (at least initially), with a combination of antibiotics.
  - Clindamycin is the antibiotic of choice to cover anaerobes. Metronidazole should not be used alone, as it has a failure rate of up to 50% when used as monotherapy.
  - Clindamycin can be combined with either amoxicillin or penicillin.
  - When the patient has a hospital- or healthcare-acquired aspiration pneumonia, it is important to consider both gram positive organisms, such as Staph and strep, and the aerobic gram negative bacilli as causes. These patients should be broadly covered with an antibiotic or combination of antibiotics, to cover the gram-positives and negatives. This usually includes vancomycin

with either a carbapenem or piperacillin/tazobactam. These regimens will also cover most pathogenic anaerobes.

- Airway obstruction from large objects needs to be relieved immediately. The preferred method is the Heimlich maneuver. If unsuccessful, a surgical airway may need to be secured.
  - Smaller objects can often be removed by bronchoscopy.

Disease Course

- Aspiration pneumonitis. The course varies considerably based upon the patient's underlying medical condition and the cause of the aspiration. The majority of patients will recover rapidly. A small percentage will go on to develop ARDS and/or bacterial superinfection. There is a significant mortality associated with both of these complications.
- Patients with bacterial aspiration pneumonia often recover fully, but when the predominant pathogens are anaerobic bacteria, a small percentage can go on to develop pulmonary abscess or empyema as complications of the primary infection. The incidence of these complications has been decreasing.
- All patients who suffer from aspiration need to be evaluated for the primary cause of their aspiration, or they remain at risk for further episodes.
- Most patients who have an airway obstruction recover uneventfully if the obstruction is relieved in a timely manner.

Related Evidence

Paper of particular interest have been highlighted as:
*** Of key importance*

Practice Guideline

Australian and New Zealand Society for Geriatric Medicine. Australian and New Zealand Society for Geriatric Medicine. Position statement - dysphagia and aspiration in older people. Australas J Ageing. 2011 Jun;30(2):98-103. https://doi.org/10.1111/j.1741-6612.2011.00537.x. PMID: 21672120. http://www.ncbi.nlm.nih.gov/pubmed/21672120 **

Review

DiBardino DM, Wunderink RG. Aspiration pneumonia: a review of modern trends. J Crit Care. 2015 Feb;30(1):40-8. https://doi.org/10.1016/j.jcrc.2014.07.011. PMID: 25129577. http://www.ncbi.nlm.nih.gov/pubmed/25129577 **

Waybright RA, Coolidge W, Johnson TJ. Treatment of clinical aspiration: a reappraisal. Am J Health Syst Pharm. 2013 Aug 1;70(15):1291-300. https://doi.org/10.2146/ajhp120319. PMID: 23867486. http://www.ncbi.nlm.nih.gov/pubmed/23867486 **

van der Maarel-Wierink CD, Vanobbergen JN, Bronkhorst EM, Schols JM, de Baat C. Risk factors for aspiration pneumonia in frail older people: a systematic literature review. J Am Med Dir Assoc. 2011 Jun;12(5):344-54. https://doi.org/10.1016/j.jamda.2010.12.099. PMID: 21450240. http://www.ncbi.nlm.nih.gov/pubmed/21450240 **

Marik PE. Pulmonary aspiration syndromes. Curr Opin Pulm Med. 2011 May;17(3):148-54. https://doi.org/10.1097/MCP.0b013e32834397d6. PMID: 21311332. http://www.ncbi.nlm.nih.gov/pubmed/21311332 **

Raghavendran K, Nemzek J, Napolitano LM, Knight PR. Aspiration-induced lung injury. Crit Care Med. 2011 Apr;39(4):818-26. https://doi.org/10.1097/CCM.0b013e31820a856b. PMID: 21263315. http://www.ncbi.nlm.nih.gov/pubmed/21263315 **

Beck-Schimmer B, Bonvini JM. Bronchoaspiration: incidence, consequences and management. Eur J Anaesthesiol. 2011 Feb;28(2):78-84. https://doi.org/10.1097/EJA.0b013e32834205a8. PMID: 21157355. http://www.ncbi.nlm.nih.gov/pubmed/21157355 **

de Benedictis FM, Carnielli VP, de Benedictis D. Aspiration lung disease. Pediatr Clin North Am. 2009 Feb;56(1):173-90, xi. https://doi.org/10.1016/j.pcl.2008.10.013. PMID: 19135587. http://www.ncbi.nlm.nih.gov/pubmed/19135587 **

Paintal HS, Kuschner WG. Aspiration syndromes: 10 clinical pearls every physician should know. Int J Clin Pract. 2007 May;61(5):846-52. PMID: 17493092. http://www.ncbi.nlm.nih.gov/pubmed/17493092 **

Janda M, Scheeren TW, Nöldge-Schomburg GF. Management of pulmonary aspiration. Best Pract Res Clin Anaesthesiol. 2006 Sep;20(3):409-27. PMID: 17080693. http://www.ncbi.nlm.nih.gov/pubmed/17080693 **

Use PubMed Clinical Queries to find the most recent evidence. Use this search strategy:

"Respiratory Aspiration"[Mesh] OR "Pneumonia, Aspiration"[Mesh] OR "Aspiration"

Chapter 11
Asthma

Charles V. Pollack, Jr., Melissa Platt, Richard M. Cantor, and Victoria G. Riese

Name and Synonyms

Asthma

Incidence/Epidemiology

- Approximately 235 million people, worldwide, are affected by asthma.
- Approximately 250,000 people die of asthma each year.
- Rates vary between countries with prevalence between 1 % and 18 %.
- There is some racial predilection (for example, asthma severity and asthma mortality is higher in US blacks than US whites). This may be more socioeconomic than clinical,

C. V. Pollack, Jr. (✉)
Department of Emergency Medicine, Thomas Jefferson University, Philadelphia, PA, USA

M. Platt
Department of Emergency Medicine, University of Louisville, Louisville, KY, USA

R. M. Cantor
Department of Emergency Medicine and Pediatrics, State University of New York Upstate Medical University, Syracuse, NY, USA

V. G. Riese
Librarian Consultant, Eldersburg, MD, USA

C. V. Pollack, Jr. (ed.), *Differential Diagnosis of Cardiopulmonary Disease*, https://doi.org/10.1007/978-3-319-63895-9_11

Population (Survey, sample size)	Poor self-rated health %[a] (95 % CI)	Impaired physical health % (95 % CI)	Impaired mental health % (95 % CI)	Limited activity % (95 % CI)
Adults (Behavioral Risk Factor Surveillance System, $N = 1{,}082{,}135$)	16.2 (16.0–16.3)	10.7 (10.6–10.8)	10.2 (10.1–10.3)	4.0 (3.9–4.1)
No asthma[b]	14.8 (14.7–15.0)	9.5 (9.4–9.7)	9.2 (9.1–9.3)	3.3 (3.3–3.4)
Former asthma[c]	15.7 (15.0–16.4)	11.1 (10.5–11.7)	12.3 (11.7–13.0)	4.4 (4.0–4.7)
Current asthma[d]	29.6 (29.0–30.2)	22.2 (21.6–22.7)	18.9 (18.3–19.5)	10.5 (10.1–10.9)
Ever-employed adults with current asthma[e] (Asthma Call-back Survey, $N = 38{,}306$)	26.9 (25.9–27.9)	20.6 (19.7–21.4)	18.2 (17.3–19.1)	10.2 (9.5–10.9)
Non-work-related asthma[f]	21.6 (20.4–22.8)	15.8 (14.8–16.8)	14.3 (13.1–15.4)	6.6 (5.9–7.2)
Possible work-related asthma[g]	31.3 (29.6–33.0)	24.5 (23.0–26.0)	21.9 (20.3–23.5)	13.3 (11.9–14.6)
HCP-diagnosed work-related asthma[h]	40.2 (36.9–43.6)	32.4 (29.2–35.6)	26.2 (23.0–29.4)	19.2 (16.5–21.9)

CI confidence interval, *HCP* health-care professional

[a] Results presented as weighted average annual estimate

[b] Behavioral Risk Factor Surveillance System participants who answered "No" to the question "Were you ever told by a doctor or other health professional that you had asthma?"

[c] Behavioral Risk Factor Surveillance System participants who answered "Yes" to the question "Were you ever told by a doctor or other health professional that you had asthma?" and "No" to the question "Do you still have asthma?"

[d] Behavioral Risk Factor Surveillance System participants who answered "Yes" to the questions "Were you ever told by a doctor or other health professional that you had asthma?" and "Do you still have asthma?"

[e] Asthma Call-back Survey participants who described current employment status as "employed full-time" or "employed part-time" or responded "yes" to the question "Have you ever been employed outside the home?"

[f] "No" to all of the following five questions: "Were you ever told by a doctor or other health professional that your asthma was related to any job you ever had?", "Was your asthma caused by chemicals, smoke, fumes, or dust in your current job?", "Was your asthma caused by chemicals, smoke, fumes, or dust in any previous job you ever had?", "Is your asthma made worse by chemicals, smoke, fumes, or dust in your current job?", and "Was your asthma made worse by chemicals, smoke, fumes, or dust in any previous job you ever had?"

[g] "No" response to the question "Were you ever told by a doctor or other health professional that your asthma was related to any job you ever had?" and "Yes" responses to any of the following four questions: "Was your asthma caused by chemicals, smoke, fumes, or dust in your current job?", "Was your asthma caused by chemicals, smoke, fumes, or dust in any previous job you ever had?", "Is your asthma made worse by chemicals, smoke, fumes, or dust in your current job?", and "Was your asthma made worse by chemicals, smoke, fumes, or dust in any previous job you ever had?"

[h] "Yes" to the question "Were you ever told by a doctor or other health professional that your asthma was related to any job you ever had?"

Estimated proportion of individuals with poor health-related quality of life among select population groups, Behavioral Risk Factor Surveillance System and Asthma Call-back Survey, 38 states and District of Columbia, 2006–2009 [Knoeller GE, Mazurek JM, Moorman JE. Health-related quality of life among adults with work-related asthma in the United States. Quality of Life Research. 2013 May;22(4): 771–80.] *Caption from original*

- Asthma is the most common chronic disease in childhood.
- Asthma occurs more frequently in boys before puberty and in girls after puberty.

Differential Diagnosis

- See chart, but includes:
    - Airway foreign body
    - Bronchitis with bronchospasm
    - Pneumonia with bronchospasm
    - Congestive heart failure
    - Bronchiolitis
    - Chronic obstructive pulmonary disease
    - Cystic fibrosis

- Pulmonary embolism
- Tracheomalacia
- Vocal cord dysfunction

Chronic bronchitis	Vocal cord dysfunction
Emphysema	Congestive heart failure
Cystic fibrosis	Pulmonary embolism
Viral bronchiolitis	Eosinophilic pneumonia
Bronchial stenosis	Drug-induced cough
Mechanical airway obstruction	β-Blockers
Aspirated foreign body	Angiotensin-converting enzyme inhibitors
Endobronchial tumor	Systemic vasculitis
Superior vena cava syndrome	Carcinoid syndrome
Substernal thyroid	Allergic bronchopulmonary aspergillosis

Differential diagnosis of asthma [Holgate S, Sewell J, Payne KD. Chapter 01. In: Crapo J, editor. Bone's atlas of pulmonary and critical care medicine. Philadelphia: Current Medicine; 2005. ISBN: 1-57340-211-7] *Caption adapted from original*

Pathophysiology and Etiology

- An inflammatory process of the airways that results in periodic, at least partially reversible airflow obstruction.
- Bronchial hyperresponsiveness.
- Family history may be pertinent for asthma diagnosis.
- Many cells and cellular elements contribute to asthma, including:
  - Neutrophils
  - Mast cells
  - Eosinophils
  - Macrophages
  - Activated T lymphocytes
  - Epithelial cells
- Many asthma triggers exist, including:
  - Environmental allergens: dust mites, molds, animal dander, cockroach allergens, fungi, etc.
  - Viral respiratory tract infections
  - Hyperventilation
  - Gastroesophageal reflux disease
  - Environmental pollutants, e.g., tobacco smoke
  - Obesity
  - Hypersensitivity to nonsteroidal anti-inflammatory drugs (NSAID)

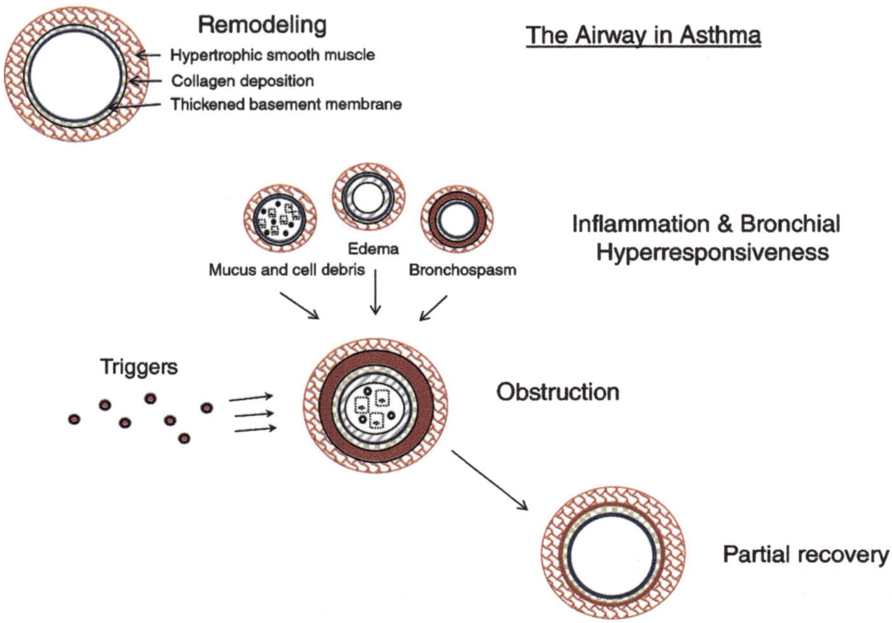

Pathophysiology of asthma at steady state and during an exacerbation. The airways of asthmatic individuals are characterized by pathological changes, including thickened basement membrane, collagen deposition and hypertrophic smooth muscle, collectively called 'airway remodeling'. Inflammation is triggered by a variety of factors, including allergens and respiratory viruses. These factors also induce hyperreactive responses in the asthmatic airways, associated with mucus and cell debris released into the lumen, oedema and bronchoconstriction, leading to airway obstruction and related acute exacerbations. Although pathophysiological changes related to asthma are generally reversible, recovery may be partial. [From article: Research needs in allergy: an EAACI position paper, in collaboration with EFA. Clinical and Translational Allergy. 2012;2(1):21.; https://doi.org/10.1186/2045-7022-2-21, at http://link.springer.com/article/10.1186%2F2045-7022-2-21/fulltext.html; by Nikolaos G Papadopoulos, Ioana Agache, Sevim Bavbek, et al., © Papadopoulos et al.; licensee BioMed Central Ltd. 2012; licensed under Creative Commons Attribution License BY 2.0 http://creativecommons.org/licenses/by/2.0] *Caption from original*

Presentation

Typical/"Classic"

- Wheezing, coughing, shortness of breath, chest tightness, tachypnea, tachycardia, respiratory distress, altered mental status.

Atypical

- Cough-variant asthma, nonasthmatic eosinophilic bronchitis, and atopic cough.
  - Approximately 30 % of cough variant asthma that go untreated will result in progression to asthma

Primary Differential Considerations

- Vocal cord dysfunction
- Allergic and environmental asthma
- Tracheal and bronchial lesions
- Foreign bodies
- Pulmonary migraine
- Congestive heart failure
- Diffuse panbronchiolitis
- Aortic arch anomalies
- Sinus disease
- Gastroesophageal reflux
- Pulmonary embolism
- Cystic fibrosis
- Eosinophilia count >8 %, consider allergic bronchoplumonary aspergillosis, Churg-Strauss syndrome, or eosinophilic pneumonia

History and Physical Exam

- Categories of asthma severity are determined by the following factors:
  - Reported symptoms over the previous 2 – 4 weeks
  - Current level of lung function: FEV_1, FEV_1 (FVC values)
  - Number of exacerbations requiring oral glucocorticoids per year
- Asthma Severity categories:
  - Intermittent
  - Mild persistent
  - Moderate persistent
  - Severe persistent
- Family history of asthma is often common for diagnoses of asthma, allergies, eczema, and/or nasal polyps.
- Social history is frequently helpful to ascertain for environmental smoke exposure. As mentioned under Incidence/Epidemiology, lower socioeconomic status may be associated with more severe asthma.

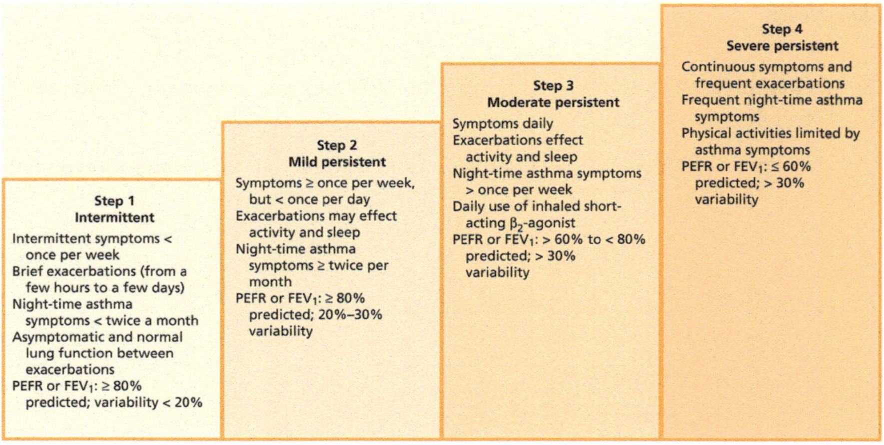

Classification of asthma severity. Severity of asthma is classified into four groups according to symptoms and lung function measurements. This method of classification is important because therapy for asthma takes a stepwise approach according to the disease severity. Generally patients have poor perception of the severity of their asthma because they tend to adapt their lifestyle to accommodate their symptoms. This in turn leads to poor control of the disease as well as poor quality of life. Classifying the disease in this stepwise fashion allows the targeting of therapy according to the severity of the disease. FEV1—forced expiratory volume in 1 second; PEFR—peak expiratory flow rate. [Gnanakumaran G, Holgate S. Asthma in Adults. In: Lieberman P, Blaiss M, editors. Atlas of Allergic Diseases, 2e. Philadelphia: Current Medicine; 2005] *Caption from original*

Findings That Confirm Diagnosis

- Arterial blood gases and pulse oximetry for severity and response to treatment.
- Eosinophil counts >4 %, absence is not exclusionary.
- Spirometry before and after short-acting bronchodilator.
- Bronchoprovocation test.
- High-resolution computed tomography (HRCT).

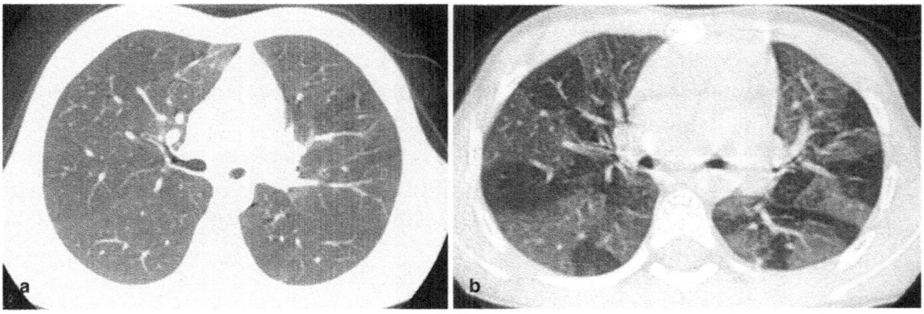

Expiratory HRCT technique. A 9-year-old girl with suspected asthma. a Normal inspiratory HRCT scan. b Expiratory HRCT shows visible differences in lung attenuation (mosaic pattern) due to obstructive small airway disease, which proved to be asthma. Air-trapping is better depicted on expiratory scans [Garcia-Peña P, Lucaya J. HRCT in children: technique and indications. European Radiology Supplements. 2004 Mar 1;14(4):L13–30.] *Caption from original*

Factors That Suggest Diagnosis

- Serum immunoglobulin E levels greater than 100 IU frequently an allergic reaction, may not be asthma but other conditions.
- Elevated blood eosinophils.
- Non-specific IgE >150IU.
- Family history.
- Allergies.

Factors That Exclude Diagnosis

- Laboratory assessments and studies are usually used to exclude other diagnoses.

Evaluation of Exacerbations

- Pulse oximetry: Inability to maintain pulse ox between above 92% suggests impending respiratory failure.
- PEFR or FEV_1 measurement: PEFR is effort-dependent but can be used to compare severity of exacerbation and response to therapy to previous care episodes. FEV_1 is more accurate but is often logistically challenging to obtain in the acute setting

Ancillary Studies

Laboratory

- ABG: progression of severity is typically hyperoxemia → hypoxemia → hypercarbia.
- Pulse oximetry.
- WBC: may be high due to stress release and/or to concomitant infection.

Electrocardiography

- Indicated in patients at risk for cardiac disease, dysrhythmias, myocardial ischemia.
- Transient ST-T wave changes in severe asthma.
- Tachycardia typical.

Imaging

- Chest x-ray is not necessary unless there is suspicion of pneumonia, pneumothorax or pneumomediastinum, foreign body aspiration, comorbid illness, diabetes, AIDS, renal failure, or cancer.

Other Studies

- Peak Flow
- Spirometry
- Lung function study
- Provocative testing
- Diffusing capacity for carbon monoxide (DLco)
- Allergy testing

Special Populations

Age

Pediatrics

- Asthma is not an uncommon cause of chest pain in children.
- Severity classification in children is key.
  - Even children with mild asthma can have severe exacerbations.
  - Controller medications are based on the severity of the symptoms and exacerbation.
- Nonspecific symptoms in infants or young children may have a history of recurrent bronchitis, bronchiolitis, or pneumonia.
- Review for family history or allergy and medical history of early injury to airway.
- Infants are vulnerable to respiratory failure.

Drug name (trade name)	Category	Components (scientific names)	Pediatric indication[a]
Accolate	Leukotriene receptor antagonist	Zafirlukast	5 years and older
Advair Diskus	Combination (ICS + LABA)	Fluticasone propionate Salmeterol xinafoate	4 years and older
Advair HFA	Combination (ICS + LABA)	Fluticasone propionate Salmeterol xinafoate	12 years and older
Albuterol oral syrup	SABA	Albuterol sulfate	2 years and older
Alvesco	Inhaled ICS	Ciclesonide	12 years and older
Asmanex Twisthaler	Inhaled ICS	Mometasone furoate	4 years and older
Atrovent HFA	Anticholinergic	Ipratropium bromide	Not established
Dulera	Combination (ICS + LABA)	Mometasone furoate Formoterol fumarate dihydrate	12 years and older
Foradil	LABA	Formoterol fumarate	5 years and older
Intal inhaler	Anti-inflammatory	Cromolyn	Discontinued in USA, available still in other countries
Intal nebulization solution	Anti-inflammatory	Cromolyn	2 years and older
Pro-Air HFA	SABA	Albuterol sulfate	4 years and older
Proventil HFA	SABA	Albuterol sulfate	4 years and older
Pulmicort Flexhaler	Inhaled ICS	Budesonide	6 years and older
Pulmicort respules	Inhaled (nebulized) ICS	Budesonide	12 months to 8 years
QVAR	Inhaled ICS	Beclomethasone dipropionate	5 years and older
Seretide Accuhaler	Combination (ICS + LABA)	Fluticasone propionate Salmeterol xinafoate	4 years and older (Australia)
Seretide MDI	Combination (ICS + LABA)	Fluticasone propionate Salmeterol xinafoate	4 years and older (Australia)
Serevent Accuhaler	LABA	Salmeterol xinafoate	4 years and older (Australia)
Serevent Diskus	LABA	Salmeterol xinafoate	4 years and older (USA)
Serevent Inhaler	LABA	Salmeterol xinafoate	4 years and older (Australia)
Singulair	Leukotriene receptor antagonist	Montelukast	12 months and older (for asthma)
Spiriva HFA	Anticholinergic	Tiotropium bromide	Not indicated in children
Symbicort HFA	Combination (ICS + LABA)	Budesonide Formoterol fumarate dihydrate	12 years and older
Tilade CFC free	Anti-inflammatory	Nedocromil sodium	2 years and older
Ventolin HFA	SABA	Albuterol sulfate	4 years and older
Xolair	Monoclonal anti-IgE	Omalizumab	12 years and older
Xopenex HFA	SABA	Levalbuterol tartrate	4 years and older
Xopenex nebulization solution	SABA	Levalbuterol HCl	6 years and older
Zyflo	Leukotriene receptor antagonist	Zileuton	12 years and older

[a] These are current pediatric age indications by the FDA or corresponding regulatory agency if drug is available elsewhere

Pediatric indications for asthma drugs [Chang C. Asthma in Children and Adolescents: A Comprehensive Approach to Diagnosis and Management. Clinical Reviews in Allergy & Immunology. 2012 Aug;43(1-2):98–137.] *Caption from original*

- The management of an acute asthmatic in a child is not substantially different than that utilized for the adult patient.
- Inhaled anticholinergics in children should be utilized as recue medications. Early administration of steroids is effective and recommended in all cases.
- The use of chest radiographs in pediatric asthma should be reserved for infants or children who present with wheezing for the first time.
- Children are more likely to have cough-variant asthma, in which coughing is a more predominant presenting symptom than wheezing. The cough generally responds to bronchodilator therapy.

Elderly

- The elderly have high prevalence of other obstructive lung disease. The elderly may have increased sensitivity to adverse effects of β_2-agonists and inhaled corticosteroids.

Pregnancy

- Treat asthma aggressively during pregnancy. The National Asthma Education and Prevention Program Working Group Report on Managing Asthma During Pregnancy: Recommendations for Pharmacologic Treatment (2004; U.S. Department of Health and Human Services) can be found at the following link:http://www.nhlbi.nih.gov/health-pro/guidelines/archive/asthma-management-pregnancy-guidelines

Co-morbidities

- Rhinitis and rhinosinusitis management
- Allergic sensitivity and allergen exposure
- Psychological dysfunction
- Paradoxical vocal cord dysfunction
- Asymptomatic gastroesophageal reflux
- Obstructive sleep apnea
- Connective tissue disease
- Dermatologic conditions
- Immunologic and hematologic disease
- Metabolic disorders
- Obesity
- Obstructive lung disease
- Pregnancy
- Respiratory infection

Pitfalls in Diagnosis

Critical Steps Not to Miss

- Altered mental status may signal respiratory failure.
- Correct use of medications such as inhalers and nebulizers.
- Monitor peak flows to assess severity and response to treatment.

Mimics

- Sinusitis
- Myocardial ischemia
- Gastrointestinal reflux
- Congestive heart failure
- Not all wheezing in infants and young children is asthma

Time-Dependent Interventions

- Immediate initiation of inhaled β_2- adrenergic agonist.
- Nebulized treatment.
- Supplemental oxygen.
- Administration of subcutaneous epinephrine unless concerned about coronary artery disease or hypertension.
- Intubation in respiratory failure.
- Corticoteroids should be given early, as they require 4–6 hours to show benefit.

Overall Principles of Treatment

- Treatment is based on asthma severity.
- Routine monitoring of symptoms and lung function.
- Patient education is essential.
- Recognize and control trigger factors (environmental factors).
- Controlling comorbid conditions that contribute to asthma severity.
- Pharmacologic therapy.
- Reduction of personal impairment and reduction of risk.
- Preventative approach with regularly scheduled check-ups and family/patient education.
- Awareness, recognition, and treatment of these atypical asthmas is important.
- Many base their management of asthma in children upon the National Asthma Education and Prevention Program (NAEPP) Expert panel guidelines (http://www.nhlbi.nih.gov/health-pro/guidelines/current/asthma-guidelines/full-report).

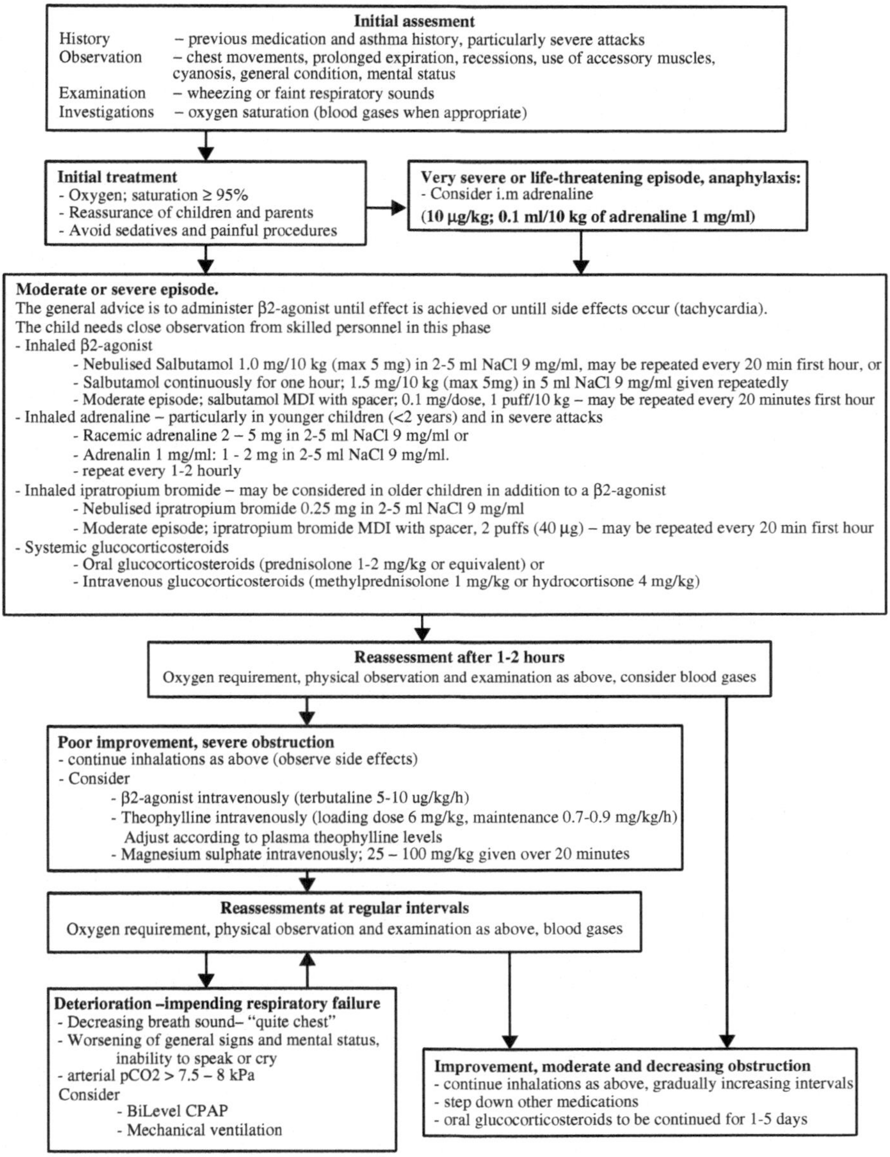

Acute exacerbation treatment: Treatment algorithm for children with moderate or severe asthma exacerbations. [From article: Emergency presentation and management of acute severe asthma in children. Scandinavian Journal of Trauma, Resuscitation and Emergency Medicine. 2009;17(1):40. https://doi.org/10.1186/1757-7241-17-40, at http://link.springer.com/article/10.1186%2F1757-7241-17-40/fulltext.html; by Knut Øymar, Thomas Halvorsen, © Øymar and Halvorsen; licensee BioMed Central Ltd.

2009; licensed under Creative Commons Attribution License BY 2.0 http://creativecommons.org/licenses/by/2.0] *Caption from original*

Disease Course

- By definition, asthma is characterized by *reversible* airflow obstruction, which means the impact of asthma on quality of life varies, from year to year, sometimes from season to season, or even day to day. There is little consensus on factors that determine disease progression versus disease stabilization.
- There is much interindividual variation is the course of asthma, and fatal exacerbations sometimes occur but are clearly unusual.
- With good control, asthmatics lead relatively normal and functional lives and have a normal lifespan. Poorer control is associated with impaired quality of life, more unscheduled healthcare visits, and more common hospitalization.

Related Evidence

Papers of particular interest have been highlighted as:
*** Of key importance*

Practice Guideline

British Thoracic Society; Scottish Intercollegiate Guidelines Network. British guideline on the management of asthma. Thorax. 2014 Nov;69 Suppl 1:1-192. PMID: 25323740. http://www.ncbi.nlm.nih.gov/pubmed/25323740 **

Lougheed MD, Leniere C, Ducharme FM, Licskai C, Dell SD, Rowe BH, FitzGerald M, Leigh R, Watson W, Boulet LP; Canadian Thoracic Society Asthma Clinical Assemby.Canadian Thoracic Society 2012 guideline update: Diagnosis and management of asthma in preschoolers, children and adults: executive summary. Can Respir J. 2012 Nov-Dec;19(6):e81-8. No abstract available. Erratum in: Can Respir J. 2013 May-Jun;20(3):185. PMID: 23248807. http://www.ncbi.nlm.nih.gov/pubmed/23248807 **

Kling S, Zar HJ, Levin ME, Green RJ, Jeena PM, Risenga SM, Thula SA, Goussard P, Gie RP; South African Childhood Asthma Working Group (SACAWG). Guideline for the management of acute asthma in children: 2013 update. S Afr Med J. 2013 Feb 5;103(3 Pt 3):199-207. https://doi.org/10.7196/samj.6658. PMID: 23656745. http://www.ncbi.nlm.nih.gov/pubmed/23656745 **

Lalloo UG, Ainslie GM, Abdool-Gaffar MS, Awotedu AA, Feldman C, Greenblatt M, Irusen EM, Mash R, Naidoo SS, O'Brien J, Otto W, Richards GA, Wong ML; South African Thoracic Society. Guideline for the management of acute asthma in adults: 2013 update. S Afr Med J. 2012 Dec 3;103(3 Pt 2):189-98. https://doi.org/10.7196/samj.6526. PMID: 23656743. http://www.ncbi.nlm.nih.gov/pubmed/236567453 **

Review

Murphy VE, Schatz M. Asthma in pregnancy: a hit for two. Eur Respir Rev. 2014 Mar 1;23(131):64-8. https://doi.org/10.1183/09059180.00008313. PMID: 24591663. http://www.ncbi.nlm.nih.gov/pubmed/24591663 **

Patadia MO, Murrill LL, Corey J. Asthma: symptoms and presentation. Otolaryngol Clin North Am. 2014 Feb;47(1):23-32. https://doi.org/10.1016/j.otc.2013.10.001. PMID: 24286676. http://www.ncbi.nlm.nih.gov/pubmed/24286676 **

Maslan J, Mims JW. What is asthma? Pathophysiology, demographics, and health care costs. Otolaryngol Clin North Am. 2014 Feb;47(1):13-22. https://doi.org/10.1016/j.otc.2013.09.010. PMID: 24286675. http://www.ncbi.nlm.nih.gov/pubmed/24286675 **

Reddy AP, Gupta MR. Management of asthma: the current US and European guidelines. Adv Exp Med Biol. 2014;795:81-103. https://doi.org/10.1007/978-1-4614-8603-9_6. PMID: 24162904. http://www.ncbi.nlm.nih.gov/pubmed/24162904 **

Shah S, Sharma G. Current clinical diagnostic tests for asthma. Adv Exp Med Biol. 2014;795:75-80. https://doi.org/10.1007/978-1-4614-8603-9_5. PMID: 24162903. http://www.ncbi.nlm.nih.gov/pubmed/24162903 **

Croisant S. Epidemiology of asthma: prevalence and burden of disease. Adv Exp Med Biol. 2014;795:17-29. https://doi.org/10.1007/978-1-4614-8603-9_2. PMID: 24162900. http://www.ncbi.nlm.nih.gov/pubmed/24162900 **

Use PubMed Clinical Queries to find the most recent evidence. Use this search strategy:
"Asthma"[Mesh] OR "Asthma"

Chapter 12
Atrial Fibrillation

Charles V. Pollack, Jr., Melissa Platt, and Victoria G. Riese

Name and Synonyms

Atrial Fibrillation (AF)

Incidence/Epidemiology

- The most common cardiac arrhythmia
  - Affects 4 % of individuals older than 60 years and 8 % of those older than 80 years.
- It is more prevalent in men, and prevalence increases with age.
- In developed countries, hypertension and coronary artery disease are the most common underlying disorders.
- Rheumatic heart disease is associated with a higher incidence of AF, but this is much less common than in the past. Other causes of mitral valve disease also may lead to AF.

C. V. Pollack, Jr. (✉)
Department of Emergency Medicine, Thomas Jefferson University, Philadelphia, PA, USA

M. Platt
Department of Emergency Medicine, University of Louisville, Louisville, KY, USA

V. G. Riese
Librarian Consultant, Eldersburg, MD, USA

C. V. Pollack, Jr. (ed.), *Differential Diagnosis of Cardiopulmonary Disease*,
https://doi.org/10.1007/978-3-319-63895-9_12

- Classified as follows:
  - Paroxysmal AF: terminates spontaneously or with intervention within 7 days of onset.
  - Persistent AF: does not terminate within 7 days.
  - Permanent AF: persists for a year or longer.
  - "Lone" AF: does not occur with any other clinical or echocardiographic cardiac problems; usually occurs in patients younger than 50.

Differential Diagnosis

- Atrial flutter
- Multifocal atrial tachycardia
- Supraventricular tachycardia

Pathophysiology and Etiology

- Instead of being coordinated, atrial contractions are irregular, disorganized, chaotic, and very rapid.
- This electrical malfunction may result in:
  - Tachypalpitations, often described by patients as a "fluttering" or "butterflies" in the chest.
  - Inadequate "topping off" of the ventricular volume prior to ventricular systole, which may result in fatigue, dizziness, or heart failure.
- Because the cardiac cycle of atrial systole followed by ventricular systole is disrupted by the lack of regularity of impulses through the atrioventricular node, the ventricles beat irregularly and often beat faster than normal.
  - This "irregularly irregular" rhythm is classified as showing a "controlled" ventricular response (rate <100 bpm) or "rapid" ventricular response (rate ≥ 100 bpm).
- The precise mechanism that causes AF is not completely understood, but AF often is seen concomitantly with other heart and metabolic diseases, including:
  - Congestive heart failure
  - Coronary artery disease
  - Valvular heart disease
  - Hypertension
  - Hyperthyroidism
- Acute alcohol abuse, especially in binges, may cause AF ("holiday heart").

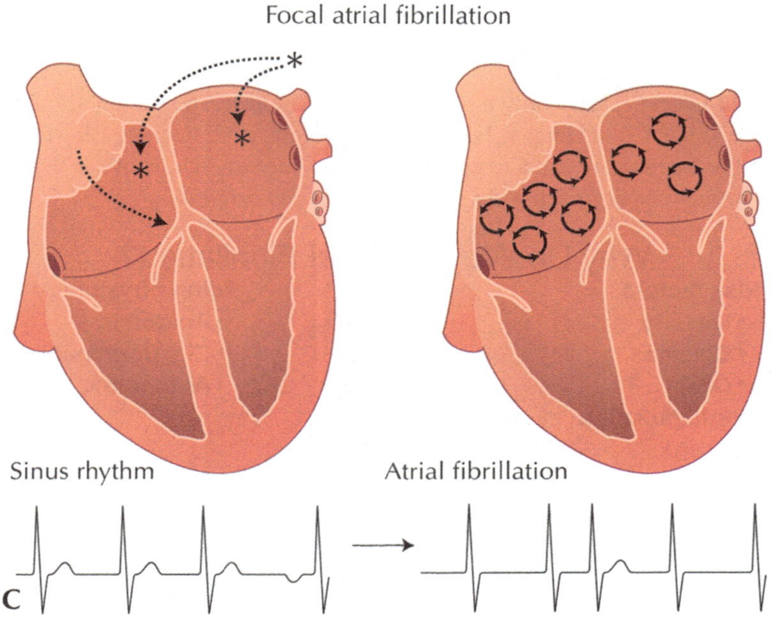

Focal atrial premature complexes usually originating from pulmonary veins can initiate AF. Ablation of these arrhythmogenic focal triggers can restore rhythm. This finding opens an exciting era in electrophysiology with the possibility of curing AF by ablation. [Grogin HR. Supraventricular tachycardia. In: Scheinman M, editor. Arrhythmias: electrophysiologic principles. Philadelphia: Current Medicine; 1996. Chapter 5 (Braunwald E, editor. Atlas of heart diseases; vol. 9).] *Caption adapted from original*

Atrial Fibrillation	
Common causes	Heart failure Hypertension Cardiac ischemia Myocardial infarction Mitral valve disease Pneumonia Hyperthyroidism Alcohol Postoperative AF
Rare causes	Cardiomyopathy Constrictive pericarditis Sick sinus syndrome Bronchial carcinoma Atrial myxoma Endocarditis Haemochromatosis Sarcoidosis

Causes of Atrial Fibrillation. [From article: Reversible atrial fibrillation secondary to a mega-oesophagus. BMC Ear Nose Throat Disord. 2006 Dec 13;6(1):15. https://doi.org/10.1186/1472-6815-6-15, at http://link.springer.com/article/10.1186%2F1472-6815-6-15; by Tahwinder Upile, Waseem Jerjes, Mohammed El Maaytah, Sandeep Singh, Colin Hopper, Jaspal Mahil, © Upile et al; licensee BioMed Central Ltd. 2006; licensed under Creative Commons Attribution License BY 2.0 http://creativecommons.org/licenses/by/2.0] *Caption from original*

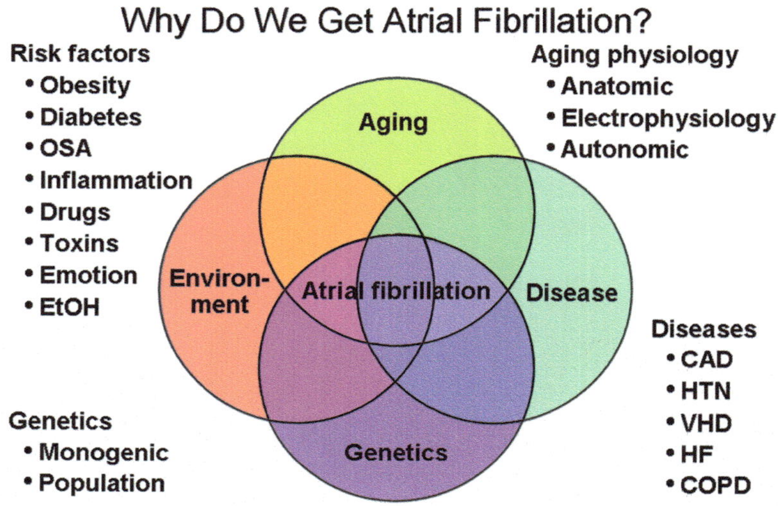

Atrial fibrillation is a multifactorial condition resulting from an interaction between cardiovascular disease effects, aging, genetics, and environmental factors. *CAD* coronary artery disease, *COPD* chronic obstructive pulmonary disease, *EtOH* alcohol use, *HF* heart failure, *HTN* hypertension, *OSA* obstructive sleep apnea, *VHD* valvular heart disease [Eleid MF, Cha Y-M, Shen W-K. Atrial fibrillation and heart failure: rate versus rhythm control. In: Bartunek J, Vanderheyden M, editors. Translational approach to heart failure [Internet]. New York: Springer; 2013 [cited 2015 Aug 13]. p. 129–44. Available from: http://link.springer.com/10.1007/978-1-4614-7345-9_6] *Caption from original*

Presentation

Typical/"Classic"

- Not all patients with AF have symptoms, but the risk of thromboembolic complications is the same, regardless.

- Typical symptoms include palpitations, tachycardia, fatigue, weakness, dizziness, lightheadedness, reduced exercise capacity, and dyspnea.

Atypical

- The first presentation of AF may be a thromboembolic complication, such as stroke or mesenteric ischemia.
- AF may present as anginal pain.
- Some patients, particularly those who are elderly, may not notice the palpitations (particularly if the ventricular rate is less than 100 bpm) and may present with completely unrelated complaints.

Primary Differential Considerations

- Atrial flutter
- Multifocal atrial tachycardia
- Supraventricular tachycardia
- Premature atrial contractions
- Premature ventricular contractions

History and Physical Exam

Findings That Confirm Diagnosis

- Although an "irregularly irregular" pulse is suggestive of AF, this also may be associated with other arrhythmias, and an ECG is required to differentiate among them.

Factors That Suggest Diagnosis

- Irregularly irregular pulse on examination
- Palpitations plus dyspnea
- Palpitations plus syncope or near-syncope
- Palpitations and generalized weakness
- Palpitations and hypotension
- Unexplained dyspnea, syncope, generalized weakness, or hypotension
- Acute ischemic stroke

Factors That Exclude Diagnosis

- ECG showing a normal sinus rhythm excludes AF "in the moment," but does not exclude paroxysmal AF.

Ancillary Studies

Laboratory

- Often obtained in search for underlying disorders or other associated disorders:
  - B-type natriuretic peptide (BNP)
  - Troponin
  - Electrolytes
  - Blood glucose
  - Thyroid-stimulating hormone (TSH)
  - Toxicology

Electrocardiography

- ECG is necessary to make the diagnosis.
- Irregular rate with an atrial rate greater than 300 bpm
- Ventricular rate may be slow, normal, or fast.
- Absent or erratic P waves are noted.
- PR interval is absent.
- QRS may be normal but may be widened if conduction delay is present.

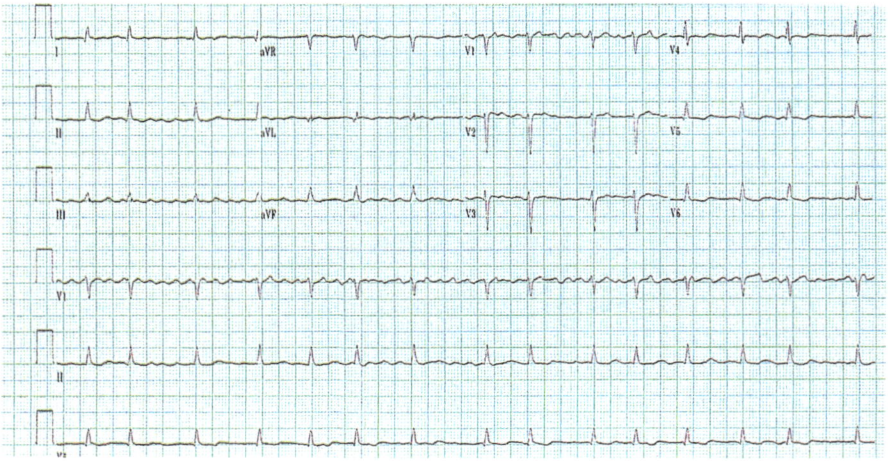

Atrial fibrillation. Atrial fibrillation is characterized by the absence of P waves, which are replaced by irregular f waves or no sign of atrial activity. The QRS complexes may be normal or irregular and varying in amplitude. The 12-lead ECG shown here demonstrates atrial fibrillation with moderate ventricular response rate. [Leung J. Electrocardiographic monitoring. In: Lichtor JL, editor. Preoperative preparation and intraoperative monitoring. Philadelphia: Current Medicine; 1997. Chapter 7. (Miller RD, editor. Atlas of anesthesia; vol. 3).] *Caption from original*

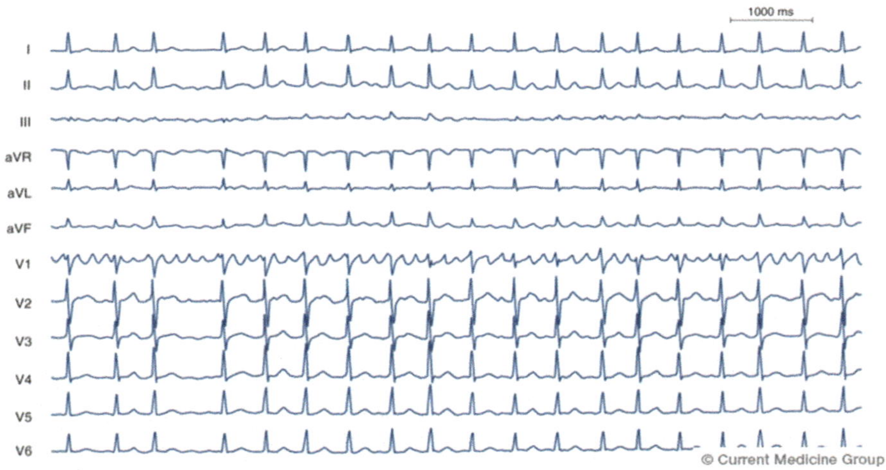

Atrial fibrillation (AF) 12-lead surface electrocardiogram. AF is the most common sustained arrhythmia and is particularly prevalent in the elderly. Characteristic of AF is an irregular ventricular response and rapid irregular oscillations or fibrillatory waves that vary in shape, amplitude, and timing. [Epstein L, Stevenson W, Steven D, Seiler J, Roberts-Thomson K, See V. Arrhythmias. In: Libby P, editor. Essential atlas of cardiovascular disease. 4th ed. Philadelphia: Current Medicine; 2009. Chapter 7.] *Caption from original*

Imaging

- Transthoracic echocardiography may be performed to evaluate the size of the right and left atria and size and function of the right and left ventricles; this also can detect valvular heart disease.
- Transesophageal echocardiography is used to identify thrombi in the left atrium or left atrial appendage.

Special Populations

Age

- Incidence of AF increases with advancing age.
- "Lone AF" more common below age 50.

Co-morbidities

- As under "Pathophysiology and Etiology," a host of other cardiac and metabolic disorders are frequent co-morbidities in patients with AF.
- Binge alcohol consumption predisposes to "holiday heart."

Pitfalls in Diagnosis

Critical Steps Not to Miss

- Complications such as blood clot formation, strokes, and heart failure may arise, but rhythm conversion reduces the chances that such complications will develop.

Mimics

- Atrial flutter
- Multifocal atrial tachycardia
- Supraventricular tachycardia

Time-Dependent Interventions

- Patients may have potentially life-threatening symptoms that need immediate intervention with electrical cardioversion, including decompensated congestive heart failure, hypotension, angina, or cardiac ischemia.

Overall Principles of Treatment

- The initial focus of AF management is rate control to minimize any perfusion stress on the ventricles.
  - The usual approach is with titrated doses of calcium channel blockers or beta-blockers.
- Once rate is controlled (or if patient presents with a controlled ventricular rate), consideration is given to converting the rhythm out of AF back into a sinus rhythm.
  - This may be approached pharmacologically with a variety of potential drugs, such as ibutilide or procainamide, or electrically via synchronized cardioversion.
- If the patient has been in AF for 24 to 48 hours or longer, anticoagulation therapy should be provided before attempting cardioversion, as clots that may have formed in the fibrillating atria or atrial appendage may dislodge and embolize when normal atrial electrical activity is restored. Therapy may be provided acutely with parenteral agents such as unfractionated or low-molecular weight heparin or with fast-acting non-warfarin oral anticoagulants (dabigatran, rivaroxaban, apixaban, edoxaban)
  - Alternatively, cardioversion may be attempted after transesophageal echocardiography that excludes atrial clots
  - Likelihood of stroke or systemic embolization may be assessed with CHA2DS2-VASc score

Risk factor	**Points**
Age over 75 years	1
Previous stroke/TIA	2
Hypertension	1
Symptoms or signs of LV dysfunction	1
Diabetes mellitus	1

CHADS$_2$VASC score points for prediction of stroke in atrial fibrillation. (Data from Gage BF, Waterman AD, Shannon W, Boechler M, Rich MW, Radford MJ. Validation of Clinical Classification Schemes for Predicting Stroke: Results From the National Registry of Atrial Fibrillation. JAMA.2001;285(22):2864-2870. https://doi.org/10.1001/jama.285.22.2864.) [Table from Verheugt FWA. The new oral anticoagulants. Netherlands Heart Journal. 2010 Jun;18(6):314–8.] *Caption adapted from original*

- Patients whose AF is resistant to cardioversion or recurs after initially successful cardioversion may be referred to electrophysiology, where the possibility of catheter ablation of the electrical source of the AF can be addressed definitively and specifically.
  - Success rates usually exceed 65–75 %

Disease Course

- The most feared complication of AF is thromboembolism to a critical vascular bed—especially stroke.
- The palpitations of AF may have a very adverse effect on quality of life. They may be symptomatic even in patients with controlled ventricular response.
- Patients with diminished pump function are particularly sensitive to the absence of consistent ventricular filling (the missing "atrial kick") and may experience persistent easy fatigability and even angina.
- Longstanding AF increases mortality.

Related Evidence

Papers of particular importance have been highlighted as:
*** Of key importance*

Practice Guideline

January CT, Wann LS, Alpert JS, Calkins H, Cigarroa JE, Cleveland JC Jr, Conti JB, Ellinor PT, Ezekowitz MD, Field ME, Murray KT, Sacco RL, Stevenson WG, Tchou PJ, Tracy CM, Yancy CW; American College of Cardiology/American Heart Association Task Force on Practice Guidelines. 2014 AHA/ACC/HRS guideline for the management of patients with atrial fibrillation: a report of the American College of Cardiology/American Heart Association Task Force on Practice Guidelines and the Heart Rhythm Society. J Am Coll Cardiol. 2014 Dec 2;64(21):e1-76. https://doi.org/10.1016/j.jacc.2014.03.022. PMID: 24685669. http://www.ncbi.nlm.nih.gov/pubmed/24685669 **

Verma A, Cairns JA, Mitchell LB, Macle L, Stiell IG, Gladstone D, McMurtry MS, Connolly S, Cox JL, Dorian P, Ivers N, Leblanc K, Nattel S, Healey JS; CCS Atrial Fibrillation Guidelines Committee. 2014 focused update of the Canadian Cardiovascular Society Guidelines for the management of atrial fibrillation. Can J Cardiol. 2014 Oct;30(10):1114-30. https://doi.org/10.1016/j.cjca.2014.08.001. PMID: 25262857. http://www.ncbi.nlm.nih.gov/pubmed/25262857 **

Steinberg BA, Beckley PD, Deering TF, Clark CL, Amin AN, Bauer KA, Cryer B, Mansour M, Scheiman JM, Zenati MA, Newby LK, Peacock WF, Bhatt DL; Society of Cardiovascular Patient Care. Evaluation and management of the atrial fibrillation patient: a report from the Society of Cardiovascular Patient Care. Crit Pathw Cardiol. 2013 Sep;12(3):107-15. https://doi.org/10.1097/HPC.0b013e31829834ed. PMID: 23892939. http://www.ncbi.nlm.nih.gov/pubmed/23892939 **

Frendl G, Sodickson AC, Chung MK, Waldo AL, Gersh BJ, Tisdale JE, Calkins H, Aranki S, Kaneko T, Cassivi S, Smith SC Jr, Darbar D, Wee JO, Waddell TK, Amar D, Adler D; American Association for Thoracic Surgery. 2014 AATS guidelines for the prevention and management of perioperative atrial fibrillation and flutter for thoracic surgical procedures. J Thorac Cardiovasc Surg. 2014 Sep;148(3):e153-93. https://doi.org/10.1016/j.jtcvs.2014.06.036. PMID: 25129609. http://www.ncbi.nlm.nih.gov/pubmed/25129609**

Review

Zoni-Berisso M, Lercari F, Carazza T, Domenicucci S. Epidemiology of atrial fibrillation: European perspective. Clin Epidemiol. 2014 Jun 16;6:213-20. https://doi.org/10.2147/CLEP.S47385. PMID: 24966695. http://www.ncbi.nlm.nih.gov/pubmed/24966695**

Ball J, Carrington MJ, McMurray JJ, Stewart S. Atrial fibrillation: profile and burden of an evolving epidemic in the 21st century. Int J Cardiol. 2013 Sep 1; 167(5):1807-24. https://doi.org/10.1016/j.ijcard.2012.12.093. PMID: 23380698. http://www.ncbi.nlm.nih.gov/pubmed/23380698

Hu YF, Chen YJ, Lin YJ, Chen SA. Inflammation and the pathogenesis of atrial fibrillation. Nat Rev Cardiol. 2015 Jan 27. https://doi.org/10.1038/nrcardio.2015.2.PMID:25622848.http://www.ncbi.nlm.nih.gov/pubmed/25622848**

Mohmand-Borkowski A, Tang WH. Atrial fibrillation as manifestation and consequence of underlying cardiomyopathies: from common conditions to genetic diseases. Heart Fail Rev. 2014 May;19(3):295-304. https://doi.org/10.1007/s10741-014-9424-0. PMID: 24531802. http://www.ncbi.nlm.nih.gov/pubmed/24531802**

Longobardo L, Todaro MC, Zito C, Piccione MC, Di Bella G, Oreto L, Khandheria BK, Carerj S. Role of imaging in assessment of atrial fibrosis in patients with atrial fibrillation: state-of-the-art review. Eur Heart J Cardiovasc Imaging. 2014 Jan;15(1):1-5. https://doi.org/10.1093/ehjci/jet116. PMID: 23798579. http://www.ncbi.nlm.nih.gov/pubmed/23798579**

Chapa DW, Akintade B, Thomas SA, Friedmann E. Gender differences in stroke, mortality, and hospitalization among patients with atrial fibrillation: A systematic review. Heart Lung. 2015 Feb 19. pii: S0147-9563(15)00009-6. https://doi.org/10.1016/j.hrtlng.2015.01.008. PMID: 25703992. http://www.ncbi.nlm.nih.gov/pubmed/25703992**

Vergara P, Della Bella P. Management of atrial fibrillation. F1000Prime Rep. 2014 Apr 1;6:22. https://doi.org/10.12703/P6-22. PMID: 24765527. http://www.ncbi.nlm.nih.gov/pubmed/24765527**

Use PubMed Clinical Queries to find the most recent evidence. Use this search strategy: "Atrial Fibrillation"[Mesh] OR "Atrial Fibrillation"

Chapter 13
Bradyarrhythmias

Christopher J. Rees, Richard M. Cantor, Charles V. Pollack, Jr., and Victoria G. Riese

Name and Synonyms

Bradyarrhythmias

- Bradycardia

Incidence/Epidemiology

- The bradyarrhythmias encompass a broad range of disorders; therefore, their incidence varies widely.
- Sinus bradycardia may be normal in up to 35 % of people younger than 25 years. It also may be normal in well-conditioned athletes at most ages.
- Sick sinus syndrome becomes more common as people age, with more than 50 % of cases occurring in people over 50, but it may occur at any age.

C. J. Rees
Emergency Department, Pennsylvania Hospital, Philadelphia, PA, USA

R. M. Cantor
Department of Emergency Medicine and Pediatrics, State University of New York Upstate Medical University, Syracuse, NY, USA

C. V. Pollack, Jr. (✉)
Department of Emergency Medicine, Thomas Jefferson University, Philadelphia, PA, USA

V. G. Riese
Librarian Consultant, Eldersburg, MD, USA

C. V. Pollack, Jr. (ed.), *Differential Diagnosis of Cardiopulmonary Disease*,
https://doi.org/10.1007/978-3-319-63895-9_13

Differential Diagnosis

- Clinically significant bradycardias may cause a wide range of symptoms, the most common of which are syncope, presyncope, chest pain, general fatigue, dyspnea on exertion, and dyspnea at rest. As such, the differential is broad and far ranging.
- Bradycardias also have a broad range of causes; therefore, the differential diagnosis of the bradycardia itself also is extensive.

Pathophysiology and Etiology

- Bradycardia is defined as a heart rate below 60 bpm.
- Bradycardia generally is caused by two different mechanisms:
  - Slowing, blocking, or failure of impulse generation in the sinus node
  - Block in the conduction system from the atrioventricular (AV) node down through the His–Purkinje system.
- Many different processes may lead to these mechanisms, including intrinsic conduction system disease, other heart diseases, other systemic diseases, and drugs, to name a few.
- When these blocks occur, alternative pacemakers within the heart take over the pacemaker function. Other conduction tissue, or even myocytes, may act as alternative pacemakers. In general, the higher within the conduction system the impulse originates, the faster the rate; if the impulse is generated within or above the bundle of His, the rate generally is enough to maintain adequate cardiac output. This association also may be used as a clue to the location of the block based on the escape rate.
- Although slow heart rates can occur with junctional or ventricular pacemakers, the bradyarrhythmias usually are classified according to the location of the block: either sinoatrial (SA) node dysfunction or AV node dysfunction.
- Sinus node dysfunction:
  - Sinus bradycardia: defined as a sinus node rate less than 60 impulses per minute.
    - An ECG will show normal sinus P waves and a fixed P-P interval that is equal to the R-R interval, with 1:1 AV conduction.
    - It may be physiologic and normal in well-conditioned athletes, in young people, and during sleep.
    - It may be secondary to excess vagal stimulation, which may even occur as a result of a necktie that is too tight.
    - Medications are a common cause, especially beta-blockers, calcium channel blockers, digoxin, and opioids.
    - It also (although less commonly) may be pathologic. Sinus bradycardia may be seen in the setting of acute inferior myocardial infarction (MI), increased intracranial pressure, carotid sinus hypersensitivity, and profound hypothyroidism.

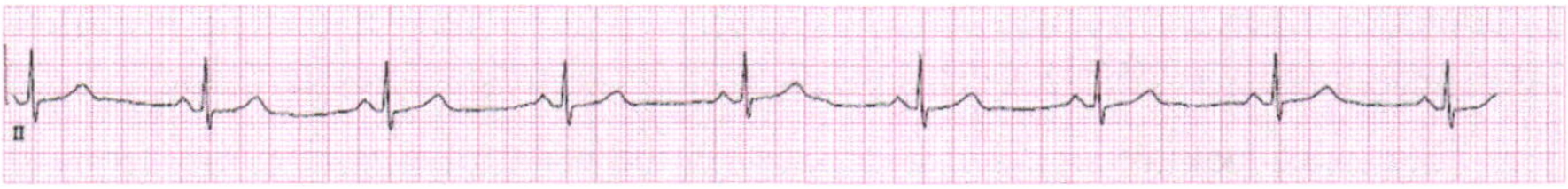

Sinus bradycardia. No other abnormalities noted here except for sinus bradycardia at 50 bpm. [Almasry IO. Evidenced-based approach to bradyarrhythmias. In: Stergiopoulos K, Brown DL, editors. Evidence-based cardiology consult [Internet]. London: Springer; 2014 [cited 2015 May 22]. p. 105–18. Available from: http://link.springer.com/10.1007/978-1-4471-4441-0_9] *Caption adapted from original*

- Sinus arrhythmia (sinus dysrhythmia): similar to sinus bradycardia except for the presence of a variable P-P interval, leading to a slightly irregular rhythm. This is a normal variant and not pathologic. It is common in children and young adults. In the most common situation, the sinus node rate increases with inspiration and decreases during expiration because of the changes in vagal tone with breathing.

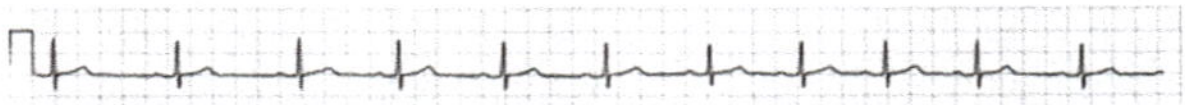

Sinus arrhythmia. Rhythmic variation in the sinus rate is noted across the rhythm strip. P-wave morphology and PR intervals remain essentially unchanged. [Foreman B. Common atrial and ventricular arrhythmias. In: Toth PP, Cannon CP, editors. Comprehensive cardiovascular medicine in the primary care setting [Internet]. Totowa, NJ: Humana Press; 2011 [cited 2015 May 22]. p. 459–96. Available from: http://link.springer.com/10.1007/978-1-60327-963-5_24] *Caption from original*

- Sinus arrest (sinus pause). In sinus arrest, the SA node fails to generate an impulse. It is recognized as a pause in the sinus rhythm. During the pause/arrest, no P waves are seen on the ECG. The P-P interval of the two complexes surrounding the pause will not be a multiple of the usual P-P interval, as would be the case if the pause were from an SA exit block. If the pause lasts long enough, there may be an escape beat from somewhere else along the conduction system or the ventricles. This may be a normal variant, but it also occurs in acute MI, intrinsic SA node disease, digitalis toxicity, stroke, and excessive vagal stimulation. Notably, frequent and prolonged sinus pauses may be seen in up to 30 % of patients with obstructive sleep apnea.

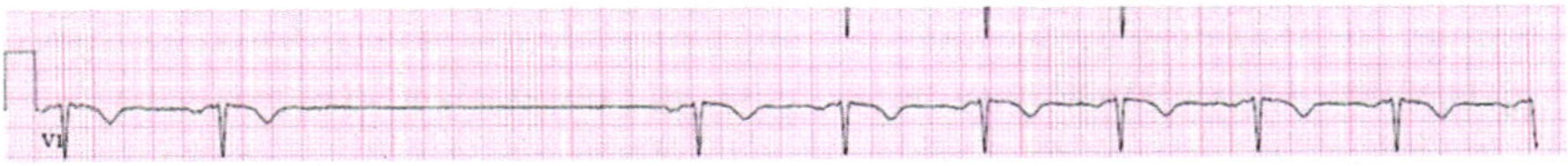

Sinus arrest. Note sudden cessation of sinus impulse for 3 s prior to resumption of normal sinus rhythm. [Almasry IO. Evidenced-based approach to bradyarrhythmias. In: Stergiopoulos K, Brown DL, editors. Evidence-based cardiology consult [Internet].

London: Springer; 2014 [cited 2015 May 22]. p. 105–18. Available from: http://link.springer.com/10.1007/978-1-4471-4441-0_9] *Caption adapted from original*

- SA exit block: recognized as a pause in the usual rhythm resulting from the absence of a normally expected P wave, usually because of blocked or slowed impulse generation within the SA node. The P-P interval of the two complexes surrounding the pause will have a P-P interval that is a multiple of the usual P-P interval. SA exit block may be subclassified as first degree; second degree, types I and II; and third degree. These usually are difficult, if not impossible, to see on a surface ECG and require electrophysiologic mapping of the sinus node discharge. These blocks may be seen following acute MI, acute rheumatic fever, and myocarditis, and secondary to drugs such as beta-blockers, calcium channel blockers, digoxin, quinidine, and salicylates. They also may be seen in well-conditioned athletes or secondary to excessive vagal stimulation. They usually are transient and not clinically significant.

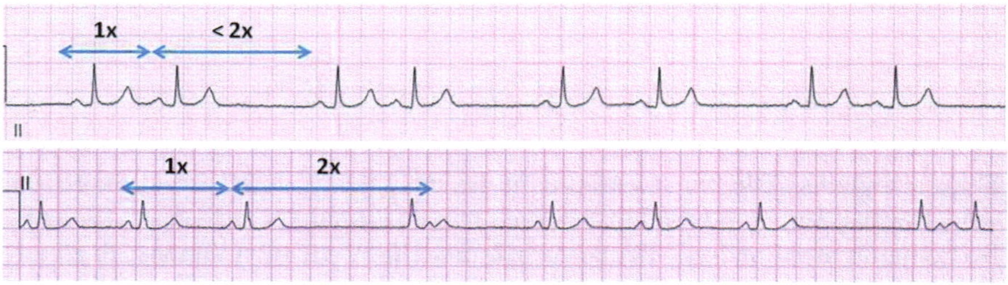

Top panel: Type I second-degree sinoatrial exit block. Note the pause that is less than two times the PP interval. Also note the group beating consistent with Wenckebach periodicity. Bottom panel: Type II second-degree sinoatrial exit block. The pause here is two times the PP interval, with the occurrence of a junctional beat prior to the return of a sinus P wave which is followed by unperturbed sinus mechanism before there is another recurrence. [Almasry IO. Evidenced-based approach to bradyarrhythmias. In: Stergiopoulos K, Brown DL, editors. Evidence-based cardiology consult [Internet]. London: Springer; 2014 [cited 2015 May 22]. p. 105–18. Available from: http://link.springer.com/10.1007/978-1-4471-4441-0_9] *Caption from original*

- Sick sinus syndrome (tachycardia–bradycardia syndrome/tachy–brady syndrome): a mixed group of disorders marked by abnormalities of supraventricular impulse formation and conduction that are associated with both tachy- and bradyarrhythmias. It usually is the result of intrinsic disease of the sinus node or the surrounding tissue, sometimes with associated AV nodal disease. The tachyarrhythmias usually are either atrial fibrillation or atrial flutter, and the bradyarrhythmias usually are marked sinus bradycardia, prolonged sinus arrest, and SA block associated with abnormal AV conduction leading to inadequate escape rhythms. On prolonged rhythm monitoring, it is typical to see long periods of tachycardia followed by profound bradycardia upon the spontaneous termination of the tachycardia. It is most common in the elderly as a result of fibrotic degeneration of conduction tissue. It also may be seen in cardiomyopathies, in connective tissue diseases, and with the use of some medications. It usually is suspected in elderly patients who present with syncope and is an indication for a permanent pacemaker.

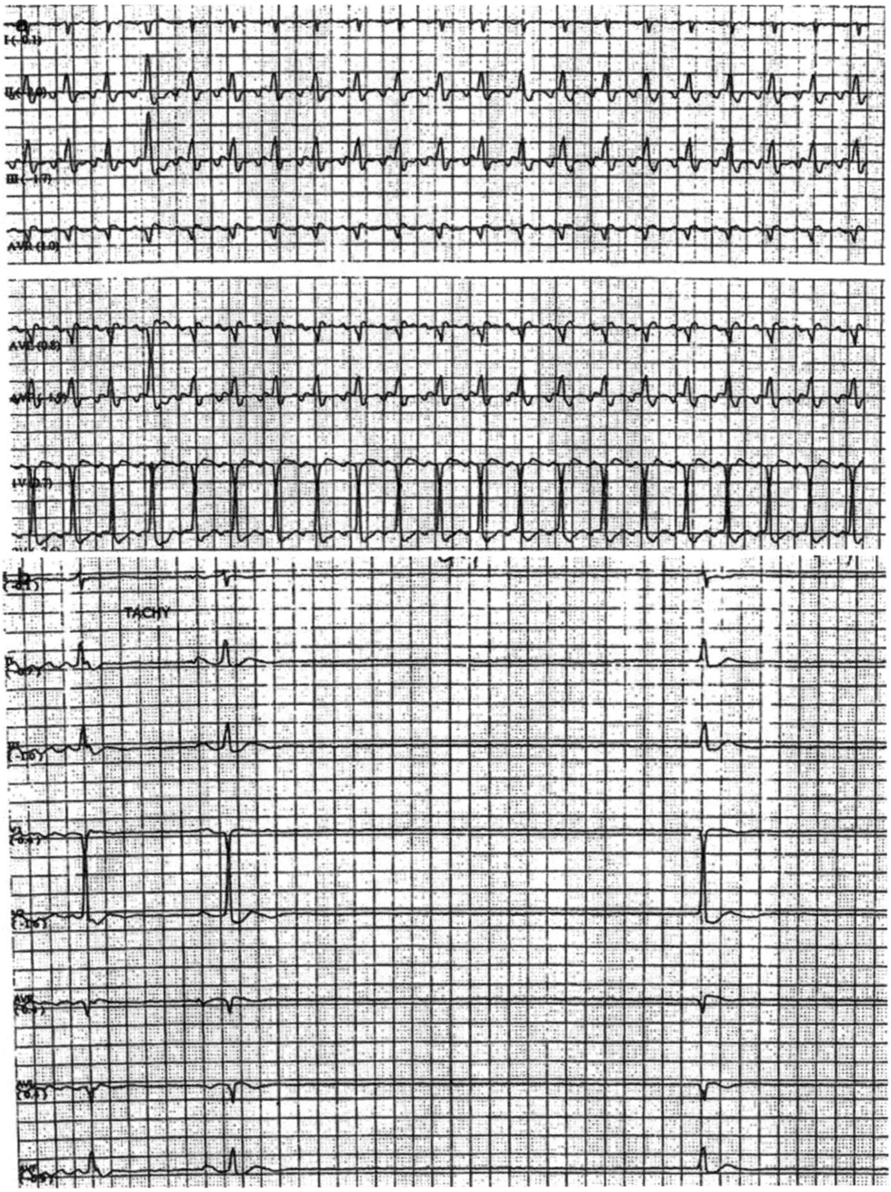

(a) Twelve-lead electrocardiogram of an 84-year-old female who presented with altered mental status. Atrial flutter with 2:1 A:V conduction is seen. (b) 12-lead electrocardiogram showing flutter termination. A 4.9-s period of asystole is noted before ventricular activity resumes. The patient had multiple sinus pauses during sinus rhythm. These rhythms are typical of Tachy–Brady syndrome and are characteristic of sick sinus syndrome [El Hage L, Badhwar N, Goldschlager N. Top ten electrocardiographic (ECG) abnormalities not to miss. In: Stergiopoulos K, Brown DL, editors. Evidence-based cardiology consult [Internet]. London: Springer; 2014 [cited 2015 May 22]. p. 133–48. Available from: http://link.springer.com/10.1007/978-1-4471-4441-0_11] *Caption from original*

- Chronotropic incompetence: failure of the heart rate to increase appropriately with exercise
- Junctional rhythms. Under typical conditions, the sinus node impulses suppress (by nature of being faster) impulse generation distally along the conduction tree. If the sinus impulse is suppressed or blocked, the AV node may take over the pacemaker function. This is termed a junctional or junctional escape rhythm. The AV node naturally discharges at a rate of 40–60 bpm, which usually is enough to maintain cardiac output and blood pressure. As the impulse is generated in the AV node, the QRS complex will be narrow, but because the sinus impulses are blocked, there will be no P waves. Junctional rhythms may be seen after acute inferior MI and in congestive heart failure, myocarditis, hypokalemia, and digoxin toxicity.

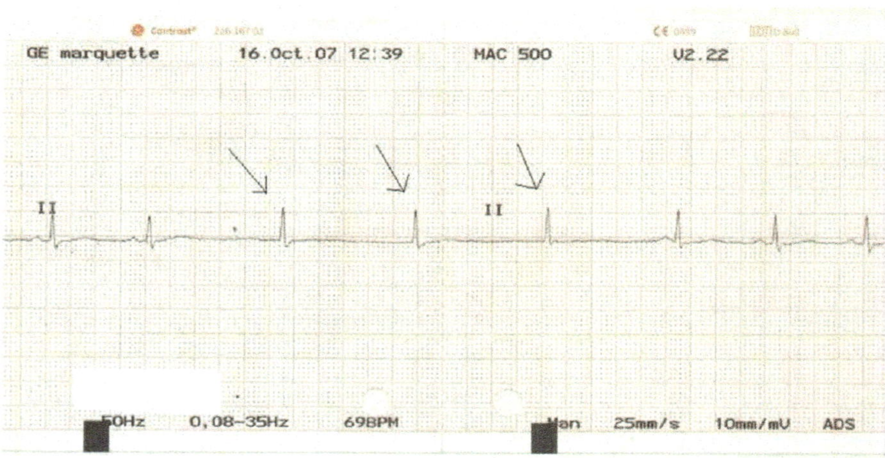

ECG shows transient sinus arrest with escape junctional rhythm. *Arrow* indicates escape junctional rhythm [Bhaskar EM, Moorthy S, Ganeshwala G, Abraham G. Cardiac conduction disturbance due to prallethrin (pyrethroid) poisoning. J Med Toxicol. 2010 Mar;6(1):27–30.] *Caption from original*

- AV node dysfunction
  - AV block is caused by either delayed or blocked conduction of impulses between the atria and the ventricles.

- AV block is classified into first-degree, second-degree (of which there are two types), and third-degree AV block (also referred to as complete heart block).
- First-degree AV block is defined as a P-R interval greater than 0.20 sec on an ECG. This indicates delayed conduction through the AV node, but all impulses are conducted to the ventricles. It may be a normal variant and generally portends no increased risk of further conduction disease or heart disease. It may be associated with increased vagal tone, digoxin toxicity, acute inferior MI, or myocarditis. When there is an underlying cause, the block usually is transient.

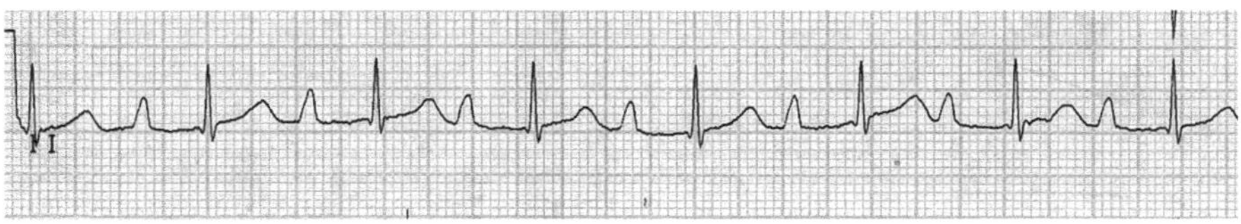

First-degree AV block [Mendoza A, Belda S, Salguero R, Granados MA. Congenital complete atrioventricular block associated with QT prolongation: description of a patient with an unusual outcome. Pediatr Cardiol. 2010 Aug;31(6):887–90.] *Caption from original*

- Second-degree AV block is marked by the failure of some sinus impulses to reach the ventricles. On an ECG, some P waves are seen without an associated QRS complex. There are two types: type I (also called Mobitz I or Wenckebach) and type II (Mobitz II).
  - Type I second-degree, Mobitz I AV (Wenckebach) block: There is progressive prolongation of AV conduction (noted as progressive lengthening of the P-R interval) until the atrial impulse is completely blocked and a QRS complex is dropped. The conduction ratio is the ratio of atrial impulses to those that are conducted into the ventricles, i.e., a 4:3 conduction ratio means that three of every four atrial impulses are conducted into the ventricles. In other words, there is a dropped QRS complex after every three sinus beats, so for four P waves, there are only three QRS complexes. This ratio usually is stable for any given patient, but some patients can manifest changing (variable) ratios of block. This block occurs at the level of the AV node. This type of block does not carry an increased risk of progression to third-degree heart block. It usually is transient, reversible, and asymptomatic. It may be seen during acute inferior MI, with myocarditis, with digoxin toxicity, and after cardiothoracic surgery.

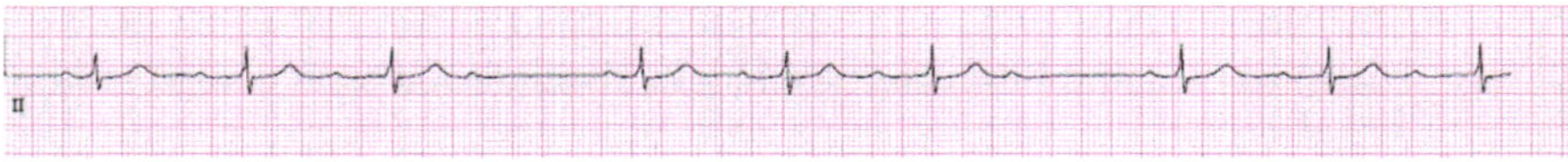

Mobitz type I (Wenckebach) Second-Degree AV block. Notice the classic form of Wenckebach in a 4:3 pattern. The PP intervals are fixed, with lengthening of each successive PR interval with progressively decreasing increments and shorter RR intervals prior to the dropped beat. The pause is less than a multiple of the shortest RR interval, the return-cycle PR interval is shorter than the PR interval prior to the dropped beat, and there is obvious group beating periodicity. [Almasry IO. Evidenced-based approach to bradyarrhythmias. In: Stergiopoulos K, Brown DL, editors. Evidence-based cardiology consult [Internet]. London: Springer; 2014 [cited 2015 May 22]. p. 105–18. Available from: http://link.springer.com/10.1007/978-1-4471-4441-0_9] *Caption from original*

- Second-degree, Mobitz II AV block: The P-R interval is constant, and there are nonconducted impulses. As with Mobitz I block, there usually is a constant conduction ratio, but it may be variable. When the conduction ratio is 2:1, it is impossible to tell the difference between Mobitz I and Mobitz II heart block, as progressive P-R prolongation cannot be appreciated. This level of block usually occurs below the AV node (infranodal). If the escape pacemaker is high enough in the conduction system, the QRS complexes may still be narrow, but if the pacemaker is lower, the QRS complexes may be wide. This type of heart block almost always indicates some structural damage to the conduction system and usually is permanent. It carries a high risk of progression to third-degree heart block, especially if it occurs in the setting of an acute anterior MI.

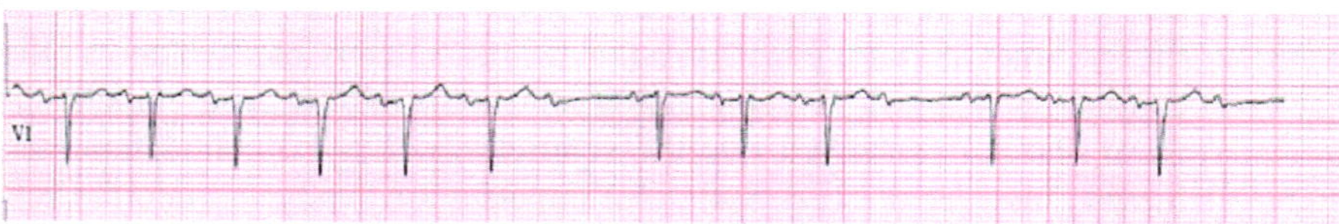

Mobitz type II second-degree AV block. Note that there is ongoing sinus rhythm with a fixed PP interval before there is a sudden failure of conduction to the ventricles demonstrated by a dropped QRS. Note that there is no change in the PR interval preceding and following the dropped QRS, and this recurs later in the strip. The resultant pause is exactly twice the PP interval. Note the narrow QRS in this example that may suggest a nodal site of conduction block. [Almasry IO. Evidenced-based approach to bradyarrhythmias. In: Stergiopoulos K, Brown DL, editors. Evidence-based cardiology consult [Internet]. London: Springer; 2014 [cited 2015 May 22]. p. 105–18. Available from: http://link.springer.com/10.1007/978-1-4471-4441-0_9] *Caption adapted from original*

- Third-degree heart block (complete heart block): All conduction between the atria and ventricles is blocked. This block is seen on an ECG as the absence of a relationship between the P waves and the QRS complexes; therefore, it also is called *AV dissociation*. The atrial rate must be greater than the escape pacemaker rate for this lack of a relationship to be appreciated. If the rates are similar, it may be difficult to determine that there is no relationship between the P waves and QRS complexes (isorhythmic dissociation). A ventricular rate greater than the atrial rate precludes the diagnosis of third-degree heart block. AV dissociation with a ventricular rate greater than the atrial rate may be seen in some accelerated junctional rhythms, as well as in ventricular tachycardia. If the escape pacemaker is within the AV node (nodal), the escape rate is usually 40 to 60 bpm, with narrow QRS complexes. If the escape pacemaker is infranodal, the escape rate may be less than 40 bpm, in which case the QRS complex usually is widened. Nodal complete heart block may be transient, especially in the setting of an acute inferior MI. Infranodal complete heart block usually is permanent and the result of intrinsic conduction system disease, acute ischemia, drugs, or, rarely, Lyme disease.

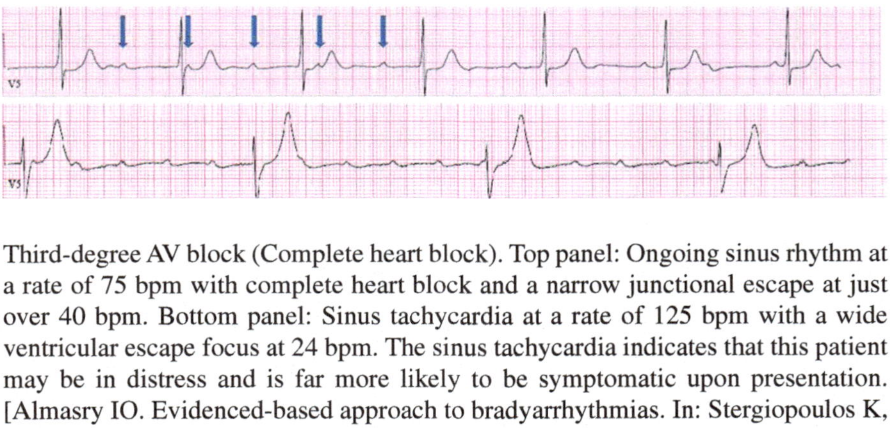

Third-degree AV block (Complete heart block). Top panel: Ongoing sinus rhythm at a rate of 75 bpm with complete heart block and a narrow junctional escape at just over 40 bpm. Bottom panel: Sinus tachycardia at a rate of 125 bpm with a wide ventricular escape focus at 24 bpm. The sinus tachycardia indicates that this patient may be in distress and is far more likely to be symptomatic upon presentation. [Almasry IO. Evidenced-based approach to bradyarrhythmias. In: Stergiopoulos K, Brown DL, editors. Evidence-based cardiology consult [Internet]. London: Springer; 2014 [cited 2015 May 22]. p. 105–18. Available from: http://link.springer.com/10.1007/978-1-4471-4441-0_9] *Caption adapted from original*

Presentation

Typical/"Classic"

- Bradyarrhythmias often are asymptomatic and sometimes are found on routine evaluation or for evaluation of other complaints. This is especially true for sinus bradycardia, sinus arrhythmia, sinus block, first-degree AV block, and type I second-degree AV (Wenckebach) block. Sinus bradycardia, sinus arrhythmia, and first-degree AV block may be normal variants. It is a common situation to find one of these abnormalities on an ECG performed for other reasons, such as preoperative clearance in an otherwise healthy person.

- These dysrhythmias also may be associated with other, more serious concerns (e.g., an acute MI or drug overdose or intoxication), and the symptoms of these disorders may predominate in the clinical presentation. In these situations, it often is difficult to discern whether the symptoms are being caused by the primary event or the dysrhythmia. However, these dysrhythmias often are transient and resolve spontaneously or with appropriate treatment of the primary event.
- Patients who have symptoms from their bradyarrhythmias often have vague and nonspecific complaints, such as fatigue, exercise intolerance, shortness of breath (especially on exertion), and feeling generally unwell.
- Most significantly, these dysrhythmias may present acutely with syncope, near-syncope, chest pain, acute dyspnea, and other signs of systemic hypoperfusion (change in mental status, hypotension, cyanosis, i.e., shock state). These presentations are much more likely with heart rates of 40 bpm or less, as well as with greater levels of block.
- Sick sinus syndrome often presents as syncope or near-syncope in elderly patients. Sometimes, however, symptoms from the tachycardia predominate, and the patient will present with palpitations and chest heaviness/pain, followed by syncope, presyncope, or generalized fatigue.

Atypical

- Because there is no "typical" presentation for bradyarrhythmias, almost all presentations are atypical.

Primary Differential Considerations

- Bradycardia is a self-evident diagnosis based on a heart rate less than 50 bpm. The differential diagnosis of *causes* of bradyarrhythmias is broad and includes:
    - Heart blocks or slow atrial fibrillation
    - Primary cardiac causes such as MI with cardiogenic shock
    - Metabolic causes such as hyperkalemia
    - Neurologic causes such as increased intracranial pressure or spinal cord injury
    - Drug toxicity (calcium channel blockers, beta-blockers, digitalis, clonidine)
    - Infections such as myocarditis, rheumatic fever, or Lyme disease
    - Malfunctioning pacemaker

History and Physical Exam

Findings That Confirm Diagnosis

- The diagnosis is considered by finding a slow pulse rate on physical exam, then confirmed by finding a bradyarrhythmia on a 12-lead ECG and/or continuous cardiac monitoring.

Factors That Suggest Diagnosis

- The diagnosis may be suggested in patients presenting with the symptoms reviewed above (syncope, near-syncope, fatigue, exercise intolerance, chest pain or heaviness, palpitations).
- Patients with any of the aforementioned symptoms should undergo 12-lead ECG and may need further, more prolonged cardiac monitoring if the ECG does not secure the diagnosis.

Factors That Exclude Diagnosis

- Because many of these arrhythmias may be both transient and intermittent, they are all difficult to exclude, and the patient may require reassessments over time for complete exclusion. Patients also may require extended cardiac monitoring and/or electrophysiologic study for any of these abnormalities to be completely excluded.

Ancillary Studies

Laboratory

- In general, there are no specific laboratory tests that are diagnostic for any of these arrhythmias.
- All patients should have their electrolyte levels checked, as hypo- and hyperkalemia may lead to or exacerbate some of these disturbances.
- Thyroid-stimulating hormone levels also should be checked, as hypothyroidism also may cause bradycardia (most commonly sinus bradycardia).
- Patients on digoxin should have their serum levels checked, as digoxin toxicity may cause many of these arrhythmias.

- Patients who present with more acute symptoms, such as chest pain/heaviness or dyspnea, should have their cardiac biomarkers checked, as many of these rhythms may occur in the setting of an acute MI, especially an inferior MI.
- Many times, the laboratory evaluation of these patients is guided by the acuity of the presentation, not the bradyarrhythmia.
- Lyme disease may cause conduction disturbances; therefore, in the correct clinical setting, a Lyme titer may need to be analyzed. Chagas disease also may cause conduction disturbances so in the correct clinical setting, also may need to be evaluated.

Imaging

- Most patients being evaluated for cardiovascular-related complaints will have a chest x-ray, which may indicate contributing issues or show evidence of other heart disease (e.g., heart failure and/or cardiomegaly).
- Echocardiogram (either transthoracic or transesophageal) usually is performed in the workup of patients with symptomatic bradycardias. These studies may help reveal any structural heart disease that may be causative or contributory (e.g., cardiomyopathy, cardiac amyloidosis).

Special Populations

Age

- Most of these arrhythmias increase in incidence as age increases, as they often are associated with underlying heart disease or medication use.
- Exceptions include sinus bradycardia, sinus arrhythmia, and low-level heart blocks, which may be normal variants in the young.
- The most common cause of bradycardia in infancy is hypoxia.
- In adolescents and young adults, the pulse rate may drop normally to 35 to 40 bpm during sleep. This also may be associated with sinus pauses of up to 2 seconds. These findings are normal in this age group and usually do not require further evaluation.
- Complete heart block may be seen in infants and children and is almost always associated with congenital heart disease.
- Children presenting with high-grade heart block and no significant medical history should be evaluated for drug ingestion (digoxin, beta-blockers, calcium channel blockers, other antiarrhythmics, and opiates). It also may be necessary to consider conduction abnormalities from cardiac Lyme disease and, if appropriate (prolonged travel or immigration from endemic areas), Chagas disease.

Co-morbidities

- There are multiple co-morbidities of interest in patients presenting with bradyarrhythmias.
- Many of these disturbances are seen in patients with underlying structural heart disease and in those with coexistent coronary artery disease. Many of these conduction disturbances may be seen with or caused by cardiac medications.
- Increased vagal tone may precipitate many of these abnormalities, so anything that increases vagal tone should be considered (e.g., carotid sinus hypersensitivity, intra-abdominal catastrophe, increased intracranial pressure, drugs).
- As noted, conduction disturbances also may be found in association with many other diseases:
  - Inflammatory: rheumatic heart disease, myocarditis, pericarditis, and collagen vascular diseases such as rheumatoid arthritis and systemic sclerosis
  - Infectious: Lyme disease and Chagas disease
  - Systemic/cardiac amyloidosis
  - Post open heart surgery
  - Post mediastinal radiation therapy
  - Chest trauma
  - Rare genetic and familial diseases, such as myotonic dystrophy

Pitfalls in Diagnosis

Critical Steps Not to Miss

- It is critical to consider the entire clinical picture when confronted with a patient who is bradycardic.
- It must be determined whether the patient is symptomatic and, if so, whether the symptoms arise from the bradycardia itself or an underlying/causative disorder.
- It is critical to look for these underlying disorders and not to stop at the diagnosis of bradycardia.
- All patients who are bradycardic should have a 12-lead ECG and, if in an appropriate clinical setting, continuous cardiac and vital sign monitoring.

Mimics

- Because bradycardia usually is defined by an absolute rate, there are no mimics; however, multiple potential etiologies must be considered in patients with bradycardia.

Time-Dependent Interventions

- Time-dependent interventions in bradycardias are necessary only in patients who have symptoms and show signs of reduced cardiac output, such as hypotension, a change in mental status, cyanosis, and syncope.
- In these situations, treatment must begin before obtaining a complete database.
- When a patient demonstrates any of these signs or symptoms, it is critical to act quickly to attempt to return cardiac output to more normal levels.
- Support of airway, breathing, and circulation is of paramount importance. All patients should have supplemental oxygen and adequate intravenous access for administration of medications and fluid. All unstable, or potentially unstable, patients with an arrhythmia should have defibrillator pads placed and attached to the defibrillator/monitor.

Overall Principles of Treatment

- As mentioned earlier, support of airway, breathing, and circulation is the most important management principle.
- All unstable, or potentially unstable, patients should have supplemental oxygen, adequate intravenous access for administration of medications and fluid, and defibrillator pads placed and attached to the defibrillator/monitor.
- In general, emergent treatment of bradycardias is not necessary unless the heart rate is less than 50 bpm and associated with signs of hypoperfusion, or if there is a risk of progression to complete heart block.
- Several urgent/emergent treatments are common and relevant to all the bradycardias:
    - Atropine. Atropine is a class II medication in the treatment of symptomatic bradycardias. It is a naturally occurring antimuscarinic drug that competitively antagonizes the effects of acetylcholine and other antimuscarinic agents. It increases the rate of sinus node firing (automaticity) and enhances AV nodal conduction. Because it blocks vagal activity, it sometimes is described as parasympatholytic or vagolytic. It is administered intravenously as 0.5-mg boluses (in situations other than bradycardia, it may be given as 1-mg boluses). It may be given every 5 minutes until the desired effect is achieved, or until a total of 3 mg (0.04 mg/kg) has been administered (this is the fully vagolytic dosage). If the conduction abnormality is an SA or AV nodal problem, it likely will respond to atropine. If the problem is infranodal or lower, the response rate decreases. Atropine's onset of action is about 2 to 4 minutes, and the effects may last for 5 to 6 hours. However, it is important to remember that the effect is temporary. Atropine must be administered with caution in settings of concurrent myocardial ischemia, as it increases the heart rate, which increases myocardial oxygen

demand, and may worsen ischemia. Atropine is not indicated in asymptomatic bradycardia. Atropine likely will have no effect on a transplanted heart, as heart transplants are denervated. Doses below 0.4 mg may cause a paradoxic bradycardia.

- Transcutaneous pacemaker. Transcutaneous pacing is a class I intervention for unstable patients with symptomatic bradycardia. All unstable patients should undergo transcutaneous pacing. Although atropine may be given as a temporizing measure, it should not replace transcutaneous pacing in unstable patients with high-grade (type II second-degree and complete) heart block. Self-adhesive pads are placed with the left pad over the left anterolateral precordial area and the right pad in the right subscapular region. Most patients have capture (i.e., when the pacing impulse results in a heartbeat) with 100 mA of output. Sometimes, however, it may require up to 200 mA of output for capture to occur. Outputs above 200 mA should not be attempted. Transcutaneous pacing may be uncomfortable and painful; therefore, all patients should receive either pain control or sedation with anxiolytics. If it is impossible to induce capture, it may be necessary to move to transvenous pacing.

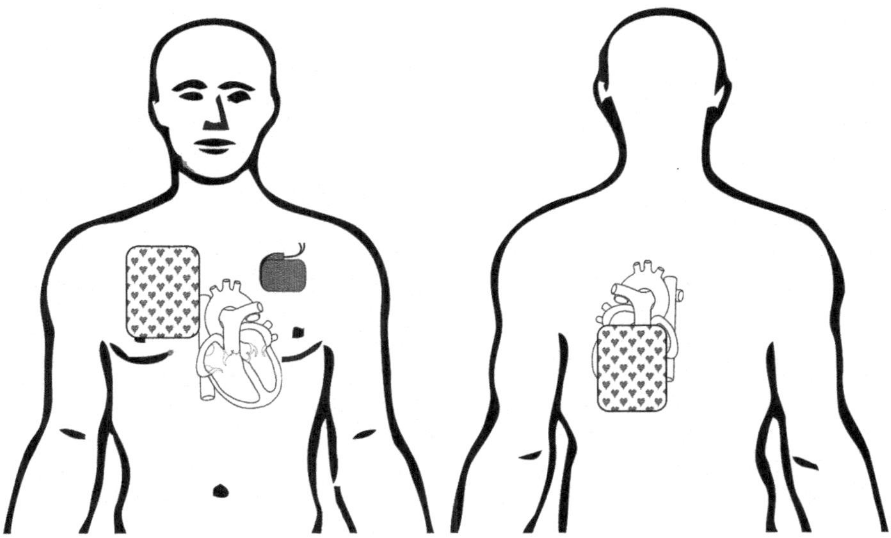

Placement of transcutaneous pacemaker pads. [Healey JS, Merchant R, Simpson C, Tang T, Beardsall M, Tung S, Fraser JA, Long L, van Vlymen JM, Manninen P, Ralley F, Venkatraghavan L, Yee R, Prasloski B, Sanatani S, Philippon F. Society position statement: Canadian Cardiovascular Society/Canadian Anesthesiologists' Society/Canadian Heart Rhythm Society joint position statement on the perioperative management of patients with implanted pacemakers, defibrillators, and neurostimulating devices. Can J Anaesth. 2012 Apr;59(4):394–407.] *Caption adapted from original*

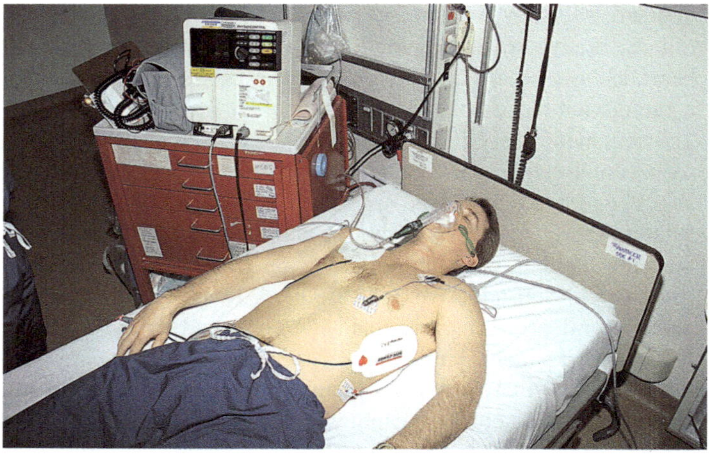

The right pad is placed in the alternative, right upper anterior chest and apex positions. [Woodcock B. Hemodynamic emergencies. In: Tremper KK, editor. Principles of anesthetic techniques and anesthetic emergencies. Philadelphia: Current Medicine; 1998. 195 p. (Miller RD, editor. Atlas of anesthesia; vol. 4).]

https://www.youtube.com/watch?v=qkSGaJkNqvg
Video demonstrating transcutaneous pacing.

- Transvenous pacing. Transvenous pacing has the same indication as transcutaneous pacing. It requires central venous access because the leads are passed through the central catheter into the heart. This is an invasive procedure, and although it may be attempted emergently at the bedside, it is best performed in conjunction with expert consultation and guidance. Currently, this technique is performed most often under fluoroscopic guidance in a cardiac catheterization laboratory as a bridge to a permanent pacemaker.
- Epinephrine and dopamine. Epinephrine and dopamine may be considered for blood pressure support if atropine and emergent pacing have been unsuccessful. Administration of these agents is only temporizing measure until the patient can be prepared for definitive therapy.
- Specific drug ingestions that lead to symptomatic and/or unstable bradycardias should be treated with specific antidotes if available, but also may be treated with atropine and pacing as required.

Following is a list of recommendations based on the specific bradycardia:

- Sinus bradycardia: generally requires no treatment unless the rate is less than 50 bpm and associated with symptoms, which may occur with profound vagal stimulation. If necessary, treatment may start with atropine and, if necessary, transcutaneous pacing.
- Sinus arrhythmia: requires no treatment.
- Sinus pauses/sinus arrest: treatment should be aimed at the underlying causes.

- Sick sinus syndrome: this is an indication for a permanent pacemaker.
- Junctional bradycardia: usually does not require treatment and is transient. If the patient is symptomatic or unstable, atropine and/or pacing may be used; however, it also is important to search for the underlying cause.
- SA block: often requires no treatment; however, the underlying cause should be evaluated.
- First-degree AV block: usually requires no treatment.
- Second-degree AV block, Mobitz type I (Wenckebach): usually does not require treatment unless the patient has symptoms. It usually is transient, and when the underlying cause is identified and treated, the block usually resolves. If treatment is necessary, most patients will respond to atropine.
- Second-degree AV block, Mobitz type II: these patients are unstable, with a high risk of progression to complete heart block. They should have pacemaker pads placed and attached for use if necessary. Atropine may be used as a temporizing measure (about 60 % of patients respond), but in most circumstances, pacing will be necessary. Because this type of block usually is associated with permanent damage to the conduction system, most patients will require a permanent pacemaker at some point in their care.
- Third-degree heart block (complete heart block): this is an inherently unstable block and usually is symptomatic and hemodynamically significant. It usually indicates permanent damage to the conduction system and requires either transcutaneous or transvenous pacing as a bridge to a permanent pacemaker. Some patients may respond to atropine if the block is higher within the His–Purkinje system.

Disease Course

- As detailed earlier, many of these rhythms/conduction problems are either normal variants or transient and can be resolved with identification and treatment of the underlying disorders.
- Higher-grade AV blocks almost always indicate some permanent damage to the conducting system and require placement of a permanent pacemaker.

Related Evidence

Papers of particular interest have been highlighted as:
*** Of key importance*

Practice Guideline

European Society of Cardiology (ESC); European Heart Rhythm Association (EHRA), Brignole M, Auricchio A, Baron-Esquivias G, Bordachar P, Boriani G, Breithardt OA, Cleland J, Deharo JC, Delgado V, Elliott PM, Gorenek B, Israel CW, Leclercq C, Linde C, Mont L, Padeletti L, Sutton R, Vardas PE. 2013 ESC guidelines on cardiac pacing and cardiac resynchronization therapy: the task force on cardiac pacing and resynchronization therapy of the European Society of Cardiology (ESC). Developed in collaboration with the European Heart Rhythm Association (EHRA). Europace. 2013 Aug;15(8):1070-118. https://doi.org/10.1093/europace/eut206. PMID: 23801827. http://www.ncbi.nlm.nih.gov/pubmed/23801827 **

Epstein AE, DiMarco JP, Ellenbogen KA, Estes NA 3rd, Freedman RA, Gettes LS, Gillinov AM, Gregoratos G, Hammill SC, Hayes DL, Hlatky MA, Newby LK, Page RL, Schoenfeld MH, Silka MJ, Stevenson LW, Sweeney MO, Tracy CM, Epstein AE, Darbar D, DiMarco JP, Dunbar SB, Estes NA 3rd, Ferguson TB Jr, Hammill SC, Karasik PE, Link MS, Marine JE, Schoenfeld MH, Shanker AJ, Silka MJ, Stevenson LW, Stevenson WG, Varosy PD; American College of Cardiology Foundation; American Heart Association Task Force on Practice Guidelines; Heart Rhythm Society. 2012 ACCF/AHA/HRS focused update incorporated into the ACCF/AHA/HRS 2008 guidelines for device-based therapy of cardiac rhythm abnormalities: a report of the American College of Cardiology Foundation/American Heart Association Task Force on Practice Guidelines and the Heart Rhythm Society. J Am Coll Cardiol. 2013 Jan 22;61(3):e6-75. https://doi.org/10.1016/j.jacc.2012.11.007. PMID: 23265327. http://www.ncbi.nlm.nih.gov/pubmed/23265327 **

Review

Tadros R, Ton AT, Fiset C, Nattel S. Sex differences in cardiac electrophysiology and clinical arrhythmias: epidemiology, therapeutics, and mechanisms. Can J Cardiol. 2014 Jul;30(7):783-92. https://doi.org/10.1016/j.cjca.2014.03.032. PMID: 24970790. http://www.ncbi.nlm.nih.gov/pubmed/24970790 **

Sohinki D, Obel OA. Newer algorithms in bradycardia management. Cardiol Clin. 2014 May;32(2):283-92. https://doi.org/10.1016/j.ccl.2014.01.004. PMID: 24793803. http://www.ncbi.nlm.nih.gov/pubmed/24793803 **

Deal N. Evaluation and management of bradydysrhythmias in the emergency department. Emerg Med Pract. 2013 Sep;15(9):1-15; quiz 15-6. PMID: 24044868. http://www.ncbi.nlm.nih.gov/pubmed/24044868 **

Semelka M, Gera J, Usman S. Sick sinus syndrome: a review. Am Fam Physician. 2013 May 15;87(10):691-6. PMID: 23939447. http://www.ncbi.nlm.nih.gov/pubmed/23939447 **

Vogler J, Breithardt G, Eckardt L. Bradyarrhythmias and conduction blocks. Rev Esp Cardiol (Engl Ed). 2012 Jul;65(7):656-67. https://doi.org/10.1016/j.recesp.2012.01.025. PMID: 22627074. http://www.ncbi.nlm.nih.gov/pubmed/22627074 **

Barnes BJ, Hollands JM. Drug-induced arrhythmias. Crit Care Med. 2010 Jun;38(6 Suppl):S188-97. https://doi.org/10.1097/CCM.0b013e3181de112a. PMID: 20502173. http://www.ncbi.nlm.nih.gov/pubmed/20502173 **

Lampert R, Ezekowitz MD. Management of arrythmias. Clin Geriatr Med. 2000 Aug;16(3):593-618. PMID: 10918649. http://www.ncbi.nlm.nih.gov/pubmed/10918649 **

Spodick DH. Normal sinus heart rate: appropriate rate thresholds for sinus tachycardia and bradycardia. South Med J. 1996 Jul;89(7):666-7. PMID: 8685750. http://www.ncbi.nlm.nih.gov/pubmed/8685750 **

Cohort Study

Udo EO, van Hemel NM, Zuithoff NP, Doevendans PA, Moons KG. Prognosis of the bradycardia pacemaker recipient assessed at first implantation: a nationwide cohort study. Heart. 2013 Nov;99(21):1573-8. https://doi.org/10.1136/heartjnl-2013-304445. PMID: 23969476. http://www.ncbi.nlm.nih.gov/pubmed/23969476

Use PubMed Clinical Queries to find the most recent evidence. Use this search strategy:

"Bradycardia"[Mesh] OR "Sick Sinus Syndrome"[Mesh] OR "Bradycardia" OR "Bradyarrhythmia"

Chapter 14
Bronchiectasis

Christopher J. Rees, Charles V. Pollack, Jr., and Victoria G. Riese

Name and Synonyms

Bronchiectasis

Incidence/Epidemiology

- It is estimated that between 100,000 and 125,000 people in the United States have bronchiectasis.
- The prevalence increases with age.
- It is more common in women than in men.
- The incidence of bronchiectasis has been decreasing in developed nations.
- The incidence of bronchiectasis may be up to three times higher in developing nations. This is likely due to a combination of environmental and genetic factors that lead to a higher incidence of recurrent pulmonary infections, especially among children and young adults.

C. J. Rees
Emergency Department, Pennsylvania Hospital, Philadelphia, PA, USA

C. V. Pollack, Jr. (✉)
Department of Emergency Medicine, Thomas Jefferson University, Philadelphia, PA, USA

V. G. Riese
Librarian Consultant, Eldersburg, MD, USA

C. V. Pollack, Jr. (ed.), *Differential Diagnosis of Cardiopulmonary Disease*,
https://doi.org/10.1007/978-3-319-63895-9_14

Differential Diagnosis

- The differential diagnosis includes all the causes of chronic cough, sputum production, and dyspnea.
- This includes chronic bronchitis, asthma, chronic obstructive pulmonary disease, chronic sinusitis, and idiopathic pulmonary fibrosis, among others.

Pathophysiology and Etiology

- Bronchiectasis refers to lung disease dominated clinically by chronic cough with sputum production. Symptoms are often present for months to years prior to diagnosis.
- The major pathophysiologic change is irreversible airway dilatation with wall thickening and scarring.

https://www.youtube.com/watch?v=uNeprw1rsgE
Video animation of the pathophysiology of bronchiectasis.

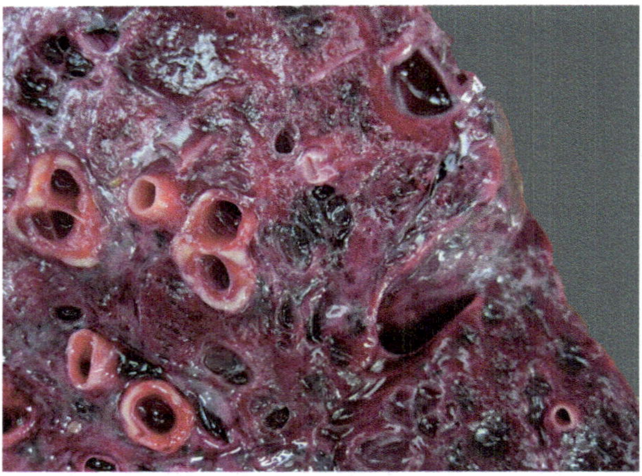

Close inspection of the cut surface of this lung in a case of mild bronchiectasis shows somewhat fibrotic-walled airways, which are dilated and congested. In addition, there is local, patchy emphysema and some cystic change and interstitial scarring. Many cases of lung disease do not show a single, pure format [Suvarna SK. Thorax: Heart, Lungs, Mediastinum, and Pleura. In: Suvarna SK, editor. Atlas of Adult Autopsy [Internet]. Cham: Springer International Publishing; 2016 [cited 2016 Nov 7]. p. 65–160. Available from: http://link.springer.com/10.1007/978-3-319-27022-7_4] *Caption from original*

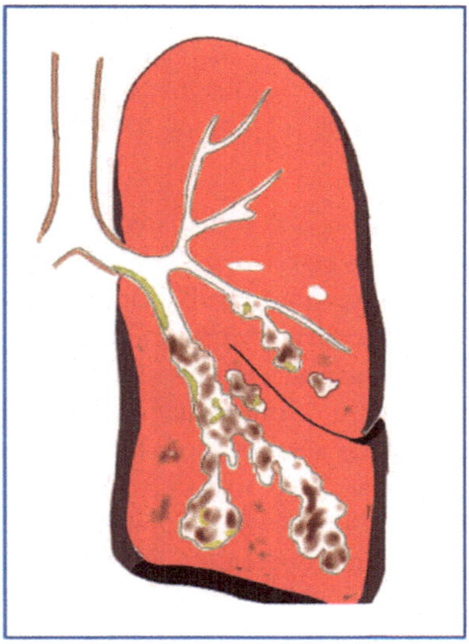

Bronchiectasis. There is dilatation of the airways with inflammation and increased mucous production [Ruggeri G, Gobbi D, Libri M, Lima M. Pediatric Bronchiectasis. In: Lima M, editor. Pediatric Thoracic Surgery [Internet]. Springer Milan; 2013 [cited 2015 May 11]. p. 351–62. Available from: http://link.springer.com/chapter/10.1007/978-88-470-5202-4_30]

- The lung changes can be focal or diffuse.

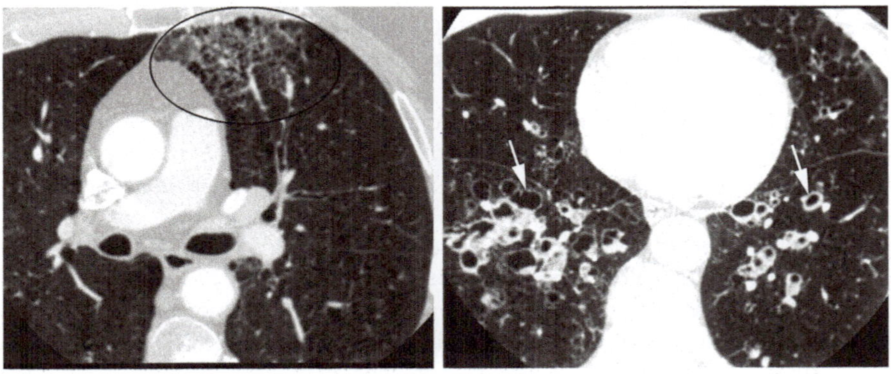

Focal bronchiectasis (circled area of upper panel) may be seen in patients with recurrent aspiration or pneumonias. Bilateral and diffuse bronchiectasis (arrows in lower panel) is typically the result of diffuse necrotizing infections in childhood, cystic fibrosis, immotile cilia syndromes, or immunoglobulinopathies, among others. [Callister T, Budoff M, Braunwald E. Atlas of Cardiovascular Computed Tomography, Volume 01, Chapter 18. In: Budoff M, Narula J, Achenbach SS, editors. Atlas of Cardiovascular Computed Tomography. Philadelphia: Current Medicine; 2007 [cited 2015 May 11]. Book DOI 978-1-57340-267-5] *Caption adapted from original.*

- These changes lead to airways that easily collapse and obstruct airflow.
- The initiation of bronchiectasis requires many factors. It is felt that there needs to be an inciting infectious insult, often in the setting of some impaired host defenses, that leads to airway obstruction that impairs drainage of inflammatory and purulent material and sets up a chronic airway inflammatory response. This leads to chronic inflammation, with permanent scarring, dilatation, and destruction of the airways (both large and small).
- The chronic inflammation leads to recurrent infections, which then lead to continued inflammation, setting up a vicious cycle.
- Many diseases and environmental issues can incite and/or worsen bronchiectasis.
- The pattern of involvement in the lungs may be a helpful clue as to etiology. Focal bronchiectasis points to foreign body aspiration or intrinsic or extrinsic airway compression as the cause.
- Causes/etiologies of bronchiectasis include:
  - Obstruction. Bronchiectasis can result from an aspirated foreign body, intrinsic compression/blockage from an endobronchial lesion or mass, or extrinsic compression from a mass.
- Infection. Can be bacterial pneumonia, atypical pneumonia such as viral or *Mycoplasma*, tuberculous, and non-tuberculous mycobacteria. *Mycobacterium avium*-intracellulare complex (MAC) is the most common non-tuberculous mycobacteria causing bronchiectasis, classically occurring in nonsmoking women over age 50.
- Immunodeficiency. Hypogammaglobulinemias, such as severe, combined immunodeficiency. These patients often have recurrent infections starting in childhood. Immunodeficiency also includes HIV infection and bronchiolitis obliterans after lung transplantation.
- Autoimmune/rheumatologic disorders. Rheumatoid arthritis, Sjogren's syndrome, inflammatory bowel disease.
- Immune-mediated diseases such as allergic bronchopulmonary aspergillosis.
- Genetic causes such as cystic fibrosis, ciliary dyskinesia (by decreasing secretion clearance), alpha-one anti-trypsin deficiency (usually causes early-onset emphysema, but bronchiectatic changes are also common).
- Recurrent aspiration.
- Idiopathic. Often represents from 25 – 50% of cases.
- Cigarette smoking.

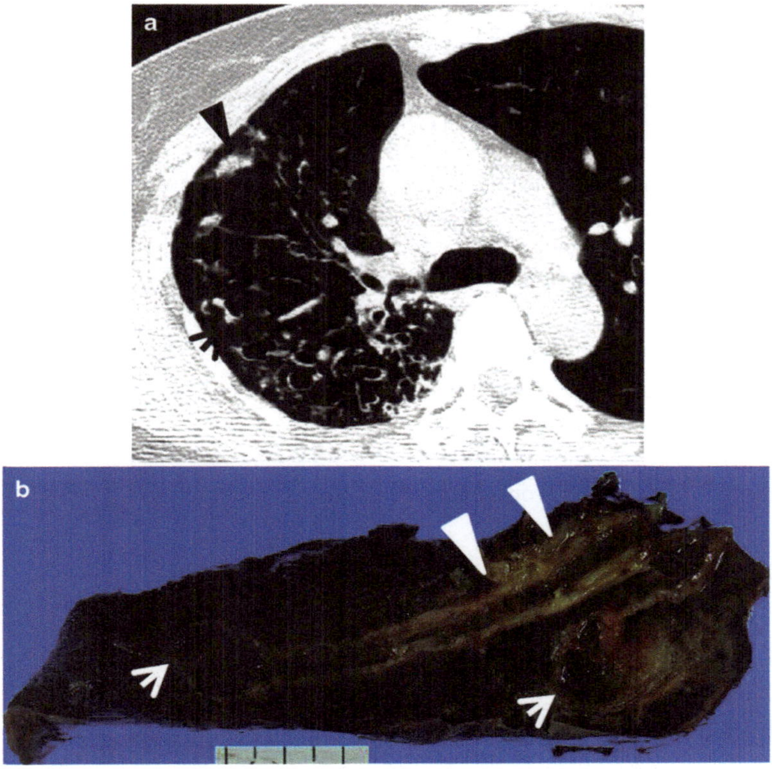

Bronchiectasis showing signet ring sign in a 44-year-old man. (a) Lung window image of CT scan (2.5-mm section thickness) obtained at level of the right upper lobar bronchus shows dilated bronchi showing signet ring sign (arrows) in right upper lobe. Also note mucus plugging (arrowhead) in dilated bronchi. (b) Gross pathologic specimen obtained with right upper lobectomy discloses cylindrical bronchiectasis and distal cystic changes (arrows, cystic bronchiectasis). Also note thickened bronchial wall (arrowheads) with active inflammation [Lee KS, Han J, Chung MP, Jeong YJ. Signet Ring Sign. Radiology Illustrated: Chest Radiology [Internet]. Berlin, Heidelberg: Springer Berlin Heidelberg; 2014 [cited 2015 Nov 19]. p. 139–42. Available from: http://link.springer.com/10.1007/978-3-642-37096-0_15] *Caption from original.*

Presentation

Typical/"Classic"

- The typical presentation of bronchiectasis is one of prolonged (months) cough that produces thick sputum. Usually there is an absence of acute infectious symptoms such as fever. Patients may also complain of dyspnea, especially on exertion. They may also exhibit wheezing.

Atypical

- Patients may present with symptoms more consistent with chronic obstructive pulmonary disease or asthma, with wheezing and shortness of breath being more prominent.
- Patients may also present with a more acutely infectious appearance with fever, associated with productive cough. This is especially common if they have been undiagnosed and are suffering from an acute infectious exacerbation from their undiagnosed bronchiectasis.

Primary Differential Considerations

- Asthma
- Acute and chronic bronchitis
- Cystic fibrosis
- GERD
- Pneumonia
- Alpha-1-antitrypsin deficiency

History and Physical Exam

Findings That Confirm Diagnosis

- A typical presentation with prolonged cough productive of thick sputum will strongly suggest the diagnosis, but the diagnosis is usually only confirmed by typical findings on CT scan of the chest.

Factors That Suggest Diagnosis

- Again, the typical symptoms should strongly suggest the diagnosis.
- This is especially true if the patient has any of the known predisposing conditions.

Factors That Exclude Diagnosis

- There are no historical or physical examination findings that can reliably exclude the diagnosis.
- Bronchiectasis may coexist with many other diseases, especially COPD.

Ancillary Studies

Laboratory

- Although there are no laboratory tests specifically needed for the diagnosis, patients will usually require a CBC with differential and basic chemistries in the evaluation. They may also require tests specific for the disorder if they need to be evaluated for any of the etiologies of bronchiectasis, such as tests for RA, SS, and alpha-one antitrypsin.
- Sputum culture may be necessary when trying to evaluate for MAC or other mycobacterial causes of bronchiectasis. Sputum culture may also be helpful for management of acute infectious exacerbations of bronchiectasis.

Imaging

- Chest CT is the diagnostic imaging study of choice for confirming the diagnosis of bronchiectasis.
- Plain chest x-ray may show findings consistent with bronchiectasis (such as dilated bronchioles), but CT is necessary to confirm the diagnosis.

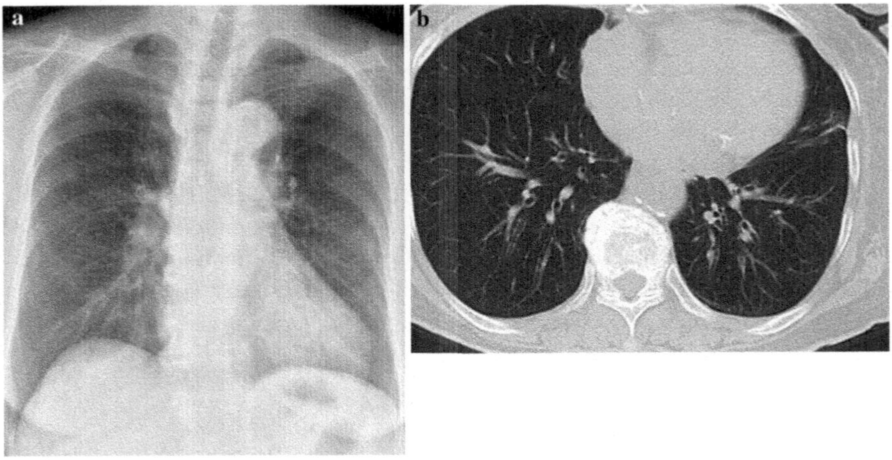

A Chest X-ray revealed clear lung fields. b High-resolution CT image through the lungs at the level of bronchus shows right lower lobe and lingular bronchiectasis. [Toyoda M, Yokomori H, Kaneko F, Yoshida H, Takahashi A, Hoshi K, Takeuchi H, Tahara K, Kondo H, Motoori T. Hepatic granulomas as primary presentation of Mycobacterium avium infection in an HIV-negative, nonimmunosuppressed patient. Clinical Journal of Gastroenterology. 2009 Dec;2(6):431–7.] *Caption adapted from original.*

- CT findings in bronchiectasis include airway dilatation, lack of bronchial tapering (usually noticed as tubular structures within 1 cm of the pleural surface), bronchial wall thickening in dilated airways, and a large amount of dried secretions (tree-in-bud pattern).
- The signet-ring sign on CT is when there is a cross-sectional airway with a diameter that is at least 1.5 times larger than an adjacent vessel.

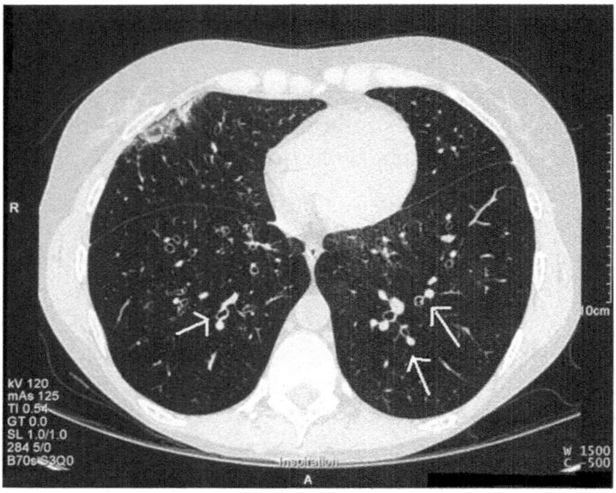

(CT Thorax): Resolution of areas of consolidation and "signet ring sign". The signet ring sign is a finding seen on CT scans of the thorax. It consists of a small circle of soft tissue attenuation that abuts a ring of soft tissue attenuation surrounding a larger low attenuating circle of air and is indicative of bronchiectasis. [From article: Invasive pulmonary aspergillosis 10 years post bone marrow transplantation: a case report. Journal of Medical Case Reports. 2009;3(1):26. https://doi.org/10.1186/1752-1947-3-26, at http://link.springer.com/article/10.1186%2F1752-1947-3-26/fulltext.html; by Rifat Rashid, David W Denning, © Rashid and Denning; licensee BioMed Central Ltd. 2009; licensed under Creative Commons Attribution License BY 2.0 http://creativecommons.org/licenses/by/2.0] *Caption adapted from original.*

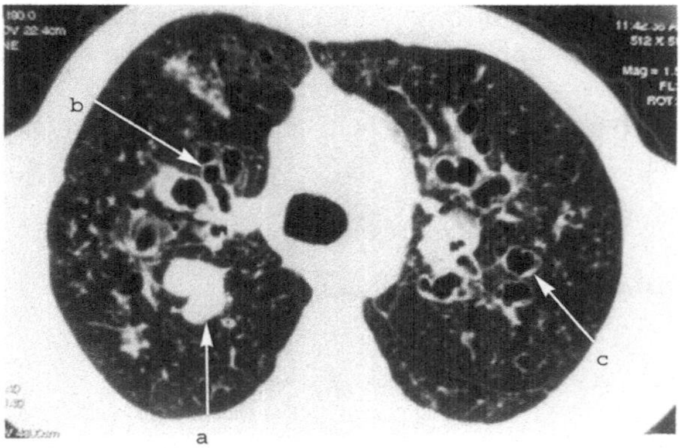

High resolution chest computed tomography scan (lung window) showing (a) mucus-filled dilated bronchi (arrow) and extensive bilateral central bronchiectasis characterised by (b) "string of pearls" and (c) "signet ring" appearances [Shah A. How to Diagnose Allergic Bronchopulmonary Aspergillosis. In: Comarú Pasqualotto A, editor. Aspergillosis: From Diagnosis to Prevention [Internet]. Dordrecht: Springer Netherlands; 2009 [cited 2015 Nov 19]. p. 725–45. Available from: http://www.springerlink.com/index/10.1007/978-90-481-2408-4_43] *Caption from original.*

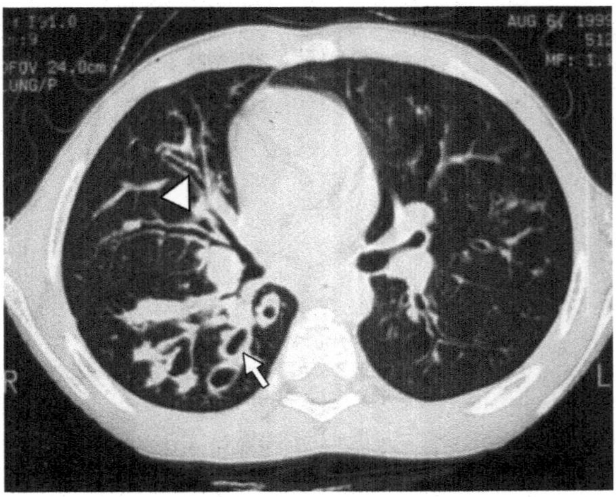

Computed tomographic image of bronchiectasis. Chest CT showing diffuse dilated bronchi (bronchiectasis), especially in the right lower lobe. Thick-walled bronchi are seen. Also present is the "signet-ring" sign (arrow), in which the diameter of the airway (lumen) is greater than that of the adjacent vessel. Apparent in the right middle lobe is "tram-tracking" (arrowhead), with absence of tapering of the peripheral bronchi. [MacLusky I, Solomon M, Laxer R, Ford-Jones EL, Friedman J, Gerstle T. Atlas of Pediatrics, Volume IA, Chapter 14. In: Laxer RM, editor. The Hospital for Sick Children: Atlas of Pediatrics. Philadelphia, PA: Current Medicine Group; 2005. 519 p. ISBN 1-57340-188-9] *Caption from original.*

- Most patients with bronchiectasis will undergo bronchoscopy during evaluation. This is most important in patients with focal bronchiectasis to exclude airway obstruction from a mass or foreign body.
- Pulmonary function testing can help in gauging the functional impairment of the patient.

Special Populations

Age

- The incidence of bronchiectasis increases with age.
- Patients with cystic fibrosis can develop clinically significant bronchiectasis in adolescence or young adulthood.

Co-morbidities

- Co-morbidities of interest include all the etiologies listed above.
- Bronchiectasis may coexist with COPD and other chronic lung diseases.
- Bronchiectasis may also coexist with causes of chronic dyspnea and cough, such as congestive heart failure.

Pitfalls in Diagnosis

Critical Steps Not to Miss

- Consideration of the diagnosis is the first critical step.
- It is important to perform appropriate imaging in patients in whom the diagnosis is being considered.
- A search for the possible etiology should be performed for all patients being evaluated for bronchiectasis.

Mimics

- Typical mimics of bronchiectasis include COPD/emphysema, asthma, and pulmonary fibrosis.

Time-Dependent Interventions

- Time-dependent interventions in bronchiectasis are rarely necessary. This is a chronic, slowly progressive disease.
- Acute exacerbations often benefit from the timely use of antibiotics, as well as from bronchial hygiene measures (help to enhance secretion clearance) such as chest physiotherapy, mucolytics, hydration, and sometimes bronchodilator therapy.

Overall Principles of Treatment

- The general treatment of bronchiectasis involves:
  - control of any active infection.
  - attempts to improve bronchial hygiene to help minimize the risk of repeated infections.
- Antibiotics are usually administered for acute exacerbations. These are suspected clinically in the presence of a worsened cough, qualitative (and often quantitative) change in the sputum, and sometimes fever. The most commonly isolated causative organisms of acute infectious exacerbations are *Haemophilus influenza*, and *Pseudomonas aeruginosa*. The typical antibiotics used are fluoroquinolones, such as ciprofloxacin and levofloxacin.
- The decision to treat *Mycobacterium avium*-intracellulare complex (MAC) is difficult. This organism can exist as a colonizer as well as a pathogen, and the treatment regimens are prolonged and often poorly tolerated. MAC, however, is the most common non-tuberculous mycobacterial cause of bronchiectasis. The diagnosis of this infection, and the decision to treat, is often guided by expert opinion.
- Multiple approaches are usually taken to try and enhance secretion clearance (bronchial hygiene) in these patients.
  - Maintaining adequate hydration and the use of mucolytics to keep secretions thin.
- Use of bronchodilators.
  - Chest physiotherapy, including chest percussion and newer mechanical devices.
- The use of systemic glucocorticoids is controversial. There has been no compelling evidence demonstrating improvements in pulmonary function or of lower exacerbation rates from their use.
  - Oral or systemic glucocorticoids may be necessary for some patients depending upon the etiology of their bronchiectasis. Patients with allergic bronchopulmonary aspergillosis, Rheumatoid arthritis, and Sjogren's

syndrome may benefit from glucocorticoids for both their bronchiectasis and their underlying disease.

- In severe or refractory cases, surgery (such as resection of involved lung tissue) may be considered. This is especially true of patients with focal bronchiectasis.
- End-stage patients may be considered for lung transplantation.
- All patients with chronic respiratory conditions should be kept up to date on vaccinations, especially influenza and pneumococcal. Appropriate use of these vaccinations can help reduce the rate of recurrent infections.
- Patients who smoke should be counseled about cessation and offered help with quitting.

Disease Course

- Bronchiectasis is a chronic, recurrent, progressive disease.
- Outcomes and course vary widely based upon the underlying etiology.
- The decline in lung function is similar to that seen in patients with COPD.

Related Evidence

Papers of particular interest have been highlighted as:
*** Of key importance*

Practice Guideline

Pasteur MC, Bilton D, Hill AT; British Thoracic Society Bronchiectasis non-CF Guideline Group. British Thoracic Society guideline for non-CF bronchiectasis. Thorax. 2010 Jul;65 Suppl 1:i1-58. https://doi.org/10.1136/thx.2010.136119. PMID: 20627931. http://www.ncbi.nlm.nih.gov/pubmed/20627931 **

Review

Sidhu MK, Mandal P, Hill AT. Bronchiectasis: an update on current pharmacotherapy and future perspectives. Expert Opin Pharmacother. 2014 Mar;15(4):505-25. https://doi.org/10.1517/14656566.2014.878330. PMID: 24410485. http://www.ncbi.nlm.nih.gov/pubmed/24410485 **

Lee AL, Burge A, Holland AE. Airway clearance techniques for bronchiectasis. Cochrane Database Syst Rev. 2013 May 31;5:CD008351. https://doi.org/10.1002/14651858.CD008351.pub2. PMID: 23728674. http://www.ncbi.nlm.nih.gov/pubmed/23728674 **

McShane PJ, Naureckas ET, Tino G, Strek ME. Non-cystic fibrosis bronchiectasis. Am J Respir Crit Care Med. 2013 Sep 15;188(6):647-56. https://doi.org/10.1164/rccm.201303-0411CI. PMID: 23898922. http://www.ncbi.nlm.nih.gov/pubmed/23898922 **

McDonnell MJ, Ward C, Lordan JL, Rutherford RM. Non-cystic fibrosis bronchiectasis. QJM. 2013 Aug;106(8):709-15. https://doi.org/10.1093/qjmed/hct109. PMID: 23728208. http://www.ncbi.nlm.nih.gov/pubmed/23728208 **

Bonavita J, Naidich DP. Imaging of bronchiectasis. Clin Chest Med. 2012 Jun;33(2):233-48. https://doi.org/10.1016/j.ccm.2012.02.007. PMID: 22640843. http://www.ncbi.nlm.nih.gov/pubmed/22640843 **

Moulton BC, Barker AF. Pathogenesis of bronchiectasis. Clin Chest Med. 2012 Jun;33(2):211-7. https://doi.org/10.1016/j.ccm.2012.02.004. PMID: 22640841. http://www.ncbi.nlm.nih.gov/pubmed/22640841 **

Singer LG, Herridge MS. Clinical year in review II: bronchiectasis, mycobacterial infections of the lung, sleep-disordered breathing, and lung transplantation. Proc Am Thorac Soc. 2010 Sep;7(5):305-11. https://doi.org/10.1513/pats.201007-051TT. PMID: 20844288. http://www.ncbi.nlm.nih.gov/pubmed/20844288 **

Goeminne P, Dupont L. Non-cystic fibrosis bronchiectasis: diagnosis and management in 21st century. Postgrad Med J. 2010 Aug;86(1018):493-501. https://doi.org/10.1136/pgmj.2009.091041. PMID: 20709772. http://www.ncbi.nlm.nih.gov/pubmed/20709772 **

Cantin L, Bankier AA, Eisenberg RL. Bronchiectasis. AJR Am J Roentgenol. 2009 Sep;193(3):W158-71. https://doi.org/10.2214/AJR.09.3053. PMID: 19696251. http://www.ncbi.nlm.nih.gov/pubmed/19696251 **

Use PubMed Clinical Queries to find the most recent evidence. Use this search strategy:

"Bronchiectasis"[Mesh] OR "Bronchiectasis"

Chapter 15
Bronchiolitis

Richard M. Cantor, Charles V. Pollack, Jr., and Victoria G. Riese

Name and Synonyms

Formally known as Respiratory Syncytial Viral (RSV) pneumonia, but many other viruses (such as metapneumovirus, adenovirus, parainfluenza virus) may cause the same clinical disease.

Incidence/Epidemiology

- Typically affects infants under 2 years of age.
- Reported peak incidence between 2 and 6 months.
- Seasonal peaks during fall and winter.
- Bronchiolitis is the leading cause of hospitalization in young children.

R. M. Cantor
Department of Emergency Medicine and Pediatrics, State University of New York Upstate Medical University, Syracuse, NY, USA

C. V. Pollack, Jr. (✉)
Department of Emergency Medicine, Thomas Jefferson University, Philadelphia, PA, USA

V. G. Riese
Librarian Consultant, Eldersburg, MD, USA

C. V. Pollack, Jr. (ed.), *Differential Diagnosis of Cardiopulmonary Disease*,
https://doi.org/10.1007/978-3-319-63895-9_15

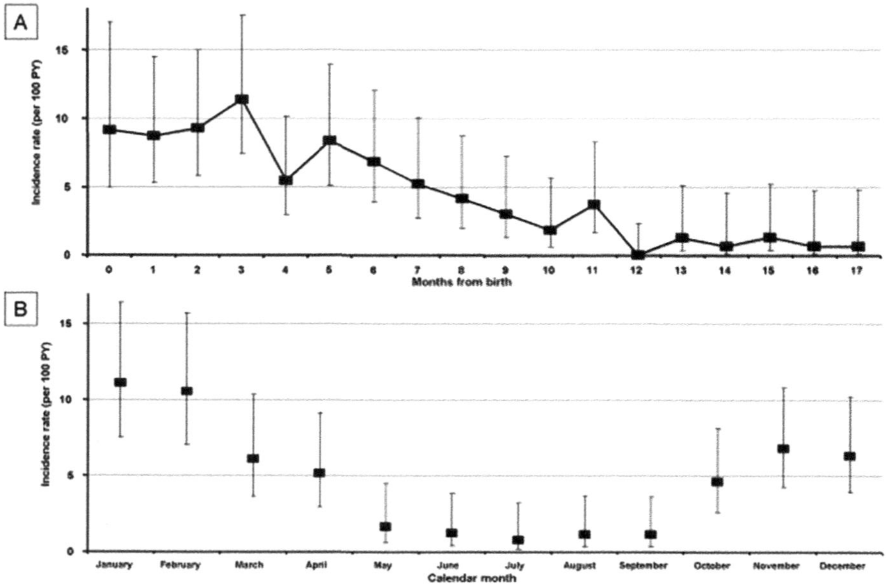

Incidence rates of hospitalizations for bronchiolitis by age (in months) (section A) and by calendar month (section B) in pre-term infants; Rome, Italy 2000-2006. [From article: Incidence and risk factors of hospitalization for bronchiolitis in preterm children: a retrospective longitudinal study in Italy. BMC Pediatrics. 2009 Sept 10; 9:56; https://doi.org/10.1186/1471-2431-9-56, at http://bmcpediatr.biomedcentral.com/articles/10.1186/1471-2431-9-56; by Patrizio Pezzotti, Jessica Mantovani, Nicoletta Benincori, Eleonora Mucchino, Domenico Di Lallo, © Pezzotti et al; licensee BioMed Central Ltd. 2009; licensed under Creative Commons Attribution License BY 2.0 http://creativecommons.org/licenses/by/2.0] *Caption from original*

Differential Diagnosis

The typical affected infant presents with fever and wheezing, and as such initially prompts these differential considerations:

- Bacterial pneumonia
- Chlamydial pneumonia
- Foreign-body aspiration
- Reactive airway disease/asthma
- Aspiration pneumonia
- Congenital heart disease
- Vascular rings

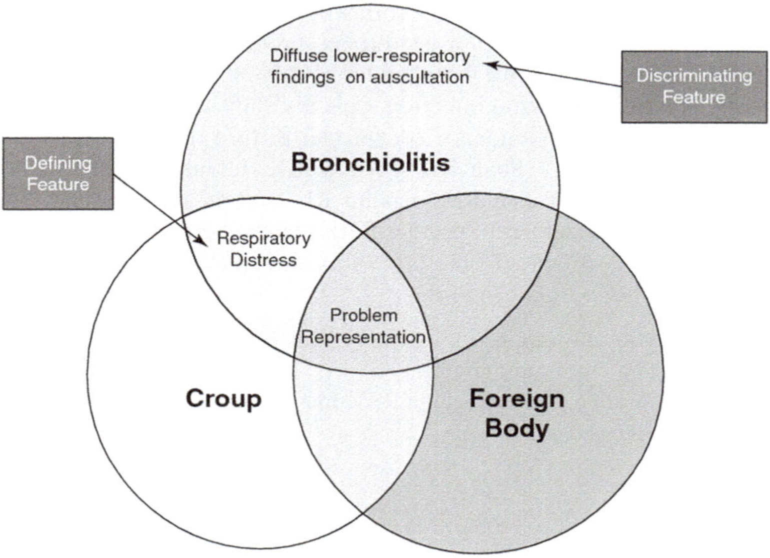

The problem representation allows identification of three illness scripts that fit the defining features of this toddler with respiratory distress case. Diffuse lower respiratory findings on auscultation is the key discriminating feature, which allows a diagnosis of bronchiolitis [Mutnick A, Barone M. Assessing and Remediating Clinical Reasoning. In: Kalet A, Chou CL, editors. Remediation in Medical Education [Internet]. New York, NY: Springer New York; 2014 [cited 2016 Jul 28]. p. 85–101. Available from: http://link.springer.com/10.1007/978-1-4614-9025-8_6] *Caption from original*

Pathophysiology and Etiology

- Viral infiltration of terminal bronchioles results in edema, increased mucous production, and sloughing of respiratory epithelial cells.

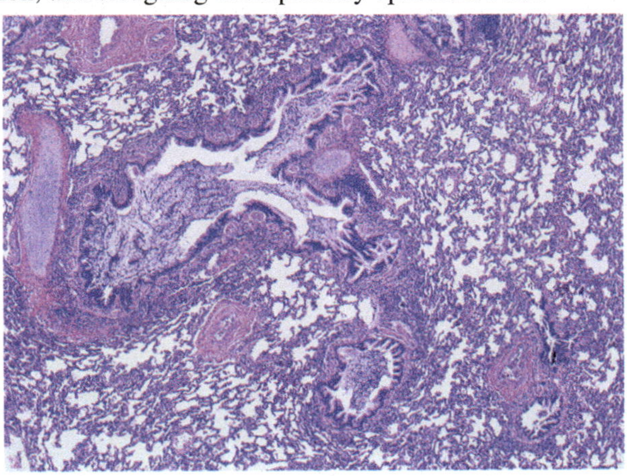

Influenza virus infection. Like other forms of respiratory viral infection, influenza may cause a lymphocytic or necrotizing bronchiolitis, in this case associated with mucus stasis in the bronchioles (H&E, 40×). Autopsy examination following fatal influenza viral infection typically shows a necrotizing bronchitis and bronchiolitis with pulmonary edema and diffuse alveolar damage in the background (not shown) [Shah KK, Dishop MK. Infantile Viral Illnesses. In: Fraire AE, Woda BA, Welsh RM, Kradin RL, editors. Viruses and the Lung [Internet]. Berlin, Heidelberg: Springer Berlin Heidelberg; 2014 [cited 2016 Jul 28]. p. 143–58. Available from: http://link.springer.com/10.1007/978-3-642-40605-8_17] *Caption from original*

- Lymphocytic infiltration causes the typical pattern of peribronchial cuffing seen on plain chest radiographs.
- Known causative viruses include RSV, metapneumovirus, rhinovirus, parainfluenza virus, and adenovirus.

Presentation

Typical/"Classic"

- There is often a 2 to 4-day prodrome consisting of cough and rhinorrhea.
- Infants present after the prodrome with fever, increasing cough, and variable degrees of respiratory distress.
- Patients manifest a wide range of work of breathing, characterized by tachypnea, expiratory prolongation, retractions, and in more severe cases, grunting.

Atypical

- In infants less than 6 weeks of age, apneic episodes may be the first sign of bronchiolitis.

Primary Differential Considerations

- Early diagnostic consideration should also be given to:
  - Asthma
  - Pneumonia
  - Croup

- Congenital heart disease
- Aspiration pneumonitis

History and Physical Exam

- Historically an infant with a mild URI (prodrome, as above) will develop a progressively worsening cough.
- At initial presentation, most infants will have signs of lower respiratory disease.
- Most infants will be febrile, increasing insensible fluid losses.
- Excessive work of breathing may severely impair the ability to feed, resulting in variable degrees of dehydration.
- Cough, retractions, tachypnea, and grunting may be present.
- Auscultation will reveal expiratory prolongation, impairment of air entry, and ronchi/wheezing.

Findings That Confirm Diagnosis

- The typical clinical syndrome, when seasonally encountered (fall and winter) makes the diagnosis obvious.
- Viral testing will further identify the particular etiologic agent.

Factors That Suggest Diagnosis

- As mentioned previously, bronchiolitis is a seasonal epidemic, providing the caregiver with obvious signs.

Factors That Exclude Diagnosis

- The presence of tachycardia with a gallop or cardiomegaly points towards congenital heart disease.
- Toxic appearance, hyperthermia, and lobar infiltrates suggest bacterial pneumonia.

Ancillary Studies

Laboratory Studies

- Viral testing is optional in atypical cases (specifically infants who present only with apnea) and in facilities that have co-bedding of pediatric inpatients.
- Blood work is not indicated.

Imaging

- Chest radiographs will demonstrate hyperinflation, interstitial disease, and peribronchial cuffing; in some instances, variable degrees of atelectasis may be present.

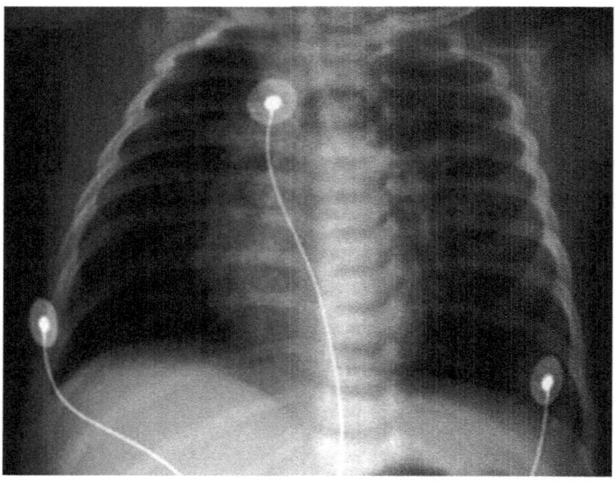

RSV-bronchiolitis. Markedly hyperinflated lungs with flattening of the diaphragm and peribronchial hilar infiltrates are demonstrated on the chest radiograph. [Staatz G. Bronchitis and Bronchiolitis in Childhood. In: Baert AL, editor. Encyclopedia of Diagnostic Imaging [Internet]. Berlin, Heidelberg: Springer Berlin Heidelberg; 2008 [cited 2016 Jul 28]. p. 203–5. Available from: http://www.springerlink.com/index/10.1007/978-3-540-35280-8_337] *Caption from original*

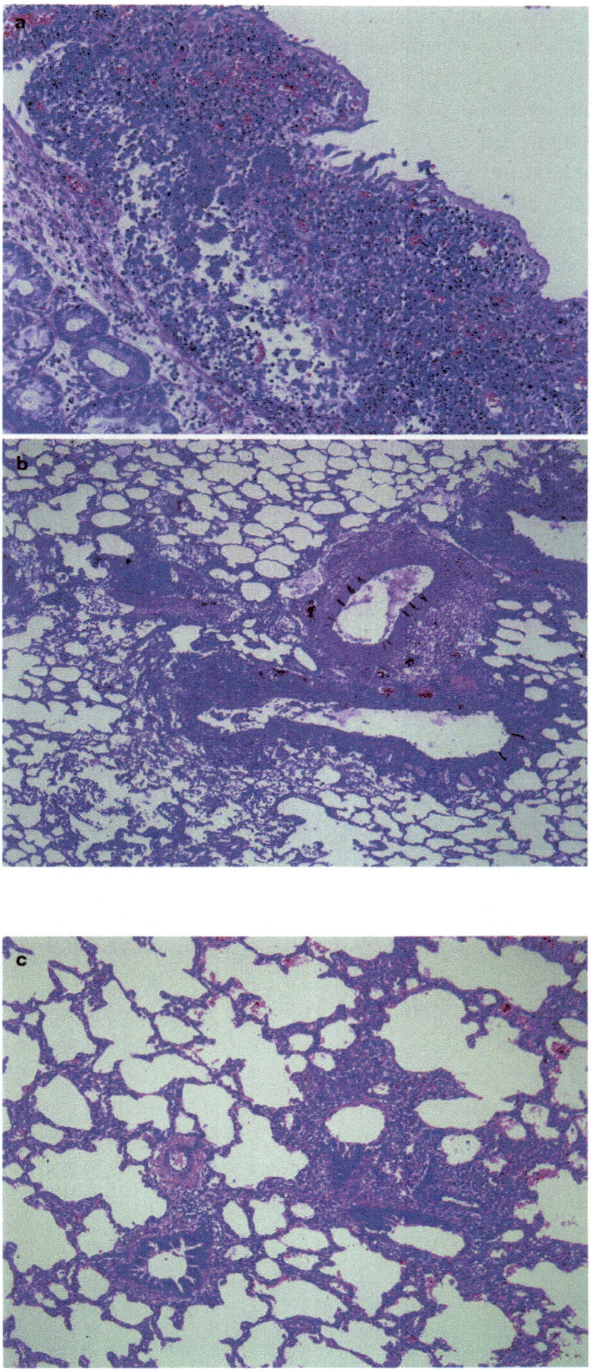
a
b
c

Respiratory syncytial virus infection in an infant. The prototypic infantile respiratory virus, RSV, causes a lymphocytic bronchitis and bronchiolitis. (a) This bronchus demonstrates a cuff of lymphocytes in the submucosa (H&E, 200×). (b) Circumferential lymphocyte infiltrates are also noted in the small airways (H&E, 100×). (c) Bronchiolitis may be accompanied by an interstitial pneumonitis, characterized by interstitial widening by lymphocyte infiltrates. Syncytial-type multinucleate cells are absent or rare in lung tissues from otherwise healthy infants but are characteristic of the viral cytopathic effect seen in culture in the diagnostic virology laboratory (H&E, 100×) [Shah KK, Dishop MK. Infantile Viral Illnesses. In: Fraire AE, Woda BA, Welsh RM, Kradin RL, editors. Viruses and the Lung [Internet]. Berlin, Heidelberg: Springer Berlin Heidelberg; 2014 [cited 2016 Jul 28]. p. 143–58. Available from: http://link.springer.com/10.1007/978-3-642-40605-8_17] *Caption from original*

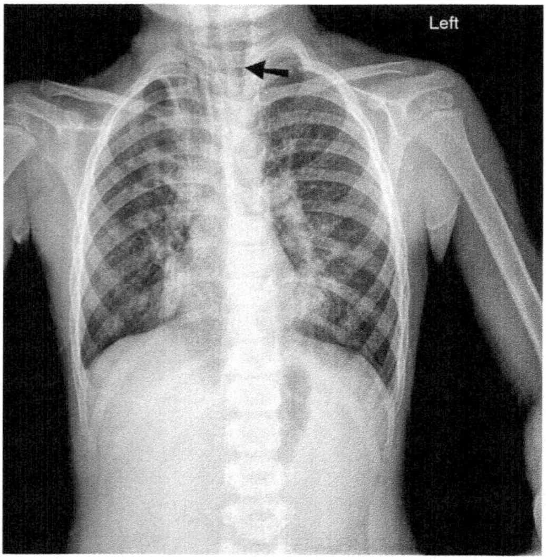

Bronchiolitis and pneumomediastinum. Frontal chest radiograph in a patient with RSV infection demonstrates a combination of bilateral perihilar atelectasis and hyperexpanded lungs. Note the presence of pneumomediastinum (arrow) with gas tracking up the neck soft tissues [Krol JJ, von Herrmann PF, Challa HR, Dillon JE. Imaging of Pediatric Emergencies. In: Singh A, editor. Emergency Radiology [Internet]. New York, NY: Springer New York; 2013 [cited 2016 Jul 28]. p. 361–73. Available from: http://link.springer.com/10.1007/978-1-4419-9592-6_26] *Caption from original*

Special Populations

Age

- Children older than 3 may contract viral infections that present identically to bronchiolitis, though RSV titers will be negative.

Co-morbidities

- Risk factors for the development of apnea include:
  - History of prematurity (less than 35 weeks)
  - Age less than 2 months
  - Presence of congenital heart disease
  - Presence of marked atelectasis

Pitfalls in Diagnosis

- Most patients present with typical symptomatology.
- Not considering bronchiolitis in infant apneic spells would be unwise.

Critical Steps Not to Miss

- Obtaining a careful birth history is mandatory.
- There is usually an older child in the home with a simple cold.

Mimics

- As previously mentioned, bacterial pneumonia may present with similar findings.
- New onset CHF will often present with respiratory distress and wheezing.

Time-Dependent Interventions

- Supplemental oxygen is often necessary.
- In dehydrated infants, IV fluids are indicated.

- Nasopharyngeal suctioning may dramatically lessen the work required to breathe.
- The use of albuterol has recently been discouraged in the literature; many practitioners, however, still favor a single albuterol treatment in an attempt to identify the rare patient with reversible bronchospasm.
- Steroids are NOT recommended.
- Severe cases may respond to aerosolized racemic epinephrine.

Overall Principles of Treatment

- Simple correction of hypoxemia and fluid deficits are important first steps.
- Unfortunately, most infants will not respond to bronchodilators.
- Hospital admission is often the only option.

Disease Course

- Studies have demonstrated that this is a 14-to-21-day illness with vacillating degrees of respiratory compromise.
- The cough may take 2 weeks to resolve

Related Evidence

Papers of particular interest have been highlighted as:
*** Of key importance*

Practice Guideline

Ralston SL, Lieberthal AS, Meissner HC, Alverson BK, Baley JE, Gadomski AM, Johnson DW, Light MJ, Maraqa NF, Mendonca EA, Phelan KJ, Zorc JJ, Stanko-Lopp D, Brown MA, Nathanson I, Rosenblum E, Sayles S 3rd, Hernandez-Cancio S; American Academy of Pediatrics. Clinical practice guideline: the diagnosis, management, and prevention of bronchiolitis. Pediatrics. 2014 Nov;134(5):e1474-502. https://doi.org/10.1542/peds.2014-2742. PMID: 25349312. http://www.ncbi.nlm.nih.gov/pubmed/25349312 **

Turner T, Wilkinson F, Harris C, Mazza D; Health for Kids Guideline Development Group. Evidence based guideline for the management of bronchiolitis. Aust Fam

Physician. 2008 Jun;37(6 Spec No):6-13. PMID: 19142264. http://www.ncbi.nlm.nih.gov/pubmed/19142264 **

American Academy of Pediatrics Subcommittee on Diagnosis and Management of Bronchiolitis. Diagnosis and management of bronchiolitis. Pediatrics. 2006 Oct;118(4):1774-93. PMID: 17015575. http://www.ncbi.nlm.nih.gov/pubmed/17015575 **

Review

Hasegawa K, Mansbach JM, Camargo CA Jr. Infectious pathogens and bronchiolitis outcomes. Expert Rev Anti Infect Ther. 2014 Jul;12(7):817-28. https://doi.org/10.1586/14787210.2014.906901. PMID: 24702592. http://www.ncbi.nlm.nih.gov/pubmed/24702592 **

Schroeder AR, Mansbach JM. Recent evidence on the management of bronchiolitis. Curr Opin Pediatr. 2014 Jun;26(3):328-33. https://doi.org/10.1097/MOP.0000000000000090. PMID: 24739493. http://www.ncbi.nlm.nih.gov/pubmed/24739493 **

Nicolai A, Ferrara M, Schiavariello C, Gentile F, Grande ME, Alessandroni C, Midulla F. Viral bronchiolitis in children: a common condition with few therapeutic options. Early Hum Dev. 2013 Oct;89 Suppl 3:S7-11. https://doi.org/10.1016/j.earlhumdev.2013.07.016. PMID: 23972293. http://www.ncbi.nlm.nih.gov/pubmed/23972293 **

Teshome G, Gattu R, Brown R. Acute bronchiolitis. Pediatr Clin North Am. 2013 Oct;60(5):1019-34. https://doi.org/10.1016/j.pcl.2013.06.005. PMID: 24093893. http://www.ncbi.nlm.nih.gov/pubmed/24093893 **

Papiris SA, Malagari K, Manali ED, Kolilekas L, Triantafillidou C, Baou K, Rontogianni D, Bouros D, Kagouridis K. Bronchiolitis: adopting a unifying definition and a comprehensive etiological classification. Expert Rev Respir Med. 2013 Jun;7(3):289-306. https://doi.org/10.1586/ers.13.21. PMID: 23734650. http://www.ncbi.nlm.nih.gov/pubmed/23734650 **

Garibaldi BT, Illei P, Danoff SK. Bronchiolitis. Immunol Allergy Clin North Am. 2012 Nov;32(4):601-19. https://doi.org/10.1016/j.iac.2012.08.002. PMID: 23102068. http://www.ncbi.nlm.nih.gov/pubmed/23102068 **

Williams C, Bartram T. Towards evidence based emergency medicine: best BETs from the Manchester Royal Infirmary. BET 4: Chest x-rays in bronchiolitis. Emerg Med J. 2012 Jun;29(6):514-5. https://doi.org/10.1136/emermed-2012-201374.5. PMID: 22635392. http://www.ncbi.nlm.nih.gov/pubmed/22635392 **

Use PubMed Clinical Queries to find the most recent evidence. Use this search strategy:

"Bronchiolitis"[Mesh] OR "Bronchiolitis"

Chapter 16
Carbon Monoxide Poisoning

Charles V. Pollack, Jr., Melissa Platt, Richard M. Cantor, Victoria G. Riese, and Jaime Friel Blanck

Name and Synonyms

Carbon Monoxide (CO) Poisoning

Incidence/Epidemiology

- CO poisoning is responsible for up to 40,000 emergency department visits and 5000 to 6000 deaths a year.
- CO poisoning is unintentional in about 500 cases annually, whereas the rate of intentional poisoning is 10 times higher.
- The case-fatality rate ranges from 0 % to 31 %.

C. V. Pollack, Jr. (✉)
Department of Emergency Medicine, Thomas Jefferson University, Philadelphia, PA, USA

M. Platt
Department of Emergency Medicine, University of Louisville, Louisville, KY, USA

R. M. Cantor
Department of Emergency Medicine and Pediatrics, State University of New York Upstate Medical University, Syracuse, NY, USA

V. G. Riese
Librarian Consultant, Eldersburg, MD, USA

J. F. Blanck
Welch Medical Library, Johns Hopkins University, Baltimore, MD, USA

C. V. Pollack, Jr. (ed.), *Differential Diagnosis of Cardiopulmonary Disease*,
https://doi.org/10.1007/978-3-319-63895-9_16

Differential Diagnosis

- Acute respiratory distress syndrome
- Depression and suicide
- Diabetic ketoacidosis
- Encephalitis
- Gastroenteritis
- Headache, tension
- Hypothyroidism and myxedema coma
- Labyrinthitis
- Lactic acidosis
- Meningitis
- Methemoglobinemia
- Migraine headache
- Pediatrics, hypoglycemia
- Toxicity, alcohols
- Toxicity, narcotics

Pathophysiology and Etiology

- CO is an odorless, tasteless, colorless, nonirritating gas formed by hydrocarbon combustion. It binds to hemoglobin and diminishes the ability to absorb oxygen.
- CO poisoning interferes with oxygen transport to the cells and possibly results in electron transport failure.
- CO combines preferentially with hemoglobin to produce carboxyhemoglobin (COHb), displacing oxygen and reducing systemic arterial oxygen.
- CO poisoning may cause tissue hypoxia and impair tissue perfusion.
- Exogenous sources of CO include the following:
    - Smoke inhalation
    - Poorly functioning heating systems
    - Improperly vented fuel-burning devices
    - Motor vehicles in poorly vented areas
    - Open-air motorboat exhaust
    - Underground electrical cable fires
    - Spray paints and solvents—methylene chloride
    - Wood stoves
    - Tobacco smoke

Presentation

Typical/"Classic"

- Highly variable and nonspecific
- Mild to moderate poisoning: headache, malaise, nausea, dizziness, weakness, vomiting, blurred vision, and shortness of breath
- Severe CO toxicity: seizures, syncope, coma, myocardial ischemia, ventricular arrhythmias, pulmonary edema, and profound lactic acidosis

Atypical

- Unexplained alteration in mental status

Primary Differential Considerations

Consistent with the presentation of CO toxicity, the following differential diagnoses also may apply:

- Sepsis
- Intoxication
- Ketoacidosis
- Hypoglycemia
- Atypical migraine
- Viral syndrome

History and Physical Exam

Findings That Confirm Diagnosis

- There are no physical exam findings that confirm the diagnosis of CO poisoning.

Factors That Suggest Diagnosis

- History and physical exam with headache, nausea, vomiting
- Acute infarction in the globus pallidus bilaterally

- Other forms of pure hypoxia produce similar findings.
- "Cherry red" appearance of lips and skin (a late finding)

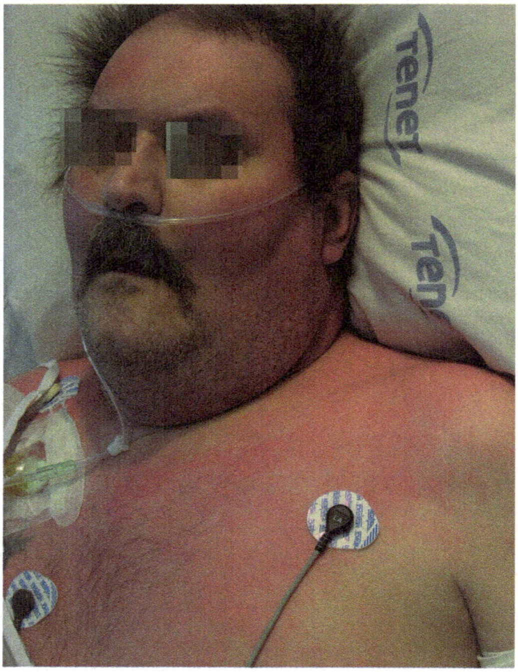

The cheeks and neck are red in this patient with carbon monoxide poisoning. [Allen HB. Dermatology terminology [Internet]. London: Springer; 2010. Chapter 8, Miscellaneous disorders; [cited 2015 Sep 9]; p. 171–85. Available from: http://link.springer.com/10.1007/978-1-84882-840-7_8] *Caption from original*

Carboxyhemoglobin saturation (%)	Signs and symptoms
5–10	Visual acuity impairment
11–20	Flushing, headache
21–30	Nausea, impaired dexterity
31–40	Vomiting, dizziness, syncope
41–50	Tachypnea, tachycardia
>50	Coma, death

Signs and symptoms of carbon monoxide poisoning [Knighton J. Nursing management of the burn-injured person. In: Jeschke MG, Kamolz L-P, Shahrokhi S, editors. Burn care and treatment [Internet]. Vienna: Springer; 2013 [cited 2015 Sep 9]. p. 111–47. Available from: http://link.springer.com/10.1007/978-3-7091-1133-8_8] *Caption from original*

COHb concentration	Symptoms
Up to 10 %	No significant symptoms (smoker)
10–15 %	Possible shortness of breath on physical exertion (heavy smoker)
15–25 %	Usually no effects when resting, but shortness of breath on physical exertion
25–35 %	Headache, dizziness, vomiting, impaired judgement, impaired vision
35–45 %	Confusion, signs of paralysis, syncope on mild exertion
45–55 %	Severely impaired consciousness or loss of consciousness, collapse, life-threatening situation after prolonged exposure
55–65 %	Cramps, apnea
From ca. 65 %	Imminent threat of death

Stages of carbon monoxide poisoning [Dettmeyer RB, Verhoff MA, Schütz HF. Forensic medicine [Internet]. Berlin, Heidelberg: Springer; 2014. Chapter 30, Forensic toxicology; [cited 2015 Sep 9]; p. 495–542. Available from: http://link.springer.com/10.1007/978-3-642-38818-7_30] *Caption from original*

Factors That Exclude Diagnosis

The only way to exclude CO toxicity definitively is with an arterial blood gas panel with co-oximetry.

Ancillary Studies

Laboratory

- Elevated COHb level
  - Nonsmokers may have up to 3 %, smokers 10 % to 15 %. Anything above these levels may be considered CO poisoning.
- In CO poisoning as a result of suicide attempt, a drug screen should also be obtained.

Electrocardiography

- Sinus tachycardia/arrhythmias/myocardial injury

Computed Tomography (CT) of the brain

- Hypoattenuation of the globus pallidus and white matter changes

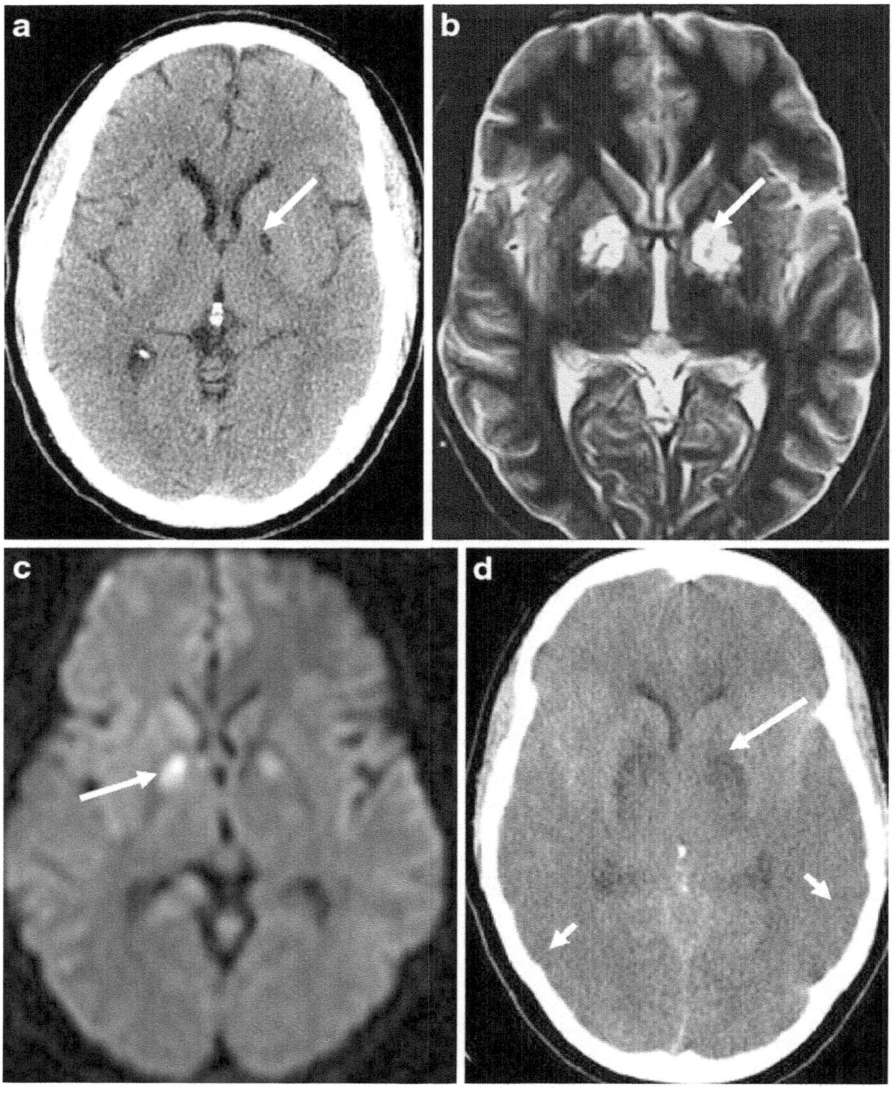

Four different patients with history of carbon monoxide poisoning. a Noncontrast head CT shows focal low density in bilateral globus pallidus (arrows). b Transaxial T2 weighted image shows bilateral symmetric hyperintensity involving globus pallidus (arrows). c DWI shows bilateral pallidal diffusion restriction (arrows). d Noncontrast head CT shows diffuse anoxic injury (short arrows) in addition to the basal ganglia hypodensities (long arrow) [Moore MJ, Vagal AS, Strub WM, Leach JL. Reducing the gray zone: imaging spectrum of hypoperfusion and hypoxic brain injury in adults. Emerg Radiol. 2010 Mar;17(2):123–30.] *Caption from original*

Special Populations

Age

- Older patients with limited cardiopulmonary reserve may develop clinical manifestations at lower CoHb levels.

Co-morbidities

- Pregnancy
  - The fetus is particularly sensitive to hypoxemia, so both mother and child are at significant risk.
- Patients with preexisting lung disease are affected more severely by CO-induced hypoxemia.

Pediatric Considerations

- Signs and symptoms may be subtle and nonspecific.
- Infants and toddlers may have fussiness and difficulty feeding.
- Signs and symptoms in older children are similar to those in adults: headache, nausea, and vomiting.
- Younger children experience problems earlier in exposure because of of higher rates of oxygen utilization and minute ventilation.

Pitfalls in Diagnosis

Critical Steps Not to Miss

- Without the patient's history, CO toxicity may be difficult to diagnosis. Standard pulse oximetry cannot screen for CO exposure.

- All individuals at a fire scene and/or with significant thermal injury should be evaluated for CO poisoning.

Mimics

- Most common misdiagnosis is viral syndrome.
- Very high or very low blood glucose levels may present similarly to CO toxicity.

Time-Dependent Interventions

- CO poisoning is associated with high morbidity and mortality. In the absence of exposure history, CO poisoning must be considered in two or more patients who present with similar symptoms simultaneously.
- Oxygen therapy should be started while COHb tests results are pending.
- Hyperbaric oxygen (HBO) therapy, if available, should be considered, especially in cases of severe exposure and in pregnant patients.

Overall Principles of Treatment

- 100 % oxygen therapy is the main treatment for CO poisoning.
- HBO is indicated in anyone who experienced unconsciousness, cardiovascular instability or ischemia, persistent mental and/or neurologic deficits, or a COHb level greater than 25 %.
    - HBO may help the late neurocognitive outcomes.
- HBO should be considered in pregnant patients with elevated COHb levels.

Disease Course

- Outcomes are difficult to predict, even when the CO level is known. Patients with cardiac arrest or coma may recover fully after treatment. The mortality rate in severe CO toxicity is 33 % or higher.

Related Evidence

Papers of particular interest have been highlighted as:
*** Of key importance*

Practice Guideline

Wolf SJ, Lavonas EJ, Sloan EP, Jagoda AS; American College of Emergency Physicians. Clinical policy: critical issues in the management of adult patients presenting to the emergency department with acute carbon monoxide poisoning. Ann Emerg Med. 2008 Feb;51(2):138-52. https://doi.org/10.1016/j.annemergmed.2007.10.012. PMID: 18206551. http://www.ncbi.nlm.nih.gov/pubmed/18206551 **

Review

Betterman K, Patel S. Neurologic complications of carbon monoxide intoxication. Handb Clin Neurol. 2014;120:971-9. https://doi.org/10.1016/B978-0-7020-4087-0.00064-4. PMID: 24365364. http://www.ncbi.nlm.nih.gov/pubmed/24365364 **

Kurt F, Bektaş Ö, Kalkan G, Öncel MY, Yakut HI, Kocabaş CN. Does age affect presenting symptoms in children with carbon monoxide poisoning? Pediatr Emerg Care. 2013 Aug;29(8):916-21. https://doi.org/10.1097/PEC.0b013e31829ec22b. PubMed PMID: 23903672. http://www.ncbi.nlm.nih.gov/pubmed/23903672

Huzar TF, George T, Cross JM. Carbon monoxide and cyanide toxicity: etiology, pathophysiology and treatment in inhalation injury. Expert Rev Respir Med. 2013 Apr;7(2):159-70. https://doi.org/10.1586/ers.13.9. PMID: 23547992. http://www.ncbi.nlm.nih.gov/pubmed/23547992 **

Guzman JA. Carbon monoxide poisoning. Crit Care Clin. 2012 Oct;28(4):537-48. https://doi.org/10.1016/j.ccc.2012.07.007. PMID: 22998990. http://www.ncbi.nlm.nih.gov/pubmed/22998990 **

Iqbal S, Clower JH, Hernandez SA, Damon SA, Yip FY. A review of disaster-related carbon monoxide poisoning: surveillance, epidemiology, and opportunities for prevention. Am J Public Health. 2012 Oct;102(10):1957-63. PMID: 22897556. http://www.ncbi.nlm.nih.gov/pubmed/22897556 **

Hampson NB, Piantadosi CA, Thom SR, Weaver LK. Practice recommendations in the diagnosis, management, and prevention of carbon monoxide poisoning. Am J Respir Crit Care Med. 2012 Dec 1;186(11):1095-101. https://doi.org/10.1164/rccm.201207-1284CI. PMID: 23087025. http://www.ncbi.nlm.nih.gov/pubmed/23087025 **

Buckley NA, Juurlink DN, Isbister G, Bennett MH, Lavonas EJ. Hyperbaric oxygen for carbon monoxide poisoning. Cochrane Database Syst Rev. 2011 Apr

13;(4):CD002041. https://doi.org/10.1002/14651858.CD002041.pub3. PMID: 21491385. http://www.ncbi.nlm.nih.gov/pubmed/21491385 **

Smollin C, Olson K. Carbon monoxide poisoning (acute). Clin Evid (Online). 2010 Oct 12;2010. pii: 2103. PMID: 21418677. http://www.ncbi.nlm.nih.gov/pubmed/21418677 **

Weaver LK. Clinical practice. Carbon monoxide poisoning. N Engl J Med. 2009 Mar 19;360(12):1217-25. https://doi.org/10.1056/NEJMcp0808891. PMID: 19297574. http://www.ncbi.nlm.nih.gov/pubmed/19297574 **

Cho CH, Chiu NC, Ho CS, Peng CC. Carbon monoxide poisoning in children. Pediatr Neonatol. 2008 Aug;49(4):121-5. https://doi.org/10.1016/S1875-9572(08)60026-1. PMID: 19054917. http://www.ncbi.nlm.nih.gov/pubmed/19054917 **

Cohort Study

Kurt F, Bektaş Ö, Kalkan G, Öncel MY, Yakut HI, Kocabaş CN. Does age affect presenting symptoms in children with carbon monoxide poisoning? Pediatr Emerg Care. 2013 Aug;29(8):916-21. https://doi.org/10.1097/PEC.0b013e31829ec22b. PMID: 23903672. http://www.ncbi.nlm.nih.gov/pubmed/23903672

Use PubMed Clinical Queries to find the most recent evidence. Use this search strategy: "Carbon Monoxide Poisoning"[Mesh] OR "carbon monoxide poisoning"

Chapter 17
Chest Neoplasms

Christopher J. Rees, Charles V. Pollack, Jr., and Victoria G. Riese

Name and Synonyms

Chest Neoplasms

Incidence/Epidemiology

- The incidence of chest neoplasm varies widely by tumor type.
- Chest neoplasms are of much higher incidence in adults.
- Over large populations, chest neoplasia incidence follows tobacco abuse patterns and therefore is more common in older males.
- In women, lung and breast tumors are most common.
- Metastases of colon cancer to the thorax are not uncommon.

Differential Diagnosis

- Many neoplasms may present as chest masses.
- They may be either benign or malignant lesions.

C. J. Rees
Emergency Department, Pennsylvania Hospital, Philadelphia, PA, USA

C. V. Pollack, Jr. (✉)
Department of Emergency Medicine, Thomas Jefferson University, Philadelphia, PA, USA

V. G. Riese
Librarian Consultant, Eldersburg, MD, USA

C. V. Pollack, Jr. (ed.), *Differential Diagnosis of Cardiopulmonary Disease*,
https://doi.org/10.1007/978-3-319-63895-9_17

- There are primary chest masses and secondary masses. Secondary masses are metastatic lesions that have primary tumors somewhere other than the chest.
- Primary tumors of the chest include:
  - Breast cancer
  - Lung cancer
  - Esophageal cancer
  - Primary cardiac tumors
  - Primary tumors of the ribs and spine
  - Soft tissue sarcomas
  - Mesothelioma
  - Multiple myeloma
  - Lymphoid tumors
- Many different types of tumors can metastasize to the chest.

Pathophysiology and Etiology

- Pathophysiology varies based on primary vs metastatic etiology, and invasive vs more benign tissue types.
- There are behavioral (e.g., smoking) and genetic (e.g., BRAC1 gene) predispositions to chest tumors.

Presentation

Typical/"Classic"

- Tumors within the chest are often asymptomatic.
- They are most commonly found during diagnostic studies for other reasons.
- Symptoms, if present, are usually the result of direct compression from tumors or direct infiltration into surrounding structures. If the surrounding structures infiltrated are blood vessels, hemoptysis may result.
- Lymphoproliferative tumors often cause constitutional symptoms.
- Bronchogenic carcinoma may present as a postobstructive pneumonia.
- Breast or chest wall tumors may be palpable or painful, prompting presentation.

Atypical

- Fulminant presentations with respiratory insufficiency or massive hemoptysis are unusual.
- Vague constitutional symptoms, such as nagging cough and weight loss, may be presenting symptoms.

Primary Differential Considerations

Prompt consideration also should be given to the possible diagnosis of:

- Pneumonia and other infectious etiologies
- Thymus enlargement
- Pneumoconiosis
- Pulmonary nodule

History and Physical Exam

Findings That Confirm Diagnosis

- The diagnosis is usually confirmed only through pathologic interpretation of biopsy specimens.

Factors That Suggest Diagnosis

- These are often asymptomatic and found incidentally when performing diagnostic imaging studies for other reasons.

Factors That Exclude Diagnosis

- Advanced imaging studies (CT, MRI) can exclude masses of significance.

Ancillary Studies

Laboratory

- Laboratory studies are sometimes helpful in evaluating chest masses. There may be evidence of lymphoproliferative disorders on a complete blood count. Multiple myeloma is often associated with anemia, renal insufficiency, hypercalcemia, and an anion gap less than 5.

Imaging

- Most chest neoplasms are found incidentally during diagnostic imaging of the chest for other reasons.

- They most often are discovered on either plain chest x-ray or CT scan of the chest.
- Primary cardiac lesions may be found on echocardiogram

Special Populations

Age

- Chest neoplasms may occur in any age group.

Co-morbidities

- There are many potential co-morbidities to consider depending on the specific type of neoplasm. COPD is often present in patients with bronchogenic carcinoma.
- Thymus mass (thymoma) is associated with myasthenia gravis in about one-half of cases.

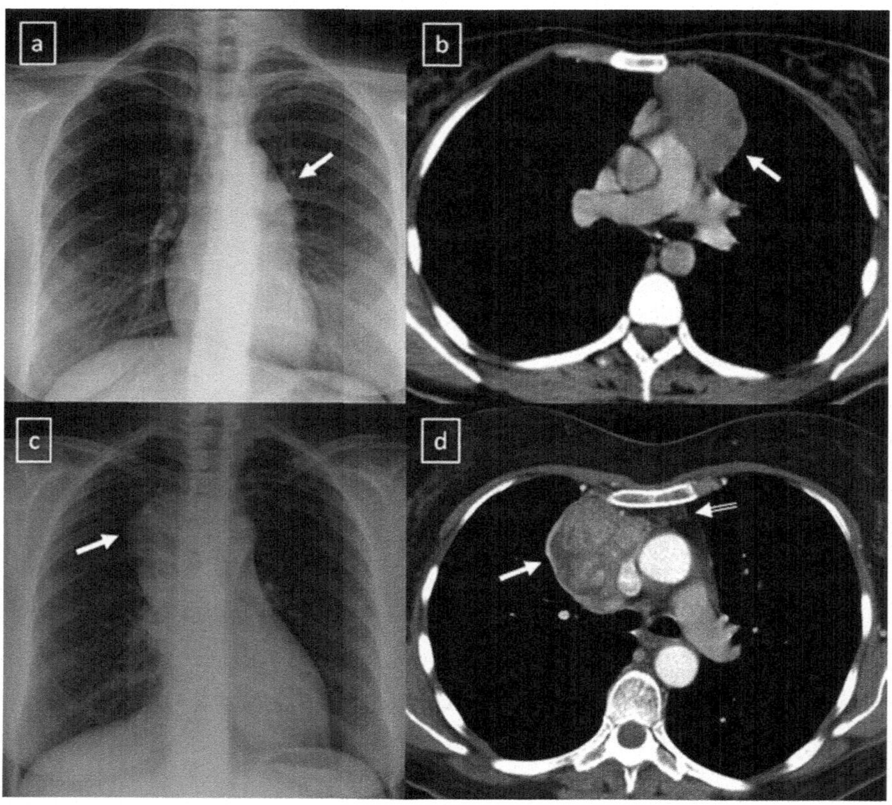

a, b Stage II thymoma (WHO type B1) in a 33-year-old woman who presented with myasthenia gravis. Frontal chest radiograph shows a hilum overlay sign (arrow) of a suggestive anterior mediastinal mass. Contrast-enhanced CT scan confirms the presence of a low-heterogeneous anterior mediastinal mass (arrow). Note the indentation of the arterial trunk pulmonary by the mass. c, d Stage III thymoma (WHO type B2) in a 54-year-old woman. Frontal chest radiograph reveals a lobulated mediastinal mass (arrow) on the right side. Contrast-enhanced CT scan demonstrates an enhanced anterior mediastinal mass (arrow) with infiltration of surrounding fat (open arrow) [From article: A diagnostic approach to the mediastinal masses. Insights into Imaging. 2013 Feb;4(1):29–52. https://doi.org/10.1007/s13244-012-0201-0, at http://link.springer.com/article/10.1007%2Fs13244-012-0201-0/fulltext.html; by Sergi Juanpere, Noemí Cañete, Pedro Ortuño, Sandra Martínez, Gloria Sanchez, Lluis Bernado, © The Author(s) 2012; licensed under Creative Commons Attribution License BY 2.0 http://creativecommons.org/licenses/by/2.0] *Caption from original*

Pitfalls in Diagnosis

Critical Steps Not to Miss

- A thorough medical history and chest imaging are essential early in the evaluation of a chest tumor

Mimics

- Infection is the primary mimic of neoplasms in the chest

Time-Dependent Interventions

- Ensuring adequate oxygenation
- Imaging to establish likely etiology

Overall Principles of Treatment

- Treatment depends on the type of neoplasm and whether any symptomatic obstruction or compression exists.

Disease Course

- Disease course depends on the specific diagnosis.

Related Evidence

Papers of particular interest have been highlighted as:
*** Of key importance*

Practice Guideline

Rivera MP, Mehta AC, Wahidi MM. Establishing the diagnosis of lung cancer: Diagnosis and management of lung cancer, 3rd ed: American College of Chest Physicians evidence-based clinical practice guidelines. Chest. 2013 May;143(5 Suppl):e142S-65S. https://doi.org/10.1378/chest.12-2353. PMID: 23649436. http://www.ncbi.nlm.nih.gov/pubmed/23649436 **

Moreau P, San Miguel J, Ludwig H, Schouten H, Mohty M, Dimopoulos M, Dreyling M; ESMO Guidelines Working Group. Multiple myeloma: ESMO Clinical Practice Guidelines for diagnosis, treatment and follow-up. Ann Oncol. 2013 Oct;24 Suppl 6:vi133-7. https://doi.org/10.1093/annonc/mdt297. PMID: 23956208. http://www.ncbi.nlm.nih.gov/pubmed/23956208 **

Senkus E, Kyriakides S, Penault-Llorca F, Poortmans P, Thompson A, Zackrisson S, Cardoso F; ESMO Guidelines Working Group. Primary breast cancer: ESMO Clinical Practice Guidelines for diagnosis, treatment and follow-up. Ann Oncol. 2013 Oct;24 Suppl 6:vi7-23. https://doi.org/10.1093/annonc/mdt284. PMID: 23970019. http://www.ncbi.nlm.nih.gov/pubmed/23970019 **

Ettinger DS, Akerley W, Borghaei H, Chang A, Cheney RT, Chirieac LR, D'Amico TA, Demmy TL, Ganti AK, Govindan R, Grannis FW, Horn L, Jahan TM, Jahanzeb M, Kessinger A, Komaki R, Kong FM, Kris MG, Krug LM, Lennes IT, Loo BW, Martins R, O'Malley J, Osarogiagbon RU, Otterson GA, Patel JD, Schenck MP, Pisters KM, Reckamp K, Riely GJ, Rohren E, Swanson SJ, Wood DE, Yang SC; National Comprehensive Cancer Network. Malignant pleural mesothelioma. J Natl Compr Canc Netw. 2012 Jan;10(1):26-41. PMID: 22223867. http://www.ncbi.nlm.nih.gov/pubmed/22223867 **

Ray CE Jr, English B, Funaki BS, Burke CT, Fidelman N, Ginsburg ME, Kinney TB, Kostelic JK, Kouri BE, Lorenz JM, Nair AV, Nemcek AA Jr, Owens CA, Saleh AG, Vatakencherry G, Mohammed TL. ACR appropriateness criteria® radiologic management of thoracic nodules and masses. J Am Coll Radiol. 2012 Jan;9(1):13-9. https://doi.org/10.1016/j.jacr.2011.09.013. PMID 22221631. http://www.ncbi.nlm.nih.gov/pubmed/22221631 **

Zelenetz AD, Abramson JS, Advani RH, Andreadis CB, Bartlett N, Bellam N, Byrd JC, Czuczman MS, Fayad LE, Glenn MJ, Gockerman JP, Gordon LI, Harris NL, Hoppe RT, Horwitz SM, Kelsey CR, Kim YH, LaCasce AS, Nademanee A, Porcu P, Press O, Pro B, Reddy N, Sokol L, Swinnen LJ, Tsien C, Vose JM, Wierda WG, Yahalom J, Zafar N. Non-Hodgkin's lymphomas. J Natl Compr Canc Netw. 2011 May;9(5):484-560. PMID: 21550968. http://www.ncbi.nlm.nih.gov/pubmed/21550968 **

Demetri GD, Antonia S, Benjamin RS, Bui MM, Casper ES, Conrad EU 3rd, DeLaney TF, Ganjoo KN, Heslin MJ, Hutchinson RJ, Kane JM 3rd, Letson GD, McGarry SV, O'Donnell RJ, Paz IB, Pfeifer JD, Pollock RE, Randall RL, Riedel RF, Schupak KD, Schwartz HS, Thornton K, von Mehren M, Wayne J; National Comprehensive Cancer Network Soft Tissue Sarcoma Panel. Soft tissue sarcoma. J Natl Compr Canc Netw. 2010 Jun;8(6):630-74. PMID: 20581298. http://www.ncbi.nlm.nih.gov/pubmed/20581298 **

Stahl M, Budach W, Meyer HJ, Cervantes A; ESMO Guidelines Working Group. Esophageal cancer: Clinical Practice Guidelines for diagnosis, treatment and follow-up. Ann Oncol. 2010 May;21 Suppl 5:v46-9. https://doi.org/10.1093/annonc/mdq163. PMID: 20555101. http://www.ncbi.nlm.nih.gov/pubmed/20555101 **

Review

Mirrielees JA, Kapur JH, Szalkucki LM, Harter JM, Salkowski LR, Strigel RM, Traynor AM, Wilke LG. Metastasis of primary lung carcinoma to the breast: a systematic review of the literature. J Surg Res. 2014 May 15;188(2):419-31. https://doi.org/10.1016/j.jss.2014.01.024. PMID: 24560348. http://www.ncbi.nlm.nih.gov/pubmed/24560348 **

Kurihara Y, Matsuoka S, Yamashiro T, Fujikawa A, Matsushita S, Yagihashi K, Nakajima Y. MRI of pulmonary nodules. AJR Am J Roentgenol. 2014 Mar;202(3):W210-6. https://doi.org/10.2214/AJR.13.11618. PMID: 24555616. http://www.ncbi.nlm.nih.gov/pubmed/24555616

Mechtler LL, Nandigam K. Spinal cord tumors: new views and future directions. Neurol Clin. 2013 Feb;31(1):241-68. https://doi.org/10.1016/j.ncl.2012.09.011. PMID: 23186903. http://www.ncbi.nlm.nih.gov/pubmed/23186903 **

Lamba G, Frishman WH. Cardiac and pericardial tumors. Cardiol Rev. 2012 Sep-Oct;20(5):237-52. https://doi.org/10.1097/CRD.0b013e31825603e7. PMID: 22447042. http://www.ncbi.nlm.nih.gov/pubmed/22447042 **

Restrepo CS, Chen MM, Martinez-Jimenez S, Carrillo J, Restrepo C. Chest neoplasms with infectious etiologies. World J Radiol. 2011 Dec 28;3(12):279-88. https://doi.org/10.4329/wjr.v3.i12.279. PMID: 22224176. http://www.ncbi.nlm.nih.gov/pubmed/22224176 **

Leja MJ, Shah DJ, Reardon MJ. Primary cardiac tumors. Tex Heart Inst J. 2011;38(3):261-2. PMID: 21720466. http://www.ncbi.nlm.nih.gov/pubmed/21720466 **

Smith SE, Keshavjee S. Primary chest wall tumors. Thorac Surg Clin. 2010 Nov;20(4):495-507. https://doi.org/10.1016/j.thorsurg.2010.07.003. PMID: 20974433. http://www.ncbi.nlm.nih.gov/pubmed/20974433 **

Cohort Study

Sakellaridis T, Gaitanakis S, Piyis A. Rib tumors: a 15-year experience. Gen Thorac Cardiovasc Surg. 2014 Jul;62(7):434-40. https://doi.org/10.1007/s11748-014-0387-9. PMID: 24615297. http://www.ncbi.nlm.nih.gov/pubmed/24615297 **

Use PubMed Clinical Queries to find the most recent evidence. Use this search strategy:

"Thoracic Neoplasms"[Mesh] OR "Breast Neoplasms"[Mesh] OR "Esophageal Neoplasms"[Mesh] OR "Spinal Neoplasms"[Mesh] OR "Sarcoma"[Mesh] OR "Mesothelioma"[Mesh] OR "Multiple Myeloma"[Mesh] OR "Lymphoma"[Mesh]

Chapter 18
Chronic Obstructive Pulmonary Disease

Christopher J. Rees, Charles V. Pollack, Jr., and Victoria G. Riese

Name and Synonyms

Chronic Obstructive Pulmonary Disease; COPD; Emphysema

Incidence/Epidemiology

- COPD affects about 5 % of the U.S. population.
- COPD is reported as the third- or fourth-leading cause of death in the U.S, depending upon the survey. COPD is directly responsible for about 120,000 deaths per year in the U.S.
- COPD is associated with a very high rate of medical resource utilization. The majority of these costs are for hospitalization of acute exacerbations of COPD.
- In the U.S., nearly 2 % of all hospital admissions are directly attributable to COPD. It is considered a major contributing factor in another 9 % of hospital admissions. In patients older than 65, the percentage of all hospital admission related to COPD approaches 20 %.
- COPD is the only major cause of death that is increasing in the U.S.

C. J. Rees
Emergency Department, Pennsylvania Hospital, Philadelphia, PA, USA

C. V. Pollack, Jr. (✉)
Department of Emergency Medicine, Thomas Jefferson University, Philadelphia, PA, USA

V. G. Riese
Librarian Consultant, Eldersburg, MD, USA

C. V. Pollack, Jr. (ed.), *Differential Diagnosis of Cardiopulmonary Disease*,
https://doi.org/10.1007/978-3-319-63895-9_18

- The incidence and mortality of COPD in women is increasing worldwide. This is likely related to the increased incidence of smoking among women during the last 50 years.
- Tobacco smoke is the major risk factor for developing COPD, but only 15 % of smokers will develop COPD.
- Alpha-1 antitrypsin deficiency accounts for less than 1 % of COPD cases.

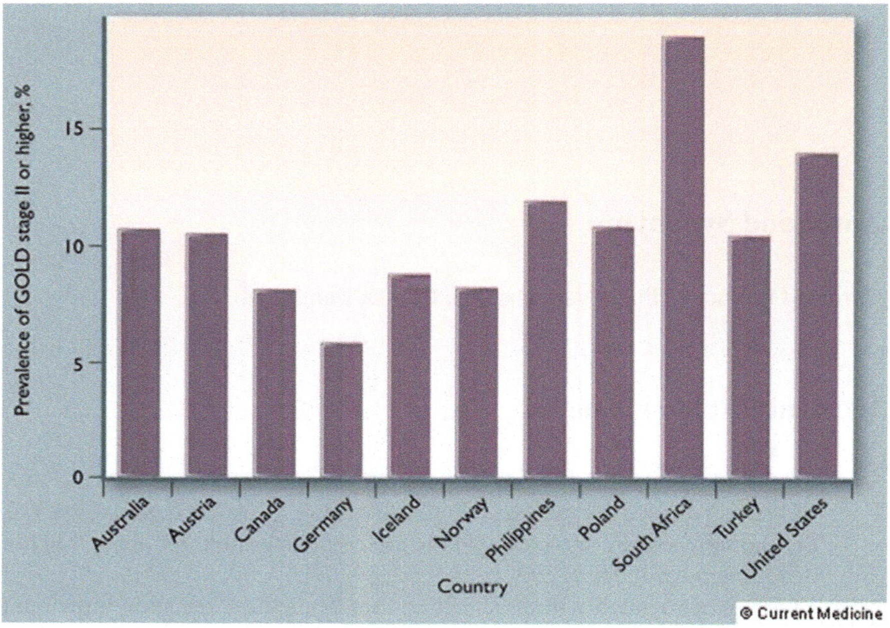

Worldwide prevalence of chronic obstructive pulmonary disease (COPD). The prevalence of COPD (in 2007) in different geographic regions based on the Burden of Obstructive Lung Disease data [Buist AS, McBurnie MA, Vollmer WM, et al. International variation in the prevalence of COPD (the BOLD Study): a population-based prevalence study. Lancet. 2007; 370:741 -750.] is presented based on results for specific cities within the countries listed. The reasons for these regional differences are not entirely clear and may be due to different environmental exposures (smoking, biomass, occupation), as well as possibly genetic factors. [Cho M, Silverman E. Genetics and Racial, Ethnic, and Gender Characteristics of COPD. In: Crapo JD, editor. Atlas of Chronic Obstructive Pulmonary Disease. Philadelphia, PA: Current Medicine Group; 2009. 160 p. ISBN: 978-1-57340-294-1] *Caption from original*

Differential Diagnosis

- The primary symptoms of COPD are dyspnea (usually exertional early in the disease course), cough, and sputum production.

- The differential diagnosis of these symptoms is broad, and includes many diseases and organ symptoms.
- Patients may present with worsening fatigue, exercise or activity intolerance, and often complain of daily cough for many months.
- In patients without a current diagnosis of COPD, the differential includes:
  - Congestive heart failure
  - Interstitial lung disease
  - Thromboembolic Disease (pulmonary embolism)
  - Asthma
  - Bronchiectasis
  - Tuberculosis
  - Bronchiolitis
  - Airway obstruction from bronchogenic or metastatic cancer, lymphadenopathy (sarcoidosis), and tracheal stenosis/scarring.
- It is important to remember that many of these disorders can occur together.
- In patients with an existing diagnosis of COPD, who present with acute dyspnea (exacerbation of COPD), the cause of the exacerbation needs to be investigated. The differential for acute dyspnea in these patients is also broad, and includes:
  - CHF/pulmonary edema
  - Acute coronary syndrome
  - Pneumonia
  - Viral respiratory infection
  - Pulmonary embolism
  - Pleural effusion
  - Pneumothorax
  - Pericardial effusion
  - Mucous plugging of bronchi
  - Rib fracture from severe coughing
  - Electrolyte imbalance (especially hypokalemia and hypocalcemia)

Pathophysiology and Etiology

- Chronic obstructive pulmonary disease (COPD) is a disease characterized by chronic, progressive airflow obstruction.
- The Global Initiative for Chronic Obstructive Lung Disease (GOLD), sponsored by the National Heart, Lung, and Blood Institute (NHLBI) and the World Health Organization (WHO), defines COPD as follows: "Chronic obstructive pulmonary disease (COPD), a common preventable and treatable disease, is characterized by airflow limitation that is usually progressive and associated with an enhanced chronic inflammatory response in the airways and the lung to noxious particles or gases. Exacerbations and comorbidities contribute to the overall severity in individual patients."

Global Initiative for Chronic Obstructive Lung Disease, GOLD [3]: $FEV_1/FVC < 70\%$		
I:	Mild COPD	$FEV_1 \geq 80\%$ predicted
II:	Moderate COPD	FEV_1 50- < 80% predicted
III:	Severe COPD	FEV_1 30- < 50% predicted
IV:	Very severe COPD	FEV_1 < 30% predicted
British Thoracic Society, BTS [2]: $FEV_1/VC < 70\%$ and $FEV_1 < 80\%$ predicted		
I:	Mild COPD	FEV_1 60- < 80% predicted
II:	Moderate COPD	FEV_1 40-59% predicted
III:	Severe COPD	FEV_1 < 40% predicted

A group labelled BTS stage 0 was created for subjects with $FEV_1 \geq 80\%$ predicted: i.e. identical with mild COPD according to the GOLD criteria.

Severity criteria of COPD. [3] BTS: BTS guidelines for the management of chronic obstructive pulmonary disease. The COPD Guidelines Group of the Standards of Care Committee of the BTS. Thorax 1997, 52:S1-28. [2] Pauwels RA, Buist AS, Calverley PMA, Jenkins CR, Hurd SS: Global strategy for the diagnosis, management, and prevention of chronic obstructive pulmonary disease: NHLBI and WHO Global Initiative for Chronic Obstructive Lung Disease (GOLD): executive summary. Respiratory Care 2001, 46:798-825. [From article: Health-related quality of life is related to COPD disease severity. Health and Quality of Life Outcomes. 2005 Sep 9;3(1):56. https://doi.org/10.1186/1477-7525-3-56, at http://link.springer.com/article/10.1186%2F1477-7525-3-56/fulltext.html; by Elisabeth Ståhl, Anne Lindberg, Sven-Arne Jansson, Eva Rönmark, Klas Svensson, Fredrik Andersson, Claes-Göran Löfdahl, Bo Lundbäck, © Ståhl et al; licensee BioMed Central Ltd. 2005; licensed under Creative Commons Attribution License BY 2.0 http://creativecommons.org/licenses/by/2.0]

- The pathophysiology of COPD involves the airways, lung parenchyma, and pulmonary vasculature.
  - Airways: The most significant pathologic change in the airways involves chronic inflammation from exposure to cigarette smoke and other pollutants, which leads to several permanent anatomic changes such as:
    - Mucous gland hyperplasia and increased numbers of goblet cells, resulting in increased mucous secretion. Increased mucous secretion and stasis leads to pathogenic bacterial colonization.
    - Increased mucous-secreting and goblet cells replace surfactant-secreting cells, which augments collapse and destruction of the small airways.
    - Increased induction of inflammatory cells with increased local protease production, accelerating tissue damage and breakdown.
    - Fibrosis with loss of elastic recoil, narrowing, collapse, and subsequent destruction and reduction in the number of small airways.
    - There is also squamous metaplasia within the airways resulting in an increased risk for cancer.

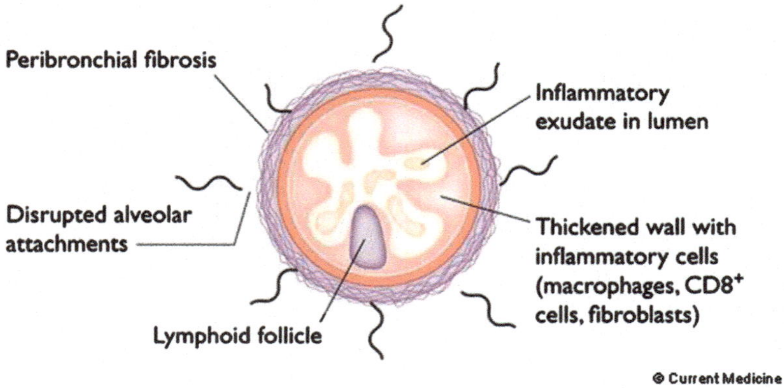

Overview of small airways in COPD: schematic view [Barnes PJ. Pathophysiology of COPD. In: Crapo JD, editor. Atlas of Chronic Obstructive Pulmonary Disease. Philadelphia, PA: Current Medicine Group; 2009. 160 p. ISBN: 978-1-57340-294-1] *Caption adapted from original*

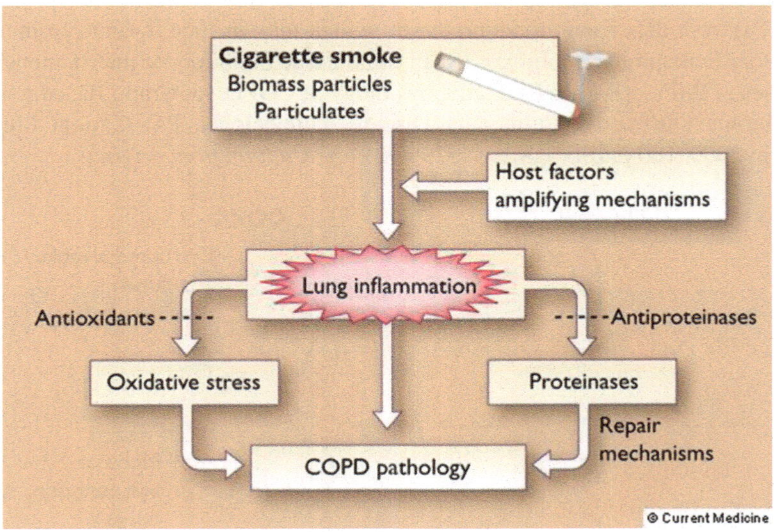

Link between inflammation and airway obstruction in chronic obstructive pulmonary disease (COPD). Chronic exposure to inhaled cigarette smoke and biomass particles (wood smoke) results in chronic inflammation of the lungs. Genetic and other unknown factors are responsible for the increased susceptibility to inhaled irritants. Inflammation generates reactive oxygen species (oxidative stress), which is normally counteracted by endogenous antioxidant mechanisms, but these may be defective in COPD. Inflammation also activates proteinases, which result in connective tissue destruction. This may be countered by antiproteinases and repair mechanisms that may also be defective in COPD.

[Barnes PJ. Pathophysiology of COPD. In: Crapo JD, editor. Atlas of Chronic Obstructive Pulmonary Disease. Philadelphia, PA: Current Medicine Group; 2009. 160 p. ISBN: 978-1-57340-294-1] *Caption from original*

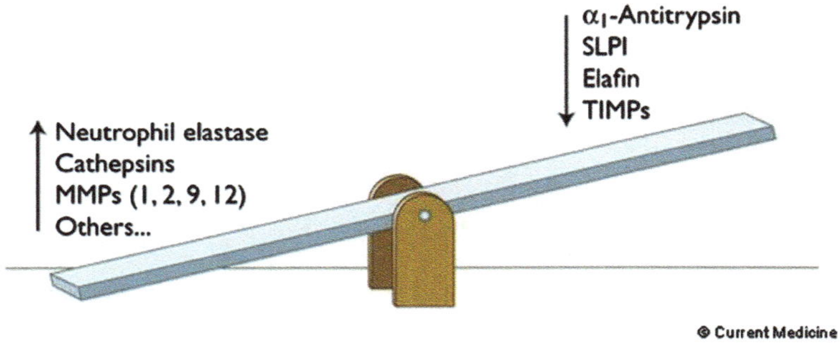

Protease-antiprotease imbalance in COPD: schematic view. Protease–antiprotease imbalance in chronic obstructive pulmonary disease (COPD). In COPD the balance appears to be tipped in favor of increased proteolysis, either because of an increase in proteases, including neutrophil elastase, cathepsins, and matrix metalloproteinases (MMPs), or a deficiency in antiproteases, which may include α_1-antitrypsin, elafin, secretory leukoprotease inhibitor (SLPI), and tissue inhibitors of matrix metalloproteinases (TIMPs). [Barnes PJ. Pathophysiology of COPD. In: Crapo JD, editor. Atlas of Chronic Obstructive Pulmonary Disease. Philadelphia, PA: Current Medicine Group; 2009. 160 p. ISBN: 978-1-57340-294-1] *Caption from original*

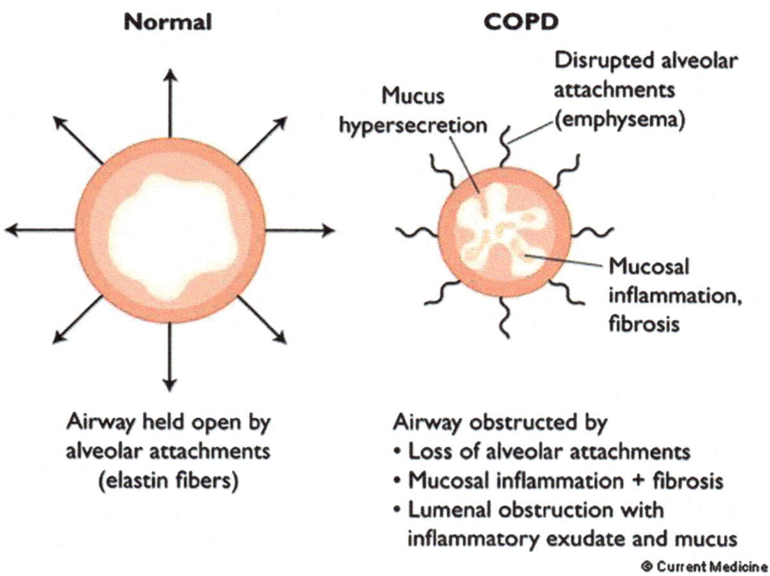

Mechanisms of airflow limitation in COPD: schematic view. Mechanisms of airflow limitation in chronic obstructive pulmonary disease (COPD). The airway in normal subjects is distended by alveolar attachments, which contain elastin fibers during expiration, allowing alveolar emptying and lung deflation. In COPD these attachments are disrupted due to emphysema, thus contributing to airway closure during expiration, trapping gas in the alveoli and resulting in hyperinflation. Peripheral airways are also obstructed and distorted by airway inflammation and peribronchiolar fibrosis (chronic obstructive bronchiolitis), and by occlusion of the airway lumen by inflammatory exudate and mucus secretions that may be trapped in the airways due to poor mucociliary clearance. [Barnes PJ. Pathophysiology of COPD. In: Crapo JD, editor. Atlas of Chronic Obstructive Pulmonary Disease. Philadelphia, PA: Current Medicine Group; 2009. 160 p. ISBN: 978-1-57340-294-1] *Caption from original*

- Lung Parenchyma. The lung parenchymal changes are also called emphysema. The changes mostly affect the acinus, the functional unit distal to the terminal bronchiole that includes the respiratory bronchiole, alveolar ducts, alveolar sacs, and alveoli. There is destruction of this unit leading initially to collapse and then subsequent enlargement as air becomes trapped within the destroyed unit. The loss of elastic recoil prevents the air from escaping. There are three subtypes of emphysema:
  - Centrilobular: This involves the proximal acinus (predominately the respiratory bronchioles.) It is the form most strongly associated with cigarette smoking.
  - Panacinar: This involves all parts of the acinus, and is mostly seen with alpha-1 ant-trypsin deficiency.
  - Distal (paraseptal): Affects predominately the alveolar ducts.
- Pulmonary vasculature. Chronic hypoxia leads to reflex vasoconstriction of the small pulmonary arteries, which results in intimal hyperplasia, smooth muscle hypertrophy and hyperplasia, and ultimately pulmonary hypertension.

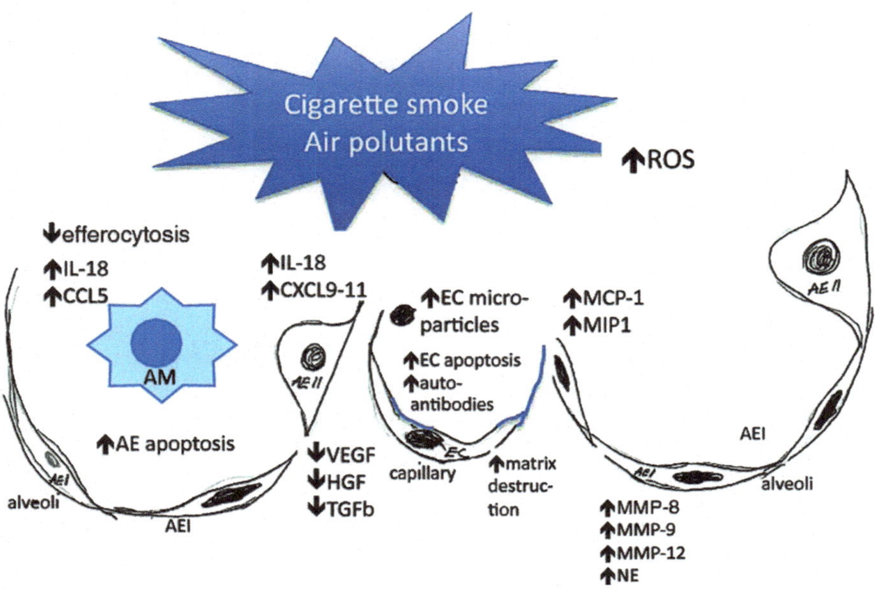

Destruction of the lung maintenance program in emphysema. Chronic exposure to cigarette smoke leads to a change in the local milieu: increased release of proinflammatory mediators (IL-8, IL-18, CCL5, IL-8, IFNgama, MIP1) that contribute to paracrine and autocrine signaling, impairment in efferocytosis, decreased levels of growth and survival factors (most notably VEGF and HGF), and extracellular matrix degradation (increased levels of matrix metalloproteases MMP-9 and MMP-12). Increased apoptosis of endothelial and epithelial cells might contribute to autoantibody formation. Reduced levels of TGF might signal delay repair processes and contribute to inflammatory cell activation. AM – alveolar macrophage; AEI – alveoli type I cell; AEII – alveoli type II cell; EC – capillary endothelial cell; ROS – reactive oxygen species [Taraseviciene-Stewart L, Voelkel NF. Immunopathology of COPD. In: Rogers TJ, Criner GJ, Cornwell WD, editors. Smoking and Lung Inflammation [Internet]. Springer New York; 2013 [cited 2016 May 16]. p. 1–27. Available from: http://link.springer.com/chapter/10.1007/978-1-4614-7351-0_1] *Caption from original*

- The single largest risk factor for the development of COPD is cigarette smoking. In the United States, nearly 80 % of patients diagnosed with COPD have history of cigarette smoking. The amount and duration of smoking are the largest predictors of disease severity. The single most reliable predictor for finding airflow obstruction on spirometric testing is a greater than 40 packs-per-year history of cigarette use.
- However, only 15 % of smokers will develop COPD.
- Smoking is the largest risk factor for the development of COPD, but not the only risk factor. Twenty percent of patients with COPD do not have a significant history of cigarette smoking. Other causes of COPD include occupational exposures (such as coal mining, gold mining, and cotton dust). There are also genetic causes, such as alpha-1 anti-trypsin deficiency, although this accounts for less than 1 % of cases of COPD.
- There is currently no strong evidence linking air pollution or second-hand smoke to the development of COPD.

Presentation

Typical/"Classic"

- The most common presenting symptoms of COPD are exertional dyspnea and chronic cough with sputum production.
- COPD is a slowly progressive disease with a prolonged asymptomatic phase. Patients are often unaware of the dyspnea, or just relate it to aging or poor fitness. They will often adjust their activities to limit the symptoms of dyspnea.
- Wheezing is often a later symptom.

- The course is one of slow progression with intermittent exacerbations of dyspnea and cough.
- Early in the course of the disease, the patient may have no physical signs of the disease.
- As the disease progresses, patients may develop the more classic signs of COPD, such as a barrel chest (increased AP diameter from air trapping), prolonged expiration with expiratory wheezing, decreased breath sounds, tachypnea, and pursed lip breathing.

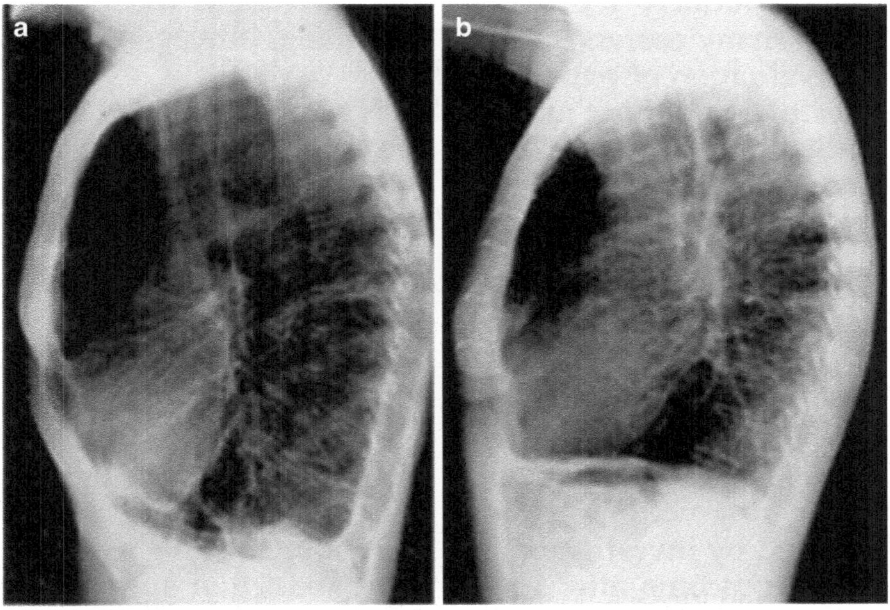

A lateral chest X-ray is shown. (a) Depicts the patient before lung volume reduction surgery (LVRS): the thorax is barrel-shaped with high transparency of the lungs, a large retrosternal air-filled space, and a flattened to concave diaphragm. The chest X-ray of the same subject (b) is shown 3 months after LVRS: the lung fields are less transparent, the air-filled retrosternal space decreased significantly, and the diaphragm exhibits an almost normal, convex shape. [Sullivan EA. Lung Volume Reduction. In: Slinger P, editor. Principles and Practice of Anesthesia for Thoracic Surgery [Internet]. Springer New York; 2011 [cited 2016 May 16]. p. 511–21. Available from: http://link.springer.com/chapter/10.1007/978-1-4419-0184-2_36] *Caption from original*

- Patients will often be noted to need to sit up and lean forward with their hands on their knees (tripod position) as this increases accessory muscle use (sternocleidomastoid, scalene, and intercostal muscles) and diaphragmatic excursion, both of which help to improve lung volumes.

- Patients with advanced disease will often have significant wasting with loss of muscle mass and subcutaneous fat. This is an independent predictor of a very poor prognosis.
- Clubbing of the digits is not a sign of COPD. If a patient with COPD develops clubbing, there is usually another cause, such as the interval development of lung cancer.

Atypical

- COPD less commonly presents initially with wheezing.
- COPD can present with chest tightness as the predominant symptom.

Primary Differential Considerations

- Initial consideration in patients with an acute presentation should be given to these differential diagnoses:
  - Asthma
  - Congestive heart failure
  - Pulmonary hypertension
  - Pulmonary embolism
  - Pneumonia

History and Physical Exam

Findings That Confirm Diagnosis

- There are no historical or physical exam findings that can confirm COPD. There is a large overlap with other disease states that cause dyspnea, such as asthma, congestive heart failure, and bronchiectasis.
- The diagnosis can be nearly confirmed when a patient presents with the typical symptoms of dyspnea on exertion with a chronic cough and sputum production associated with findings on spirometry of a forced expiratory volume in one second (FEV_1) less than 80 % of predicted and a ratio of FEV_1 to the forced vital capacity (FVC) of <0.7.

Assess and Monitor Disease: Key Points
Consider a diagnosis of COPD in any patient with a cough, dyspnea, or exposure to risk factors and confirm with spirometry.
Spirometry is the gold standard for the diagnosis and assessment of COPD and a postbronchodilator $FEV_1/FVC < 0.70$ confirms the presence of airflow limitation that is not fully reversible.
Health care workers involved in the diagnosis and management of COPD should have access to spirometry.
Severity of COPD is determined by symptoms, spirometric abnormalities, and complications. Changes in therapy should also be based on these factors.
Blood gas measurements should be made in patients with $FEV_1 < 50\%$ predicted or in those with evidence for right heart failure.
Comorbidities are common in COPD and are often the cause of death. They should be actively identified.

Assessment of COPD. [Dransfield MT. Diagnosis of COPD and the GOLD Guidelines. In: Crapo JD, editor. Atlas of Chronic Obstructive Pulmonary Disease. Philadelphia, PA: Current Medicine Group; 2009. 160 p. ISBN: 978-1-57340-294-1] *Caption adapted from original*

Factors That Suggest Diagnosis

- A patient who presents with the typical symptoms of dyspnea, cough, and sputum production, and has a greater than 40 pack-per-year history of cigarette smoking, has a high likelihood of having COPD.

Factors That Exclude Diagnosis

- Normal spirometric findings can exclude the diagnosis in a patient with the classic symptoms.

Ancillary Studies

Laboratory

- There are no lab tests that are diagnostic for COPD. However, many lab tests are helpful in the evaluation of the dyspneic patient to evaluate for other causes of the dyspnea.
- A complete blood count can help assess for anemia as the cause of dyspnea. Patients with advanced COPD may demonstrate polycythemia induced by chronic hypoxemia.

- A BNP (brain natriuretic peptide) level may help to distinguish between COPD and congestive heart failure as the cause of dyspnea. It is important to remember, however, that these diseases may often be present in the same patient.
- An alpha-1 anti-trypsin level should be measured in any patient with early-onset (before age 45) COPD, a non-smoker with COPD, or a family history of premature development of COPD.

Imaging

- Plain chest x-rays are unreliable in the diagnosis of COPD. Only about one-half of patients with moderate COPD will have any findings of COPD on a chest x-ray.
- The classic CXR findings of COPD include flattened diaphragms, an increased antero-posterior diameter of the chest, and increased radiolucency of the lungs. These are usually only seen in moderate-to-severe COPD, and are due to hyperinflation and air trapping.
- CXR can also be used to evaluate for alternative diagnoses (such as lung cancer, CHF, bronchiectasis), co-morbidities (the list also includes lung cancer, CHF, and bronchiectasis), and complications (such as pneumonia, pneumothorax) of COPD that are apparent on chest x-ray.
- CT is more sensitive at detecting the pathologic changes of COPD, but is not often needed to make the diagnosis. CT can be very helpful in the evaluation for alternative diagnoses, co-morbidities, and complications of COPD.

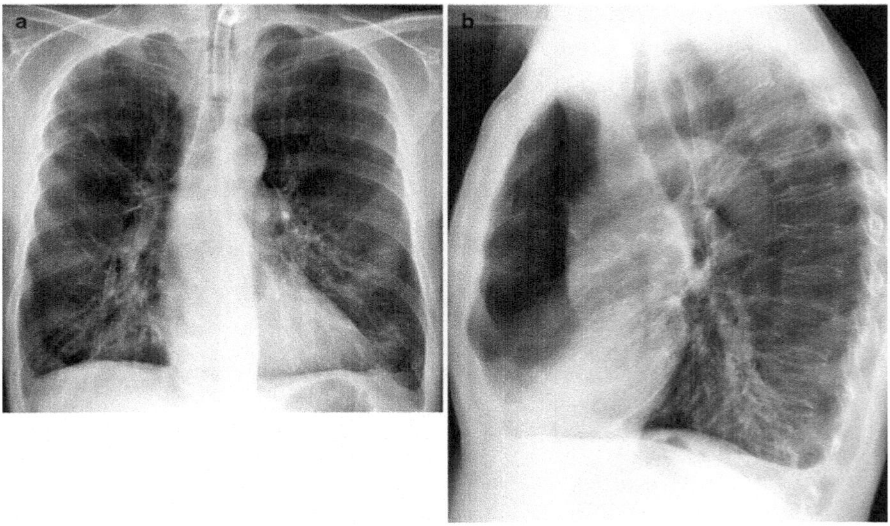

Chest X-rays of a 75-year-old patient with a clinical diagnosis of COPD. Posteroanterior (a) and lateral views (b) show radiographic signs consistent with pulmonary emphysema. Thickening of the bronchial wall is also evident in the lung bases. Tracheostomy was previously placed due to respiratory failure [Larici AR, Franchi P, Occhipinti M, Devicienti E, Mereu M, del Ciello A, Bonomo L. Airway Disease. In: Guglielmi G, Peh WCG, Guermazi A, editors. Geriatric Imaging [Internet]. Berlin, Heidelberg: Springer Berlin Heidelberg; 2013 [cited 2016 May 16]. p. 319–52. Available from: http://link.springer.com/10.1007/978-3-642-35579-0_14] *Caption from original*

Pulmonary Function Tests

- PFT's, especially spirometry, are the most helpful studies in diagnosing COPD. They are also useful in assessing the severity of disease, response to treatment, and for following progression.
- Spirometry (the measuring of breathing) is the most useful pulmonary function test in diagnosing and following COPD. Specifically, the forced expiratory volume in one second (FEV1), and the forced vital capacity and their ratio are the most helpful diagnostic tests for COPD.
- Spirometry performed both before and after inhaled bronchodilator use can determine whether airflow limitation is present, and whether it is at all reversible. Airflow limitation that is reversible is characteristic of asthma; airflow that is only partially reversible or is irreversible is consistent with COPD.
- Generally, COPD is felt to be present in a patient with an FEV1 less than 80 % of predicted, and and FEV1/FVC ratio of less than 0.7.

https://www.youtube.com/watch?v=s8pXdtp_Duw
Video demonstrating spirometry procedure, including the patient interview.

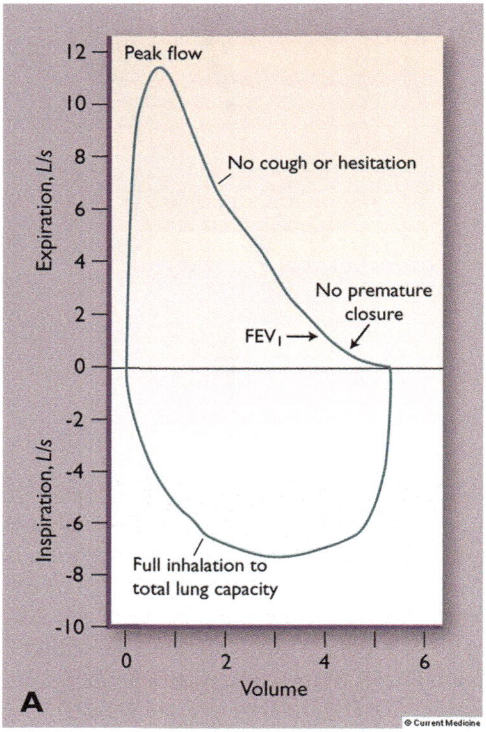

Spirometry in diagnosis of COPD [Hegewald M, Crapo R, Jensen R. Clinical Physiology of COPD. In: Crapo JD, editor. Atlas of Chronic Obstructive Pulmonary Disease. Philadelphia, PA: Current Medicine Group; 2009. 160 p. ISBN: 978-1-57340-294-1] *Caption adapted from original*

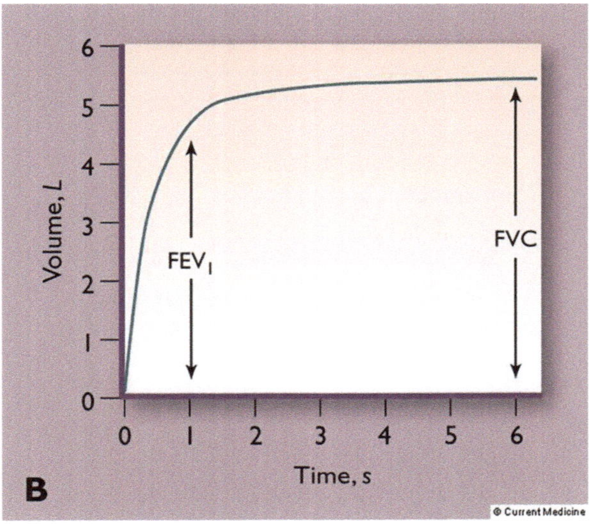

Spirometry in diagnosis of COPD [Hegewald M, Crapo R, Jensen R. Clinical Physiology of COPD. In: Crapo JD, editor. Atlas of Chronic Obstructive Pulmonary Disease. 2009 edition. Philadelphia, PA: Current Medicine Group; 2009. 160 p. ISBN: 978-1-57340-294-1] *Caption adapted from original*

Special Populations

Age

- COPD is a slowly progressive disease that often presents later in life. It is uncommon to diagnose before the sixth decade of life.
- Patients who are diagnosed with COPD before the age of 45 need to be evaluated for alpha-one antitrypsin deficiency.

Co-morbidities

- As a disease of older patients, COPD is often is seen in combination with other diseases, such as coronary artery disease, congestive heart failure, and cancer.

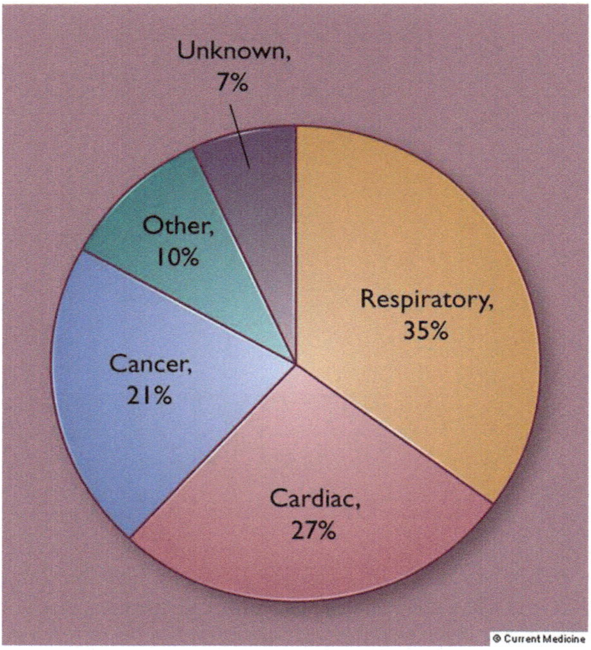

Causes of death in patients with COPD [Make BJ, Crapo JD. The Worldwide Epidemic of COPD: Clinical Phenotypes. In: Crapo JD, editor. Atlas of Chronic Obstructive Pulmonary Disease. Philadelphia, PA: Current Medicine Group; 2009. 160 p. ISBN: 978-1-57340-294-1] *Caption adapted from original*

Pitfalls in Diagnosis

Critical Steps Not to Miss

- It is imperative to consider the diagnosis, especially early in the course of the disease when the symptoms may be non-specific and subtle. Interventions such as smoking cessation can help to slow and stop the progression of disease if instituted early in the course.
- It is imperative to consider to alternative diagnoses, such as lung cancer and congestive heart failure.

Mimics

- Any disease that causes dyspnea can mimic COPD.
- Early COPD can sometimes be confused with atypical angina, as COPD, like angina, can cause chest tightness and dyspnea. Smoking is a significant risk factor for both diseases.
- Early in the course it is easily mimicked by asthma (although asthma has reversible airflow obstruction and COPD has irreversible airflow obstruction).
- Later in the course, COPD can mimic CHF, lung cancer with airway obstruction, bronchiectasis, pulmonary fibrosis, and other disorders causing dyspnea and cough.

Time-Dependent Interventions

- COPD cannot be reversed, so it is important to initiate treatment as early as possible to try and prevent progression of symptoms and pathology.
- Smoking cessation is critically important to these patients. It is also very difficult and may require a multi-modal treatment approach that includes pharmacologic and behavioral interventions.

Overall Principles of Treatment

- Therapy for compensated COPD involves numerous modalities including: oxygen therapy when indicated, bronchodilators, corticosteroids, reducing mucous secretion, smoking cessation, and pulmonary rehabilitation.
- Oxygen therapy in chronically hypoxic patients reduces mortality. The goal is to keep the PaO2 $\leq$60 mmHg of oxygen saturation $\geq$90 % at rest. The generally accepted criteria for oxygen therapy are: PaO2 $\leq$55 mmHg, an oxygen saturation of $\leq$88 % on room air, or a PaO2 of 56–59 mmHg in the presence of pulmonary hypertension, cor pulmonale, and polycythemia.
- Bronchodilator therapy does not affect the progression of the disease, but it can provide symptomatic relief and control and reduce exacerbations. Bronchodilator therapy also can improve quality of life. Patients would typically be maintained on long-acting inhaled beta agonists such as salmeterol and formoterol. Short-acting beta agonists such as albuterol are usually reserved for symptom control and for use during acute exacerbations. Inhaled anticholinergics (ipratropium) also cause bronchodilatation. The use of inhaled beta agonists combined with an inhaled anticholinergic improves FEV1 and symptoms better than either of these alone.

- Systemic corticosteroids can be useful in helping to control acute exacerbations, but most authorities don't recommend their long-term use. Only about 20–30 % of patients will note any improvement with the use of oral steroids. Some patients may improve with the use of inhaled steroids, especially those with an FEV1 <50 % of predicted.
- The only measures shown to help with mucous handling are adequate hydration and room humidification. Antitussives, antihistamines, and decongestants are all drying agents, and their use should be limited. Mucolytics and expectorants are of no clear benefit.
- Smoking cessation is the only intervention proven to reduce the rate of disease progression. Smoking cessation also reduces mortality. A multi-modal approach is often necessary and may include both pharmacologic and behavioral therapies.
- Pulmonary rehabilitation can increase exercise tolerance and improve quality of life, and is indicated for moderate-to-severe COPD.
- It is important that patients with COPD receive a pneumococcal vaccine, and also receive yearly influenza vaccination.

Disease Course

- COPD is a chronic, slowly progressive disease. It is marked by periods of relative stability interrupted by acute exacerbations, and a slow, steady decline in lung function.
- The frequency of exacerbations is a surrogate marker for disease progression.

Related Evidence

Papers of particular interest have been highlighted as:
*** Of key importance*

Practice Guideline

Rennard S, Thomashow B, Crapo J, Yawn B, McIvor A, Cerreta S, Walsh J, Mannino D. Introducing the COPD Foundation Guide for Diagnosis and Management of COPD, recommendations of the COPD Foundation. COPD. 2013 Jun;10(3):378-89. https://doi.org/10.3109/15412555.2013.801309. PMID: 23713598. http://www.ncbi.nlm.nih.gov/pubmed/23713598 **

Russi EW, Karrer W, Brutsche M, Eich C, Fitting JW, Frey M, Geiser T, Kuhn M, Nicod L, Quadri F, Rochat T, Steurer-Stey C, Stolz D; Swiss Respiratory Society.

Diagnosis and management of chronic obstructive pulmonary disease: the Swiss guidelines. Official guidelines of the Swiss Respiratory Society. Respiration. 2013;85(2):160-74. https://doi.org/10.1159/000346025. PMID: 23406723. http://www.ncbi.nlm.nih.gov/pubmed/23406723 **

Qaseem A, Wilt TJ, Weinberger SE, Hanania NA, Criner G, van der Molen T, Marciniuk DD, Denberg T, Schünemann H, Wedzicha W, MacDonald R, Shekelle P; American College of Physicians; American College of Chest Physicians; American Thoracic Society; European Respiratory Society. Diagnosis and management of stable chronic obstructive pulmonary disease: a clinical practice guideline update from the American College of Physicians, American College of Chest Physicians, American Thoracic Society, and European Respiratory Society. Ann Intern Med. 2011 Aug 2;155(3):179-91. https://doi.org/10.7326/0003-4819-155-3-201108020-00008. PMID: 21810710. http://www.ncbi.nlm.nih.gov/pubmed/21810710 **

National Clinical Guideline Centre (UK). Chronic Obstructive Pulmonary Disease: Management of Chronic Obstructive Pulmonary Disease in Adults in Primary and Secondary Care. London: Royal College of Physicians (UK); 2010 Jun. PMID: 22319804 http://www.ncbi.nlm.nih.gov/pubmed/22319804 **

O'Donnell DE, Hernandez P, Kaplan A, Aaron S, Bourbeau J, Marciniuk D, Balter M, Ford G, Gervais A, Lacasse Y, Maltais F, Road J, Rocker G, Sin D, Sinuff T, Voduc N. Canadian Thoracic Society recommendations for management of chronic obstructive pulmonary disease - 2008 update - highlights for primary care. Can Respir J. 2008 Jan-Feb;15 Suppl A:1A-8A. PMID: 18292855. http://www.ncbi.nlm.nih.gov/pubmed/18292855 **

Review

Postma DS, Bush A, van den Berge M. Risk factors and early origins of chronic obstructive pulmonary disease. Lancet. 2015 Mar 7;385(9971):899-909. https://doi.org/10.1016/S0140-6736(14)60446-3. PMID: 25123778. http://www.ncbi.nlm.nih.gov/pubmed/25123778 **

Johns DP, Walters JA, Walters EH. Diagnosis and early detection of COPD using spirometry. J Thorac Dis. 2014 Nov;6(11):1557-69. https://doi.org/10.3978/j.issn.2072-1439.2014.08.18. PMID: 25478197. http://www.ncbi.nlm.nih.gov/pubmed/25478197 **

Casaburi R, Duvall K. Improving early-stage diagnosis and management of COPD in primary care. Postgrad Med. 2014 Jul;126(4):141-54. https://doi.org/10.3810/pgm.2014.07.2792. PMID: 25141252. http://www.ncbi.nlm.nih.gov/pubmed/25141252 **

Diaz-Guzman E, Mannino DM. Epidemiology and prevalence of chronic obstructive pulmonary disease. Clin Chest Med. 2014 Mar;35(1):7-16. https://doi.org/10.1016/j.ccm.2013.10.002. PMID: 24507833. http://www.ncbi.nlm.nih.gov/pubmed/24507833 **

Washko GR. The role and potential of imaging in COPD. Med Clin North Am. 2012 Jul;96(4):729-43. https://doi.org/10.1016/j.mcna.2012.05.003. PMID: 22793941. http://www.ncbi.nlm.nih.gov/pubmed/22793941
Washko GR. Diagnostic imaging in COPD. Semin Respir Crit Care Med. 2010 Jun;31(3):276-85. https://doi.org/10.1055/s-0030-1254068. PMID: 20496297. http://www.ncbi.nlm.nih.gov/pubmed/20496297 **

Use PubMed Clinical Queries to find the most recent evidence. Use this search strategy:
"Pulmonary Disease, Chronic Obstructive"[Mesh] OR "COPD" OR "Chronic Obstructive Pulmonary Disease"

Chapter 19
Cor Pulmonale

Christopher J. Rees, Richard M. Cantor, Charles V. Pollack, Jr., and Jaime Friel Blanck

Name and Synonyms

Cor Pulmonale; Right Heart Failure; Pulmonary Heart Disease

Incidence/Epidemiology

- The true incidence and prevalence of cor pulmonale are unknown, as there are no standard diagnostic guidelines, and no definitive diagnostic tests for this condition.
- COPD (Chronic Obstructive Pulmonary Disease) causes about half of all cases of cor pulmonale in North America. Up to one-third of patients with COPD will develop cor pulmonale at some point during the course of their illness.
- Up to 20% of patients with obstructive sleep apnea (OSA) will develop cor pulmonale.
- Pulmonary vascular disorders (primary pulmonary hypertension, chronic thromboembolic disease, and scleroderma lung disease) are rare diseases, but cor pulmonale is a common end-stage complication of these diseases.

C. J. Rees
Emergency Department, Pennsylvania Hospital, Philadelphia, PA, USA

R. M. Cantor
Department of Emergency Medicine and Pediatrics, State University of New York Upstate Medical University, Syracuse, NY, USA

C. V. Pollack, Jr. (✉)
Department of Emergency Medicine, Thomas Jefferson University, Philadelphia, PA, USA

J. F. Blanck
Welch Medical Library, Johns Hopkins University, Baltimore, MD, USA

C. V. Pollack, Jr. (ed.), *Differential Diagnosis of Cardiopulmonary Disease*,
https://doi.org/10.1007/978-3-319-63895-9_19

- Interstitial lung diseases (ILD), especially idiopathic pulmonary fibrosis (IPF), often lead to cor pulmonale.

Differential Diagnosis

- The differential diagnosis of cor pulmonale is broad, and encompasses all diseases that present with dyspnea, fatigue, and exercise intolerance, such as COPD, asthma, PE, CHF, acute and chronic coronary syndromes, interstitial lung disease, and pulmonary vascular diseases, among many others.
- Also, cor pulmonale does not exist in isolation; it occurs as a complication of other disease processes with the common denominator being the presence of significant pulmonary hypertension.
- It is important in the differential diagnosis of these patients to consider worsening of the underlying disease as a cause of worsening dyspnea.
- It is also important to evaluate these patients for left heart failure from cardiac causes.

Pathophysiology and Etiology

- Cor pulmonale is defined as an alteration in the structure and function of the right ventricle in the presence of underlying chronic lung disease.
- Right-sided heart failure that results from left heart failure is not considered cor pulmonale.
- Cor pulmonale is triggered by the development of pulmonary hypertension.
- There are many diseases that can lead to pulmonary hypertension, and subsequently cor pulmonale. These are reviewed in the section on pulmonary hypertension.
- Pulmonary hypertension (either acutely or chronically) causes changes in right ventricular structure (dilatation with or without hypertrophy) and function (decreased contractility). If present chronically, pulmonary hypertension causes the pulmonary vascular bed to undergo vasoconstriction, remodeling, fibrosis, and ultimately destruction. This leads to further increases in pulmonary artery pressure (the normal PA pressure is about 15 mm Hg), increasing the work of the RV to pump against higher pressures (increased RV afterload), leading to decreases in left ventricular filling and cardiac output, but usually with preservation of left ventricular ejection fraction.
- Chronic cor pulmonale is a chronic, slowly progressive condition that leads to worsening pulmonary hypertension, right ventricular hypertrophy, and dilatation.
- Cor pulmonale can also occur acutely, in the absence of right ventricular hypertrophy. A large pulmonary embolism can cause acute increase in right

ventricular and pulmonary artery pressure, leading to right ventricular dilatation and failure.

Presentation

Typical/"Classic"

- Dyspnea is the most common symptom of cor pulmonale. As many of these patients have significant underlying pulmonary disease, they often note a worsening of chronic dyspnea.
- Other symptoms often attributed to cor pulmonale include:
    - dyspnea on exertion
    - fatigue
    - lethargy
    - exertional syncope
    - exertional angina (even in the absence of coronary artery disease)
- Abdominal pain, ascites, and peripheral edema are also frequently seen in patients with cor pulmonale. These are related more to the left heart changes caused by cor pulmonale.
- Patients often present with worsening dyspnea, often with worsening edema and ascites. They will likely exhibit some degree of hypoxia.

Atypical

- Patients with no history of underlying pulmonary disease may present with acute cor pulmonale.
- These patients usually will have profound dyspnea and be hypoxemic and hypotensive. The most common cause for this will be a large, central pulmonary embolism.

Primary Differential Considerations

- The primary differential diagnoses for cor pulmonale are pulmonary hypertension, pulmonary embolism, constrictive pericarditis, and biventricular heart failure.

History and Physical Exam

Findings That Confirm Diagnosis

- There are no historical or physical examination findings that are pathognonomic for cor pulmonale, as many of the symptoms and signs of right heart failure are shared with left heart failure. These symptoms and signs include dyspnea, tachypnea, hypoxia, elevated jugular venous distension, hepatomegaly, and peripheral edema.

Factors That Suggest Diagnosis

- A patient with a history of known, chronic pulmonary disease, and who presents with worsening dyspnea, is a primary candidate for this diagnosis. However, it is important to remember that there are many other causes of worsening dyspnea in these patients (pneumonia, CHF, pulmonary embolism, pneumothorax, profound anemia, and others).
- Physical exam findings that suggest the diagnosis include:
  - A right ventricular third heart sound.
  - Prominent v-waves in the jugular venous pulse. This results from acute tricuspid regurgitation.

https://www.youtube.com/watch?v=ceX3KmZCZhY

An example showing a prominent v-wave in the jugular venous pulse associated with tricuspid regurgitation.

- A right ventricular heave at the left sternal border.
- Carvallo's Sign is an increase in the intensity of the holosystolic murmur of tricuspid regurgitation upon inspiration. This can often be noted with acute cor pulmonale. This finding becomes less apparent as right ventricular failure worsens.
- Central and peripheral cyanosis can be noted, but they are often late signs.
- Patients with end-stage cor pulmonale often have signs of cardiogenic shock such as hypotension, tachycardia, decreased urine output, and peripheral and central cyanosis.

Factors That Exclude Diagnosis

- Cor pulmonale cannot be diagnosed in the presence of left heart failure.

Ancillary Studies

Laboratory

- There are no laboratory studies that are specific for cor pulmonale.
- B-type natriuretic peptide levels should be checked, as they will be elevated. These levels will also be elevated in left heart failure, so they cannot help to distinguish between left heart failure and right heart failure.
- It is helpful to send routine laboratory studies, such as basic chemistries, a complete blood count, thyroid function, and cardiac biomarkers, to evaluate for other causes for the patient's symptoms.

Electrocardiography

- The ECG in cor pulmonale and severe pulmonary hypertension can show a right axis deviation, right ventricular hypertrophy, right atrial enlargement (p pulmonale), and a right bundle branch block. These ECG changes are almost always present in pulmonary hypertension, but can also be present in many other disease states (they are specific but not sensitive).

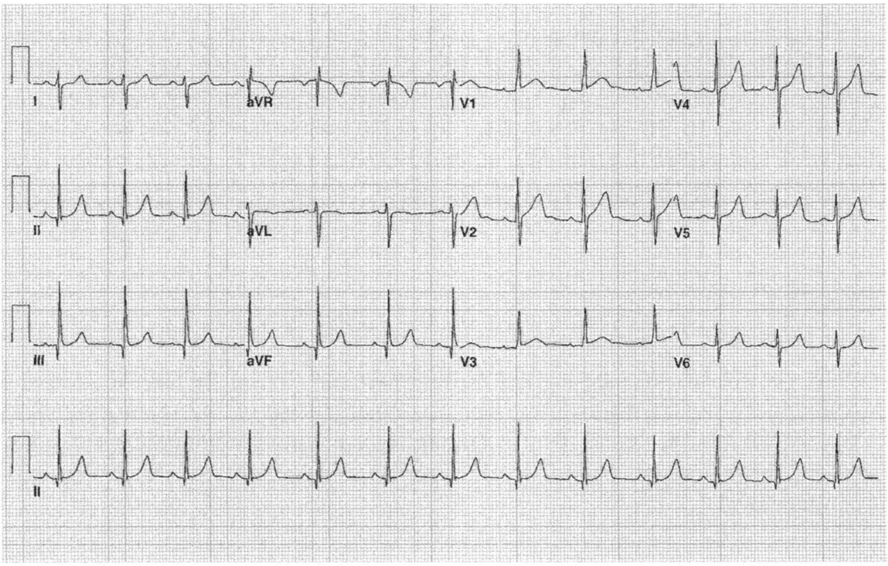

Electrocardiogram showing the signs of right hypertrophy and right deviation of the cardiac axis in a patient with cor pulmonale [Massimi L, Di Rocco

C. Complications Specific to the Type of CSF Shunt: Atrial Shunt. In: Di Rocco C, Turgut M, Jallo G, Martínez-Lage JF, editors. Complications of CSF Shunting in Hydrocephalus [Internet]. Cham: Springer International Publishing; 2015 [cited 2015 Sep 3]. p. 177–85. Available from: http://link.springer.com/10.1007/978-3-319-09961-3_12] *Caption from original*

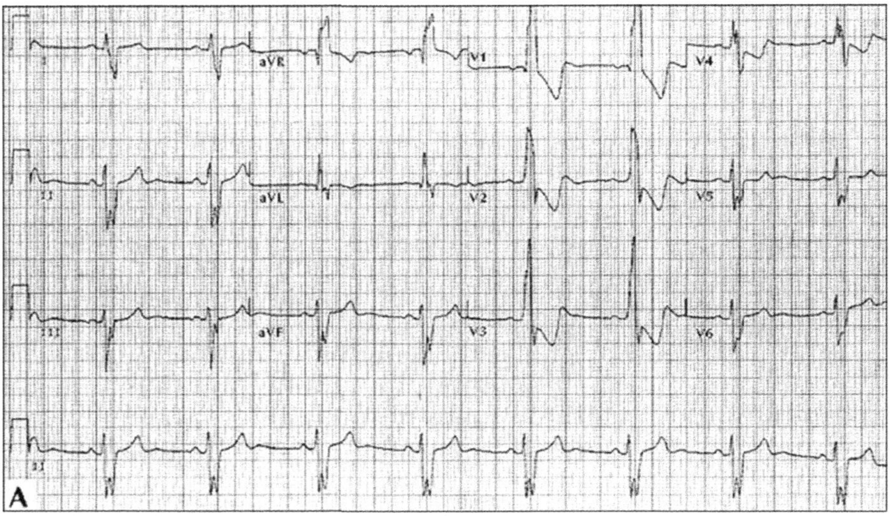

Electrocardiographic finding with advanced cor pulmonale. Note the complete right bundle branch pattern with an RR′ in lead V1. This tracing demonstrates pressure and volume overload of the right ventricle, consistent with cor pulmonale. [Loh E. Chapter 01. In: Goldhaber S, editor. Cardiopulmonary Diseases and Cardiac Tumors. Philadelphia: Current Medicine; 1995 (Braunwald E, editor. Atlas of heart diseases; vol. 3.)] *Caption adapted from original*

Imaging

- The chest x-ray may be helpful in the evaluation for cor pulmonale. Chronic pulmonary hypertension often leads to enlargement of the main pulmonary artery, hilar vessels, and the descending right pulmonary artery. On the lateral view, there may be loss of the retrosternal air space due to right ventricular enlargement.

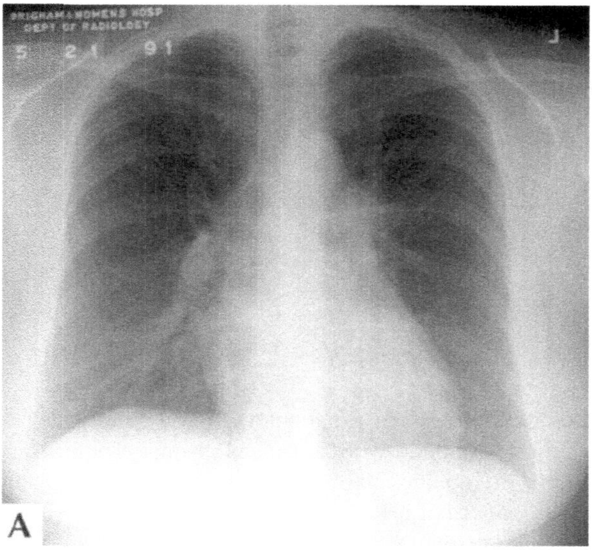

Chest radiograph demonstrating features of advanced cor pulmonale secondary to pulmonary hypertension. Typical radiograph of a patient with primary pulmonary hypertension and cor pulmonale. Note the peripheral oligemia of the pulmonary vessels with mild bilateral enlargement of the main pulmonary arteries.[Loh E. Chapter 01. In: Goldhaber S, editor. Cardiopulmonary Diseases and Cardiac Tumors. Philadelphia: Current Medicine; 1995 (Braunwald E, editor. Atlas of heart diseases; vol. 3.)] *Caption adapted from original*

- Transthoracic echocardiography (TTE) can be very helpful in the evaluation for and diagnosis of cor pulmonale and pulmonary hypertension. Pulmonary hypertension alone is associated only with signs of elevated right ventricular pressure. In chronic cor pulmonale there is a thickened (hypertrophied) right ventricular wall and right ventricular dilatation (early in the course of the disease, only hypertrophy may be appreciated). The right ventricular dilatation usually leads to tricuspid regurgitation. Acute cor pulmonale may lead to right ventricular dilatation in the absence of right ventricular hypertrophy. Reduced function of the right ventricle can also often be appreciated on TTE.

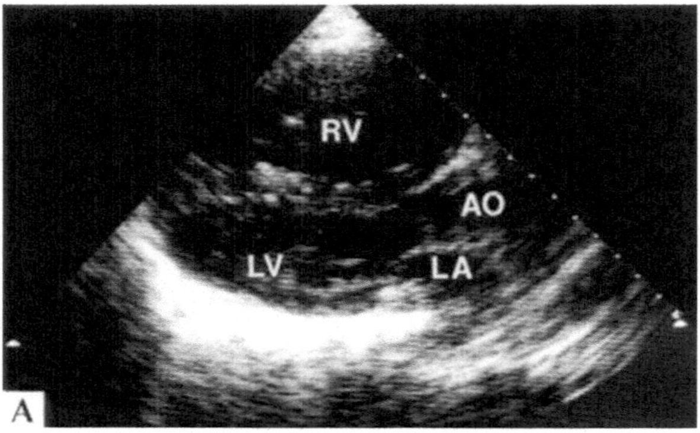

Echocardiographic features of the heart in a patient with cor pulmonale. A, Parasternal long-axis view from a patient with advanced primary pulmonary hypertension complicated by cor pulmonale. Note the abnormal flattening of the interventricular septum and its abnormal bulging into the left ventricle (LV), consistent with volume and pressure overload of the right ventricle (RV). [Loh E. Chapter 01. In: Goldhaber S, editor. Cardiopulmonary Diseases and Cardiac Tumors. Philadelphia: Current Medicine; 1995 (Braunwald E, editor. Atlas of heart diseases; vol. 3.)] *Caption from original*

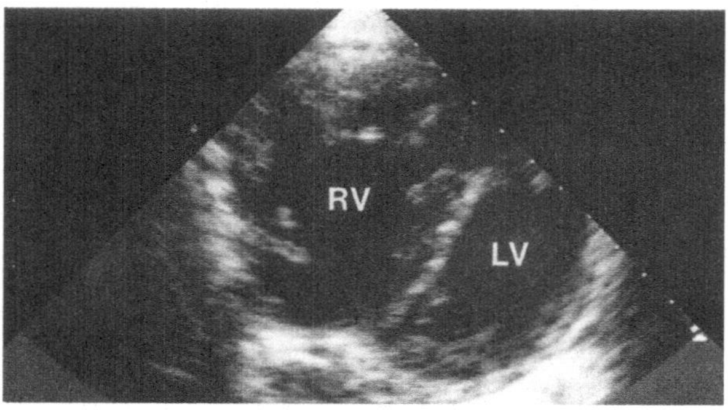

Short-axis view demonstrating a markedly enlarged RV with RV hypertrophy. Abnormal bowing of the interventricular septum into the LV gives a characteristic D configuration of the LV, consistent with volume and pressure overload of the RV. [Loh E. Chapter 01. In: Goldhaber S, editor. Cardiopulmonary Diseases and Cardiac Tumors. Philadelphia: Current Medicine; 1995 (Braunwald E, editor. Atlas of heart diseases; vol. 3.)] *Caption from original*

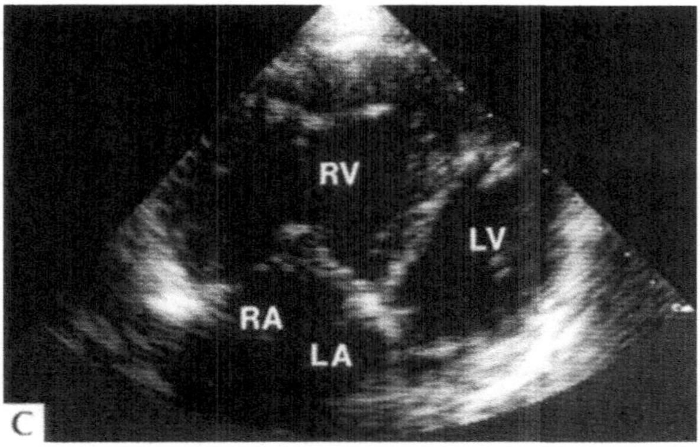

Apical four-chamber view also demonstrating RV hypertrophy and abnormal septal bowing as described in panels A and B. AO—aorta; LA—left atrium; RA—right atrium. [Loh E. Chapter 01. In: Goldhaber S, editor. Cardiopulmonary Diseases and Cardiac Tumors. Philadelphia: Current Medicine; 1995 (Braunwald E, editor. Atlas of heart diseases; vol. 3.)] *Caption from original*

- Cardiac magnetic resonance imaging (MRI), if available, is superior to transthoracic echocardiography in the evaluation of right ventricular structure and function.
- Right heart catheterization is considered the best diagnostic test for cor pulmonale and pulmonary hypertension. Patients with cor pulmonale will have right ventricular dysfunction as evidenced by an elevated central venous pressure and elevated right ventricular end-diastolic pressure, pulmonary hypertension (PA pressure greater than 25 mmHg), and no evidence of left heart disease, as evidenced by either a normal (less than 15 mmHg) left ventricular end-diastolic pressure. All chamber dimensions and pressures can be directly measured.

Special Populations

Age

- Cor pulmonale is a disease of adults starting in middle-age.
- Most patients with chronic cor pulmonale will have had severe, underlying pulmonary disease for many years prior to the onset of cor pulmonale.
- In the pediatric patient, the vast majority of cases are secondary to cystic fibrosis.
- Neonates with severe bronchopulmonary dysplasia are also susceptible to the development of cor pulmonale.

Co-morbidities

- Many co-morbid conditions can worsen the prognosis, and make the diagnosis of cor pulmonale difficult. These include, but are not limited to, cardiac diseases, other pulmonary diseases, liver disease, and kidney disease.

Pitfalls in Diagnosis

Critical Steps Not to Miss

- It is imperative that all patients be evaluated for left ventricular dysfunction. The most common cause of right heart failure is left heart failure, and left heart failure precludes a diagnosis of cor pulmonale.
- It is also important to consider all alternative diagnoses that may cause worsening or acute dyspnea in patients with chronic pulmonary and heart disease. This list includes, but is not limited to, pneumonia, CHF, pulmonary embolism, pneumothorax, significant pleural effusion, and acute metabolic issues that can cause dyspnea.

Mimics

- Left heart failure can mimic right heart failure.
- Other diseases that can present in a similar fashion include acute liver failure, acute kidney failure, and others.

Time-Dependent Interventions

- The most important intervention is to decrease the work of breathing by correcting hypoxemia and respiratory acidosis. Correcting these will decrease pulmonary vascular resistance and thereby reduce demands on the right ventricle.

Overall Principles of Treatment

- Optimizing treatment of the underlying lung disease can help improve hemodynamics and lessen the symptoms and progression of cor pulmonale.

- Specific treatment for cor pulmonale consists of managing three physiologic parameters—pulmonary artery pressure; right ventricular pressure; and right ventricular contractility—as follows:
  - Reduce pulmonary artery pressure (reduce right ventricular afterload). This pressure can be reduced by the use of supplemental oxygen to decrease the effect of hypoxia-induced vasoconstriction. This is particularly necessary in hypoxic patients.
  - Reduce right ventricular pressure. Diuretic use has shown some utility in improving hemodynamics in patients with markedly elevated right ventricular pressure. Diuresis must be performed carefully, as over-diuresis can lead to reduced right ventricular filling and a decrease in cardiac output.
  - Improve right ventricular contractility. This therapy is generally reserved for patients with severe cor pulmonale who have resistant hypotension and are in shock. The most common inotropic agents used are dobutamine and milrinone.
- Patients should be evaluated for any underlying or acute issues that, if treated, can help improve the symptoms of cor pulmonale. These include such issues as pulmonary embolism, pneumonia, pneumothorax, and pleural effusions.

Disease Course

- Cor pulmonale is a chronic, progressive disease that occurs only when other underlying pulmonary diseases have progressed and are severe.
- As noted above, acute cor pulmonale is less common but can occur.
- The overall long-term prognosis once cor pulmonale has been diagnosed is poor. Mortality in the first year after the diagnosis of cor pulmonale is around 35%.
- Survival is significantly lessened once cor pulmonale complicates pre-existing lung disease.

Related Evidence

Papers of particular interest have been highlighted as:
    *** Of key importance*

Practice Guideline

King C, May CW, Williams J, Shlobin OA. Management of right heart failure in the critically ill. Crit Care Clin. 2014 Jul;30(3):475-98. https://doi.org/10.1016/j.ccc.2014.03.003. Review. PubMed PMID: 24996606. http://www.ncbi.nlm.nih.gov/pubmed/24996606 **

Rudski LG, Lai WW, Afilalo J, Hua L, Handschumacher MD, Chandrasekaran K, Solomon SD, Louie EK, Schiller NB. Guidelines for the echocardiographic assessment of the right heart in adults: a report from the American Society of Echocardiography endorsed by the European Association of Echocardiography, a registered branch of the European Society of Cardiology, and the Canadian Society of Echocardiography. J Am Soc Echocardiogr. 2010 Jul;23(7):685-713; quiz 786-8. https://doi.org/10.1016/j.echo.2010.05.010. PubMed PMID: 20620859. http://www.ncbi.nlm.nih.gov/pubmed/20620859 **

Review

Repessé X, Charron C, Vieillard-Baron A. Acute cor pulmonale in ARDS: rationale for protecting the right ventricle. Chest. 2015 Jan;147(1):259-65. https://doi.org/10.1378/chest.14-0877. Review. PubMed PMID: 25560864. http://www.ncbi.nlm.nih.gov/pubmed/25560864 **

Gomez-Arroyo J, Sandoval J, Simon MA, Dominguez-Cano E, Voelkel NF, Bogaard HJ. Treatment for pulmonary arterial hypertension-associated right ventricular dysfunction. Ann Am Thorac Soc. 2014 Sep;11(7):1101-15. https://doi.org/10.1513/AnnalsATS.201312-425FR. Review. PubMed PMID: 25079379. http://www.ncbi.nlm.nih.gov/pubmed/25079379 **

King C, May CW, Williams J, Shlobin OA. Management of right heart failure in the critically ill. Crit Care Clin. 2014 Jul;30(3):475-98. https://doi.org/10.1016/j.ccc.2014.03.003. Review. PubMed PMID: 24996606. http://www.ncbi.nlm.nih.gov/pubmed/24996606 **

Vonk-Noordegraaf A, Haddad F, Chin KM, Forfia PR, Kawut SM, Lumens J, Naeije R, Newman J, Oudiz RJ, Provencher S, Torbicki A, Voelkel NF, Hassoun PM. Right heart adaptation to pulmonary arterial hypertension: physiology and pathobiology. J Am Coll Cardiol. 2013 Dec 24;62(25 Suppl):D22-33. https://doi.org/10.1016/j.jacc.2013.10.027. Review. PubMed PMID: 24355638. http://www.ncbi.nlm.nih.gov/pubmed/24355638 **

Forfia PR, Vaidya A, Wiegers SE. Pulmonary heart disease: The heart-lung interaction and its impact on patient phenotypes. Pulm Circ. 2013 Jan;3(1):5-19. https://doi.org/10.4103/2045-8932.109910. PubMed PMID: 23662171; PubMed Central PMCID: PMC3641739. http://www.ncbi.nlm.nih.gov/pubmed/23662171

Madsen PH, Hess S, Høilund-Carlsen PF, Alavi A. Positron emission tomography in chronic obstructive pulmonary disease. Hell J Nucl Med. 2013

May-Aug;16(2):121-4. Review. PubMed PMID: 23865084. http://www.ncbi.nlm.nih.gov/pubmed/23865084

Greyson CR. Right heart failure in the intensive care unit. Curr Opin Crit Care. 2012 Oct;18(5):424-31. https://doi.org/10.1097/MCC.0b013e3283577070. Review. PubMed PMID: 22889868. http://www.ncbi.nlm.nih.gov/pubmed/?term=22889868 **

Hoeper MM, Granton J. Intensive care unit management of patients with severe pulmonary hypertension and right heart failure. Am J Respir Crit Care Med. 2011 Nov 15;184(10):1114-24. https://doi.org/10.1164/rccm.201104-0662CI. Review. PubMed PMID: 21700906. http://www.ncbi.nlm.nih.gov/pubmed/21700906 **

Barr RG. The epidemiology of vascular dysfunction relating to chronic obstructive pulmonary disease and emphysema. Proc Am Thorac Soc. 2011 Nov;8(6):522-7. https://doi.org/10.1513/pats.201101-008MW. Review. PubMed PMID: 22052931; PubMed Central PMCID: PMC3359073. http://www.ncbi.nlm.nih.gov/pubmed/22052931

Healy F, Hanna BD, Zinman R. Clinical practice. The impact of lung disease on the heart and cardiac disease on the lungs. Eur J Pediatr. 2010 Jan;169(1):1-6. https://doi.org/10.1007/s00431-009-1027-8. Epub 2009 Jul 29. Review. PubMed PMID: 19639339. http://www.ncbi.nlm.nih.gov/pubmed/19639339

Jardin F, Vieillard-Baron A. Acute cor pulmonale. Curr Opin Crit Care. 2009 Feb;15(1):67-70. Review. PubMed PMID: 19186411. http://www.ncbi.nlm.nih.gov/pubmed/19186411 **

Weitzenblum E, Chaouat A. Cor pulmonale. Chron Respir Dis. 2009;6(3):177-85. https://doi.org/10.1177/1479972309104664. Review. PubMed PMID: 19643833. http://www.ncbi.nlm.nih.gov/pubmed/19643833 **

Han MK, McLaughlin VV, Criner GJ, Martinez FJ. Pulmonary diseases and the heart. Circulation. 2007 Dec 18;116(25):2992-3005. Review. PubMed PMID: 18086941. http://www.ncbi.nlm.nih.gov/pubmed/18086941 **

Shujaat A, Minkin R, Eden E. Pulmonary hypertension and chronic cor pulmonale in COPD. Int J Chron Obstruct Pulmon Dis. 2007;2(3):273-82. Review. PubMed PMID: 18229565; PubMed Central PMCID: PMC2695205. http://www.ncbi.nlm.nih.gov/pubmed/18229565

Carbone R, Bossone E, Bottino G, Monselise A, Rubenfire M. Secondary pulmonary hypertension--diagnosis and management. Eur Rev Med Pharmacol Sci. 2005 Nov-Dec;9(6):331-42. Review. PubMed PMID: 16479737. http://www.ncbi.nlm.nih.gov/pubmed/16479737

Meyer FJ, Schoene AM, Borst MM. Pathophysiological aspects of cardiopulmonary interaction. Clin Nephrol. 2003 Jul;60 Suppl 1:S75-80. Review. PubMed PMID: 12940537. http://www.ncbi.nlm.nih.gov/pubmed/12940537

Lehrman S, Romano P, Frishman W, Rashid A, Dobkin J, Reichel J. Primary pulmonary hypertension and cor pulmonale. Cardiol Rev. 2002 Sep-Oct;10(5):265-78. Review. PubMed PMID: 12215190. http://www.ncbi.nlm.nih.gov/pubmed/12215190 **

Romano PM, Peterson S. The management of cor pulmonale. Heart Dis. 2000 Nov-Dec;2(6):431-7. Review. PubMed PMID: 11728294. http://www.ncbi.nlm.nih.gov/pubmed/11728294

Clinical Trial

Liu WH, Luo Q, Liu ZH, Zhao Q, Xi QY, Zhao ZH. Differences in exercise capacity in patients with chronic left heart failure and chronic right heart failure. Heart Lung Circ. 2014 Nov;23(11):1036-40. https://doi.org/10.1016/j.hlc.2014.05.003. Epub 2014 May 27. PubMed PMID: 24931066. http://www.ncbi.nlm.nih.gov/pubmed/24931066

Comparative Study

Kawut SM, Poor HD, Parikh MA, Hueper K, Smith BM, Bluemke DA, Lima JA, Prince MR, Hoffman EA, Austin JH, Vogel-Claussen J, Barr RG. Cor pulmonale parvus in chronic obstructive pulmonary disease and emphysema: the MESA COPD study. J Am Coll Cardiol. 2014 Nov 11;64(19):2000-9. https://doi.org/10.1016/j.jacc.2014.07.991. Epub 2014 Nov 3. PubMed PMID: 25440095; PubMed Central PMCID: PMC4347835. http://www.ncbi.nlm.nih.gov/pubmed/25440095

Gao Y, Du X, Liang L, Cao L, Yang Q, Li K. Evaluation of right ventricular function by 64-row CT in patients with chronic obstructive pulmonary disease and cor pulmonale. Eur J Radiol. 2012 Feb;81(2):345-53. https://doi.org/10.1016/j.ejrad.2010.11.004. Epub 2010 Nov 27. PubMed PMID: 21112711. http://www.ncbi.nlm.nih.gov/pubmed/21112711 **

Park JH, Park YS, Kim YJ, Lee IS, Kim JH, Lee JH, Choi SW, Jeong JO, Seong IW. Differentiation between acute and chronic cor pulmonales with midventricular systolic strain of the right ventricle in the emergency department. Heart Vessels. 2011 Jul;26(4):435-9. https://doi.org/10.1007/s00380-010-0072-6. Epub 2010 Nov 26. PubMed PMID: 21110197. http://www.ncbi.nlm.nih.gov/pubmed/21110197

Use PubMed Clinical Queries to find the most recent evidence. Use this search strategy:

("Pulmonary Heart Disease"[Majr] OR "pulmonary heart disease"[tiab] OR "cor pulmonale"[tiab] OR "right heart failure"[tiab])

Chapter 20
Costochondritis

Christopher J. Rees, Richard M. Cantor, Charles V. Pollack, Jr., and Victoria G. Riese

Name and Synonyms

Costochondritis; Costosternal Syndrome; Tietze's Syndrome; Chest Wall Pain Syndrome

Incidence/Epidemiology

- Chest pain is a common presenting complaint to both Emergency Departments and primary care offices.
- There are an estimated six million emergency department visits a year for chest pain.
- The evaluation of chest pain utilizes a substantial amount of health care resources, primarily with the goal of excluding life-threatening diagnoses.
- Musculoskeletal causes of chest pain account for up to one-third of all causes in the outpatient evaluation of chest pain.
- The true incidence of costochondritis and other musculoskeletal chest pain syndromes is unknown, as many cases don't present for evaluation.

C. J. Rees
Emergency Department, Pennsylvania Hospital, Philadelphia, PA, USA

R. M. Cantor
Department of Emergency Medicine and Pediatrics, State University of New York Upstate Medical University, Syracuse, NY, USA

C. V. Pollack, Jr. (✉)
Department of Emergency Medicine, Thomas Jefferson University, Philadelphia, PA, USA

V. G. Riese
Librarian Consultant, Eldersburg, MD, USA

C. V. Pollack, Jr. (ed.), *Differential Diagnosis of Cardiopulmonary Disease*,
https://doi.org/10.1007/978-3-319-63895-9_20

Differential Diagnosis

- The initial differential diagnosis of chest pain must include all the serious and potentially life-threatening diseases, such as acute coronary syndromes, aortic dissection, pulmonary embolism, and pneumothorax.
- The differential diagnosis of musculoskeletal causes of chest pain is broad. It includes, primarily, inflammatory musculoskeletal pain syndromes such as costochondritis (and others as below), and rheumatic musculoskeletal syndromes such as fibromyalgia, rheumatoid arthritis, ankylosing spondylitis, and psoriatic arthritis.
- Primary (inflammatory) musculoskeletal chest pain syndromes include:
  - Costochondritis. Costochondritis typically affects those over age 40, and usually involves pain to palpation over the costochondral junctions of the third, fourth, and fifth ribs. Costochondritis is diagnosed more often in women.
  - Tietze's Syndrome. In Tietze's syndrome there is painful swelling of usually one (but sometimes several), costochondral joints. It usually involves either the second or third costochondral junctions. There must be obvious physical signs of inflammation, such as erythema, swelling, and warmth over the affected joint, for the diagnosis to be considered. It is a rare disorder of unknown etiology. Tietze's syndrome is more common in those under 40, and affects both sexes equally.

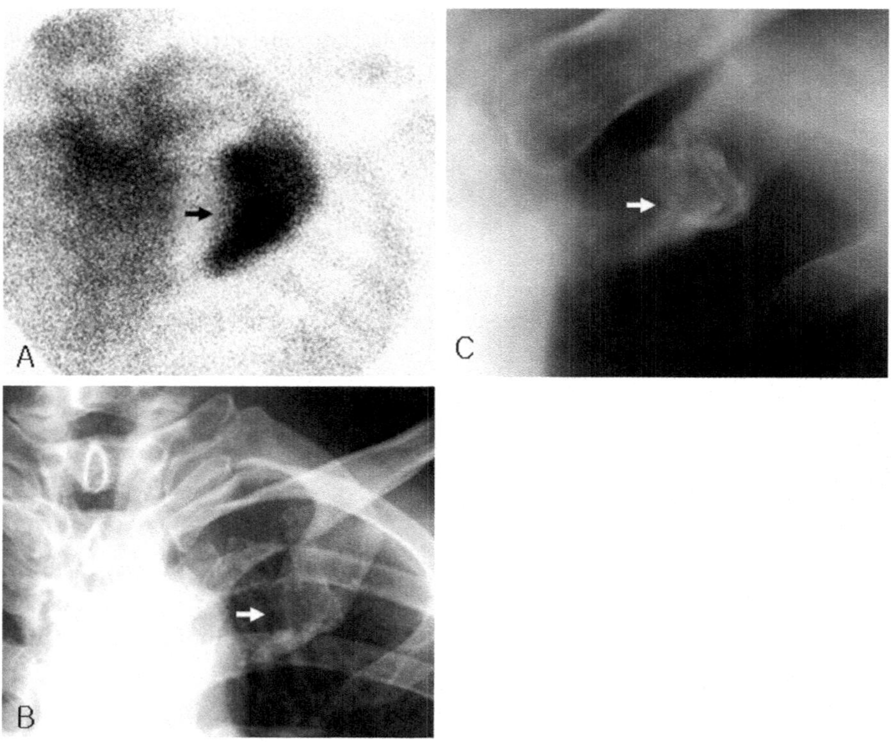

Inverted C-shape tracer uptake in chronic Tietze's disease. **A** Anterior pinhole scan in a 63-year-old man with tender swelling for 2 months in the left first costochondral junction shows inverted C-shape tracer uptake (*arrow*). **B** Posteroanterior radiograph shows nonspecific calcification (*arrow*). **C** Conventional X-ray tomograph shows inverted C-shape ossification in the costochondral junction (*arrow*) [Bahk Y-W. Infective and Infl ammatory Diseases of Bone. In: Combined Scintigraphic and Radiographic Diagnosis of Bone and Joint Diseases [Internet]. Berlin, Heidelberg: Springer Berlin Heidelberg; 2013 [cited 2016 Nov 7]. p. 75–106. Available from: http://link.springer.com/10.1007/978-3-642-25144-3_6] *Caption from original*

- Xiphodynia/xiphalgia. Sharp, pleuritic chest pain that is reproduced by light palpation of the xyphoid process.
- Precordial catch syndrome (sometimes called texidor twinge). Fleeting (lasting seconds to minutes), lancinating episodes of chest pain, often precipitated by deep inspiration.
- Slipped rib syndrome. Pain and often a feeling of fullness usually along the inferior margin of the anterior tenth rib. There is often point tenderness and reproduction of the symptoms with pressure. Thought to be secondary to hypermobility of the distal costal cartilage that occurs after lifting or twisting. More commonly diagnosed in women.
- Sternalis syndrome. Localized tenderness over the sternum thought secondary to inflammation of the overlying sternalis muscle. Rare, more common in women, and often causes bilateral pain, especially with palpation.
- Sternoclavicular subluxation. Another rare diagnosis, marked by spontaneous or traumatic subluxation of a sternoclavicular joint. More commonly noted on the side of the dominant hand, and worsens with pulling and lifting motions. Mostly seen in women 40 – 60 years old, and associated with moderately heavy repetitive tasks.

Pathophysiology and Etiology

- The pathophysiology of costochondritis is felt to primarily involve inflammation of the costochondral junctions. The inflammation may be spontaneous and idiopathic, or may be related to injuries cause by trauma or overuse.

Presentation

Typical/"Classic"

- Chest pain that that is highly localized, and consistently reproducible by light palpation over a small area.
- Usually described as sharp and pleuritic, and often worsens when changing positions, coughing, and sneezing.
- Onset can be sudden, but is more often gradual and insidious.

Atypical

- May present as dull, diffuse pain that is poorly localized.

Primary Differential Considerations

- Initial consideration to patients presenting with these symptoms should be given to the following differential diagnoses:
  - Acute coronary syndrome
  - Pulmonary embolism
  - Pericarditis
  - Pleurisy
  - GERD
  - Herpes zoster (shingles)

History and Physical Exam

Findings That Confirm Diagnosis

- It must be stressed that all the life-threatening causes of chest pain must always be considered in patients presenting with a complaint of chest pain.
- It must also be stressed that reproducibility and chest wall tenderness are not sensitive or specific signs, and they can also occur with acute coronary syndromes.
- The diagnosis can usually be confirmed, after more serious causes of have chest pain have been excluded (either by history and physical or testing), when there is a discrete area of tenderness in which the pain is consistently reproduced by light palpation.

Factors That Suggest Diagnosis

- Chest pain that is sharp, localized, and consistently reproducible by light palpation.

Factors That Exclude Diagnosis

- Chest wall pain syndromes can coexist with many other causes of chest pain, and as such can only be excluded when there is no complaint of chest pain.

Ancillary Studies

Laboratory

- Laboratory studies are inly useful in excluding other diagnoses. There are no laboratory studies that help in the diagnosis of costochondritis or other chest wall pain syndromes.

Imaging

- Imaging studies are only helpful in the exclusion of other diagnoses.

Special Populations

Age

- Costochondritis is more common above the age of 40, but can be diagnosed in any adult age group.
- Costochondritis can affect children as well as adults.
- In some studies of musculoskeletal chest pain in children, costochondritis accounted for nearly 15 percent of final diagnoses.

Co-morbidities

- Costrochondritis can coexist with any other diagnosis. There are no co-morbidities of significance.

Pitfalls in Diagnosis

Critical Steps Not to Miss

- It is critically important to first consider the life-threatening causes of chest pain.

Mimics

- Costochondritis can present similarly to other, more serious causes of chest pain, such as pulmonary embolism and acute coronary syndrome.

Time-Dependent Interventions

- There are no time-dependent interventions.

Overall Principles of Treatment

- Costochondritis and the other musculoskeletal chest pain syndromes are usually self-limited conditions.
- Treatment is usually conservative, and starts with reassurance that no more serious condition exists.
- Treatment is usually with simple analgesics such as acetaminophen. If acetaminophen is unsuccessful, a trial of NSAIDs may be appropriate.
- In situations where the precipitating event is felt to be trauma or overuse, a short period of rest may be helpful.
- In situations where the pain is well localized, a trial of capsaicin cream, NSAID creams or patches, or lidocaine patches may be helpful.
- In resistant cases, it may be necessary to refer to a pain center for local injections of a glucocorticoid/local anesthetic mixture.

Disease Course

- The course of costochondritis and the other chest wall pain syndromes is generally benign and self-limited and will resolve spontaneously within 2–3 weeks or a month.

Related Evidence

Papers of particular interest have been highlighted as:
*** Of key importance*

Practice Guideline

Woodard PK, White RD, Abbara S, Araoz PA, Cury RC, Dorbala S, Earls JP, Hoffmann U, Hsu JY, Jacobs JE, Javidan-Nejad C, Krishnamurthy R, Mammen L, Martin ET, Ryan T, Shah AB, Steiner RM, Vogel-Claussen J, White CS. ACR Appropriateness

Criteria chronic chest pain-low to intermediate probability of coronary artery disease. J Am Coll Radiol. 2013 May;10(5):329-34. https://doi.org/10.1016/j.jacr.2013.01.018. PMID: 23542027. http://www.ncbi.nlm.nih.gov/pubmed/23542027 **

Review

King JE, Magdic KS. Chest pain: a time for concern? AACN Adv Crit Care. 2014 Jul-Sep;25(3):279-83. https://doi.org/10.1097/NCI.0000000000000039. PMID: 25054533. http://www.ncbi.nlm.nih.gov/pubmed/25054533 **

Ayloo A, Cvengros T, Marella S. Evaluation and treatment of musculoskeletal chest pain. Prim Care. 2013 Dec;40(4):863-87, viii. https://doi.org/10.1016/j.pop.2013.08.007. PMID: 24209723. http://www.ncbi.nlm.nih.gov/pubmed/24209723 **

Proulx AM, Zryd TW. Costochondritis: diagnosis and treatment. Am Fam Physician. 2009 Sep 15;80(6):617-20. PMID: 19817327. http://www.ncbi.nlm.nih.gov/pubmed/19817327 **

Cohort Study

Bösner S, Bönisch K, Haasenritter J, Schlegel P, Hüllermeier E, Donner-Banzhoff N. Chest pain in primary care: is the localization of pain diagnostically helpful in the critical evaluation of patients?--A cross sectional study. BMC Fam Pract. 2013 Oct 18;14:154. https://doi.org/10.1186/1471-2296-14-154. PMID: 24138299. http://www.ncbi.nlm.nih.gov/pubmed/24138299

Case Study

Cubuk R, Tasali N. Medical image. Tietze's syndrome. N Z Med J. 2009 Feb 13;122(1289):87-8. PMID: 19305456. http://www.ncbi.nlm.nih.gov/pubmed/19305456

Volterrani L, Mazzei MA, Giordano N, Nuti R, Galeazzi M, Fioravanti A. Magnetic resonance imaging in Tietze's syndrome. Clin Exp Rheumatol. 2008 Sep-Oct;26(5):848-53. PMID: 19032818. http://www.ncbi.nlm.nih.gov/pubmed/19032818 **

Use PubMed Clinical Queries to find the most recent evidence. Use this search strategy:
"Tietze's Syndrome"[Mesh] OR "Costochondritis"

Chapter 21
Cyanide Poisoning

Charles V. Pollack, Jr., Melissa Platt, Richard M. Cantor, and Victoria G. Riese

Name and Synonyms

Cyanide Poisoning

Incidence/Epidemiology

- Rare occurrence
- Usually in association with smoke inhalation from a residential or industrial fire
- Occasionally seen as suicidal ingestion

Differential Diagnosis

- Myocardial infarction

C. V. Pollack, Jr. (✉)
Department of Emergency Medicine, Thomas Jefferson University, Philadelphia, PA, USA

M. Platt
Department of Emergency Medicine, University of Louisville, Louisville, KY, USA

R. M. Cantor
Department of Emergency Medicine and Pediatrics, State University of New York Upstate Medical University, Syracuse, NY, USA

V. G. Riese
Librarian Consultant, Eldersburg, MD, USA

C. V. Pollack, Jr. (ed.), *Differential Diagnosis of Cardiopulmonary Disease*,
https://doi.org/10.1007/978-3-319-63895-9_21

- Meningitis and encephalitis
- Hemlock poisoning
- Pulmonary embolism
- Cardiogenic shock
- Ischemic stroke
- Carbon monoxide toxicity
- Hydrogen sulfide toxicity
- Iron toxicity
- Isoniazid toxicity
- Nonsteroidal anti-inflammatory drug toxicity
- Azide toxicity
- Methanol toxicity
- Strychnine toxicity

Pathophysiology and Etiology

- Mitochondrial toxicity by binding cyanide to ferric ion ($Fe3^{+}$). Oxidative phosphorylation ceases, leading to anaerobic metabolism.
- Rapidly absorbed through gastrointestinal tract and skin
- Rapidly lethal
- Exposure may be
  - From smoke inhalation/fire
    - Formed when structures containing both carbon and nitrogen (such as polyurethane) burn
  - Industrial
    - From metal extraction, electroplating
  - Medical
    - Use of some antineoplastic agents (such as amygdalin) and other infusions (such as nitroprusside) may result in accumulation of toxic levels of cyanide.
  - Diet
    - Fruit pits and bitter almond contain cyanogenic glycosides
  - Tobacco abuse
    - At baseline, chronic smokers have significantly higher blood levels of cyanide than nonsmokers

Presentation

Typical/"Classic"

- Symptoms depend on severity and route of poisoning.
- Central nervous system symptoms, including headache, anxiety, confusion, vertigo, coma, and seizures, are most prominent.
- Also prominent are cardiovascular symptoms, including tachycardia, hypertension then bradycardia and hypotension, atrioventricular block, and ventricular dysrhythmias.
- Skin and lip flushing also may be seen.

Atypical

- Lower-level exposure may delay the onset of the aforementioned signs and symptoms.
- Nausea and vomiting
- Muscular twitching

Primary Differential Considerations

- Because of the wide range of signs and symptoms, the differential is quite large and includes exposure to tricyclic antidepressants, organophosphates, methemoglobin, strychnine, carbon monoxide, or arsine.

History and Physical Exam

Findings That Confirm Diagnosis

- There is no clinical confirmation of cyanide toxicity. This is a laboratory diagnosis in a challenging clinical setting in which early testing of arterial blood gas and lactate levels is important.

Factors That Suggest Diagnosis

- Bright red venous blood
  - Despite hypotension, apnea, or bradycardia, cyanosis usually is not present.
- After hydrogen cyanide inhalation:

  - Bitter almond odor
  - Headache, anxiety, nausea, and metallic taste
- After cyanogen chloride inhalation:
  - Eye and mucous membrane irritation, bronchorrhea, cough, and dyspnea
- After dermal exposure/ingestion:
  - Delayed symptoms: minutes to hours
- After parental exposure:
  - Confusion and combativeness initially may be mistaken as intensive care unit (ICU) syndrome
- After ingestion
  - Nausea and vomiting
  - Large quantities of such foods may result in toxicity

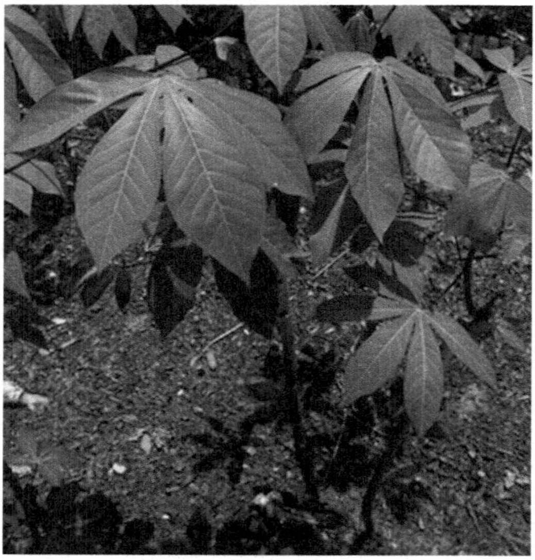

The starchy roots of the cassava plant (*Manihot esculenta*) contain cyanide. The roots are a staple in the diet of people living in the tropics, and inadequate processing of the roots can lead to cyanide poisoning [Lottermoser BG. Mine wastes [Internet]. Berlin, Heidelberg: Springer; 2010. Chapter 5, Cyanidation wastes of gold-silver ores; [cited 2015 Aug 13]; p. 243-262. Available from: http://link.springer.com/10.1007/978-3-642-12419-8_5] *Caption from original*

Factors That Exclude Diagnosis

- There is no clinical exclusion for cyanide poisoning when the presentation is suggestive.

Ancillary Studies

Laboratory

- Basic metabolic panel to assess for anion gap metabolic acidosis
- Serum lactate:
  - Closely correlates with severity of cyanide toxicity
  - A normal level casts doubt on true cyanide poisoning.
  - Levels may be used to monitor treatment progress.
- Central venous blood gas to assess venous arterial PO2 gradient
- Carboxyhemoglobin and methemoglobin levels in concomitant carbon monoxide exposure
- Cyanide levels:
  - May be obtained for diagnostic confirmation, but results will not be available in time to be clinically useful and may be unreliable
  - Levels do not correlate directly with survivability.

Special Populations

Age

- Sodium nitrite–induced 20–30 % level of methemoglobinemia may be lethal in children or anemic patients and should not be given to pregnant patients.
- Pediatric patients are thought to be vulnerable to cyanide exposure because of their higher respiratory rates and immature detoxification systems.

Co-morbidities

- Patients with limited cardiopulmonary reserve who are exposed to cyanide have a poorer prognosis.

Pregnancy

- Fetal demise is possible in cyanide poisoning. Aggressive support and antidotal treatment of the mother are essential.

Pitfalls in Diagnosis

Critical Steps Not to Miss

- The presentation of carbon monoxide poisoning from smoke inhalation is similar to that of cyanide poisoning; thus, clinicians often focus on carboxyhemoglobin levels, neglecting coexistent cyanide toxicity.

Mimics

- Mimics of cyanide poisoning include those listed as differential considerations, especially
    - Carbon monoxide poisoning
    - Phosgene exposure
    - Hydrogen sulfide poisoning
    - Arsine exposure
    - Inert gas exposure

Time-Dependent Interventions

- If clinical history and exam suggest cyanide poisoning, antidotal therapy must be given immediately.

Overall Principles of Treatment

- Decontaminate as soon as possible, removing patient from cyanide source.
    - Rescuers should wear protective suits and respirators until proper decontamination is complete.
- Antidotal treatment involves three strategies: binding of cyanide, use of sulfur donors, and induction of methemoglobinemia.
    - Hydroxocobalamin, a precursor of vitamin B_{12}, contains a cobalt moiety that avidly binds to intracellular cyanide, forming cyanocobalamin.

    - Cyanocobalamin is excreted in urine.
- Sodium thiosulfate
    - Sulfur donor excreted renally
- +/− Sodium nitrite
    - Induces methemoglobinemia, with the goal of a 20–30 % methemoglobin level if tolerated
    - It is CONTRAINDICATED in cases of potential carbon monoxide toxicity.
    - May cause hypotension and tachycardia, vasodilation

Disease Course

- Prognosis depends on level of exposure and extent of symptoms at presentation.
- Even in patients with severe symptoms such as seizures at presentation, prompt administration of antidote improves prognosis.
    - The exception is cardiac arrest, in which even early antidote administration is unlikely to reverse the very poor prognosis.
- Patients who survive cyanide poisoning sometimes have long-term central nervous system complications, such as movement disorders and neuropsychiatric problems.
- Suicide attempts with cyanide often are successful because of the deliberately high toxin load.

Related Evidence

Papers of particular interest have been highlighted as:
*** Of key importance*

Practice Guideline

Anseeuw K, Delvau N, Burillo-Putze G, De Iaco F, Geldner G, Holmström P, Lambert Y, Sabbe M. Cyanide poisoning by fire smoke inhalation: a European expert consensus. Eur J Emerg Med. 2013 Feb;20(1):2-9. https://doi.org/10.1097/MEJ.0b013e328357170b. PMID: 22828651. http://www.ncbi.nlm.nih.gov/pubmed/22828651 **

Review

Huzar TF, George T, Cross JM. Carbon monoxide and cyanide toxicity: etiology, pathophysiology and treatment in inhalation injury. Expert Rev Respir Med. 2013 Apr;7(2):159-70. https://doi.org/10.1586/ers.13.9. PMID: 23547992. http://www.ncbi.nlm.nih.gov/pubmed/23547992 **

Dries DJ, Endorf FW. Inhalation injury: epidemiology, pathology, treatment strategies. Scand J Trauma Resusc Emerg Med. 2013 Apr 19;21:31. https://doi.org/10.1186/1757-7241-21-31. PMID: 23597126. http://www.ncbi.nlm.nih.gov/pubmed/23597126 **

Reade MC, Davies SR, Morley PT, Dennett J, Jacobs IC; Australian Resuscitation Council. Review article: management of cyanide poisoning. Emerg Med Australas. 2012 Jun;24(3):225-38. https://doi.org/10.1111/j.1742-6723.2012.01538.x. PMID: 22672162. http://www.ncbi.nlm.nih.gov/pubmed/22672162 **

O'Brien DJ, Walsh DW, Terriff CM, Hall AH. Empiric management of cyanide toxicity associated with smoke inhalation. Prehosp Disaster Med. 2011 Oct;26(5):374-82. https://doi.org/10.1017/S1049023X11006625. PMID: 22336184. http://www.ncbi.nlm.nih.gov/pubmed/22336184 **

Barillo DJ. Diagnosis and treatment of cyanide toxicity. J Burn Care Res. 2009 Jan-Feb;30(1):148-52. https://doi.org/10.1097/BCR.0b013e3181923b91. PMID: 19060738. http://www.ncbi.nlm.nih.gov/pubmed/19060738 **

Geller RJ, Barthold C, Saiers JA, Hall AH. Pediatric cyanide poisoning: causes, manifestations, management, and unmet needs. Pediatrics. 2006 Nov;118(5):2146-58. PMID: 17079589. http://www.ncbi.nlm.nih.gov/pubmed/17079589 **

Beasley DM, Glass WI. Cyanide poisoning: pathophysiology and treatment recommendations. Occup Med (Lond). 1998 Oct;48(7):427-31. PMID: 10024740. http://www.ncbi.nlm.nih.gov/pubmed/10024740 **

Use PubMed Clinical Queries to find the most recent evidence. Use this search strategy:
"Cyanide Poisoning" OR "Cyanide Toxicity"

Chapter 22
Cyanotic Congenital Heart Disease

Richard M. Cantor, Charles V. Pollack, Jr., and Jaime Friel Blanck

Name and Synonyms

Cyanotic Congenital Heart Disease

- Refers to a subset of congenital cardiac malformations that favor the development of variable degrees of cyanosis.
- The vast majority of malformations will present in the newborn period and will be diagnosed in the neonatal setting.
- There are, however, variant forms which will "escape" neonatal diagnosis and have their initial cyanotic presentations in the Emergency Department.
- Late presentations are usually encountered in infants with ductus-dependent lesions necessary for pulmonary blood flow (generally left sided outflow obstructions such as hypoplastic left ventricle or coarctation of the aorta).

Incidence/Epidemiology

- Fifteen to 20 percent of all congenital heart disease cases are of the cyanotic variety.
- Cyanotic forms account for nearly 30 percent of fatal cases.

R. M. Cantor
Department of Emergency Medicine and Pediatrics, State University of New York Upstate Medical University, Syracuse, NY, USA

C. V. Pollack, Jr. (✉)
Department of Emergency Medicine, Thomas Jefferson University, Philadelphia, PA, USA

J. F. Blanck
Welch Medical Library, Johns Hopkins University, Baltimore, MD, USA

C. V. Pollack, Jr. (ed.), *Differential Diagnosis of Cardiopulmonary Disease*,
https://doi.org/10.1007/978-3-319-63895-9_22

Differential Diagnosis

- Should be considered in the differential diagnosis of cyanotic congenital heart disease, often represented by the "5 T's":
  - Truncus Arteriosus
  - Transposition of the Great Arteries
  - Tricuspid Atresia
  - Tetralogy of Fallot
  - Total Anomalous Pulmonary Venous Return
- There are other causes of cyanosis in young infants, most traditionally classified into pulmonary insults and hemoglobinopathies (i.e., Methemoglobinemia)

Pathophysiology and Etiology

- The essential common pathway that serves as the basis for all congenital cyanotic cardiac lesions is an inability to deliver oxygen to the general circulation and therefore peripheral target organs.
- The predominant pathophysiology involves variable degrees of right-to-left shunting. Systemic (deoxygenated) blood is unable to access the alveoli, returning to the left side of the heart without being oxygenated. In most cases of cyanotic heart disease, the shunt is intracardiac.

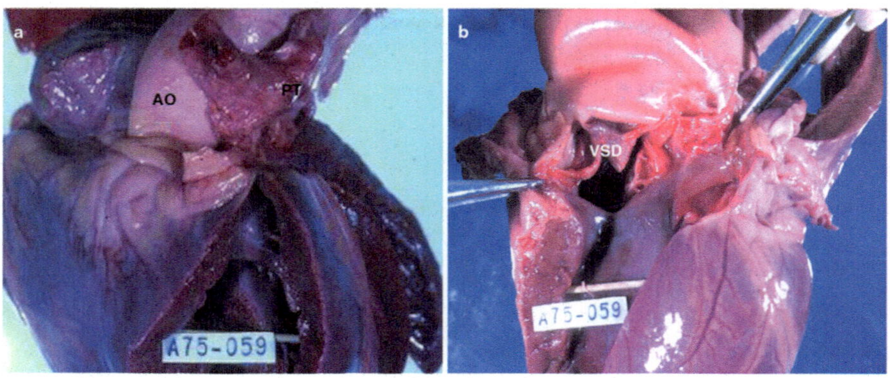

Tetralogy of Fallot. (a, b) Tetralogy of Fallot, the most common cause of cyanotic congenital heart disease, consists of a membranous VSD right ventricular outflow obstruction, rightward displacement of the aorta (AO), and secondary right ventricular hypertrophy. The right ventricular outflow obstruction may take the form of hypoplasia of the pulmonary trunk (PT), pulmonary valvular malformation and stenosis, outflow tract (infundibular) hypoplasia and narrowing, or a combination of all three components, as seen in this case [Buja LM, Cheong B. Cardiovascular Pathology. In: Krueger GRF, Buja LM, editors. Atlas of Anatomic Pathology with Imaging [Internet]. London: Springer London; 2013 [cited 2016 Jul 29]. p. 43–104. Available from: http://link.springer.com/10.1007/978-1-4471-2846-5_2] *Caption from original*

Presentation

Typical/"Classic"

- Most entities will present within the first few hours of life, with diagnosis made before discharge from the newborn unit.
- Other entities, specifically those with ductal dependency, will only present when the duct closes. The infants will present with varying degrees of shock and/or cyanosis (usually left sided outflow obstructive lesions such as an interrupted aortic arch).

Atypical

- Infants with Tetrology of Fallot may "escape" diagnosis in the first few days of life, presenting to the ED with what are known as "Tet (hypercyanotic) Spells."
- Management of Hypercyanotic Spells:
  - Provision of supplemental oxygen.
  - Placement in the knee chest position.
    - Sedation with morphine (0.1 mg/kg/dose)
    - Administration of 10-20 cc/kg of normal saline
    - Immediate consultation with a pediatric cardiologist

Primary Differential Considerations

- These specific diagnoses should be considered in patients who present with signs and symptoms of congenital cyanotic heart disease:
  - tricuspid atresia
  - Ebstein's malformation of the tricuspid valve
  - severe pulmonic stenosis with intact ventricular septum
  - complete transposition of the great vessels
  - truncus arteriosus.

History and Physical Exam

- As previously described, the majority of cyanotic congenital lesions will be diagnosed and treated within the first few days of life.
- In some patients, cyanotic presentations may be quite dramatic, unresponsive to any degree of supplemental oxygen (the hyperoxia test).
- Other patients will present with hypoperfusion and frank hypotension. Administration of isotonic volume replacement will often worsen the clinical status, alerting the clinician to the possibility of a cardiogenic etiology as the cause of shock.
- Each particular malformation has a specific set of physical and radiographic findings.
- The presence or absence of a murmur is variable and often not integral in making the diagnosis.

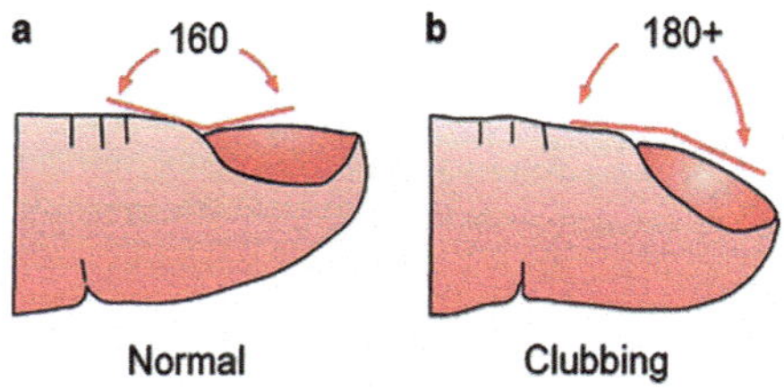

Clubbing. (**a**) The angle at the junction of skin with the nail at the dorsal surface of digits is normally around 160°. (**b**) In children with cyanotic congenital heart diseases this angle becomes wider and may exceed 180°. This is the result of hypoxia in peripheral tissue, which causes the opening of normally collapsed capillaries to better perfuse the hypoxic tissue. Perfusion of these collapsed capillaries will result in expansion of the volume of these peripheral tissues (tips of digits) resulting in clubbing. This phenomenon is seen in other lesions causing hypoxia of peripheral tissue, such as with chronic lung disease and chronic anemia (causing hypoxia through reduction of level of hemoglobin and therefore reduction of oxygen carrying capacity) such as with ulcerative colitis, Crohn's disease, and chronic liver disease [Thompson WR, Mehrotra SM. Cardiac History and Physical Examination. In: Abdulla R, editor. Heart Diseases in Children [Internet]. Boston, MA: Springer US; 2011 [cited 2016 Jul 29]. p. 3–16. Available from: http://link.springer.com/10.1007/978-1-4419-7994-0_1] *Caption from original*

Findings That Confirm Diagnosis

- Echocardiography remains the gold standard.

Factors That Suggest Diagnosis

- The use of the hyperoxia test is traditionally employed to differentiate between pulmonary, cardiac, and hematologic causes of cyanosis in infancy.
- Administer supplemental oxygen.
- If OSAT rises, it is most likely pulmonary disease.
- If OSAT does not rise, consider Cyanotic Heart Disease *or* Methemoglo binemia.
- With the patient on 100% supplemental O_2, and the pO_2 is high and OSAT is low, consider Methemoglobinemia as an etiology,
- With the patient on 100% supplemntalO_2, and the pO_2 is low *and* the OSAT is low, consider cyanotic heart disease as an etiology.

Factors That Exclude Diagnosis

- A normal echocardiogram.

Ancillary Studies

Imaging

- There are certain classic radiographic findings associated with specific forms of cyanotic heart disease in infants:
  - Cardiomegaly is seen with left-sided outflow obstructive lesions.
  - A boot-shaped heart is seen with Tetralogy.
  - An "egg-on-a-string" pattern is seen with Transposition.

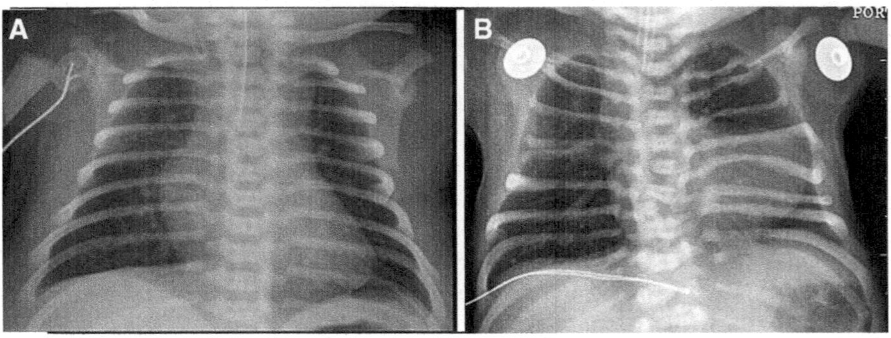

Utility of chest radiography in CHD. A: Chest radiograph of a neonate with d-transposition of the great arteries, appearing as an "egg on a string" appearance of the heart and mediastinum. This pattern-based approach to cardiac morphology is inaccurate and is rarely helpful for clinical management. Cardiac morphology is determined by echocardiography in the neonatal period while the chest radiograph sheds light on physiology. B: Neonate with complex cyanotic congenital heart disease, including mitral atresia, total anomalous pulmonary venous connection to the coronary sinus, double outlet right ventricle, and pulmonary stenosis. The chest radiograph demonstrated decreased pulmonary vascularity, which enabled decision-making regarding initial palliative treatment. The pulmonary blood flow was augmented using a modified Blalock–Taussig shunt. [Krishnamurthy R, Chitkara P. Evidence-Based Approach to Imaging of Congenital Heart Disease. In: Medina LS, Applegate KE, Blackmore CC, editors. Evidence-Based Imaging in Pediatrics [Internet]. New York, NY: Springer New York; 2010 [cited 2016 Jul 29]. p. 339–58. Available from: http://link.springer.com/10.1007/978-1-4419-0922-0_24] *Caption from original*

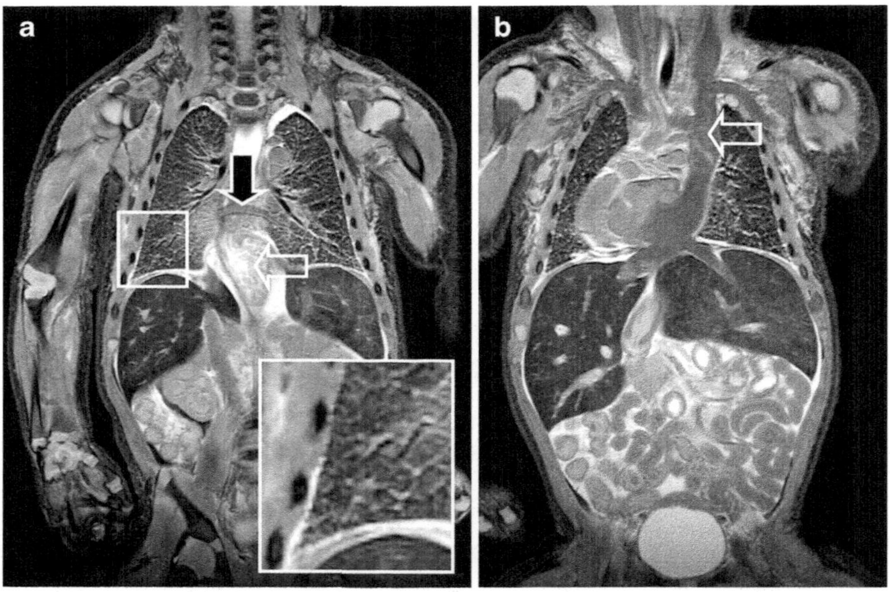

A neonate with a congenital cyanotic heart disease born at 39 weeks. Maximum support and 100% oxygen did not lead to clinical improvement and the child died. T2-W coronal MRI shows a complete anomalous venous return (arrow) with pulmonary interstitial oedema (insert). A central tendon defect is seen (open arrow) (slice thickness: 2 mm, TR: 5500, TE: 54, FA: 180°). **b** T2-W coronal MRI shows a persistent left superior caval vein (arrow), a dextrocardia and situs intermedius of the liver. Asplenia was also noted [From article: Current techniques in postmortem imaging with specific attention to paediatric applications. Pediatric Radiology. 2010

Feb;40(2):141–52. https://doi.org/10.1007/s00247-009-1486-0, at http://link.springer.com/article/10.1007/s00247-009-1486-0; by Tessa Sieswerda-Hoogendoorn, Rick R. van Rijn, © The Author(s) 2009; licensed under Creative Commons Attribution License BY 2.0 http://creativecommons.org/licenses/by/2.0] *Caption from original*

Electrocardiography

ECG finding	Likely CCHD	Remarks
RAD with RVH	TOF	Early & sudden R to S transition from V_1 to V_2
	ccTGA with VSD with PS	CHB, absent septal q in V_{5-6}
	Critical PS with IVS	RV strain (ST- T changes in V_{1-3}, II, III, aVF)
	TGA with IVS	
LAD	AVSD with PS	RVH
	Tricuspid atresia	LVH
Monomorphic QRS in V_{1-6}	Single ventricle with PS	
IRBBB	Ebstein's anomaly	Polyphasic QRS complexes

Typical ECG findings in various cyanotic congenital heart diseases [Gupta SK. Clinical Approach to a Neonate with Cyanosis. The Indian Journal of Pediatrics. 2015 Nov;82(11):1050–60.] *Caption from original*

- Cardiac Enzymes
- Not indicated.

Special Populations

Age

- As discussed, most cases are diagnosed in the first few days of life.

Co-morbidities

- TAPVR is associated with asplenia or polysplenia.

Pitfalls in Diagnosis

- Cyanotic variant
  - Emergency pediatric cardiology consultation is warranted.
- Acyanotic variety
  - Adherence to strict algorhythmic workups of neonatal CHF or respiratory distress will eventually uncover the lesion.

Critical Steps Not to Miss

- Provision of supplemental oxygen
- Early ventilator support
- Immediate PICU or Pediatric Cardiology consultation

Mimics

- Any congenital cardiac lesion causing cyanosis and/or CHF

Time-Dependent Interventions

- All interventions are emergent.

Overall Principles of Treatment

- Support oxygenation.
- Urgent echocardiography.
- Arrange specialty consultation to evaluate for surgical management.

Disease Course

- Surgical correction is almost always indicated—the earlier the better.
- Long-term outcomes are dramatically improved after full correction (less than 5%).

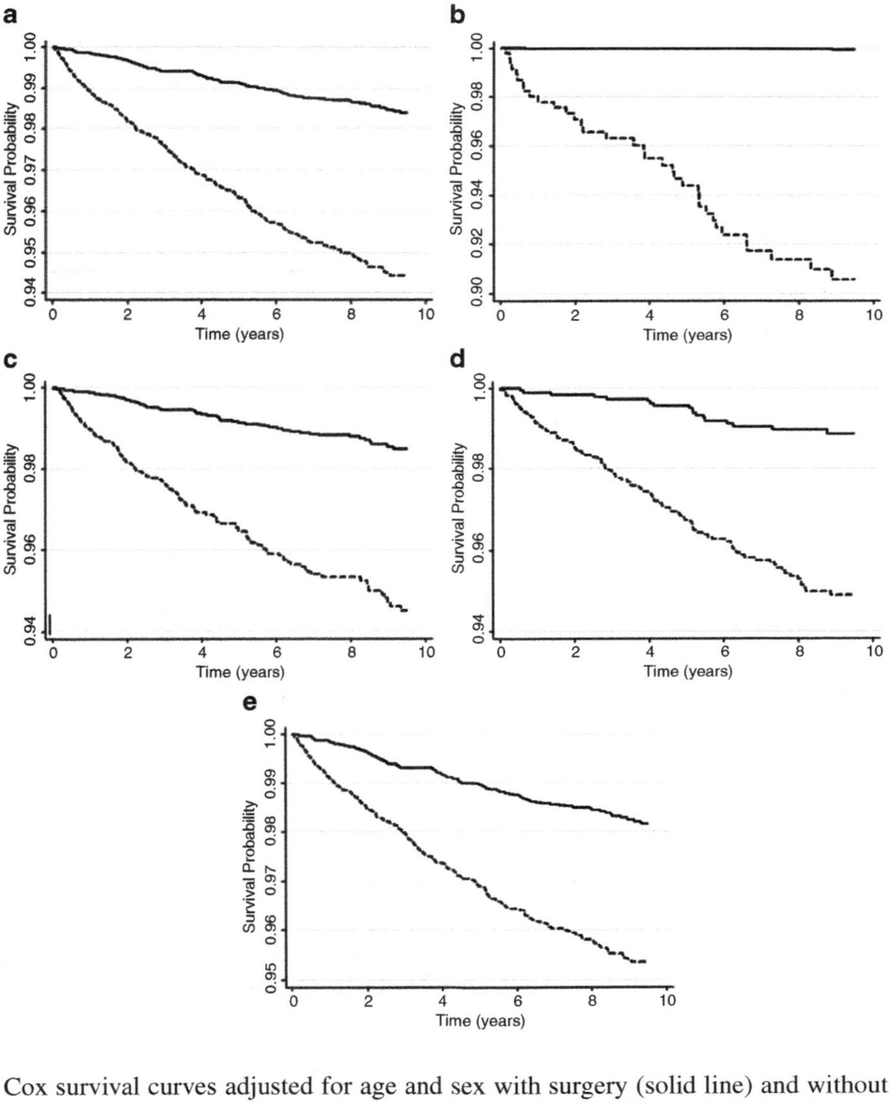

Cox survival curves adjusted for age and sex with surgery (solid line) and without surgery (dashed line) of congenital heart diseases patients. Time = 0, time at one and half year of follow-up. (A) Overall congenital heart diseases; (B) Cyanotic congenital heart diseases; (C) Noncyanotic congenital heart diseases; (D) ventricular septal defect; (E)ostium or secundum type atrial septal defect. [From article: Major adverse cardiovascular events in adult congenital heart disease: a population-based follow-up study from Taiwan. BMC Cardiovascular Disorders. 2014 Dec;14:38. https://doi.org/10.1186/1471-2261-14-38, at http://link.springer.com/article/10.1186/1471-2261-14-38; by Yu-Sheng Lin, Pi-Hua Liu, Lung-Sheng Wu, Yu-Ming Chen, Chee-Jen Chang, Pao-Hsien Chu, © Lin et al.; licensee BioMed Central Ltd. 2014; licensed under Creative Commons Attribution License BY 2.0 http://creativecommons.org/licenses/by/2.0] *Caption from original*

Related Evidence

Papers of particular interest have been highlighted as:
*** Of key importance*

Practice Guideline

Mahle WT, Sable CA, Matherne PG, Gaynor JW, Gewitz MH; American Heart Association Congenital Heart Defects Committee of the Council on Cardiovascular Disease in the Young. Key concepts in the evaluation of screening approaches for heart disease in children and adolescents: a science advisory from the American Heart Association. Circulation. 2012 Jun 5;125(22):2796-801. https://doi.org/10.1161/CIR.0b013e3182579f25. Epub 2012 Apr 30. PubMed PMID: 22547669. http://www.ncbi.nlm.nih.gov/pubmed/?term=22547669 **

Review

Strobel AM, Lu le N. The Critically Ill Infant with Congenital Heart Disease. Emerg Med Clin North Am. 2015 Aug;33(3):501-18. https://doi.org/10.1016/j.emc.2015.04.002. PubMed PMID: 26226862. http://www.ncbi.nlm.nih.gov/pubmed/26226862 **

Sorantin E, Heinzl B. What every radiologist should know about paediatric echocardiography. Eur J Radiol. 2014 Sep;83(9):1519-28. https://doi.org/10.1016/j.ejrad.2014.05.030. Epub 2014 May 29. PubMed PMID: 24938668. http://www.ncbi.nlm.nih.gov/pubmed/?term=24938668 **

Schranz D, Michel-Behnke I. Advances in interventional and hybrid therapy in neonatal congenital heart disease. Semin Fetal Neonatal Med. 2013 Oct;18(5):311-21. https://doi.org/10.1016/j.siny.2013.05.005. Epub 2013 Jun 10. PubMed PMID: 23759171. http://www.ncbi.nlm.nih.gov/pubmed/?term=23759171 **

Barata IA. Cardiac emergencies. Emerg Med Clin North Am. 2013 Aug;31(3):677-704. https://doi.org/10.1016/j.emc.2013.04.007. PubMed PMID: 23915599. http://www.ncbi.nlm.nih.gov/pubmed/?term=23915599 **

Sharkey AM, Sharma A. Tetralogy of Fallot: anatomic variants and their impact on surgical management. Semin Cardiothorac Vasc Anesth. 2012 Jun;16(2):88-96. https://doi.org/10.1177/1089253211434566. Epub 2012 Jan 24. PubMed PMID: 22275348. http://www.ncbi.nlm.nih.gov/pubmed/?term=22275348 **

Dolbec K, Mick NW. Congenital heart disease. Emerg Med Clin North Am. 2011 Nov;29(4):811-27, vii. https://doi.org/10.1016/j.emc.2011.08.005. PubMed PMID: 22040709. http://www.ncbi.nlm.nih.gov/pubmed/?term=22040709 **

Skold A, Cosco DL, Klein R. Methemoglobinemia: pathogenesis, diagnosis, and management. South Med J. 2011 Nov;104(11):757-61. https://doi.org/10.1097/SMJ.0b013e318232139f. PubMed PMID: 22024786. http://www.ncbi.nlm.nih.gov/pubmed/?term=22024786

Richards AA, Garg V. Genetics of congenital heart disease. Curr Cardiol Rev. 2010 May;6(2):91-7. https://doi.org/10.2174/157340310791162703. PubMed PMID: 21532774; PubMed Central PMCID: PMC2892081. http://www.ncbi.nlm.nih.gov/pubmed/?term=21532774

Kornosky JL, Salihu HM. Getting to the heart of the matter: epidemiology of cyanotic heart defects. Pediatr Cardiol. 2008 May;29(3):484-97. https://doi.org/10.1007/s00246-007-9185-9. Epub 2008 Jan 10. PubMed PMID: 18185949. http://www.ncbi.nlm.nih.gov/pubmed/?term=18185949 **

Silberbach M, Hannon D. Presentation of congenital heart disease in the neonate and young infant. Pediatr Rev. 2007 Apr;28(4):123-31. PubMed PMID: 17400823. http://www.ncbi.nlm.nih.gov/pubmed/?term=17400823 **

Marino BS, Bird GL, Wernovsky G. Diagnosis and management of the newborn with suspected congenital heart disease. Clin Perinatol. 2001 Mar;28(1):91-136. PubMed PMID: 11265513. http://www.ncbi.nlm.nih.gov/pubmed/?term=11265513 **

Nouri S. Congenital heart defects: cyanotic and acyanotic. Pediatr Ann. 1997 Feb;26(2):92, 95-8. PubMed PMID: 9121846. http://www.ncbi.nlm.nih.gov/pubmed/?term=9121846

Kelley MJ, Jaffe CC, Shoum SM, Kleinman CS. A radiographic and echocardiographic approach to cyanotic congenital heart disease. Radiol Clin North Am. 1980 Dec;18(3):411-40. PubMed PMID: 7005931. http://www.ncbi.nlm.nih.gov/pubmed

Clinical Trial

Dilli D, Aydin B, Zenciroğlu A, Özyazici E, Beken S, Okumuş N. Treatment outcomes of infants with cyanotic congenital heart disease treated with synbiotics. Pediatrics. 2013 Oct;132(4):e932-8. https://doi.org/10.1542/peds.2013-1262. Epub 2013 Sep 16. PubMed PMID: 24043284. http://www.ncbi.nlm.nih.gov/pubmed/?term=24043284

General

Patra S, Rama Sastry UM, Mahimaiha J, Subramanian AP, Shankarappa RK, Nanjappa MC. Spectrum of cyanotic congenital heart disease diagnosed by echocardiographic evaluation in patients attending paediatric cardiology clinic of a tertiary cardiac care centre. Cardiol Young. 2015 Jun;25(5):861-7. https://doi.org/10.1017/S1047951114000882. Epub 2014 Jun 10. PubMed PMID: 24914874. http://www.ncbi.nlm.nih.gov/pubmed/?term=24914874

Donofrio MT, Moon-Grady AJ, Hornberger LK, Copel JA, Sklansky MS, Abuhamad A, Cuneo BF, Huhta JC, Jonas RA, Krishnan A, Lacey S, Lee W, Michelfelder EC Sr, Rempel GR, Silverman NH, Spray TL, Strasburger JF, Tworetzky W, Rychik J; American Heart Association Adults With Congenital Heart Disease Joint Committee of the Council on Cardiovascular Disease in the Young and Council on Clinical Cardiology, Council on Cardiovascular Surgery and Anesthesia, and Council on Cardiovascular and Stroke Nursing. Diagnosis and treatment of fetal cardiac disease: a scientific statement from the American Heart Association. Circulation. 2014 May 27;129(21):2183-242. https://doi.org/10.1161/01.cir.0000437597.44550.5d. Epub 2014 Apr 24. Erratum in: Circulation. 2014 May 27;129(21):e512. PubMed PMID: 24763516. http://www.ncbi.nlm.nih.gov/pubmed/?term=24763516 **

Tibbles CD, Bouton M, Lucas JM, Harper M, Horwitz C, Fisher J. Emergency department management of pediatric patients with cyanotic heart disease and fever. J Emerg Med. 2013 Mar;44(3):599-604. https://doi.org/10.1016/j.jemermed.2012.09.030. Epub 2012 Dec 23. PubMed PMID: 23267753. http://www.ncbi.nlm.nih.gov/pubmed/?term=23267753

Use PubMed Clinical Queries to find the most recent evidence. Use this search strategy: ("Cyanosis"[Mesh:NoExp] OR "cyanosis" OR "cyanotic") AND ("Heart Defects, Congenital"[Mesh] OR "congenital heart defect" OR "congenital heart defects" OR "heart abnormalities" OR "congenital heart disease")

Chapter 23
Cystic Fibrosis

Richard M. Cantor, Charles V. Pollack, Jr., and Jaime Friel Blanck

Name and Synonyms

Cystic Fibrosis; CF

- The most common autosomal dominant longevity-reducing disorder among Caucasian groups.

Incidence/Epidemiology

- Cystic fibrosis has a reported incidence of 1 in 2,500 live births.
- Although it is most commonly reported in Caucasian children, due to enhanced diagnostic testing, recognition of cases in non-white populations are on the rise.
- The median predicted survival rate is approximate 37 – 38 years.

R. M. Cantor
Department of Emergency Medicine and Pediatrics, State University of New York Upstate Medical University, Syracuse, NY, USA

C. V. Pollack, Jr. (✉)
Department of Emergency Medicine, Thomas Jefferson University, Philadelphia, PA, USA

J. F. Blanck
Welch Medical Library, Johns Hopkins University, Baltimore, MD, USA

C. V. Pollack, Jr. (ed.), *Differential Diagnosis of Cardiopulmonary Disease*,
https://doi.org/10.1007/978-3-319-63895-9_23

Differential Diagnosis

- Any immune deficiency disorder may present with pulmonary findings commonly seen in CF.

Pathophysiology and Etiology

- CF is transmitted genetically in an autosomal dominant pattern.

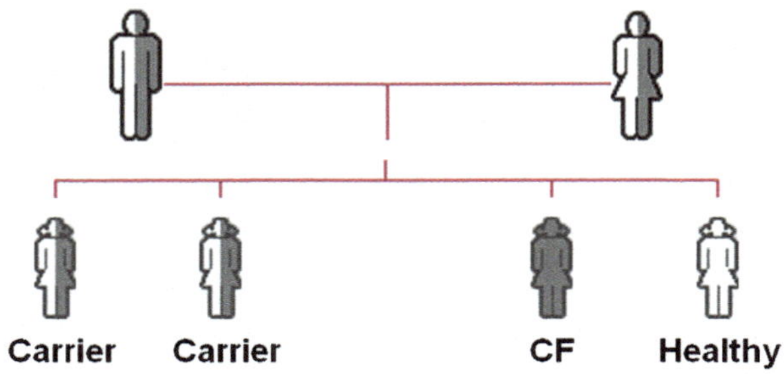

Cystic fibrosis inheritance pattern. This figure shows the inheritance pattern for children born with cystic fibrosis. If both the mother and father are carriers of the gene then they have a one in four chances of having a child with cystic fibrosis [Murphy AJ, Davies PSW. Anthropometry in Children with Cystic Fibrosis. In: Preedy VR, editor. Handbook of Anthropometry [Internet]. New York, NY: Springer New York; 2012 [cited 2015 Sep 14]. p. 1571–83. Available from: http://link.springer.com/10.1007/978-1-4419-1788-1_96] *Caption from original*

- The disorder is secondary to mutations in the cystic fibrosis trans membrane conductance regulator (CFTR) protein.
- The mutation impairs normal transport of chloride and other ions, leading to the production of thick viscous secretions commonly seen in target organs such as the lungs, liver, pancreas, and reproductive tract.

Presentation

Typical/"Classic"

- Most cases are detected by newborn screening and performance of sweat chloride testing in identified infants and children.
- There is a myriad of clinical manifestations of CF, including:

- Respiratory
  - Chronic cough
  - Sinusitis
  - Asthma
  - Bacterial colonization of the respiratory tract
- Clubbing of the digits

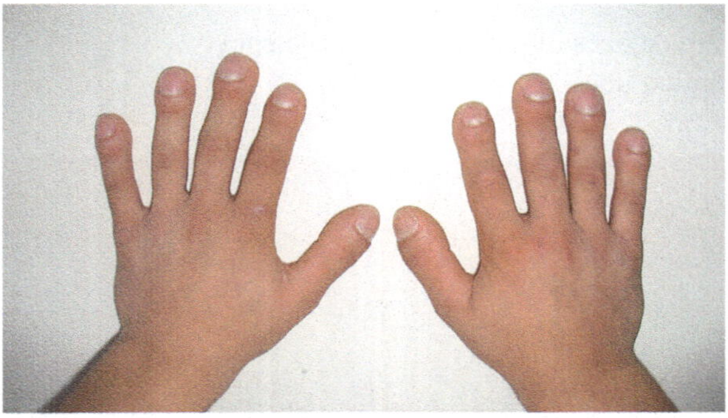

Clubbing of the fingers [Karkucak M, Erturk E, Capkin E, Akyazi H, Ozden G, Tosun M. Primary hypertrophic osteoarthropathy (pachydermoperiostosis): a case report. Rheumatology International. 2007 Jan 11;27(4):403–5.] *Caption from original*

- Nasal polyps

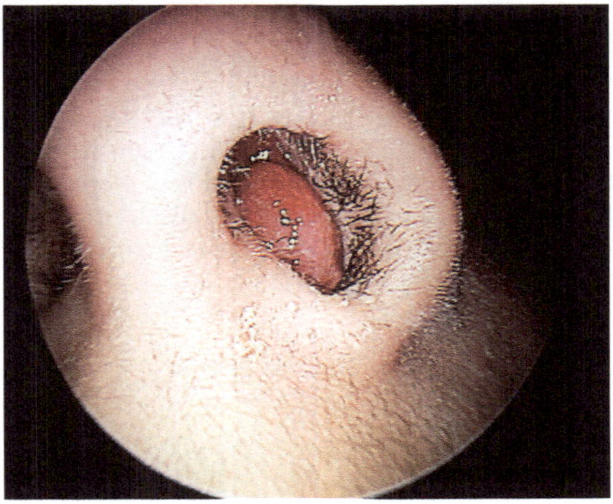

A pedunculated nasal polyp in a patient with cystic fibrosis. The polyp is obstructing the left nostril. Polyps commonly arise from the maxillary antrum. Chronic inflammation results in vasodilatation and edema of the mucosa. This initially causes mucosal hypertrophy, resulting in irregular folds within the mucosa. As the mucosa enlarges, it may herniate into the nasal cavity, creating a pedunculated polyp that may completely occlude the middle meatus. [MacLusky I, Solomon M, Laxer R, Ford-Jones EL, Friedman J, Gerstle T. Atlas of Pediatrics, Volume IA, Chapter 14. In: Laxer RM, editor. The Hospital for Sick Children: Atlas of Pediatrics. Philadelphia, PA: Current Medicine Group; 2005. 519 p. ISBN 1-57340-188-9] *Caption from original*

- Gastrointestinal
  - Varying degrees of pancreatic insufficiency
  - Meconium ileus

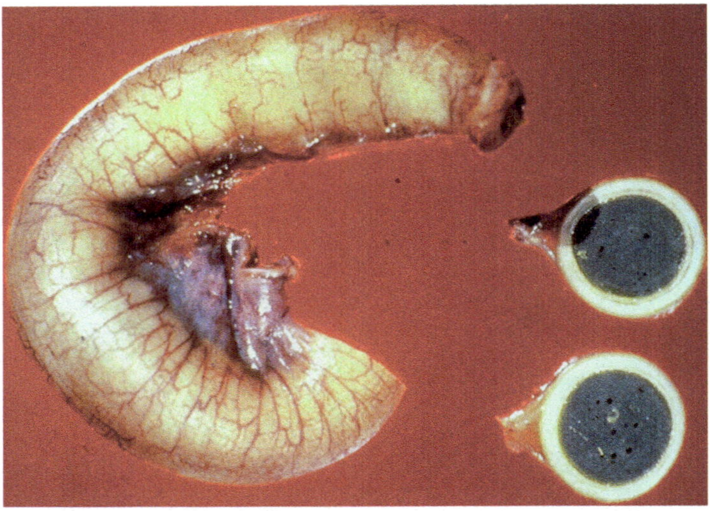

Meconium ileus in cystic fibrosis. The bowel lumen is plugged with meconium [Gilbert-Barness E, Spicer DE, Steffensen TS. Gastrointestinal (GI) System. Handbook of Pediatric Autopsy Pathology [Internet]. New York, NY: Springer New York; 2014 [cited 2015 Sep 14]. p. 355–75. Available from: http://link.springer.com/10.1007/978-1-4614-6711-3_10] *Caption from original*

- Secondary diabetes
- Pancreatitis
- Vitamin deficiencies
- Rectal prolapse

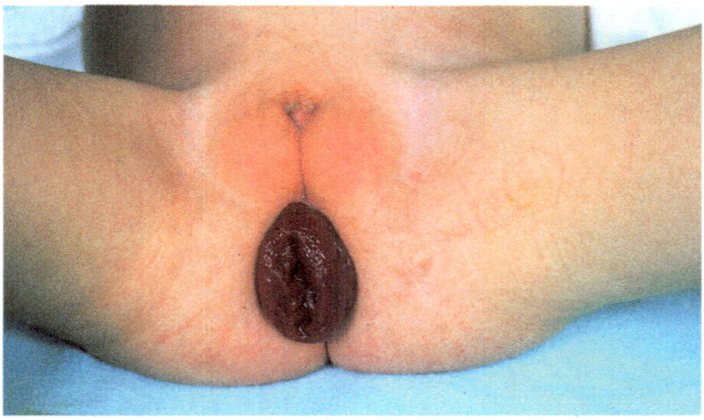

Rectal prolapse, which usually occurs during passage of a large bowel motion, can be a frightening condition for parents of young children. It is hardly ever associated with major medical complications and is easily reduced manually. This condition usually resolves spontaneously by 3 to 4 years of age. Surgical intervention is not advocated, unless the condition is persistent. [Durie P. Chapter 09. In: Hyman P, editor. Gastroenterology and Hepatology, Volume 04. Philadelphia: Current Medicine; 1996 (Feldman M, series editor) ISBN: 0-443-07852-1] *Caption from original*

- Genitourinary
    - Male infertility

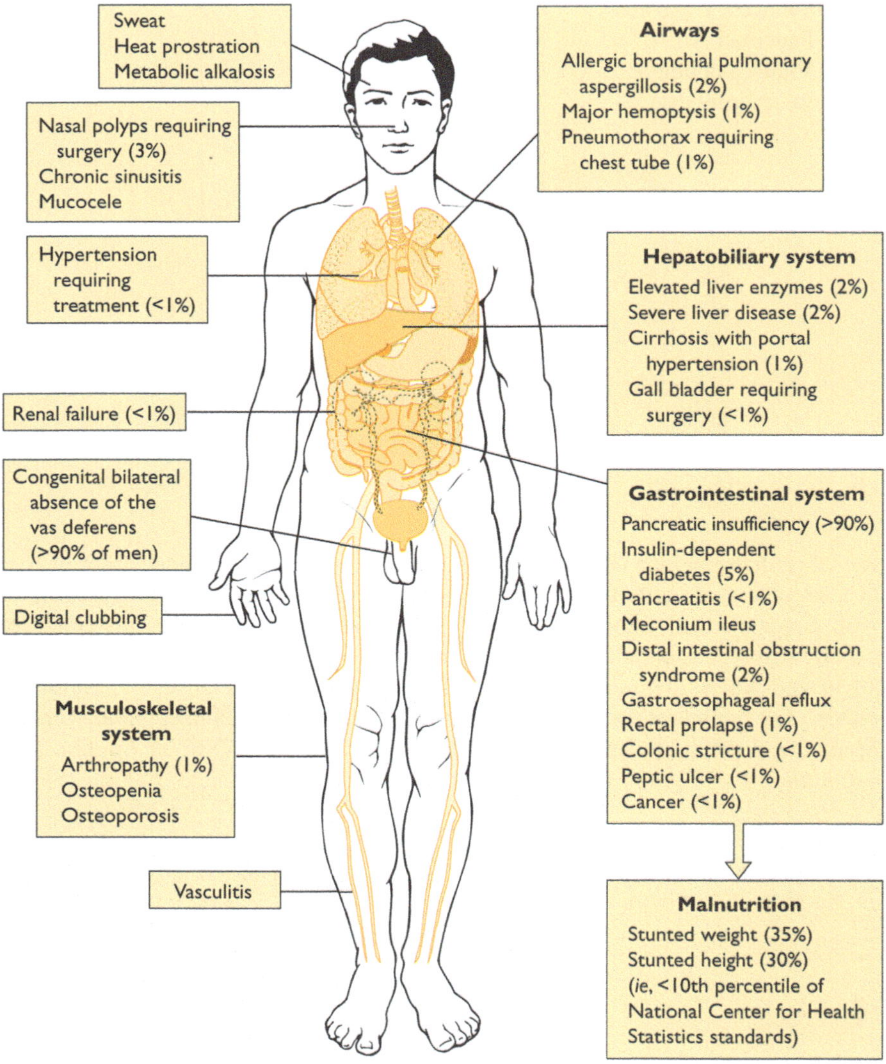

Clinical manifestations and co-morbidity of cystic fibrosis. Cystic fibrosis is associated with numerous complications and co-morbid conditions. As indicated in the figure, almost every patient with cystic fibrosis who lives long enough will eventually develop pulmonary symptoms. However, the age of onset, the rate at which cystic fibrosis progresses, and the incidence of co-morbid conditions are extremely variable. The 1999 incidence of some of these manifestations and co-morbid conditions, obtained from the Cystic Fibrosis Foundation Registry, are provided in parentheses. It is important to note that the incidence of most of these conditions increases significantly with age and disease progression. Thus, the prevalence of some conditions (e.g., liver disease and diabetes mellitus) in a clinical setting that includes adolescents and young adults may be significantly higher than these figures suggest. [Coakley R. Boucher R. Fiel S. Schidlow D. Chapter 04. In: Crapo J, editor. Bone's Atlas of Pulmonary and Critical Care Medicine. 3rd ed. Philadelphia: Current Medicine; 2005. ISBN: 1-57340-211-7] *Caption adapted from original*

- The most common clinical presentations are overwhelmingly pulmonary in nature, including chromic cough with sputum production, dyspnea, and signs of respiratory insufficiency.

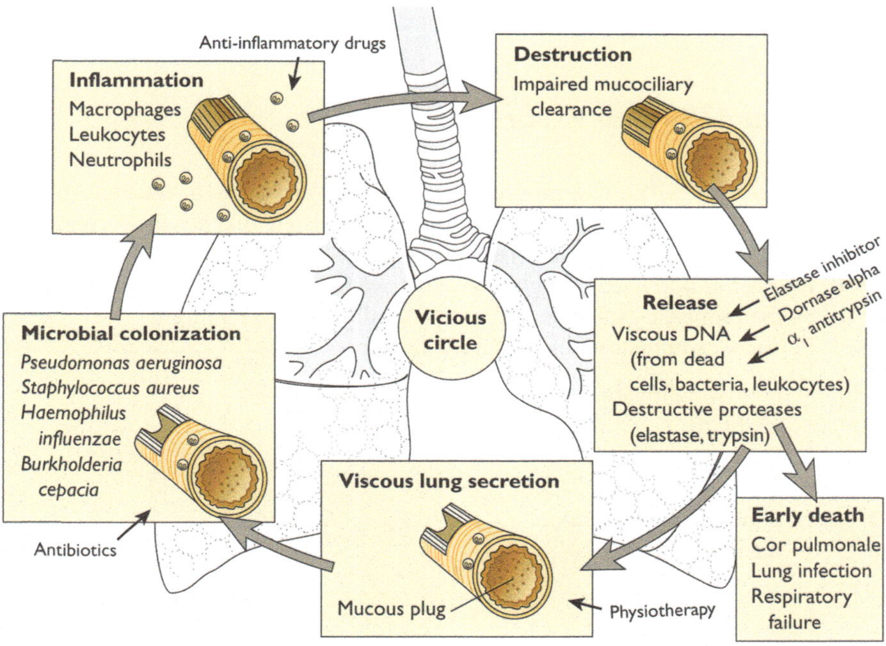

The "vicious circle" of lung disease in cystic fibrosis. Cystic fibrosis is a genetic form of chronic bronchitis characterized by a vicious circle of obstruction, infection, and inflammation related to impaired local host-defense mechanisms. This produces progressive bronchiectasis and, ultimately, respiratory failure. Despite the identification of the CFTR gene and characterization of its role as an ion channel, intense efforts are still under way to understand how defective transepithelial electrolyte transport leads to the devastating consequences seen throughout the airways. [Coakley R. Boucher R. Fiel S. Schidlow D. Chapter 04. In: Crapo J, editor. Bone's Atlas of Pulmonary and Critical Care Medicine. 3rd ed. Philadelphia: Current Medicine; 2005. ISBN: 1-57340-211-7] *Caption from original*

- Most infants and children will have already been diagnosed in the first few months of life.

Atypical

- Any of the aforementioned symptoms and signs may present.

Primary Differential Considerations

- Cystic fibrosis is a distinctive syndrome, but in early stages it may be confused with acute lung or sinus infections. Asthma and metabolic/nutritional disorders may also be differential considerations.

History and Physical Exam

- The history will reveal progressive symptoms and signs of respiratory compromise. The patient will most often have been diagnosed by abnormal screening and confirmatory testing.
- In older children, the cough is productive. In infancy, this finding is masked by the propensity of these children to swallow their secretions.
- Physical examination findings may include:
  - Poor weight gain
  - Clubbing
  - Dyspnea
  - Wheezing
  - Signs of pneumonia
  - Steatorrhea

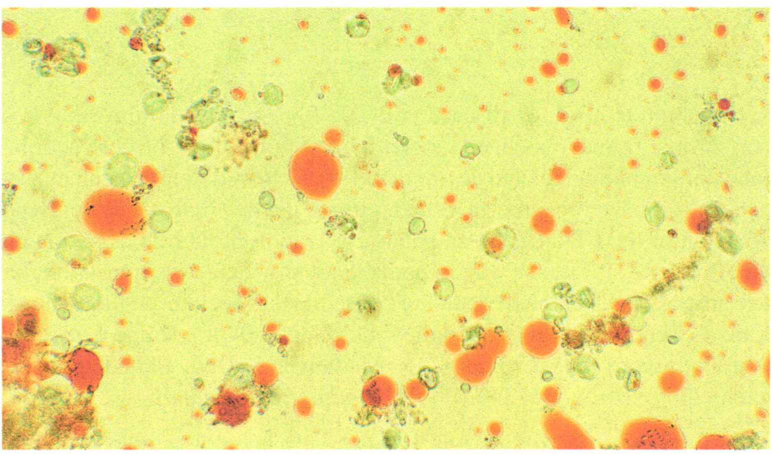

Steatorrhea by fecal Sudan stain. This photomicrograph stool sample demonstrates the presence of large amounts of fat by Sudan stain. This test is qualitative and should only be used as a screening tool for gross steatorrhea, but in this particular patient it reveals the presence of a large amount of fat in the stool. [Vanderhoof J. Chapter 06. In: Hyman P, editor. Gastroenterology and Hepatology, Volume 04. Philadelphia: Current Medicine; 1996 (Feldman M, series editor) ISBN: 0-443-07852-1] *Caption from original*

- Increased AP diameter
  - Typical symptoms suggesting the presence of CF include:
    - Meconeum ileus (25% of patients)
    - Respiratory symptoms (50% of patients)
    - Failure to thrive (25% of patients)

Findings That Confirm Diagnosis

- Abnormal sweat chloride and genetic testing

Factors That Suggest Diagnosis

- Any infant or child with failure to thrive and the early development of pulmonary compromise.

Factors That Exclude Diagnosis

- Normal screening tests

Ancillary Studies

Imaging

- Initial radiographs may be normal, with the eventual development of hyperinflation. Inevitably, the chronic nature of the disease will result in the development of bronchiectasis and cyst formation. In addition, pneumothoraces may develop.

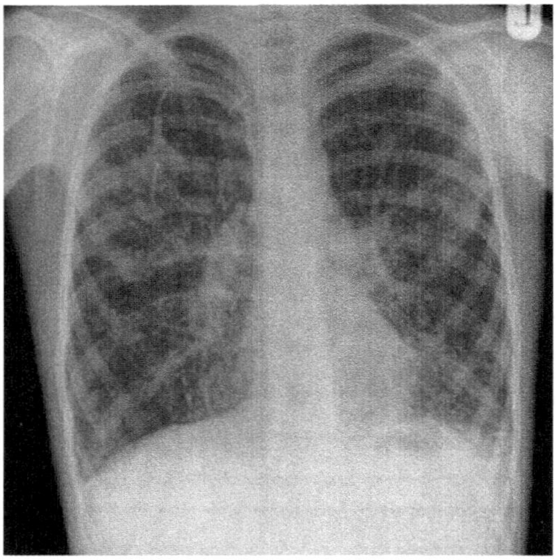

Advanced cystic fibrosis (CF). This is a chest radiograph of a 14-year-old boy with advanced CF. It demonstrates the typical changes of end-stage CF. There is marked generalized hyperinflation. Both lungs demonstrate diffuse bronchial wall thickening, with "tram tracking" (parallel lines due to thickening and absence of tapering of the bronchial walls), most evident in the left lower lobe, indicative of bronchiectasis. There are also scattered peripheral acinar infiltrates, especially in the left apex and in both lung bases, as well as blunting of the left costrophenic sulcus, due to recurrent, long-standing pneumonia. The heart size is within normal limits given the degree of lung hyperinflation. A central line is in place to provide antibiotics. [MacLusky I, Solomon M, Laxer R, Ford-Jones EL, Friedman J, Gerstle T. Atlas of Pediatrics, Volume IA, Chapter 14. In: Laxer RM, editor. The Hospital for Sick Children: Atlas of Pediatrics. Philadelphia, PA: Current Medicine Group; 2005. 519 p. ISBN 1-57340-188-9] *Caption from original*

Electrocardiography

- With the development of chronic lung disease, signs of right-sided strain/ hypertrophy will be evident.

Cardiac Enzymes

- Not indicated.

Special Populations

Age

- As discussed under Presentation, most cases are diagnosed in the first few weeks of life.

Co-morbidities

- The gene mutation in CF damages the hepatobiliary system. Diabetes may develop.

Pitfalls in Diagnosis

- Consider CF in all cases of chronic, progressive pulmonary dysfunction.

Critical Steps Not to Miss

- Early administration of bronchodilators
- Radiographic monitoring
- Cultures of expressed sputum
- Consultation with pediatric pulmonology

Mimics

- Any chronic lung disease

Time-Dependent Interventions

- Acute reversal of bronchospasm
- Provision of targeted antibiotics

Overall Principles of Treatment

- The primary goal in CF management is to maintain the patient's lung function to as high a level as possible, for as long as possible. Nutritional support is also important to both quality and quantity of life for patients with CF. Sound and prudent use of antibiotics both treats acute exacerbations and helps protect against antimicrobial resistance.

Organ System	Assessment	Therapy
Pulmonary	Clinical	Daily physiotherapy
	Routine spirometry	Antibiotics: based on sputum culture
	Chest radiography	Daily (inhaled vs oral)
	Routine sputum cultures	For acute exacerbations (oral vs IV)
	Throat swabs in infants or toddlers	Oxygen (if hypoxemic)
		Lung transplant for end - stage disease
Nutrition	Regular growth assessment: height vs weight	Pancreatic enzyme supplementation; high - protein; high-fat diet; caloric supplementation (nasogastric or gastrostomy tube feeds) if persisting malnutrition
	Skin-fold measurement	
	Fecal fat % (dietary intake)	
Gastroenterologic		
Meconium ileus	Clinical: neonate with vomiting, failure to pass meconium	Medical: N-acetylcysteine enema
	Abdominal radiography: gastric and small bowel distention ± "soap bubble" appearance in small bowel	Surgical: decompression - resection of obstructed segment, defunctioning ileostomy
	Contrast enema: meconium obstruction of terminal ileum	
DIOS	Clinical: symptoms or signs of chronic partial distal ileal or cecal obstruction	Exclude surgical complication (appendicitis, intussusception, volvulus)
	Mass in right lower quadrant	Daily mineral oil, balanced intestinal lavage (Golytely, Peglyte®)
	Radiologic: obstructing stool mass in distal ileum or cecum	
Hepatobiliary	Liver function tests	Pancreatic enzymes (increases enterohepatic circulation)
	Abdominal ultrasound (cirrhosis, portal hypertension)	Ursodeoxycholic acid therapy
		Sclerosis of esophageal varices
		Liver transplant for end - stage liver failure
Metabolic		
CF-related diabetes	Glucose tolerance test (ketosis rare unless type 1 diabetes)	Low-dose insulin (potential for hypoglycemia)
		Maintain adequate caloric intake
Sodium chloride depletion	Hyponatremia or metabolic alkalosis: blood electrolytes and gases; urinary electrolytes	Sodium chloride – water repletion
		Prevention: daily electrolyte supplements in hot weather or in high -risk populations (infants and athletes)

Clinical management of cystic fibrosis (CF). [MacLusky I, Solomon M, Laxer R, Ford-Jones EL, Friedman J, Gerstle T. Atlas of Pediatrics, Volume IA, Chapter 14. In: Laxer RM, editor. The Hospital for Sick Children: Atlas of Pediatrics.

Philadelphia, PA: Current Medicine Group; 2005. 519 p. ISBN 1-57340-188-9]
Caption from original

Disease Course

- Unfortunately, most patients will develop irreversible lung disease in early adulthood.

Related Evidence

Papers of particular interest have been highlighted as:
*** Of key importance*

Practice Guideline

Smyth AR, Bell SC, Bojcin S, Bryon M, Duff A, Flume P, Kashirskaya N, Munck A, Ratjen F, Schwarzenberg SJ, Sermet-Gaudelus I, Southern KW, Taccetti G, Ullrich G, Wolfe S; European Cystic Fibrosis Society. European Cystic Fibrosis Society Standards of Care: Best Practice guidelines. J Cyst Fibros. 2014 May;13 Suppl 1:S23-42. https://doi.org/10.1016/j.jcf.2014.03.010. Review. PubMed PMID: 24856775. http://www.ncbi.nlm.nih.gov/pubmed/24856775 **

Tangpricha V, Kelly A, Stephenson A, Maguiness K, Enders J, Robinson KA, Marshall BC, Borowitz D; Cystic Fibrosis Foundation Vitamin D Evidence-Based Review Committee. An update on the screening, diagnosis, management, and treatment of vitamin D deficiency in individuals with cystic fibrosis: evidence-based recommendations from the Cystic Fibrosis Foundation. J Clin Endocrinol Metab. 2012 Apr;97(4):1082-93. https://doi.org/10.1210/jc.2011-3050. Epub 2012 Mar 7. PubMed PMID: 22399505. http://www.ncbi.nlm.nih.gov/pubmed/22399505 **

Cystic Fibrosis Foundation, Borowitz D, Robinson KA, Rosenfeld M, Davis SD, Sabadosa KA, Spear SL, Michel SH, Parad RB, White TB, Farrell PM, Marshall BC, Accurso FJ. Cystic Fibrosis Foundation evidence-based guidelines for management of infants with cystic fibrosis. J Pediatr. 2009 Dec;155(6 Suppl):S73-93. https://doi.org/10.1016/j.jpeds.2009.09.001. PubMed PMID: 19914445. http://www.ncbi.nlm.nih.gov/pubmed/19914445 **

Flume PA, Mogayzel PJ Jr, Robinson KA, Goss CH, Rosenblatt RL, Kuhn RJ, Marshall BC; Clinical Practice Guidelines for Pulmonary Therapies Committee. Cystic fibrosis pulmonary guidelines: treatment of pulmonary exacerbations. Am J Respir Crit Care Med. 2009 Nov 1;180(9):802-8. https://doi.org/10.1164/rccm.200812-1845PP. Epub 2009 Sep 3. Review. PubMed PMID: 19729669. http://www.ncbi.nlm.nih.gov/pubmed/19729669 **

Castellani C, Southern KW, Brownlee K, Dankert Roelse J, Duff A, Farrell M, Mehta A, Munck A, Pollitt R, Sermet-Gaudelus I, Wilcken B, Ballmann M, Corbetta C, de Monestrol I, Farrell P, Feilcke M, Férec C, Gartner S, Gaskin K, Hammermann J, Kashirskaya N, Loeber G, Macek M Jr, Mehta G, Reiman A, Rizzotti P, Sammon A, Sands D, Smyth A, Sommerburg O, Torresani T, Travert G, Vernooij A, Elborn S. European best practice guidelines for cystic fibrosis neonatal screening. J Cyst Fibros. 2009 May;8(3):153-73. https://doi.org/10.1016/j.jcf.2009.01.004. Epub 2009 Feb 26. PubMed PMID: 19246252. http://www.ncbi.nlm.nih.gov/pubmed/19246252 **

Southern KW, Mérelle MM, Dankert-Roelse JE, Nagelkerke AD. Newborn screening for cystic fibrosis. Cochrane Database Syst Rev. 2009 Jan 21;(1):CD001402. https://doi.org/10.1002/14651858.CD001402.pub2. Review. PubMed PMID: 19160197. http://www.ncbi.nlm.nih.gov/pubmed/19160197 **

Farrell PM, Rosenstein BJ, White TB, Accurso FJ, Castellani C, Cutting GR, Durie PR, Legrys VA, Massie J, Parad RB, Rock MJ, Campbell PW 3rd; Cystic Fibrosis Foundation. Guidelines for diagnosis of cystic fibrosis in newborns through older adults: Cystic Fibrosis Foundation consensus report. J Pediatr. 2008 Aug;153(2):S4-S14. https://doi.org/10.1016/j.jpeds.2008.05.005. PubMed PMID: 18639722; PubMed Central PMCID: PMC2810958. http://www.ncbi.nlm.nih.gov/pubmed/18639722 **

Flume PA, O'Sullivan BP, Robinson KA, Goss CH, Mogayzel PJ Jr, Willey-Courand DB, Bujan J, Finder J, Lester M, Quittell L, Rosenblatt R, Vender RL, Hazle L, Sabadosa K, Marshall B; Cystic Fibrosis Foundation, Pulmonary Therapies Committee. Cystic fibrosis pulmonary guidelines: chronic medications for maintenance of lung health. Am J Respir Crit Care Med. 2007 Nov 15;176(10):957-69. Epub 2007 Aug 29. PubMed PMID: 17761616. http://www.ncbi.nlm.nih.gov/pubmed/17761616 **

LeGrys VA, Yankaskas JR, Quittell LM, Marshall BC, Mogayzel PJ Jr; Cystic Fibrosis Foundation. Diagnostic sweat testing: the Cystic Fibrosis Foundation guidelines. J Pediatr. 2007 Jul;151(1):85-9. PubMed PMID: 17586196. http://www.ncbi.nlm.nih.gov/pubmed/17586196 **

Review

Stoltz DA, Meyerholz DK, Welsh MJ. Origins of cystic fibrosis lung disease. N Engl J Med. 2015 Jan 22;372(4):351-62. https://doi.org/10.1056/NEJMra1300109. Review. PubMed PMID: 25607428. http://www.ncbi.nlm.nih.gov/pubmed/25607428

Martiniano SL, Hoppe JE, Sagel SD, Zemanick ET. Advances in the diagnosis and treatment of cystic fibrosis. Adv Pediatr. 2014 Aug;61(1):225-43. https://doi.org/10.1016/j.yapd.2014.03.002. Epub 2014 May 3. Review. PubMed PMID: 25037130. http://www.ncbi.nlm.nih.gov/pubmed/25037130 **

Tiddens HA, Stick SM, Davis S. Multi-modality monitoring of cystic fibrosis lung disease: the role of chest computed tomography. Paediatr Respir Rev. 2014 Mar;15(1):92-7. https://doi.org/10.1016/j.prrv.2013.05.003. Epub 2013 Jul 2. Review. PubMed PMID: 23830321. http://www.ncbi.nlm.nih.gov/pubmed/23830321

Ehre C, Ridley C, Thornton DJ. Cystic fibrosis: an inherited disease affecting mucin-producing organs. Int J Biochem Cell Biol. 2014 Jul;52:136-45. https://doi.org/10.1016/j.biocel.2014.03.011. Epub 2014 Mar 28. Review. PubMed PMID: 24685676; PubMed Central PMCID: PMC4449140. http://www.ncbi.nlm.nih.gov/pubmed/24685676

Chen DL, Atkinson JJ, Ferkol TW. FDG PET imaging in cystic fibrosis. Semin Nucl Med. 2013 Nov;43(6):412-9. https://doi.org/0.1053/j.semnuclmed.2013.06.002. Review. PubMed PMID: 24094708. http://www.ncbi.nlm.nih.gov/pubmed/24094708

Wielpütz MO, Eichinger M, Puderbach M. Magnetic resonance imaging of cystic fibrosis lung disease. J Thorac Imaging. 2013 May;28(3):151-9. https://doi.org/10.1097/RTI.0b013e31828d40d4. Review. PubMed PMID: 23545948. http://www.ncbi.nlm.nih.gov/pubmed/23545948

Schram CA. Atypical cystic fibrosis: identification in the primary care setting. Can Fam Physician. 2012 Dec;58(12):1341-5, e699-704. Review. PubMed PMID: 23242890; PubMed Central PMCID: PMC3520658. http://www.ncbi.nlm.nih.gov/pubmed/23242890

Dijk FN, Fitzgerald DA. The impact of newborn screening and earlier intervention on the clinical course of cystic fibrosis. Paediatr Respir Rev. 2012 Dec;13(4):220-5. https://doi.org/10.1016/j.prrv.2012.05.003. Epub 2012 Jul 10. Review. PubMed PMID: 23069119. http://www.ncbi.nlm.nih.gov/pubmed?term=23069119

Wagener JS, Zemanick ET, Sontag MK. Newborn screening for cystic fibrosis. Curr Opin Pediatr. 2012 Jun;24(3):329-35. https://doi.org/10.1097/MOP.0b013e328353489a. Review. PubMed PMID: 22491493. http://www.ncbi.nlm.nih.gov/pubmed/22491493 **

O'Sullivan BP, Freedman SD. Cystic fibrosis. Lancet. 2009 May 30;373(9678):1891-904. https://doi.org/10.1016/S0140-6736(09)60327-5. Epub 2009 May 4. Review. PubMed PMID: 19403164. http://www.ncbi.nlm.nih.gov/pubmed/19403164

McKay K, Wilcken B. Newborn screening for cystic fibrosis offers an advantage over symptomatic diagnosis for the long term benefit of patients: the motion for. Paediatr Respir Rev. 2008 Dec;9(4):290-4. https://doi.org/10.1016/j.prrv.2008.09.004. Epub 2008 Oct 31. Review. PubMed PMID: 19026370. http://www.ncbi.nlm.nih.gov/pubmed/19026370

Paranjape SM, Zeitlin PL. Atypical cystic fibrosis and CFTR-related diseases. Clin Rev Allergy Immunol. 2008 Dec;35(3):116-23. https://doi.org/10.1007/s12016-008-8083-0. Review. PubMed PMID: 18493878. http://www.ncbi.nlm.nih.gov/pubmed/18493878

Voter KZ, Ren CL. Diagnosis of cystic fibrosis. Clin Rev Allergy Immunol. 2008 Dec;35(3):100-6. https://doi.org/10.1007/s12016-008-8078-x. Review. PubMed PMID: 18506640. http://www.ncbi.nlm.nih.gov/pubmed/18506640 **

Robinson TE. Computed tomography scanning techniques for the evaluation of cystic fibrosis lung disease. Proc Am Thorac Soc. 2007 Aug 1;4(4):310-5. Review. PubMed PMID: 17652492. http://www.ncbi.nlm.nih.gov/pubmed/17652492

Green A, Kirk J; Guidelines Development Group. Guidelines for the performance of the sweat test for the diagnosis of cystic fibrosis. Ann Clin Biochem. 2007 Jan;44(Pt 1):25-34. Review. PubMed PMID: 17270089. http://www.ncbi.nlm.nih.gov/pubmed/17270089

Grosse SD, Rosenfeld M, Devine OJ, Lai HJ, Farrell PM. Potential impact of newborn screening for cystic fibrosis on child survival: a systematic review and analysis. J Pediatr. 2006 Sep;149(3):362-6. Review. PubMed PMID: 16939748. http://www.ncbi.nlm.nih.gov/pubmed/?term=16939748

General

Kopp BT, Nicholson L, Paul G, Tobias J, Ramanathan C, Hayes D Jr. Geographic variations in cystic fibrosis: An analysis of the U.S. CF Foundation Registry. Pediatr Pulmonol. 2015 Aug;50(8):754-62. https://doi.org/10.1002/ppul.23185. Epub 2015 Mar 30. PubMed PMID: 25825016. http://www.ncbi.nlm.nih.gov/pubmed/25825016

Ooi CY, Castellani C, Keenan K, Avolio J, Volpi S, Boland M, Kovesi T, Bjornson C, Chilvers MA, Morgan L, van Wylick R, Kent S, Price A, Solomon M, Tam K, Taylor L, Malitt KA, Ratjen F, Durie PR, Gonska T. Inconclusive diagnosis of cystic fibrosis after newborn screening. Pediatrics. 2015 Jun;135(6):e1377-85. https://doi.org/10.1542/peds.2014-2081. Epub 2015 May 11. PubMed PMID: 25963003. http://www.ncbi.nlm.nih.gov/pubmed/25963003

Woś H, Sankiewicz-Szkółka M, Więcek S, Kordys-Darmolińska B, Grzybowska-Chlebowczyk U, Kniażewska M. Diagnostic problems in cystic fibrosis - specific characteristics of a group of infants and young children diagnosed positive through neonatal screening, in whom cystic fibrosis had not been diagnosed. Dev Period Med. 2015 Jan-Mar;19(1):25-31. PubMed PMID: 26003067. http://www.ncbi.nlm.nih.gov/pubmed/26003067

MacKenzie T, Gifford AH, Sabadosa KA, Quinton HB, Knapp EA, Goss CH, Marshall BC. Longevity of patients with cystic fibrosis in 2000 to 2010 and beyond: survival analysis of the Cystic Fibrosis Foundation patient registry. Ann Intern Med. 2014 Aug 19;161(4):233-41. https://doi.org/10.7326/M13-0636. PubMed PMID: 25133359. http://www.ncbi.nlm.nih.gov/pubmed/25133359

Use PubMed Clinical Queries to find the most recent evidence. Use this search strategy: (“Cystic Fibrosis”[Majr] OR “cystic fibrosis[tiab]”)

Chapter 24
Diabetic Ketoacidosis

Christopher J. Rees, Richard M. Cantor, Charles V. Pollack, Jr., and Jaime Friel Blanck

Name and Synonyms

Diabetic Ketoacidosis; DKA

Incidence/Epidemiology

- Diabetic ketoacidosis (DKA) is classically thought to occur only with type 1 diabetes mellitus, but it can also occur with type 2 diabetes in the setting of severe physiologic stress (infection, trauma, acute MI, or acute CVA).
- It can also occur as a presenting syndrome of type 2 DM, especially in patients of Hispanic or African American origin.
- It is more common in children and young adults than in adults.
- The annual incidence ranges from 4–8 cases per 1,000 patients with diabetes.

C. J. Rees
Emergency Department, Pennsylvania Hospital, Philadelphia, PA, USA

R. M. Cantor
Department of Emergency Medicine and Pediatrics, State University of New York Upstate Medical University, Syracuse, NY, USA

C. V. Pollack, Jr. (✉)
Department of Emergency Medicine, Thomas Jefferson University, Philadelphia, PA, USA

J. F. Blanck
Welch Medical Library, Johns Hopkins University, Baltimore, MD, USA

C. V. Pollack, Jr. (ed.), *Differential Diagnosis of Cardiopulmonary Disease*,
https://doi.org/10.1007/978-3-319-63895-9_24

- Hospital admissions for DKA have been increasing. There were about 80,000 discharge diagnoses of DKA in 1989, in 2009 there were 140,000 discharge diagnoses of DKA, an increase of 50 %.
- Hospital length of stay for DKA has fallen in the same period from about 6 days to 3.5 days.
- Overall mortality has been declining for the last 20 years and now averages less than 5 % for all patients. This is likely due to improved recognition and care.
- Mortality is still much higher for the extremes of age and illness. Mortality is greater than 20 % in the elderly.

Differential Diagnosis

- The differential diagnosis of DKA includes all the causes of an elevated anion gap metabolic acidosis. The classic mnemonic for the causes of an elevated anion gap acidosis is MUD PILES:
  - **M**ethanol
  - **U**remia (renal failure)
  - **DKA,** alcoholic ketoacidosis, and starvation acidosis
  - **P**araldehyde/phenformin ingestion (medications that are no longer available)
  - **I**ron/INH overdose
  - **L**actic acidosis (from multiple causes such as sepsis, metformin overdose)
  - **E**thylene glycol ingestion
  - **S**alicylate overdose
  - Paraldehyde and phenformin are medications that are no longer marketed.
  - Other ingestions/exposures that should be included in this list are: carbon monoxide, cyanide, and toluene.
  - Other diagnoses to consider in the setting of hyperglycemia include: hyperglycemic, hyperosmolar, and nonketotic (HHNK) coma (also referred to as hyperosmolar hyperglycemic state [HHS] or diabetic hyperosmolar state [DHS]). In this disorder the hyperglycemia tends to be more severe (>600 mg/dl), with little or no elevation in the anion gap. It tends to occur in older patients, have a more prolonged onset and course, and is usually associated with more pronounced mental status changes than DKA. The mortality in HHNK is also higher than in DKA.

Finding	Mild DKA	Moderate DKA	Severe DKA	HHS
Plasma glucose (mg/dL)	>250	>250	>250	>600
Arterial pH	7.25–7.30	7.00–7.24	<7.00	>7.30
Serum HCO_3^- (mEq/L)	15–18	10–15	<10	>15
Serum or urine ketones	Positive	Positive	Positive	Small
Beta-hydroxybutyrate	High	High	High	Normal or high
Effective serum osmolality[a] (mOsm/kg)	Variable	Variable	Variable	>320
Anion gap[b]	Upper limits of normal or > normal	>Normal	Significantly > normal	Variable
Sensorium	Alert	Alert or drowsy	Stupor/coma	Stupor/coma

[a]Effective serum osmolality = 2 × measured Na^+ (mEq/L) + BUN (mg/dL)/2.8 + glucose (mg/dL)/18, >320–330 mOsm/kg associated with neurologic deterioration
[b]Anion gap = $(Na^+ + K^+) - (Cl^- + HCO_3^-)$

Diagnostic criteria in DKA and HHS [Shah SJ. Diabetic Ketoacidosis in the Urgent Anesthesia Setting. In: Benumof JL, editor. Clinical Anesthesiology [Internet]. New York, NY: Springer New York; 2014 [cited 2015 Nov 5]. p. 407–14. Available from: http://link.springer.com/10.1007/978-1-4614-8696-1_49] *Caption from original*

- The differential diagnosis prior to the identification of the metabolic abnormalities is much broader and based upon the presenting symptoms. These may include: sepsis/shock/hypovolemic syndromes, abdominal pain associated with nausea and vomiting, change in mental status, and tachypnea.

Pathophysiology and Etiology

- The primary pathophysiologic mechanism behind the development of DKA is an insulin deficiency, especially a lack of an appropriate insulin release to hyperglycemia.
- Cells require insulin to utilize glucose as a fuel source. In the absence of insulin, the body will seek alternative fuel sources. Catabolic (counterregulatory) hormones will be released that help break down and utilize protein and fat stores as fuel.
- The primary counterregulatory hormone is glucagon, but other involved counterregulatory hormones include catecholamines, cortisone, and growth hormone.
- The effect of these catabolic hormones is to increase gluconeogenesis and glycogenolysis, which in turn increases production of glucose and worsens hyperglycemia. Increasing both these processes also raises the production of byproducts and precursors such as free fatty acids and glycerol.

- Theses catabolic hormones also increase proteolysis. This boosts the amount of free glucogenic amino acids, which can be used with glycerol to produce glucose and worsen hyperglycemia.
- The free fatty acids that are produced during gluconeogenesis bind to albumin, and then are taken up by the liver, where they are converted to ketone bodies (beta-hydroxybutyrate [βHB], acetoacetic acid [AcAc], and acetone).
- Some body tissues can utilize ketone bodies for energy, but inefficiently. A low insulin level reduces the ability of brain, cardiac, and skeletal muscle to utilize ketones as an energy source, which increases the ketonemia.
- These ketone bodies are responsible for the metabolic acidosis of DKA.
- Under normal physiologic conditions, βHB and AcAc exist in a 1:1 equilibrium. During the increased lipolysis and ketogenesis of DKA, this ratio will approach 10:1. It is important to remember, however, that during insulin therapy, βHB will be metabolized at a faster rate than AcAc. This has important implications for monitoring therapy that will be discussed under the treatment section.
- Hyperglycemia causes an osmotic diuresis, resulting in profound fluid losses and volume depletion, which exacerbates hyperglycemia and ketonemia.
- The volume deficits can be profound and can lead to hypotension and shock.
- The osmotic diuresis also results in profound electrolyte losses (K, Na, Cl, PO2, Ca, Mg, and N).
- The acidosis causes a shift in potassium from intracellular to extracellular exacerbating total body potassium losses.
- In the setting of marked ketonemia, the kidney will exchange chloride for ketones, allowing the ketones to be excreted. The excretion of ketones leads to a decrease in potential bicarbonate, which leads in turn to less buffering capacity and then to worsening of the acidosis, which can lead to a hyperchloremic metabolic acidosis, in addition to the ketoacidosis.
- The breakdown of adipose tissue leads to an inflammatory response with the release of prostaglandins I2 and E2. These cause a peripheral vasodilation that can worsen hypotension and shock.
- Multiple factors and conditions are known to precipitate DKA. Many acute illnesses, as well as physiologic stress, can lead to hyperglycemia, and in the setting of insulin deficiency this leads to DKA.
- It is important to attempt to identify cause when a patient presents with DKA.
- In a significant minority of patients, no precipitating cause can be identified.
- The following list contains some of the common causes of DKA, but any acute illness and/or period of physiologic stress can initiate DKA, so this list is not exhaustive.

  - Reduction of or lack of daily insulin injections
  - Malfunction of insulin pump
  - Any acute infectious process
  - Acute MI
  - Stroke
  - Acute GI bleed

- Pregnancy
- Medications (especially steroids)
- Substance abuse (multifactorial, e.g., cocaine can cause hyperglycemia directly and then these patients forget or have no insulin available)
- Severe, acute illness or trauma

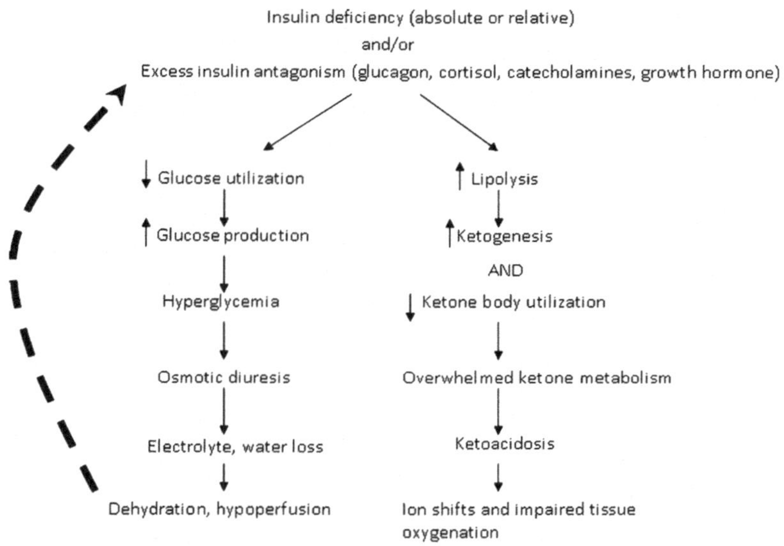

DKA pathophysiology. DKA is shown as unchecked lipolysis occurring alongside progressive water and electrolyte loss. Osmotic diuresis, progressive hypovolemia, and further reductions in glucose and ketone clearance in the absence of insulin creates a feed-forward loop that increases concentrations of antagonistic hormones and perpetuates the cycle [Steenkamp DW, Alexanian SM, McDonnell ME. Adult Hyperglycemic Crisis: A Review and Perspective. Current Diabetes Reports. 2013 Feb;13(1):130–7.] *Caption from original*

Presentation

Typical/"Classic"

- DKA develops acutely over a period of 24–48 hours.
- The early symptoms are often related directly to hyperglycemia with resultant osmotic diuresis and worsening volume loss (polydipsia/polyuria).
- As the metabolic abnormalities worsen and acidosis develops, tachypnea occurs as physiologic compensation to try and decrease the pCO2 to reduce the acidosis. Kussmaul respirations (a profound increase in the rate and depth of breathing) may develop.

- Diffuse, nonspecific abdominal pain associated with nausea and vomiting are common symptoms at presentation (especially in children). They are often related directly to DKA (prostaglandin release is felt to play a role) but can also indicate an underlying cause for the DKA.
- Vomiting contributes to the development of metabolic abnormalities, electrolyte losses, and the development of volume depletion and dehydration.
- As volume depletion worsens, the patient may develop clinical signs of shock with tachycardia, hypotension, and signs of poor perfusion (poor skin turgor, dry mucous membranes, peripheral cyanosis).
- Profound ketonemia (especially acetone) can cause a fruity odor on the breath.
- A change in mental status may occur, but is more common in HHNK. It is felt to be multifactorial and related to volume depletion, metabolic acidosis, hyperosmolarity, and hemodynamic abnormalities.

Atypical

- DKA is associated with multi-organ dysfunction. As such, it is associated with multiple, varying symptoms and presentations as above.
- Fever may be present due to an underlying infection, but it is important to remember that the absence of fever does not exclude underlying infection as a cause for DKA.
- DKA may present with the symptoms of the underlying causative disorder.
- Hypothermia may be present due to peripheral vasodilation from prostaglandin release.
- Abdominal pain with nausea and vomiting are frequent presenting symptoms of DKA as discussed in Typical/"Classic", above. However, abdominal pain and other abdominal symptoms may be due to the underlying cause. Acute pancreatitis can be both a cause and an effect of DKA. Lipase may be elevated in both situations, so it is often difficult to make the distinction.
- An alteration of decrease in the level of consciousness may occur, but is more commonly seen in HHNK. An altered level of consciousness seems to be more associated hyperosmolarity than with acidosis.

Primary Differential Considerations

- DFKA is a rather distinctive clinical entity. It is most likely to be confused with hyperosmolar nonketoic coma and alcoholic ketoacidosis. Other initial differential considerations might include:
  - Lactic academia
  - Septic shock
  - Acute pancreatitis
  - Salicylate toxicity

History and Physical Exam

Findings That Confirm Diagnosis

- There are no historical or physical examination findings that are confirmatory for DKA.
- The diagnosis of DKA requires laboratory confirmation.

Factors That Suggest Diagnosis

- A history of reduced or no insulin use should suggest the diagnosis.
- Any patient with diabetes who presents with an acute illness or severe injury should have the diagnosis of DKA considered.
- Patients being treated for other acute illnesses need to have their metabolic status monitored and controlled to avoid precipitating DKA.

Factors That Exclude Diagnosis

- There are no historical or physical exam findings that can reliably exclude the diagnosis of DKA.
- DKA is only excluded by laboratory analysis documenting the lack of ketonemia.
- It is important to remember that while most patients with DKA will have marked hyperglycemia (400–800 mg/dL), it is possible to have DKA with only modest elevations in glucose (250–500 mg/dL).

Ancillary Studies

Laboratory

- The diagnosis of DKA requires laboratory confirmation.
- Patients with suspected or confirmed DKA need to have a complete laboratory analysis of electrolytes and acid-base status. This includes measurement of glucose, sodium, potassium, chloride, bicarbonate, calcium, phosphate, magnesium, renal function, liver function, arterial or venous pH, calculation of the anion gap, and determination of ketonemia. A urine dipstick should also be performed for ketonuria and glucosuria, and for evidence of urinary infection.

- These patients may also need further laboratory evaluation for a precipitating cause for DKA. This may require evaluation of cardiac biomarkers, pancreatic enzymes, and thyroid function.
- The diagnosis is generally confirmed by the presence of all the following findings:
  - a blood glucose >250 mg/dL
  - an anion gap >11 (usually greater than 20)
  - a bicarbonate <15 mEq/L, an arterial or venous pH<7.3
  - at least moderate ketonemia
- All diabetic patients should have a fingerstick glucose determination performed when being evaluated for any acute illness.
- The glucose in DKA is usually between 400 and 800 mg/dL. Higher levels, especially those above 1,000 mg/dL are more common in HHNK. Lower levels (250–500 mg/dL) may be seen, especially in the presence of starvation/inadequate food intake due to nausea or vomiting, alcohol abuse, and other intercurrent illnesses. It may also be lower in the presence of pregnancy, liver disease, and if insulin was given within several hours prior to evaluation.
- In DKA, the anion gap increases due to the presence of the unmeasured anions, beta-hydroxybutyrate (βHB) and acetoacetate (AcAc). When calculating the anion gap, use the measured serum sodium, not the corrected sodium (see sodium below).
- Venous blood gases can be used to assess the serum pH. There is a high degree of correlation between venous and arterial pH in DKA. The venous pH is about 0.03 lower than the arterial pH. Arterial blood gases are painful, and can cause severe complications such as arterial injury and thrombosis, so venous blood gases are currently recommended.
- The degree of acidosis can be assessed by both the serum pH and bicarbonate concentration. The pH and serum bicarbonate are usually both reduced. This is consistent with the metabolic acidosis. Patients with protracted, severe vomiting may also develop a metabolic alkalosis and have normal or slightly elevated bicarbonate levels. In this setting, an elevated anion gap may be the only indication that an underlying acidosis exists.
- Historically, serum and urine ketones were assessed by the use of the nitroprusside reagent. This is mostly a qualitative assay, but the strength of reaction (color change) may give an indication of the amount of ketone present. This reagent only reacts with AcAc, it does not detect βHB. In DKA, βHB is the predominant ketone body. βHB and AcAc exist in an equilibrium that favors βHB in acidic environments. So early in the course, if using the nitroprusside reagent, the level of ketonemia or ketonuria may seem lower than it actually is. As the patient is appropriately treated, and the acidosis improves, the equilibrium will favor the conversion of βHB to AcAc (prior to clearance of the ketone bodies). When using the nitroprusside reagent, there may seem to be a paradoxical increase in ketonemia or ketonuria as the patient improves.

Most hospital laboratories now have a direct, enzymatic assay for βHB that is reliable and quantitative. This is the preferred assay.

- Patients with DKA often have profound total body potassium deficits. Acidosis causes intracellular potassium to shift into the extracellular space. The osmotic diuresis causes the potassium to then be excreted in the urine. However, measured potassium is often normal or even elevated prior to treatment. This is due to the extracellular shift of potassium with acidosis, and the hemoconcentration/increased serum osmolarity associated with hyperglycemia. During the first several hours of treatment, the serum potassium can drop precipitously.
- Osmotic diuresis also leads to renal losses of sodium chloride. Hyperglycemia causes an increase in the measured serum sodium that is factitious. The serum sodium should be corrected for the level of hyperglycemia. The classic correction factor for serum sodium in the presence of hyperglycemia is 1.6. For every elevation of 100 mg of glucose above 100 mg/dL, you add 1.6 to the measured serum sodium for the true sodium concentration. Some authorities believe that the correction factor should be 2.4 when the serum glucose exceeds 400 mg/dL.
- The osmotic diuresis causes increased urinary losses and total body depletion of all electrolytes (including phosphorus, calcium, and magnesium). However, just like potassium, hemoconcentration may cause the initial levels to be elevated. And as with potassium, treatment can cause precipitous drops in these electrolytes.
- Serum creatinine is often elevated due to intravascular volume depletion from the osmotic diuresis.
- Liver functions and lipase are often elevated in DKA even the absence of significant liver or pancreas pathology. These values often improve with treatment. However, they can be associated with an underlying condition that may have precipitated the episode of DKA.
- DKA is often associated with leukocytosis, due to physiologic stress and hemoconcentration. However, significant bandemia (above 10 %) often accompanies an infectious process that may have precipitated DKA.

Electrocardiography

- An ECG should be performed on all patients with suspected or confirmed DKA.
- It can help in the identification of electrolyte abnormalities such as hypo- or hyperkalemia.
- Also, as DKA can be precipitated by an acute myocardial infarction, an ECG should be reviewed for any signs of ischemia or infarction.

Imaging

- Imaging is not helpful in the diagnosis of DKA.
- However, imaging is often necessary in the work-up, evaluation, and treatment of DKA to search for the cause of DKA.
- Most of these patients should have chest x-ray to assess for pneumonia, congestive heart failure, or other issues that can help explain the occurrence of DKA, or help in the safe and appropriate management of DKA.
- Abdominal pain is a difficult complaint to evaluate in DKA. It may be due to the DKA itself, but an abdominal issue may also be the precipitant of DKA. Many patients presenting in DKA with predominant abdominal complaints or with marked abdominal tenderness will require abdominal imaging to evaluate for an intra-abdominal process precipitating DKA. The usual study would be an abdominal/pelvic CT scan. Many of these patients will not tolerate oral contrast due to profound nausea and vomiting, and IV contrast will often be contraindicated due to an elevated creatinine from intravascular volume depletion. A completely non-contrast-enhanced CT scan can be useful in these patients to help exclude an intra-abdominal catastrophe.

Special Populations

Age

Children

- 30–40% of cases of new-onset diabetes in children will present with DKA.
- DKA as a presenting manifestation is more common in younger children (<5), and in those from socioeconomically disadvantaged backgrounds.
- Children are more likely to present initially with diffuse abdominal pain associated with nausea and vomiting.
- DKA in children is defined by the following biochemical abnormalities:
  - Blood glucose greater than 200 mg/dL; AND
  - A venous pH less than 7.3 or plasma bicarbonate less than 15 mEg/L; AND
  - Ketosis (presence of ketones in the urine).
  - Measurements of serum beta-hydroxybutyrate are more sensitive are more accurate indicators of ketosis (levels greater than 3 mmol/L)
- Other clues to the presence of new-onset diabetes in children include polyuria, polydipsia, increased nocturia, and especially daytime enuresis.
- Decreased urine output from dehydration is often not appreciated in children, due to the profound osmotic diuresis associated with DKA.
- DKA is the leading cause of morbidity and mortality in children with type 1 diabetes.

The Elderly

- The elderly are more likely to present with HHS/HHNK than DKA.
- The elderly are also more likely to present with mental status changes.
- Morbidity and mortality are also higher among the elderly.

During Pregnancy

- DKA occurring during pregnancy is associated with a fetal mortality rate approaching 30%.
- DKA can be precipitated by lower sugar levels during pregnancy.
- Several "normal" physiologic changes of pregnancy make pregnant women more likely to develop DKA.
  - Pregnant women have lower fasting plasma glucose levels. This leads to lower baseline insulin levels (a relative insulin deficiency) and increased baseline free fatty acid levels.
  - This is also an associated increase in counter-regulatory hormone levels.
  - There is a decrease in bicarbonate levels from the chronic respiratory alkalosis in pregnancy. This leads to a decreased buffering capacity.
- All the fluid and electrolyte changes that occur in the mother occur in the fetus. Maternal hyperglycemia causes fetal hyperglycemia with resultant osmotic diuresis. Maternal acidosis leads to fetal acidosis. Maternal hyperglycemia, diuresis, volume contraction, and acidosis cause decreased uterine blood flow and decreased fetal oxygenation. Fetal hypokalemia can cause fetal arrhythmias. All these changes lead to the increase in fetal mortality.
- Treatment priorities remain the same: fluids, correction of acidosis and hyperglycemia, and electrolyte repletion.

Co-morbidities

- Any significant medical co-morbidity can increase the morbidity and mortality associated with DKA.
- Significant cardiac, pulmonary, renal, and liver disease can complicate both the diagnosis and treatment of DKA. Any significant disorder of these systems can make fluid therapy challenging.
- Patients with history of severe CHF or end-stage renal disease may need central venous pressure monitoring for appropriate fluid management.

Pitfalls in Diagnosis

Critical Steps Not to Miss

- It is important to consider the diagnosis in acutely ill patient with a history of diabetes.
- It is also important to consider the diagnosis in patients presenting acutely ill who are found to be academic and hyperglycemic even in the absence of a history of diabetes, as DKA can be the presenting issue with diabetes.
- It is critical to measure the all electrolytes, pH (a venous blood gas is often sufficient), and evaluate for ketosis.
- Appropriate resuscitative measures (especially fluid replacement) may need to be started prior to adequate confirmation of the diagnosis.
- A thorough search for a precipitating cause needs to be performed.

Mimics

- Many processes can mimic the presentation of DKA, as it is a multi-system disorder in which patients are critically ill.
- HHNK (hyperglycemic, hyperosmolar, non-ketosis) is an important mimic of DKA. Patients have ketosis, but usually little or no elevation in the anion gap. The glucose tends to be much higher (usually above 600) than those seen with DKA. These patients are usually older and have more profound mental status changes.
- Other causes of ketosis (such as alcoholic and starvation ketosis) can present similarly, but the glucose is usually normal or low at presentation.
- Patients with SIRS (systemic inflammatory response syndrome) can also present acutely ill with hypotension, acidosis (usually from lactate), and the two processes can co-exist. An acute infection can precipitate DKA.

Time-Dependent Interventions

- It is critically important to initiate fluid resuscitation early in the course of evaluation and treatment. Fluids should usually be started at the time of consideration of the diagnosis rather than after waiting for full laboratory confirmation.
- Immediate interventions on consideration of the diagnosis include aggressive fluid replacement, full monitoring including cardiac monitoring, continuous pulse ox, and frequent vital sign monitoring (blood pressure every 5 minutes

or more frequently). There should be a bedside, finger stick blood glucose check, a urine dipstick for ketones, at least two large-bore IV's, and a 12-lead ECG should be performed.

Overall Principles of Treatment

- Treatment should initially address three issues in the following order:
  - Fluid repletion
  - Potassium repletion
  - Insulin administration
- Fluid.
  - Adult patients with DKA usually have anywhere from a 5–10 liter free water deficit at presentation.
  - The first 2 liters of replacement should be given over the first 30–120 minutes of treatment. Continuing fluids can then be slowed with about 50 % of the total water deficit replaced over the first 12 hours and then subsequent 50 % over the next 12 hours.
  - Normal saline (NS) is the preferred fluid for initial resuscitation. NS helps increase intravascular volume and helps to prevent too rapid a fall in extracellular osmolarity. Too rapid a fall in extracellular osmolarity can lead to rapid transfer of free water into brain cells and cerebral edema.
  - After the initial resuscitation with 2 liters NS, most authorities recommend changing to 0.45 % (half normal) saline, if the corrected serum sodium is normal or elevated.
  - When the blood glucose falls below 250 mg/dl, the fluid should be changed to 5 % dextrose in 0.45 % NS to allow the continuation of insulin therapy.
- Potassium.
  - Patients with DKA almost universally have severe total body potassium deficits. Usually on the order of 3–5 mEq/kg.
  - The development of profound hypokalemia can be a life-threatening complication during the resuscitation and treatment of a patient with DKA.
  - However, the initial measured serum potassium is usually normal or high, due to the shift of intracellular potassium into the extracellular space in the presence of acidosis. Hypokalemia on presentation is urgently life-threatening and requires rapid and careful correction.
  - The primary goals of potassium replacement are to maintain normal extracellular potassium concentration during the acute phases of therapy when the most significant shifts are expected to occur. The intracellular deficit may be corrected over days instead of hours.
  - During initial resuscitation of DKA, the serum potassium may fall quickly due to the resolution of acidosis and insulin therapy, which both cause an

intracellular shift of potassium. This can lead to the precipitous development of profound extracellular hypokalemia with resulting cardiac arrhythmias, rhabdomyolysis, respiratory muscle paralysis, and paralytic ileus.

- The most rapid changes in potassium concentration occurs during the first several hours of therapy, so the potassium concentration needs to be measured frequently during this period (at least every 2 hours.)
- It is recommended that if the initial potassium concentration (prior to any fluids/insulin) is between 3.0 mEq/L and 5.5 mEq/L, then potassium replacement should be initiated at about 10 mEq/hour.
- If the initial potassium is below 3.0 mEq/L, the initial rate of replacement should be about 15 mEq/hour.
- If the initial serum potassium concentration is below 3.3–3.5 mEq/L, it is recommended that potassium replacement occur prior to initiation of insulin therapy, as insulin administration will cause the potassium to shift intracellularly and can precipitate profound, life-threatening extracellular hypokalemia.
- Potassium is usually given as potassium chloride in IV fluid. Potassium phosphate use is discouraged, as it can lead to profound hypocalcemia and the precipitation of calcium phosphate salt in tissues.

- Insulin.
  - There is nearly universal agreement that the administration of low dose (0.1 unit/kg/hour) intravenous short-acting insulin is the safest method for administering insulin in patients with DKA.
  - This method of insulin administration allows for a gradual reduction in plasma glucose of about 50 mg/dL/hour.
  - Multiple studies document that this method of insulin administration is associated with fewer complications (such as profound hypokalemia, hypophosphatemia, and hypoglycemia).
  - In adults, it is acceptable to give a loading dose of insulin at a dose of 1 unit/kg.
  - Children should not have a bolus dose of insulin. An IV-push loading dose has been shown to lead to more complications in children.
  - In general, insulin infusions should not be started until after an initial fluid bolus of 1–2 liters has been given.
  - Insulin therapy should be withheld in the setting of profound hypokalemia (initial serum potassium concentration less than 3.3–3.5 mEq/L) until potassium repletion has commenced. In this setting, insulin can cause profound hypokalemia by causing an intracellular shift of extracellular potassium.
  - In the first hours of treatment, the serum glucose should be measured at least every 2 hours.
  - The insulin infusion should be continued until the anion gap returns to normal and ketonemia resolves.

  - Hyperglycemia often resolves before the anion gap normalizes and ketonemia resolves. It is recommended that the IV fluid be switched to fluid containing 5% dextrose when the serum glucose concentration falls below 250 mg/dL.
  - Therapy with subcutaneous insulin should be initiated prior to stopping the insulin infusion. Subcutaneous insulin should be administered at least one hour prior to stopping the insulin infusion.

- Other electrolytes.

  - Phosphorus. Phosphorus (like potassium) is primarily intracellular, but shifts to the extracellular compartment in the setting of acidosis. As such, initial phosphorus concentrations are usually elevated in DKA but are not reflective of total body phosphorus. In DKA, total body phosphorus is usually depleted due to increased renal losses from the osmotic diuresis. However, phosphorus levels usually fall more gradually than potassium, and the levels often don't decrease until 24–48 hours into therapy. Intravenous replacement is not recommended unless the serum phosphorus falls below 1.0 mg/dL.
  - Magnesium. Magnesium concentrations may fall from the osmotic diuresis of DKA. Magnesium concentration doesn't usually fall until 24 hours into therapy. Magnesium repletion is recommended when the serum concentration falls below 2.0 mg/dL. Magnesium may be given intravenously as magnesium sulfate 2.0 grams over one hour. If the patient is tolerating orals, it can be given orally as magnesium oxide.
  - Calcium. Calcium homeostasis usually remains intact during DKA, but severe hypomagnesemia can lead to hypocalcemia (due to decreased parathyroid secretion). Patients with severe hypomagnesemia should have calcium levels followed and restored as necessary.
  - Bicarbonate. The administration of supplemental bicarbonate is contraindicated in the vast majority of cases of DKA. The acidosis will resolve spontaneously with resolution of ketogenesis. Bicarbonate therapy can be associated with and cause severe hypokalemia, worsen intracellular acidosis, worsen central nervous system acidosis, shift the oxyhemoglobin dissociation curve to the left, prolong ketogenesis, and precipitate cerebral edema.

Laboratory evaluation
After a brief history and physical examination, initial laboratory evaluation should include determination of complete blood count, blood glucose, serum electrolytes, blood urea nitrogen, creatinine, serum ketones, osmolality, arterial blood gases, and urinalysis. Admission ECG, chest radiograph, and cultures of blood, urine, and sputum may be ordered if clinically indicated. During therapy, capillary blood glucose should be determined every 1–2 hours at the bedside using a glucose oxidase reagent strip; and blood should be drawn every 4 hours for determination of serum electrolytes, glucose, blood urea nitrogen, creatinine, phosphorus, and venous pH
Fluids
1000 mL normal saline (0.9% sodium chloride) first hour, then normal or 0.45% saline at 250–500 mL per hour depending on serum sodium concentration and hydration status. When plasma glucose < 250 mg/dL, change to D5%1/2NS saline to allow continued insulin administration until ketonemia is controlled, while avoiding hypoglycemia
Insulin
0.1 U/kg body weight as intravenous bolus followed by 0.1 U/kg/h as a continuous infusion. The goal is to achieve a rate of decline of glucose between 50–100 mg per hour. When plasma glucose is < 250 mg/dL, reduce insulin rate to 0.05 U/kg per hour. Thereafter, adjust insulin rate to maintain glucose levels between 150–200 mg/dL until ketoacidosis is resolved. In patients with mild to moderate diabetic ketoacidosis, subcutaneous regular insulin or rapid-acting insulin analogs may be an alternative to intravenous insulin [037], [038]
Potassium
Serum K^+ > 5.0 mEq/L; no supplementation is required.
Serum K^+ = 4–5 mEq/L; add 20 mEq/L to each L of replacement fluid
Serum K^+ = 3–4 mEq/L; add 40 mEq/L to each L of replacement fluid
Serum K^+ < 3 mEq/L; hold insulin and give 10–20 mEq per hour until K^+ > 3.3, then add 40 mEq/L to each L of replacement fluid
Bicarbonate
Arterial pH < 7.0 or bicarbonate < 5 mEq; 50 mEq/L in 200 ml of H_2O over 1 hour until pH increases to > 7.0. Do not give bicarbonate if pH > 7.0
Phosphate
If indicated (serum levels < 1 mg/dL), 20–30 mmol potassium phosphate over 24 hours. Monitor serum calcium level
Transition to subcutaneous insulin
Insulin infusion should be continued until resolution of ketoacidosis (glucose < 200 mg/dL, bicarbonate > 18 mEq/L, pH > 7.30). When this occurs, start subcutaneous insulin regimen.
To prevent recurrence of diabetic ketoacidosis during the transition period to subcutaneous insulin, intravenous insulin should be continued for 1–2 hours after subcutaneous insulin is given [028]

Summary of management of patients with diabetic ketoacidosis, (028). Fisher JN, Shahshahani MN, Kitabchi AE. Diabetic ketoacidosis: low-dose insulin therapy by various routes. N Engl J Med. 1977; 297:238 -247. (037). Umpierrez GE, Cuervo R, Karabell A, et al. Treatment of diabetic ketoacidosis with subcutaneous insulin aspart. Am J Med. 2004; 117:291 -296. (038). Umpierrez GE, Latif K, Stoever J, et al. Efficacy of subcutaneous insulin lispro versus continuous intravenous regular insulin for treatment of diabetic ketoacidosis. Diabetes Care. 2004; 27:1873 -1878. [Kitabchi AE, Murphy MB. Consequences of Insulin Deficiency. In: Skyler J, editor. Atlas of Diabetes. 3rd edition. Philadelphia: Current Medicine Group; 2006. ISBN 1-57340-222-2] *Caption from original*

$CO2$—carbon dioxide; IV—intravenous; K+—potassium ion; NaCl—sodium chloride; NaHCO3—sodium bicarbonate; SQ—subcutaneous.

Insulin	Fluid Administration	Potassium repletion	Alkali
1. Give initial IV bolus of 0.2 U/kg actual body weight.	Shock absent: Normal saline (0.9% NaCl) at 7 mL/kg/h for 4 h, and half this rate thereafter	Potassium chloride should be added to the third liter of IV infusion and subsequently if urinary output is at least 30–60 mL/h and plasma [K^+] < 5 mEq/L.	Half-normal saline (0.45% NaCl) plus 1–2 ampules (44–88 mEq) $NaHCO_3$ per liter when blood pH < 7.0 or total CO_2 < 5 mmol/L; in hyperchloremic acidosis, add $NaHCO_3$ when pH < 7.20; discontinue $NaHCO_3$ in IV infusion when total CO_2>8–10 mmol/L.
2. Add 100 U of regular insulin to 1 L of normal saline (0.1 U/mL), and follow with continuous IV drip of 0.1 U/kg actual body weight per h until correction of ketosis.	Shock present: Normal saline and plasma expanders (*ie*, albumin, low molecular weight dextran) at maximal possible rate		
3. Give double rate of infusion if the blood glucose level does not decrease in a 2-h interval (expected decrease is 40–80 mg/dL/h or 10% of the initial value.)	Start a glucose-containing solution (*eg*, 5% dextrose in water) when blood glucose level decreases to 250 mg/dL.	Add K^+ to the initial 2 L of IV fluids if initial plasma [K^+] < 4 mEq/L and adequate diuresis is secured.	
4. Give SQ dose (10–30 U) of regular insulin when ketosis is corrected and the blood glucose level decreases to 300 mg/dL, and continue with SQ insulin injection every 4 h on a sliding scale (*ie*, 5 U if below 150, 10 U if 150–200, 15 U if 200–250, and 20 U if 250–300 mg/dL).			

Diabetic ketoacidosis (DKA) and nonketotic hyperglycemia (NKH) management. Administration of insulin is the cornerstone of management for both DKA and NKH. Replacement of the prevailing water, sodium, and potassium deficits is also required. Alkali are administered only under certain circumstances in DKA and virtually never in NKH, in which ketoacidosis is generally absent. Because the fluid deficit is generally severe in patients with NKH, many of whom have preexisting heart disease and are relatively old, safe fluid replacement may require monitoring of central venous pressure, pulmonary capillary wedge pressure, or both (001), Adrogué HJ, Madias NE. Management of life-threatening acid-base disorders. N Engl J Med. 1998; 338:26 -34, 107–111. (017), AdroguÈ HJ. Diabetic ketoacidosis and hyperosmolar nonketotic syndrome. In: Suki WN, Massry SG, eds. Therapy of Renal Diseases and Related Disorders. Boston: Kluwer Academic Publishers; 1997; 233 -251. (018). Adrogué HJ, Barrero J, Eknoyan G. Salutary effects of modest fluid replacement in the treatment of adults with diabetic ketoacidosis. JAMA. 1989; 262:2108 -2113. [Adrogué HJ, Madias NE, Disorders of Acid-Base Balance.

In: Berl T. Bonventre JV, editors. Volume 1: Disorders of Water, Electrolytes, and Acid-Base; Acute Renal Failure. 1 edition. Philadelphia: Current Medicine Group; 1999. (Schrier RW, editor. Atlas of Diseases of the Kidney). ISBN: 0-632-04385-7] *Caption from original*

Disease Course

- With appropriate and aggressive treatment, most cases of DKA resolve over 24–72 hours.
- Advances in knowledge leading to improved and more aggressive treatment has reduced the mortality of DKA to less than 5 %.
- Currently, most mortality is seen in the very young and the very old.
- Overwhelming infection and acute myocardial infarction precipitating DKA are associated with increased mortality.
- In general, the sicker a patient is at presentation, the higher the mortality.
- Some complications related to therapy for DKA have previously been discussed (hypokalemia, hypophosphatemia, and hypoglycemia). Other complications of therapy include the adult respiratory distress syndrome, and cerebral edema.
- Adult respiratory distress syndrome (ARDS): This is a rare complication, generally felt to result in over-aggressive fluid repletion especially in patients with underlying pulmonary or cardiac disease.
- Cerebral edema. Cerebral edema is a feared complication of DKA in children. It tends to occur 4–24 hours after the initiation of therapy, and patients usually appear to be improving prior to its onset. Cerebral edema is associated with high morbidity and mortality. It is thought to result from free water diffusing into brain cells at a fast rate, causing cells to swell. The only known risk factors are young age and DKA being the presenting manifestation of diabetes. There are currently no identified presenting or treatment issues that reliably predict the onset of cerebral edema. Symptoms may include headache, incontinence, change in mental status, seizures, or other changes in autonomic or neurologic function. If the diagnosis of cerebral edema is being considered, therapy with intravenous mannitol (1–2 grams/kg IV) should be started immediately, without awaiting confirmatory studies.

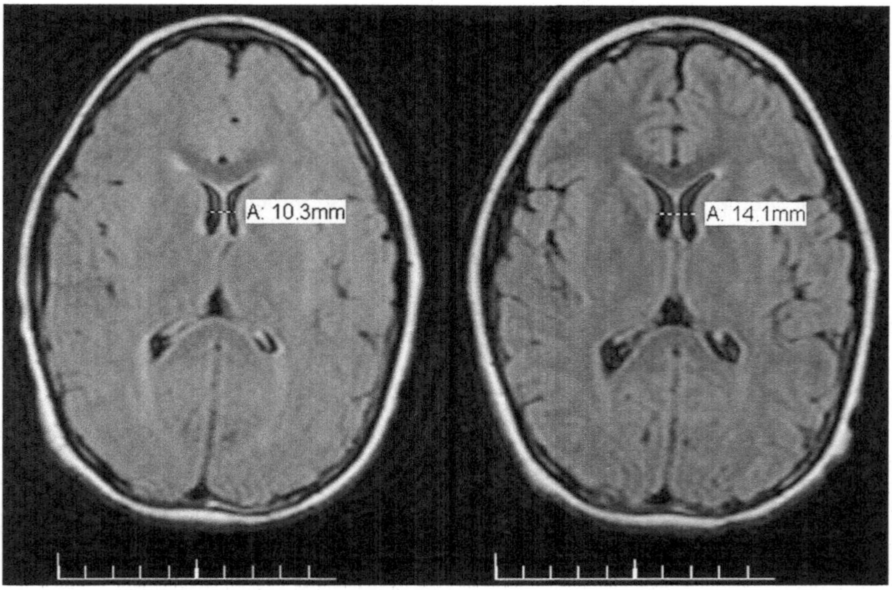

A 12-year-old boy in DKA (left) and following recovery from the DKA episode (right). Axial FLAIR images (1.5 T) demonstrate that the intercaudate distance is smaller during DKA than after recovery, suggesting mild diffuse brain swelling. [Wootton-Gorges SL, Glaser NS. Imaging of the brain in children with type I diabetes mellitus. Pediatric Radiology. 2007 Jul 27;37(9):863–9.] *Caption adapted from original*

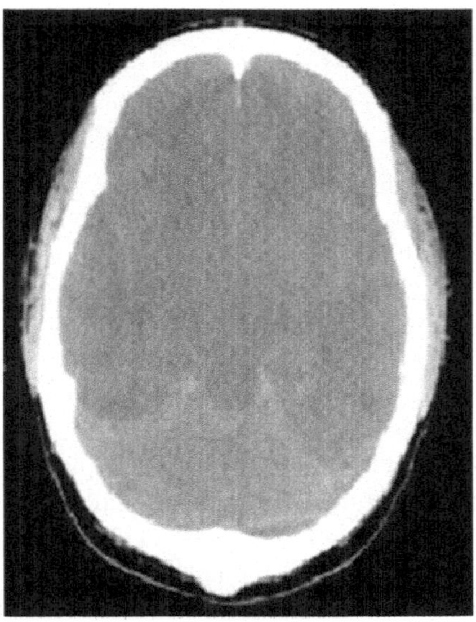

Computerized Tomography (CT) head showing diffuse cerebral edema with effacement of basal cisterns and generalized loss of gray-white differentiation [From article: Dialysis Disequilibrium Syndrome: Brain death following hemodialysis for metabolic acidosis and acute renal failure–A case report. BMC Nephrology. 2004 Aug 19;5(1):9. https://doi.org/10.1186/1471-2369-5-9, at http://link.springer.com/article/10.1186%2F1471-2369-5-9/fulltext.html; by Sean M Bagshaw, Adam D Peets, Morad Hameed, Paul JE Boiteau, Kevin B Laupland, Christopher J Doig, © Bagshaw et al; licensee BioMed Central Ltd. 2004; licensed under Creative Commons Attribution License BY 2.0 http://creativecommons.org/licenses/by/2.0] *Caption from original*

- Metabolic acidosis that does not respond to usual therapy is often due to lactic acidosis from unrecognized infection.
- Hypotension/shock refractory to fluid administration should prompt a consideration of concurrent gram-negative sepsis or myocardial infarction with cardiogenic shock.
- Venous thromboembolism (VTE) can occur as a late complication.
- Rhinocerebral mucormycosis is a rare, late, complication of DKA. It is an infection of the sinuses, nasal passages, oral cavity, and brain caused by saprophytic, aerobic fungi. It is associated with a very high mortality.

Related Evidence

Papers of particular interest have been highlighted as:
*** Of key importance*

Practice Guideline

Wolfsdorf JI, Allgrove J, Craig ME, Edge J, Glaser N, Jain V, Lee WW, Mungai LN, Rosenbloom AL, Sperling MA, Hanas R; International Society for Pediatric and Adolescent Diabetes. ISPAD Clinical Practice Consensus Guidelines 2014. Diabetic ketoacidosis and hyperglycemic hyperosmolar state. Pediatr Diabetes. 2014 Sep;15 Suppl 20:154-79. https://doi.org/10.1111/pedi.12165. Epub 2014 Jul 12. PMID:25041509. http://www.ncbi.nlm.nih.gov/pubmed/25041509 **

Canadian Diabetes Association Clinical Practice Guidelines Expert Committee, Goguen J, Gilbert J. Hyperglycemic emergencies in adults. Can J Diabetes. 2013 Apr;37 Suppl 1:S72-6. https://doi.org/10.1016/j.jcjd.2013.01.023. Epub 2013 Mar 26. PMID:24070967. http://www.ncbi.nlm.nih.gov/pubmed/24070967 **

Savage MW, Dhatariya KK, Kilvert A, Rayman G, Rees JA, Courtney CH, Hilton L, Dyer PH, Hamersley MS; Joint British Diabetes Societies. Joint British Diabetes Societies guideline for the management of diabetic ketoacidosis. Diabet Med.

2011 May;28(5):508-15. https://doi.org/10.1111/j.1464-5491.2011.03246.x. PMID:21255074. http://www.ncbi.nlm.nih.gov/pubmed/21255074 **

Wolfsdorf J, Craig ME, Daneman D, Dunger D, Edge J, Lee WR, Rosenbloom A, Sperling MA, Hanas R; International Society for Pediatric and Adolescent Diabetes. Diabetic ketoacidosis. Pediatr Diabetes. 2007 Feb;8(1):28-43. PMID:17341289. http://www.ncbi.nlm.nih.gov/pubmed/17341289 **

Meta-Analysis

Mukhopadhyay A, Farrell T, Fraser RB, Ola B. Continuous subcutaneous insulin infusion vs intensive conventional insulin therapy in pregnant diabetic women: a systematic review and metaanalysis of randomized, controlled trials. Am J Obstet Gynecol. 2007 Nov;197(5):447-56. Epub 2007 Aug 6. Review. PMID: 17678864. http://www.ncbi.nlm.nih.gov/pubmed/17678864

Review

Jefferies CA, Nakhla M, Derraik JG, Gunn AJ, Daneman D, Cutfield WS. Preventing Diabetic Ketoacidosis. Pediatr Clin North Am. 2015 Aug;62(4):857-71. https://doi.org/10.1016/j.pcl.2015.04.002. Epub 2015 May 30. Review. PubMed PMID: 26210621. http://www.ncbi.nlm.nih.gov/pubmed/26210621

Misra S, Oliver NS. Utility of ketone measurement in the prevention, diagnosis and management of diabetic ketoacidosis. Diabet Med. 2015 Jan;32(1):14-23. https://doi.org/10.1111/dme.12604. Epub 2014 Nov 19. Review. PMID: 25307274. http://www.ncbi.nlm.nih.gov/pubmed/25307274

Gosmanov AR, Gosmanova EO, Dillard-Cannon E. Management of adult diabetic ketoacidosis. Diabetes Metab Syndr Obes. 2014 Jun 30;7:255-64. https://doi.org/10.2147/DMSO.S50516. eCollection 2014. Review. PMID: 25061324. http://www.ncbi.nlm.nih.gov/pubmed/25061324 **

Corwell B, Knight B, Olivieri L, Willis GC. Current diagnosis and treatment of hyperglycemic emergencies. Emerg Med Clin North Am. 2014 May;32(2):437-52. https://doi.org/10.1016/j.emc.2014.01.004. Epub 2014 Feb 19. Review. PMID: 24766942. http://www.ncbi.nlm.nih.gov/pubmed/24766942

Maletkovic J, Drexler A. Diabetic ketoacidosis and hyperglycemic hyperosmolar state. Endocrinol Metab Clin North Am. 2013 Dec;42(4):677-95. https://doi.org/10.1016/j.ecl.2013.07.001. Review. PubMed PMID: 24286946. http://www.ncbi.nlm.nih.gov/pubmed/24286946 **

Van Ness-Otunnu R, Hack JB. Hyperglycemic crisis. J Emerg Med. 2013 Nov;45(5):797-805. https://doi.org/10.1016/j.jemermed.2013.03.040. Epub 2013 Jun 18. Review. PubMed PMID: 23786780. http://www.ncbi.nlm.nih.gov/pubmed/23786780

Vincent M, Nobécourt E. Treatment of diabetic ketoacidosis with subcutaneous insulin lispro: a review of the current evidence from clinical studies. Diabetes Metab. 2013 Sep;39(4):299-305. https://doi.org/10.1016/j.diabet.2012.12.003. Epub 2013 Apr 30. Review. PMID: 23642642. http://www.ncbi.nlm.nih.gov/pubmed/23642642

de Veciana M. Diabetes ketoacidosis in pregnancy. Semin Perinatol. 2013 Aug;37(4):267-73. https://doi.org/10.1053/j.semperi.2013.04.005. Review. PMID:23916025. http://www.ncbi.nlm.nih.gov/pubmed/23916025

Olivieri L, Chasm R. Diabetic ketoacidosis in the pediatric emergency department. Emerg Med Clin North Am. 2013 Aug;31(3):755-73. https://doi.org/10.1016/j.emc.2013.05.004. Epub 2013 Jul 6. Review. PMID: 23915602. http://www.ncbi.nlm.nih.gov/pubmed/23915602

Klocker AA, Phelan H, Twigg SM, Craig ME. Blood β-hydroxybutyrate vs. urine acetoacetate testing for the prevention and management of ketoacidosis in Type 1 diabetes: a systematic review. Diabet Med. 2013 Jul;30(7):818-24. https://doi.org/10.1111/dme.12136. Review. PMID: 23330615. http://www.ncbi.nlm.nih.gov/pubmed/23330615

Usher-Smith JA, Thompson MJ, Sharp SJ, Walter FM. Factors associated with the presence of diabetic ketoacidosis at diagnosis of diabetes in children and young adults: a systematic review. BMJ. 2011 Jul 7;343:d4092. https://doi.org/10.1136/bmj.d4092. Review. PMID: 21737470. http://www.ncbi.nlm.nih.gov/pubmed/21737470

Nyenwe EA, Kitabchi AE. Evidence-based management of hyperglycemic emergencies in diabetes mellitus. Diabetes Res Clin Pract. 2011 Dec;94(3):340-51. https://doi.org/10.1016/j.diabres.2011.09.012. Epub 2011 Oct 5. Review. PMID: 21978840. http://www.ncbi.nlm.nih.gov/pubmed/21978840

Wilson JF. In clinic. Diabetic ketoacidosis. Ann Intern Med. 2010 Jan 5;152(1):ITC1-1, ITC1-2, ITC1-3,ITC1-4, ITC1-5, ITC1-6, ITC1-7, ITC1-8, ITC1-9, ITC1-10, ITC1-11, ITC1-12, ITC1-13, ITC1-14, ITC1-15, table of contents; quiz ITC1-16. https://doi.org/10.7326/0003-4819-152-1-201001050-01001. Review. PMID:20048266. http://www.ncbi.nlm.nih.gov/pubmed/20048266 **

Kitabchi AE, Umpierrez GE, Miles JM, Fisher JN. Hyperglycemic crises in adult patients with diabetes. Diabetes Care. 2009 Jul;32(7):1335-43. https://doi.org/10.2337/dc09-9032. Review. PMID: 19564476. http://www.ncbi.nlm.nih.gov/pubmed/19564476 **

Davis SN, Umpierrez GE. Diabetic ketoacidosis in type 2 diabetes mellitus--pathophysiology and clinical presentation. Nat Clin Pract Endocrinol Metab. 2007 Nov;3(11):730-1. Epub 2007 Sep 11. Review. PMID:17848925. http://www.ncbi.nlm.nih.gov/pubmed/17848925 **

Parker JA, Conway DL. Diabetic ketoacidosis in pregnancy. Obstet Gynecol Clin North Am. 2007 Sep;34(3):533-43, xii. Review. PMID: 17921013. http://www.ncbi.nlm.nih.gov/pubmed/17921013

Hardern RD, Quinn ND. Emergency management of diabetic ketoacidosis in adults. Emerg Med J. 2003 May;20(3):210-3. Review. PMID: 12748130. http://www.ncbi.nlm.nih.gov/pubmed/12748130

Case Study

Pollock F, Funk DC. Acute diabetes management: adult patients with hyperglycemic crises and hypoglycemia. AACN Adv Crit Care. 2013 Jul-Sep;24(3):314-24. https://doi.org/10.1097/NCI.0b013e31829b7d38. PMID:23880754. http://www.ncbi.nlm.nih.gov/pubmed/23880754 **

Use PubMed Clinical Queries to find the most recent evidence. Use this search strategy: "Diabetic ketoacidosis"[mesh] OR "Diabetic ketoacidosis"

Chapter 25
Duchenne Muscular Dystrophy

Richard M. Cantor, Charles V. Pollack, Jr., and Victoria G. Riese

Name and Synonyms

Duchenne Muscular Dystrophy (DMD)

- A member of a group of diseases termed dystrophinopathies (includes Duchenne and Becker Muscular Dystrophy)
- Duchenne's is the most severe form

Incidence/Epidemiology

- Caused by a defective gene on the X chromosome.
- An X linked recessive trait.
- A population-based surveillance study of males 5–24 years old in four states found the overall prevalence of DMD/Becker muscular dystrophy (BMD) to be from 1.3 to 1.8 per 10,000.

R. M. Cantor
Department of Emergency Medicine and Pediatrics, State University of New York Upstate Medical University, Syracuse, NY, USA

C. V. Pollack, Jr. (✉)
Department of Emergency Medicine, Thomas Jefferson University, Philadelphia, PA, USA

V. G. Riese
Librarian Consultant, Eldersburg, MD, USA

C. V. Pollack, Jr. (ed.), *Differential Diagnosis of Cardiopulmonary Disease*,
https://doi.org/10.1007/978-3-319-63895-9_25

Differential Diagnosis

- The differential diagnosis of infants and children with muscle weakness is large.
- Some helpful clinical findings include:
  - Cranial nerve deficits are seen in neuromuscular junction dysfunction (myasthenia gravis, botulism, and tick paralysis).
  - Spinal cord dysfunction is heralded by loss of function below the level of the lesion (poor rectal tone, decreased cremasteric reflexes).
- Hyperesthesias are common in peripheral nerve disorders.
- The presence of ataxia and cerebellar signs favors a central anomaly.
- Hyporeflexia is common in Guillain-Barré syndrome, tick paralysis, and botulism.

Pathophysiology and Etiology

- The result of a defective gene located on the X chromosome that is responsible for the production of dystrophin.
- Dystrophin is responsible for stabilization of muscle proteins, protecting them from degradation.
- Damage to these proteins results in muscle fiber degeneration.

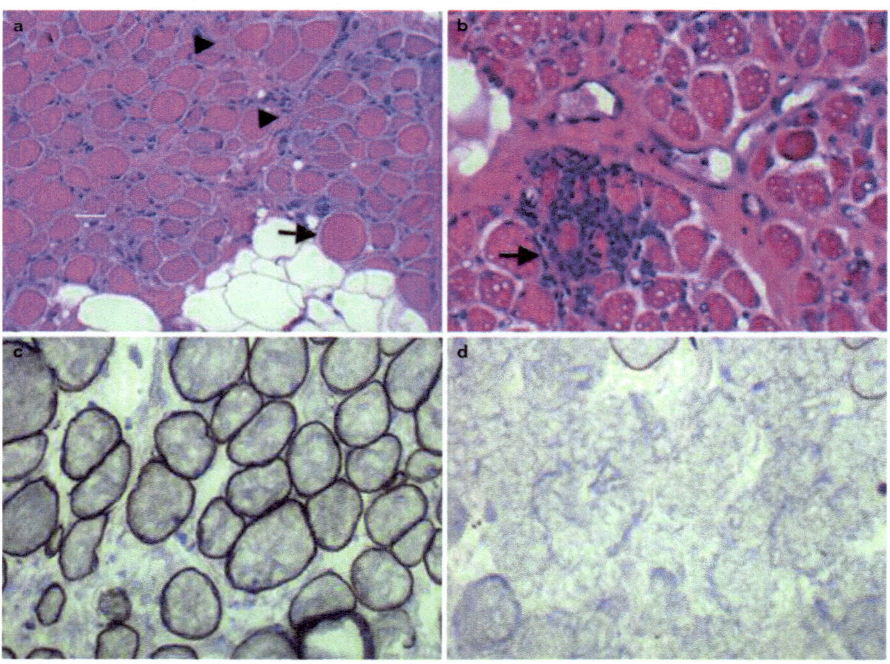

Duchenne muscular dystrophy. (a) On hematoxylin and eosin (H&E) staining, considerable fiber-type variation, including an occasional hypertrophic fiber (arrow) and fibrosis with fatty infiltration (arrow heads), is noted. (b) Also on H&E staining, lymphocytic infiltrates are demonstrated (arrow). (c) Normal dystrophin staining. (d) Loss of dystrophin staining in DMD [Russell JW, Weiss MD, Distad BJ, Castellani RJ. Muscle and Myotonic Diseases. In: Feldman EL, Grisold W, Russell JW, Löscher WN, editors. Atlas of Neuromuscular Diseases [Internet]. Vienna: Springer Vienna; 2014 [cited 2016 Aug 1]. p. 247–81. Available from: http://link.springer.com/10.1007/978-3-7091-1605-0_11] *Caption from original*

Presentation

Typical/"Classic"

- Neuromuscular presentation is most common.
- Obvious clinical signs of weakness occur between 2 and 3 years of age.
- Lower extremity muscles are initially affected, specifically proximal limb musculature.

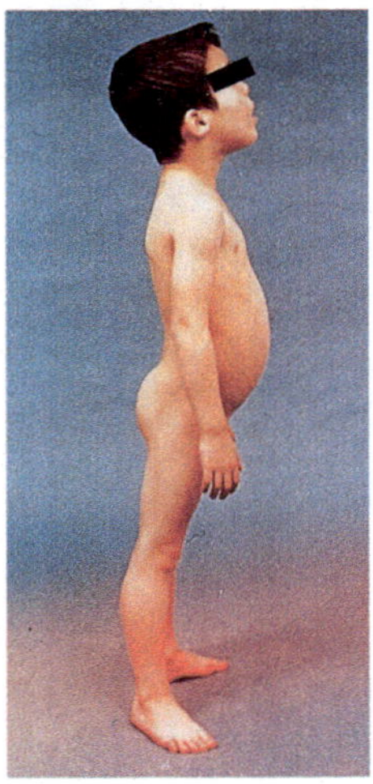

Duchenne dystrophy. Duchenne dystrophy is an X-linked progressive myopathy of childhood caused by mutations of the dystrophin gene. A,Lateral photograph of a boy with Duchenne dystrophy. Note the lumbar lordosis and enlarged calves [Pleasure D, Bird S, Scherer S, Sladky J, Schotland D. Neuromuscular Disease. In: Rosenberg RN, editor. Atlas of Clinical Neurology [Internet]. Current Medicine Group; 2003 [cited 2016 Aug 1]. p. 385–401. Available from: http://link.springer.com/chapter/10.1007/978-1-4757-4552-8_11] *Caption from original.*

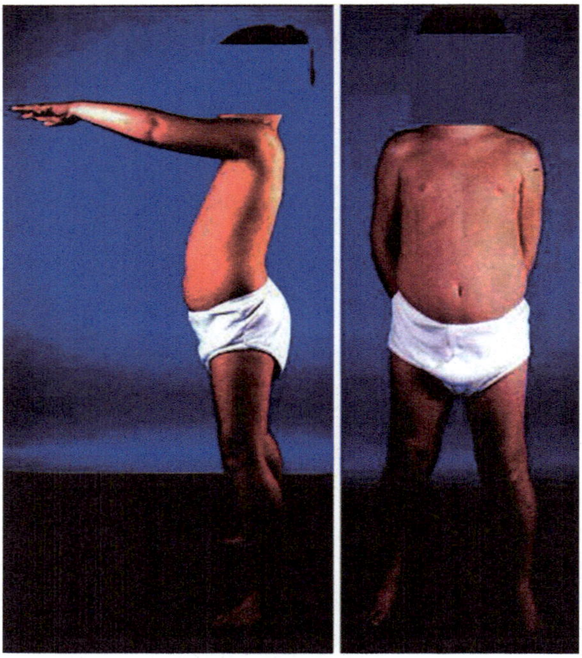

Duchenne muscular dystrophy. Note the prominent abdomen and lumbar lordosis, calf pseudohypertrophy, and equinus at the ankles [Bleck EE, Robb JE. Hereditary and Developmental Neuromuscular Disorders. In: Benson M, Fixsen J, Macnicol M, Parsch K, editors. Children's Orthopaedics and Fractures [Internet]. London: Springer London; 2010 [cited 2016 Aug 1]. p. 249–64. Available from: http://link.springer.com/10.1007/978-1-84882-611-3_16] *Caption from original*

- There is impairment of running, jumping, and climbing stairs. Fractures from falls are common,
- Look for Gower's Sign—children will have to actively push up with their hands to attain a standing position.

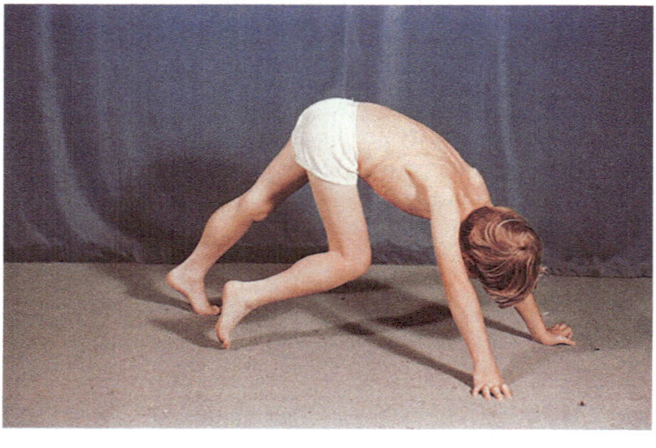

Duchenne's dystrophy, Gower maneuver [MacGregor DL. Neurology. In: Laxer R, Ford-Jones EL, Friedman J, Gerstle T, editors. The Hospital for Sick Children: atlas of pediatrics. Philadelphia: Current Medicine; 2005. Atlas of Pediatrics, Volume IA, Chapter 05;. ISBN: 1-57340-188-9] *Caption from original*

- Most patients are wheelchair-bound by early adolescence.

Atypical

- There may also be variable degrees of global developmental deficits.
- Cardiac presentations are less common than neuromuscular presentations.
- DMD causes a dilated cardiomyopathy.

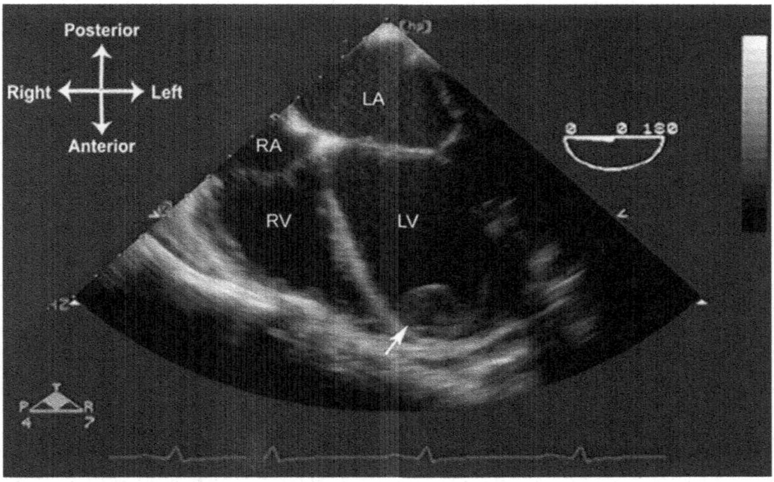

Thrombus (arrow) in the left ventricular apex of a patient with Duchenne muscular dystrophy and dilated cardiomyopathy. Mid-esophageal four-chamber view, multiplane angle 0°. LA left atrium, LV left ventricle, RA right atrium, RV right ventricle [Wong PC. Additional Applications of Transesophageal Echocardiography. In: Wong PC, Miller-Hance WC, editors. Transesophageal Echocardiography for Congenital Heart Disease [Internet]. London: Springer London; 2014 [cited 2016 Aug 1]. p. 399–436. Available from: http://link.springer.com/10.1007/978-1-84800-064-3_16] *Caption from original*

- Conduction abnormalities may be present (resulting in mostly supraventricular disorders).
- The progression of cardiac disease is gradual, with full expression after 18 years of age.
- Most children, by virtue of their lack of strenuous activity, are asymptomatic.
- Most children with DMD develop scoliosis.

Primary Differential Considerations

- Other muscular dystrophies must be considered; the most common is Becker muscular dystrophy. Muscle biopsy can differentiate among these and other diagnoses.

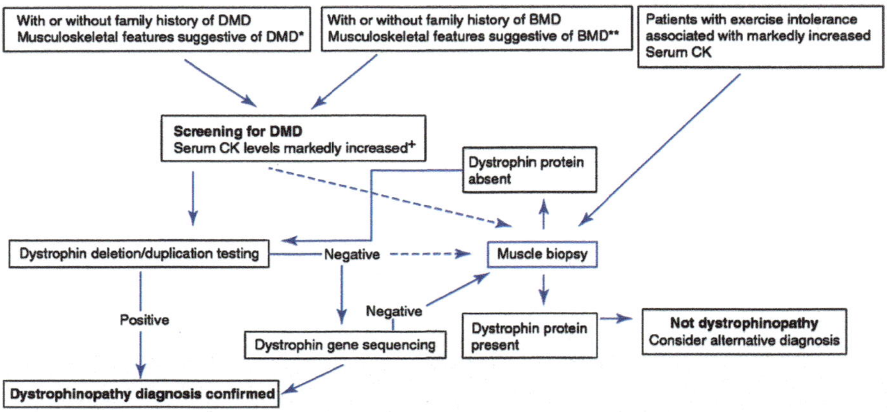

Algorithm to guide diagnostic workup in suspected DMD/BMD patients for confirmation of dystrophinopathy diagnosis. For patients diagnosed by muscle biopsy, dystrophin genetic testing is also necessary. For patients diagnosed by genetic testing, muscle biopsy is not necessary, and if at all possible, defer muscle biopsy until patient participates in a later clinical trial. DMD Duchenne muscular dystrophy, BMD Becker muscular dystrophy, CK creatine kinase [Sahenk Z, Rodino-Klapac LR. Dystrophinopathies. In: Katirji B, Kaminski HJ, Ruff RL, editors. Neuromuscular Disorders in Clinical Practice [Internet]. New York, NY: Springer New York; 2014 [cited 2016 Aug 1]. p. 1207–29. Available from: http://link.springer.com/10.1007/978-1-4614-6567-6_56] *Caption adapted from original*

History and Physical Exam

Findings That Confirm Diagnosis

- Common findings include a wide-based gait, lumbar lordosis, pseudohypertrophy of the calf muscles, shortening of the Achilles tendons, and hyporeflexia or areflexia.
- Depending on the degree of scoliosis, respiratory function may be compromised.

Factors That Suggest Diagnosis

- Most children will have already been diagnosed prior to their first Emergency Department encounter.

Factors That Exclude Diagnosis

- No clinical findings can exclude DMD in patients with suggestive findings. A muscle biopsy is required.

Ancillary studies

Electrocardiography

- As previously mentioned, a variety of arrhythmias may occur, particular supraventricular.

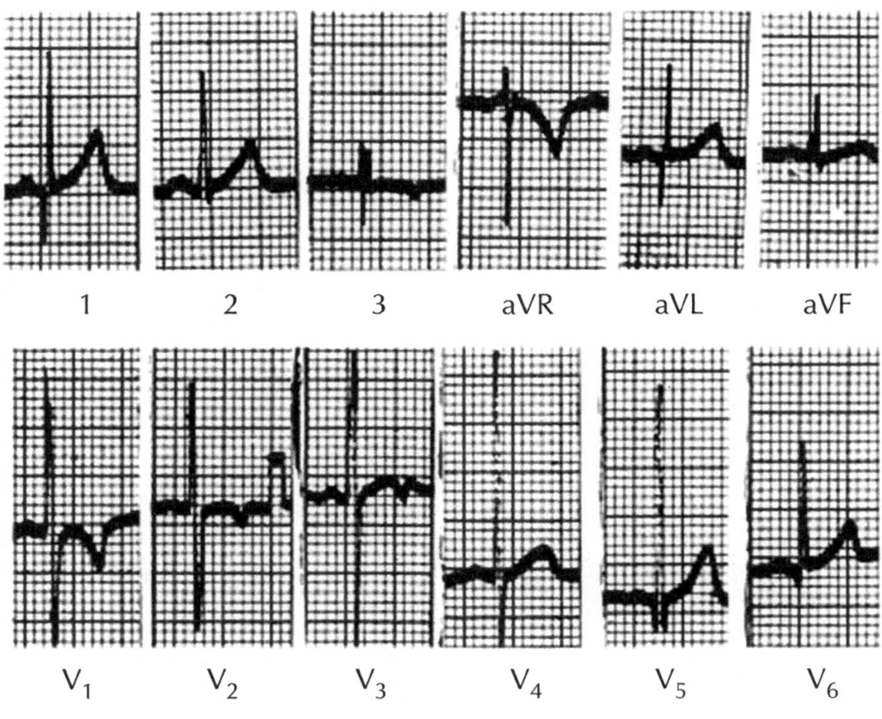

Electrocardiogram of female carrier of Duchenne dystrophy gene [Perloff J, Abelmann W. Chapter 6. In: Lee RT, Braunwald E, editors. Atlas of cardiac imaging. Philadelphia: Current Medicine; 1998. ISBN: 0-443-07567-0] *Caption from original*

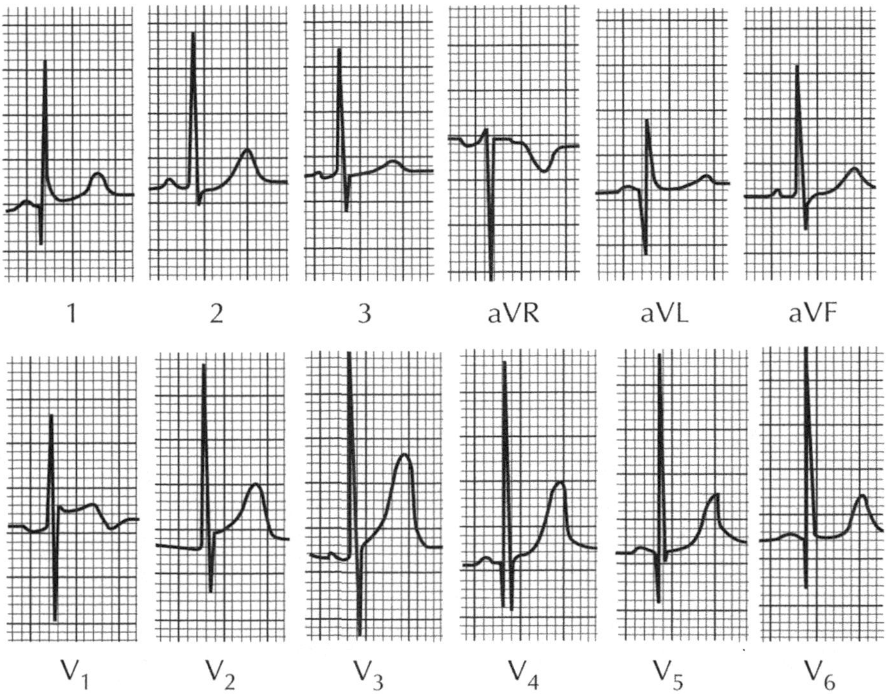

Electrocardiogram of Duchenne dystrophy in 10-year-old boy [Perloff J, Abelmann W. Chapter 6. In: Lee RT, Braunwald E, editors. Atlas of cardiac imaging. Philadelphia: Current Medicine; 1998. ISBN: 0-443-07567-0] *Caption from original*

Laboratory

- Patients with DMD will have elevated levels of serum creatine kinase.
- These elevations may occur prior to the appearance of clinical disease.
- Levels peak in early childhood but may actually normalize as damaged muscle fibers are replaced by fibrotic change.

Special Populations

Age

- DMD is identified in early life. The usual life expectancy of patients with DMD is about 25 years.

Co-morbidities

- None significant

Pitfalls in Diagnosis

Critical Steps Not to Miss

- It is most important to anticipate the variable forms of target organ dysfunction that accompany DMD patients.
- Complications of respiratory compromise are the most frequent etiologies of emergency department visits.
- Aspiration pneumonia and cases of primary bacterial pneumonia are commonly encountered.
- Use extreme caution when providing sedation and analgesia to DMD patients.
- DMD patients are susceptible to the development of malignant hyperthermia, specifically associated with administration of succinylcholine and inhalational agents.

Mimics

- In general, these patients are already diagnosed prior to ED presentation.

Time-Dependent Interventions

- Depending on the particular complication, early administration of fluids and broad-spectrum antibiotics are indicated.

Overall Principles of Treatment

- As mentioned, most ED cases necessitate pulmonary support and attention to obvious complications.

Disease Course

- Sadly, most children with DMD are confined to a wheelchair by early adolescence.
- Death usually occurs by early adulthood, and is caused by cardiopulmonary insufficiency.

Related Evidence

Papers of particular interest have been highlighted as:
*** Of key importance*

Practice Guideline

Bushby K, Finkel R, Birnkrant DJ, Case LE, Clemens PR, Cripe L, Kaul A, Kinnett K, McDonald C, Pandya S, Poysky J, Shapiro F, Tomezsko J, Constantin C; DMD Care Considerations Working Group. Diagnosis and management of Duchenne muscular dystrophy, part 1: diagnosis, and pharmacological and psychosocial management. Lancet Neurol. 2010 Jan;9(1):77-93. https://doi.org/10.1016/S1474-4422(09)70271-6. PMID: 19945913. http://www.ncbi.nlm.nih.gov/pubmed/19945913 **

Bushby K, Finkel R, Birnkrant DJ, Case LE, Clemens PR, Cripe L, Kaul A, Kinnett K, McDonald C, Pandya S, Poysky J, Shapiro F, Tomezsko J, Constantin C; DMD Care Considerations Working Group. Diagnosis and management of Duchenne muscular dystrophy, part 2: implementation of multidisciplinary care. Lancet Neurol. 2010 Feb;9(2):177-89. https://doi.org/10.1016/S1474-4422(09)70272-8. PMID: 19945914. http://www.ncbi.nlm.nih.gov/pubmed/19945914 **

Birnkrant DJ, Panitch HB, Benditt JO, Boitano LJ, Carter ER, Cwik VA, Finder JD, Iannaccone ST, Jacobson LE, Kohn GL, Motoyama EK, Moxley RT, Schroth MK, Sharma GD, Sussman MD. American College of Chest Physicians consensus statement on the respiratory and related management of patients with Duchenne muscular dystrophy undergoing anesthesia or sedation. Chest. 2007 Dec;132(6):1977-86. PMID: 18079231. http://www.ncbi.nlm.nih.gov/pubmed/18079231 **

American Academy of Pediatrics Section on Cardiology and Cardiac Surgery. Cardiovascular health supervision for individuals affected by Duchenne or Becker muscular dystrophy. Pediatrics. 2005 Dec;116(6):1569-73. PMID: 16322188. http://www.ncbi.nlm.nih.gov/pubmed/16322188 **

Review

Annexstad EJ, Lund-Petersen I, Rasmussen M. Duchenne muscular dystrophy. Tidsskr Nor Laegeforen. 2014 Aug 5;134(14):1361-4. https://doi.org/10.4045/tidsskr.13.0836. PMID: 25096430. http://www.ncbi.nlm.nih.gov/pubmed/25096430 **

Chelly J, Desguerre I. Progressive muscular dystrophies. Handb Clin Neurol. 2013;113:1343-66. https://doi.org/10.1016/B978-0-444-59565-2.00006-X. PMID: 23622359. http://www.ncbi.nlm.nih.gov/pubmed/23622359 **

Verma S, Anziska Y, Cracco J. Review of Duchenne muscular dystrophy (DMD) for the pediatricians in the community. Clin Pediatr (Phila). 2010 Nov;49(11):1011-7. https://doi.org/10.1177/0009922810378738. PMID: 20724320. http://www.ncbi.nlm.nih.gov/pubmed/20724320 **

Centers for Disease Control and Prevention (CDC). Prevalence of Duchenne/Becker muscular dystrophy among males aged 5-24 years - four states, 2007. MMWR Morb Mortal Wkly Rep. 2009 Oct 16;58(40):1119-22. PMID: 19834452. http://www.ncbi.nlm.nih.gov/pubmed/19834452

Hayes J, Veyckemans F, Bissonnette B. Duchenne muscular dystrophy: an old anesthesia problem revisited. Paediatr Anaesth. 2008 Feb;18(2):100-6. https://doi.org/10.1111/j.1460-9592.2007.02302.x. PMID: 18184239. http://www.ncbi.nlm.nih.gov/pubmed/18184239

Manzur AY, Kuntzer T, Pike M, Swan A. Glucocorticoid corticosteroids for Duchenne muscular dystrophy. Cochrane Database Syst Rev. 2008 Jan 23;(1):CD003725. https://doi.org/10.1002/14651858.CD003725.pub3. PMID: 18254031. http://www.ncbi.nlm.nih.gov/pubmed/18254031

Deconinck N, Dan B. Pathophysiology of duchenne muscular dystrophy: current hypotheses. Pediatr Neurol. 2007 Jan;36(1):1-7. PMID: 17162189. http://www.ncbi.nlm.nih.gov/pubmed/17162189 **

Sanger TD, Chen D, Delgado MR, Gaebler-Spira D, Hallett M, Mink JW; Taskforce on Childhood Motor Disorders. Definition and classification of negative motor signs in childhood. Pediatrics. 2006 Nov;118(5):2159-67. PMID: 17079590. http://www.ncbi.nlm.nih.gov/pubmed/17079590 **

Nowak KJ, Davies KE. Duchenne muscular dystrophy and dystrophin: pathogenesis and opportunities for treatment. EMBO Rep. 2004 Sep;5(9):872-6. PMID: 15470384. http://www.ncbi.nlm.nih.gov/pubmed/15470384 **

Emery AE. The muscular dystrophies. Lancet. 2002 Feb 23;359(9307):687-95. PMID: 11879882. http://www.ncbi.nlm.nih.gov/pubmed/11879882

Use PubMed Clinical Queries to find the most recent evidence. Use this search strategy:
"Muscular Dystrophy, Duchenne"[Mesh] OR "Duchenne muscular dystrophy"

Chapter 26
Epiglottitis

Richard M. Cantor, Charles V. Pollack, Jr., and Victoria G. Riese

Name and Synonyms

- Epiglottitis (Supraglottitis)

Incidence/Epidemiology

- There has been a marked decrease in cases since the introduction of the Hib vaccine.
- According to current estimates, in the United States 1.6 cases occur per 100,000 adults, and 0.5 cases occur per 100,000 children.
- As a result of immunization practices, the median age of children presenting with epiglottitis has increased from 3 years to 6–12 years of age.

R. M. Cantor
Department of Emergency Medicine and Pediatrics, State University of New York Upstate Medical University, Syracuse, NY, USA

C. V. Pollack, Jr. (✉)
Department of Emergency Medicine, Thomas Jefferson University, Philadelphia, PA, USA

V. G. Riese
Librarian Consultant, Eldersburg, MD, USA

C. V. Pollack, Jr. (ed.), *Differential Diagnosis of Cardiopulmonary Disease*,
https://doi.org/10.1007/978-3-319-63895-9_26

Differential Diagnosis

- Other causes of acute upper airway obstruction must be considered:
  - Croup
  - Bacterial tracheitis
  - Peritonsillar abscess
  - Retropharyngeal abscess
  - Upper airway foreign body
  - Congenital upper airway anomalies

	Croup	**Epiglottitis**
Cause	Viral	Bacterial
Age	6 mo to 3 y	4–6 y
Site of obstruction	Subglottic	Supraglottic
Clinical features		
Onset	Gradual (days)	Sudden (hours)
Fever	With or without low grade fever	High fever (> 102°F)
Dysphagia, drooling		Present
Cough	Barking, dry cough	Not common
Respiratory rate	↑	Normal
Position	Normal	Sitting upright
Appearance	Mild distress	Toxic appearing
Quality of voice	Hoarseness	Muffled
Primary Treatment	Supportive:	Secure airway:
Hydration	Needed	Needed
Antibiotics	Not Needed	Needed to treat *Haemophilus* influenza
Airway support	Not Needed	Always needed
Extubation	Not Needed	When temperature decreases and with leak around the endotracheal tube

Differential diagnosis of croup vs epiglottitis. The two most common infectious causes of upper airway obstruction in children, croup and epiglottitis, differ in etiology, patient demographics, and symptomatology. [Rasmussen G, Deshpande J. Pediatric anesthesia. In: Muravchick S, editor. Subspecialty care. Philadelphia: Current Medicine; 1998. 236 p. (Miller RD editor, Atlas of anesthesia; vol. 5). ISBN: 0-443-07905-6] *Caption from original*

Pathophysiology and Etiology

- Epiglottitis is essentially a cellulitic process secondary to bacteremic spread.
- The onset of edema is rapid and usually does not involve subglottic structures.

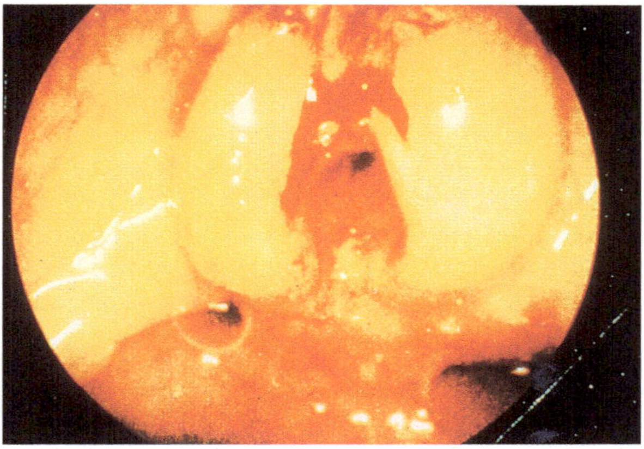

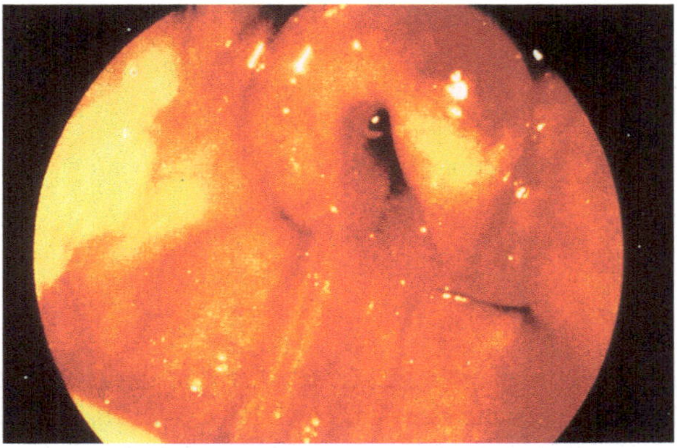

Severe epiglottitis. Two patients with severe epiglottitis. A, The characteristic edema of the epiglottis and laryngeal structures and purulent material. B, Extent that advanced edema can become, so that by the time many patients present, they are breathing through an extremely small aperture. [Rasmussen G, Deshpande J. Pediatric anesthesia. In: Muravchick S, editor. Subspecialty care. Philadelphia: Current Medicine; 1998. 236 p. (Miller RD editor, Atlas of anesthesia; vol. 5). ISBN: 0-443-07905-6] *Caption from original*

- Most cases are bacterial in origin, usually from *Haemophilus influenza* type b (Hib).
- Other causes in children include streptococci and *Staphylococcus aureus* (including MRSA strains).

Presentation

Typical/"Classic"

- Look for the "3 D's": distress, drooling, and dysphagia.
- Unlike croup, there is generally no prodromal URI.
- Most children become ill within 24 hours, often with a toxic appearance.
- Younger children will assume a "sniffing posture," in which the chin is thrust forward and the neck hyperextended in order to maximize airway patency.

	Children	Adults
Age at acquisition	3–5 yrs	—
Location of pathology	Supraglottic	Supraglottic
Onset	Rapid	Most have a mild illness with prolonged course, painful dysphagia, and pharyngitis
Fever	High	Variable
Appearance	Toxic	Usually not toxic
Stridor	+++	Not usual
Cough	Not usual	—
Drooling	Often	—

Clinical features of acute epiglottitis [Tristram D. Chapter 07. In: Brook I, editor. Atlas of Upper Respiratory and Head and Neck Infections, 2e. Philadelphia: Current Medicine; 2000. (Mandell GL, editor. Atlas of infectious diseases; vol. 4). ISBN: 1-57340-140-4]

Atypical

- Older children and adults may only complain of a sore throat, and generally do not appear toxic

Primary Differential Considerations

- Early consideration in patients with symptoms referable to epiglottitis should also be given to the following differential diagnoses:
  - Peritonsillar or retropharyngeal abscess
  - Angioedema
  - Laryngitis
  - Tonsillitis
  - Laryngeal diphtheria

History and Physical Exam

Findings That Confirm Diagnosis

- In the purest sense, the diagnosis is confirmed by direct visualization of the epiglottis in the operating room.

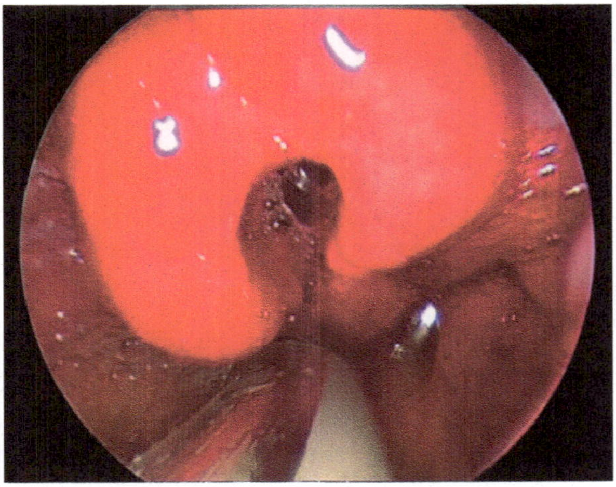

Direct laryngoscopy findings in a 10-year-old presenting with epiglottitis [Hughes AL, Karter N, Swanson DS. Laryngeal Infections. In: Valdez T, Vallejo J, editors. Infectious Diseases in Pediatric Otolaryngology [Internet]. Cham: Springer International Publishing; 2016 [cited 2016 Aug 3]. p. 151–61. Available from: http://link.springer.com/10.1007/978-3-319-21744-4_11] *Caption from original*

- Indirect diagnosis may be obtained by visualization of a swollen epiglottis on lateral neck radiographs ("thumb print sign").

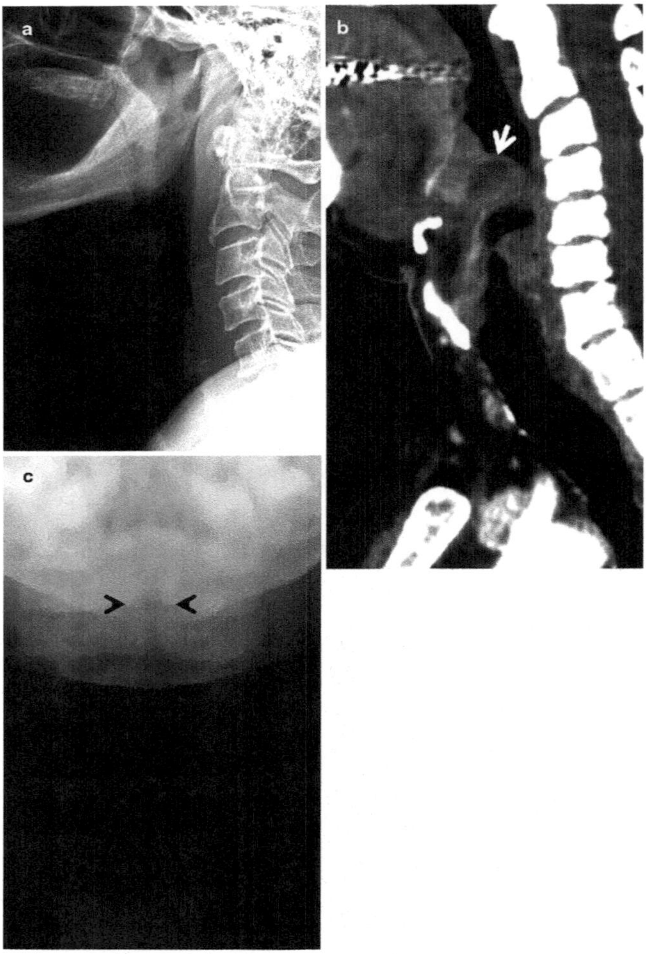

(a, b) Acute epiglottitis. Note the swollen epiglottis with a thumb-like appearance. Radiography is unnecessary in acute epiglottitis and must not be undertaken lightly but occasionally may be performed to exclude a foreign body. It is best performed with the patient in a sitting position to keep the airway open. Epiglottitis can be life-threatening and resources to secure the airway must be available at all times. The CT image shows an edematous epiglottis containing an abscess (arrow). CT is unnecessary for acute epiglottitis. (c) Croup – "steeple" like narrowing of the subglottic airway (arrowheads) [Raghavan P, Shonka DC, Wintermark M, Mukherjee S. Larynx and Hypopharynx. In: Raghavan P, Mukherjee S, Jameson MJ, Wintermark M. Manual of Head and Neck Imaging [Internet]. Berlin, Heidelberg: Springer Berlin Heidelberg; 2014 [cited 2016 Aug 2]. p. 109–36. Available from: http://link.springer.com/10.1007/978-3-642-40377-4_5] *Caption from original*

Factors That Suggest Diagnosis

- Many studies have highlighted the following findings:
  - Difficulty breathing (80 %)
  - Stridor (80 %)
  - Muffled or hoarse voice (79 %)
  - Pharyngitis (73 %)
  - Fever (57 %)
  - Sore throat (50 %)
  - Difficulty swallowing (26 %)
  - Change in voice (20 %)

Symptom	No. of patients	Percent
Sore throat	272	94
Dysphagia	252	88
Odynophagia	178	62
Fever	118	41
Dyspnea	85	30
Hoarseness	40	14
Foreign body sensation	23	8
Cough	19	7
Muffled voice	18	6
Otalgia	11	4
Stridor	4	1
Drooling	4	1
Heartburn	4	1
Vomiting	2	1
Tripod position	0	0

Patients may have more than one presenting symptom

Presenting symptoms and signs in 288 acute supraglottitis adult patients [Ovnat Tamir S, Marom T, Barbalat I, Spevak S, Goldfarb A, Roth Y. Adult supraglottitis: changing trends. European Archives of Oto-Rhino-Laryngology. 2015 Apr;272(4):929–35.] *Caption from original*

Factors That Exclude Diagnosis

- A normal epiglottitis on direct view in the surgical suite is the only way to exclude the diagnosis fully in patients suspected of having epiglottitis.

Ancillary Studies

Laboratory

- Note: It is advisable to wait until definitive equipment and personnel are at the bedside (or in the OR) before negatively stimulating the child.
- Although the diagnosis is a clinical one, leukocytosis is common, as are positive blood cultures.

Imaging

- Radiographs should only be obtained at no risk to the child.
- No patient should leave the Emergency Department without adequate airway personnel and equipment.

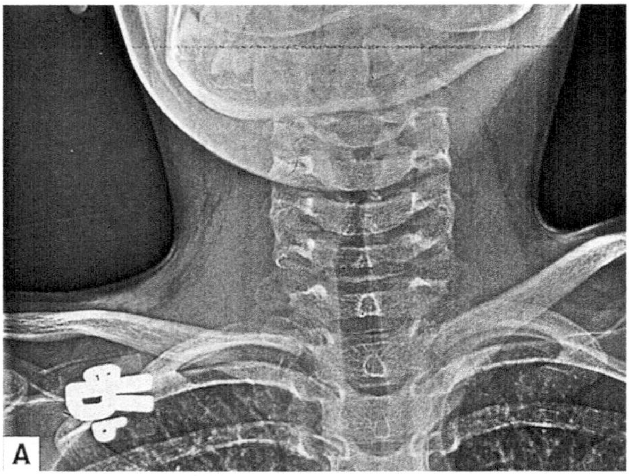

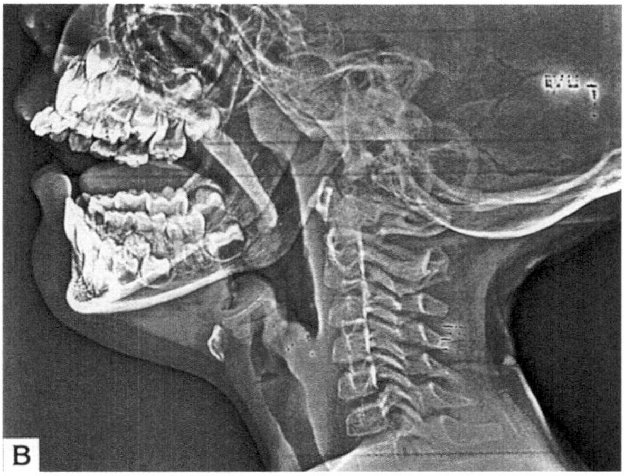

Epiglottitis as seen by xeroradiography. A, Anteroposterior view of the neck of a child with documented epiglottitis shows narrowing in the diameter of the trachea, which can be confused with acute viral croup. The lateral neck view is preferable because it can demonstrate the enlarged epiglottis, or "thumb sign." B, Xeroradiograph showing a lateral neck view of the same child demonstrates the acute epiglottic and aryepiglottic swelling seen in acute epiglottitis. Direct visualization in the operating room revealed a markedly swollen epiglottis. [Tristram D. Chapter 07. In: Brook I, editor. Atlas of Upper Respiratory and Head and Neck Infections, 2e. Philadelphia: Current Medicine; 2000. (Mandell GL, editor. Atlas of infectious diseases; vol. 4). ISBN: 1-57340-140-4] *Caption from original*

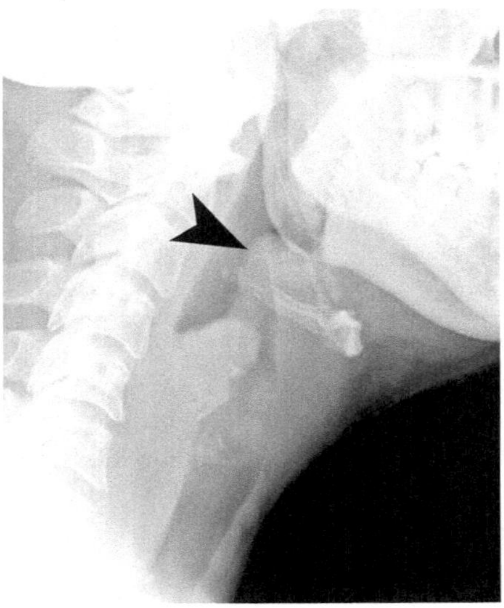

Epiglottitis. Lateral radiograph of the neck demonstrates gross enlargement of the epiglottis (arrowhead) as well as the aryepiglottic fold, resulting in narrowing of the supraglottic laryngeal airway [Singh A. Imaging of Neck Emergencies. In: Singh A, editor. Emergency Radiology [Internet]. New York, NY: Springer New York; 2013 [cited 2016 Aug 2]. p. 183–98. Available from: http://link.springer.com/10.1007/978-1-4419-9592-6_15] *Caption from original*

Special Populations

Age

- Epiglottitis can present at all ages. Adult epiglottitis is generally less acute and is certainly less life-threatening than the pediatric issue.
- Pediatric epiglottitis is much less common in areas where the Hib vaccine is widely given; kids who are not immunized are at higher risk.

Co-morbidities

- Immune-compromised patients are at higher risk of developing epiglottitis. This is particularly true in adult cases.

Co-morbidity	Number of patients	Percent
None	108	38
Smoking	121	42
Cardiovascular disease	87	30
Gastroesophageal reflux	37	13
Diabetes mellitus	29	10
Immunosuppression	20	7
Others	124	43

Patients may present with several co-morbidities

Most common co-morbidities among 288 acute supraglottitis adult patients [Ovnat Tamir S, Marom T, Barbalat I, Spevak S, Goldfarb A, Roth Y. Adult supraglottitis: changing trends. European Archives of Oto-Rhino-Laryngology. 2015 Apr;272(4):929–35.*] Caption from original*

Pitfalls in Diagnosis

- The two most significant pitfalls in diagnosis are:
  - failing to consider the diagnosis altogether
  - being cavalier in the workup and sending a child suspected of epiglottitis to radiology without definitive airway assistance.
- Failing to consider significant differential diagnoses such as peritonsillar abscess is a problem.

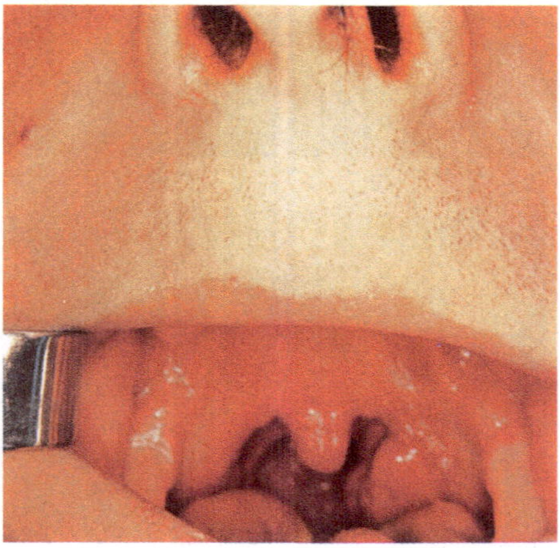

Peritonsillar abscess [Endicott J, Seper J. Chapter 10. In: Brook I, editor. Atlas of Upper Respiratory and Head and Neck Infections, 2e. Philadelphia: Current Medicine; 2000. (Mandell GL, editor. Atlas of infectious diseases; vol. 4). ISBN: 1-57340-140-4]

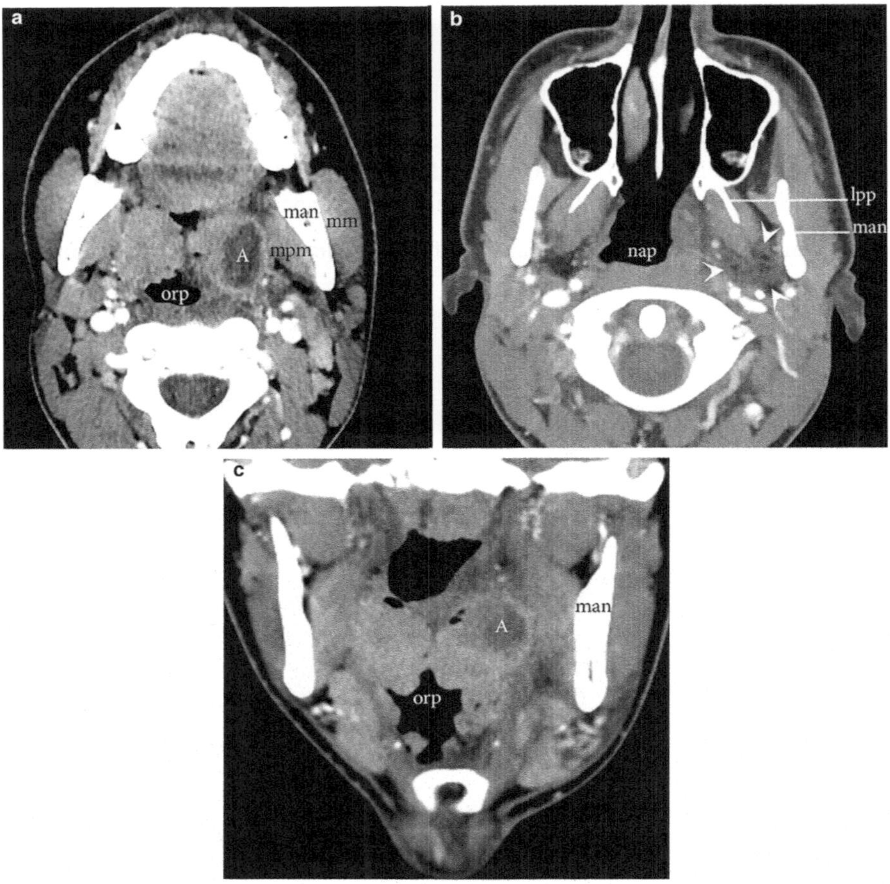

Peritonsillar abscess. Axial (***a***, ***b***) and coronal (***c***) CECT images demonstrate a rim-enhancing left-sided peritonsillar abscess (A) in this child with odynophagia and fever. There is resultant narrowing of pharynx and "kissing" appearance of the enlarged tonsils. There is infiltration of left parapharyngeal fat (white arrows). Medial pterygoid muscle (mpm, ***a***), mandible (man, ***a***, ***b***, ***c***), masseter muscle (mm, ***a***), oropharynx (orp, ***a***, ***c***), lateral pterygoid plate (lpp, ***b***), nasopharynx (nap, ***b***) [Pawha P, Jiang N, Shpilberg K, Luttrull M, Govindaraj S. Gross and Radiographic Anatomy. In: Levine AI, Govindaraj S, DeMaria, S, editors. Anesthesiology and Otolaryngology [Internet]. New York, NY: Springer New York; 2013 [cited 2016 Aug 2]. p. 3–33. Available from: http://link.springer.com/10.1007/978-1-4614-4184-7_2] *Caption from original*

Critical Steps Not to Miss

- If a diagnosis of epiglottitis is suspected, all efforts should be directed toward obtaining the personnel and equipment necessary for intubation.
- Without question, intubation is best carried out in the OR by medical caregivers expert in Pediatric airway management (i.e., ENT or Anesthesia).

Mimics

- Most other causes of upper airway disease in children do not present in a manner similar to that of epiglottitis.

Time-Dependent Interventions

- Early confirmation of the diagnosis and expectant airway management by expert operators is essential to good outcomes in acute epiglottitis.

Overall Principles of Treatment

- The management of epiglottitis has 3 phases:
    - Recognition
    - Intubation
    - Intravenous antibiotics

Disease Course

- The prognosis is excellent if surgical correction is carried out.

Related Evidence:

Papers of particular interest have been highlighted as:
*** Of key importance*

Cohort Study

Hermansen MN, Schmidt JH, Krug AH, Larsen K, Kristensen S. Low incidence of children with acute epiglottis after introduction of vaccination. Dan Med J. 2014 Apr;61(4):A4788. PMID: 24814584. http://www.ncbi.nlm.nih.gov/pubmed/24814584

Shah RK, Stocks C. Epiglottitis in the United States: national trends, variances, prognosis, and management. Laryngoscope. 2010 Jun;120(6):1256-62. https://doi.org/10.1002/lary.20921. PMID: 20513048. http://www.ncbi.nlm.nih.gov/pubmed/20513048 **

Acevedo JL, Lander L, Choi S, Shah RK. Airway management in pediatric epiglottitis: a national perspective. Otolaryngol Head Neck Surg. 2009 Apr;140(4):548-51. https://doi.org/10.1016/j.otohns.2008.12.037. PMID: 19328345. http://www.ncbi.nlm.nih.gov/pubmed/19328345 **

Briem B, Thorvardsson O, Petersen H. Acute epiglottitis in Iceland 1983-2005. Auris Nasus Larynx. 2009 Feb;36(1):46-52. https://doi.org/10.1016/j.anl.2008.03.012. PMID: 18502071. http://www.ncbi.nlm.nih.gov/pubmed/18502071 **

Guldfred LA, Lyhne D, Becker BC. Acute epiglottitis: epidemiology, clinical presentation, management and outcome. J Laryngol Otol. 2008 Aug;122(8):818-23. PMID: 17892608. http://www.ncbi.nlm.nih.gov/pubmed/17892608 **

Glynn F, Fenton JE. Diagnosis and management of supraglottitis (epiglottitis). Curr Infect Dis Rep. 2008 May;10(3):200-4. PMID:18510881. http://www.ncbi.nlm.nih.gov/pubmed/18510881 **

Shah RK, Roberson DW, Jones DT. Epiglottitis in the Hemophilus influenzae type B vaccine era: changing trends. Laryngoscope. 2004 Mar;114(3):557-60. PMID: 15091234. http://www.ncbi.nlm.nih.gov/pubmed/15091234 **

McEwan J, Giridharan W, Clarke RW, Shears P. Paediatric acute epiglottitis: not a disappearing entity. Int J Pediatr Otorhinolaryngol. 2003 Apr;67(4):317-21. PMID: 12663101. http://www.ncbi.nlm.nih.gov/pubmed/12663101 **

Mayo-Smith MF, Spinale JW, Donskey CJ, Yukawa M, Li RH, Schiffman FJ. Acute epiglottitis. An 18-year experience in Rhode Island. Chest. 1995 Dec;108(6):1640-7. PMID: 7497775. http://www.ncbi.nlm.nih.gov/pubmed/7497775 **

Comparative Study

Comparative Study. McVernon J, Slack MP, Ramsay ME. Changes in the epidemiology of epiglottitis following introduction of Haemophilus influenzae type b (Hib) conjugate vaccines in England: a comparison of two data sources. Epidemiol Infect. 2006 Jun;134(3):570-2. PMID: 16288684. http://www.ncbi.nlm.nih.gov/pubmed/16288684 **

Use PubMed Clinical Queries to find the most recent evidence. Use this search strategy:
"Epiglottitis"[Mesh] OR "Epiglottitis" OR "Supraglottitis"

Chapter 27
Esophageal Rupture

Christopher J. Rees, Charles V. Pollack, Jr., and Victoria G. Riese

Name and Synonyms

Esophageal Rupture

- Esophageal Perforation, Boerhaave's Syndrome

Incidence/Epidemiology

- Esophageal rupture is a rare but life-threatening event.
- Current mortality of 30 %.
- There are many causes of esophageal rupture (described below). Iatrogenic causes are the most common, accounting for about half of all cases. Classic Boerhaave's syndrome accounts for another 15 %, foreign bodies for 14 %, trauma (penetrating, blunt, caustic ingestion) for 10 %, and other miscellaneous causes for the remainder of cases seen.

C. J. Rees
Emergency Department, Pennsylvania Hospital, Philadelphia, PA, USA

C. V. Pollack, Jr. (✉)
Department of Emergency Medicine, Thomas Jefferson University, Philadelphia, PA, USA

V. G. Riese
Librarian Consultant, Eldersburg, MD, USA

C. V. Pollack, Jr. (ed.), *Differential Diagnosis of Cardiopulmonary Disease*,
https://doi.org/10.1007/978-3-319-63895-9_27

Differential Diagnosis

- Esophageal rupture usually causes acute onset of chest pain, so all the causes of acute chest pain need to be considered in the differential. These include; acute coronary syndrome, aortic dissection, pulmonary embolism, pneumonia, pneumothorax, other intra-abdominal catastrophes, amongst others.
- Esophageal rupture has many causes. Usually the history will lead to recognition of the cause of the rupture once identified.

Pathophysiology and Etiology

- Rupture of the esophagus allows for the direct contamination/communication of esophageal contents into the mediastinum. The esophagus has no serosal mucosal covering, so there is no anatomic mechanism for containment. The parietal pleura is very thin and weak, so the local inflammatory response allows for easy disruption of the parietal pleura and passage of contents into the pleural space.
- The left, posterior, distal esophagus just above the esophagogastric junction is the weakest point in the esophagus and the most common place for spontaneous rupture and rupture from gastrointestinal endoscopic procedures.
- Complications from tracheal and pharyngeal procedures may lead to rupture of the cervical esophagus at the level of the cricopharyngeal muscle just distal to the esophageal introitus, an anatomic narrowing point of the esophagus. Cervical ruptures often are better localized and not as serious as distal ruptures.
- There are multiple causes of esophageal rupture.
    - Iatrogenic, which is the most common, accounting for about 50 % of cases
        - Esophageal rupture complicates about 0.2–1 % of endoscopies. It is more likely in the setting of pre-existing esophageal disease such as caustic burns, tumors, eosinophilic esophagitis, and other causes of esophageal scarring.
        - Esophageal dilatation.
        - Endotracheal procedures/intubations, and with esophageal obturator airway placement.
    - Spontaneous "Boerhaave's syndrome"
        - Causes about 15 % of all cases.
        - First described by Boerhaave in the early 1700s.
        - Very high mortality if not recognized early. The forces required to rupture the esophagus also force the spread of esophageal contents throughout the mediastinal space, leading to massive mediastinal contamination.

  - The usual site of perforation is the distal esophagus in the left posterior region, just above the gastroesophageal junction.
  - Usually occurs after episodes of sudden, forceful vomiting (about 75 % of these cases), but also may occur after severe coughing, straining, seizures, and childbirth (25 % of cases). Therefore, 25 % of cases do not have the typical history of forceful vomiting.
  - A history of alcoholism, recent heavy drinking, and/or overindulging in food is found in most of the cases due to forceful vomiting.

- Foreign bodies

  - Cause 10 % of esophageal perforations.
  - Usually from pills, batteries, buttons.
  - Caused by either direct laceration or pressure or chemical necrosis.
  - Usually occurs at either the cervical or lower esophagus.

- Trauma

  - Causes about 10 % of cases.
  - May be from caustic (alkali or acid) burns, penetrating trauma, or blunt trauma.
  - Perforation more likely from alkali burns than acid burns.
  - Penetrating wounds to the neck, chest, and abdomen associated with only about a 0.5 % incidence of esophageal perforation.
  - Often overlooked initially as more obvious injuries are treated.
  - Blunt trauma is a very rare cause.
  - Miscellaneous causes (remaining 15 %)
  - Esophageal tumors, esophageal disease (achalasia, Barrett's esophagus, eosinophilic esophagitis), infectious (rare), aortic pathology (aortic aneurysm, aberrant right subclavian artery).

Presentation

Typical/"Classic"

- Acute onset of severe, constant, sharp, substernal chest pain immediately following an appropriate procedure or an episode of forceful vomiting. Pain is often pleuritic and radiates in an esophageal pattern (neck into chest and upper abdomen). Pain often worsens with swallowing.
- Usually the patient appears ill and uncomfortable. He or she also may complain of shortness of breath and be diaphoretic.
- If the patient presents early in the course, physical exam findings may be normal.
- If presenting 1–2 hours into the course, the patient may appear septic, with fever, tachycardia, hypotension, and hypoxia.

- "Hamman crunch": crunching sound heard on auscultation during systole as the result of air in the mediastinum surrounding the pericardium.
- Classically described subcutaneous emphysema (feeling of crunchiness [crepitus] under skin due to air tracking through subcutaneous tissues) in neck is present in only about 25 % at time of presentation.
- Chest x-ray (CXR) may be normal early in course, but over time pneumomediastinum, left more often than right pleural effusion, pneumothorax, hydropneumothorax, and/or a widened mediastinum may develop. CXR also may demonstrate subcutaneous air.

Atypical

- About one-third of cases will present atypically.
- May present as back pain only.
- Remember that about 25 % of patients with spontaneous esophageal rupture do not give a history of forceful vomiting.
- Many of the classically described physical and radiologic findings may not develop until several hours into the clinical course, so a high index of suspicion must be maintained by the treating physician.
- Pneumomediastinum is demonstrated in only about 40 % on plain CXR, even well into the clinical course.

Primary Differential Considerations

- Patients who present with signs and symptoms consistent with esophageal rupture also should be evaluated for these differential diagnoses:
  - Acute coronary syndrome
  - Aortic dissection
  - Peptic ulcer disease
  - Acute pancreatitis

History and Physical Exam

Findings That Confirm Diagnosis

- Esophageal rupture is a rare disease, and a high index of suspicion must be maintained by the treating physician.
- CT is the most common confirmatory study.

- Contrast esophagoscopy and endoscopy also may be used, but less commonly.
- Endoscopy may be falsely negative.
- The combination of contrast esophagoscopy and endoscopy approaches 100 % sensitivity for diagnosis.

Factors That Suggest Diagnosis

- The development of severe chest or upper abdominal pain after an ENT or GI procedure, after an episode forceful vomiting, after penetrating trauma, or in a patient with known esophageal disease should suggest the diagnosis, and a high index of suspicion should be maintained by the treating physician.
- Finding a pneumomediastinum on CXR in the appropriate clinical setting (s/p procedure, or after forceful vomiting) makes the diagnosis likely enough that appropriate treatment can proceed while confirmation is sought.
- It is important to remember that pneumomediastinum takes 1–2 hours to develop, especially in perforation of the lower esophagus, so its absence does not exclude the diagnosis.
- Pneumomediastinum may be present in only about 40 % of cases.
- Other suggestive findings on CXR include pleural effusions (left-sided more common than right), pneumothorax, hydropneumothorax, subcutaneous emphysema, or pneumoperitoneum.

Factors That Exclude Diagnosis

- The finding of another cause for the acute chest pain (e.g., acute myocardial infarction, aortic dissection) essentially excludes the diagnosis.
- Radiographic studies may all be normal early (first 1-4 hours) in the course of the disease, so in an appropriate clinical setting, suspicion must be maintained even if initial studies are unrevealing.

Ancillary Studies

Laboratory

- There are no laboratory tests that are specific to the diagnosis.
- Patients often manifest laboratory values consistent with an acute, severe, infectious, or inflammatory condition, such as leukocytosis, acidosis, or elevated lactate.

Imaging

- The plain CXR often is normal early in the disease course.
- Classically, the CXR may show multiple findings (alone or in combination):
  - Pneumomediastinum (seen in 40 %) with or without subcutaneous emphysema

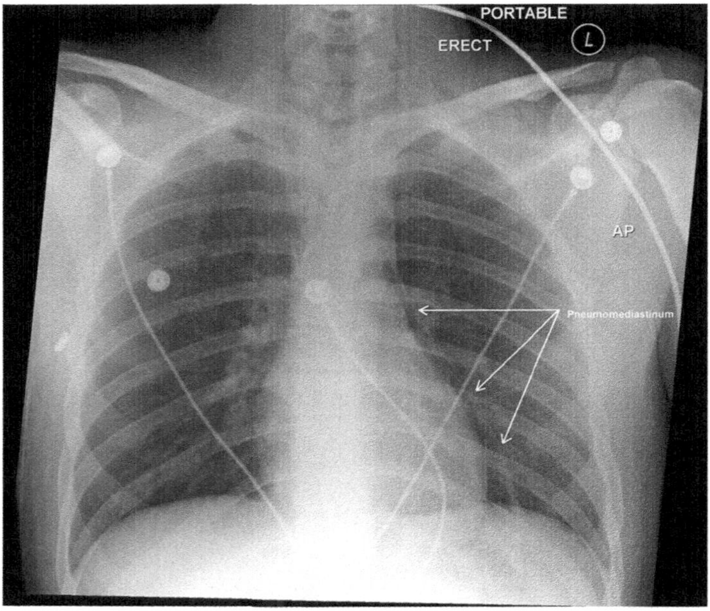

Chest X-ray showing pneumomediastinum. [From article: Pneumomediastinum from nasal insufflation of cocaine. International Journal of Emergency Medicine. 2010 Dec;3(4):435–7. https://doi.org/10.1007/s12245-010-0205-9, at http://link.springer.com/article/10.1007%2Fs12245-010-0205-9; by Brian T. Kloss, Claire E. Broton, Elliot Rodriguez, © Springer-Verlag London Ltd 2010; licensed under Creative Commons Attribution License BY 2.0 http://creativecommons.org/licenses/by/2.0] *Caption adapted from original*

- Left-sided pleural effusion

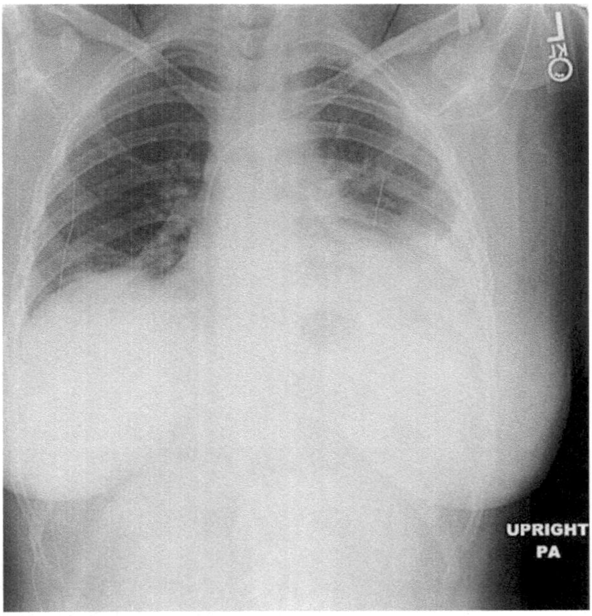

CXR demonstrating a left-sided pleural effusion. [Kohler JA, Ellis AR. Libman-Sacks Endocarditis in Pediatric Patient With Systemic Lupus Erythematosus. Pediatric Cardiology. 2012 Dec;33(8):1466–8.]

- Pneumothorax or hydropneumothorax
- Widened mediastinum
- CT scan of the chest often demonstrates the esophageal perforation and is more sensitive than CXR for detecting mediastinal air. Chest CT is the diagnostic study of choice.

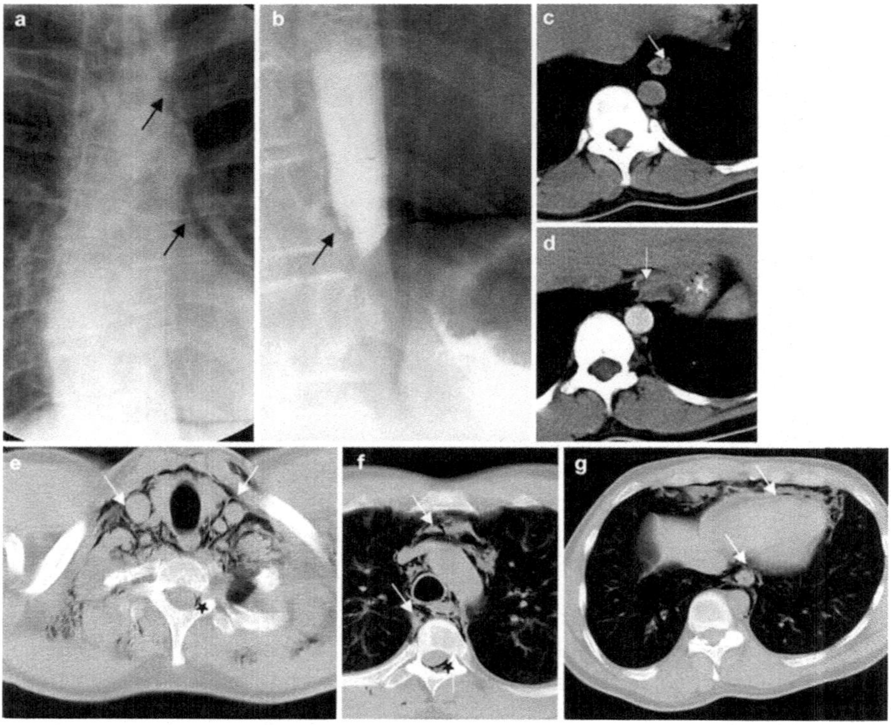

a Chest radiography demonstrating pneumomediastinum (arrows). There were no infiltrates, atelectasis, or pleural effusion apart from the subcutaneous emphysema. b Esophagography with water-soluble contrast medium depicted a small but visible right-sided submucosal tear representing a contained esophageal perforation (arrow). No contrast medium extravasation through the esophagus was seen. c Nonenhanced CT demonstrated high attenuation of the supradiaphragmatic wall at a typical site, suggesting an intramural hematoma. c, d Nonenhanced and contrast-enhanced CT revealed an esophageal wall thickening which is a nonspecific finding. e–g CT at the level of the thyroid gland showed extensive pneumomediastinum and subcutaneous emphysema. Intraspinal air collections were seen at multiple levels in the spinal canal as visualization of air tracks (*). In addition to a large quantity of air in the anterior and posterior mediastinum, local periesophageal extraluminal air collections were observed indicating extraluminal complications of Boerhaave's syndrome. CT scan depicted air tracks (arrows) extending from the esophagus into the anterior lower mediastinum (g). [Radiological findings in Boerhaave's syndrome - Springer. [cited 2015 May 19]; Available from: http://link.springer.com/article/10.1007%2Fs10140-002-0264-1/fulltext.html] *Caption adapted from original*

- Contrast esophagoscopy also may demonstrate the esophageal defect. It should be performed initially with a water-soluble contrast agent (Gastrograffin), as barium-containing contrast agents, if extruded into the surrounding tissues, may incite an inflammatory response. However, water-soluble contrast has a higher false-negative rate, so a negative water-soluble study should then be confirmed by a barium contrast study if the clinical suspicion remains high.

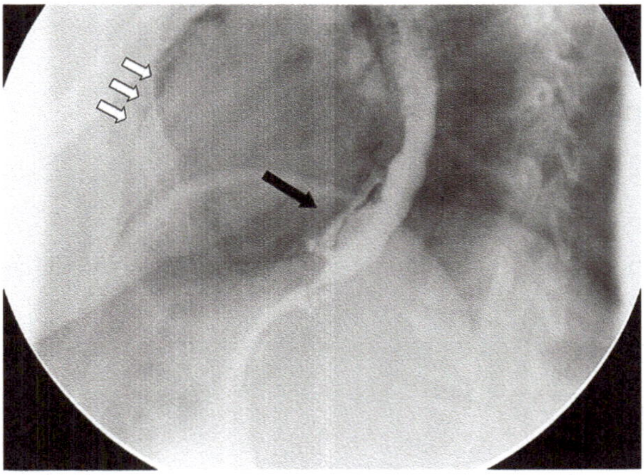

Water-soluble contrast radiograph of a patient with a distal esophageal perforation. The white arrows indicate free air in the mediastinum; the black arrow indicates extravasation of esophageal contrast. [Sánchez-Pernaute A, Aguirre EP, Talavera P, Valladares LD, de la Serna JP, Mantilla CS, de León AR, Torres A. Laparoscopic approach to esophageal perforation secondary to pneumatic dilation for achalasia. Surgical Endoscopy. 2009 May;23(5):1106–9.] *Caption from original*

- Esophagogastroduodenoscopy (EGD, upper endoscopy) also can directly demonstrate the esophageal defect. However, endoscopy may also miss a small defect. The combination of contrast esophagoscopy and endoscopy approaches 100 % sensitivity for the diagnosis.

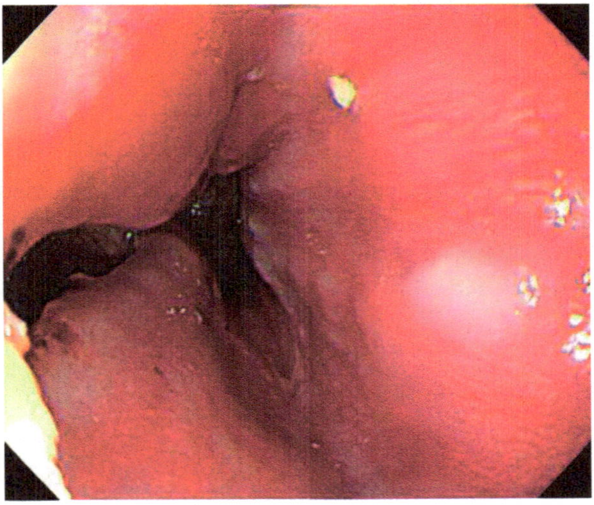

Boerhaave syndrome. Perforation site was observed in the left side of the esophagus. [Park JM. Miscellaneous Esophageal Diseases. In: Chun HJ, Yang S-K, Choi M-G, editors. Clinical Gastrointestinal Endoscopy [Internet]. Berlin, Heidelberg: Springer Berlin Heidelberg; 2014 [cited 2015 May 19]. p. 87–98. Available from: http://link.springer.com/10.1007/978-3-642-35626-1_7] *Caption from original*

Special Populations

Age

- Esophageal rupture is slightly more common inmiddle-aged and older populations.

Co-morbidities

- Esophageal rupture is associated with chronic alcohol use and with other esophageal diseases that cause strictures or scarring of the esophagus.

Pitfalls in Diagnosis

Critical Steps Not to Miss

- Consideration of the diagnosis is the critical step. It also is critical to continue to consider the diagnosis, as physical and radiographic findings may take several hours to develop after the rupture.

Mimics

- Anything that causes acute chest or upper abdominal pain can mimic esophageal rupture. These include but are not limited to acute myocardial infarction, pulmonary embolism, aortic dissection, spontaneous pneumothorax, perforated peptic ulcer, pancreatitis, acute cholecystitis, and mesenteric thrombosis.

Time-Dependent Interventions

- Early diagnosis is important. Time is critical in decreasing morbidity and mortality. If primary closure of the defect occurs within the first 24 hours, there is 80–90 % survival. If repair occurs greater than 24 hours after rupture, survival falls below 50 % and may reach 30 %.
- Any patient with hemodynamic instability should be resuscitated, as would any patient in shock.

Overall Principles of Treatment

- Rapid resuscitation with intravenous fluids, empiric broad-spectrum antibiotics, and appropriate management of complications such as pneumothorax or hydropneumothorax should begin as appropriate, even if the diagnosis is not certain.
- Early primary surgical repair of the defect is definitive treatment. Some contained cervical esophageal ruptures may be managed conservatively and nonoperatively.

Disease Course

- Esophageal rupture may be rapidly fatal if not identified and treated early.
- Patients often present in extremis or have a rapidly progressive course.

Related Evidence

Papers of particular interest have been highlighted as:
*** Of key importance*

Practice Guideline

ASGE Standards of Practice Committee, Ben-Menachem T, Decker GA, Early DS, Evans J, Fanelli RD, Fisher DA, Fisher L, Fukami N, Hwang JH, Ikenberry SO, Jain R, Jue TL, Khan KM, Krinsky ML, Malpas PM, Maple JT, Sharaf RN, Dominitz JA, Cash BD. Adverse events of upper GI endoscopy. Gastrointest Endosc. 2012 Oct;76(4):707-18. https://doi.org/10.1016/j.gie.2012.03.252. PMID: 22985638. http://www.ncbi.nlm.nih.gov/pubmed/22985638 **

Review

Nirula R. Esophageal perforation. Surg Clin North Am. 2014 Feb;94(1):35-41. https://doi.org/10.1016/j.suc.2013.10.003. PMID: 24267495. http://www.ncbi.nlm.nih.gov/pubmed/24267495 **

Blencowe NS, Strong S, Hollowood AD. Spontaneous oesophageal rupture. BMJ. 2013 May 31;346:f3095. https://doi.org/10.1136/bmj.f3095. PMID: 23729218. http://www.ncbi.nlm.nih.gov/pubmed/23729218 **

Biancari F, D'Andrea V, Paone R, Di Marco C, Savino G, Koivukangas V, Saarnio J, Lucenteforte E. Current treatment and outcome of esophageal perforations in adults: systematic review and meta-analysis of 75 studies. World J Surg. 2013 May;37(5):1051-9. https://doi.org/10.1007/s00268-013-1951-7. PMID: 23440483. http://www.ncbi.nlm.nih.gov/pubmed/23440483

Gomez-Esquivel R, Raju GS. Endoscopic closure of acute esophageal perforations. Curr Gastroenterol Rep. 2013 May;15(5):321. https://doi.org/10.1007/s11894-013-0321-9. PMID: 23558969. http://www.ncbi.nlm.nih.gov/pubmed/23558969

Carrott PW Jr, Low DE. Advances in the management of esophageal perforation. Thorac Surg Clin. 2011 Nov;21(4):541-55. https://doi.org/10.1016/j.thorsurg.2011.08.002. PMID: 22040636. http://www.ncbi.nlm.nih.gov/pubmed/22040636 **

Søreide JA, Viste A. Esophageal perforation: diagnostic work-up and clinical decision-making in the first 24 hours. Scand J Trauma Resusc Emerg Med. 2011 Oct 30;19:66. https://doi.org/10.1186/1757-7241-19-66. PMID: 22035338. http://www.ncbi.nlm.nih.gov/pubmed/22035338 **

Sepesi B, Raymond DP, Peters JH. Esophageal perforation: surgical, endoscopic and medical management strategies. Curr Opin Gastroenterol. 2010 Jul;26(4):379-83. https://doi.org/10.1097/MOG.0b013e32833ae2d7. PMID: 20473156. http://www.ncbi.nlm.nih.gov/pubmed/20473156

Butler KH, Swencki SA. Chest pain: a clinical assessment. Radiol Clin North Am. 2006 Mar;44(2):165-79, vii. PMID: 16500201. http://www.ncbi.nlm.nih.gov/pubmed/16500201 **

Use PubMed Clinical Queries to find the most recent evidence. Use this search strategy:

"Esophageal Perforation"[Mesh] OR "esophageal perforation" OR "esophageal rupture"

Chapter 28
Esophagitis

Charles V. Pollack, Jr., Richard M. Cantor, and Victoria G. Riese

Name and Synonyms

Esophagitis

Incidence/Epidemiology

- Esophagitis has been implicated as the cause of chest pain in 20–60 % of patients with chest pain not having an acute myocardial infarction.

Differential Diagnosis

- Esophagitis may cause acute chest pain, so the initial differential diagnostic considerations include all the acute causes of chest pain.
- Once the esophagus is believed to be the source of the chest pain, the differential diagnosis may focus on the causes of acute esophagitis, including inflammatory and infectious esophagitis, each of which has multiple causes.

C. V. Pollack, Jr. (✉)
Department of Emergency Medicine, Thomas Jefferson University, Philadelphia, PA, USA

R. M. Cantor
Department of Emergency Medicine and Pediatrics, State University of New York Upstate Medical University, Syracuse, NY, USA

V. G. Riese
Librarian Consultant, Eldersburg, MD, USA

C. V. Pollack, Jr. (ed.), *Differential Diagnosis of Cardiopulmonary Disease*,
https://doi.org/10.1007/978-3-319-63895-9_28

Pathophysiology and Etiology

- The final common pathway of pathophysiology is inflammation of the esophageal mucosa. The pathologic changes may progress to include inflammation and ulceration of both the mucosal and muscular layers of the esophagus. Both may lead to permanent scarring with strictures and narrowing of the esophagus.
  - This inflammation may result from multiple insults:
    - Inflammatory:
      - The best example is severe gastroesophageal reflux leading to inflammation, ulceration, scarring, and strictures.
      - "Pill" esophagitis results from pills remaining in contact with the esophageal mucosa. The most common location for pills to get stuck is at the level of the aortic arch, an anatomic narrow point in the esophagus. This may occur with any medication, but the most commonly implicated are nonsteroidal drugs; potassium tablets; antibiotics, such as clindamycin, doxycycline, and tetracycline; and bisphosphonates. Pill esophagitis usually causes dysphagia and odynophagia in addition to chest pain. Risk factors for the development of pill esophagitis include poor pill-taking practices, such as incorrect head position and insufficient water intake with the medication; swallowing of large tablets; and the extremes of age.

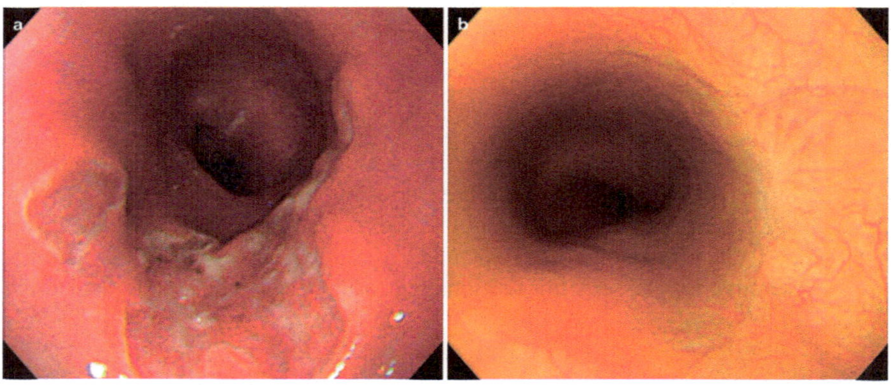

Pill-induced esophagitis. (a) Three days after ingestion of an unknown medication, a small and a neighboring, large well-demarcated ulcer with intact surrounding mucosa are noted at mid-esophagus. (b) Scar change of the ulcer after 2 months [Park KS. Infectious and Noninfectious Esophagitis. In: Chun HJ, Yang S-K, Choi M-G, editors. Clinical Gastrointestinal Endoscopy [Internet]. Berlin, Heidelberg:

Springer Berlin Heidelberg; 2014 [cited 2015 May 14]. p. 17–30. Available from: http://link.springer.com/10.1007/978-3-642-35626-1_3] *Caption from original*

- Eosinophilic esophagitis. Caused by sequestration and localization of eosinophils within the esophageal mucosa, leading to inflammation and narrowing of the esophageal lumen, with subsequent fibrosis and scarring. Usually causes dysphagia and odynophagia, and is a common cause of esophageal food impaction. Believed to be the result of an allergic response within the esophageal mucosa.

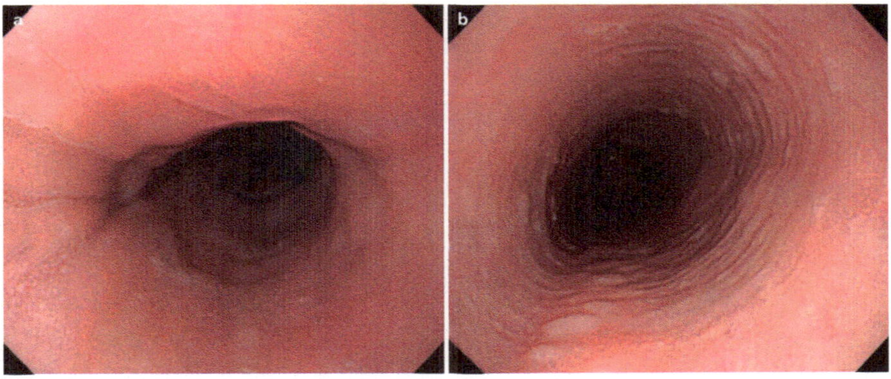

Eosinophilic esophagitis. (a) Linear furrows, (b) multiple rings [Park KS. Infectious and Noninfectious Esophagitis. In: Chun HJ, Yang S-K, Choi M-G, editors. Clinical Gastrointestinal Endoscopy [Internet]. Berlin, Heidelberg: Springer Berlin Heidelberg; 2014 [cited 2015 May 14]. p. 17–30. Available from: http://link.springer.com/10.1007/978-3-642-35626-1_3] *Caption from original*

- Corrosive esophagitis. Occurs after alkali (or less likely, acid) ingestion, with initial inflammation and ulceration and subsequent scarring and stricture formation.
- Radiation esophagitis. A long-term sequela of mantle radiotherapy for cancer.
- Infectious: Infectious esophagitis usually is associated with underlying immunosuppression (such as from HIV, cancer, severe diabetes). Diagnosing infectious esophagitis in an otherwise healthy patient should prompt a search for underlying immunosuppression.
- Candida albicans is the most common cause.

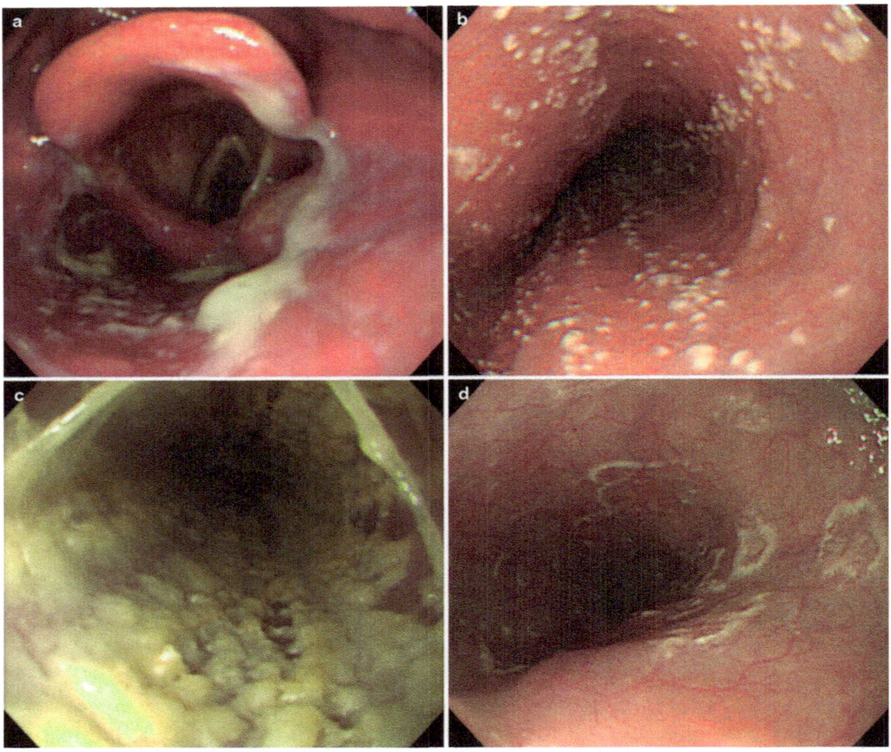

Candida esophagitis. (a) Coexisting pharyngeal lesions help to diagnose Candida esophagitis. (b) Multiple white plaques. (c) Diffuse membranous white material. (d) Atypical lesions which resemble herpetic esophagitis [Park KS. Infectious and Noninfectious Esophagitis. In: Chun HJ, Yang S-K, Choi M-G, editors. Clinical Gastrointestinal Endoscopy [Internet]. Berlin, Heidelberg: Springer Berlin Heidelberg; 2014 [cited 2015 May 14]. p. 17–30. Available from: http://link.springer.com/10.1007/978-3-642-35626-1_3] *Caption from original*

- Viral causes include cytomegalovirus and herpes simplex virus.

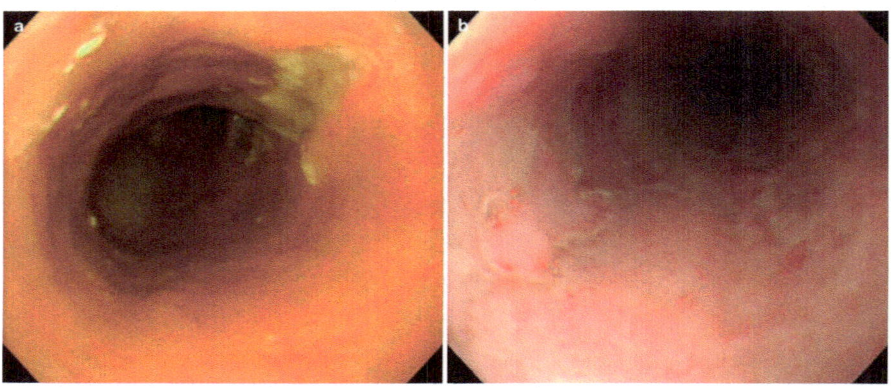

CMV esophagitis. (a) Longitudinal deep ulcer, (b) multiple shallow ulcers mimicking herpes esophagitis [Park KS. Infectious and Noninfectious Esophagitis. In: Chun HJ, Yang S-K, Choi M-G, editors. Clinical Gastrointestinal Endoscopy [Internet]. Berlin, Heidelberg: Springer Berlin Heidelberg; 2014 [cited 2015 May 14]. p. 17–30. Available from: http://link.springer.com/10.1007/978-3-642-35626-1_3] *Caption from original*

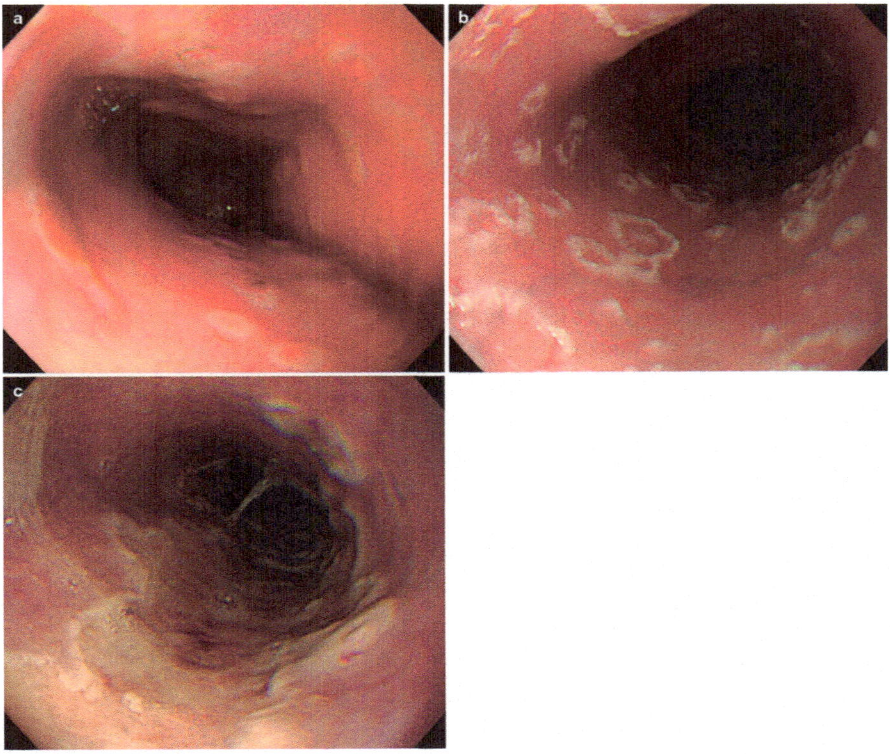

Herpes esophagitis. (a) Multiple vesicular lesions, (b) shallow ulcers with prominent demarcation, (c) large ulcer formation by confluence of small ulcers [Park KS. Infectious and Noninfectious Esophagitis. In: Chun HJ, Yang S-K, Choi M-G, editors. Clinical Gastrointestinal Endoscopy [Internet]. Berlin, Heidelberg: Springer Berlin Heidelberg; 2014 [cited 2015 May 14]. p. 17–30. Available from: http://link.springer.com/10.1007/978-3-642-35626-1_3] *Caption from original*

Presentation

Typical/"Classic"

- Chest pain, often described as burning. There is no historical or examination feature sensitive or specific enough to exclude cardiac causes of chest pain; therefore, a cardiac workup should be performed before or during evaluation for esophagitis.

- Certain symptoms may be helpful if present:
  - Odynophagia: pain with swallowing or pain exacerbated by swallowing
  - Dysphagia: difficulty swallowing. It may be described as a sensation of food or liquid getting stuck.

Atypical

- Any complaint of chest pain may be caused by esophagitis, so there is no typical or atypical presentation.

Primary Differential Considerations

Early in the evaluation of patients with symptoms of esophagitis, consider the following important differential diagnoses:

- Acute coronary syndrome
- Aortic dissection
- Acute pericarditis
- Pneumothorax
- Pleurisy
- Pneumonia
- Esophageal rupture
- Peptic ulcer disease

History and Physical Exam

Findings That Confirm Diagnosis

- The only findings that can completely confirm the diagnosis are typical findings on esophagogastroduodenoscopy (EGD/endoscopy).

Factors That Suggest Diagnosis

- Chest pain associated with pain with swallowing (odynophagia) and/or difficulties swallowing (dysphagia) strongly suggest the diagnosis.

Factors That Exclude Diagnosis

- A normal EGD excludes esophagitis.

Ancillary Studies

Laboratory

- No laboratory studies are helpful in suggesting or confirming the diagnosis of esophagitis. Laboratory studies may help exclude the diagnosis, e.g., positive cardiac biomarkers in a patient with chest pain. Remember that esophagitis may coexist with other diagnoses.

Imaging

- Plain chest x-ray usually is unremarkable.
- CT of the chest may demonstrate esophageal wall thickening, but this is often an incidental finding during studies performed for other reasons, such as evaluation for pulmonary embolism. It also may suggest the diagnosis, but it does not confirm the diagnosis.

Special Populations

Age

- Esophagitis may occur at any age. Certain diagnoses within the category may have age predilections, such as eosinophilic esophagitis, which is more likely in children and young adults.
- Clinical manifestations in children include:
  - Emesis
  - Feeding problems
  - Dysphagia
  - Abdominal pain
  - Food impaction
- In the pediatric population, there is a definite association with other forms of allergic disease (asthma, allergic rhinitis, urticaria, eczema)

Co-morbidities

- Common co-morbidities include obesity, diabetes, immunosuppression, alcohol abuse, and cigarette smoking.

Pitfalls in Diagnosis

Critical Steps Not to Miss

- Consideration of the diagnosis is important.
- However, it is more important to make sure the cause of chest pain is not a more immediately life-threatening condition.

Mimics

- The entire constellation of diagnoses underlying chest pain syndrome can mimic the pain and overall presentation of esophagitis.
- Esophagitis is more often considered a "mimic" of cardiac causes of chest pain.

Time-Dependent Interventions

- Check the ECG immediately for signs of acute myocardial ischemia. Remember that a normal ECG does not exclude acute coronary syndrome!
- If the patient has signs of GI bleeding, initiate stabilization and resuscitation immediately.

Overall Principles of Treatment

- Treatment depends on identifying the underlying cause of the esophagitis.
- Inflammatory causes of esophagitis often improve with acid suppression, usually from proton-pump inhibitors.
- Infectious causes need to be treated with the appropriate anti-infective agents.
- Eosinophilic esophagitis may be treated with elimination diets for removal of putative causative agents or with topical or systemic corticosteroids.
- The use of acid suppression with proton-pump inhibitors is prescribed nearly universally for all causes of esophagitis.

- If the esophagus becomes scarred or develops strictures, endoscopically guided esophageal dilatation may be necessary.

Disease Course

- Most cases of esophagitis from almost any cause will improve within several weeks of initiation of appropriate treatment.

Related Evidence

Papers of particular interest have been highlighted as:
*** Of key importance*

Practice Guideline

Papadopoulou A, Koletzko S, Heuschkel R, Dias JA, Allen KJ, Murch SH, Chong S, Gottrand F, Husby S, Lionetti P, Mearin ML, Ruemmele FM, Schäppi MG, Staiano A, Wilschanski M, Vandenplas Y; ESPGHAN Eosinophilic Esophagitis Working Group and the Gastroenterology Committee. Management guidelines of eosinophilic esophagitis in childhood. J Pediatr Gastroenterol Nutr. 2014 Jan;58(1):107-18. https://doi.org/10.1097/MPG.0b013e3182a80be1. PMID: 24378521. http://www.ncbi.nlm.nih.gov/pubmed/24378521 **

ACG clinical guideline: Evidenced based approach to the diagnosis and management of esophageal eosinophilia and eosinophilic esophagitis (EoE). Dellon ES, Gonsalves N, Hirano I, Furuta GT, Liacouras CA, Katzka DA; American College of Gastroenterology. Am J Gastroenterol. 2013 May;108(5):679-92; quiz 693. https://doi.org/10.1038/ajg.2013.71. PMID: 23567357. http://www.ncbi.nlm.nih.gov/pubmed/23567357 **

Review

Segal D, Chande N. The management of eosinophilic esophagitis in adults. J Clin Gastroenterol. 2013 Aug;47(7):570-7. https://doi.org/10.1097/MCG.0b013e318288a3c2. PMID: 23507765. http://www.ncbi.nlm.nih.gov/pubmed/23507765

Dellon ES. Eosinophilic esophagitis. Gastroenterol Clin North Am. 2013 Mar;42(1):133-53. https://doi.org/10.1016/j.gtc.2012.11.008. PMID: 23452635. http://www.ncbi.nlm.nih.gov/pubmed/23452635

Rosołowski M, Kierzkiewicz M. Etiology, diagnosis and treatment of infectious esophagitis. Prz Gastroenterol. 2013;8(6):333-7. https://doi.org/10.5114/pg.2013.39914. PMID: 24868280. http://www.ncbi.nlm.nih.gov/pubmed/24868280

Dellon ES. Eosinophilic esophagitis: diagnostic tests and criteria. Curr Opin Gastroenterol. 2012 Jul;28(4):382-8. https://doi.org/10.1097/MOG.0b013e328352b5ef. PMID: 22450900. http://www.ncbi.nlm.nih.gov/pubmed/22450900 **

Liacouras CA, Furuta GT, Hirano I, Atkins D, Attwood SE, Bonis PA, Burks AW, Chehade M, Collins MH, Dellon ES, Dohil R, Falk GW, Gonsalves N, Gupta SK, Katzka DA, Lucendo AJ, Markowitz JE, Noel RJ, Odze RD, Putnam PE, Richter JE, Romero Y, Ruchelli E, Sampson HA, Schoepfer A, Shaheen NJ, Sicherer SH, Spechler S, Spergel JM, Straumann A, Wershil BK, Rothenberg ME, Aceves SS. Eosinophilic esophagitis: updated consensus recommendations for children and adults. J Allergy Clin Immunol. 2011 Jul;128(1):3-20.e6; quiz 21-2. https://doi.org/10.1016/j.jaci.2011.02.040. PMID: 21477849. http://www.ncbi.nlm.nih.gov/pubmed/21477849 **

Canalejo Castrillero E, García Durán F, Cabello N, García Martínez J. Herpes esophagitis in healthy adults and adolescents: report of 3 cases and review of the literature. Medicine (Baltimore). 2010 Jul;89(4):204-10. https://doi.org/10.1097/MD.0b013e3181e949ed. PMID: 20616659. http://www.ncbi.nlm.nih.gov/pubmed/20616659

Noffsinger AE. Update on esophagitis: controversial and underdiagnosed causes. Arch Pathol Lab Med. 2009 Jul;133(7):1087-95. https://doi.org/10.1043/1543-2165-133.7.1087. PMID: 19642735. http://www.ncbi.nlm.nih.gov/pubmed/19642735 **

Orlando RC. Pathogenesis of reflux esophagitis and Barrett's esophagus. Med Clin North Am. 2005 Mar;89(2):219-41, vii. PMID: 15656926. http://www.ncbi.nlm.nih.gov/pubmed/15656926

Case Study

Brncić N, Mijandrusić-Sincić B, Visković I. Candida esophagitis. Wien Klin Wochenschr. 2005 Aug;117(15-16):520. PMID: 1616080. http://www.ncbi.nlm.nih.gov/pubmed/16160801

Use PubMed Clinical Queries to find the most recent evidence. Use this search strategy:

"Esophagitis"[Mesh] OR "Esophagitis"

Chapter 29
Foreign Body Aspiration

Charles V. Pollack, Jr., Richard M. Cantor, and Victoria G. Riese

Name and Synonyms

Foreign Body Aspiration (esophageal/tracheal)

Incidence/Epidemiology

- Swallowed and inhaled foreign bodies both may cause chest pain with or without shortness of breath.
- Both swallowed and inhaled foreign bodies are more common among young children, but esophageal food bolus impaction may occur at any age and is more common in the elderly, often presenting as chest pain.
- Foreign body aspiration may be life threatening at any age; cases in which food is the aspirated agent are referred to as "café coronary."

C. V. Pollack, Jr. (✉)
Department of Emergency Medicine, Thomas Jefferson University,
Philadelphia, PA, USA

R. M. Cantor
Department of Emergency Medicine and Pediatrics, State University of New York Upstate
Medical University, Syracuse, NY, USA

V. G. Riese
Librarian Consultant, Eldersburg, MD, USA

C. V. Pollack, Jr. (ed.), *Differential Diagnosis of Cardiopulmonary Disease*,
https://doi.org/10.1007/978-3-319-63895-9_29

Symptoms can include choking, coughing, wheezing, upper airway obstructive breathing, and if severe, cyanosis.
The foreign body can be lodged in the esophagus and compress the trachea, it can lie in the trachea itself, or it can lie in a mainstem bronchus.
The foreign body may be of various materials, including chunks of food, pieces of toys, coins, and—worst of all—a peanut, which may increase in size as it absorbs secretions.
Bronchoscopy usually is performed to remove the foreign body. The anesthetic plan must be tailored to the type of foreign body and the amount of the patient's distress.
Anesthetic induction: An inhalational technique may need to be performed to avoid muscle relaxation and prevent the foreign body from changing position with relaxation. The dilemma is inducing the patient having a full stomach with an inhalational technique. If intravenous access has been obtained, rapid sequence induction may be considered; however, avoid cricoid pressure, which may compress the object and cause tracheal or esophageal lacerations.

Features associated with aspiration of a foreign body. This is a common emergency situation in a child with a foreign body that becomes lodged in either the trachea or the esophagus that can result in airway compromise. The patients undergo bronchoscopy to retrieve the foreign body and are generally kept spontaneously ventilating in order to remove the object. [Rasmussen G, Deshpande J. Pediatric anesthesia. In: Muravchick S, editor. Subspecialty care. Philadelphia: Current Medicine; 1998. 236 p. (Miller RD editor, Atlas of anesthesia; vol. 5). ISBN: 0-443-07905-6] *Caption from original*

	Case	Sex		Percentage (%)
		Male	Female	
Age (years)				
32–39	9	6	3	7.44
40–49	11	7	4	9.09
50–59	49	34	15	40.50
60–69	47	31	16	38.84
Over 70	5	4	1	4.13
Duration of the foreign body impacted in the esophagus				
Within 3 days	17	10	7	14.05
3–5 days	42	31	11	34.71
5–7 days	54	35	19	44.63
7–14 days	8	6	2	6.61
Clinical manifestations				
Dysphagia	121	82	39	100
Odynophagia	121	82	39	100
Polysialia	121	82	39	100
Hematemesis	13	8	5	10.74
Dyspnea	24	11	13	19.83
High fever	45	14	31	37.19
Aerodermectasia	68	39	29	56.20
Cervical abscess	67	43	24	55.37
Cervical and mediastinum abscess	21	16	5	17.36
Mediastinitis	15	10	5	12.40
Mediastinum abscess	17	12	5	14.05
Hemopneumothorax[a]	6	6	0	4.96
Location of the foreign body				
Entrance of the esophagus	67	44	23	55.37
The junction of the cervical esophagus and thoracic esophagus	21	14	7	17.36
The region where the aortic arch is across the esophagus	29	21	8	23.97
The region where the left bronchus is across the anterior wall of the esophagus	4	3	1	3.30
Types of foreign bodies				
Pork bone	6	4	2	4.96[b]
Fishbone	53	34	19	43.80[b]
Chicken bone	21	11	10	17.36[b]
Duck bone	9	6	3	7.44[b]
Dental prosthesis	21	17	4	17.36[b]
Metal articles	7	6	1	5.79[b]
Glass	1	1	0	0.82[b]
Blade	3	3	0	2.48[b]
Total	121	82	39	

[a] Means the patients are with hemopneumothorax and mediastinum abscess simultaneously

[b] Stands for the percentage of one kind of the foreign body

Foreign bodies, sex, age and clinical manifestations of 121 cases with dangerous esophageal foreign bodies. [Peng A, Li Y, Xiao Z, Wu W. Study of clinical treatment of esophageal foreign body-induced esophageal perforation with lethal complications. Eur Arch Otorhinolaryngol. 2012 Sep;269(9):2027–36.] *Caption from original*

Differential Diagnosis

- The differential diagnosis is limited in cases of acute presentation, because the patient usually reports what has happened. Large foreign body aspiration in an unresponsive patient may be identified during direct laryngoscopy for rescue endotracheal intubation. Patients with an esophageal food bolus impaction may present with lower chest pain and retching, suggesting an atypical acute coronary syndrome.

Pathophysiology and Etiology

- Foreign body aspiration in patients above toddler age generally is accidental. Symptoms are driven by the size of the foreign body, which in turn determines the location of "lodging."
- Esophageal food bolus impaction generally is associated with inadequate chewing and often occurs in the setting of concomitant alcohol consumption.

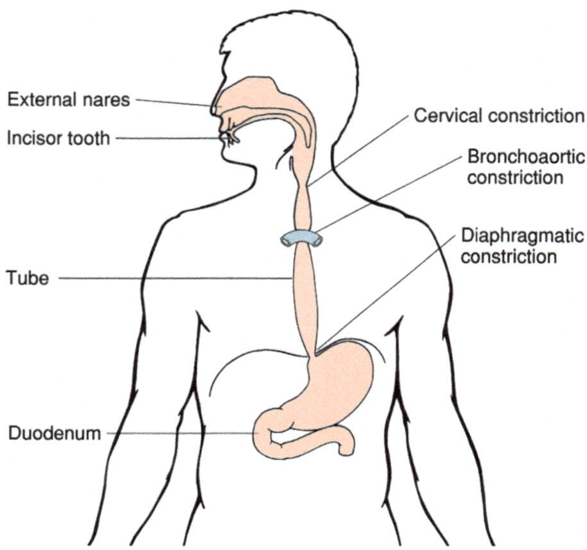

Esophageal foreign bodies. In the last several decades, endoscopy has become the method of choice in the management of esophageal foreign bodies, although a trial of sublingual nitroglycerin and intravenous glucagon is warranted. At times this will allow the offending bolus to pass. The most common location of the impaction is the distal esophagus at the level of the diaphragm; however, compressions at the level of the cricopharyngeus, aortic arch, and left main-stem bronchus may also be the site of impaction. It is also helpful to identify foreign bodies as sharp or dull, pointed or blunt, and toxic or nontoxic (eg, batteries). Also, food-related impactions should be distinguished. If the foreign body is known, in vitro simulation may be helpful in choosing the right accessory for use during the procedure. [Bozymski EM, Kenney CM. Esophageal therapeutics. In: Orlando RC, editor. Atlas of esophageal diseases. 2nd ed. Philadelphia: Current Medicine; 2002. 248 p. ISBN: 1-57340-181-1] *Caption from original*

Type of foreign body	
Coin	553 (84 %)
Penny	317
Nickel	29
Dime	32
Quarter	94
Other/unknown	81
Impacted food	42 (6 %)
Others	60 (9 %)
Unknown	2 (<1 %)
Location of FB	
Proximal 1/3	510 (78 %)
Middle 1/3	64 (10 %)
Distal 1/3	75 (11 %)
Stomach/bowel	8 (1 %)

Type and location of esophageal foreign bodies. [Russell R, Lucas A, Johnson J, Yannam G, Griffin R, Beierle E, Anderson S, Chen M, Harmon C. Extraction of esophageal foreign bodies in children: rigid versus flexible endoscopy. Pediatr Surg Int. 2014 Apr;30(4):417–22.] *Caption from original*

Presentation

Typical/"Classic"

- Aspirated foreign bodies typically present as choking, coughing, and/or shortness of breath

- Dyspnea
- Audible wheezes may be present.
- Large proximal aspirated foreign bodies may present as cardiac arrest.

- Esophageal foreign bodies typically present as lower chest pain and an inability to swallow; the patient often is spitting out saliva.
  - There often is a history of achalasia or previous similar episodes.

Atypical

- Especially in children, no reliable history may be available, making the etiology of typical symptoms more obscure.
- Smaller aspirated foreign bodies may not cause symptoms until days or week later, when secondary inflammation or infection has developed.

Primary Differential Considerations

- For aspirated foreign bodies, consider:
  - Epiglottitis
  - Retropharyngeal or peritonsillar abscess
  - Caustic ingestion
  - Anxiety
- For esophageal foreign bodies, consider:
  - Esophageal injury
  - Anxiety ("globus hystericus")
  - Caustic ingestion

History and Physical Exam

- Except in toddlers, the history usually is very helpful.
- On physical exam, assessing patency of the airway and adequacy of oxygenation is the priority.

Findings That Confirm Diagnosis

- Visualization of the foreign body
- History of aspiration and subsequent coughing/gagging/choking

- History of swallowing incompletely chewed food and subsequent inability to handle oral secretions

Factors That Suggest Diagnosis

- Suggestive history

Factors That Exclude Diagnosis

- Clinically difficult to exclude, even with few symptoms; passage of time with diminishing symptoms is helpful.

Ancillary Studies

Laboratory

- No diagnostic laboratory findings

Electrocardiography

- Useful only if myocardial ischemia is a diagnostic consideration

Imaging

- Aspirated foreign bodies:
  - Plain chest radiography may be helpful in patients with bronchial foreign bodies, when asymmetric lung volumes may be appreciated.
  - Chest CT may be helpful in localizing more distal foreign bodies.

Radiological findings	No of cases; *n* (%)
Obstructive emphysema	15 (20.5%)
Collapse	34 (41.65%)
Normal	20 (24.3%)
Pneumonitis	6 (7.3%)
Consolidation	4 (5%)
Foreign body visualised	2 (2.43%)
Abscess	1 (1.25%)

Radiographic findings in patients with airway foreign body. [Jaswal A, Jana U, Maiti PK. Tracheo-bronchial foreign bodies: a retrospective study and review of literature. Indian J Otolaryngol Head Neck Surg. 2014 Jan;66(S1):156–60.] *Caption from original*

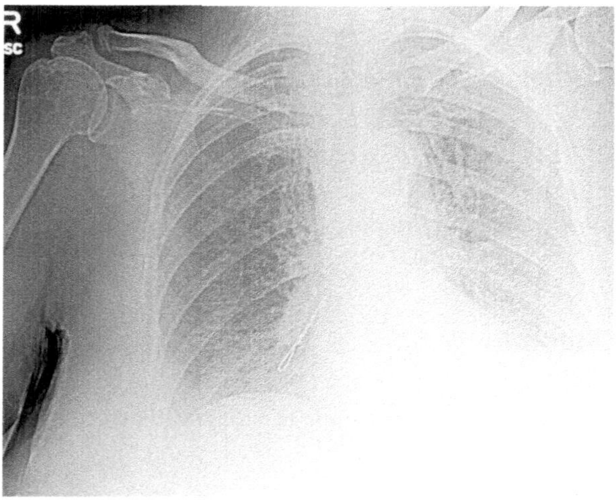

Foreign body in right main bronchus. [Tsikoudas A, Sheikh S. An interesting case of a wandering foreign body in the tracheobronchial tree. Eur Arch Otorhinolaryngol. 2005 May;262(5):426–7.] *Caption from original*

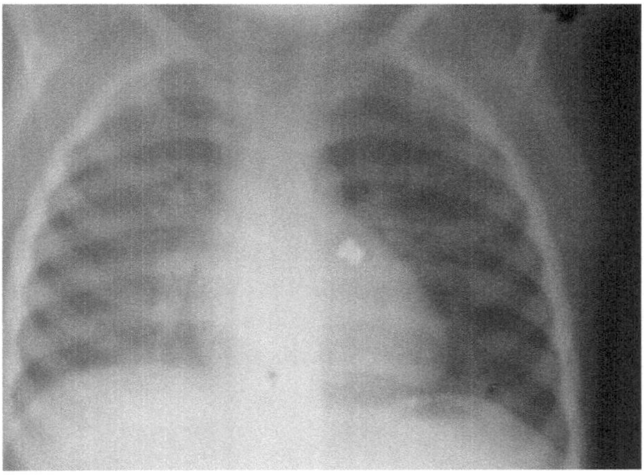

Chest radiograph showing foreign body in left main bronchus with obstructive emphysema of left lung. [Jaswal A, Jana U, Maiti PK. Tracheo-bronchial foreign bodies: a retrospective study and review of literature. Indian J Otolaryngol Head Neck Surg. 2014 Jan;66(S1):156–60.] *Caption from original*

- Esophageal foreign bodies:
  - Plain chest radiography is not useful for food bolus impactions.
  - Barium swallow may be challenging for the patient but will be diagnostic.
  - More proximal foreign bodies may be visualized on plain radiography.

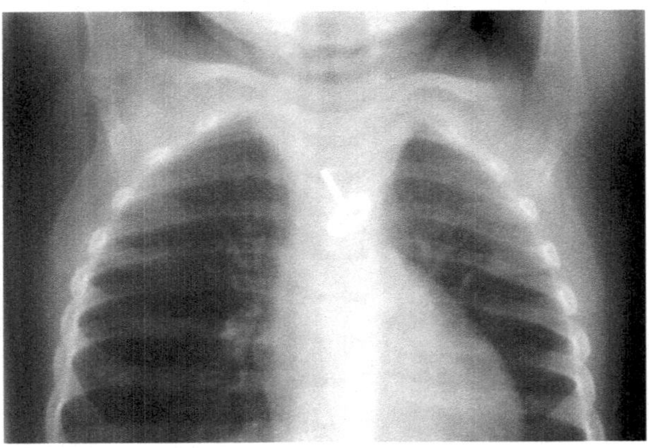

Esophageal foreign bodies (FBs). Ingested FBs may become impacted at any level but are typically held up at the three sites of natural narrowing: the cricopharyngeus muscle, the level of the aortic arc, and the gastroesophageal junction. The most common esophageal FBs are coins. They usually lodge at the cricopharyngeus, resulting in marked dysphagia even for liquids. Anteroposterior (from base of skull to pelvic outlet) and lateral radiographs are recommended if a coin ingestion is suspected because the presence of multiple coins may not be appreciated on a single anteroposterior view. Sharp FBs are particularly treacherous because they may perforate the esophagus, resulting in mediastinitis or major vessel injury and life-threatening hemorrhage. This radiograph shows a metallic foreign body lodged in the midesophagus of a 4-year-old boy who had stopped eating solid foods 2 months previously, precisely at the time his older brother's toy tractor steering wheel disappeared. Removal at esophagoscopy was complicated because the foreign body was deeply embedded in the esophageal wall. [Papsin BC, James A, Friedberg J, Forte V, Crysdale WS. Otolaryngology—head and neck surgery. In: Laxer RM, editor. The Hospital for Sick Children: atlas of pediatrics. Philadelphia: Current Medicine; 2005. p. 231-250.] *Caption from original*

Other Studies

- Endoscopy often is indicated.

Special Populations

Age

- Aspiration of foreign bodies may occur at any age but is most common in toddlers.

Dysphagia
Sedative or hypnotic drug use
Poor dentition
Altered Sensorium
Chronic aspiration
Parkinson's disease
Primary neurologic disorders with impairment of swallowing or mental status
Trauma with loss of consciousness
Seizure
General anesthesia
Alcohol intoxication
Polypharmacy and difficulty swallowing large pills
Eating while lying supine or just before falling asleep

Risk factors for foreign body aspiration in elderly patients. [Folch E, Majid A. Foreign body aspiration in the elderly patient. Curr Geriatr Rep. 2015 Jun;4(2):192–201.] *Caption from original*

- Esophageal food bolus impaction is more common in older patients.
- Commonly aspirated FBs in children include nuts, seeds, popcorn, food particles, hardware, and fragments of playthings.
- Coins are aspirated more commonly by older children.
- Fatal aspirations usually involve toy balloons or similar items.
- In one study, common anatomic sites in childhood aspiration included the larynx (3 %), trachea/carina (13 %), right hemithorax (60 %), left hemithorax (23 %), and bilateral bronchial tree (2 %).
- In the pediatric patient, the diagnosis often is delayed. Children may present with wheezing, dyspnea, recurrent pneumonia, or chronic cough. Aggressive investigations beyond plain radiography, especially bronchoscopy, are warranted in patients with recurrent or otherwise unexplained symptoms.

Co-morbidities

- Achalasia

Pitfalls in Diagnosis

Critical Steps Not to Miss

- Evaluation for satisfactory airway
- Evaluation for satisfactory oxygenation

Mimics

- Asthma

Time-Dependent Interventions

- Immediate evaluation for adequate airway and gas exchange

Overall Principles of Treatment

- Identify and remove foreign body.
- In cases of esophageal food bolus impaction, consider using glucagon before endoscopy; the use of meat tenderizer, advocated in the past, no longer is recommended.

Disease Course

- The course is determined by the acuity of presentation and underlying etiology, as well as the rapidity with which the foreign body is removed.
- The vast majority of foreign body cases are not life threatening.

Related Evidence

Papers of particular interest have been highlighted as:
*** Of key importance*

Review

Sehgal IS, Dhooria S, Ram B, Singh N, Aggarwal AN, Gupta D, Behera D, Agarwal R. Foreign body inhalation in the adult population: experience of 25,998 bronchoscopies and systematic review of the literature. Respir Care. 2015 May 12. pii: respcare.03976. PMID: 25969517. http://www.ncbi.nlm.nih.gov/pubmed/25969517 **

Hegde SV, Hui PK, Lee EY. Tracheobronchial foreign bodies in children: imaging assessment. Semin Ultrasound CT MR. 2015 Feb;36(1):8-20. https://doi.org/10.1053/j.sult.2014.10.001. Epub 2014 Oct 18. PMID: 25639173. http://www.ncbi.nlm.nih.gov/pubmed/25639173 **

Pinto A, Lanza C, Pinto F, Grassi R, Romano L, Brunese L, Giovagnoni A. Role of plain radiography in the assessment of ingested foreign bodies in the pediatric patients. Semin Ultrasound CT MR. 2015 Feb;36(1):21-7. https://doi.org/10.1053/j.sult.2014.10.008. PMID: 25639174. http://www.ncbi.nlm.nih.gov/pubmed/25639174

Prather AD, Smith TR, Poletto DM, Tavora F, Chung JH, Nallamshetty L, Hazelton TR, Rojas CA. Aspiration-related lung diseases. J Thorac Imaging. 2014 Sep;29(5):304-9. https://doi.org/10.1097/RTI.0000000000000092. PMID: 24911122. http://www.ncbi.nlm.nih.gov/pubmed/24911122 **

Rodríguez H, Passali GC, Gregori D, Chinski A, Tiscornia C, Botto H, Nieto M, Zanetta A, Passali D, Cuestas G. Management of foreign bodies in the airway and oesophagus. Int J Pediatr Otorhinolaryngol. 2012 May 14;76 Suppl 1:S84-91. https://doi.org/10.1016/j.ijporl.2012.02.010. PMID: 22365376. http://www.ncbi.nlm.nih.gov/pubmed/22365376 **

Gang W, Zhengxia P, Hongbo L, Yonggang L, Jiangtao D, Shengde W, Chun W. Diagnosis and treatment of tracheobronchial foreign bodies in 1024 children. J Pediatr Surg. 2012 Nov;47(11):2004-10. https://doi.org/10.1016/j.jpedsurg.2012.07.036. PMID: 23163990. http://www.ncbi.nlm.nih.gov/pubmed/23163990 **

Ambe P, Weber SA, Schauer M, Knoefel WT. Swallowed foreign bodies in adults. Dtsch Arztebl Int. 2012 Dec;109(50):869-75. https://doi.org/10.3238/arztebl.2012.0869. PMID: 23293675. http://www.ncbi.nlm.nih.gov/pubmed/23293675 **

Cutrone C, Pedruzzi B, Tava G, Emanuelli E, Barion U, Fischetto D, Sari M, Narne S, Zadra N, Martini A. The complimentary role of diagnostic and therapeutic endoscopy in foreign body aspiration in children. Int J Pediatr Otorhinolaryngol. 2011 Dec;75(12):1481-5. https://doi.org/10.1016/j.ijporl.2011.08.014. PMID: 21924505. http://www.ncbi.nlm.nih.gov/pubmed/21924505 **

Paintal HS, Kuschner WG. Aspiration syndromes: 10 clinical pearls every physician should know. Int J Clin Pract. 2007 May;61(5):846-52. PMID: 17493092. http://www.ncbi.nlm.nih.gov/pubmed/17493092 **

Swanson KL, Edell ES. Tracheobronchial foreign bodies. Chest Surg Clin N Am. 2001 Nov;11(4):861-72. PMID: 11780300. http://www.ncbi.nlm.nih.gov/pubmed/11780300 **

Case Study

Bain A, Barthos A, Hoffstein V, Batt J. Foreign-body aspiration in the adult: presentation and management. Can Respir J. 2013 Nov-Dec;20(6):e98-9. PMID: 24137576. http://www.ncbi.nlm.nih.gov/pubmed/24137576 **

Use PubMed Clinical Queries to find the most recent evidence. Use this search strategy:

"Foreign Bodies"[Mesh] OR "Foreign bodies"

Chapter 30
Gastroesophageal Reflux Disease

Christopher J. Rees, Richard M. Cantor, Charles V. Pollack, Jr., and Victoria G. Riese

Name and Synonyms

Gastroesophageal Reflux Disease

- GERD, Reflux, Indigestion, Heartburn, Pyrosis

Incidence/Epidemiology

- Six to 7 % of the US population reports daily, persistent heartburn.
- Twenty to 40 % report monthly heartburn.
- GERD is responsible for a significant amount of morbidity and has substantial economic consequences.

C. J. Rees
Emergency Department, Pennsylvania Hospital, Philadelphia, PA, USA

R. M. Cantor
Department of Emergency Medicine and Pediatrics, State University of New York Upstate Medical University, Syracuse, NY, USA

C. V. Pollack, Jr. (✉)
Department of Emergency Medicine, Thomas Jefferson University, Philadelphia, PA, USA

V. G. Riese
Librarian Consultant, Eldersburg, MD, USA

C. V. Pollack, Jr. (ed.), *Differential Diagnosis of Cardiopulmonary Disease*,
https://doi.org/10.1007/978-3-319-63895-9_30

Differential Diagnosis

- GERD may present with the acute onset of chest pain similar to acute cardiac pain, so acute myocardial infarction (MI) and the other causes of acute chest pain have to be considered in the differential diagnosis.
- The presentation of GERD also may be similar to that of esophagitis, peptic ulcer disease (PUD), biliary disease, pancreatitis, hepatitis, and gastrointestinal motility disorders.

Pathophysiology and Etiology

- Reflux of gastric contents into the esophagus occurs several times a day in most people as a normal physiologic event. It becomes abnormal, and considered GERD, when it is associated with symptoms or pathologic changes within the gastrointestinal or respiratory tracts. The Montreal Classification defines GERD as "A condition that develops when the reflux of stomach contents causes troublesome symptoms and/or complications."
- The lower esophageal sphincter (LES) is the main physiologic barrier to reflux.
- When reflux does occur, both mechanical (gravity) and physiologic (peristalsis, saliva, esophageal secretions) forces can help push gastric contents back into the stomach.
- GERD may be caused or worsened by anything that reduces LES pressure, decreases esophageal motility or gastric emptying time, or directly irritates the esophageal mucosa, as well as by mechanical means.
- Factors that may reduce LES pressure include drugs (anticholinergic agents, benzodiazepines, calcium-channel blockers, progesterone), foods (chocolate, caffeine, high-fat foods, peppermint, nitrates), nicotine, and alcohol.
- Conditions that decrease esophageal motility include achalasia, diabetes, and scleroderma.
- Factors and conditions that may decrease gastric emptying time include anticholinergic medications, diabetic gastroparesis, and gastric outlet obstruction.
- Substances that may act as direct irritants to the gastric mucosa include caffeine, citrus products, and tomato-based products.
- Mechanical factors include stooping, bending forward, the Valsalva maneuver, and the supine position.
- GERD is much more common in obese patients.
- Hiatal hernia (prolapse of a portion of the stomach through the diaphragmatic esophageal hiatus) also is considered a risk factor for GERD.

Presentation

Typical/"Classic"

- The most common complaint is heartburn, a burning sensation from the sub-xyphoid region radiating into the neck or pharynx.
- Typically, symptoms worsen after large meals or with recumbency.
- Symptoms usually are relieved with antacids; however, this effect is not pathognomonic and does not reliably exclude cardiac causes of pain.
- Other common presenting complaints include regurgitation and nausea, but usually these are associated with heartburn.
- An uncommon but somewhat specific symptom of GERD is water brash, a vagally mediated increase in saliva production often perceived by patients as "foaming at the mouth."
- GERD also may cause extraesophageal symptoms, including asthma (or worsening asthma) from reflux associated with aspiration, chronic cough, hoarse voice, recurrent laryngitis or sore throat, frequent throat clearing, and dental problems.

Atypical

- It is important to remember that GERD symptoms can mimic those of acute MI. Patients may describe the acute onset of chest pressure, dull chest pain, or squeezing. The radiation pattern can mimic that of acute MI and radiate to the back, jaw, or arm.
- Dysphagia (difficulty swallowing) and odynophagia (painful swallowing) are uncommon symptoms for GERD and should prompt further evaluation for other causes.
- Globus is a perception of fullness or a lump in the throat, unrelated to swallowing. It is not a usual symptom of GERD, and its presence should prompt a search for other causes. It often is thought to be related to emotional stress or to have a functional basis.

Primary Differential Considerations

- Prompt consideration also should be given to the possible diagnosis of:
  - Acute coronary syndrome
  - Esophageal spasm
  - Biliary colic
  - Gastritis
  - Hiatal hernia

History and Physical Exam

Findings That Confirm Diagnosis

- Because the diagnosis of GERD can be applied only for symptoms, there are no tests that are confirmatory. A classic history of heartburn, worse after large meals, and recumbency relieved by antacids is enough to make a presumptive diagnosis of GERD.
- The physical exam is often unremarkable and not helpful in making the diagnosis.

Factors That Suggest Diagnosis

- A classic presentation as above suggests the diagnosis.
- The diagnosis of GERD should be kept within the differential when evaluating a patient for new-onset or worsening asthma not explained by other factors, as a cause of chronic cough or laryngitis, and for patients with unexplained hoarseness.

Factors That Exclude Diagnosis

- GERD may exist even in the absence of symptoms; there is no factor that excludes the diagnosis.
- Normal endoscopy does not exclude the diagnosis of GERD.

Ancillary Studies

Laboratory

- Lab tests are unhelpful in the diagnosis of GERD and often are used only to evaluate for other causes of the patient's symptoms.

Imaging

- Imaging usually is not helpful or indicated for the diagnosis of GERD.
- Patients may need imaging or endoscopy to exclude other diagnoses.

- Patients with symptoms such as dysphagia, odynophagia, weight loss, or other constitutional symptoms may need endoscopy to exclude malignancy and other serious causes of their symptoms.

Special Populations

Age

- GERD occurs in all age groups, including infants and children.
- In children, the term *gastroesophogeal reflux disease* applies when the reflux results in untoward complications, such as esophagitis, respiratory events, or growth failure.
  - There is some evidence that severe reflux in infancy predisposes children to GERD later in life.
- GERD and asthma often overlap in children and adolescents, but current data do not suggest that control of one has a significant clinical impact on the other.

Co-morbidities

- GERD may coexist with any other condition.
- Conditions that may make GERD more likely include obesity, diabetes, achalasia, motility disorders, and hiatal hernia.

Pitfalls in Diagnosis

Critical Steps Not to Miss

- It is critical to consider the more immediately life-threatening causes of chest and abdominal pain.

Mimics

- GERD is a classic mimic of acute MI.
- GERD also can mimic PUD, all the causes of esophagitis, biliary disease, pancreatitis, and esophageal and gastric motility disorders.

Time-Dependent Interventions

- The only time-dependent intervention is to exclude more serious causes of pain.

Overall Principles of Treatment

- Patients with a suggestive history, as well as those in whom more serious causes of the symptoms have been excluded, often are treated empirically with acid suppression and lifestyle changes.
- Lifestyle changes include decreasing or stopping known exacerbating substances, weight loss, and elevating the head of the bed.
- Acid suppression usually is attempted with either H2-blockers or proton-pump inhibitors (PPIs). H2-blockers have been shown to promote esophageal healing in mild esophagitis. PPIs suppress acid more effectively than H2-blockers and are more efficacious both in relieving symptoms and in promoting esophageal mucosal healing. However, PPIs are much more expensive than H2-blockers.
- Anywhere from 40–90 % of patients will report symptom improvement from PPIs.
- However, symptom improvement is not a diagnostic criterion for GERD.
- Patients whose symptoms are refractory to treatment may need further evaluation, although this group of patients usually constitutes a small minority. This is especially true for patients with worrisome symptoms such as dysphagia and odynophagia.
- Further evaluation may include esophagogastroduodenoscopy (EGD), esophageal manometry, and ambulatory pH monitoring.
- It is worth remembering that EGD may be normal in GERD, and this study usually is performed to exclude other diagnoses.
- Esophageal manometry and ambulatory pH monitoring are invasive tests; patients should be evaluated by a specialist before undergoing these studies.

Disease Course

- GERD is a chronic condition. It often requires long-term medical therapy for control.
- A minority of patients have long-term relief from lifestyle changes.
- GERD may be associated with several long-term complications, many of them serious.

- GERD may be associated with chronic esophageal mucosal changes, starting with thinning and inflammation and then scarring. These events may lead to esophageal strictures, which may cause dysphagia, odynophagia, food impactions, etc.
- The most serious complication of GERD is damage to the normal esophageal stratified squamous epithelium by acid, leading to replacement with metaplastic columnar epithelium. This condition, known as *Barrett's esophagus*, is associated with a higher incidence of esophageal adenocarcinoma. Currently, it is believed that 1–10 % of people with Barrett's esophagus will develop esophageal adenocarcinoma. Patients with Barrett's esophagus require endoscopic surveillance with biopsies to look for cancerous changes.

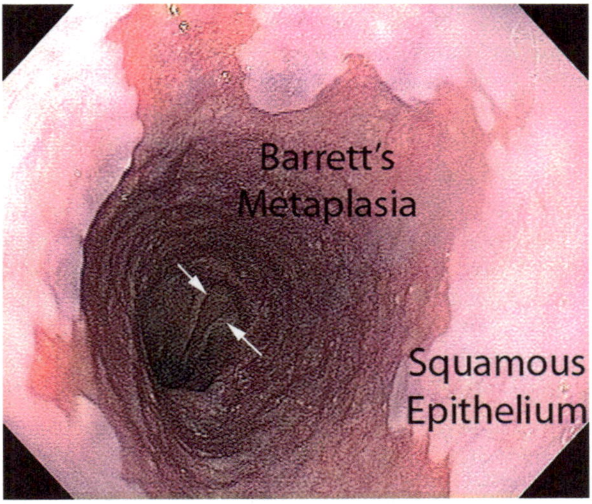

Endoscopic photograph of long-segment Barrett's esophagus. The arrows mark the proximal extent of the gastric folds, which is the location of the gastroesophageal junction. Note that Barrett's metaplasia extends well above the GEJ to line the distal esophagus. The reddish-pink (salmon) color and velvet-like texture of Barrett's epithelium contrasts sharply with the pale and glossy appearance of the esophageal squamous epithelium. [Spechler SJ. Barrett's Esophagus. In: Shaker R, Belafsky PC, Postma GN, Easterling C, editors. Principles of Deglutition [Internet]. New York, NY: Springer New York; 2013 [cited 2015 May 14]. p. 723–38. Available from: http://link.springer.com/10.1007/978-1-4614-3794-9_49] *Caption from original*

Related Evidence

Papers of particular interest have been highlighted as:
*** Of key importance*

Practice Guideline

Davies I, Burman-Roy S, Murphy MS; Guideline Development Group. Gastro-oesophageal reflux disease in children: NICE guidance. BMJ. 2015 Jan 14;350:g7703. https://doi.org/10.1136/bmj.g7703. PMID: 25591811. http://www.ncbi.nlm.nih.gov/pubmed/25591811 **

Katz PO, Gerson LB, Vela MF. Guidelines for the diagnosis and management of gastroesophageal reflux disease. Am J Gastroenterol. 2013 Mar;108(3):308-28; quiz 329. https://doi.org/10.1038/ajg.2012.444. PMID: 2341938. http://www.ncbi.nlm.nih.gov/pubmed/23419381 **

Shaheen NJ, Weinberg DS, Denberg TD, Chou R, Qaseem A, Shekelle P; Clinical Guidelines Committee of the American College of Physicians. Upper endoscopy for gastroesophageal reflux disease: best practice advice from the clinical guidelines committee of the American College of Physicians. Ann Intern Med. 2012 Dec 4;157(11):808-16. https://doi.org/10.7326/0003-4819-157-11-201212040-00008. PMID: 23208168. http://www.ncbi.nlm.nih.gov/pubmed/23208168 **

Vandenplas Y, Rudolph CD, Di Lorenzo C, Hassall E, Liptak G, Mazur L, Sondheimer J, Staiano A, Thomson M, Veereman-Wauters G, Wenzl TG, North American Society for Pediatric Gastroenterology Hepatology and Nutrition, European Society for Pediatric Gastroenterology Hepatology and Nutrition. Pediatric gastroesophageal reflux clinical practice guidelines: joint recommendations of the North American Society for Pediatric Gastroenterology, Hepatology, and Nutrition (NASPGHAN) and the European Society for Pediatric Gastroenterology, Hepatology, and Nutrition (ESPGHAN). J Pediatr Gastroenterol Nutr. 2009 Oct;49(4):498-547. https://doi.org/10.1097/MPG.0b013e3181b7f563. PMID: 19745761. http://www.ncbi.nlm.nih.gov/pubmed/19745761 **

Review

Spechler SJ. Barrett esophagus and risk of esophageal cancer: a clinical review. JAMA. 2013 Aug 14;310(6):627-36. https://doi.org/10.1001/jama.2013.226450. PMID: 23942681. http://www.ncbi.nlm.nih.gov/pubmed/23942681

Lee YY, McColl KE. Pathophysiology of gastroesophageal reflux disease. Best Pract Res Clin Gastroenterol. 2013 Jun;27(3):339-51. https://doi.org/10.1016/j.bpg.2013.06.002. PMID: 23998973. http://www.ncbi.nlm.nih.gov/pubmed/23998973 **

Chandra S, Gorospe EC, Leggett CL, Wang KK. Barrett's esophagus in 2012: updates in pathogenesis, treatment, and surveillance. Curr Gastroenterol Rep. 2013 May;15(5):322. https://doi.org/10.1007/s11894-013-0322-8. PMID: 23605564. http://www.ncbi.nlm.nih.gov/pubmed/23605564

McConaghy JR, Oza RS. Outpatient diagnosis of acute chest pain in adults. Am Fam Physician. 2013 Feb 1;87(3):177-82. PMID: 23418761. http://www.ncbi.nlm.nih.gov/pubmed/23418761 **

Gill RS, Collins JS, Talley NJ. Management of noncardiac chest pain in women. Womens Health (Lond Engl). 2012 Mar;8(2):131-43; quiz 144-5. https://doi.org/10.2217/whe.12.3. PMID: 22375717. http://www.ncbi.nlm.nih.gov/pubmed/22375717

Smith JA, Abdulqawi R, Houghton LA. GERD-related cough: pathophysiology and diagnostic approach. Curr Gastroenterol Rep. 2011 Jun;13(3):247-56. https://doi.org/10.1007/s11894-011-0192-x. PMID: 21465223. http://www.ncbi.nlm.nih.gov/pubmed/21465223 **

Lacy BE, Weiser K, Chertoff J, Fass R, Pandolfino JE, Richter JE, Rothstein RI, Spangler C, Vaezi MF. The diagnosis of gastroesophageal reflux disease. Am J Med. 2010 Jul;123(7):583-92. https://doi.org/10.1016/j.amjmed.2010.01.007. PMID: 20493461. http://www.ncbi.nlm.nih.gov/pubmed/20493461

Oranu AC, Vaezi MF. Noncardiac chest pain: gastroesophageal reflux disease. Med Clin North Am. 2010 Mar;94(2):233-42. https://doi.org/10.1016/j.mcna.2010.01.001. PMID: 20380953. http://www.ncbi.nlm.nih.gov/pubmed/20380953 **

Use PubMed Clinical Queries to find the most recent evidence. Use this search strategy:

"Gastroesophageal Reflux"[Mesh] OR "Gastroesophageal Reflex" OR "GERD"

Chapter 31
Goiter

Christopher J. Rees, Charles V. Pollack, Jr., and Jaime Friel Blanck

Name and Synonyms

Goiter

Incidence/Epidemiology

- Dietary deficiency of iodine is the most common cause of goiter worldwide. There are estimated to be about 200 million cases of iodine-deficient goiter worldwide.
- In the United States (where significant dietary deficiency of iodine only occurs in new immigrants), the most common cause of goiter is multinodular goiter.
- The female: male ratio is 4:1.
- Goiter is distributed equally among races.
- The incidence of goiter increases with age.

C. J. Rees
Emergency Department, Pennsylvania Hospital, Philadelphia, PA, USA

C. V. Pollack, Jr. (✉)
Department of Emergency Medicine, Thomas Jefferson University, Philadelphia, PA, USA

J. F. Blanck
Welch Medical Library, Johns Hopkins University, Baltimore, MD, USA

C. V. Pollack, Jr. (ed.), *Differential Diagnosis of Cardiopulmonary Disease*,
https://doi.org/10.1007/978-3-319-63895-9_31

Differential Diagnosis

- Goiters often present as an anterior neck mass on physical examination. The differential diagnosis of anterior neck masses is broad, but generally falls into several categories:
  - Inflammatory masses (such as lymphadenopathy)
  - Neoplastic masses (both primary and metastatic)
  - Congenital (vascular anomalies, thyroglossal duct cysts)
- Some goiters extend into the thoracic cavity (substernal goiters) and present as mediastinal masses (most often anterior mediastinal masses) found on an imaging study (CXR, CT chest) performed for other reasons. The most common causes of a mediastinal mass (in decreasing order of frequency) are:
  - Substernal goiter
  - Neurogenic tumors
  - Thymoma
  - Pericardial or bronchogenic cysts
  - Lymphoma
  - Teratoma

Pathophysiology and Etiology

- A goiter refers to an abnormally enlarged thyroid gland.
- Goiters can be classified as diffuse or nodular, toxic or non-toxic, and either benign or malignant. A toxic goiter overproduces thyroid hormone.
- The most common pathophysiologic reason for goiter formation is increased secretion of thyroid stimulating hormone (TSH) by the anterior pituitary gland. This occurs as the thyroid becomes unable to synthesize adequate amounts of T3 and T4. This can have multiple causes, such as iodine deficiency and thyroid cell inflammation and destruction from autoimmune thyroiditis (Hashimoto's Thyroiditis).
- Goiters can also form when TSH secretion is normal. This can result from the action of multiple growth factors acting on thyroid cells over a long period of time, usually in the presence of a genetic predisposition to goiter formation. This leads to nontoxic, multinodular goiters.
- Patients with Graves' disease produce TSH receptor antibodies. These autoantibodies stimulate the TSH receptor and lead to thyroid growth and overproduction of thyroid hormones.
- As stated in the Incidence/Epidemiology section, iodine deficiency is the leading cause of goiter worldwide. However, iodine deficiency is mostly unheard of in the United States and Western Europe. In these areas iodine deficiency is usually only found among recent immigrants.

- In most Western countries, multinodular goiter, Hashimoto's disease (autoimmune thyroiditis), and Graves' disease are the most common causes of goiter.
- Less common causes of goiter include thyroiditis (of any cause), thyroid tumors, and infiltrative diseases of the thyroid.

Presentation

Typical/"Classic"

- It is important to review the anatomy of the thyroid gland, as the presenting symptoms of goiter can be related to compression of neighboring structures.
    - The thyroid sits just below the larynx; it has 2 lobes connected by a small bridge of thyroid tissue termed the isthmus. The thyroid partially encircles the anterolateral aspects of the trachea. It is bordered posteriorly by the trachea and esophagus, and laterally by the carotid sheaths. Anteriorly, the thyroid is covered only by the thin strap muscles anterolaterally, and then connective tissue, subcutaneous tissue, and skin. As a result of this minimal anterior anatomic coverage, the thyroid mostly enlarges outward and does not usually compress any lateral or posterior structures.

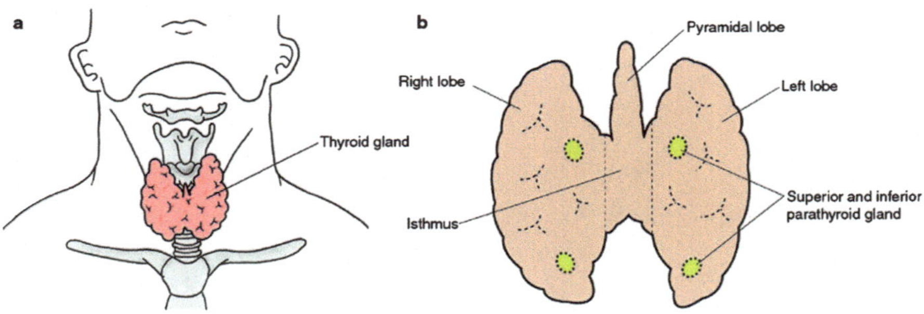

Position and anatomy of the thyroid gland. (**a**) Normal position of the thyroid gland, (**b**) anatomy of the thyroid gland. [Youn Y-K, Lee KE, Choi JY. Surgical Anatomy of the Thyroid Gland. Color Atlas of Thyroid Surgery [Internet]. Berlin, Heidelberg: Springer Berlin Heidelberg; 2014 [cited 2015 Dec 4]. p. 1–10. Available from: http://link.springer.com/10.1007/978-3-642-37262-9_1] *Caption from original*

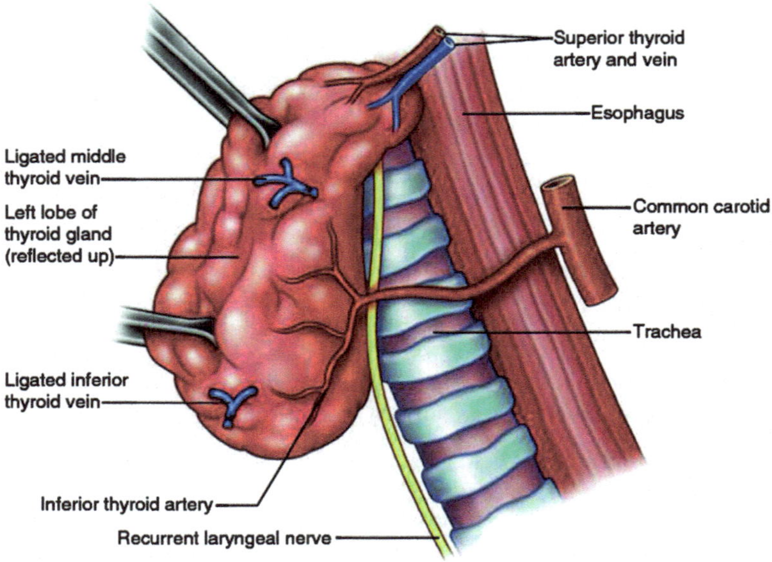

Surgical anatomy during thyroidectomy: trachea, esophagus, common carotid artery, superior thyroid artery, superior thyroid vein, middle thyroid vein, inferior thyroid artery, inferior thyroid vein, and recurrent laryngeal nerve [Sarpel U. Thyroidectomy. Surgery [Internet]. New York, NY: Springer New York; 2014 [cited 2015 Dec 4]. p. 195–205. Available from: http://link.springer.com/10.1007/978-1-4939-0903-2_18] *Caption from original*

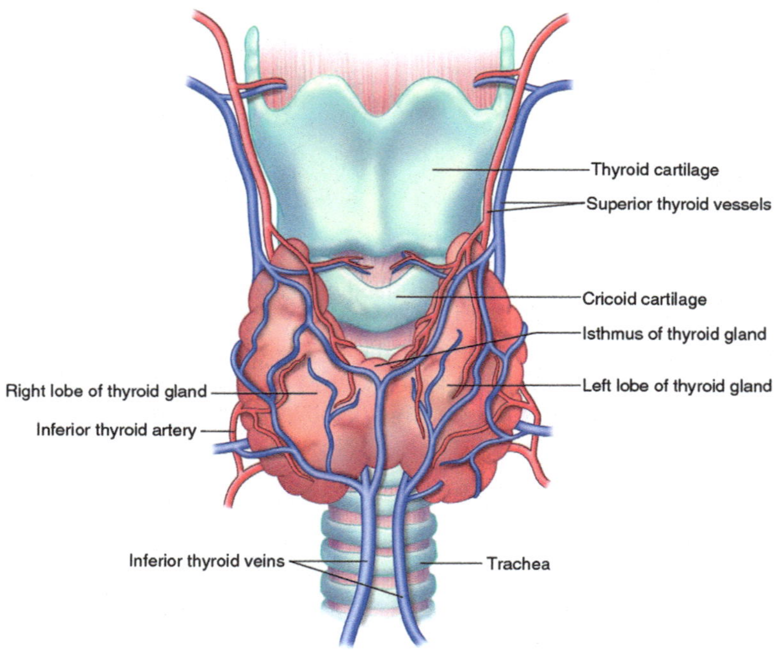

Thyroid gland anatomy and blood supply [Porter S, Schwartz A, DeMaria S, Genden EM. Thyroid, Parathyroid, and Parotid Surgery. In: Levine AI, Govindaraj S, DeMaria, S, editors. Anesthesiology and Otolaryngology [Internet]. New York, NY: Springer New York; 2013 [cited 2015 Dec 4]. p. 217–40. Available from: http://link.springer.com/10.1007/978-1-4614-4184-7_14] *Caption from original*

- In goiters that grow asymmetrically, however, enlargement of one lobe is predominant. Asymmetrical goiters can also enlarge circumferentially around the trachea, which can cause compression of the jugular veins, tracheal narrowing, and/or impingement of the esophagus.
- Goiters can also extend caudally into the thoracic inlet. The thoracic inlet is an oval-shaped area about 5 cm (anteroposteriorly) by 10 cm (laterally). It is bordered anteriorly by the sternum, laterally by the first ribs, and posteriorly by the first thoracic vertebra. Structures within the thoracic include the trachea, esophagus, and major vascular structures. As the borders of the thoracic inlet are all bony, there is no room for expansion. If a goiter extends caudad through the thoracic inlet, the goiter is referred to as substernal (or retrosternal). Substernal goiters are more likely to cause compression than purely cervical goiters. Substernal goiters are thought to account for anywhere from 2–20 % of all goiters.
- Most goiters grow very slowly, do not cause thyroid dysfunction, and are asymptomatic. They are usually found on routine physical examination, and on imaging studies being performed for other reasons.
- Most goiters are painless.
- Once a goiter is detected, an evaluation should be performed with three major goals:
  - Identify the underlying cause.
  - Evaluate for the presence of obstructive symptoms.
  - Evaluate for the presence of features suspicious for malignancy.

Atypical

- As most goiters are asymptomatic, any symptomatic goiter can be considered the "atypical" presentation of goiter.
- However, goiters may be associated with either hypo- or hyperthyroidism, and patients can present with symptoms of those disorders.
  - Hypothyroidism. A goiter due to long-standing, burned-out Hashimoto's (autoimmune) thyroiditis, and severe iodine deficiency, can be associated with hypothyroidism. Those symptoms are protean and can include profound fatigue, unintentional weight gain, constipation, and cold intolerance.
  - Hyperthyroidism. Some causes of goiter can be associated with hyperfunctioning thyroid tissue (multinodular goiter with autonomously functioning nodules), and Graves' disease. Patients with goiter from these conditions may present with symptoms of hyperthyroidism, such as unexplained weight loss, palpitations, and dyspnea on exertion.

- Goiters may present with symptoms of obstruction or compression of neighboring structures. This occurs most commonly from substernal goiters, but can also occur from large cervical goiters. It can also happen acutely, if there is acute enlargement of the thyroid. This can happen from acute thyroiditis, and also, rarely, from hemorrhage into a thyroid nodule (these situations are also associated with pain in the thyroid.)
  - Exertional dyspnea is the most common compressive symptom from goiters, present in 30–60 % that have compressive symptoms. The development of exertional dyspnea usually indicates that the tracheal diameter has been reduced to less than 8 mm. When the tracheal diameter is reduced below 5 mm, patients will typically have wheezing or stridor.
    - In the early stages, the dyspnea may be intermittent and positional, occurring when lying down, or when reaching or bending (reaching and bending force the thyroid further into the thoracic inlet.)
  - Cough is also a common symptom of obstruction, present in 10–30 % of patients with compressive symptoms.
  - Other, less common obstructive/compressive symptoms include:
    - Dysphagia from extrinsic narrowing of the esophagus.
    - Hoarseness from compression of the recurrent laryngeal nerve with vocal cord paralysis (can be transient or permanent).
    - Venous engorgement of the face, neck, and upper anterior chest from jugular vein compression. This can also lead to thrombosis of the jugular vein.

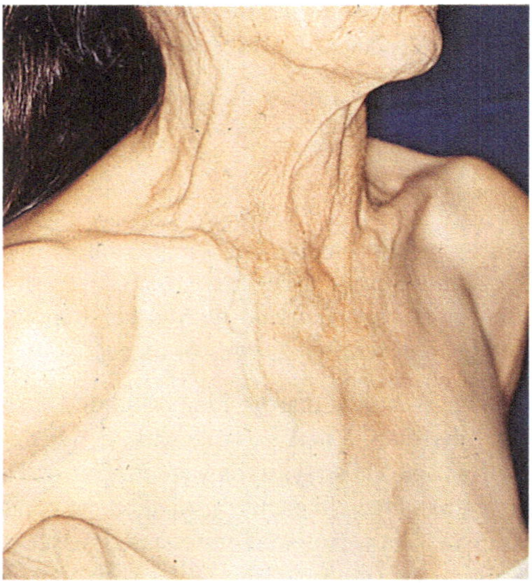

Photograph of a woman who has a large retrosternal goiter with signs of compression of the venous system. She has engorged superficial veins on her anterior neck and chest. [Medeiros-Neto G. Chapter 3. In: Surks MI, editor. Volume 1: Thyroid Diseases. 1 edition. Philadelphia: Current Medicine Group; 1999. (Korenman SG, editor. Atlas of Clinical Endocrinology). ISBN: 0-632-04397-0]

- Horner's syndrome. Horner's syndrome results when the goiter causes compression of the cervical sympathetic nerve supply to the eye. Horner's syndrome is rare, and it is especially rarely caused by goiter. The classic triad of Horner's consists of (all on the affected side);
  - Miosis (constricted pupil).
  - Partial ptosis, drooping eyelid from partial paralysis of the superior tarsal muscle.
  - Hemifacial anhidrosis, loss of sweating on the affected half of the face.

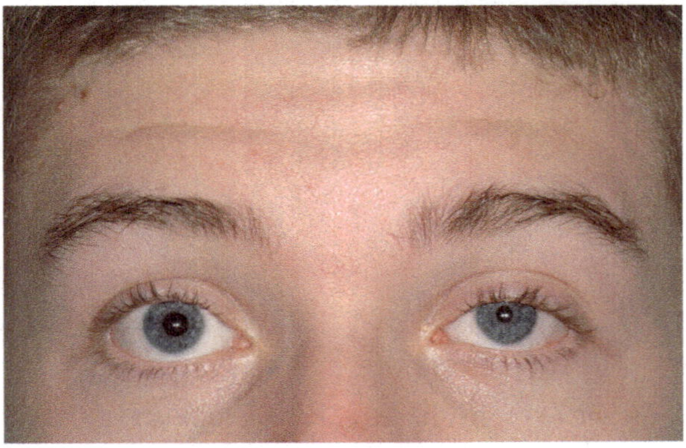

Photograph of the eyes showing the left ptosis and miosis of Horner's syndrome. [Mutalib M, Vandervelde C, Varghese A, Sallomi DF, Silva P de, Casey JMH, Howlett DC. Horner's syndrome secondary to asymptomatic pneumothorax in an adolescent. Eur J Pediatr. 2006 Sep 19;166(5):507–8.] *Caption from original*

Primary Differential Considerations

- Patients who present with an exam consistent with goiter should be also be evaluated for other possible diagnoses, including:
  - Other thyroid pathology, such as nodules, thyroiditis, or malignancy
  - Parathyroid cyst or malignancy
  - Lipoma or fibroma
  - Branchial cleft cyst or cystic hygroma

History and Physical Exam

Findings That Confirm Diagnosis

- The diagnosis can be confirmed by the direct palpation of the goiter. A goiter can usually be distinguished from other anterior neck masses (such as fatty tissue, redundant skin, etc.) as the thyroid will go up and down with swallowing. It is often helpful to ask the patient to swallow a sip of water and just observe the anterior neck for this up and down motion.

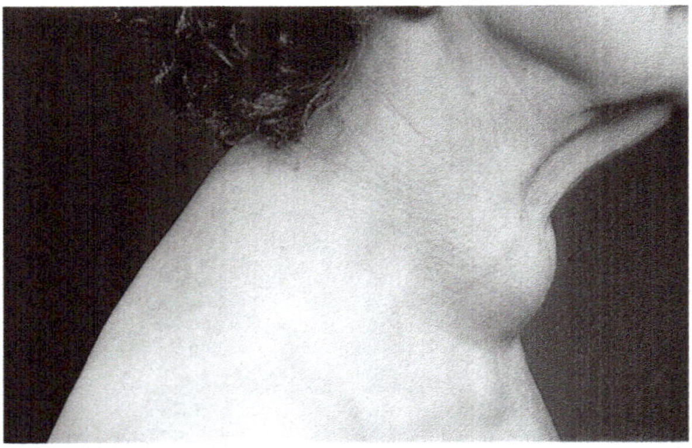

Diffuse goiter: Hashimoto's thyroiditis [Gharib H. Chapter 4. In: Surks MI, editor. Volume 1: Thyroid Diseases. 1 edition. Philadelphia: Current Medicine Group; 1999. (Korenman SG, editor. Atlas of Clinical Endocrinology). ISBN: 0-632-04397-0] *Caption adapted from original*

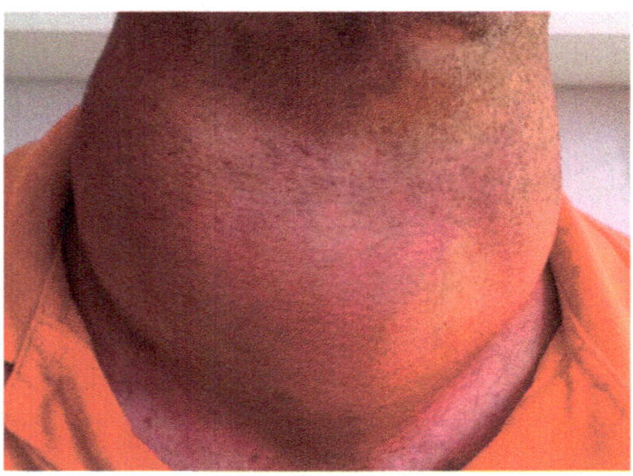

Large goiter in a 57-year-old man. [Giovanella L. Nontoxic Multinodular Goiter. In: Giovanella L, Treglia G, Valcavi R, editors. Atlas of Head and Neck Endocrine Disorders [Internet]. Cham: Springer International Publishing; 2016 [cited 2015 Dec 17]. p. 67–72. Available from: http://link.springer.com/10.1007/978-3-319-22276-9_10] *Caption adapted from original*

- In patients with short and thick necks it can be difficult to adequately palpate the thyroid. These patients may require some form of imaging to be certain a goiter is present.

Factors That Suggest Diagnosis

- Patients with a family history of thyroid disease, recent immigrants from areas of the world considered iodine-deficient, those with a history of head and neck irradiation, or other radiation exposure, should be considered to be at higher risk for goiter.
- All patients in whom the diagnosis is being considered should be directly questioned about the presence of hyper- or hypothyroid symptoms, and for the presence or absence of obstructive symptoms.
- The presence of a substernal thyroid can be suggested by:
  - The inability to directly palpate the inferior thyroid margin on either side.
  - Pemberton's maneuver. In this provocative physical exam test, the examiner holds the patient's arms directly above the head for about one minute. This maneuver forces the thyroid into the thoracic inlet and can exacerbate obstructive symptoms and signs. These include dyspnea, distension of the neck veins, facial flushing or cyanosis, or the inability to swallow.

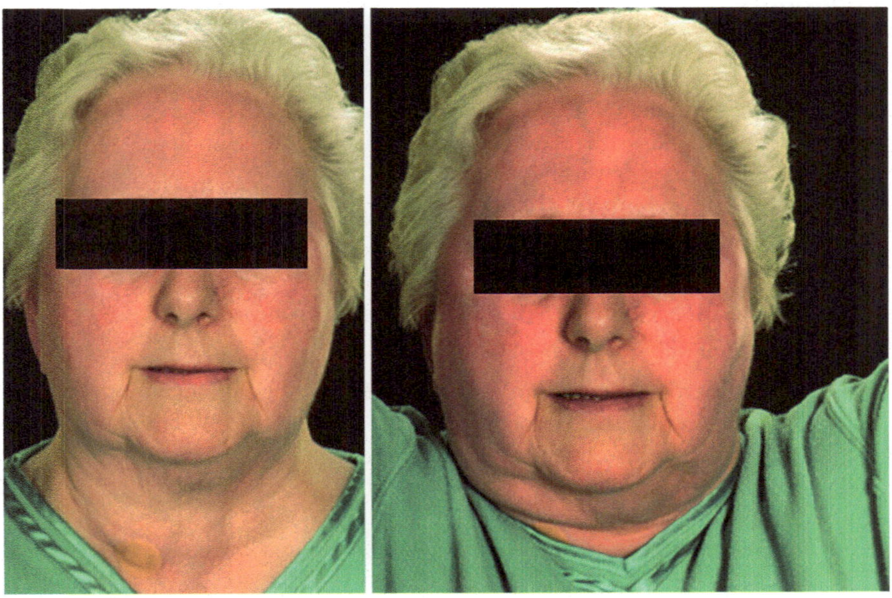

Pemberton's sign. The presence of a retrosternal goiter causes facial flushing and distended superficial veins. Mild flushing is noted with the arms by the side indicating some baseline obstruction at rest. [Sharma N, Watkinson JC. Retrosternal Goiter.

In: Watkinson JC, Scott-Coombes DM, editors. Tips and Tricks in Endocrine Surgery [Internet]. London: Springer London; 2014 [cited 2015 Dec 17]. p. 161–6. Available from: http://link.springer.com/10.1007/978-1-4471-2146-6_20] *Caption from original*

- Kocher's test. This is a physical examination maneuver that can be used to test for the presence of tracheal compression. In a positive test, compression of the lateral lobes of the thyroid will produce stridor from tracheal compression.

Factors That Exclude Diagnosis

- No historical or physical examination factors can adequately exclude the diagnosis.
- In patients with short and thick necks it can be difficult to adequately palpate the thyroid. These patients may require some form of imaging to be certain a goiter is either present or absent.

Ancillary Studies

Laboratory

- Thyroid stimulating hormone (TSH). All patients with goiter should have their thyroid function evaluated by measurement of their serum TSH. Serum TSH is often normal (euthyroid), but can also be low (suppressed) with hyperthyroidism, and high with hypothyroidism.
  - If the TSH is low, the serum-free thyroxine (T4) and total triiodothyronine (T3) should also be measured to assess for an autonomously functioning multinodular goiter or Graves' disease.
  - If the TSH is high, free T4 should be measured as part of the evaluation for likely Hashimoto's disease.
- Thyroid peroxidase antibodies (TPO). Patients with Hashimoto's (autoimmune) thyroiditis almost always have elevated TPO. Patients with goiter and hypothyroidism in the United States will most likely have Hashimoto's thyroiditis as the cause of their goiter. This can be confirmed by elevated TPO.
- TSH receptor antibodies. These should be measured when Graves' disease is being considered in the differential diagnosis of the goiter. This is mostly in the setting of a goiter associated with hyperthyroidism.

Imaging

- Thyroid ultrasound should be obtained in most patients with goiter. Thyroid ultrasound can be used to evaluated thyroid size and volume; it can also help assess thyroid function. Thyroid ultrasound can also help in the evaluation of a goiter with features that may be consistent with thyroid cancer. These "worrisome" features include a rapidly growing goiter, asymmetric thyroid enlargement, firm consistency to focal areas of the thyroid, and tenderness to palpation.
- Chest x-ray. Substernal goiters are often found incidentally on a CXR being performed for other reasons. They can appear as a mass that causes tracheal deviation or narrowing, or as superior mediastinal widening, or a mediastinal mass.

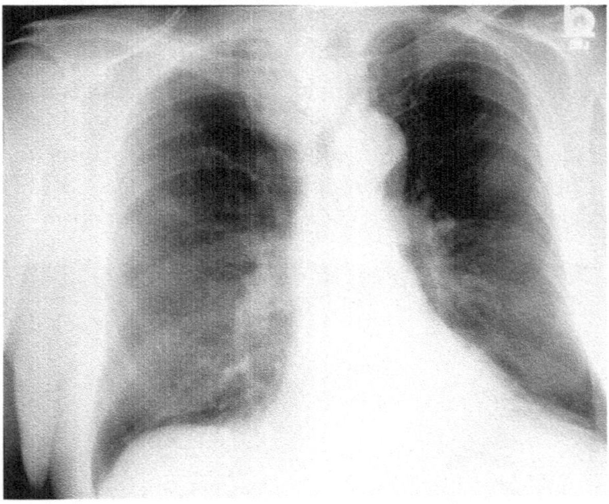

Chest radiograph in substernal goiter. There is an anterior mediastinal mass, which was thought to be compatible with a substernal goiter. Note the deviation of the trachea to the left and the presence of a mass in the upper anterior mediastinum. [Singer P. Chapter 12. In: Surks MI, editor. Volume 1: Thyroid Diseases. 1 edition. Philadelphia: Current Medicine Group; 1999. (Korenman SG, editor. Atlas of Clinical Endocrinology). ISBN: 0-632-04397-0] *Caption adapted from original*

- CT scan. Goiters may be incidentally noted on CT scans of the neck and chest being performed for other reasons, but a CT chest can also be an important test in the evaluation of large cervical goiters and suspected substernal goiters. CT can help delineate the extent of the goiter. To fully evaluate the goiter, a CT of the neck and chest may be necessary.

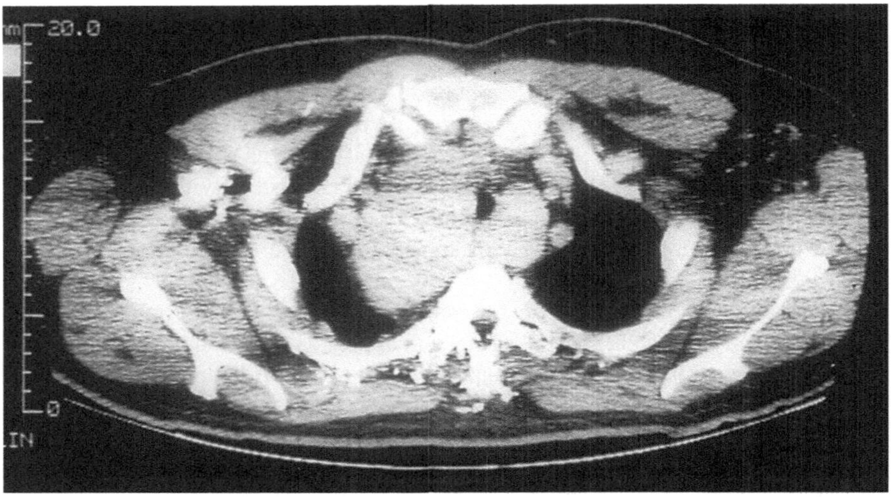

Computed tomography in substernal goiter. Note the predominantly right-sided mass with tissue to the left of the trachea as well. The trachea is not significantly narrowed. [Singer P. Chapter 12. In: Surks MI, editor. Volume 1: Thyroid Diseases. 1 edition. Philadelphia: Current Medicine Group; 1999. (Korenman SG, editor. Atlas of Clinical Endocrinology). ISBN: 0-632-04397-0] *Caption adapted from original*

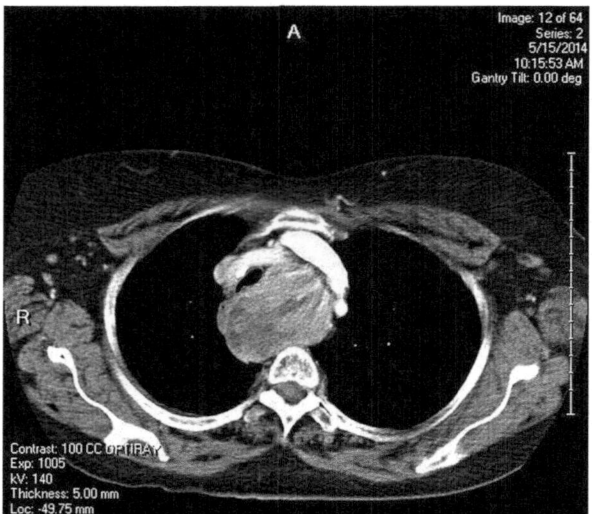

Substernal goiter Substernal goiter (SG) leading to significant tracheal deviation and compression with symptomatic dyspnea on exertion[Wilhelm SM. Multinodular Goiter. In: Pasieka JL, Lee JA, editors. Surgical Endocrinopathies [Internet]. Cham:

Springer International Publishing; 2015 [cited 2015 Dec 17]. p. 57–63. Available from: http://link.springer.com/10.1007/978-3-319-13662-2_11] *Caption from original*

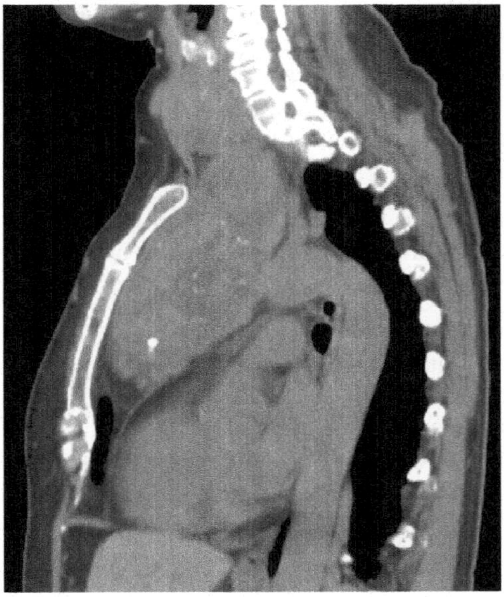

Image from a computed tomography of a patient with a massive intrathoracic goiter. The goiter is clearly below the aortic arch[Rolighed L, Rønning H, Christiansen P. Sternotomy for substernal goiter: retrospective study of 52 operations. Langenbeck's Archives of Surgery. 2015 Apr;400(3):301–6.] *Caption from original*

- Thyroid radionuclide imaging may be necessary to identify any nodules or areas of autonomous functioning within the thyroid.

Other

- Flow-Volume Loop. Any patient with symptoms or signs consistent with an obstructive goiter should have pulmonary function tests with a flow-volume loop. If another imaging study reports a tracheal diameter less than 10 mm, the patient should also have a flow-volume loop performed. A fixed, mechanical obstruction in the trachea will show a blunted or "notched" flow-volume loop. A positive flow-volume loop may influence treatment and suggest the need for surgery.
- Fine needle aspiration (FNA) biopsy. FNA biopsy may be necessary to evaluate suspicious areas of goiter, or suspicious nodules for cancer. Suspicious findings include:
  - Rapid growth of the goiter
  - Pain or tenderness
  - Asymmetry in the consistency of the thyroid on examination

Special Populations

Age

- Goiter is most common in the middle-aged to older adult population. The incidence of goiter rises with age.
- Although rare, goiters can occur in infants and children. They can be congenital or acquired.
    - Congenital Goiter. Goiters can occur in infants from congenital causes. Congenital goiters may not be evident at birth, but will usually develop over the first several months of life. The causes of congenital goiter include:
        - Inborn errors of thyroid hormone production
        - Mother's with Hashimoto's or Graves' can have transplacental transfer of maternal antibody leading to goiter
        - Maternal ingestion of antithyroid drugs
        - Inborn mutations of thyroid hormones and receptors
        - Thyroid tumors
    - Acquired Goiter. Acquired goiters in children follow a similar distribution as adults. In iodine-deficient parts of the world, iodine-deficient goiters are the most common cause. In areas of the world where iodine-deficiency is uncommon, common causes of goiter include:
        - Hashimoto's Thyroiditis
        - Graves' Disease
- Colloid Goiter. This is a unique form of goiter that occurs in adolescent girls. The cause is unknown. Thyroid function is usually normal. It usually improves over time with no treatment.

Co-morbidities

- Goiters can occur in patients with multiple other co-morbid illnesses. Significant cardiac and pulmonary disease can complicate the management of goiters. As one of the primary treatments for goiter may be surgical, patients with multiple co-morbid conditions may not be good candidates for surgery.

Pitfalls in Diagnosis

Critical Steps Not to Miss

- It is critical to take a complete history, including a family history and exposure to radiation history, to help determine the cause for a goiter and to guide the appropriate work-up and treatment.
- It is critical to assess for a substernal goiter, by asking about obstructive symptoms, performing a thorough examination, and ordering appropriate imaging studies.

Mimics

- There are no significant mimics of goiter.
- There are other causes of anterior neck masses, but thorough physical examination, and/or an appropriate imaging study, can determine the etiology of the mass.

Time-Dependent Interventions

- Goiters are usually very slow-growing and can be dealt with over time.
- Substernal goiters may cause acute symptoms from tracheal compression. This can be due to continued growth of the thyroid, acute hemorrhage into a large nodule, or from acute swelling from thyroiditis. These symptoms usually include dyspnea, associated with wheezing or stridor.
- In these situations, an adequate airway must be obtained. Temporary measures can include humidified oxygen, positive pressure ventilation such as continuous positive airway pressure (CPAP), and use of heliox (a helium/oxygen mixture). All of these are temporizing measures however, and a secure airway will need to be obtained. This usually requires the involvement of a surgeon with experience in these matters.

Overall Principles of Treatment

- The treatment goals for goiters differ based upon the cause of the goiter, whether the goiter is symptomatic or asymptomatic, and whether the goiter is cervical or substernal.

- Goiters that are not associated with hyperthyroidism and are non-obstructive (such as Hashimoto's): The primary goals are to treat any underlying hypothyroidism, decrease the size of the goiter, and prevent further growth. If there is significant hypothyroidism, treatment with thyroid replacement hormone can decrease the size of the goiter. If the patient is asymptomatic, the goiter can be followed. If the goiter is large, surgery or radioiodine ablation (RIA) may be appropriate. Surgery is indicated for large goiters, especially those that are continuing to grow over time. RIA can be an alternative to surgery for those patients that are not good surgical candidates.
- Substernal (or cervical) Goiter with obstructive symptoms:
  - Once obstructive symptoms occur, the patient requires treatment. There is a small incidence of spontaneous hemorrhage into an enlarged thyroid. This can cause an acute increase in thyroid size leading to acute compression that can be fatal.
  - The usual treatment is surgical resection of the thyroid gland.
  - If the patient is unable or unwilling to have surgery, RIA can be considered.
- Asymptomatic Substernal Goiter:
  - These patients can be observed over time for the development of obstructive symptoms.
  - These patients can also be offered definitive surgical treatment.
  - Early, definitive surgical treatment should be considered, for the following reasons:
    - Most goiters will continue to enlarge.
    - Surgery will become more technically difficult as the goiter enlarges.
    - A significant minority (up to 40%) of patients with asymptomatic substernal goiter have abnormal flow-volume loops.
    - There is a small risk of cancer developing in the goiter. The risk of cancer developing in a goiter is about the same as the risk of cancer developing in any thyroid nodule.
    - There is a small risk of acute hemorrhage into the thyroid with potentially fatal acute airway obstruction.
  - Patients are considered safe to observe, rather than to undergo surgery, when any of the following conditions is met:
    - They have a normal flow-volume loop.
    - The substernal component ends at or above the brachiocephalic vein.
    - The patient is a poor surgical candidate.
  - Patients being observed should be followed closely for the development of obstructive symptoms, and should have a CT scan every year until stability is documented.

  - Goiters with associated hyperthyroidism: These are usually associated with Graves' disease. These patients need to have their primary disease process treated. Goiters associated with Graves' will often become smaller owing to treatment of the Graves'.
- Any goiter or thyroid nodule that has features or findings concerning for malignancy should have a fine needle aspiration (FNA) biopsy performed.
- Radioiodine ablation works best in large, hyperfunctioning (hyperthyroid), multinodular goiters. In this setting there can be a 30–40% reduction in the size of the goiter.

Disease Course

- Goiters usually grow slowly.
- Most will continue to increase in size over time, but a minority may remain stable in size.

Related Evidence

Papers of particular interest have been highlighted as:
*** Of key importance*

Practice Guideline

Chen AY, Bernet VJ, Carty SE, Davies TF, Ganly I, Inabnet WB 3rd, Shaha AR; Surgical Affairs Committee of the American Thyroid Association. American Thyroid Association statement on optimal surgical management of goiter. Thyroid. 2014 Feb;24(2):181-9. https://doi.org/10.1089/thy.2013.0291. Epub 2014 Jan 20. PubMed PMID: 24295043. http://www.ncbi.nlm.nih.gov/pubmed/24295043 **

Gharib H, Papini E, Paschke R, Duick DS, Valcavi R, Hegedüs L, Vitti P; AACE/AME/ETA Task Force on Thyroid Nodules. American Association of Clinical Endocrinologists, Associazione Medici Endocrinologi, and EuropeanThyroid Association Medical Guidelines for Clinical Practice for the Diagnosis and Management of Thyroid Nodules. Endocr Pract. 2010 May-Jun;16 Suppl 1:1-43. https://doi.org/10.4158/10024.GL. PubMed PMID: 20497938. http://www.ncbi.nlm.nih.gov/pubmed/20497938 **

Meta-Analysis

Malboosbaf R, Hosseinpanah F, Mojarrad M, Jambarsang S, Azizi F. Relationship between goiter and gender: a systematic review and meta-analysis. Endocrine. 2013 Jun;43(3):539-47. https://doi.org/10.1007/s12020-012-9831-8. Epub 2012 Dec 14. Review. PubMed PMID: 23238875. http://www.ncbi.nlm.nih.gov/pubmed/23238875

Review

Carlé A, Krejbjerg A, Laurberg P. Epidemiology of nodular goitre. Influence of iodine intake. Best Pract Res Clin Endocrinol Metab. 2014 Aug;28(4):465-79. https://doi.org/10.1016/j.beem.2014.01.001. Epub 2014 Jan 10. Review. PubMed PMID: 25047199. http://www.ncbi.nlm.nih.gov/pubmed/25047199 **

Fiore E, Tonacchera M, Vitti P. Influence of iodization programmes on the epidemiology of nodular goitre. Best Pract Res Clin Endocrinol Metab. 2014 Aug;28(4):577-88. https://doi.org/10.1016/j.beem.2014.04.002. Epub 2014 May 14. Review. PubMed PMID: 25047207. http://www.ncbi.nlm.nih.gov/pubmed/25047207

Rago T, Vitti P. Diagnostic role of ultrasound and elastosonography in nodular goiter. Best Pract Res Clin Endocrinol Metab. 2014 Aug;28(4):519-29. https://doi.org/10.1016/j.beem.2014.02.003. Epub 2014 Mar 20. Review. PubMed PMID: 25047203. http://www.ncbi.nlm.nih.gov/pubmed/25047203

Watt T, Cramon P, Frendl DM, Ware JE Jr; ThyQoL Group. Assessing health-related quality of life in patients with benign non-toxic goitre. Best Pract Res Clin Endocrinol Metab. 2014 Aug;28(4):559-75. https://doi.org/10.1016/j.beem.2014.01.009. Epub 2014 Jan 28. Review. PubMed PMID: 25047206. http://www.ncbi.nlm.nih.gov/pubmed/25047206

Sørensen JR, Hegedüs L, Kruse-Andersen S, Godballe C, Bonnema SJ. The impact of goitre and its treatment on the trachea, airflow, oesophagus and swallowing function. A systematic review. Best Pract Res Clin Endocrinol Metab. 2014 Aug;28(4):481-94. https://doi.org/10.1016/j.beem.2014.03.002. Epub 2014 Apr 4. Review. PubMed PMID: 25047200. http://www.ncbi.nlm.nih.gov/pubmed/25047200 **

Medeiros-Neto G, Camargo RY, Tomimori EK. Approach to and treatment of goiters. Med Clin North Am. 2012 Mar;96(2):351-68. https://doi.org/10.1016/j.mcna.2012.01.010. Review. PubMed PMID: 22443980. http://www.ncbi.nlm.nih.gov/pubmed/22443980

Bahn RS, Castro MR. Approach to the patient with nontoxic multinodular goiter. J Clin Endocrinol Metab. 2011 May;96(5):1202-12. https://doi.org/10.1210/jc.2010-2583. Review. PubMed PMID: 21543434. http://www.ncbi.nlm.nih.gov/pubmed/21543434

Luster M, Verburg FA, Scheidhauer K. Diagnostic imaging work up in multi-nodular goiter. Minerva Endocrinol. 2010 Sep;35(3):153-9. Review. PubMed PMID: 20938418. http://www.ncbi.nlm.nih.gov/pubmed/20938418

Tonacchera M, Pinchera A, Vitti P. Assessment of nodular goitre. Best Pract Res Clin Endocrinol Metab. 2010 Feb;24(1):51-61. https://doi.org/10.1016/j.beem.2009.08.008. Review. PubMed PMID: 20172470. http://www.ncbi.nlm.nih.gov/pubmed/20172470 **

Moalem J, Suh I, Duh QY. Treatment and prevention of recurrence of multinodular goiter: an evidence-based review of the literature. World J Surg. 2008 Jul;32(7):1301-12. https://doi.org/10.1007/s00268-008-9477-0. Review. PubMed PMID: 18305998. http://www.ncbi.nlm.nih.gov/pubmed/18305998

Porterfield JR Jr, Thompson GB, Farley DR, Grant CS, Richards ML. Evidence-based management of toxic multinodular goiter (Plummer's Disease). World J Surg. 2008 Jul;32(7):1278-84. https://doi.org/10.1007/s00268-008-9566-0. Review. PubMed PMID: 18357484. http://www.ncbi.nlm.nih.gov/pubmed

White ML, Doherty GM, Gauger PG. Evidence-based surgical management of substernal goiter. World J Surg. 2008 Jul;32(7):1285-300. https://doi.org/10.1007/s00268-008-9466-3. PubMed PMID: 18266028. http://www.ncbi.nlm.nih.gov/pubmed/18266028

Kotwal A, Priya R, Qadeer I. Goiter and other iodine deficiency disorders: A systematic review of epidemiological studies to deconstruct the complex web. Arch Med Res. 2007 Jan;38(1):1-14. Review. Erratum in: Arch Med Res. 2007 Apr;38(3):366. PubMed PMID: 17174717. http://www.ncbi.nlm.nih.gov/pubmed/17174717

Use PubMed Clinical Queries to find the most recent evidence. Use this search strategy: “Goiter”[Mh] OR “goiter”[tiab] OR “goiters”[tiab]

Chapter 32
Heart Failure

Charles V. Pollack, Jr. and Victoria G. Riese

Name and Synonyms

Heart Failure; Congestive Heart Failure

Incidence/Epidemiology

- Heart failure is a clinical state in which perfusion of tissues and/or venous return to the heart is impaired because of inadequate pumping functionality of the cardiac muscle, or when perfusion can only be maintained from an abnormally high diastolic volume.
- There are multiple ways to characterize heart failure:
  - Systolic vs diastolic
    - In systolic failure, the ventricles are unable to contract normally.
    - In diastolic failure, the ventricles fail to relax and fill properly.
    - Patients who have both dilated and hypertrophic ventricles may have both systolic and diastolic failure
  - Right-sided vs left-sided
    - Left-sided heart failure leaves blood in the lungs and therefore usually presents as pulmonary edema.

C. V. Pollack, Jr. (✉)
Department of Emergency Medicine, Thomas Jefferson University, Philadelphia, PA, USA

V. G. Riese
Librarian Consultant, Eldersburg, MD, USA

C. V. Pollack, Jr. (ed.), *Differential Diagnosis of Cardiopulmonary Disease*,
https://doi.org/10.1007/978-3-319-63895-9_32

    - Right-sided heart failure leaves blood in the periphery and therefore usually presents with edema and liver congestion.
    - Long-standing heart failure usually manifests findings of both left- and right-sided failure

- Acute vs chronic

    - Acute heart failure usually develops immediately after a large myocardial infarction or rupture of a heart valve.
    - Chronic heart failure develops more slowly and is often due to systemic hypertension, dilated cardiomyopathy, or multivalvular disease.

Chronic heart failure	Chronic heart failure is a clinical syndrome characterized by complex and variable symptoms and signs. The cardinal manifestations of heart failure are dyspnea and fatigue, which may limit exercise tolerance, and fluid retention, which may lead to pulmonary congestion and peripheral edema. Chronic heart failure is often punctuated by acute decompensation.
Acute heart failure	New onset of decompensated heart failure or decompensation of chronic, established heart failure with symptoms sufficient to warrant hospitalization. Cardiac dysfunction can be related to systolic or diastolic dysfunction, to abnormalities in cardiac rhythm, or to preload and after-load mismatch.
Heart failure with reduced LVEF (also referred to as systolic heart failure or heart failure with reduced systolic function)	A clinical syndrome characterized by signs and symptoms of heart failure and reduced LVEF. Most commonly associated with left ventricular chamber dilation.
Heart failure with preserved LVEF (also referred to as diastolic heart failure or heart failure with preserved systolic function)	A clinical syndrome characterized by signs and symptoms of heart failure with preserved LVEF. Most commonly associated with a nondilated left ventricle. May be the result of valvular disease or other causes.

Classification of the heart failure syndrome. Heart failure is often classified as heart failure with abnormal systolic function versus heart failure with preserved systolic function. These classifications often consider normal systolic function and normal ejection fraction to be the same. Heart failure with preserved left ventricular ejection fraction (LVEF) is variably defined as an LVEF greater than 40%, greater than 45%, or greater than 50%. Heart failure with preserved LVEF is not a distinct condition, but rather a syndrome with numerous possible causative or comorbid conditions, including hypertension, diabetes mellitus, vascular stiffness, renal impairment, and atrial fibrillation. There is no current consensus about nomenclature for heart failure with preserved systolic function. The clinical classification of patients with acute decompensated heart failure continues to evolve and reflects ongoing changes in the understanding of the pathophysiology of this syndrome. Worsening renal function, persistent neurohormonal activation, and progressive deterioration in myocardial function all seem to play a role. Decompensation also commonly occurs without a fundamental worsening of underlying cardiac structure or function. Failure to adhere to prescribed medications or an inadequate medical regimen may lead to hospitalization without a worsening of underlying circulatory function. Other descriptive terms used for heart failure include right- and left-sided heart failure referring to syndromes presenting predominately with congestion of the systemic or pulmonary vascular beds. Mild, moderate, and severe heart failure are used as clinical symptomatic descriptions instead of or in addition to New York Heart Association functional classification. [Kittleson MM, Fonarow GC. Clinical Syndromes of Acute and Chronic Heart Failure. In: Colucci WS, editor. Atlas of heart failure, 5th ed. Philadelphia: Current Medicine Group; 2008. 344 p. ISBN: 1-57340-261-3] *Caption adapted from original*

- Black males have the highest incidence of heart failure per capita.

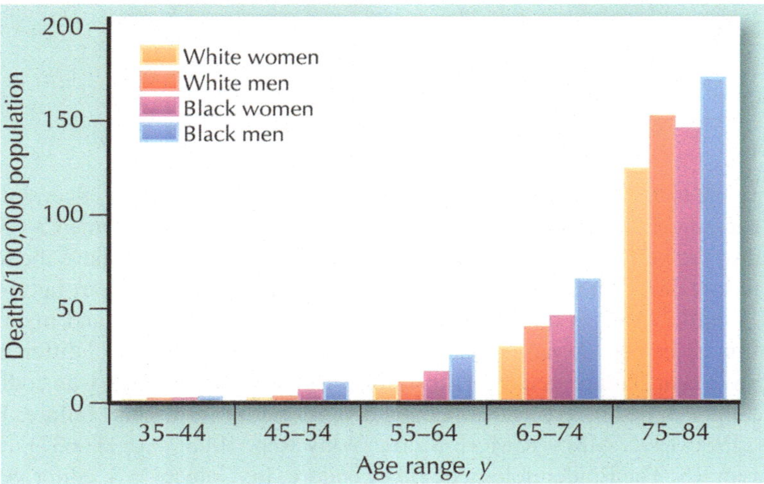

US heart failure deaths by age, sex, and race. Among all age groups, black men experienced the highest rates of heart failure death. In all age groups except ages 75 to 84 years, black women experienced the next highest rates of heart failure death followed by white men. In the age group of 75 to 84 years, white men had higher rates of heart failure—related death than black women. In all age groups, white women experienced the least heart failure–related mortality (American Heart Association: Heart Disease and Stroke Statistics —2007 Update.. Dallas: American Heart Association; 2007). [Parikh NI, Vasan RS. The Epidemiology of Heart Failure. In: Colucci WS, editor. Atlas of heart failure, 5th ed. Philadelphia: Current Medicine Group; 2008. 344 p. ISBN: 1-57340-261-3] *Caption from original*

- There is a "heart failure belt" across middle America

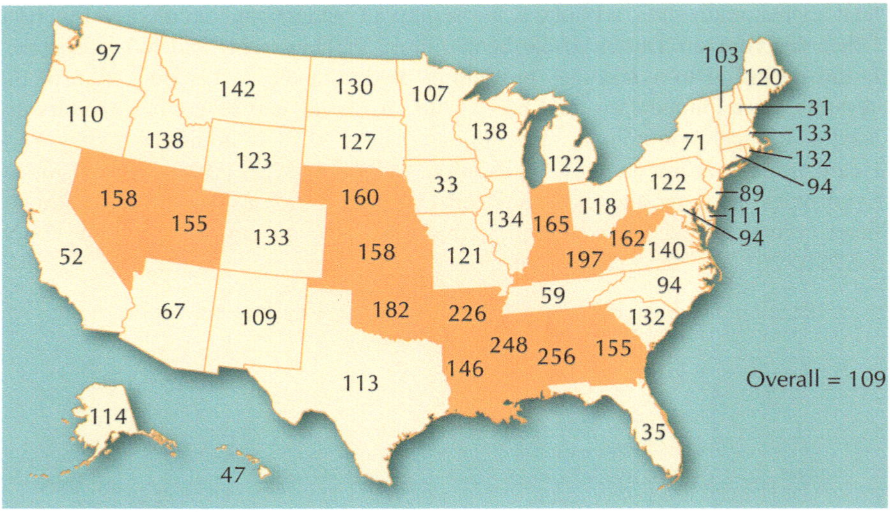

Geographic heterogeneity in US heart failure death rates. Numbers reflect state-specific, age-adjusted death rates per 100,000 persons for men and women > 65 years of age for the period from 1990 to 1996. The 13 highlighted states have the highest heart failure death rates. Possible explanations for the apparent "heart failure belt" across middle-America are 1) higher prevalence of hypertension and myocardial infarction in the belt, 2) varying access to early diagnosis, 3) regional differences in congestive heart failure treatment, or 4) differing practices of diagnostic coding for heart failure in death certificates (Changes in mortality from heart failure: United States, 1980-1995. MMWR Morb Mortal Wkly Rep. 1998; 47:633 -637). [Parikh NI, Vasan RS. The Epidemiology of Heart Failure. In: Colucci WS, editor. Atlas of heart failure, 5th ed. Philadelphia: Current Medicine Group; 2008. 344 p. ISBN: 1-57340-261-3] *Caption from original*

- Heart failure is classified by multiple scales, but the most commonly used is from the New York Heart Association (NHYA) and is symptom-driven.

Class I	No limitation of daily physical activity.
Class II	Slight limitation of activity. Comfortable at rest but ordinary physical activity produces fatigue and dyspnea.
Class III	Marked limitation of physical activity. Fatigue and dyspnea results from minimal physical activity.
Class IV	Severe physical limitation. Dyspnea at rest and unable to carry on physical activity without severe symptoms.

New York Heart Association classification of heart failure. The functional classification of patients with congestive heart failure developed by the New York Heart Association is based on the amount of activity tolerated by patients before the onset of symptoms. Despite the limitations of this subjective classification, it is a useful descriptive system and remains the standard by which patients with heart failure are compared (Boston: Little, Brown; 1964; 114). [O'Connor C, Tuman K. Chapter 7. In: Miller RD, Reves JG, editors. Atlas of Anesthesia: Cardiothoracic Anesthesia, Volume 8, 1e. Philadelphia: Current Medicine Group; 1999. 256 p. ISBN: 0-443-07974-9] *Caption from original*

Differential Diagnosis

- The differential diagnosis of heart failure is to some extent dependent upon the type of failure being manifest. In general, the differential includes:
  - Acute exacerbation of COPD

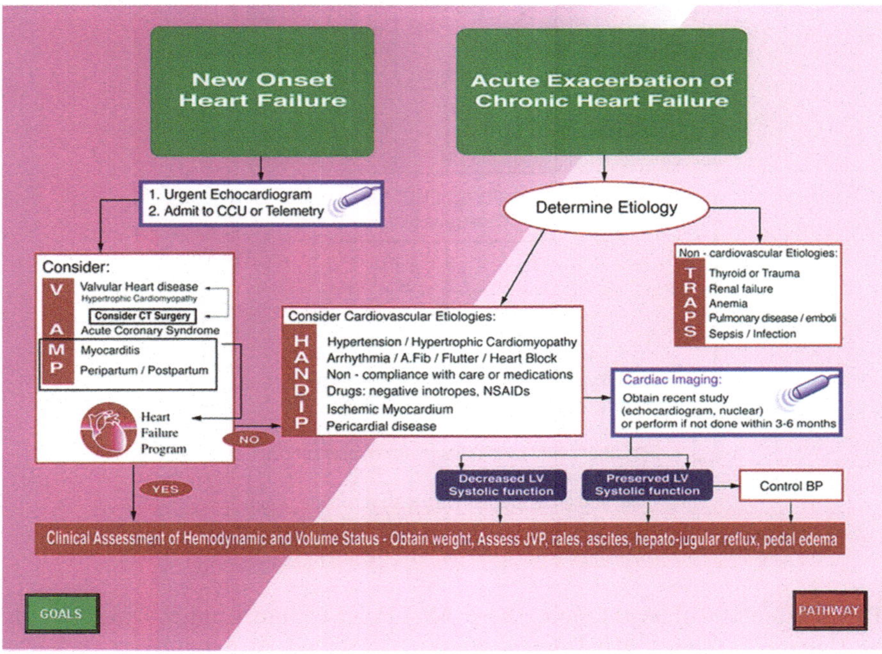

Differential diagnosis between new onset heart failure and acute exacerbation of chronic heart failure with timing of imaging and consideration of precipitating pathophysiology. [Wild D, Herzog E, Aziz E, Kukin M. Pathway for the Management of Heart Failure Complicating Acute Coronary Syndrome. In: Herzog E, Chaudhry F, editors. Echocardiography in Acute Coronary Syndrome [Internet]. London: Springer London; 2009 [cited 2015 Jun 4]. p. 365–76. Available from: http://link.springer.com/10.1007/978-1-84882-027-2_25] *Caption from original*

- Pulmonary embolism
- Pneumonia
- Acute renal failure
- Noncardiogenic pulmonary edema
- Myocardial infarction
- Respiratory failure

Pathophysiology and Etiology

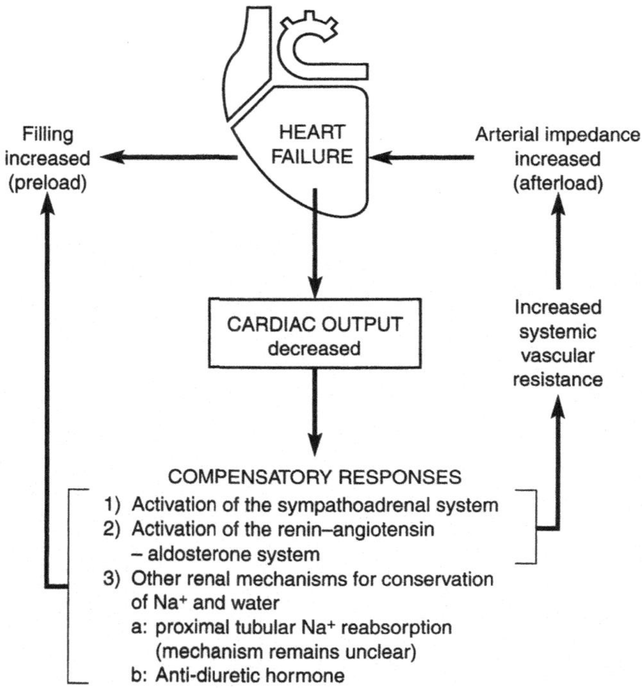

Pathophysiology of heart failure. [Khan MG. Heart Failure. Cardiac Drug Therapy, 8e [Internet]. Totowa, NJ: Humana Press; 2015 [cited 2015 Jun 4]. p. 369–421. Available from: http://link.springer.com/10.1007/978-1-61779-962-4_12] *Caption from original*

Common
Coronary heart disease
Hypertension
Idiopathic
Diabetes mellitus
Valvular disease
Less common
Anemia
Connective tissue disease
Viral myocarditis
Hemochromatosis
Human immunodeficiency virus infection
Hyperthyroidism, hypothyroidism
Hypertrophic cardiomyopathy
Infiltrative disease (including amyloidosis and sarcoidosis)
Mediastinal radiation
Peripartum cardiomyopathy
Restrictive pericardial disease
Tachyarrhythmia
Toxins (including drugs and alcohol)
Trypanosomiasis (Chagas' disease)

Etiologies of heart failure. [Marín-García J. Diagnosis of Heart Failure: Evidence-Based Perspective. Heart Failure [Internet]. Totowa, NJ: Humana Press; 2010 [cited 2015 Jun 4]. p. 353–63. Available from: http://link.springer.com/10.1007/978-1-60761-147-9_18] *Caption from original*

- There are many contributing factors to the development of heart failure, including:
  - Increased metabolic demand on the heart, such as:
    - Infection
    - Anemia
  - Other demand for increased cardiac output, such as:
    - Pregnancy
    - Thyrotoxicosis
    - Sepsis
    - Hypovolemia
  - Physical demand on the heart, such as:
    - Hypertension
    - Endocarditis
    - Pulmonary embolism
    - Salt and volume retention

- Injury to heart muscle, such as:
  - Myocardial infarction
  - Myocarditis
- Arrhythmia
- Toxic exposures
- Chagas' disease

Presentation

Typical/"Classic"

- Most patients with acute heart failure present with shortness of breath.
- Dyspnea on exertion and orthopnea are common.
- Chest pain and palpitations are not uncommon.
- Patients with right-sided failure only will complain of dependent edema, weight gain, and swelling of the abdomen.

Atypical

- Patients may present only with weight gain or nocturia.
- Chest pain or palpitations without dyspnea would be unusual.

Primary Differential Considerations

- Patients who present with signs and symptoms of heart failure should also be evaluated for these potential diagnoses:
  - Acute coronary syndrome
  - Pulmonary embolism
  - COPD exacerbation
  - Pneumonia

History and Physical Exam

- In the history, focus on symptoms of fluid overload and pump failure, such as:
  - Dyspnea (specifically asking about dyspnea at rest vs only with exertion, and about nocturnal dyspnea/orthopnea)

  - Peripheral edema and ascites (socks leaving indentations, having to loosen belt)
  - Nocturia and insomnia
  - Fatigue
  - Generalized weakness
  - Abdominal pain (which may result from hepatic congestion)

- On physical examination, there are a number of findings associated with heart failure that should be sought:

  - Pulmonary rales

http://www.easyauscultation.com/rales

Rales. [Rales Lung Sounds; Easy Auscultation; www.easyauscultation.com; copyright 2015, MedEdu LLC]

- Peripheral edema
- Hepatomegaly
- Orthopnea
- Third heart sound (S3 gallop)

https://www.youtube.com/watch?v=xbLMC0kPQ-E

Audio of the third heart sound.

- Fourth heart sound

https://www.youtube.com/watch?v=r-HqK7NRL8I

Audio of the fourth heart sound with animated diagram.

- Neck vein distention

Findings that Confirm Diagnosis

- More than two or three of the signs and symptoms are strongly suggestive of heart failure. Confirmation of the diagnosis (and important prognostic information) is obtained by echocardiography.

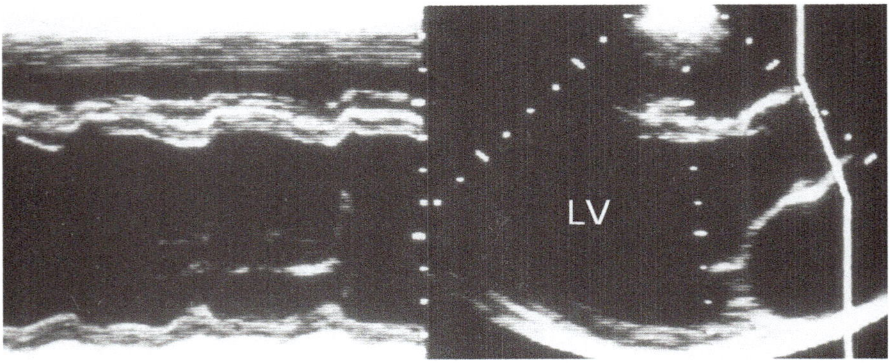

M-mode echocardiogram (left) and parasternal long-axis view from a patient with marked alcohol consumption and heart failure. The echocardiographic pattern is that of dilated cardiomyopathy with reduced contraction. [Nihoyannopoulos P. Cardiomyopathies. In: Nihoyannopoulos P, Kisslo J, editors. Echocardiography [Internet]. London: Springer London; 2009 [cited 2015 Jun 4]. p. 399–434. Available from: http://link.springer.com/10.1007/978-1-84882-293-1_20] *Caption from original*

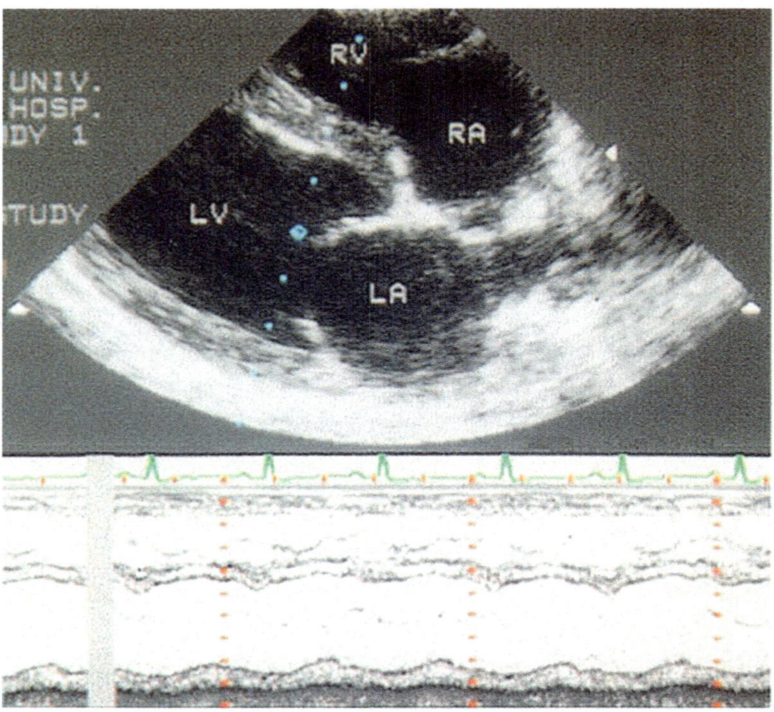

Two-dimensional M-mode echocardiogram of a dog with congestive heart failure induced by rapid pacing. Note the generalized cardiac dilatation and decreased left ventricular shortening fraction. LA—left atrium; LV—left ventricle; RA—right atrium; RV—right ventricle. [Gwathmey J, Abelmann W. Chapter 11. In: Lee RT, Braunwald E, editors. Atlas of Cardiac Imaging, 1e. Philadelphia: Current Medicine; 1998. 248 p. ISBN: 0-443-07567-0] *Caption from original*

Factors that Suggest Diagnosis

- More than two of the signs and symptoms listed above are suggestive and warrant specific evaluation

Factors that Exclude Diagnosis

- A normal echocardiogram and a normal brain-type natriuretic peptide (BNP level) exclude heart failure. It may not be possible to exclude the diagnosis fully on clinical grounds alone.

Ancillary Studies

Laboratory

- Baseline CBC (to exclude anemia) and renal function should be evaluated
- Urine should be checked for protein, blood, and glucose
- Serum electrolytes (especially potassium) should be checked
- A BNP level should be checked

Electrocardiography

- Electrocardiogram should be obtained to evaluate rhythm and to look for left ventricular hypertrophy or Q-waves. There are no pathognomonic findings for heart failure on ECG.

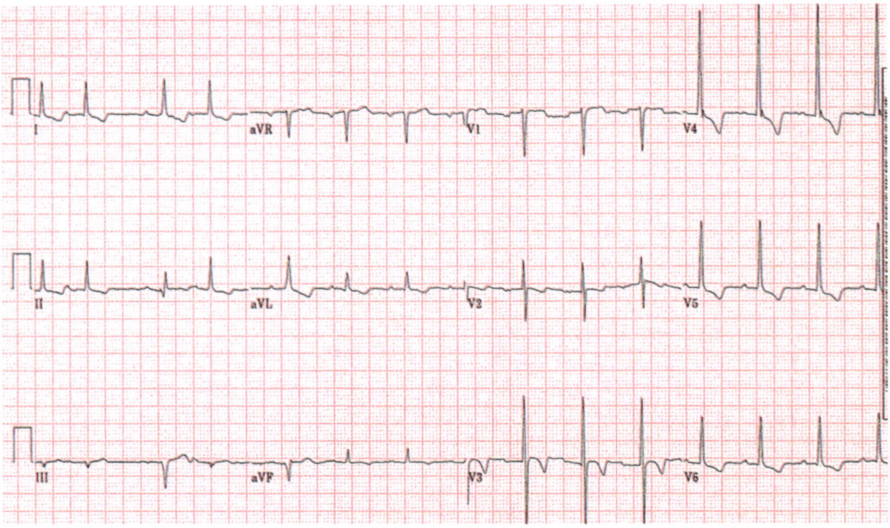

A 12-lead electrocardiogram demonstrating left ventricular hypertrophy with a "strain" pattern. [Fleisher L. Chapter 3. In: Miller RD, Lichtor JL, editors. Atlas of Anesthesia: Preoperative Preparation and Intraoperative Monitoring, Volume 3, 1e. Philadelphia: Current Medicine; 1997. 251 p. ISBN: 0-443-07902-1] *Caption adapted from original*

Imaging

- Chest x-ray should be obtained to look for cardiac enlargement, pleural effusion, signs of pulmonary edema, COPD, or pneumonia.

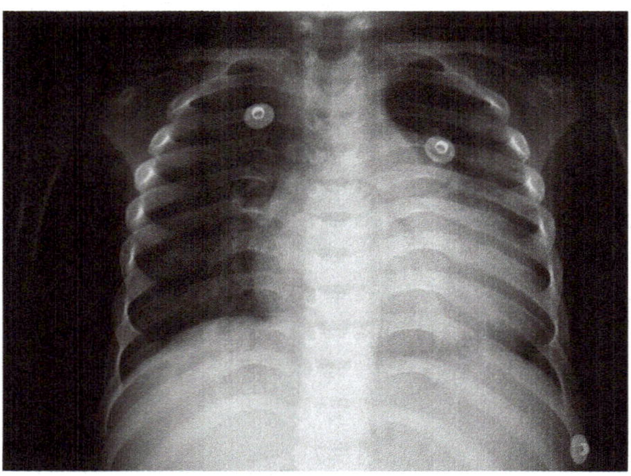

Cardiomegaly on chest X-ray. [Yıldırım SV, Durmaz C, Pourbagher MA, Erkan AN. A case of achondroplasia with severe pulmonary hypertension due to obstructive sleep apnea. European Archives of Oto-Rhino-Laryngology. 2006 Aug;263(8):775–7.] *Caption from original*

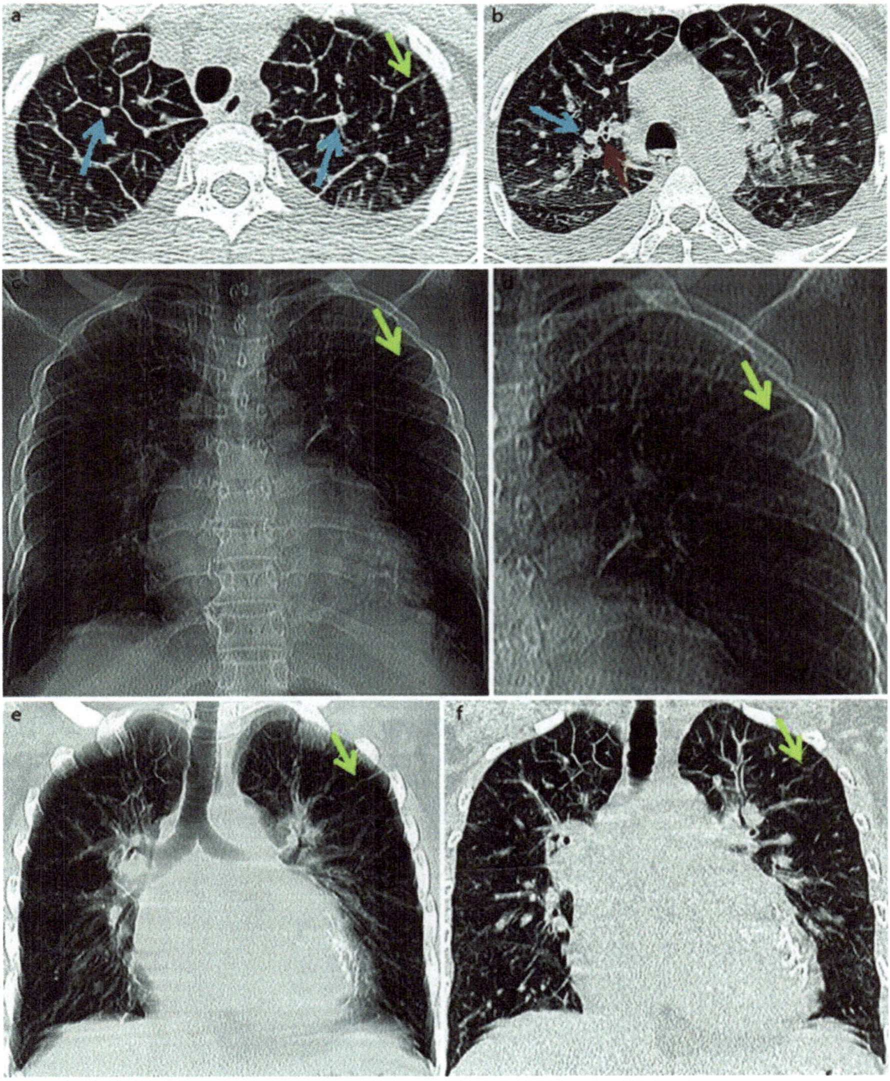

Hydrostatic pulmonary edema in a patient with congestive heart failure. Two successsive axial computed tomography slices (a and b) demonstrate a nodular thickening of the interlobular septa reflecting the enlarged pulmonary veins (blue arrows) with bilateral pleural effusion. Note the peribronchial cuffing on (b; orange arrow). The chest radiograph equivalent (c) and the focused view on the left upper lobe (d) show a loss of definition of vascular markings throughout both lungs associated with Kerley lines (yellow arrows), reminiscent of interstitial edema. Note the enlargement of the cardiac silhouette. By viewing average coronal slabs (c–f) of decreasing slice thickness, Kerley A lines seen on (f) corresponding to septal thickening are perfectly understood. [Ilsen B, Gosselin R, Delrue L, Duyck P, de Mey J, Beigelman-Aubry C. Interstitial Lung Disease. In: Coche EE, Ghaye B, de Mey J, Duyck P, editors. Comparative Interpretation of CT and Standard Radiography of the Chest [Internet]. Berlin, Heidelberg: Springer Berlin Heidelberg; 2011 [cited 2015 Jun 4]. p. 195–220. Available from: http://link.springer.com/10.1007/978-3-540-79942-9_8] *Caption from original*

- Echocardiography is helpful in diagnosing, staging, and following heart failure.

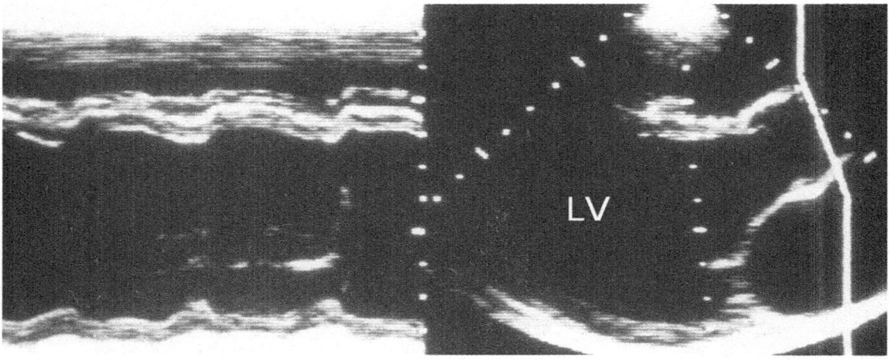

M-mode echocardiogram (left) and parasternal long-axis view from a patient with marked alcohol consumption and heart failure. The echocardiographic pattern is that of dilated cardiomyopathy with reduced contraction. [Nihoyannopoulos P. Cardiomyopathies. In: Nihoyannopoulos P, Kisslo J, editors. Echocardiography [Internet]. London: Springer London; 2009 [cited 2015 Jun 4]. p. 399–434. Available from: http://link.springer.com/10.1007/978-1-84882-293-1_20] *Caption from original*

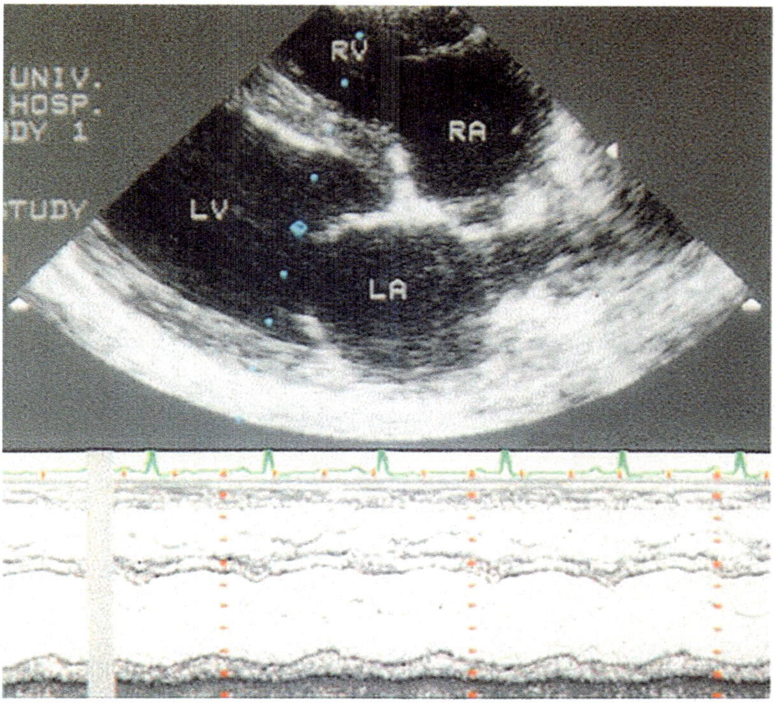

Two-dimensional M-mode echocardiogram of a dog with congestive heart failure induced by rapid pacing. Note the generalized cardiac dilatation and decreased left ventricular shortening fraction. LA—left atrium; LV—left ventricle; RA—right atrium; RV—right ventricle. [Gwathmey J, Abelmann W. Chapter 11. In: Lee RT, Braunwald E, editors. Atlas of Cardiac Imaging, 1e. Philadelphia: Current Medicine; 1998. 248 p. ISBN: 0-443-07567-0] *Caption from original*

Other Studies

- None indicated in initial evaluation.

Special Populations

Age

- With rare exception, heart failure is a disease of older patients, with the incidence increasing with increasing age.

Co-morbidities

- Co-morbidities may include:
  - Hypertension
  - Renal disease
  - Cardio- and cerebrovascular disease
  - Drug and alcohol abuse

Pitfalls in Diagnosis

Critical Steps Not to Miss

- Recognition of acute heart failure that may precipitate circulatory collapse or severe pulmonary

Mimics

- Potential mimics include:
  - Pneumonia
  - COPD
  - Acute coronary syndrome
  - Pulmonary embolism

Time-Dependent Interventions

- Provide ventilatory and circulatory support as needed.
- Noninvasive ventilation should be attempted before intubation and mechanical ventilation unless the patient is already in ventilatory failure.
- Initiation of diuresis.

Overall Principles of Treatment

- Relief of fluid overload and improvement in ventilatory and circulatory status are paramount.
- Diuresis with attention to electrolyte levels will improve symptoms.

- ACE inhibitors and beta-blockers will improve long-term management.
- Diet and exercise counseling will help patients manage their symptoms better.

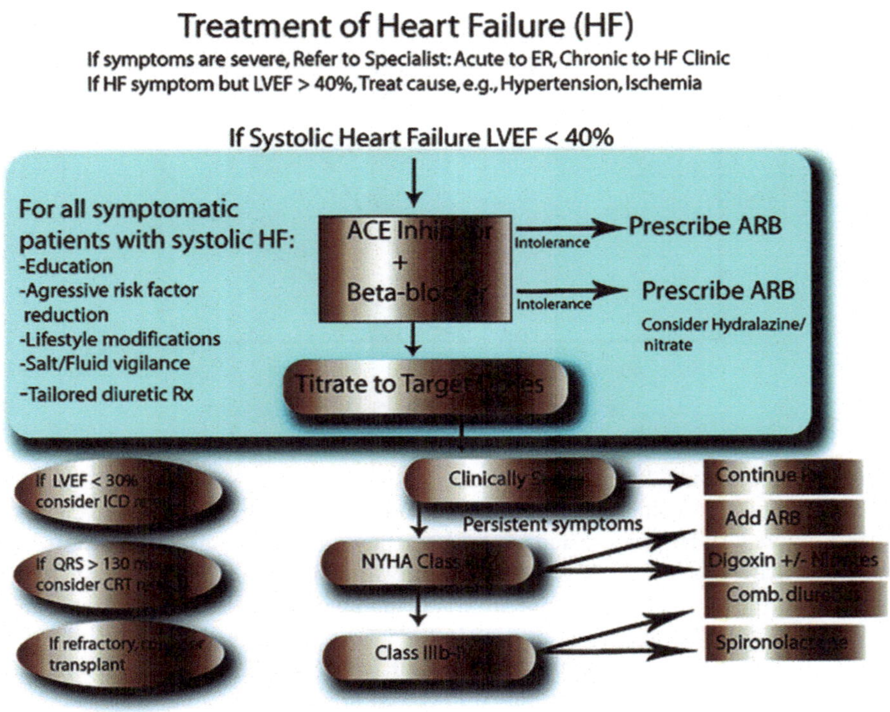

Treatment algorithm of patients with chronic heart failure. [Marín-García J. Treatment of Chronic Heart Failure. Heart Failure [Internet]. Totowa, NJ: Humana Press; 2010 [cited 2015 Jun 4]. p. 379–92. Available from: http://link.springer.com/10.1007/978-1-60761-147-9_20] *Caption from original*

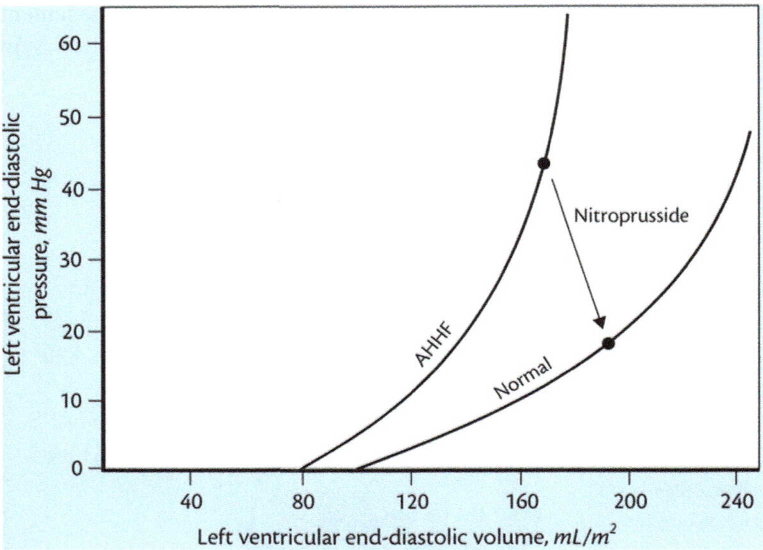

Treatment of acute hypertensive heart failure. The left ventricular (LV) end-diastolic pressure-volume relationships (compliance curves) in acute hypertensive heart failure (AHHF) before and after treatment with sodium nitroprusside are represented schematically. In AHHF, the pressure-volume curve is shifted up and to the left, reflecting an acute decrease in LV compliance caused by severe systemic hypertension. In this setting, a higher than normal LV end-diastolic pressure (LVEDP) is required to achieve any given level of LV end-diastolic volume (LVEDV). Normal LV systolic function (ejection fraction and cardiac output) is maintained but at the expense of a very high wedge pressure that results in acute pulmonary edema. Treatment with sodium nitroprusside causes a reduction in the elevated systemic vascular resistance, with a concomitant decrease in impedance to LV ejection. As a result, LV compliance improves. Pulmonary edema resolves owing to a reduction in LVEDP, despite the fact that LVEDV actually increases during treatment. Sodium nitroprusside is the preferred drug for treatment of AHHF. There is no absolute blood pressure goal. The infusion should be titrated until signs and symptoms of pulmonary edema resolve or the blood pressure decreases to hypotensive levels. Rarely is it necessary to lower the blood pressure to this extent, however, because reduction to levels still within the hypertensive range is usually associated with dramatic clinical improvement. Although hemodynamic monitoring is not always required, it is essential in patients in whom concomitant myocardial ischemia or compromised cardiac output is suspected. After the hypertensive crisis has been controlled and pulmonary edema has resolved, oral antihypertensive therapy can be substituted as the patient is weaned from the nitroprusside infusion. As in the treatment of hypertensive patients with chronic congestive heart failure symptoms owing to isolated diastolic dysfunction, agents such as β-blockers, angiotension-converting enzyme inhibitors, or calcium channel blockers may represent logical first-line therapy. These agents directly improve diastolic function in addition to reducing systemic blood pressure. In patients with malignant hypertension or resistant hypertension, however, adequate control of blood pressure may require therapy with more than one drug. Potent direct-acting vasodilators such as hydralazine or minoxidil may be used in conjunction with a β-blocker to control reflex tachycardia and a diuretic to prevent reflex salt and water retention. [Nolan CR. Hypertensive Crises. In: Schrier RW, Wilcox CS. Atlas of Diseases of the Kidney, Volume 3: Hypertension and the Kidney. Philadelphia: Current Medicine Group; 1999. 182 p.] *Caption from original*

Goals of Treatment in Decompensated Heart Failure

Clinical goals	**Hemodynamic goals**
Resolution of dyspnea and orthopnea	Systolic blood pressure ≥ 80 mm Hg
Resolution of ascites and peripheral edema	Right atrial pressure ≤ 8 mm Hg
Jugular venous pressure ≤ 8 cm H_2O	Pulmonary capillary wedge pressure ≤ 16 mm Hg
Control of hypertension	Systemic vascular resistance ≤ 1200 dynes/s/cm-5
Minimize adverse effects of treatment, reduce duration and cost of stay	
Initiate treatments that improve long-term outcome	

Goals of treatment in decompensated heart failure. Goals of in-patient therapy. The early goal of treatment is to improve symptoms while maintaining or improving the hemodynamic status. Progress may be tracked by following body weights and fluid intake and output while monitoring vital signs, electrolytes, and renal function. Consideration also should be given to identifying precipitating factors and etiology, and patients who may benefit from coronary revascularization. [Givertz MM, Colucci WS. Heart Failure. In: Libby P, editor. Essential Atlas of Cardiovascular Disease. 4th ed. Philadelphia: Current Medicine Group; 2009. 432 p.] Caption adapted from original

Drug	Dosing	Potential Advantage	Potential Disadvantages
Nitroglycerin	Sublingual: 1 tablet (or 1–2 sprays) three or four times at 5-minute intervals; IV: 0.4 μg/kg/min initially (increase as needed)	Favorable effect on coronary vasculature and in myocardial ischemia/infarction; preload reduction > afterload	Tolerance during prolonged infusion; inadequate afterload reduction in catastrophic cardiovascular disorders (*eg*, acute valvular insufficiency, ventricular rupture)
Nitroprusside	IV: 0.1 μg/kg/min initially; increase as needed	Relatively powerful preload and afterload reduction	Less favorable effects on coronary vasculature and myocardial ischemia; administration must be closely monitored to avoid marked hypotension; thiocyanate or cyanide toxicity during high-dose or prolonged infusions, particularly in patients with renal or hepatic dysfunction
Nesiritide	0.005–0.01 μg/kg/min initially, ± bolus; increase as needed	Preload and afterload reduction; possible facilitative effect on diuresis	Hypotension; meta-analysis of clinical trials suggests adverse effects on mortality and renal function

Principal preload- and afterload-reducing drugs for acute or severe heart failure. Nesiritide, nitroglycerin, and nitroprusside are the primary vasodilators used to reduce excessive preload and afterload in acute or severe heart failure. Nitroglycerin is used most often, particularly in conditions caused by occlusive atherosclerotic coronary artery disease. Nitroprusside is the drug of choice when more aggressive afterload and preload reduction are needed; examples include catastrophic cardiovascular events (eg, acute, severe mitral, or aortic regurgitation), hypertensive emergencies (eg, aortic dissection, pulmonary edema), and inadequate response to nesiritide or nitroglycerin. [Ooi H, Colucci WS. Management of the Hospitalized Patient. In: Colucci WS, editor. Atlas of heart failure, 5th ed. Philadelphia: Current Medicine Group; 2008. 344 p. ISBN: 1-57340-261-3] *Caption adapted from original*

Disease Course

- Prognosis depends on type and severity of failure.
- With aggressive medical therapy, ventricular assist devices, and even cardiac transplant, even severe heart disease is no longer a short-term mortality diagnosis.
- Patient compliance with management is an important predictor of both outcomes and quality of life.

Related Evidence

Papers of particular interest have been highlighted as:
*** Of key importance*

Practice Guideline

Moe GW, Ezekowitz JA, O'Meara E, Lepage S, Howlett JG, Fremes S, Al-Hesayen A, Heckman GA, Abrams H, Ducharme A, Estrella-Holder E, Grzeslo A, Harkness K, Koshman SL, McDonald M, McKelvie R, Rajda M, Rao V, Swiggum E, Virani S, Zieroth S, Arnold JM, Ashton T, D'Astous M, Chan M, De S, Dorian P, Giannetti N, Haddad H, Isaac DL, Kouz S, Leblanc MH, Liu P, Ross HJ, Sussex B, White M; Canadian Cardiovascular Society. The 2014 Canadian Cardiovascular Society Heart Failure Management Guidelines Focus Update: anemia, biomarkers, and recent therapeutic trial implications. Can J Cardiol. 2015 Jan;31(1):3-16. https://doi.org/10.1016/j.cjca.2014.10.022. PMID: 25532421. http://www.ncbi.nlm.nih.gov/pubmed/25532421 **

Dworzynski K, Roberts E, Ludman A, Mant J; Guideline Development Group of the National Institute for Health and Care Excellence. Diagnosing and managing acute heart failure in adults: summary of NICE guidance. BMJ. 2014 Oct 8;349:g5695. https://doi.org/10.1136/bmj.g5695. PMID: 25296764. http://www.ncbi.nlm.nih.gov/pubmed/25296764 **

National Clinical Guideline Centre (UK). Acute Heart Failure: Diagnosing and Managing Acute Heart Failure in Adults. London: National Institute for Health and Care Excellence (UK); 2014 Oct. PMID: 25340219. http://www.ncbi.nlm.nih.gov/pubmed/25340219 **

Page K, Marwick TH, Lee R, Grenfell R, Abhayaratna WP, Aggarwal A, Briffa TG, Cameron J, Davidson PM, Driscoll A, Garton-Smith J, Gascard DJ, Hickey A, Korczyk D, Mitchell JA, Sanders R, Spicer D, Stewart S, Wade V; National Heart Foundation of Australia. A systematic approach to chronic heart failure care: a consensus statement. Med J Aust. 2014 Aug 4;201(3):146-50. PMID: 25128948. http://www.ncbi.nlm.nih.gov/pubmed/25128948 **

Yancy CW, Jessup M, Bozkurt B, Butler J, Casey DE Jr, Drazner MH, Fonarow GC, Geraci SA, Horwich T, Januzzi JL, Johnson MR, Kasper EK, Levy WC, Masoudi FA, McBride PE, McMurray JJ, Mitchell JE, Peterson PN, Riegel B, Sam F, Stevenson LW, Tang WH, Tsai EJ, Wilkoff BL; American College of Cardiology Foundation/American Heart Association Task Force on Practice Guidelines. 2013 ACCF/AHA guideline for the management of heart failure: a report of the American College of Cardiology Foundation/American Heart Association Task Force on practice guidelines. Circulation. 2013 Oct 15;128(16):e240-327. https://doi.org/10.1161/CIR.0b013e31829e8776. PMID: 23741058. http://www.ncbi.nlm.nih.gov/pubmed/23741058 **

White RD, Patel MR, Abbara S, Bluemke DA, Herfkens RJ, Picard M, Shaw LJ, Silver M, Stillman AE, Udelson J; American College of Radiology; American College of Cardiology Foundation. 2013 ACCF/ACR/ASE/ASNC/SCCT/SCMR appropriate utilization of cardiovascular imaging in heart failure: an executive summary: a joint report of the ACR Appropriateness Criteria ® Committee and the ACCF Appropriate Use Criteria Task Force. J Am Coll Radiol. 2013 Jul;10(7):493-500. https://doi.org/10.1016/j.jacr.2013.05.002. PMID: 23827001. http://www.ncbi.nlm.nih.gov/pubmed/23827001 **

Review

Oktay AA, Shah SJ. Diagnosis and management of heart failure with preserved ejection fraction: 10 key lessons. Curr Cardiol Rev. 2015;11(1):42-52. PMID: 24251461. http://www.ncbi.nlm.nih.gov/pubmed/24251461 **

Ferrero P, Iacovoni A, D'Elia E, Vaduganathan M, Gavazzi A, Senni M. Prognostic scores in heart failure - Critical appraisal and practical use. Int J Cardiol. 2015 Mar 26;188:1-9. https://doi.org/10.1016/j.ijcard.2015.03.154. PMID: 25880571. http://www.ncbi.nlm.nih.gov/pubmed/25880571 **

Use PubMed Clinical Queries to find the most recent evidence. Use this search strategy:

"Heart Failure"[Mesh] OR "Heart Failure"

Chapter 33
Hemoptysis

Charles V. Pollack, Jr., Richard M. Cantor, and Victoria G. Riese

Name and Synonyms

Hemoptysis

Incidence/Epidemiology

- Hemoptysis is the expectoration of blood from the respiratory tract with cough. Because coughing sometimes leads to vomiting (tussive emesis), it is important to distinguish between hemoptysis and hematemesis.
- Hemoptysis may range in severity from scant blood-streaked mucous that is self-limited to life-threatening airway obstruction from blood clots or diminished gas exchange in blood-filled alveoli.
- Because there are so many varied causes of hemoptysis, epidemiologic data are not meaningful. Smokers and those with chronic lung or sinus disease are more likely to have hemoptysis.

C. V. Pollack, Jr. (✉)
Department of Emergency Medicine, Thomas Jefferson University, Philadelphia, PA, USA

R. M. Cantor
Department of Emergency Medicine and Pediatrics, State University of New York Upstate Medical University, Syracuse, NY, USA

V. G. Riese
Librarian Consultant, Eldersburg, MD, USA

C. V. Pollack, Jr. (ed.), *Differential Diagnosis of Cardiopulmonary Disease*,
https://doi.org/10.1007/978-3-319-63895-9_33

Hemoptysis	Massive	Exsanguinating
One expectoration (mL)		>300
mL by hour	>25	>150
mL by 24 h	>600	>1,000

Definition of hemoptysis. [Bussières JS. Massive hemoptysis. In: Slinger P, editor. Principles and practice of anesthesia for thoracic surgery [Internet]. New York: Springer; 2011 [cited 2015 May 28]. p. 485–96. Available from: http://link.springer.com/10.1007/978-1-4419-0184-2_34] *Caption from original*

Differential Diagnosis

- The important first differential issue to address is whether the bleeding is a result of a respiratory or gastrointestinal (GI) cause. The possibility of epistaxis as a cause should also be evaluated. Beyond that, the differential concerns regard the *cause* of hemoptysis, which generally may be divided into these categories:
  - Infectious
  - Vascular
  - Iatrogenic
  - Coagulopathic
  - Traumatic
  - Neoplastic
  - Pulmonary miscellaneous

Infections • Mycobacteria, particularly tuberculosis • Fungal infections (mycetoma) • Lung abscess • Necrotising pneumonia (Klebsiella, Staphylococcus, Legionella)	Vascular • Pulmonary embolism and infarction • Mitral stenosis • Arteriobronchial fistula • Arteriovenous malformations • Bronchial telangiectasia • Left ventricular failure
Iatrogenic • Bronchoscopy • Swan–Ganz catheterization • Transbronchial biopsy • Transtracheal aspirate	Coagulopathy • Von Willebrand's disease • Hemophilia • Anticoagulant therapy • Thrombocytopenia • Platelet dysfunction • Disseminated intravascular coagulation • Vasculitis • Behcet's disease • Wegener's granulomatosis
Parasitic • Hydatid cyst • Paragonimiasis	
Trauma • Blunt/penetrating injury • Suction ulcers • Tracheoarterial fistula	
Neoplasm • Bronchogenic carcinoma • Bronchial adenoma • Pulmonary metastases • Sarcoma	Pulmonary • Bronchiectasis (including cystic fibrosis) • Chronic bronchitis • Emphysematous bullae
Hemoptysis in children • Foreign body aspiration • Bronchial adenoma • Vascular anomalies	Miscellaneous • Lymphangioleiomyometosis • Catamenial (endometriosis) • Pneumoconiosis • Broncholith • Idiopathic
	Spurious • Epistaxis • Hematemesis

Causes of hemoptysis. [Subramanian S, Kate AH, Chhajed PN. Role of bronchoscopy in hemoptysis. In: Mehta A, Jain P, editors. Interventional bronchoscopy [Internet]. Totowa, NJ: Humana Press; 2013 [cited 2015 May 28]. p. 245–56. Available from: http://link.springer.com/10.1007/978-1-62703-395-4_14] *Caption from original*

Pathophysiology and Etiology

- Hemoptysis may result from several different processes.
- The two most common causes are bronchitis and other lung infections and endobronchial carcinoma with erosion into a bronchial vessel.
- Many patients may never have a definitive cause identified.
- Hemoptysis may result from inflammation/infection or from physical injury to a bronchial vessel.

- Hemoptysis may also result from the high pulmonary venous pressure that results from severe mitral valve stenosis
- The mnemonic "BATTLE CAMP" may be helpful in remembering common etiologies of hemoptysis:

B	Bronchitis, bronchiectasis
A	Aspergillosis, alveolar hemorrhage
T	Tumor, trauma
T	Tuberculosis
L	Lung abscess
E	Emboli
C	Coagulopathy
A	Autoimmune, AVM
M	Mitral stenosis
P	Pneumonia
Others	Tracheostomy related, foreign bodies, aortopulmonary collaterals

Causes of hemoptysis—"Battlecamp." [Hogan MJ. Bronchial artery interventions in children. In: Temple M, Marshalleck FE, editors. Pediatric interventional radiology [Internet]. New York: Springer; 2014 [cited 2015 May 28]. p. 71–83. Available from: http://link.springer.com/10.1007/978-1-4419-5856-3_6] Caption from original

Presentation

Typical/"Classic"

- Patients who present "coughing up blood" usually are hemodynamically stable (massive hemoptysis that causes shock is a medical emergency).
- Patients may not be able to distinguish among cough with expectoration of blood caused by pulmonary sources, posterior epistaxis, and GI bleeding with hematemesis.
- The amount of blood loss should be quickly assessed, and that will drive the pace of evaluation and management.

Atypical

- "Rusty"-colored sputum may not be recognized as hemoptysis.

Primary Differential Considerations

- Primary differential considerations for hemoptysis are limited to:
- Epistaxis
- Hematemesis
  - To help differentiate, remember that blood from the GI tract likely has been exposed to the acidic pH of the stomach and will be darker, whereas blood from the respiratory tract tends to be a brighter red, although chronic infection/tumor may result in expectoration of "older" blood that is darker in color.
- Airway foreign bodies

History and Physical Exam

- Expectoration of even small amounts of blood may provoke significant anxiety in patients, and their quantification of the amount of blood loss may be exaggerated.
- The first historical factors to be established include:
  - Timeframe—how long has hemoptysis been occurring?
  - Course—is it getting worse or better?
  - Character of hemoptysis—is it blood-streaked sputum or is it frank blood?
  - Associated issues—fever and chills? Night sweats? Weight loss? Using an anticoagulant or antiplatelet drug? Any chronic lung disease?
  - Is there pleuritic chest pain with or without dyspnea, suggesting a pulmonary embolism? Are there any signs of deep venous thrombosis?
  - Is the patient a smoker?
- On physical examination, the lungs should be auscultated for evidence of bronchospasm, consolidation, or pleural friction.
- Check the heart sounds for a murmur of mitral stenosis.

Mitral stenosis murmur. [Mitral stenosis (diastolic murmur); Easy Auscultation; www.easyauscultation.com; copyright 2015, MedEdu LLC]
http://www.easyauscultation.com/cases?coursecaseorder=14&courseid=31

Bronchiectasis	Pulmonary tuberculosis
Fungal infections in cavities—aspergilloma	Bronchogenic carcinoma
Severe mitral stenosis	Coagulopathies
Foreign bodies	Trauma
Vasculitis	Pulmonary embolism

Causes of severe hemoptysis. [Bansal A, Kantroo V. Massive hemoptysis. In: Chawla R, Todi S, editors. ICU protocols [Internet]. India: Springer India; 2012 [cited 2015 May 28]. p. 65–70. Available from: http://www.springerlink.com/index/10.1007/978-81-322-0535-7_8] *Caption from original*

Findings That Confirm Diagnosis

- Witnessed expectoration of blood confirms the diagnosis; without firsthand evidence, it is difficult to know with certainty that there is a respiratory tract source.

Factors That Suggest Diagnosis

- A reported history of hemoptysis in a patient at risk for one or more common etiologies of hemoptysis (acute or chronic lung infection, chronic obstructive pulmonary disease [COPD], mitral stenosis, coagulopathy, or pulmonary embolism) should prompt diagnostic evaluation for one of these causes.

Factors That Exclude Diagnosis

- Clinically, hemoptysis cannot be excluded. The history of blood expectoration should be evaluated thoroughly on the supposition that the patient's history is accurate.

Ancillary Studies

Laboratory

- Patients with active hemoptysis and those with a history of repeated or chronic episodes should be evaluated with a complete blood count (CBC).
- Patients on warfarin anticoagulation should be checked for international normalized ratio (INR); patients on unfractionated heparin should be evalu-

ated for activated partial thromboplastin time (aPTT); patients taking an injectable low-molecular-weight heparin should be checked for renal function, and the time of last dose should be noted.

- D-dimer testing may be helpful in determining possible pulmonary embolism.
- Sputum evaluation may be helpful.

Electrocardiography

- In general, ECG should be performed in ill patients but is unlikely to be particularly helpful in the evaluation of hemoptysis.

Imaging

- Chest x-ray is an essential first step in evaluating hemoptysis. Look for mass lesions, infection, signs of chronic lung disease, or evidence of a foreign body.
- A computed tomographic pulmonary angiogram is indicated if pulmonary embolism is suspected.

Other Studies

- Bronchoscopy may be indicated.

Special Populations

Age

- Older patients have a higher risk of lung cancer, COPD, pulmonary embolism, and pneumonia.
- Hemoptysis in children is less common than in adults and has a different differential diagnosis. Infection of the lungs is less likely to manifest as hemoptysis in children. Instead, consider foreign body aspiration or
  - bronchial adenoma
  - congenital vascular anomalies

Co-morbidities

- COPD
- Lung cancer
- Bronchitis
- Pneumonia
- Therapeutic anticoagulation
- Tobacco abuse

Pitfalls in Diagnosis

Critical Steps Not to Miss

- Evaluation for satisfactory oxygenation
- Evaluation for hemodynamic stability
- Evaluation for correctable coagulopathy
- Altered mental status may signal respiratory failure.
- Chest x-ray should be done early.

Mimics

- Upper GI bleed
- Posterior epistaxis

Time-Dependent Interventions

- Immediate evaluation for adequate gas exchange and hemodynamic stability
- Chest x-ray early

Overall Principles of Treatment

- Stabilize hemodynamic and ventilatory status.
- Evaluate for etiology.
- Treat accordingly with antibiotics, bronchoscopic intervention, reversal of anticoagulation, etc.

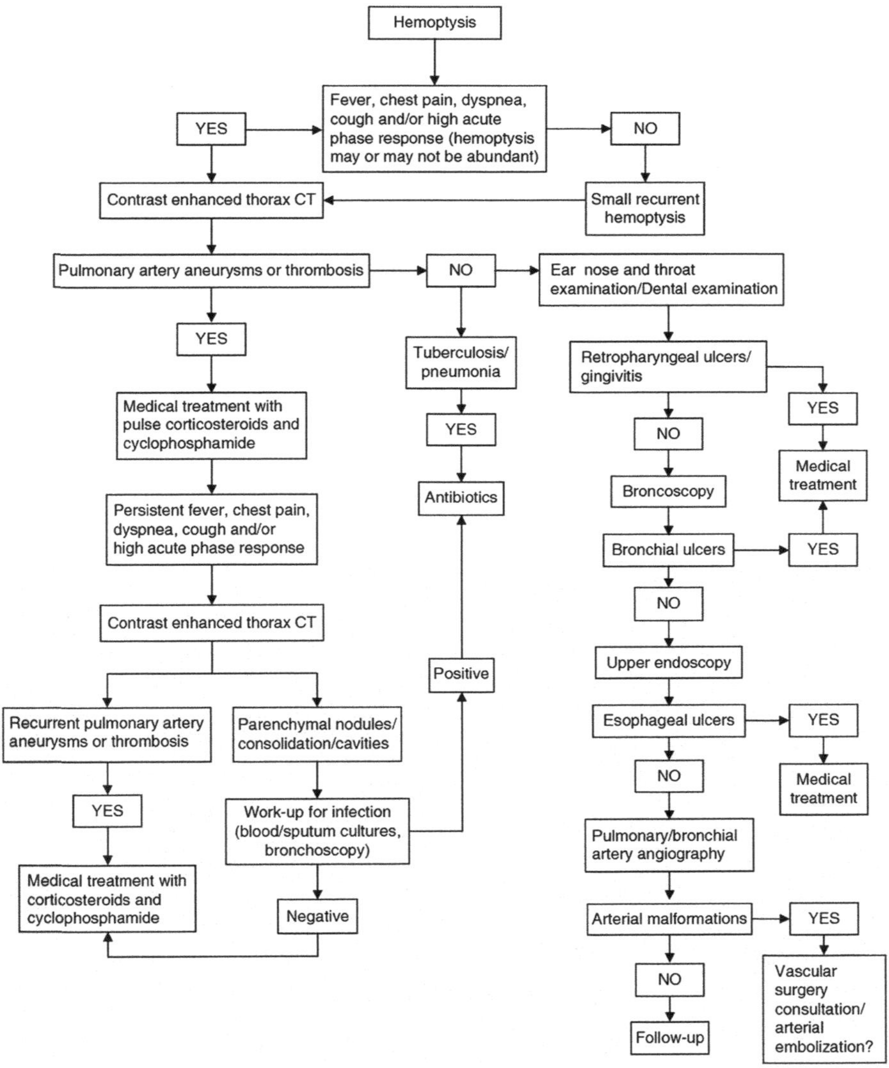

Algorithm for diagnosis and management of hemoptysis due to Behçet's syndrome. [Seyahi E, Tascilar K, Yazici H. Behçet's syndrome: clinical presentations affecting prognosis and survival. In: Khamashta MA, Ramos-Casals M, editors. Autoimmune diseases [Internet]. London: Springer; 2011 [cited 2015 May 28]. p. 163–84. Available from: http://link.springer.com/10.1007/978-0-85729-358-9_11] *Caption from original*

Disease Course

- Course is determined by acuity of presentation and underlying etiology.
- The vast majority of hemoptysis cases are not life threatening, although the underlying etiology may be significant.

Related Evidence

Papers of particular interest have been highlighted as:
*** Of key importance*

Review

Ketai LH, Mohammed TL, Kirsch J, Kanne JP, Chung JH, Donnelly EF, Ginsburg ME, Heitkamp DE, Henry TS, Kazerooni EA, Lorenz JM, McComb BL, Ravenel JG, Saleh AG, Shah RD, Steiner RM, Suh RD; Expert Panel on Thoracic Imaging. ACR appropriateness criteria® hemoptysis. J Thorac Imaging. 2014 May;29(3):W19-22. https://doi.org/10.1097/RTI.0000000000000084. PMID: 24717602. http://www.ncbi.nlm.nih.gov/pubmed/24717602 **

Singh D, Bhalla AS, Veedu PT, Arora A. Imaging evaluation of hemoptysis in children. World J Clin Pediatr. 2013 Nov 8;2(4):54-64. https://doi.org/10.5409/wjcp.v2.i4.54. eCollection 2013 Nov 8. PMID: 25254175. http://www.ncbi.nlm.nih.gov/pubmed/25254175 **

Jaroszewski DE, Webb BJ, Leslie KO. Diagnosis and management of lung infections. Thorac Surg Clin. 2012 Aug;22(3):301-24. https://doi.org/10.1016/j.thorsurg.2012.05.002. PMID: 22789595. http://www.ncbi.nlm.nih.gov/pubmed/22789595 **

Hurt K, Bilton D. Haemoptysis: diagnosis and treatment. Acute Med. 2012;11(1):39-45. PMID: 22423349. http://www.ncbi.nlm.nih.gov/pubmed/22423349 **

Kapur S, Louie BE. Hemoptysis and thoracic fungal infections. Surg Clin North Am. 2010 Oct;90(5):985-1001. https://doi.org/10.1016/j.suc.2010.06.006. PMID: 20955879. http://www.ncbi.nlm.nih.gov/pubmed/20955879 **

Dudha M, Lehrman S, Aronow WS, Rosa J. Hemoptysis: diagnosis and treatment. Compr Ther. 2009 Fall-Winter;35(3-4):139-49. PMID: 20043609. http://www.ncbi.nlm.nih.gov/pubmed/20043609 **

Fartoukh M, Parrot A, Khalil A. Aetiology, diagnosis and management of infective causes of severe haemoptysis in intensive care units. Curr Opin Pulm Med. 2008 May;14(3):195-202. https://doi.org/10.1097/MCP.0b013e3282f79663. PMID: 18427242. http://www.ncbi.nlm.nih.gov/pubmed/18427242 **

Bidwell JL, Pachner RW. Hemoptysis: diagnosis and management. Am Fam Physician. 2005 Oct 1;72(7):1253-60. PMID: 16225028. http://www.ncbi.nlm.nih.gov/pubmed/16225028 **

Use PubMed Clinical Queries to find the most recent evidence. Use this search strategy:
"Hemoptysis"[Mesh] OR "Hemoptysis"

Chapter 34
Herpes Zoster

Christopher J. Rees, Charles V. Pollack, Jr., and Victoria G. Riese

Name and Synonyms

Herpes Zoster; Shingles

Incidence/Epidemiology

- The Centers for Disease Control and Prevention (CDC) estimates that up to one-third of the adult population in the United States will be diagnosed with shingles at some point in their lives.
- There are about 1 million to 1.2 million cases annually in the United States.
- It may occur in all adult age groups, but the incidence increases dramatically after age 50.
- It is unusual in children.
- Shingles has a very low mortality and is rarely life threatening but has substantial morbidity, mostly as the result of postherpetic neuralgia (PHN).
- Most cases occur in healthy individuals, but the incidence increases among the immunocompromised.

C. J. Rees
Emergency Department, Pennsylvania Hospital, Philadelphia, PA, USA

C. V. Pollack, Jr. (✉)
Department of Emergency Medicine, Thomas Jefferson University, Philadelphia, PA, USA

V. G. Riese
Librarian Consultant, Eldersburg, MD, USA

C. V. Pollack, Jr. (ed.), *Differential Diagnosis of Cardiopulmonary Disease*,
https://doi.org/10.1007/978-3-319-63895-9_34

Differential Diagnosis

- Coxsackievirus and herpes simplex virus also may cause a vesicular rash in a dermatomal distribution.

Pathophysiology and Etiology

- The varicella-zoster virus (VZV) causes shingles.
- Primary infection with VZV causes chickenpox.
- After primary infection, the virus may become dormant in the dorsal root ganglia of the spinal cord. It may lie dormant for decades, but in response to immunosuppression, or the waning of innate immunity due to aging, the virus may reactivate. The virus travels down the corresponding sensory nerve of the involved dorsal root ganglion to cause the rash along those sensory dermatomes. Reactivation usually involves just one dermatome, but may involve several or many dermatomes, especially if there is an underlying immunosuppression.
- The exact mechanisms and causes of reactivation are unknown.

Presentation

Typical/"Classic"

- Symptoms usually start with pain in one sensory dermatome. Patients also often note paresthesias or itching in the area of pain. The dermatomal distribution of the pain sometimes is not recognized by either the patient or the physician.
- In retrospect, most patients also describe a prodrome of malaise with a mild headache.
- The rash classically erupts within 1-10 days (most typically 3) of symptom onset.
- The skin lesions often start as an erythematous maculopapular rash. Vesicles then erupt. The vesicles are generally small and closely grouped into clusters of lesions. The grouped vesicles remain on an erythematous base. The vesicles initially contain clear fluid, but the fluid becomes cloudy and appears more purulent over the next several days. Ultimately the lesions dry, ulcerate, and crust over. It may be 2 weeks until the lesions crust, and then another 2 weeks for the scabs to fall off.
- The lesions do not cross the midline.
- The vesicles may be of differing sizes, and they may be of differing stages in the same areasimialr to primary chicken pox.
- The thorax and face are the most commonly affected areas, but shingles may occur anywhere on the body.

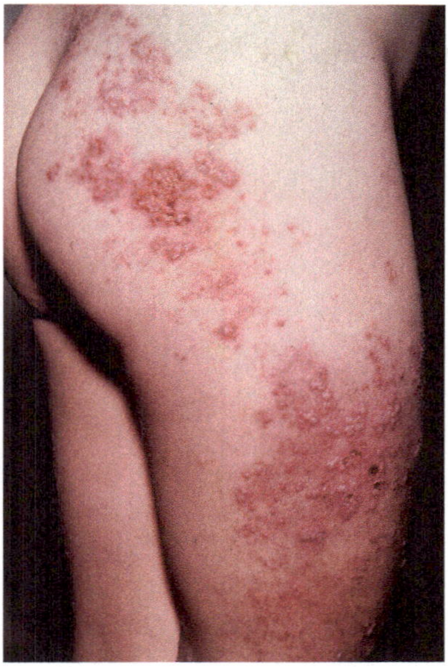

Vesicles in a dermatomal distribution represent herpes zoster. [Allen HB. Vesiculobullous Disorders (Including Dermatitis/Eczema). In: Dermatology Terminology [Internet]. London: Springer London; 2010 [cited 2016 Aug 22]. p. 15–32. Available from: http://link.springer.com/10.1007/978-1-84882-840-7_2] *Caption from original*

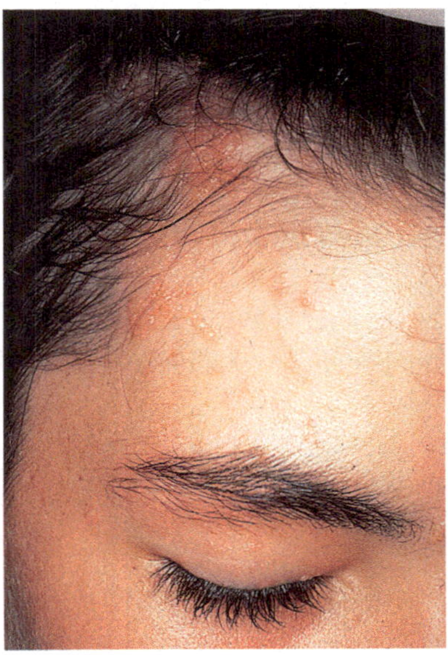

Early stage of shingles with clear vesicles on an erythematous base. [Gilsdorf J, Shope T. Viral exanthems of childhood. In: Fekety R, editor. External manifestations of systemic infections. Philadelphia: Current Medicine; 1996. 237 p. (Mandell GL, editor. Atlas of infectious diseases; vol. 6.) ISBN: 0-443-07760-6]

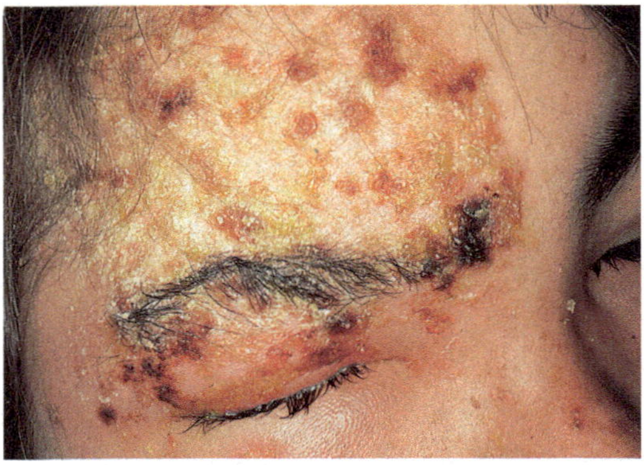

More developed stage of shingles with crusting. [Gilsdorf J, Shope T. Viral exanthems of childhood. In: Fekety R, editor. External manifestations of systemic infections. Philadelphia: Current Medicine; 1996. 237 p. (Mandell GL, editor. Atlas of infectious diseases; vol. 6.) ISBN: 0-443-07760-6]

Atypical

- Shingles may occur less commonly in more than one dermatome, or be generalized.
- There is some thought and evidence that zoster may cause a syndrome of dermatomal pain without a rash: zoster sine herpetica.

Primary Differential Considerations

- Pain from shingles may precede the appearance of the rash, making early diagnosis more challenging. Differential diagnoses that should be considered include:
  - Acute coronary syndrome
  - Pulmonary embolism
  - Pleurisy

History and Physical Exam

Findings That Confirm Diagnosis

- Shingles is a clinical diagnosis. A full classic presentation of prodromal pain with development of the classic rash confirms the diagnosis.

Factors That Suggest Diagnosis

- Any rash or pain in a dermatomal distribution should suggest the diagnosis.

Factors That Exclude Diagnosis

- There are no historical or physical exam findings that can exclude the diagnosis.

Ancillary Studies

Laboratory

- Laboratory studies often are not required to make the diagnosis.
- Confirmatory testing may include antigen testing, viral culture, and polymerase chain reaction (PCR) on vesicular fluid. Culture and PCR generally are not available clinically; they usually are research techniques.
- The diagnosis may be suggested by performing a Tzanck smear. A fresh vesicle is unroofed, the bottom of the lesion is superficially scraped, and a slide is made of the scraped material. The presence of multinucleated giant cells may confirm the diagnosis; however, the false negative rate is high.

Imaging

- There are no diagnostic imaging findings that are helpful in the diagnosis of shingles.

Special Populations

Age

- It may occur in all adult age groups, but the incidence increases dramatically after age 50.
- It is unusual in children.

Co-morbidities

- Co-morbidities of importance are any type of immune compromise, including:
  - iatrogenic, from immune suppressive therapy for organ transplants, and long-term glucocorticoid therapy
  - lymphoproliferative disorders (especially leukemia and Hodgkin's lymphoma) and HIV
- The incidence of shingles increases with immune suppression, as does the risk for complications.
- Patients who have undergone hematopoietic stem cell transplantation are at particularly increased risk for shingles and its complications.

Pitfalls in Diagnosis

Critical Steps Not to Miss

- Always consider this diagnosis.

Mimics

- Coxsackievirus and herpes simplex virus also may cause a vesicular rash in a dermatomal distribution.
- Shingles may cause severe pain and can mimic many other causes of acute, severe pain if the patient presents before the rash develops.

Time-Dependent Interventions

- The only time-dependent intervention in shingles is to start treatment with antivirals within 3 days of the eruption of the rash.
- Treatment within this timeframe has been shown to reduce the incidence of developing PHN, especially in those over 50.

Overall Principles of Treatment

- The primary goal of treatment is to reduce the incidence and severity of PHN.
- This is accomplished by starting antivirals (typically valacyclovir) within 72 hours of the onset of the rash.
- Immunocompromised patients should be treated regardless of the timing from the onset of rash.
- Adjunctive corticosteroids may be considered for severe pain or for older patients with no contraindications to their use.
- Administering the shingles vaccine in those over 65 may help reduce the incidence and severity of shingles, and also reduces the incidence of PHN by up to two-thirds.
- Admission for intravenous antivirals is often indicated for disseminated shingles, central nervous system (CNS) shingles, and severely immunocompromised patients.

Disease Course

- The rash usually dries and crusts within 2 weeks. Crusts fall off over the next 2 weeks.
- Recurrence occurs in only 1–4 %. Recurrence should make one consider underlying immunocompromise.
- Complications may be serious and debilitating, and they account for most of the morbidity associated with shingles.
- PHN is the continuation of pain (often severe) for more than 30 days after the rash resolves. PHN is the most common complication of shingles. It is more common in older and immunocompromised patients. The incidence rises from 5 % in those under 60 to greater than 20 % in those over 80. The pain from PHN may be debilitating and may last for months to years. At least 50 % of affected patients over age 50 report some pain in the involved dermatome even months after resolution of rash. Many patients with PHN also describe sensory changes over the affected dermatome. The incidence may be reduced by the appropriate use of the shingles vaccine.
- Multidermatomal (disseminated zoster) is much more common in the immunocompromised. If shingles disseminates, the risk for other complications rises by 5–10 %. If an otherwise young, healthy person presents with shingles in three or more dermatomes, it is important to consider underlying immunosuppression (such as HIV).
- Shingles occurring along the ophthalmic division of the trigeminal nerve may cause zoster ophthalmicus. Shingles involving the eye may lead to severe retinitis and blindness. Patients with zoster in this distribution should be evaluated and followed up by an ophthalmologist. Vesicles present on the tip of the nose should increase suspicion of zoster ophthalmicus.

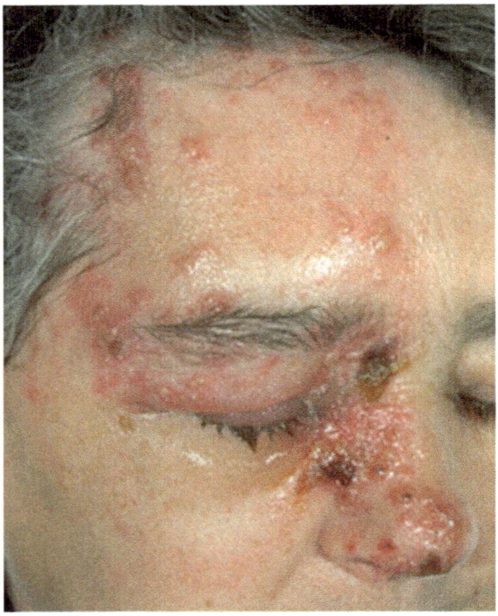

Zoster ophthalmicus. Note lesions on tip of nose. [Wassilew SW, Wutzler P. Schutz vor zoster: impfung blockiert virusreaktivierung. Präv Gesundheitsf. 2010 Jun;5(S1):23–7.]

- Ramsay-Hunt syndrome (zoster oticus) may occur when shingles involves the sensory branch of the facial nerve. The classic triad of Ramsay-Hunt is pain and vesicles in the external auditory canal, loss of taste on the anterior two-thirds of the tongue, and ipsilateral facial palsy. The facial palsy may be prolonged and severe. The presence of Ramsay-Hunt is a risk factor for CNS zoster.

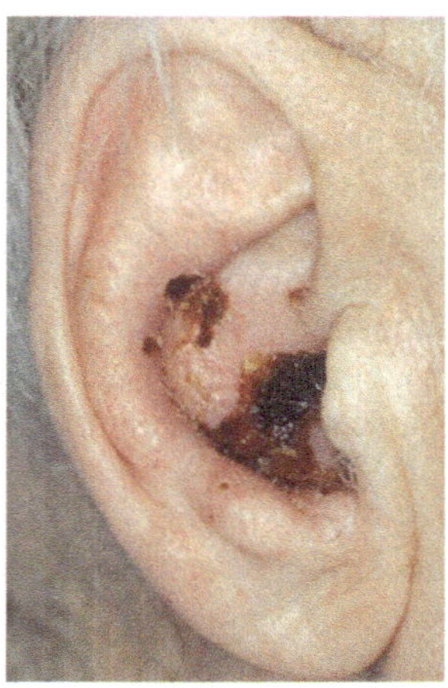

Zoster oticus. Note lesions in the external auditory canal. [Weisshaar E, Kallen U, Klintworth N, Zenk J. Pruritus, erytheme & co: das ohr aus dermatologischer sicht. HNO. 2011 Mar;59(3):301–10.]

- Shingles rarely may involve the CNS. CNS involvement can manifest as meningoencephalitis, transverse myelitis (with or without motor involvement), or, very rarely, granulomatous angiitis.

Related Evidence

Papers of particular interest have been highlighted as:
*** Of key importance*

Practice Guideline

Dworkin RH, Johnson RW, Breuer J, Gnann JW, Levin MJ, Backonja M, Betts RF, Gershon AA, Haanpaa ML, McKendrick MW, Nurmikko TJ, Oaklander AL, Oxman MN, Pavan-Langston D, Petersen KL, Rowbotham MC, Schmader KE, Stacey BR, Tyring SK, van Wijck AJ, Wallace MS, Wassilew SW, Whitley RJ. Recommendations for the management of herpes zoster. Clin Infect Dis. 2007 Jan 1;44 Suppl 1:S1-26. PMID: 17143845. http://www.ncbi.nlm.nih.gov/pubmed/17143845 **

Review

Gershon AA, Gershon MD. Pathogenesis and current approaches to control of varicella-zoster virus infections. Clin Microbiol Rev. 2013 Oct;26(4):728-43. https://doi.org/10.1128/CMR.00052-13. PMID: 24092852. http://www.ncbi.nlm.nih.gov/pubmed/24092852 **

Cohen JI. Clinical practice: Herpes zoster. N Engl J Med. 2013 Jul 18;369(3):255-63. https://doi.org/10.1056/NEJMcp1302674. PMID: 23863052. http://www.ncbi.nlm.nih.gov/pubmed/23863052 **

O'Connor KM, Paauw DS. Herpes zoster. Med Clin North Am. 2013 Jul;97(4):503-22, ix. https://doi.org/10.1016/j.mcna.2013.02.002. PMID: 23809711. http://www.ncbi.nlm.nih.gov/pubmed/23809711 **

Bader MS. Herpes zoster: diagnostic, therapeutic, and preventive approaches. Postgrad Med. 2013 Sep;125(5):78-91. https://doi.org/10.3810/pgm.2013.09.2703. PMID: 24113666. http://www.ncbi.nlm.nih.gov/pubmed/24113666 **

Yawn BP, Gilden D. The global epidemiology of herpes zoster. Neurology. 2013 Sep 3;81(10):928-30. https://doi.org/10.1212/WNL.0b013e3182a3516e. PMID: 23999562. http://www.ncbi.nlm.nih.gov/pubmed/23999562 **

Gagliardi AM, Gomes Silva BN, Torloni MR, Soares BG. Vaccines for preventing herpes zoster in older adults. Cochrane Database Syst Rev. 2012 Oct 17;10:CD008858. https://doi.org/10.1002/14651858.CD008858.pub2. PMID: 23076951. http://www.ncbi.nlm.nih.gov/pubmed/23076951 **

Wilson JF. Herpes zoster. Ann Intern Med. 2011 Mar 1;154(5):ITC31-15; quiz ITC316. https://doi.org/10.7326/0003-4819-154-5-201103010-01003. PMID: 21357905. http://www.ncbi.nlm.nih.gov/pubmed/21357905 **

Adams EN, Parnapy S, Bautista P. Herpes zoster and vaccination: a clinical review. Am J Health Syst Pharm. 2010 May 1;67(9):724-7. https://doi.org/10.2146/ajhp090118. PMID: 20410546. http://www.ncbi.nlm.nih.gov/pubmed/20410546 **

Gershon AA, Gershon MD, Breuer J, Levin MJ, Oaklander AL, Griffiths PD. Advances in the understanding of the pathogenesis and epidemiology of herpes zoster. J Clin Virol. 2010 May;48 Suppl 1:S2-7. https://doi.org/10.1016/S1386-6532(10)70002-0. PMID: 20510263. http://www.ncbi.nlm.nih.gov/pubmed/20510263 **

Use PubMed Clinical Queries to find the most recent evidence. Use this search strategy: "Herpes Zoster"[Mesh] OR "Shingles"

Chapter 35
Hiatal Hernia

Christopher J. Rees, Charles V. Pollack, Jr., and Victoria G. Riese

Name and Synonyms

Hiatal Hernia

- Hiatus Hernia

Incidence/Epidemiology

- Hiatal hernias commonly are found incidentally when patients undergo imaging for other reasons, or during endoscopy.
- Most hiatal hernias are asymptomatic.
- The true incidence is unknown, as they often are asymptomatic and only incidentally found.
- The incidence increases with age, obesity, and pregnancy.
- Hiatal hernias (especially type 1) significantly increase the risk for gastroesophageal reflux disease (GERD).

C. J. Rees
Emergency Department, Pennsylvania Hospital, Philadelphia, PA, USA

C. V. Pollack, Jr. (✉)
Department of Emergency Medicine, Thomas Jefferson University, Philadelphia, PA, USA

V. G. Riese
Librarian Consultant, Eldersburg, MD, USA

C. V. Pollack, Jr. (ed.), *Differential Diagnosis of Cardiopulmonary Disease*,
https://doi.org/10.1007/978-3-319-63895-9_35

Differential Diagnosis

- Because hiatal hernias usually are found incidentally during either chest or abdominal imaging to evaluate another issue, there is no specific differential diagnosis. However, it is important to determine the type of hiatal hernia that exists.
- If the patient has symptoms, they usually are the symptoms of GERD; therefore, the differential is that of GERD, including:
  - Esophagitis
  - Gastritis
  - Peptic ulcer disease
  - Esophageal motility disorders
  - Functional dyspepsia

Pathophysiology and Etiology

- A hiatal hernia is a structural disorder of the esophagus marked by the herniation of intra-abdominal contents (most often the cardia of the stomach) through the esophageal hiatus of the diaphragm.
- The esophagus is anchored to the diaphragm by the phrenoesophageal membrane (PEM) or ligament. The PEM is composed mostly of elastic connective tissue and inserts circumferentially into the esophageal musculature at the diaphragmatic hiatus. A defect or laxity of the PEM allows for the herniation of abdominal contents.
- It most commonly is thought to be caused by age-related degeneration of the PEM.
- Longstanding acid reflux also may lead to tonic contracture of the longitudinal muscle layer of the esophagus, resulting in increased stress on and degeneration of the PEM.
- Types II through IV are recognized complications of surgery involving the hiatus.
- There are four distinct anatomic types of hiatal hernia.
- Type I, or sliding hiatal hernia:
  - These account for about 95 % of all hiatal hernias.
  - Laxity of the PEM allows the gastric cardia to "slide" through the diaphragmatic hiatus. It is not a true hernia; there is no defect in the PEM and no true hernia sac.
  - The likelihood of symptomatic GERD increases with the size of the hernia.
  - It is felt that a hiatal hernia impairs the function of the gastroesophageal (GE) junction and prolongs clearance of esophageal contents, leading to symptoms of GERD.

- However, many asymptomatic patients are found to have a type I hiatal hernia.

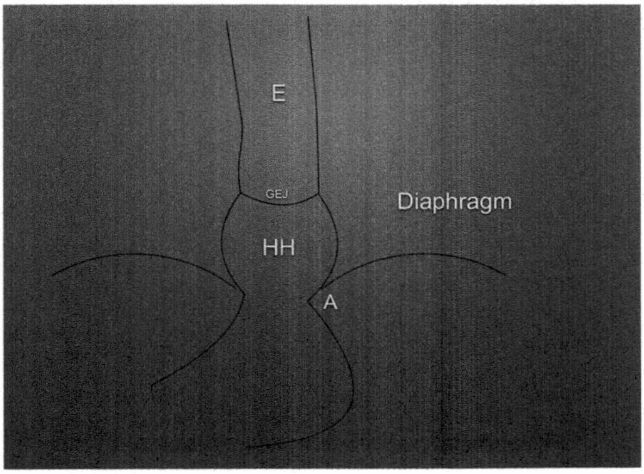

Diagram of a type I (sliding) hiatal hernia (HH). The gastroesophageal junction (GEJ) has migrated above the diaphragm into the chest. The Angle of HIS (A) is blunted, reducing its ability to protect against gastroesophageal reflux [Belafsky PC, Kuhn MA. The clinician's guide to swallowing fluoroscopy [Internet]. New York: Springer; 2014. Chapter 11, Abnormal esophageal fluoroscopy; [cited 2015 Aug 14]; p. 95–123. Available from: http://link.springer.com/10.1007/978-1-4939-1109-7_11] *Caption from original*

- Type II through IV:
  - Types II through IV are all paraesophageal hernias. They are true hernias with defects in the PEM and true hernia sacs, and include viscera other than the gastric cardia.
  - In a type II hernia, the gastric fundus also herniates, but the GE junction remains fixed at the hiatus.
  - Type III hernia is a combination of types I and II: it is both a sliding and a paraesophageal hernia.
  - Types II and III may lead to gastric volvulus and ischemia. As the defect enlarges, more of the stomach may herniate through. Because the stomach remains fixed at the GE junction, it may invert, leading to an upside down, intrathoracic stomach. This may interrupt the blood supply and cause ischemia, resulting in a mechanical gastric volvulus.
  - Type IV hiatal hernias are associated with the largest defects in the PEM, and they involve herniation of abdominal contents other than the stomach, most commonly the colon.
  - Type III is the most common type of paraesophageal hiatal hernia, accounting for about 90 % of paraesophageal hernias. Type II is the least common.

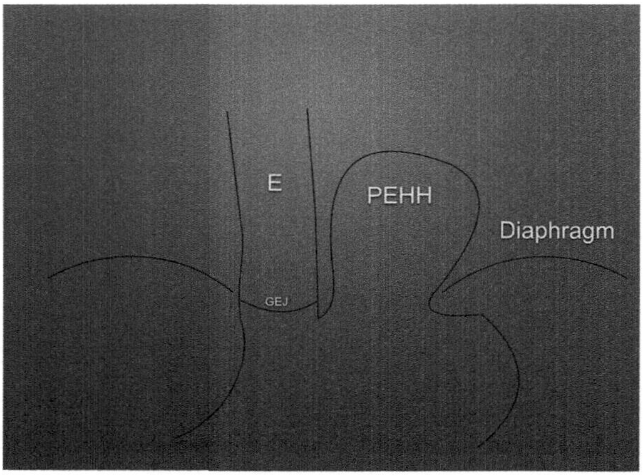

Diagram of a type II hiatal hernia. A type II hernia is a pure paraesophageal hiatal hernia (PEHH) and the gastroesophageal junction (GEJ) remains at or below the level of the diaphragm [Belafsky PC, Kuhn MA. The clinician's guide to swallowing fluoroscopy [Internet]. New York: Springer; 2014. Chapter 11, Abnormal esophageal fluoroscopy; [cited 2015 Aug 14]; p. 95–123. Available from: http://link.springer.com/10.1007/978-1-4939-1109-7_11] *Caption from original*

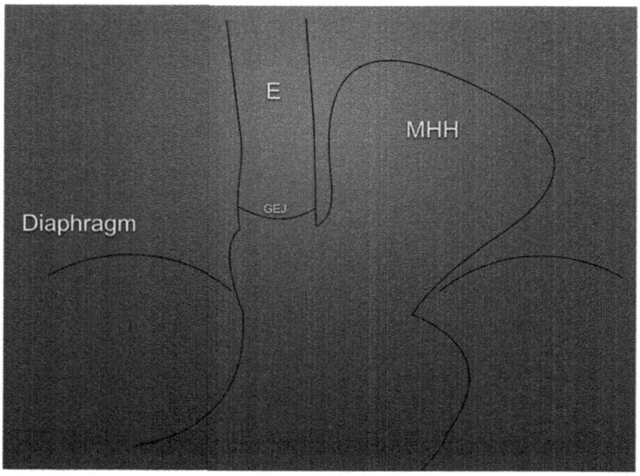

Diagram of a type III (mixed) hiatal hernia (MHH). A type III hiatal hernia is a mixed hernia in which the fundus and gastroesophageal junction (GEJ) have herniated alongside each other above the diaphragm into the chest. The majority of paraesophageal hiatal hernias are type III [Belafsky PC, Kuhn MA. The clinician's guide to swallowing fluoroscopy [Internet]. New York: Springer; 2014. Chapter 11, Abnormal esophageal fluoroscopy; [cited 2015 Aug 14]; p. 95–123. Available from: http://link.springer.com/10.1007/978-1-4939-1109-7_11] *Caption from original*

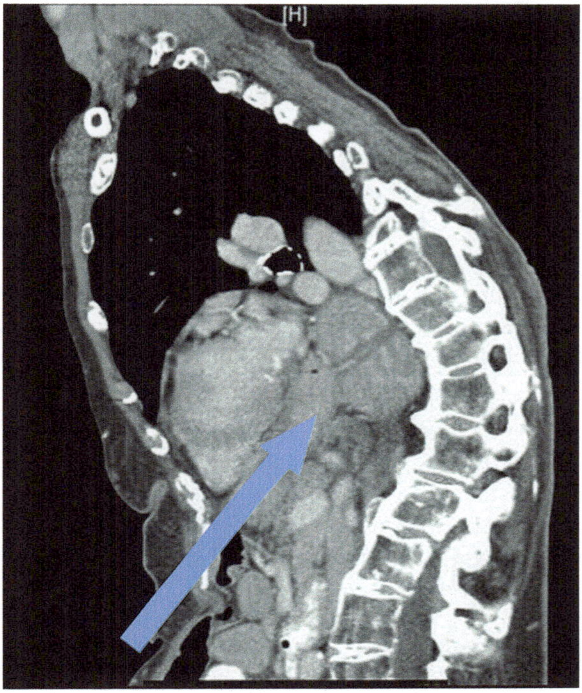

Sagittal CT scan images of a patient with a large Type IV hiatal hernia; note the retrocardiac herniation of small bowel [Sarpel U. Surgery: an introductory guide [Internet]. New York: Springer; 2014. Chapter 4, Fundoplication; [cited 2015 Aug 14]; p. 27–35. Available from: http://link.springer.com/10.1007/978-1-4939-0903-2_4] *Caption from original*

Presentation

Typical/"Classic"

- Most are asymptomatic.
- Type I (sliding) hiatal hernias often are associated with symptomatic GERD.
- Type II through IV (paraesophageal) hernias often have ambiguous symptoms. They may be asymptomatic, or patients may describe epigastric or chest pain, early satiety, excessive fullness after eating, nausea, or retching. GERD is a less common complaint for these types.

Atypical

- Because most hiatal hernias are asymptomatic, there are no typical or atypical features.

Primary Differential Considerations

- Chest pain resulting from hiatal hernia often is nonspecific. Other diagnoses that should be considered early in the evaluation of patients with similar symptoms include:
  - Acute coronary syndrome
  - GERD
  - Peptic ulcer disease
  - Pneumonia
  - Gastric outlet obstruction
  - Esophageal food bolus impaction or other foreign body

History and Physical Exam

Findings That Confirm Diagnosis

- The diagnosis can be confirmed only by imaging, most likely by CT scan but also by barium study of the upper gastrointestinal tract.
- There are no confirmatory historical or physical examination findings.

Factors That Suggest Diagnosis

- Sliding hiatal hernias are suggested in patients with symptoms of GERD and increasing age.
- Paraesophageal hernias are suggested in patients who have vagus upper abdominal symptoms have had a previous surgical procedure involving the diaphragmatic hiatus.

Factors That Exclude Diagnosis

- Paraesophageal hernias can be excluded by a normal CT scan.
- Small sliding hiatal hernias may be missed on endoscopy and imaging and therefore cannot be excluded, but their clinical significance remains in question.

Ancillary Studies

Laboratory

- Laboratory studies are not helpful in the diagnosis of hiatal hernia.

Imaging

- Sliding hiatal hernias often are diagnosed incidentally on imaging studies (chest x-ray, chest and abdominal CT). They also may be found on other imaging studies, such as endoscopy, barium swallow or upper gastrointestinal series, or esophageal manometry. However, sliding hiatal hernias less than 2 cm long may be missed by all the aforementioned studies.
- Paraesophageal hernias usually are diagnosed by CT of the chest and abdomen. Although barium swallow is performed less frequently, it is more sensitive in detecting paraesophageal hernias.

Special Populations

Age

- The incidence of sliding hiatal hernias increases with age.

Co-morbidities

- Sliding hiatal hernia may coexist with any other diagnosis.
- Paraesophageal hernias are found mostly in patients who have had prior thoracic or abdominal surgery involving manipulation of the diaphragmatic hiatus.

Pitfalls in Diagnosis

Critical Steps Not to Miss

- A critical mistake would be attributing a patient's symptoms (especially chest pain, epigastric pain, nausea and/or vomiting, and shortness of breath) to a sliding hiatal hernia and not continuing diagnostic evaluation for other causes.

Mimics

- Because hiatal hernias usually are asymptomatic, no significant mimics exist, and they typically do not mimic any other diseases.
- The appearance on imaging studies, especially plain radiographs, may sometimes mimic that of an elevated hemidiaphragm or a cavitary lung lesion.

Time-Dependent Interventions

- There are no time-dependent interventions.

Overall Principles of Treatment

- There is no specific treatment for a sliding hiatal hernia; treatment often is aimed at symptomatic treatment of GERD.
- It is important to stress that atypical symptoms, such as chest pain, abdominal pain, and shortness of breath, should not be attributed to a sliding hiatal hernia.
- Asymptomatic paraesophageal hernias often are treated conservatively with only follow-up.
- Symptomatic or very large paraesophageal hernias may need to be repaired surgically.

Disease Course

- Sliding hiatal hernias often grow and worsen in radiologic appearance as the patient ages, which may increase the likelihood of symptomatic GERD, although the true clinical significance is unknown.

Related Evidence

Papers of particular interest have been highlighted as:
*** Of key importance*

Practice Guideline

Kohn GP, Price RR, DeMeester SR, Zehetner J, Muensterer OJ, Awad Z, Mittal SK, Richardson WS, Stefanidis D, Fanelli RD; SAGES Guidelines Committee. Guidelines for the management of hiatal hernia. Surg Endosc. 2013 Dec;27(12):4409-28. https://doi.org/10.1007/s00464-013-3173-3. PMID: 24018762. http://www.ncbi.nlm.nih.gov/pubmed/24018762 **

Review

Furnée E, Hazebroek E. Mesh in laparoscopic large hiatal hernia repair: a systematic review of the literature. Surg Endosc. 2013 Nov;27(11):3998-4008. https://doi.org/10.1007/s00464-013-3036-y. PMID: 23793804. http://www.ncbi.nlm.nih.gov/pubmed/23793804 **

Lee YY, McColl KE. Pathophysiology of gastroesophageal reflux disease. Best Pract Res Clin Gastroenterol. 2013 Jun;27(3):339-51. https://doi.org/10.1016/j.bpg.2013.06.002. PMID: 23998973. http://www.ncbi.nlm.nih.gov/pubmed/23998973 **

Andrici J, Tio M, Cox MR, Eslick GD. Hiatal hernia and the risk of Barrett's esophagus. J Gastroenterol Hepatol. 2013 Mar;28(3):415-31. https://doi.org/10.1111/j.1440-1746.2012.07199.x. PMID: 22694245. http://www.ncbi.nlm.nih.gov/pubmed/22694245 **

Antoniou SA, Antoniou GA, Koch OO, Pointner R, Granderath FA. Lower recurrence rates after mesh-reinforced versus simple hiatal hernia repair: a meta-analysis of randomized trials. Surg Laparosc Endosc Percutan Tech. 2012 Dec;22(6):498-502. https://doi.org/10.1097/SLE.0b013e3182747ac2. PMID: 23238375. http://www.ncbi.nlm.nih.gov/pubmed/23238375

Dean C, Etienne D, Carpentier B, Gielecki J, Tubbs RS, Loukas M. Hiatal hernias. Surg Radiol Anat. 2012 May;34(4):291-9. https://doi.org/10.1007/s00276-011-0904-9. PMID: 22105688. http://www.ncbi.nlm.nih.gov/pubmed/22105688 **

Weber C, Davis CS, Shankaran V, Fisichella PM. Hiatal hernias: a review of the pathophysiologic theories and implication for research. Surg Endosc. 2011 Oct;25(10):3149-53. https://doi.org/10.1007/s00464-011-1725-y. PMID: 21528392. http://www.ncbi.nlm.nih.gov/pubmed/21528392 **

Comparative Study

Khajanchee YS, Cassera MA, Swanström LL, Dunst CM. Diagnosis of Type-I hiatal hernia: a comparison of high-resolution manometry and endoscopy. Dis Esophagus. 2013 Jan;26(1):1-6. https://doi.org/10.1111/j.1442-2050.2011.01314.x. PMID: 22320417. http://www.ncbi.nlm.nih.gov/pubmed/22320417

Use PubMed Clinical Queries to find the most recent evidence. Use this search strategy:

"Hernia, Hiatal"[Mesh] OR "Hiatal Hernia" OR "Hiatus Hernia"

Chapter 36
Hypertension

Charles V. Pollack, Jr., Richard M. Cantor, and Victoria G. Riese

Name and Synonyms

Hypertension

- High blood pressure, "high blood"

Incidence/Epidemiology

- Hypertension is the most prevalent disease state in the world.
- There are many definitions and staging systems for hypertension, but in general, a diastolic blood pressure greater than 90 mm Hg and/or a systolic blood pressure greater than 150 mm Hg are associated with the incidence of cardiovascular and cerebrovascular disease, and with benefit from chronic pressure-lowering therapy.
- Most cases of hypertension are "primary" (also called "essential"), but there are secondary causes, such as renal disease, pheochromocytoma, hyperaldosteronism, and Cushing's syndrome. Pregnancy is also often associated with hypertension.

C. V. Pollack, Jr. (✉)
Department of Emergency Medicine, Thomas Jefferson University,
Philadelphia, PA, USA

R. M. Cantor
Department of Emergency Medicine and Pediatrics, State University of New York Upstate
Medical University, Syracuse, NY, USA

V. G. Riese
Librarian Consultant, Eldersburg, MD, USA

C. V. Pollack, Jr. (ed.), *Differential Diagnosis of Cardiopulmonary Disease*,
https://doi.org/10.1007/978-3-319-63895-9_36

- Many adjectives frequently are associated with hypertension, such as *controlled* or *uncontrolled*, *resistant* for hard-to-treat hypertension, and *accelerated* or *malignant* for hypertension that is severe and acute.
- Prevalence is higher among African American populations than white populations.

Hypertension is highly prevalent
Hypertension is associated with an increased risk of heart disease, stroke, renal failure, and death
The treatment of moderate and severe hypertension reduces the risk of hypertensive complications
The treatment of mild hypertension decreases the incidence of strokes and probably reduces the incidence of CHD
The treatment of hypertension is widespread, and approximately $10 billion/y is spent on therapy

The epidemiology and rationale for cost-effectiveness analysis of the treatment of hypertension. CHD—coronary heart disease. [Heidenreich P, Krumholz H. Cost-effectiveness of risk factors. In: Grundy SM, editor. Atlas of atherosclerosis. 4th ed. Philadelphia: Current Medicine; 2005. ISBN: 1-57340-224-9] *Caption from original*

Blood pressure, mmHg	NICE 2011 [3]	ESH/ESC 2013 [4]	AHA/ACC/CDC 2013 [6]	ASH/ISH 2013 [5]	JSH 2014 [7]	JNC 8 [2]
Definition of hypertension	≥140/90 and daytime ABPM (or home BP) ≥135/85	≥140/90	≥140/90	≥140/90	≥140/90 and home BP ≥135/85	Not addressed
In mild hypertension at low to moderate risk, lifestyle management without drugs can be considered	Not addressed	Not addressed	3 months	Some months	3 months	Not addressed
Initiate drug therapy in low-risk patients	≥160/100 or daytime ABPM ≥150/95	≥140/90	≥140/90	≥140/90	≥140/90	≥140/90 for <60 years ≥150/90 for ≥60 years
Blood pressure targets						
Diabetes	Not addressed	<140/85	<140/90 Lower targets may be appropriate	<140/90	<130/80	<140/90
CKD with proteinuria	Not addressed	SBP <130 may be considered	<140/90 Lower targets may be appropriate	<130/80	<130/80	<140/90
Elderly	<150/90 for ≥80 years	SBP 140–150 for ≥80 years	<140/90 Lower targets may be appropriate	<150/90 for ≥80 years	<150/90 for >75 years, <140/90, if tolerated	<150/90 for ≥60 years

NICE the National Institute for Health and Clinical Excellence, *ESH/ESC* the European Society of Hypertension and the European Society of Cardiology, *AHA/ACC/CDC* the American Heart Association, the American College of Cardiology, and the Centers for Disease Control and Prevention, *ASH/ISH* the American Society of Hypertension and the Internal Society of Hypertension, *JSH* the Japanese Society of Hypertension, *JNC-8* the Eighth Joint National Committee, *ABPM* ambulatory blood pressure monitoring, *BP* blood pressure, *CKD* chronic kidney disease, *SBP* systolic blood pressure

Comparison of hypertension guidelines regarding definition of hypertension and blood pressure targets 2011–2014. [Kokubo Y, Iwashima Y, Kamide K. Hypertension: introduction, types, causes, and complications. In: Jagadeesh G, Balakumar P, Maung-U K, editors. Pathophysiology and pharmacotherapy of cardiovascular disease [Internet]. Cham, Switzerland: Springer; 2015 [cited 2015 Jun 22]. p. 635–53. Available from: http://link.springer.com/10.1007/978-3-319-15961-4_30] *Caption from original*

Differential Diagnosis

- Hypertension is a quantitatively defined disease. Consideration of differentials is more limited to possible causes of secondary disease. Hypertension may also be a cardinal aspect of the presentation of acute coronary syndrome, acute heart failure, acute renal failure, and acute stroke. Acute presentations also may be prompted by anxiety, stimulant use, or steroid use.

Primary care	Cause of resistant hypertension	Tertiary center
Problems with BP measurement		
20–30%	White-coat hypertension	10–20%
Medication-related causes		
~5%	Suboptimal medication regimen	30–60%
~10%	Drug-drug interaction	<5
<2%	Objective medication intolerance[a]	<2%
Interfering substances		
1–5%	Excessive dietary sodium	1–10%
1–7%	Ethanol or illicit substances	1–12%
Secondary hypertension		
<5%	Sleep apnea/aldosterone excess	1–83%
<5%	Traditional secondary causes[b]	5–28%
Psychological causes		
1–2%	Anxiety/panic disorder/depression	1–2%
1–2%	Subjective medication intolerance[a]	1–5%

[a] Objective and subjective medication intolerance are distinguished based on whether or not, respectively, the patient's reported adverse effect is mentioned in the prescribing information approved by the US Food and Drug Administration.

[b] Traditional secondary causes include renovascular hypertension, primary hyperaldosteronism, pheochromocytoma, Cushing's syndrome, etc.

BP blood pressure.

Differential diagnosis of resistant hypertension, with relative proportion of each, depending on the population studied. [Elliott WJ. Management of resistant hypertension. Curr Cardiovasc Risk Rep. 2011 Oct;5(5):373–82.] *Caption from original*

Pathophysiology and Etiology

- Hypertension is a pleomorphic disease, the etiology of which may be inapparent (although even in these cases, a genetic contribution is likely)
- Other defined causes include
  - Renal (renal artery stenosis, chronic pyelonephritis, polycystic kidney disease)
  - Endocrine (adrenocortical hyperfunction, pheochromocytoma)
  - Neurogenic (dysautonomia)
  - Vascular (such as coarctation of the aorta or polyarteritis nodosa)
- Factors contributing to hypertension are varied and include
  - Obesity
  - Salt intake
  - Alcohol intake
  - Medication use
  - Drug abuse
  - Tobacco use

Age Group	Etiology
Newborn	Renal artery or venous thrombosis Renal artery stenosis Congenital renal abnormalities Coarctation of the aorta Bronchopulmonary dysplasia History of Prematurity
First Year	Renovascular disease Renal parenchymal disease Coarctation of the aorta Iatrogenic (medication, volume) Tumor History of Prematurity
1 to 6 years	Renal parenchymal disease Renovascular disease Coarctation of the aorta Tumor History of Prematurity
	Endocrine causes* Iatrogenic Essential hypertension
Age 6 to 10 years	Renal parenchymal disease Essential hypertension Renovascular disease Coarctation of the aorta
	Endocrine causes Tumor Iatrogenic
Adolescence, *Age 12 to 18 years*	Essential hypertension Iatrogenic
	Renal parenchymal disease Endocrine causes Coarctation of the aorta

**Shaded areas* are uncommon for category

Most Common Causes of Secondary Hypertension: By Age. [Samuel JP, Swinford RD, Portman RJ. Evaluation of hypertension in pediatric patients. In: Flynn JT, Ingelfinger JR, Portman RJ, editors. Pediatric hypertension [Internet]. Totowa, NJ: Humana Press; 2013 [cited 2015 Jun 22]. p. 491–504. Available from: http://link.springer.com/10.1007/978-1-62703-490-6_32] *Caption from original*

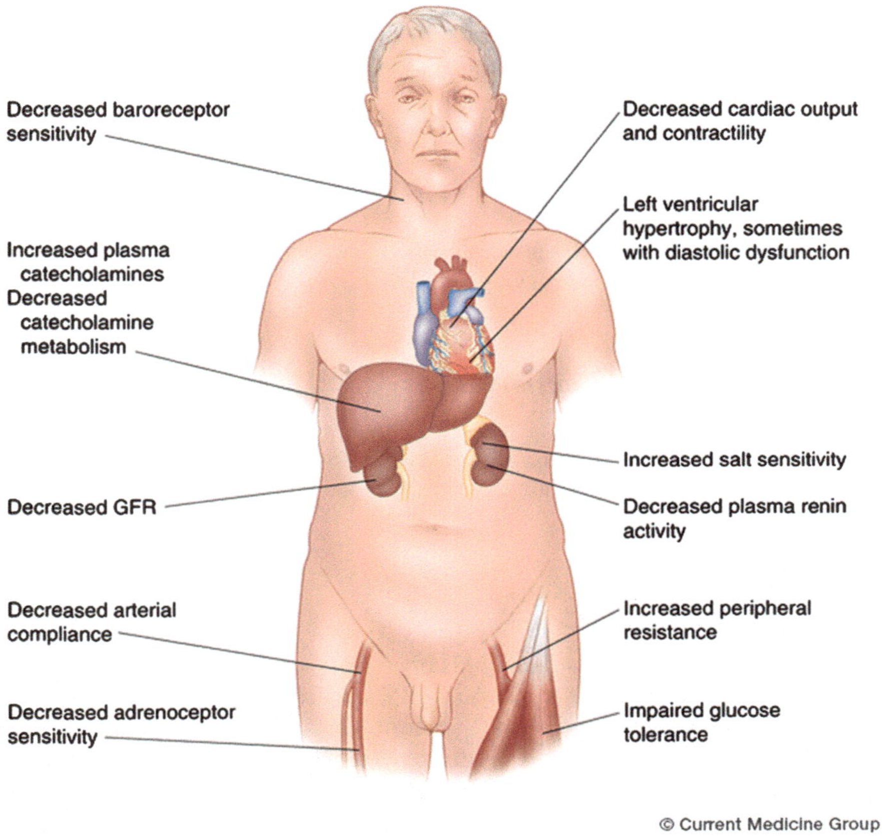

Some of the pathophysiologic features of hypertension in the elderly. Although some features are common in many elderly patients with elevated blood pressure, it is unusual for all of these features to be present in any one patient. GFR—glomerular filtration rate. [Elliott WJ, Black HR. Special situations in the management of hypertension. In: Hollenberg NK, editor. Atlas of hypertension. 6th ed. Philadelphia, PA: Springer; 2009. 334 p. ISBN: 978-1-57340-308-5] *Caption from original*

Presentation

Typical/"Classic"

- Most patients with hypertension are asymptomatic, and their elevated blood pressure is discovered incidentally.
- Moderate to severe hypertension may prompt presentation with headache, dizziness, epistaxis, or hematuria. Anxiety also is common.

- Severe hypertension may present as headache, dizziness, epistaxis, chest pain, dyspnea and heart failure, syncope, or stroke.
- There may be a history of stimulant use/abuse.

Atypical

- Health care providers often are surprised that patients with (chronically) very high blood pressures are asymptomatic.

Primary Differential Considerations

- As above, differential considerations usually apply to the symptoms that manifest with hypertension, not the elevated blood pressure itself.

History and Physical Exam

- In the history, focus on family history, age of onset, medication use (especially steroids and oral contraceptives), alcohol and drug abuse, history of renal disease, and signs and symptoms of other cardiovascular disease.
- On physical examination, note the patient's general appearance and overall health. Blood pressure should be checked in both upper extremities. Note height and weight. A thorough funduscopic exam should be performed to look for hypertensive changes. Check for neck and abdominal bruits. Listen for a fourth heart sound.

Fourth heart sound. [Fourth Heart Sound; Easy Auscultation; www.easyauscultation.com; copyright 2015, MedEdu LLC]
http://www.easyauscultation.com/cases-listing-details?caseID=42

Findings that Confirm Diagnosis

- Elevated blood pressure in both upper extremities should be documented in confirmation of the diagnosis. To make a new diagnosis of hypertension, the blood pressure should be elevated on at least two separate evaluations.

Factors that Suggest Diagnosis

- A history of elevated blood pressure and suggestive symptoms as above.

Factors that Exclude Diagnosis

- Repeatedly normal blood pressure excludes acute hypertension but may not fully exclude chronic disease.

Ancillary Studies

Laboratory

- Baseline CBC (to exclude anemia) and renal function should be evaluated.
- Urine should be checked for protein, blood, and glucose.
- Serum electrolytes (especially potassium) should be checked.
- Lipid profile may be helpful.
- Serum calcium, phosphate, and uric acid should be checked.

Electrocardiography

- Should be obtained to evaluate rhythm and to look for left ventricular hypertrophy or Q waves.

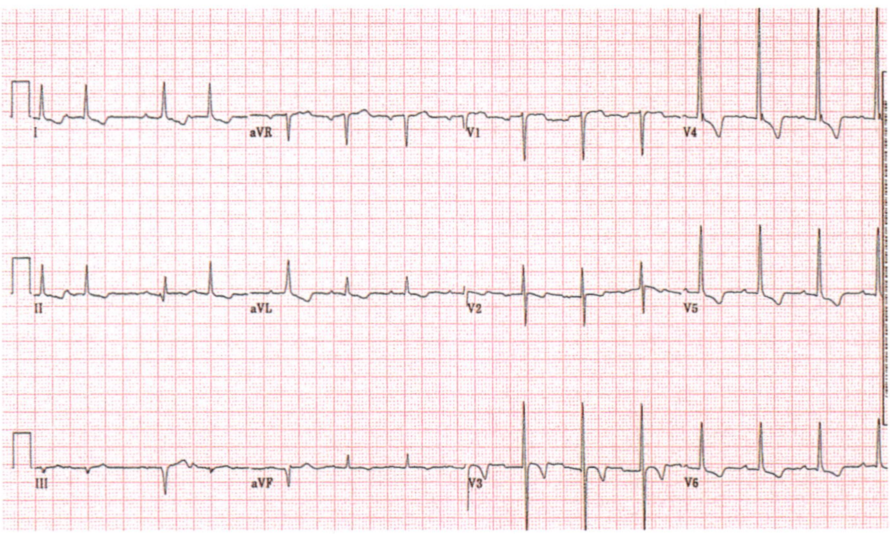

A 12-lead electrocardiogram demonstrating left ventricular hypertrophy with a "strain" pattern. [Fleisher L. Chapter 3. In: Lichtor JL, editor. Preoperative preparation and intraoperative monitoring. Philadelphia: Current Medicine; 1997. 251 p.

(Miller RD, editor. Atlas of anesthesia; vol. 3.) ISBN: 0-443-07902-1] *Caption adapted from original*

Imaging

- Chest x-ray should be obtained to look for cardiac enlargement, aortic dilation, rib notching from aortic coarctation, or signs of pulmonary edema.

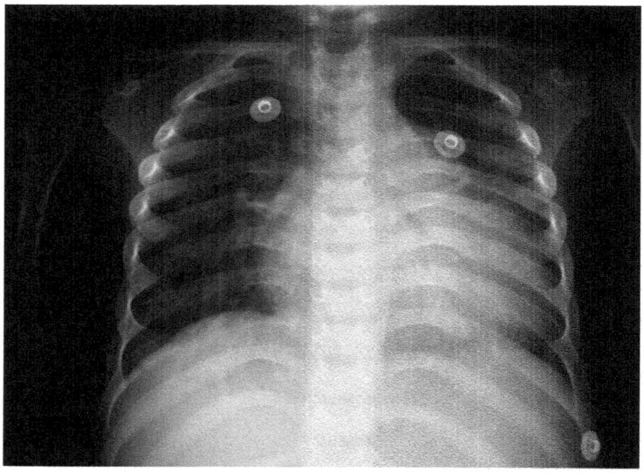

Cardiomegaly on chest X-ray. [Yıldırım SV, Durmaz C, Pourbagher MA, Erkan AN. A case of achondroplasia with severe pulmonary hypertension due to obstructive sleep apnea. Eur Arch Otorhinolaryngol. 2006 Aug;263(8):775–7.] *Caption from original*

- Concern for aortic disease should prompt more sophisticated imaging.

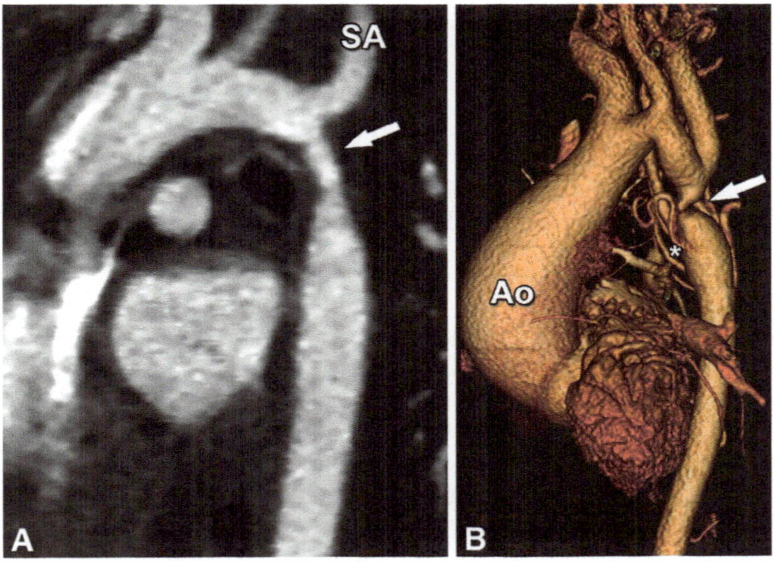

Aortic coarctation in two patients. Panel A is a double-oblique image from a prospectively ECG-triggered CT scan showing coarctation in a 2-year-old patient (arrow) just distal to the takeoff of the left subclavian artery (SA). The high-pitch CT scan was performed during free breathing with an acquisition time of 0.25 s and a dose-length product of 6 Gy.cm. The patient underwent subsequent repair of coarctation with an end-to-end anastomosis. Panel B shows a three-dimensional reconstruction of a CT scan performed for evaluation of severe aortic coarctation (arrow) in an 11-year-old patient who presented for evaluation of a murmur. His ascending aorta (Ao) was dilated and the murmur was secondary to aortic insufficiency. He was noted to be hypertensive with a blood pressure gradient of 30 mmHg between the right arm and leg. Note the collateral vessels supplying the descending aorta (asterisk). He underwent surgical repair of aortic coarctation and has since been followed clinically for aortic insufficiency and aortic root dilation [Ley S, Han BK, Arnold R, Lesser JR. Congenital and acquired heart disease. In: Dewey M, editor. Cardiac CT [Internet]. Berlin, Heidelberg: Springer; 2014 [cited 2015 Jun 22]. p. 393–414. Available from: http://link.springer.com/10.1007/978-3-642-41883-9_26] *Caption from original*

Other Studies

- Echocardiography or renal ultrasound imaging may be indicated

Special Populations

Age

- Essential hypertension rarely occurs in children. Younger patients with hypertension should be evaluated for secondary causes.
- The most common causes of hypertensive emergencies by age are listed in the table below:

Infancy	**Childhood**	**Adolescence**
Renal vascular disease	Renal disease	Primary hypertension
Congenital renal anomaly	Renal vascular disease	Nonadherence to meds
Coarctation	Pheochromocytoma	Renal disease
Volume overload	Increased intracranial pressure	Toxemia
Renal disease	Drug induced	Pheochromocytoma
Renal vein thrombosis		Illicit drug use
Congenital adrenal hyperplasia		

Co-morbidities

- May include:
  - Renal disease
  - Cardio- and cerebrovascular disease
  - Drug and alcohol abuse
  - Endocrine disorders such as diabetes, metabolic syndrome, Cushing's syndrome, or primary hyperaldosteronism

Pitfalls in Diagnosis

Critical Steps Not to Miss

- Recognition of "hypertensive emergency," as this requires parenteral treatment. Hypertensive emergency is defined as acute hypertension plus end-organ damage, such as acute heart failure, acute coronary syndrome, acute aortic dissection, or acute stroke.

Definitions of Hypertensive Emergencies and Urgencies
Hypertensive emergency
Severe elevation in blood pressure with signs or symptoms of acute, severe target organ damage, which must be reduced within minutes (typically using parenteral therapy)
Hypertensive urgency
Severe elevation in blood pressure with mild or no acute target organ damage, which must be reduced within hours (typically with oral therapy)

Definitions of hypertensive emergencies and hypertensive urgencies (Chobanian AV, Bakris GL, Black HR, et al. The seventh report of the Joint National Committee on Prevention, Detection, Evaluation, and Treatment of High Blood Pressure: The JNC 7 Report. JAMA. 2003;289:2560–72; Chobanian AV, Bakris GL, Black HR, et al. Seventh report of the Joint National Committee on Prevention, Detection, Evaluation and Treatment of High Blood Pressure. National High Blood Pressure Education Program Coordinating Committee. Hypertension. 2003;42:1206–52). Note that the older terms *accelerated hypertension* and *malignant hypertension* have been eliminated (with the exception of the terminology used by hospital administrators, as mandated by the Federal Diagnosis-Related Groups Handbook). Severe hypertension without acute target organ damage is never an emergency and does not require parenteral therapy. [Elliott WJ, Black HR. Special situations in the management of hypertension. In: Hollenberg NK, editor. Atlas of hypertension. 6th ed. Philadelphia, PA: Current Medicine Group; 2009. 334 p. ISBN: 978-1-57340-308-5] *Caption from original*

- Essential or accelerated hypertension
- Acute aortic dissection
- Preeclampsia and eclampsia
- Acute myocardial infarction or ischemia
- Endocrine disorders
  - Pheochromocytoma (excess catecholamines)
  - Aldosteronism
  - Renin-secreting tumors
  - Glucocorticoid excess
- Renal diseases
  - Chronic pylonephritis
  - Renal parenchymal disease (glomerulonephritis)
  - Renovascular disease
- Drugs
  - Cocaine
  - Amphetamines
  - Clonidine and methyldopa withdrawal
  - Monoamine oxidase inhibitor interactions
- Central nervous system injury/trauma

Causes of hypertensive emergencies. [Brennan KJ, Goldman J, D'Alonzo GE. Hypertensive crisis. In: Criner GJ, Barnette RE, D'Alonzo GE, editors. Critical care study guide 2e [Internet]. New York, NY: Springer; 2010 [cited 2015 Jun 22].

p. 1060–75. Available from: http://link.springer.com/10.1007/978-0-387-77452-7_53] *Caption from original*

Mimics

- Anxiety
- Intoxication

Time-Dependent Interventions

- In true hypertensive emergency, rapid reduction of the blood pressure (by no more than 20 %), with accompanying treatment as needed for reflex tachycardia, is required

*These doses may vary from those in the Physicians Desk Reference, 51st edition.†Hypotension may occur with all agents.‡Requires special delivery system.

DRUG	DOSE	ONSET OF ACTION	DURATION OF ACTION	ADVERSE EFFECTS†	SPECIAL INDICATIONS
Vasodilators					
Sodium nitroprusside	0.25–10 μg/kg/min as IV infusion‡	Immediate	1–2 min	Nausea, vomiting, muscle twitching, sweating, thiocyanate and cyanide intoxication	Most hypertensive emergencies; caution with high intracranial pressure or azotemia
Nicardipine hydrochloride	5–15 mg/h IV	5–10 min	15–30 min, may exceed 4 h	Tachycardia, headache, flushing, local phlebitis	Most hypertensive emergencies, except acute heart failure; caution with coronary ischemia
Fenoldopam mesylate	0.1–0.3 μg/kg/min IV infusion	< 5 min	30 min	Tachycardia, headache, nausea, flushing	Most hypertensive emergencies; caution with glaucoma
Nitroglycerin	5–100μg/min as IV infusion	2–5 min	5–10 min	Headache, vomiting, methemoglobinemia, tolerance with prolonged use	Coronary ischemia
Enalaprilat	1.25–5 mg every 6 h IV	15–30 min	6–12 h	Precipitous fall in pressure in high-renin states; variable response	Acute left ventricular failure; avoid in acute myocardial infarction
Hydralazine hydrochloride	10–20 mg IV	10–20 min IV	1–4 h IV	Tachycardia, flushing, headache, vomiting, aggravation of angina	Eclampsia
	10–40 mg IM	20–30 min IM	4–6 h IM		
Adrenergic inhibitors					
Labetalol hydrochloride	20–80 mg IV bolus every 10 min	5–10 min	3–6 h	Vomiting, scalp tingling, bronchoconstriction, dizziness, nausea, heart block, orthostatic hypotension	Most hypertensive emergencies, except acute heart failure
	0.5–2.0 mg/min IV infusion				
Esmolol hydrochloride	250–500μg/kg/min IV bolus	1–2 min	10–30 min	Hypotension, nausea, asthma, first-degree heart block, heart failure	Aortic dissection, perioperative
Phentolamine	5–15 mg IV bolus	1–2 min	10–30 min	Tachycardia, flushing, headache	Catecholamine excess

Parenteral drugs for treatment of hypertensive emergencies. IM—intramuscular; IV—intravenous. [Hollenberg NK. Recommendations of the JNC 7 report. In: Hollenberg NK, editor. Atlas of hypertension. 5th ed. Philadelphia, PA: Current Medicine Group; 2005. 383 p. ISBN: 1-57340-220-6] *Caption from original*

Overall Principles of Treatment

- Do not treat chronic hypertension aggressively; it may have taken years for the patient to develop hypertension; there is no physiologic reason to try to correct it in days, much less hours.
- Be alert for signs of end-organ damage in patients with acute hypertension.

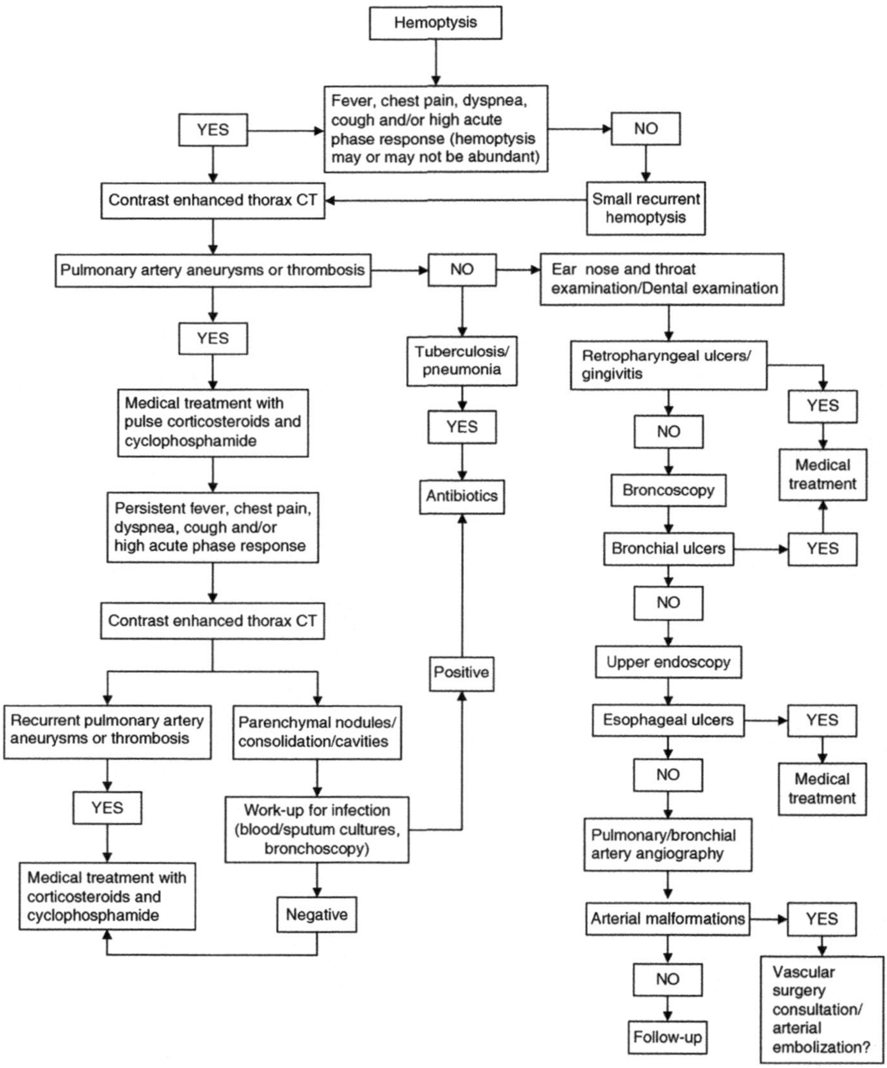

Algorithm for diagnosis and management of hemoptysis due to Behçet's syndrome [Seyahi E, Tascilar K, Yazici H. Behçet's syndrome: clinical presentations affecting prognosis and survival. In: Khamashta MA, Ramos-Casals M, editors. Autoimmune diseases [Internet]. London: Springer; 2011 [cited 2015 Jun 22]. p. 163–84. Available from: http://link.springer.com/10.1007/978-0-85729-358-9_11] *Caption from original*

Situations	Systolic blood pressure (mm Hg)	Diastolic blood pressure (mm Hg)
Uncomplicated hypertension	140	90
Elderly	140–150	90
Diabetes mellitus	140	85
Stroke	140	90
Coronary artery disease	140	90
Chronic kidney disease		
Without albuminuria[a]	140	90
With albuminuria	130	80

[a]Microalbuminuria or macroalbuminuria.

Target blood pressures in hypertension treatment. [From article: 2013 Korean Society of Hypertension guidelines for the management of hypertension. Part II—treatments of hypertension. Clin Hypertens. 2015 Dec;21(1). https://doi.org/10.1186/s40885-014-0013-2, at http://link.springer.com/article/10.1186%2Fs40885-014-0013-2; by Jinho Shin, Jeong Bae Park, Kwang-il Kim, Ju Han Kim, Dong Heon Yang, Wook Bum Pyun, Young Gweon Kim, Gheun-Ho Kim, Shung Chull Chae, The Guideline Committee of the Korean Society of Hypertension, © Shin et al.; licensee BioMed Central. 2015; licensed under Creative Commons Attribution License BY 4.0 http://creativecommons.org/licenses/by/4.0] *Caption from original*

Risk factor	Blood pressure (mm Hg)		
	Stage 2 prehypertension (130–139/85–89)	Stage 1 hypertension (140–159/90–99)	Stage 2 hypertension (≥160/100)
Risk factors 0	Lifestyle modification	Lifestyle modification[a] or drug therapy	Lifestyle modification or drug therapy[†]
Risk factors 1–2 other than DM	Lifestyle modification	Lifestyle modification[a] or drug therapy	Lifestyle modification and drug therapy
Risk factors ≥3, subclinical organ damage	Lifestyle modification	Lifestyle modification and drug therapy	Lifestyle modification and drug therapy
DM, cardiovascular disease, chronic kidney disease	Lifestyle modification or drug therapy[b]	Lifestyle modification and drug therapy	Lifestyle modification and drug therapy

DM diabetic mellitus.
[a]Lifestyle modification is carried within several weeks to 3 months. [†]Drug therapy may be begun immediately according to the height of BPs.
[b]Drug therapy may be begun as target blood pressure determined.

Treatment for hypertension according to the risk. [From article: 2013 Korean Society of Hypertension guidelines for the management of hypertension. Part II—treatments of hypertension. Clin Hypertens. 2015 Dec;21(1). https://doi.org/10.1186/s40885-014-0013-2, at http://link.springer.com/article/10.1186%2Fs40885-014-0013-2; by Jinho Shin, Jeong Bae Park, Kwang-il Kim, Ju Han Kim, Dong Heon Yang, Wook Bum Pyun, Young Gweon Kim, Gheun-Ho Kim, Shung Chull Chae, The Guideline

 Caption from original

Disease Course

- Patients with hypertension die prematurely, most often of heart disease, stroke, or renal failure
- Treatment is positively correlated with outcomes.

Related Evidence

Papers of particular interest have been highlighted as:
*** Of key importance*

Practice Guidelines

Marwick TH, Gillebert TC, Aurigemma G, Chirinos J, Derumeaux G, Galderisi M, Gottdiener J, Haluska B, Ofili E, Segers P, Senior R, Tapp RJ, Zamorano JL. Recommendations on the use of echocardiography in adult hypertension: a report from the European Association of Cardiovascular Imaging (EACVI) and the American Society of Echocardiography (ASE)†. Eur Heart J Cardiovasc Imaging. 2015 Jun;16(6):577-605. PMID: 25995329. http://www.ncbi.nlm.nih.gov/pubmed/25995329 **

Piper MA, Evans CV, Burda BU, Margolis KL, O'Connor E, Smith N, Webber E, Perdue LA, Bigler KD, Whitlock EP. Screening for High Blood Pressure in Adults: A Systematic Evidence Review for the U.S. Preventive Services Task Force. Rockville (MD): Agency for Healthcare Research and Quality (US); 2014 Dec. PMID: 25632496. http://www.ncbi.nlm.nih.gov/pubmed/25632496 **

Parati G, Stergiou G, O'Brien E, Asmar R, Beilin L, Bilo G, Clement D, de la Sierra A, de Leeuw P, Dolan E, Fagard R, Graves J, Head GA, Imai Y, Kario K, Lurbe E, Mallion JM, Mancia G, Mengden T, Myers M, Ogedegbe G, Ohkubo T, Omboni S, Palatini P, Redon J, Ruilope LM, Shennan A, Staessen JA, vanMontfrans G, Verdecchia P, Waeber B, Wang J, Zanchetti A, Zhang Y; European Society of Hypertension Working Group on Blood Pressure Monitoring and Cardiovascular Variability. European Society of Hypertension practice guidelines for ambulatory blood pressure monitoring. J Hypertens. 2014 Jul;32(7):1359-66. https://doi.org/10.1097/HJH.0000000000000221. PMID: 24886823. http://www.ncbi.nlm.nih.gov/pubmed/24886823 **

Dasgupta K, Quinn RR, Zarnke KB, Rabi DM, Ravani P, Daskalopoulou SS, Rabkin SW, Trudeau L, Feldman RD, Cloutier L, Prebtani A, Herman RJ, Bacon SL, Gilbert RE, Ruzicka M, McKay DW, Campbell TS, Grover S, Honos G, Schiffrin EL, Bolli P, Wilson TW, Lindsay P, Hill MD, Coutts SB, Gubitz G, Gelfer M, Vallée M, Prasad GV, Lebel M, McLean D, Arnold JM, Moe GW, Howlett JG, Boulanger JM, Larochelle P, Leiter LA, Jones C, Ogilvie RI, Woo V, Kaczorowski J, Burns KD, Petrella RJ, Hiremath S, Milot A, Stone JA, Drouin D, Lavoie KL, Lamarre-Cliche M, Tremblay G, Hamet P, Fodor G, Carruthers SG, Pylypchuk GB, Burgess E, Lewanczuk R, Dresser GK, Penner SB, Hegele RA, McFarlane PA, Khara M, Pipe A, Oh P, Selby P, Sharma M, Reid DJ, Tobe SW, Padwal RS, Poirier L; Canadian Hypertension Education Program. The 2014 Canadian Hypertension Education Program recommendations for blood pressure measurement, diagnosis, assessment of risk, prevention, and treatment of hypertension. Can J Cardiol. 2014 May;30(5):485-501. https://doi.org/10.1016/j.cjca.2014.02.002. PMID: 24786438. http://www.ncbi.nlm.nih.gov/pubmed/24786438 **

James PA, Oparil S, Carter BL, Cushman WC, Dennison-Himmelfarb C, Handler J, Lackland DT, LeFevre ML, MacKenzie TD, Ogedegbe O, Smith SC Jr, Svetkey LP, Taler SJ, Townsend RR, Wright JT Jr, Narva AS, Ortiz E. 2014 evidence-based guideline for the management of high blood pressure in adults: report from the panel members appointed to the Eighth Joint National Committee (JNC 8). JAMA. 2014 Feb 5;311(5):507-20. https://doi.org/10.1001/jama.2013.284427. Erratum in: JAMA. 2014 May 7;311(17):1809. PMID: 24352797. http://www.ncbi.nlm.nih.gov/pubmed/24352797 **

Weber MA, Schiffrin EL, White WB, Mann S, Lindholm LH, Kenerson JG, Flack JM, Carter BL, Materson BJ, Ram CV, Cohen DL, Cadet JC, Jean-Charles RR, Taler S, Kountz D, Townsend R, Chalmers J, Ramirez AJ, Bakris GL, Wang J, Schutte AE, Bisognano JD, Touyz RM, Sica D, Harrap SB. Clinical practice guidelines for the management of hypertension in the community a statement by the American Society of Hypertension and the International Society of Hypertension. J Hypertens. 2014 Jan;32(1):3-15. https://doi.org/10.1097/HJH.0000000000000065. PMID: 24270181. http://www.ncbi.nlm.nih.gov/pubmed/24270181 **

ESH/ESC Task Force for the Management of Arterial Hypertension. 2013 Practice guidelines for the management of arterial hypertension of the European Society of Hypertension (ESH) and the European Society of Cardiology (ESC): ESH/ESC Task Force for the Management of Arterial Hypertension. J Hypertens. 2013 Oct;31(10):1925-38. https://doi.org/10.1097/HJH.0b013e328364ca4c. PMID: 24107724. http://www.ncbi.nlm.nih.gov/pubmed/24107724 **

Review

Poulter NR, Prabhakaran D, Caulfield M. Hypertension. Lancet. 2015 Mar 27. pii: S0140-6736(14)61468-9. https://doi.org/10.1016/S0140-6736(14)61468-9. PMID: 25832858. http://www.ncbi.nlm.nih.gov/pubmed/25832858 **

Griffin BR, Schinstock CA. Thinking beyond new clinical guidelines: update in hypertension. Mayo Clin Proc. 2015 Feb;90(2):273-9. https://doi.org/10.1016/j.mayocp.2014.07.016. PMID: 25659243. http://www.ncbi.nlm.nih.gov/pubmed/25659243 **

Use PubMed Clinical Queries to find the most recent evidence. Use this search strategy:

"Hypertension"[Mesh] OR "hypertension" OR "high blood pressure"

Chapter 37
Hypertrophic Cardiomyopathy

Charles V. Pollack, Jr., Richard M. Cantor, and Victoria G. Riese

Name and Synonyms

Hypertrophic cardiomyopathy (HCM)

- Obstructive cardiomyopathy, idiopathic hypertrophic subaortic stenosis (IHSS)

Incidence/Epidemiology

- HCM is defined by hypertrophy of the left ventricle, usually in the absence of dilation of the chamber itself.
- At least half the cases of HCM are hereditary.
- It occurs in well under 1 % of the US population.

C. V. Pollack, Jr. (✉)
Department of Emergency Medicine, Thomas Jefferson University, Philadelphia, PA, USA

R. M. Cantor
Department of Emergency Medicine and Pediatrics, State University of New York Upstate Medical University, Syracuse, NY, USA

V. G. Riese
Librarian Consultant, Eldersburg, MD, USA

C. V. Pollack, Jr. (ed.), *Differential Diagnosis of Cardiopulmonary Disease*,
https://doi.org/10.1007/978-3-319-63895-9_37

Differential Diagnosis

- The primary differential considerations for chest pain due to HCM include valvular aortic stenosis and other types of obstructive or restrictive cardiomyopathy.
- Simple left ventricular hypertrophy (LVH) may be identified on electrocardiogram or chest radiography, and is much more common than HCM. LVH is usually the result of systemic hypertension.
- The entire constellation of differential considerations for unstable angina, aortic dissection, and pulmonary embolism should be considered, and may coexist with HCM.
- HCM may also present as syncope or near-syncope, which has broad differentials, including cardiac, neurologic, metabolic, psychiatric, and toxicologic etiologies.

Pathophysiology and Etiology

- The hallmark of HCM is that it occurs in the absence of typical inciting factors for LVH.

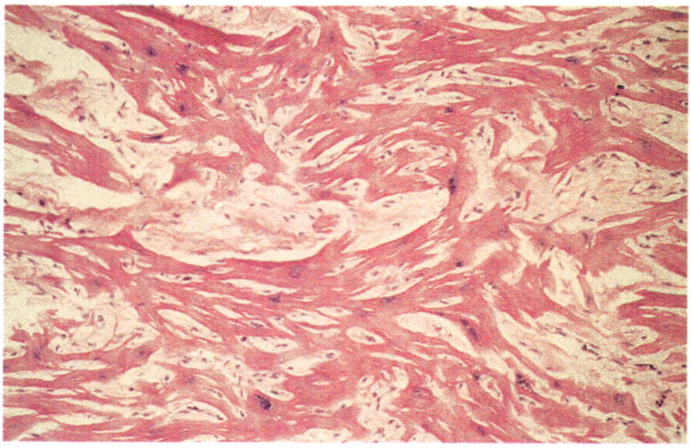

Hypertrophic cardiomyopathy. Typical histologic appearance in hypertrophic cardiomyopathy. Histologically, the left ventricle in hypertrophic cardiomyopathy exhibits disarray of myofibers and often extensive interstitial fibrosis. [Saffitz J, Zimmerman F, Lindsay B. Pathology of cardiac arrhythmias. In: McManus B, Braunwald E, editors. Atlas of cardiovascular pathology for the clinician. Philadelphia: Current Medicine; 2000. Chapter 16. ISBN: 1-57340-160-9; 2002-01-21] *Caption adapted from original*

- It is often hereditary.
- Abnormal calcium metabolism in the myocardium may lie at the root of HCM. As intracellular calcium concentrations rise, the muscle hypertrophies.
- The hypertrophy is often asymmetric. As the interventricular septum hypertrophies, there is often narrowing of the LV outflow tract, resulting in "stenosis" below the aortic valve itself (hence the term *hypertrophic subaortic stenosis*). Reduction in flow may result in anginal chest pain.

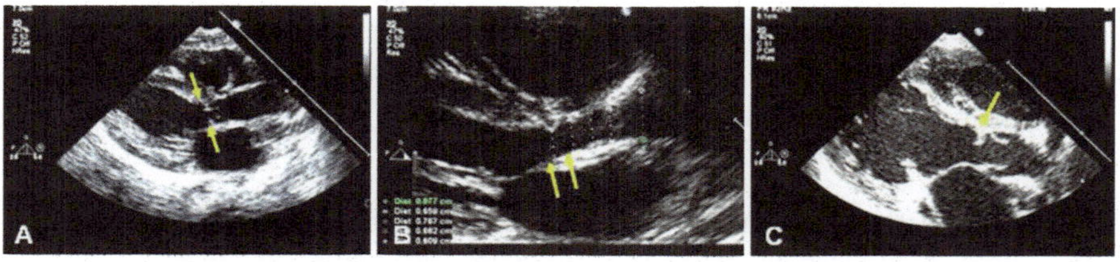

Subaortic stenosis diagnosed by echocardiography. (**a**) Parasternal left ventricular long-axis sectional view showing circumferential membranous subaortic stenosis. (**b**) Parasternal left ventricular long-axis sectional view showing tunnel-type subaortic narrowing. (**c**) Parasternal left ventricular long-axis sectional view showing an asymmetric obstructive fibrous ridge at the interventricular septum side of the left ventricular outflow tract below the aortic valve. [Ma X, Huang G, Liang X, Liu X, Jia B. Atypical Shone's complex diagnosed by echocardiography. Pediatr Cardiol. 2011 Apr;32(4):442-8. https://doi.org/10.1007/s00246-011-9886-y; 2011-03-19] *Caption from original*

Presentation

Typical/"Classic"

- Many patients with HCM are asymptomatic, and the diagnosis is discovered incidentally on imaging studies.
- Symptomatic patients may present with:
  - Dyspnea, the most common presentation of symptomatic HCM, probably occurs because stiffness of the LV walls limits LV filling.
  - Anginal chest pain, thought to be due to inadequate cardiac output for the level of the patient's exertion.
  - Sudden cardiac death, usually due to ventricular fibrillation.
  - Syncope ("black-outs") and near-syncope ("gray-outs"), due to inadequate cardiac output for the level of the patient's exertion.
  - Palpitations, due to both ventricular and atrial ectopic beats.

Atypical

- Anginal chest pain (especially with dyspnea) and sudden cardiac death often present without known antecedent. These presentations may distract the clinician from the potential diagnosis of HCM.
- Syncope and near-syncope, especially in younger patients, have a broad differential and may often have a component of anxiety. This should not distract the clinician from completing a thorough cardiovascular examination.

Primary Differential Considerations

- In the patient presenting with signs and symptoms of HCM, early consideration should also be given to the following differential diagnoses:
  - Valvular aortic stenosis
  - Restrictive cardiomyopathy

History and Physical Exam

Findings That Confirm Diagnosis

- History and physical examination are not diagnostic for HCM.

Factors That Suggest Diagnosis

- A family history of known HCM is helpful.
- Confirming that symptoms are related to exertion (especially chest pain, palpitations, dyspnea, and syncope/near-syncope) is helpful.
- A fourth heart sound (S4) is often present.

https://www.youtube.com/watch?v=r-HqK7NRL8I
Video about the fourth heart sound

- A harsh, crescendo-decrescendo systolic murmur, heard best at the apex and lower left sternal border.

https://www.youtube.com/watch?v=2OK4-vWRlWo
Systolic Murmur video with color flow Doppler

- Mitral regurgitation is common in HCM, so the murmur may sound more blowing in nature.

https://www.youtube.com/watch?v=k3ubxo-JATU
Mitral regurgitation video providing sound and depiction of anatomy

- A double carotid pulse (pulsus bisferiens) is common.
- The 12-lead ECG shows LVH.

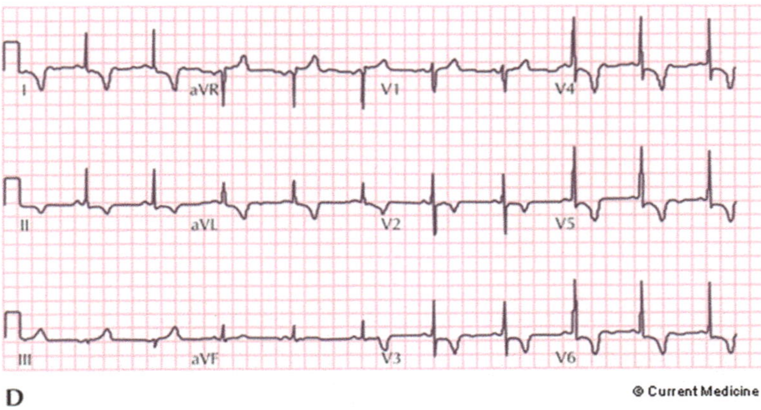

Echocardiogram of apical hypertrophic cardiomyopathy. Apical HCM is often associated with giant negative T waves on ECG, present in the lateral precordial leads (D). [Ho C, Maron B. Hypertrophic cardiomyopathy. In: Solomon SD, Braunwald E, editors. Atlas of echocardiography. Philadelphia: Current Medicine; 2008. Chapter 13. ISBN: 1-57340-217-6; 2008-10-22;] *Caption adapted from original*

Factors That Exclude Diagnosis

- There are no history or physical findings that conclusively exclude HCM.

Ancillary Studies

Laboratory

- There are no diagnostic laboratory studies for HCM.

Imaging

- The diagnosis of HCM is confirmed on 2D echocardiography.

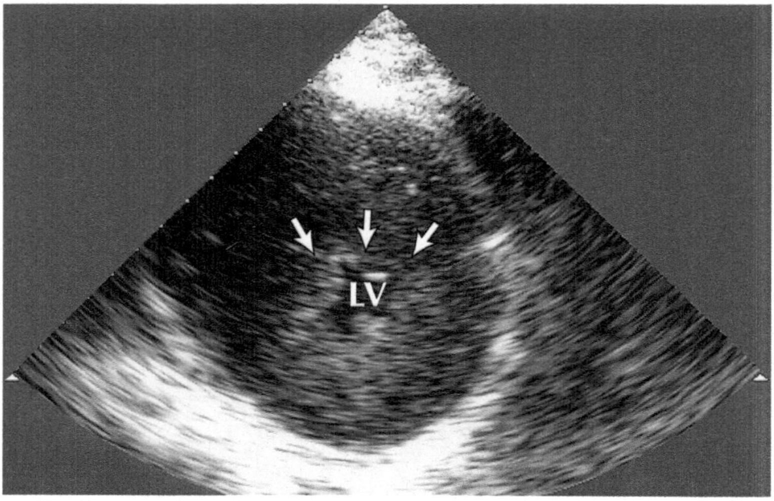

Hypertrophic cardiomyopathy. [Reimold S, Lee R. Echocardiography in acquired heart disease. In: Lee R, Braunwald E, editors. Atlas of cardiac imaging. Philadelphia: Current Medicine; 1998. Chapter 1. ISBN: 0-443-07567-0; 2002-01-23; Braunwald, Eugene]

- Cardiac MRI also demonstrates HCM.

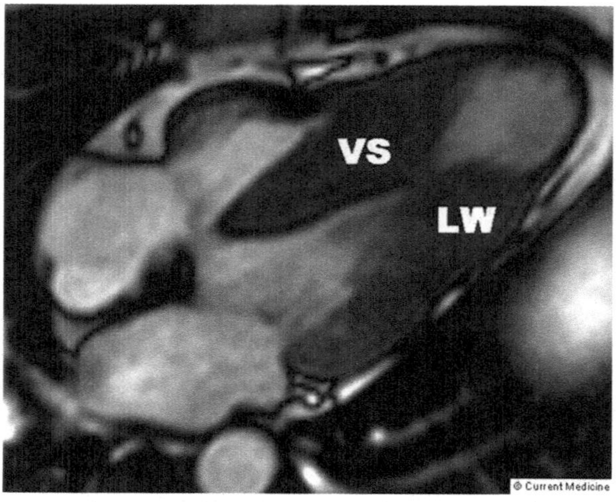

Cardiac MRI: hypertrophic cardiomyopathy with left ventricular aneurysm. Hypertrophic cardiomyopathy (HCM) patients with left ventricular (LV) apical aneurysm represent an important but fairly uncommon subgroup of the HCM disease spectrum. HCM patients with apical aneurysms also commonly demonstrate midventricular obstruction because of midsystolic apposition of the hypertrophied ventricular septum (VS) and LV free wall. It was proposed that long-standing increased LV systolic pressures created by midventricular obstruction may contribute to apical aneurysmal formation in select susceptible HCM patients in the absence of coronary artery disease. A, HCM patient with an LV apical aneurysm and characteristic midventricular hypertrophy with apposition to the septum and LV free wall in midsystole, creating midventricular obstruction. [Maron M. Dilated cardiomyopathy. In: Manning WJ, Braunwald E, editors. Atlas of cardiovascular magnetic resonance. Philadelphia: Current Medicine; 2009. Chapter 13. ISBN: 978-1-57340-299-6; 2009-01-16] *Caption from original*

- If cardiac catheterization is performed (perhaps in the evaluation of anginal chest pain), HCM may be detected as an elevated LV diastolic pressure.

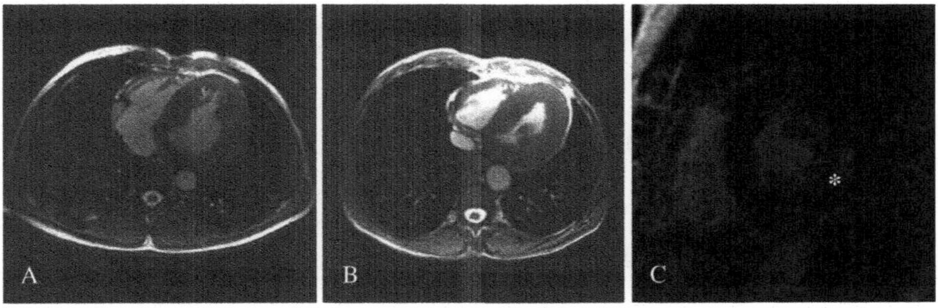

Cardiac MRI for the assessment of left ventricular hypertrophy and fibrosis: A: Left ventricular hypertrophy in a 51-year-old male patient with cerebrovascular involvement and end stage renal disease (dialysis). B: Hypertrophic cardiomyopathy in a 56-year-old male patient with arrythmya, leukoareiosis and kidney transplant. C: Late enhancement after gadolinium in a 63-year-old female patient with end stage renal disease (dialysis). [From article: Fabry disease. Orphanet J Rare Dis. 2010 Nov;5(1):30. https://doi.org/10.1186/1750-1172-5-30, at http://link.springer.com/article/10.1186/1750-1172-5-30; by Dominique P Germain, © Germain; licensee BioMed Central Ltd. 2010; licensed under Creative Commons Attribution License BY 2.0 http://creativecommons.org/licenses/by/2.0] *Caption from original*

Special Populations

Age and Gender

- HCM occurs slightly more often in males than in females.
- In females, HCM often presents at a younger age and tends to be more symptomatic.

- HCM is most commonly diagnosed in either the first or the third decade of life.
- HCM may present in infancy, but most pediatric cases present during the growth spurt associated with the onset of puberty.
- When it occurs in younger patients, it is most common for LVH to develop during the pubertal growth spurt.
- Wall thickness measurements generally do not change once adulthood is reached.

Co-morbidities

- A hereditary pattern is seen in about half the cases of HCM, but there are no typical co-morbidities.

Pitfalls in Diagnosis

Critical Steps Not to Miss

- Consideration of the diagnosis is the first critical step. Echocardiography is required to confirm the diagnosis.

Mimics

- The entire constellation of diagnoses that underlies chest pain syndrome, especially those often accompanied by dyspnea, can mimic the pain and overall presentation of HCM.
- Sudden cardiac death may mimic or be a presentation of HCM.
- Syncope or near-syncope may mimic or be a presentation of HCM.

Time-Dependent Interventions

- There are usually no time-dependent interventions in the management of HCM, unless the presentation is dramatic (angina, heart failure, arrhythmia/sudden death).

Overall Principles of Treatment

- Treatment of HCM is multimodal, with abstention from strenuous activities, beta-blockers, and calcium blockers often being used in maintenance care.

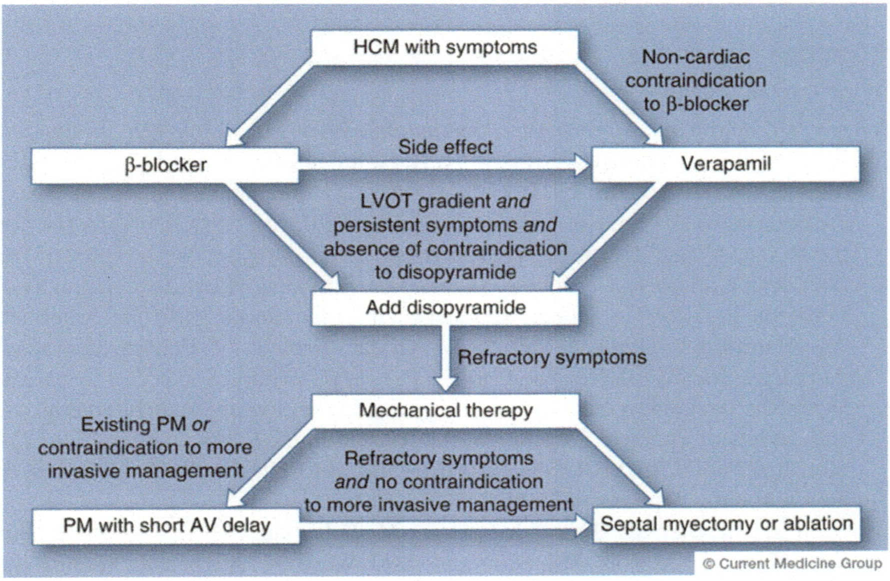

Treatment algorithm for hypertrophic cardiomyopathy. Proposed algorithm for the medical, mechanical, and surgical/interventional ablative treatment of patients with hypertrophic cardiomyopathy. Only 20% to 30% of patients with hypertrophic cardiomyopathy have outflow obstruction and would be candidates for the addition of disopyramide pacemaker therapy, or septal ablation [15]. AV—atrial ventricular; HCM—hypertrophic cardiomyopathy; LVOT—left ventricular outflow tract; PM—pacemaker. [Baughman K. Cardiomyopathy, myocarditis, and pericardial disease. In Libby P, editor. Essential atlas of cardiovascular disease. Philadelphia: Current Medicine; 2009. Chapter 6. ISBN: 978-1-57340-309-2; 2009-05-21;] *Caption from original*

Disease Course

- HCM may improve or stabilize over time.
- The risk of sudden cardiac death is always present and, even in less symptomatic patients, is justification for limited strenuous/athletic activities.
- There are limited surgical options for severe cases.

Related Evidence

Papers of particular interest have been highlighted as:
*** Of key importance*

Practice Guideline

Gersh BJ, Maron BJ, Bonow RO, Dearani JA, Fifer MA, Link MS, Naidu SS, Nishimura RA, Ommen SR, Rakowski H, Seidman CE, Towbin JA, Udelson JE, Yancy CW; American College of Cardiology Foundation/American Heart Association Task Force on Practice Guidelines. 2011 ACCF/AHA Guideline for the Diagnosis and Treatment of Hypertrophic Cardiomyopathy: a report of the American College of Cardiology Foundation/American Heart Association Task Force on Practice Guidelines. Developed in collaboration with the American Association for Thoracic Surgery, American Society of Echocardiography, American Society of Nuclear Cardiology, Heart Failure Society of America, Heart Rhythm Society, Society for Cardiovascular Angiography and Interventions, and Society of Thoracic Surgeons. J Am Coll Cardiol. 2011 Dec 13;58(25):e212–60. https://doi.org/10.1016/j.jacc.2011.06.011. PMID: 22075469. http://www.ncbi.nlm.nih.gov/pubmed/22075469 **

Nagueh SF, Bierig SM, Budoff MJ, Desai M, Dilsizian V, Eidem B, Goldstein SA, Hung J, Maron MS, Ommen SR, Woo A; American Society of Echocardiography; American Society of Nuclear Cardiology; Society for Cardiovascular Magnetic Resonance; Society of Cardiovascular Computed Tomography; American Society of Echocardiography clinical recommendations for multimodality cardiovascular imaging of patients with hypertrophic cardiomyopathy: Endorsed by the American Society of Nuclear Cardiology, Society for Cardiovascular Magnetic Resonance, and Society of Cardiovascular Computed Tomography. J Am Soc Echocardiogr. 2011 May;24(5):473–98. https://doi.org/10.1016/j.echo.2011.03.006. PMID: 21514501. http://www.ncbi.nlm.nih.gov/pubmed/21514501 **

Review

Efthimiadis GK, Pagourelias ED, Gossios T, Zegkos T. Hypertrophic cardiomyopathy in 2013: Current speculations and future perspectives. World J Cardiol. 2014 Feb 26;6(2):26–37. https://doi.org/10.4330/wjc.v6.i2.26. PMID: 24575171. http://www.ncbi.nlm.nih.gov/pubmed/24575171

Jacoby DL, DePasquale EC, McKenna WJ. Hypertrophic cardiomyopathy: diagnosis, risk stratification and treatment. CMAJ. 2013 Feb 5;185(2):127–34. https://

doi.org/10.1503/cmaj.120138. PMID: 23109605. http://www.ncbi.nlm.nih.gov/pubmed/23109605 **

Sen-Chowdhry S, Tomé Esteban MT, McKenna WJ. Insights and challenges in hypertrophic cardiomyopathy, 2012. Herzschrittmacherther Elektrophysiol. 2012 Sep;23(3):174–85. https://doi.org/10.1007/s00399-012-0227-5. PMID: 23008086. http://www.ncbi.nlm.nih.gov/pubmed/23008086

Review. Moak JP, Kaski JP. Hypertrophic cardiomyopathy in children. Heart. 2012 Jul;98(14):1044–54. https://doi.org/10.1136/heartjnl-2011-300531. PMID: 22591735. http://www.ncbi.nlm.nih.gov/pubmed/22591735

Yetman AT, McCrindle BW. Management of pediatric hypertrophic cardiomyopathy. Curr Opin Cardiol. 2005 Mar;20(2):80–3. PMID: 15711191. http://www.ncbi.nlm.nih.gov/pubmed/15711191

Cohort Study

Maron BJ, Casey SA, Poliac LC, Gohman TE, Almquist AK, Aeppli DM. Clinical course of hypertrophic cardiomyopathy in a regional United States cohort. JAMA. 1999 Feb 17;281(7):650–5. Erratum in: JAMA 1999 Jun 23–30;281(24):2288. PubMed PMID: 10029128. http://www.ncbi.nlm.nih.gov/pubmed/10029128

Use PubMed Clinical Queries to find the most recent evidence. Use this search strategy:

("Cardiomyopathy, Hypertrophic"[Mesh] OR "hypertrophic cardiomyopathy")

Chapter 38
Idiopathic Pulmonary Fibrosis

Christopher J. Rees, Charles V. Pollack, Jr., and Victoria G. Riese

Name and Synonyms

Idiopathic Pulmonary Fibrosis (IPF)

- Cryptogenic Fibrosing Alveolitis

Incidence/Epidemiology

- IPF is the most common interstitial lung disease (ILD). It accounts for 25–35 % of all diagnoses of ILD.
- The diagnosis usually is not considered in those under 40.
- It is typically seen in those over 55 years of age.

Differential Diagnosis

- The differential diagnosis of IPF is broad and includes all the diagnoses encompassing the ILDs, of which there are more than 200.

C. J. Rees
Emergency Department, Pennsylvania Hospital, Philadelphia, PA, USA

C. V. Pollack, Jr. (✉)
Department of Emergency Medicine, Thomas Jefferson University, Philadelphia, PA, USA

V. G. Riese
Librarian Consultant, Eldersburg, MD, USA

C. V. Pollack, Jr. (ed.), *Differential Diagnosis of Cardiopulmonary Disease*,
https://doi.org/10.1007/978-3-319-63895-9_38

- The differential also includes all the causes of chronic dyspnea and cough, especially chronic obstructive pulmonary disease (COPD) and congestive heart failure (CHF).

Pathophysiology and Etiology

- IPF is a chronic, progressive disease of the lower respiratory tract; so far, no precipitating cause has been identified.
- It is predominately a fibrotic disease, with abnormal fibroblast proliferation and abnormal collagen metabolism.
- Chronic inflammation, once thought to play a role in the pathogenesis, is now known to be less important than fibrosis in the pathophysiology of IPF. When biopsies are performed for diagnosis, there often is little inflammation present.
- The classic histologic pattern is termed *usual interstitial pneumonia* (UIP). Although UIP is not pathognomonic to IPF, it may be seen in other lung diseases marked by fibrosis, such as diseases associated with connective tissue disorders, chronic hypersensitivity pneumonitis, and asbestosis.
- UIP is characterized by the presence of "honeycomb cysts." These are subpleural, cystic airspaces in which there are an abnormal proliferation of mesenchymal cells, varying degrees of fibrosis, and overproduction and disorganized deposition of collagen and extracellular matrix.
- Another characteristic feature of UIP is the presence of fibroblast foci, clusters of fibroblasts and myofibroblasts found next to areas of established fibrosis. The presence and number of fibroblastic foci correlate with disease severity and mortality.

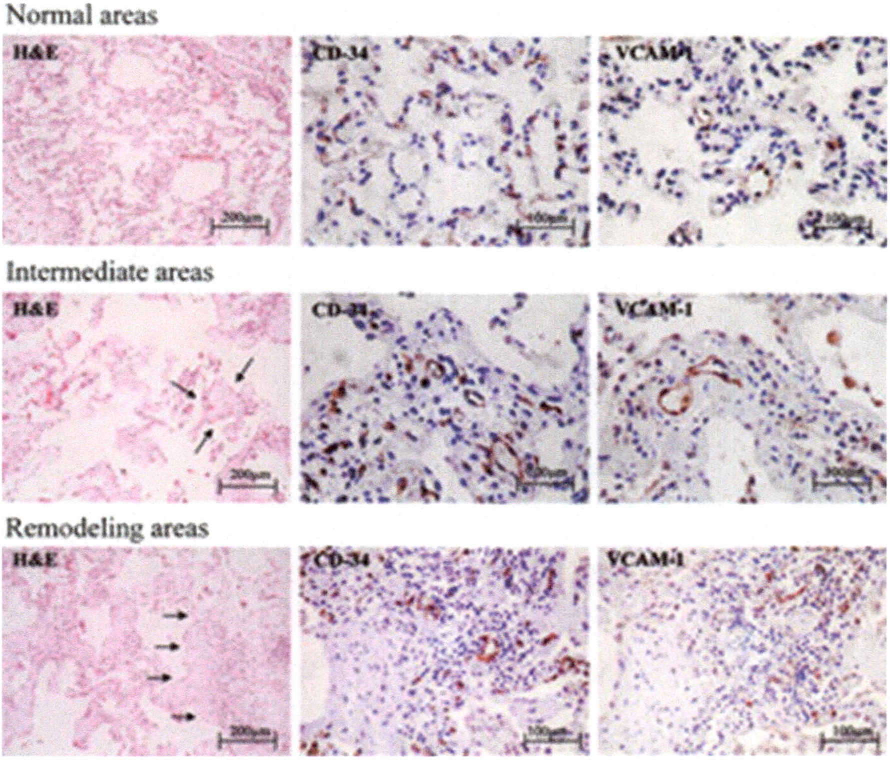

UIP (usual interstitial pneumonia) lungs showing nonhomogeneous CD34-positive and VCAM-1-positive immunostaining in alveolar capillaries. In normal parenchyma areas (H&E) (×100), a diffuse decrease of CD34 immunolocalization and endothelial cells of increased capillaries strongly immunoreactive with VCAM-1 can be appreciated (×200). Collapsed and mural organizing fibrosis areas present in UIP are shown at H&E staining (×100). In a high magnification of the area with arrows, CD34 decreases gradually toward more severe mural fibrosis. In contrast, increased VCAM-1 is shown in inflammatory septal thickening (nonorganizing fibrosis) and mural organizing fibrosis areas (200). [Parra ER, da Costa LRS, Ab'Saber A, de Carvalho CRR, Kairalla RA, Fernezlian SM, Teixeira LR, Capelozzi VL. Nonhomogeneous density of CD34 and VCAM-1 alveolar capillaries in major types of idiopathic interstitial pneumonia. Lung. 2005 Oct;183(5):363–73.] *Caption from original*

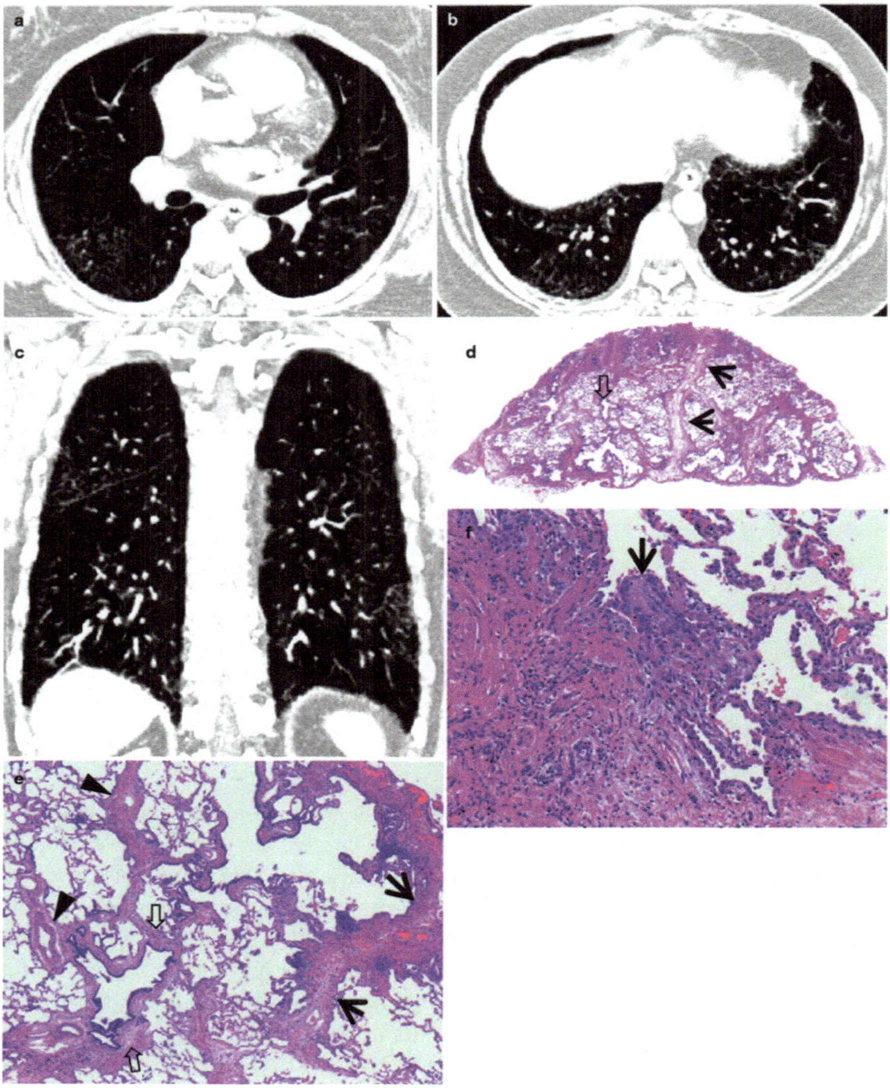

Interstitial fibrosis of usual interstitial pneumonia pattern in a 59-year-old woman with progressive systemic sclerosis. (a, b) Lung window of CT scans (3.0-mm section thickness) obtained at levels of bronchus intermedius (a) and liver dome (b), respectively, show patchy and extensive areas of reticulation and ground-glass opacity in both lungs. (c) Coronal reformatted image (3.0-mm section thickness) demonstrate similar pattern of reticulation and ground-glass opacity extensively in both lungs. (d) Low-magnification (×4) photomicrograph of surgical lung biopsy specimen obtained from right lower lobe exhibits dense fibrosis along interlobular septum (arrows) and around bronchiole (open arrow). (e) High-magnification (×100) photomicrograph depicts dense fibrosis in interlobular septum (arrows) and around bronchiole (open arrows). Also note thick fibrotic vessel wall (arrowheads). (f) High-magnification (×200) photomicrograph discloses area of focal active fibrosis (arrow) [Lee KS, Han J, Chung MP, Jeong YJ. *Radiology illustrated: chest radiology [Internet]. Berlin, Heidelberg: Springer; 2014. Chapter 28,* Interstitial *lung disease in collagen vascular disease;* [cited 2015 Aug 21]*;* p. 275–83. Available from: http://link.springer.com/10.1007/978-3-642-37096-0_28] *Caption from original*

- The end result is an abnormal fibrotic response within the lung that distorts and destroys lung tissue from the pleura into the lung parenchyma.

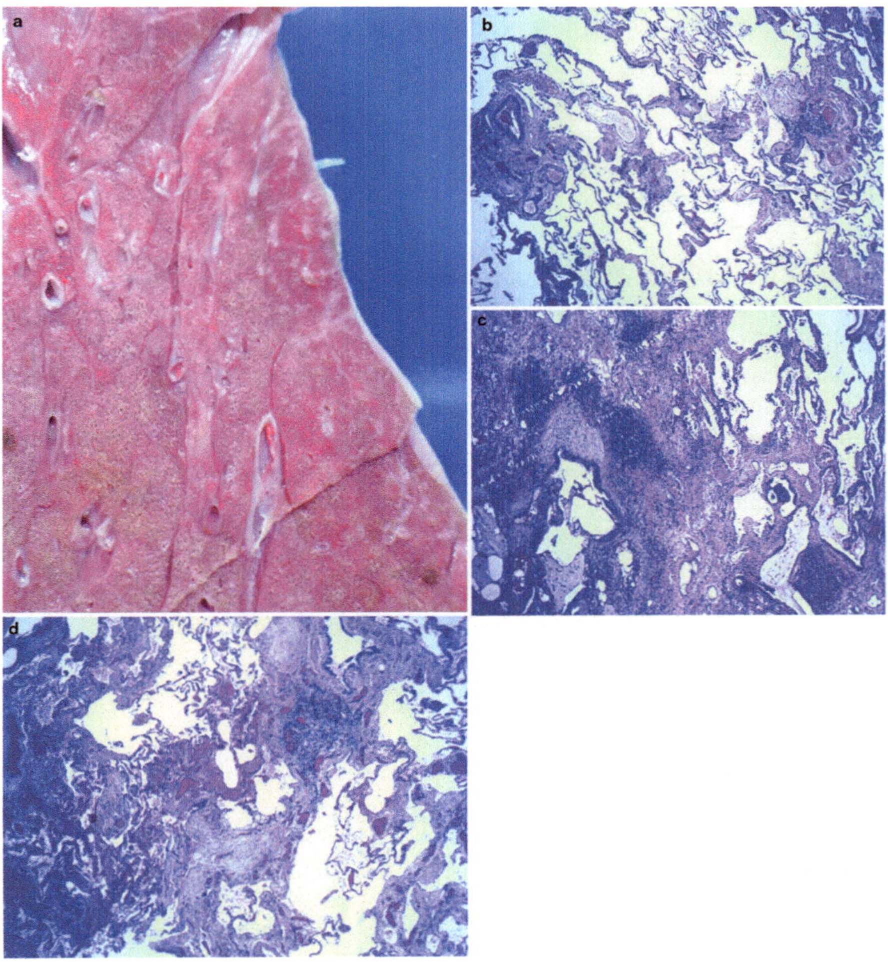

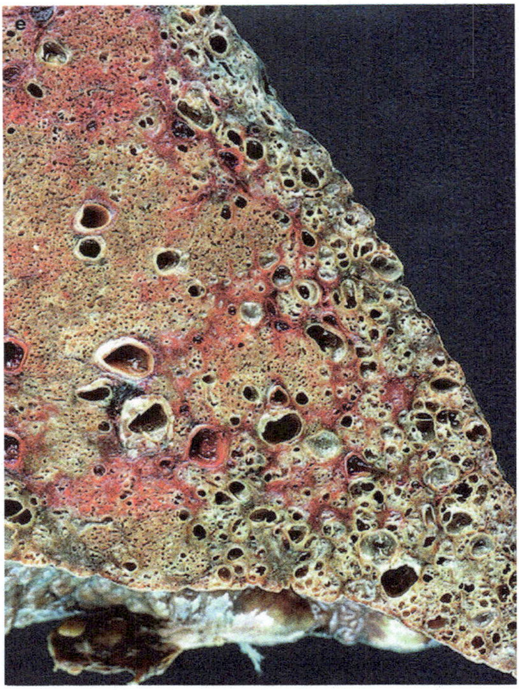

Idiopathic pulmonary fibrosis (interstitial lung disease, idiopathic interstitial pneumonias) with varying alveolar and interstitial inflammatory infiltrates, progressive interstitial fibrosis, secondary hypertensive vascular disease, and a final stage with honeycombing of the lungs. Note the fleshy gross appearance of the lungs in earlier stages (a), with various microscopic interstitial infiltrates (b–d) and gross honeycombing at the end stage (e). [Krueger GRF, Wagner M, Oldham SAA. Pathology of the respiratory tract. In: Krueger GRF, Buja LM, Chandrasekhar C, editors. Atlas of anatomic pathology with imaging [Internet]. London: Springer; 2013 [cited 2015 May 28]. p. 105–89. Available from: http://link.springer.com/10.1007/978-1-4471-2846-5_3] *Caption adapted from original*

- Causative factors currently are unknown.
- There are, however, some known risk factors, including:
  - Cigarette smoking
  - Viral infection
  - Environmental pollutants
  - Chronic aspiration
  - Genetic predisposition
  - Drugs
- None of these risk factors can explain the pathogenesis of IPF. It is felt that these risks precipitate the process in those who are susceptible.

- Several mutations have been found that may increase the risk. These mutations have been identified in both sporadic cases and in familial clusters. They include mutations of surfactant proteins, gel-forming mucin, and telomerase.

Presentation

Typical/"Classic"

- The typical presentation is chronic cough with progressive dyspnea associated with decreased lung function, as measured by a decrease in the forced vital capacity in one second (FVC1) and a decrease in the diffusing capacity to carbon monoxide (DLCO).
- High-resolution CT scan (HRCT) of the lungs will reveal typical findings of UIP, including:
  - Reticular opacities in a peripheral and basal lung distribution
  - Traction bronchiectasis
  - Honeycombing (clustered, abnormal, enlarged airspaces 3 to 10 mm in diameter) in subpleural distribution
  - Ground-glass opacities may be present but usually are less extensive than reticular opacities.
- A thorough search must be undertaken for other contributing factors that may lead to an alternative diagnosis. This includes a search for asbestos exposure, hypersensitivity pneumonitis, systemic sclerosis, and rheumatoid arthritis.

Atypical

- Some patients may present with a typical clinical syndrome of chronic cough, dyspnea, and decreased lung function but have atypical findings on HRCT. In this situation, it may be necessary to proceed to lung biopsy for a confirmation of the diagnosis.
- Patients may present with more focus on either the cough or dyspnea, but both usually are present.

Primary Differential Considerations

- In patients presenting with signs and symptoms suggesting IPF, other diagnoses warranting early consideration include:

- Acute and chronic pneumonias
- "Exposure" lung disease such as asbestosis, farmer's lung, coal worker's lung, and tobacco worker's lung
- Fungal disease such as histoplasmosis

History and Physical Exam

Findings That Confirm Diagnosis

- A full classic presentation with chronic cough, chronic progressive dyspnea, and decreased lung function, with the usual findings of UIP on HRCT, usually confirms the diagnosis.
- However, no historical or physical exam findings are pathognomonic for IPF. For example, digital clubbing is present in only 30 % of patients with IPF.

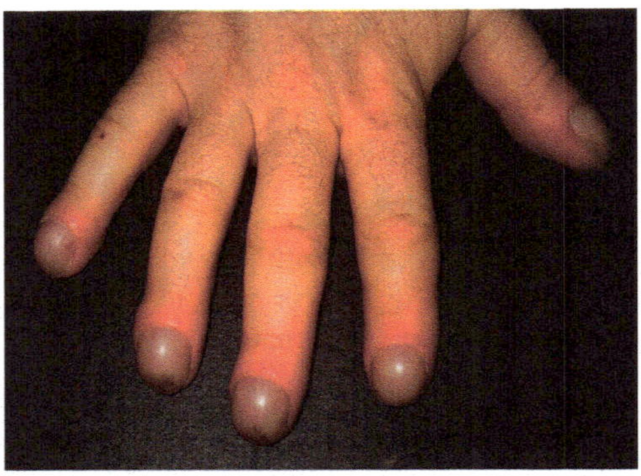

An example of digital clubbing. [Siddiqui M, Melia MT. Clinical image: clubbed with a reminder to test for HIV. J Gen Intern Med. 2014 Sep;29(9):1308–1308.] *Caption adapted from original.*

Factors That Suggest Diagnosis

- The diagnosis should be considered in any person with chronic cough and dyspnea, especially if he or she is over 55 years of age and no other causes for the cough and dyspnea are easily identified.
- On lung exam, patients often have bilateral basilar (sometimes diffuse) "dry" crackles, although this finding is not specific to IPF.

http://en.wikipedia.org/wiki/File:IPF_Lung_Sound.ogg

Dry or "Velcro" crackles in a patient with IPF. [File:IPF Lung Sound.ogg [Internet]. Wikipedia, the free encyclopedia. [cited 2015 Jun 11]. Available from: http://en.wikipedia.org/wiki/File:IPF_Lung_Sound.ogg; licensed under the Creative Commons Attribution-Share Alike 3.0 Unported license.]

Factors That Exclude Diagnosis

- It is difficult to completely exclude the diagnosis with either historical or physical exam findings. However, if another easily identified cause for the symptoms is found, the diagnosis becomes less likely.

Ancillary Studies

Laboratory

- Laboratory studies are not useful in the diagnosis and confirmation of IPF, but they are helpful in seeking alternative and complicating diagnoses.
- It is useful to check laboratory studies to evaluate for abnormalities such as significant anemia, infectious issues (leukocytosis, eosinophilia, etc.), rheumatologic disorders (rheumatoid arthritis, systemic sclerosis), cardiac issues (such as brain natriuretic peptide for CHF), and other alternative and complicating diagnoses.

Imaging

- Imaging is a necessary part of the evaluation of patients with suspected IPF, indeed for any suspected ILD.
- Nearly all patients with unexplained chronic cough and dyspnea will require HRCT of the lungs as part of their diagnostic evaluation.
- HRCT showing the typical changes of UIP (peripheral and basal reticular opacities, traction bronchiectasis, honeycombing) in a patient with chronic cough and dyspnea associated with decreased lung function is nearly diagnostic of IPF, as long as alternative diagnoses (e.g., asbestos exposure, hypersensitivity pneumonitis, systemic sclerosis, and rheumatoid arthritis) have been considered and excluded.

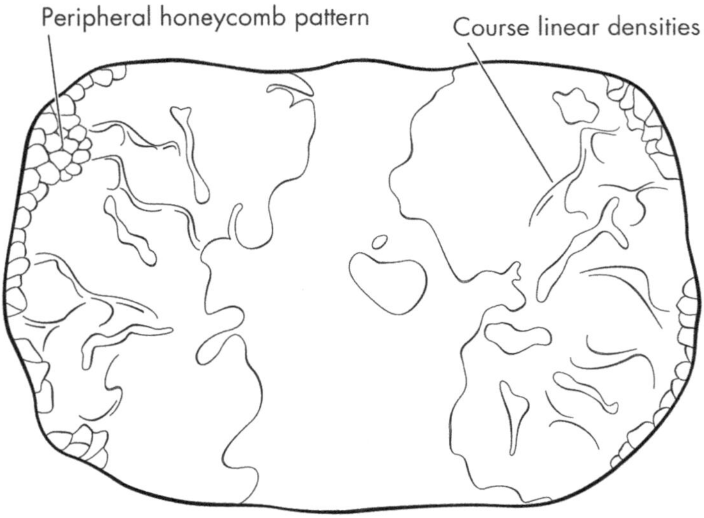

Schematic representation of chest computed tomography in IPF, showing coarse linear densities and a peripheral honeycomb pattern. [Smith M, Grichnik K. Anesthetic considerations for lung transplant and thoracic aortic surgery. In: Reves JG, editor. Cardiothoracic anesthesia. Philadelphia: Current Medicine; 1999. (Miller RD, editor. Atlas of anesthesia; vol. 8) ISBN: 0-443-07974-9] *Caption adapted from original*

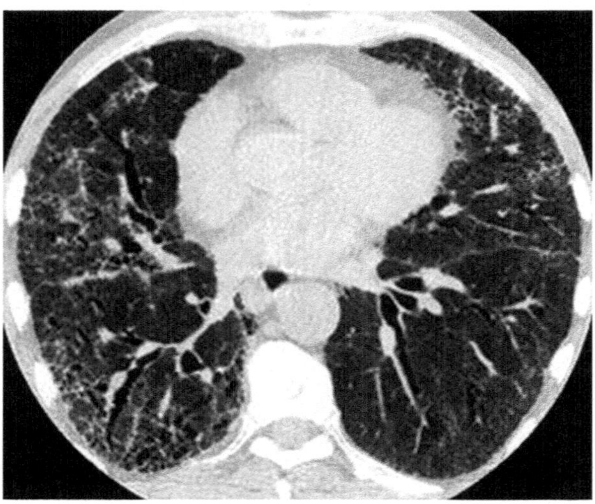

Idiopathic pulmonary fibrosis. HRCT at the level of the lower lobes shows a subpleural "reticular pattern" characterized by thickened interlobular septae, thickened intralobular interstitium, traction bronchiolectasis and bronchiectasis and minimal honeycombing. [From article: Mimics in chest disease: interstitial opacities. Insights into Imaging. 2013 Feb;4(1):9–27; https://doi.org/10.1007/s13244-012-0207-7, at http://link.springer.com/article/10.1007%2Fs13244-012-0207-7/fulltext.html; by Anastasia Oikonomou, Panos Prassopoulos, © The Author(s) 2012; licensed under Creative Commons Attribution License BY 2.0 http://creativecommons.org/licenses/by/2.0] *Caption from original*

- HRCT also is helpful in staging the severity of the disease.
- HRCT and chest x-ray also are helpful during periods of acute exacerbation to help identify and exclude complicating and alternative diagnoses and causes for the worsening dyspnea, as well as to evaluate new and advancing changes of UIP.

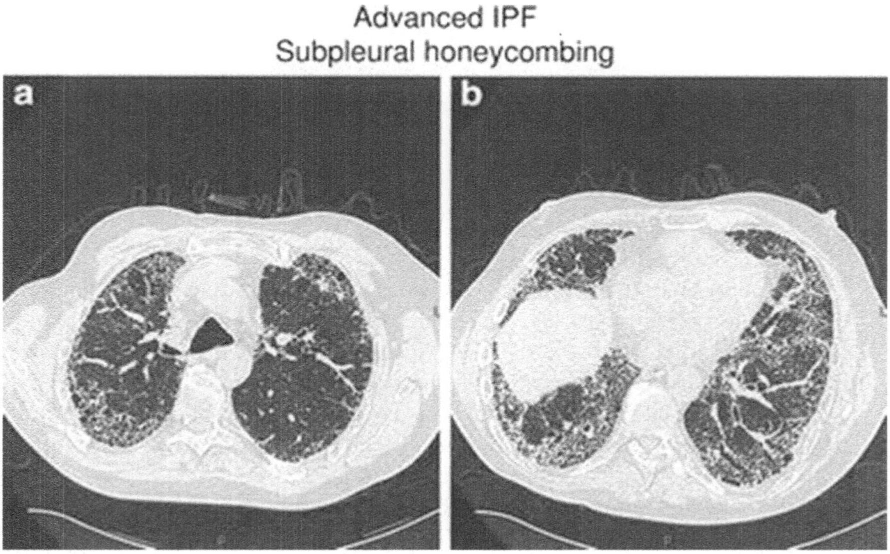

Patient with idiopathic pulmonary fibrosis. Subpleural honeycombing is identified. Disease is more extensive at the base of the lung (b) than in mid lung (a). [Baughman R, Pirozynski M. Health effects of nanoparticles (inhalation) from medical point of view/type of diseases. In: Marijnissen JC, Gradon L, editors. Nanoparticles in medicine and environment [Internet]. Dordrecht: Springer; 2010 [cited 2015 Jun 11]. p. 187–202. Available from: http://www.springerlink.com/index/10.1007/978-90-481-2632-3_10] *Caption from original*

Lung Biopsy

- Lung biopsy may be necessary when the findings on HRCT are equivocal. Transbronchial biopsy is not recommended, as the specimen usually is too small for examination. The usual approach is video-assisted thoracoscopic or open surgical biopsy.

Special Populations

Age

- IPF is a disease of middle-aged and older adults. It is typically diagnosed after age 55 and usually is not even considered a diagnostic possibility before age 40.

Co-morbidities

- Important co-morbid conditions to consider include all diseases and conditions that may worsen dyspnea and accelerate the course of IPF. Most importantly, given the population most at risk for IPF (older than 50), both COPD and CHF are important diseases to consider. However, any condition that may worsen dyspnea (e.g., anemia, coronary vascular disease, pneumonia, lung cancer, pulmonary embolism (PE), pneumothorax) must be considered in the evaluation of both newly diagnosed IPF and IPF exacerbations.
- Gastroesophageal reflux disease (GERD) is an important co-morbid condition to consider in patients diagnosed with IPF. Up to 90 % of patients with IPF also have GERD. Treatment of GERD in those with IPF has been associated with a decrease in the radiographic findings of IPF and may even be associated with improved survival.
- Pulmonary hypertension. Development of pulmonary hypertension is relatively common in patients with IPF, especially as the disease advances, and is a poor prognostic sign.

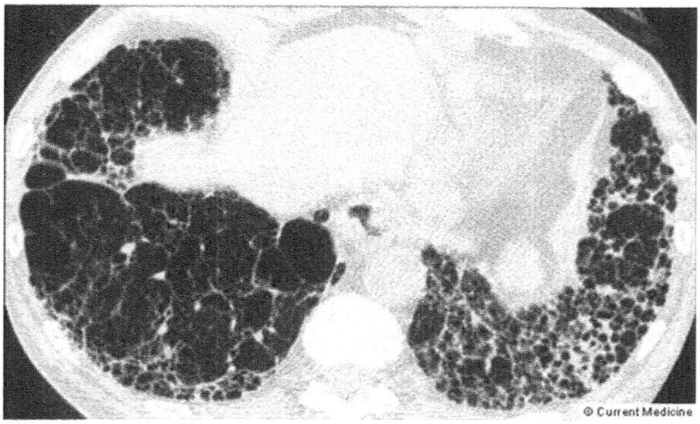

Emphysema associated with idiopathic pulmonary fibrosis in a heavy smoker. Axial thin slices of the chest, showing advanced emphysema predominantly distributed in the upper lobes. Honeycombing, as typically present in usual interstitial pneumonia-idiopathic pulmonary fibrosis, involves the subpleural regions of the lung bases. It is identified as clustered, cystic airspaces usually measuring 2 mm to 10 mm in diameter and having well-defined walls. The cysts appear to share walls and occur in several layers. [Grenier P, Beigelman-Aubry C. Radiologic phenotypes of COPD. In: Crapo JD, editor. Atlas of chronic obstructive pulmonary disease. Philadelphia: Current Medicine; 2009. ISBN: 978-1-57340-294-1] *Caption adapted from original*

Pitfalls in Diagnosis

Critical Steps Not to Miss

- Consideration of the diagnosis is the first critical step, next is establishing the diagnosis.
- More than 200 diseases encompass the diagnosis of ILD. Many of them have more and better treatment options than currently exist for IPF, so an accurate diagnosis is important for the patient to obtain the best available information about treatment and prognosis.

Mimics

- The diagnosis category of ILD includes more than 200 different diseases, many of which present similarly to IPF, with chronic cough, dyspnea, and decreased lung function.

- In addition, several other diseases may have a similar clinical syndrome and show signs of UIP on HRCT, including asbestosis, hypersensitivity pneumonitis, and lung disease associated with systemic sclerosis and rheumatoid arthritis.

Time-Dependent Interventions

- There are no time-dependent interventions in most cases of IPF. The disease is chronic and progressive.
- As with all diseases that cause dyspnea, hypoxemia must be promptly and aggressively treated and avoided.
- In the setting of an acute exacerbation of IPF, it is important and somewhat time sensitive to evaluate and rule out the presence of an emergent complication such as acute coronary syndrome, CHF, PE, pneumothorax, or infection.

Overall Principles of Treatment

- The treatment of IPF has been changing dramatically during the past several years. In 2014, the US Food and Drug Administration approved two new agents: pirfenidone and nintedanib. In clinical trials, both drugs slowed the progression of disease, and they may even confer a mortality benefit.
- In the past, many different anti-inflammatory treatments were attempted, most without success. This is not surprising considering the pathophysiology of IPF, in which biopsy samples show progressive fibrosis with little to no inflammation.
- Treatment has been mostly supportive, including:
  - Patient education
  - Oxygen therapy if hypoxemia is present
  - Pulmonary rehabilitation
  - Appropriate vaccination
  - Identification and treatment of all co-morbidities
  - Prevention and treatment of GERD
  - Lung transplantation as the disease progresses
- Pirfenidone is an antifibrotic agent that inhibits transforming growth factor-β (TGF-β). TGF-β stimulates collagen synthesis as well as fibroblast proliferation; therefore, blocking this protein decreases the extracellular matrix and fibroblast proliferation, two of the major pathophysiologic mechanisms of IPF. Side effects may include rash, photosensitivity, nausea, diarrhea, abdominal discomfort, anorexia, fatigue, and elevation in liver function tests (LFTs). It is recommended that LFTs be checked before and during treatment.

- Nintedanib is a monoclonal antibody that blocks multiple tyrosine kinase receptors. Tyrosine kinases are known to stimulate production of multiple fibrogenic growth factors. As with pirfenidone, this agent may cause LFT elevations; therefore, liver tests should be performed before and during treatment. Nintedanib also may increase the risk of bleeding from anticoagulation. Other common adverse effects include diarrhea, nausea, and vomiting.
- In severe cases complicated by pulmonary hypertension, some authorities add phosphodiesterase inhibitors (or other vasodilators) to the treatment regimen. These agents, however, are used primarily to treat pulmonary hypertension; their use in IPF is under study.
- Currently, IPF is the second most frequent diagnosis for which lung transplantation is performed. Because IPF is a chronically progressive disease associated with numerous co-morbidities, it generally is believed that lung transplantation is better and more safely performed earlier in the course of the illness.

Disease Course

- IPF is a relentlessly progressive disease. All patients have progression; no spontaneous remissions have been reported.
- The overall prognosis is poor, with a 5-year mortality rate of about 75 %.
- Multiple factors are associated with more rapidly progressive disease and shortened survival:
  - Older age at diagnosis
  - History of prolonged tobacco use
  - Lower weight
  - More severe disease at diagnosis
  - The presence of a co-morbid condition that may worsen and complicate the clinical course of IPF, such as COPD, CHF, pulmonary hypertension, coronary artery disease, or lung cancer.
- At the time of diagnosis, it is important to try to pinpoint the severity of the disease.
- Currently no validated staging system exists for IPF; its classification is based mainly on clinical grounds, including symptoms, pulmonary function test (PFT) findings, and results of HRCT.
- A typical assessment of severity is based on the following guidelines:
  - Mild or early disease
    - Patient may be asymptomatic or have only a mild cough.
    - Patient may have dyspnea on exertion (DOE), but it may be mild and unnoticed or thought to be related to some other cause.
    - Radiographic changes (reticular opacities and honeycombing) typically involve less than 10 % of the lungs.

    - PFTs may be normal or demonstrate only mild decreases in FVC1 and DLCO.
  - Moderate disease
    - Cough and DOE are more pronounced and noticeable.
    - Radiographic changes involve 20–30 % of the lungs.
    - On PFTs, the FVC1 is 50–70 % predicted and DLCO is about 50 % predicted.
  - Severe/advanced disease
    - DOE is severe; patient cannot climb one flight of stairs without stopping to rest.
    - Patient usually requires supplemental oxygen.
    - Extensive honeycombing is seen on HRCT.
    - FVC1 and DLCO are less than 50 % predicted.
- Acute exacerbations of IPF. The clinical course of IPF may be complicated by acute exacerbations in up to 60 % of patients. The term *exacerbation* is somewhat misleading, as patients often do not return to their "pre-exacerbation" level of functioning. These acute exacerbations also are known as *accelerated phases of rapid clinical deterioration*. They are associated with a poor prognosis, with in-hospital mortality approaching 80 %. Recurrences are common.
  - Accepted definition of an acute exacerbation of IPF includes:
    - Known diagnosis of IPF
    - An unexplained worsening of dyspnea within the past 30 days
    - HRCT demonstrating new bilateral ground-glass opacities and/or consolidation on a background of UIP (honeycombing and reticular opacities)
    - No evidence of pulmonary infection by endotracheal aspirate or bronchoalveolar lavage
    - The exclusion of alternative causes of worsened dyspnea, especially pneumonia, heart failure, PE, and pneumothorax
  - Treatment usually involves the administration of antibiotics for presumed superinfection and glucocorticoids for acute inflammation; however, there is no evidence that either of these agents is helpful.

Related Evidence

Papers of particular interest have been highlighted as:
*** Of key importance*

Practice Guideline

Cottin V, Crestani B, Valeyre D, Wallaert B, Cadranel J, Dalphin JC, Delaval P, Israel-Biet D, Kessler R, Reynaud-Gaubert M, Aguilaniu B, Bouquillon B, Carré P, Danel C, Faivre JB, Ferretti G, Just N, Kouzan S, Lebargy F, Marchand-Adam S, Philippe B, Prévot G, Stach B, Thivolet-Béjui F, Cordier JF; French National Reference Centre; Network of Competence Centres for Rare Lung Diseases. Diagnosis and management of idiopathic pulmonary fibrosis: French practical guidelines. Eur Respir Rev. 2014 Jun;23(132):193-214. https://doi.org/10.1183/09059180.00001814. PMID: 24881074. http://www.ncbi.nlm.nih.gov/pubmed/24881074 **

Travis WD, Costabel U, Hansell DM, King TE Jr, Lynch DA, Nicholson AG, Ryerson CJ, Ryu JH, Selman M, Wells AU, Behr J, Bouros D, Brown KK, Colby TV, Collard HR, Cordeiro CR, Cottin V, Crestani B, Drent M, Dudden RF, Egan J, Flaherty K, Hogaboam C, Inoue Y, Johkoh T, Kim DS, Kitaichi M, Loyd J, Martinez FJ, Myers J, Protzko S, Raghu G, Richeldi L, Sverzellati N, Swigris J, Valeyre D; ATS/ERS Committee on Idiopathic Interstitial Pneumonias. An official American Thoracic Society/European Respiratory Society statement: Update of the international multidisciplinary classification of the idiopathic interstitial pneumonias. Am J Respir Crit Care Med. 2013 Sep 15;188(6):733-48. https://doi.org/10.1164/rccm.201308-1483ST. PMID: 24032382. http://www.ncbi.nlm.nih.gov/pubmed/24032382 **

Diagnosis and Management of Suspected Idiopathic Pulmonary Fibrosis: Idiopathic Pulmonary Fibrosis. National Clinical Guideline Centre (UK). London: Royal College of Physicians (UK); 2013 Jun. PMID: 25340234. http://www.ncbi.nlm.nih.gov/pubmed/25340234 **

Raghu G, Collard HR, Egan JJ, Martinez FJ, Behr J, Brown KK, Colby TV, Cordier JF, Flaherty KR, Lasky JA, Lynch DA, Ryu JH, Swigris JJ, Wells AU, Ancochea J, Bouros D, Carvalho C, Costabel U, Ebina M, Hansell DM, Johkoh T, Kim DS, King TE Jr, Kondoh Y, Myers J, Müller NL, Nicholson AG, Richeldi L, Selman M, Dudden RF, Griss BS, Protzko SL, Schünemann HJ; ATS/ERS/JRS/ALAT Committee on Idiopathic Pulmonary Fibrosis. An official ATS/ERS/JRS/ALAT statement: idiopathic pulmonary fibrosis: evidence-based guidelines for diagnosis and management. Am J Respir Crit Care Med. 2011 Mar 15;183(6):788–824. https://doi.org/10.1164/rccm.2009-040GL. PMID: 21471066. http://www.ncbi.nlm.nih.gov/pubmed/21471066 **

Review

Kim HJ, Perlman D, Tomic R. Natural history of idiopathic pulmonary fibrosis. Respir Med. 2015 Jun;109(6):661-670. https://doi.org/10.1016/j.rmed.2015.02.002. PMID: 25727856. http://www.ncbi.nlm.nih.gov/pubmed/25727856 **

Renzoni E, Srihari V, Sestini P. Pathogenesis of idiopathic pulmonary fibrosis: review of recent findings. F1000Prime Rep. 2014 Aug 1;6:69. https://doi.org/10.12703/P6-69. eCollection 2014. PMID: 25165568. http://www.ncbi.nlm.nih.gov/pubmed/25165568 **

Oldham JM, Noth I. Idiopathic pulmonary fibrosis: early detection and referral. Respir Med. 2014 Jun;108(6):819-29. https://doi.org/10.1016/j.rmed.2014.03.008. PMID: 24746629. http://www.ncbi.nlm.nih.gov/pubmed/24746629 **

Kekevian A, Gershwin ME, Chang C. Diagnosis and classification of idiopathic pulmonary fibrosis. Autoimmun Rev. 2014 Apr-May;13(4-5):508-12. https://doi.org/10.1016/j.autrev.2014.01.037. PMID: 24424167. http://www.ncbi.nlm.nih.gov/pubmed/24424167 **

Woodcock HV, Maher TM. The treatment of idiopathic pulmonary fibrosis. F1000Prime Rep. 2014 Mar 3;6:16. doi: 10.12703/P6-16. eCollection 2014. PMID: 24669297. http://www.ncbi.nlm.nih.gov/pubmed/24669297 **

Walsh SL, Hansell DM. High-resolution CT of interstitial lung disease: a continuous evolution. Semin Respir Crit Care Med. 2014 Feb;35(1):129-44. https://doi.org/10.1055/s-0033-1363458. PMID: 24481766. http://www.ncbi.nlm.nih.gov/pubmed/24481766 **

Ley B, Collard HR. Epidemiology of idiopathic pulmonary fibrosis. Clin Epidemiol. 2013 Nov 25;5:483-92. https://doi.org/10.2147/CLEP.S54815. PMID: 24348069. http://www.ncbi.nlm.nih.gov/pubmed/24348069

Use PubMed Clinical Queries to find the most recent evidence. Use this search strategy:

"Idiopathic Pulmonary Fibrosis"[Mesh] OR "idiopathic pulmonary fibrosis" OR "cryptogenic fibrosing alveolitis"

Chapter 39
Infective Endocarditis

Christopher J. Rees, Charles V. Pollack, Jr., and Jaime Friel Blanck

Name and Synonyms

Infective Endocarditis

Incidence/Epidemiology

- Infective endocarditis (IE) has an estimated annual incidence of between 3 to 9 cases per 100,000 people per year in developed nations. Incidence rates can vary widely based upon predisposing conditions, risk factors, and geographic area.
- Predisposing conditions include the presence of a prosthetic heart valve, the presence of an intracardiac device, unrepaired cyanotic congenital heart disease, a prior history of infective endocarditis, chronic rheumatic heart disease, age-related degenerative valvular lesions, hemodialysis, diabetes, HIV infections, and intravenous drug use, dental infections, and poor dental hygiene. Age greater than 65 and male sex are also risk factors for IE.
- Rheumatic heart disease is now an uncommon cause of IE in developed nations, but remains a significant cause of IE in developing nations.
- Incidence has been increasing among and shifting toward those greater than 65 years old.

C. J. Rees
Emergency Department, Pennsylvania Hospital, Philadelphia, PA, USA

C. V. Pollack, Jr. (✉)
Department of Emergency Medicine, Thomas Jefferson University, Philadelphia, PA, USA

J. F. Blanck
Welch Medical Library, Johns Hopkins University, Baltimore, MD, USA

C. V. Pollack, Jr. (ed.), *Differential Diagnosis of Cardiopulmonary Disease*,
https://doi.org/10.1007/978-3-319-63895-9_39

- Increasing proportions (up to one-third) of cases of IE are now health-care associated.
- The male-to-female ratio is about 2:1.
- About 10,000–15,000 cases per year are diagnosed in the United States.

Differential Diagnosis

- The differential diagnosis for IE is exceptionally broad, and a high index of suspicion needs to be maintained.
    - Many diseases can present with fever and diffuse/multi-organ symptoms, including many infections, vasculitides, connective tissue diseases, and malignant diseases.
    - Many diseases can be associated with bacteremia, such as skin and soft tissue infections, osteomyelitis, pneumonia, meningitis, and others. All patients with bacteremia, even if there is an associated cause as above, should have an evaluation for valvular vegetations with echocardiography, as all causes of bacteremia can coexist with IE, and many are known predisposing factors for IE or complications of IE.

Pathophysiology and Etiology

- The majority of cases of endocarditis (80 %) are caused by Streptococci and Staphylococci.
- Staphylococci are the most frequent cause of health-care associated IE.
- Ten percent of cases of IE are blood culture negative. This generally results from either exposure to antibiotics prior to the diagnosis of IE, or when IE is due to slow-growing, fastidious organisms.
    - These slow-growing, fastidious organisms include bartonella species, brucella species, Coxiella burnetii, Tropheryma whippelii, and bacteria in the HACEK group. The HACEK group of organisms includes haemophilus species, Aggregatibacter actinomycetemcomitans, Cardiobacterium hominis, Eikenella corrodens, and Kingella kingae.
- The classic model of the pathogenesis of native-valve infectious endocarditis involves valvular endothelial damage that allows colonization by bacteria.
    - Endothelial damage may result from turbulent blood flow around the valve, direct trauma from the repeated injection of particulate contaminants in those who inject intravenous drugs, or by direct trauma from electrodes or catheters used during cardiac procedures.

- The bacteria that are most likely to cause IE often have specific adherence factors that facilitate their adherence and formation of vegetations.
- Vegetations are the characteristic pathologic lesions of IE. They are a mass of platelets, fibrin, organisms, and inflammatory cells that adhere to damaged endothelium or myocardium. Vegetations are most commonly found on heart valves, but can also attach to any area of myocardial damage or scarring, such as an atrial septal defect, ventricular septal defect, or endocardium damaged by foreign bodies (pacemakers, automatic implantable cardiac defibrillators [AICD]).

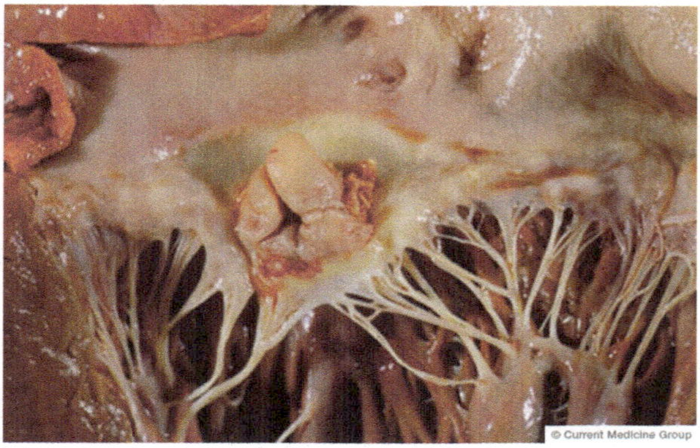

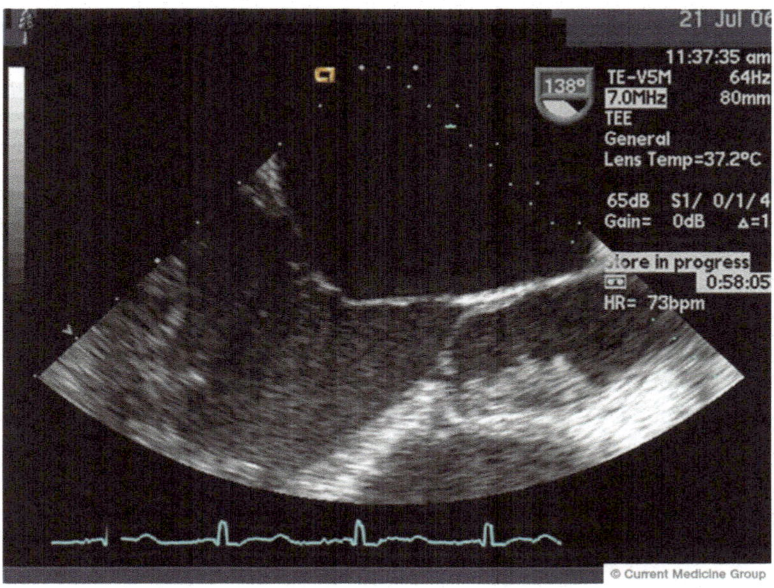

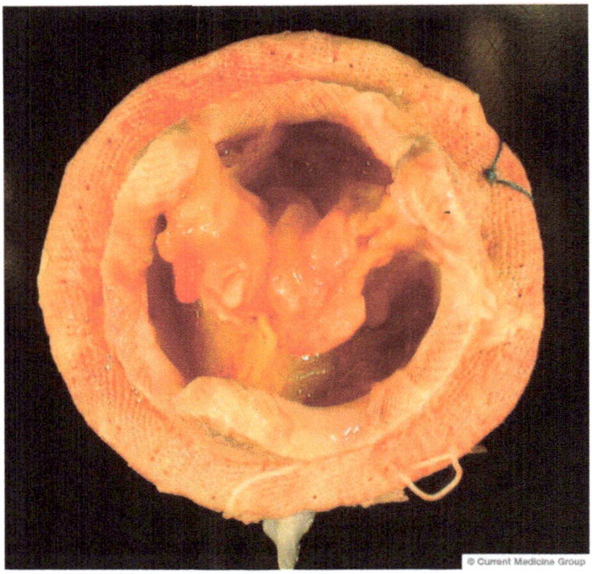

Infective endocarditis. **A**, Large, multilobulated vegetation on the anterior leaflet of the mitral valve from a patient with *Staphylococcus lugdunensis* endocarditis who died of a rupture mycotic cerebral aneurysm. **B**, Transesophageal echocardiographic image showing a cluster of vegetative material adherent to and above the anterior leaflet of the aortic valve. TEE is more sensitive than transthoracic echocardiogram (TTE) for the detection and characterization of vegetation and abscess in patients with suspected infective endocarditis. **C**, Gross operative specimen from a patient with prosthetic valve endocarditis affecting the valve leaflets, but sparing the sewing ring. [O'Gara P. Chapter 9. In: Libby P, editor. Essential Atlas of Cardiovascular Disease. 4th ed. Philadelphia: Current Medicine Group; 2009. 432 p.] *Caption adapted from original*

- Chronic inflammation of valvular tissue can also lead to endothelial damage and bacterial colonization. This is the case in rheumatic heart disease and degenerative valve disease.
- Several microorganisms are felt to cause endocarditis from a maladaptive host immune response. C. burnetii, bartonella species, and T. Whippelii are all intracellular pathogens, and when they infect valvular tissue they can cause a host immune response that can damage valvular tissue.

Presentation

Typical/"Classic"

- The classic presentation is a patient with a known predisposing factor with a fever and a new or worsened murmur.
- Fever is the most common symptom. It is present in up to 80 % of patients.
- The majority of patients will have one of the predisposing conditions noted in the etiology section.
- About half of all patients will have new murmur; about a quarter will have worsening of a known prior murmur.
- There is usually no other obvious source for the fever.

Atypical

- Infective endocarditis frequently presents atypically, especially early in the course of the disease.
- Symptoms may be non-specific, and the diagnosis may not be considered until there is fever or a complication secondary to IE.
- Patients may initially present with a complication of IE, especially from embolic infected vegetations. These complications include:
  - Pulmonary embolism, pneumonia, or pulmonary abscess from septic pulmonary emboli.
  - Stroke (both ischemic and hemorrhagic), TIA, brain abscess, and meningitis.
  - Renal failure.
  - Peripheral arterial occlusion.
  - Sepsis.
- IE caused by S. aureus, especially involving the mitral valve, is the most common cause of systemic embolic complications.
- It is important to know that embolic complications (for example, septic pulmonary emboli, cerebrovascular emboli) can occur before the diagnosis of IE is made, and may be a clue to the diagnosis.
- IE associated with injection drug use is limited to the tricuspid valve about half the time, and as such usually has no murmur that can be appreciated by auscultation, and will have no peripheral manifestations of IE. There is a higher incidence of septic pulmonary emboli in IE among injection drug users, so the diagnosis of pulmonary abscess should lead one to suspect and evaluate for the diagnosis of IE.

Primary Differential Considerations

Other diagnoses to consider in patients with signs and symptoms suggestive of IE include:

- Fever of unknown origin
- Septic pulmonary emboli
- Vasculitis
- Connective tissue diseases

History and Physical Exam

Findings That Confirm Diagnosis

- There are no completely confirmatory historical or physical examination findings for IE.
- The Duke Criteria is the current reference standard for the diagnosis of IE. They are a series of clinical, microbiologic, and echocardiographic findings that together have a sensitivity and specificity of greater than 80% for the diagnosis of IE.

Definite IE any of (1) or (2)	(1) Pathologic criteria: Microorganisms demonstrated by culture or histologic examination of a vegetation, a vegetation that has embolized, or an intracardiac abscess specimen, or pathologic lesions – vegetation or intracardiac abscess confirmed by histologic examination showing active endocarditis
	(2) Clinical criteria: Any of two major criteria, or one major criterion and three minor criteria, or five minor criteria
Possible IE	One major criterion and one minor criterion or three minor criteria
Rejected	Firm alternative diagnosis explaining evidence of IE, or resolution of IE syndrome with antibiotic treatment for 4 or less days, or no pathologic evidence of IE at surgery or autopsy with antibiotic therapy for 4 or less days, or does not meet criteria for possible IE
Major criteria:	(1) Positive blood culture for IE: (a) Typical microorganisms consistent with IE from two separate blood cultures: Viridans streptococci, *Streptococcus bovis*, HACEK group; *Staphylococcus aureus* or community-acquired enterococci in the absence of a primary focus (b) Microorganisms consistent with IE from persistently positive blood cultures defined as: At least two positive blood cultures drawn more than 12 h apart, or all of three, or a majority of four or more blood cultures with first and last sample drawn at least 1 h apart (c) Single positive blood culture for *Coxiella burnetii* or antiphase I IgG antibody titer >1:800
	(2) Evidence of endocardial involvement: (a) Positive echocardiogram for IE: Oscillating intracardiac mass on valve or supporting structures, in the path of regurgitant jets, or on implanted material in the absence of an alternative anatomic explanation, or abscess, or new partial dehiscence of prosthetic valve, or new valvular regurgitation (worsening or changing of preexisting murmur not sufficient)
Minor criteria:	(1) Predisposition – predisposing heart condition or injection drug use
	(2) Fever – temperature of 38 °C or more
	(3) Vascular phenomena – major arterial embolism, septic pulmonary infarcts, mycotic aneurysm, intracranial hemorrhage, conjunctival hemorrhages, Janeway lesions
	(4) Immunological phenomena – glomerulonephritis, Osler nodes, Roth spots, rheumatoid factor
	(5) Microbiological evidence – positive blood culture but does not meet a major criterion as noted above or serological evidence of active infection with organism consistent with IE

Modified Duke Criteria for the Diagnosis of Infective Endocarditis (IE) [Rodriguez ER, Tan CD. Cardiovascular Pathology. In: Cheng L, Bostwick DG, editors. Essentials of Anatomic Pathology [Internet]. Cham: Springer International Publishing; 2016 [cited 2016 Aug 8]. p. 1295–351. Available from: http://link.springer.com/10.1007/978-3-319-23380-2_27]

- The Duke criteria require microbiologic and echocardiographic results and as such are not particularly helpful early in the course of evaluation. A high index of suspicion is necessary for the early diagnosis of IE.

Factors That Suggest Diagnosis

- The presence of a fever with no obvious source, with any of the predisposing factors discussed in the etiology section, or with a new or worsened murmur suggests the diagnosis.
- The classic physical examination findings associated with IE have become uncommon, but their presence should suggest the diagnosis.
  - Splinter hemorrhages (linear petechiae in the center of the nail bed, as opposed to traumatic petechiae which are usually in the distal nail bed) are found in only about 5 –8% of patients.

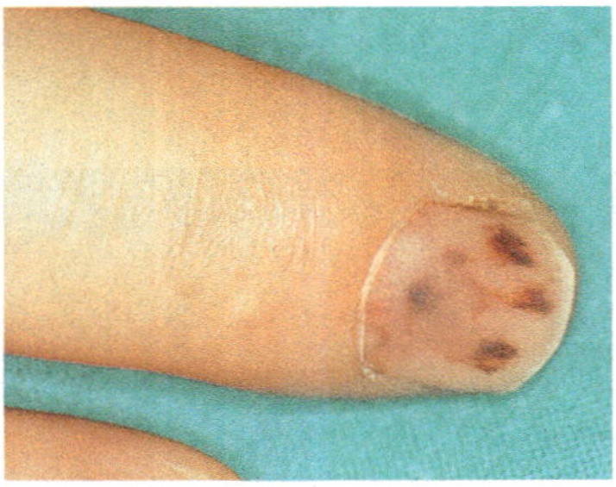

Splinter hemorrhages in a fingernail. Splinter hemorrhages may be due to simple trauma, but when multiple nails are involved in a patient with infective endocarditis, they represent a vasculitic component of the infection. [Miró J, Wilson W, Chapter 01. In: Korzeniowski O, editor. Cardiovascular Infections, 1e. Philadelphia: Current Medicine; 1998. (Mandell GL, editor. Atlas of infectious diseases; vol. 10). ISBN: 0-443-07750-9] *Caption adapted from original*

- Janeway lesions (non-tender, palpable hemorrhages on the palms and soles) in about 5%.

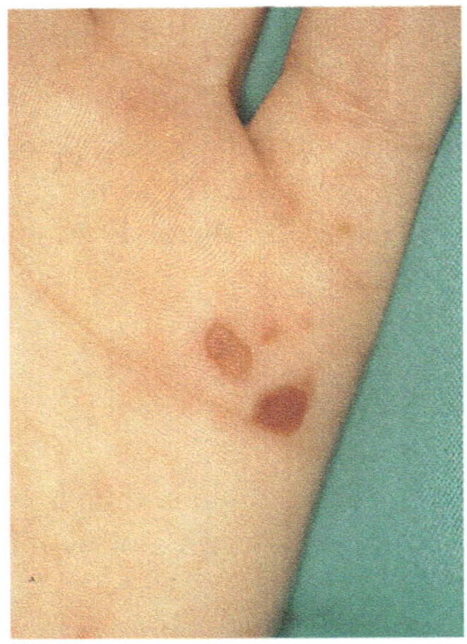

Janeway lesions in *Staphylococcus aureus* left-sided endocarditis [Miró J, Wilson W, Chapter 01. In: Korzeniowski O, editor. Cardiovascular Infections, 1e. Philadelphia: Current Medicine; 1998. (Mandell GL, editor. Atlas of infectious diseases; vol. 10). ISBN: 0-443-07750-9] *Caption from original*

- Osler's nodes are painful, purple nodules found on fingerpads and toepads, and are very rarely seen.

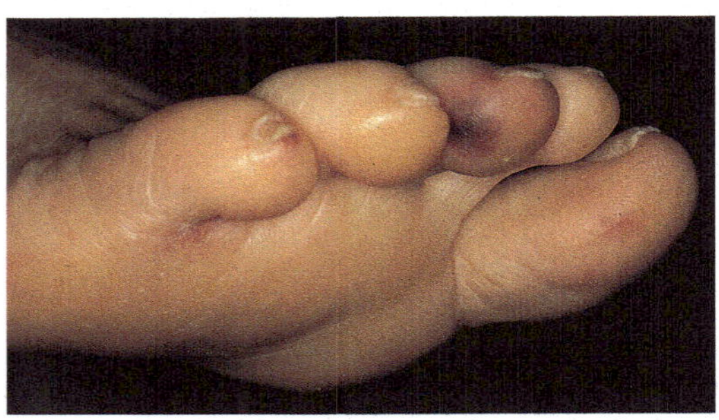

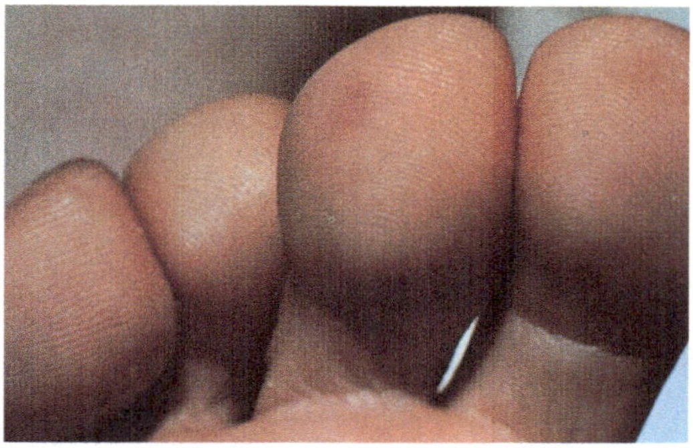

A and **B**, Osler's nodes in patients with infective endocarditis. These lesions usually occur in the tufts of the fingers or toes and are painful and evanescent. They likely are mediated by immunopathologic factors. [Scheld MW. Chapter 02. In: Fekety R, editor. External manifestations of systemic infections. Philadelphia: Current Medicine; 1997. 237 p. (Mandell GL, editor. Atlas of infectious diseases; vol. 8.) ISBN: 0-443-07760-6] *Caption from original*

- Roth's spots (white centered retinal hemorrhages) in 5%.

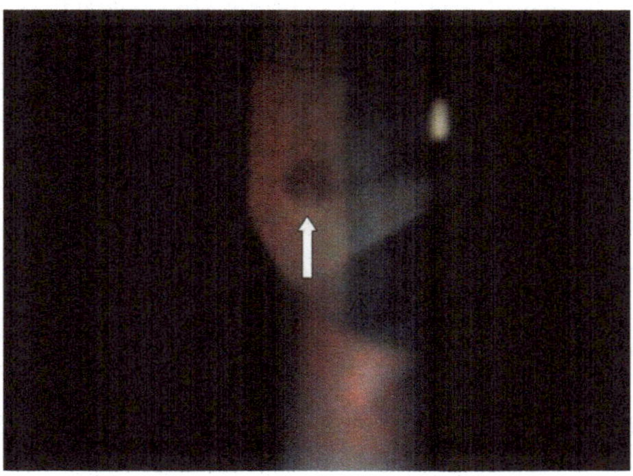

Roth's spot on the retina of the left eye. [From article: Case report: Infective endocarditis caused by *Brevundimonas vesicularis*. BMC Infectious Diseases. 2006 Dec;6(1). https://doi.org/10.1186/1471-2334-6-179, at http://link.springer.com/article/10.1186%2F1471-2334-6-179/fulltext.html; by Mei-Li Yang, Yen-Hsu Chen, Tun-Chieh Chen, Wei-Ru Lin, Chun-Yu Lin, Po-Liang Lu, © Yang et al; licensee BioMed Central Ltd. 2006; licensed under Creative Commons Attribution License BY 2.0 http://creativecommons.org/licenses/by/2.0] *Caption from original*

- Conjunctival hemorrhages in 5%.

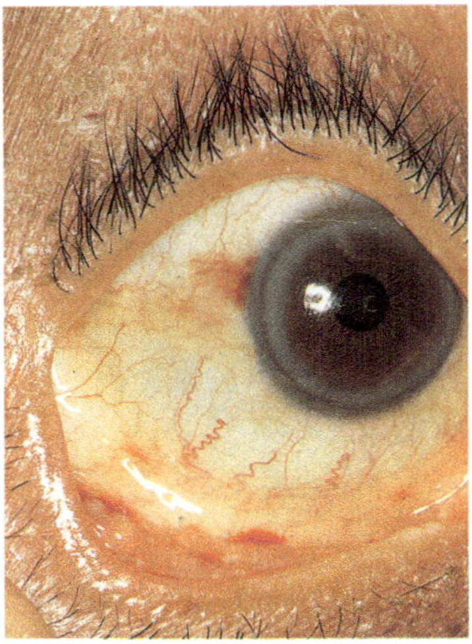

Conjunctival hemorrhages in a patient with *Staphylococcus aureus*endocarditis. [Scheld MW. Chapter 02. In: Fekety R, editor. External manifestations of systemic infections. Philadelphia: Current Medicine; 1997. 237 p. (Mandell GL, editor. Atlas of infectious diseases; vol. 8.) ISBN: 0-443-07760-6] *Caption from original*

- Patients with prosthetic heart valves are at increased risk for IE, and the diagnosis should always be considered when these patients have unexplained fever or other constitutional symptoms (such as unexplained weight loss, night sweats, loss of appetite).
- Hospitalization, especially prolonged hospitalization with indwelling venous access or recent intravascular procedures, also increases the risk for IE.

Factors That Exclude Diagnosis

- There are historical or physical examination findings that can reliably exclude the diagnosis.
- Negative blood cultures also do not reliably exclude the diagnosis, as 10% of cases of IE will have negative blood cultures (see pathophysiology and etiology section).
- The diagnosis can be rejected as per the Duke Criteria.

Ancillary Studies

Laboratory

- Blood cultures are imperative for the diagnosis of IE. All patients with suspected IE should have three sets of blood cultures drawn. Each individual blood culture should be from a separate venipuncture site (not from a vascular catheter), and include at least 10 ml of blood for adults (5 ml for each bottle), 0.5 ml for infants, and 5 ml for children. If the patient is acutely ill, the cultures should be obtained over a one-hour period. All cultures should be obtained prior to the initiation of antibiotic therapy.
  - When three sets of appropriately drawn blood cultures are performed, the causative microorganism is identified in about 90 % of cases of IE.
- Multiple other laboratory studies are often abnormal in the setting of IE, but they are also very nonspecific.
- Patients with either acute Streptococcal or Staphylococcal IE often have elevated white blood cell counts and a thrombocytopenia.
  - In sub-acute presentations, the WBC count may be normal.
- Other laboratory markers of inflammation and infection may be elevated, such as the erythrocyte sedimentation rate (ESR), and the c-reactive protein (CRP).
- IE can cause interference with and abnormal results on multiple serologic and immune tests. In fact, an elevated rheumatoid factor in a patient without a known prior history of a rheumatologic disorder is a minor criterion for the diagnosis of IE in the Duke criteria.
- The majority of patients with IE will have an abnormal urinalysis. There may be proteinuria, pyuria, and either microscopic or gross hematuria. All of these findings are nonspecific. However, glomerulonephritis, often manifested with red blood cell casts on a microscopic urinalysis, is a minor criterion for the diagnosis of IE in the Duke criteria.

Echocardiography

- Echocardiography is indispensible in the diagnosis of IE, and should be performed as soon as reasonably possible when the diagnosis of IE is considered. Echocardiography can show valvular vegetations, valve dysfunction, and para-valvular abscesses.
- In general, trans-thoracic echocardiography (TTE) should be performed first. It is less sensitive and less specific than trans-esophageal echocardiography (TEE), but it is also less invasive and doesn't require sedation to perform.

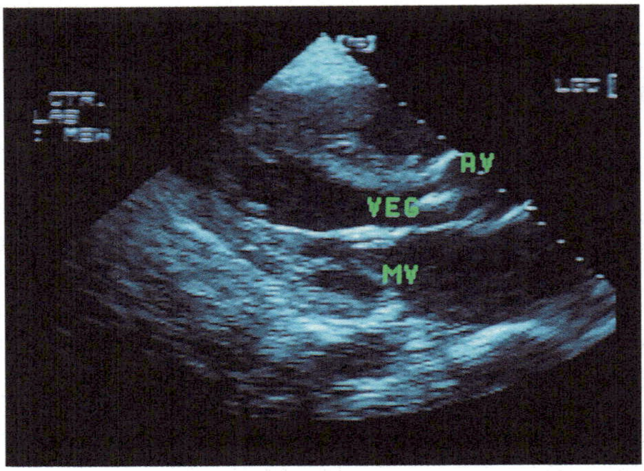

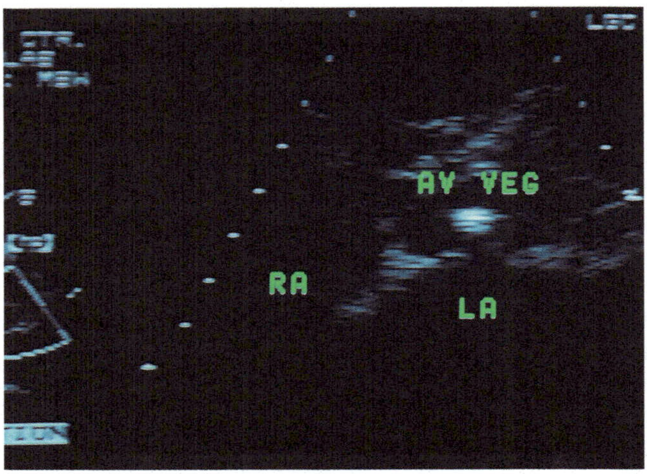

Transthoracic echocardiographic views of aortic valve endocarditis. **A**, Parasternal long-axis view shows an aortic valve vegetation prolapsing into the left ventricular outflow tract. **B**, Short axis view of the aortic valve shows a prominent vegetation in the same patient.[Scheld MW. Chapter 02. In: Fekety R, editor. External manifestations of systemic infections. Philadelphia: Current Medicine; 1997. 237 p. (Mandell GL, editor. Atlas of infectious diseases; vol. 8.) ISBN: 0-443-07760-6] *Caption from original*

- TEE is more sensitive and specific for the diagnosis of IE and should be performed in multiple situations:

- After a negative or technically difficult TTE when the clinical concern for IE is moderate-to-high.
- After a positive TTE (demonstrating a valvular vegetation) when there is also a concern for an intracardiac complication such as para-valvular abscess, significant valvular regurgitation, and in the assessment for the need for surgery.
- In patients with a prosthetic valve.
- In patients with a known history of valvular disorder (including a prior history of IE).

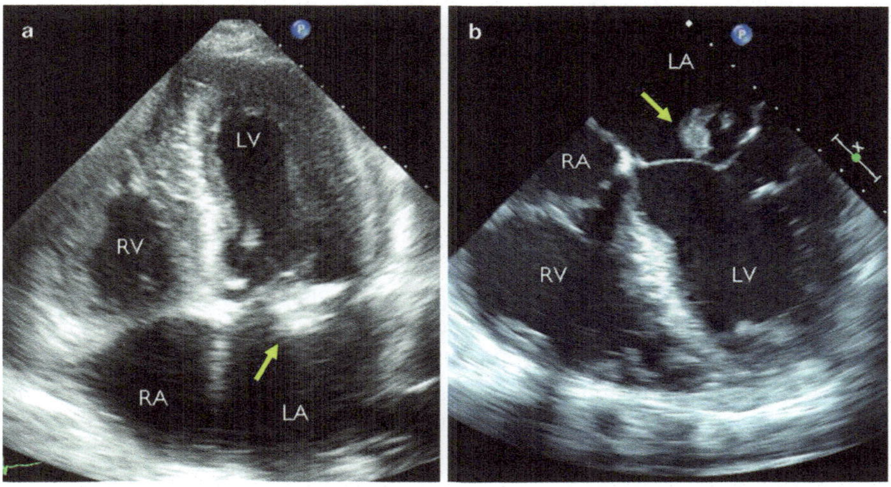

Representative images acquired by transthoracic echocardiography (TTE,**a**) and transesophageal echocardiography (TEE, **b**) in the same patient with mitral valve endocarditis (arrowhead points to bacterial vegetation adherent to the anterior leaflet). The proximity of the mitral valve to the esophagus and superior acoustic window results in improved spatial resolution of TEE over TTE. RA right atrium, RV right ventricle, LA left atrium, LV left ventricle [Michelis KC, Choi BG. Cardiovascular Imaging in Global Health Radiology. In: Mollura DJ, Lungren MP, editors. Radiology in Global Health [Internet]. New York, NY: Springer New York; 2014 [cited 2016 Aug 8]. p. 189–203. Available from: http://link.springer.com/10.1007/978-1-4614-0604-4_18] *Caption from original*

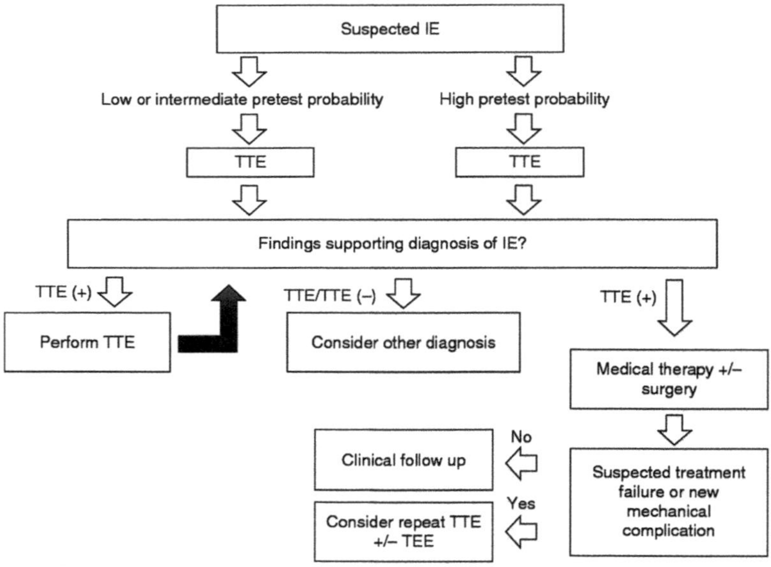

Algorithm for the use of echocardiography in the diagnosis and management of infective endocarditis [Kiefer TL, Wang A. Infective Endocarditis. In: Stergiopoulos K, Brown DL, editors. Evidence-Based Cardiology Consult [Internet]. London: Springer London; 2014 [cited 2016 Aug 8]. p. 71–8. Available from: http://link.springer.com/10.1007/978-1-4471-4441-0_6] *Caption from original*

- The combination of TTE and TEE demonstrates valvular vegetations in 90% of cases of IE.
- Echocardiography may need to be repeated if the initial study was unrevealing but the clinical suspicion remains high (for example, known risk factor in setting of positive blood cultures.)
- Echocardiography also may need to be repeated if there is a new or suspected complication of IE, clinical worsening, and at the end of therapy.

Imaging

- Chest X-ray. There are no specific findings of IE on CXR. CXR may, however, reveal complications of OE such as infiltrates or pulmonary abscess from septic pulmonary emboli.
- Other imaging studies, such as CT scan or MRI, have no specific findings for IE, but may also demonstrate, or be used to search for, complications of IE such as vertebral osteomyelitis with MRI of the spine, solid organ or other intraperitoneal collection with CT scan of the abdomen and pelvis, and any intracranial complication with either CT scan or MRI of the brain.

Special Populations

Age

- Greater than 50% of cases of IE occur in patients above the age of 65.
- IE is uncommon in children, but the incidence has been reported to be increasing over the last several decades due to the increased rate of successful surgery for congenital heart disease, and the increased use of central venous catheters. Correspondingly, these are the two biggest risk factors for IE in children.
  - As in adults, Streptococci and Staphylococci are the most common causative organisms.
  - The presentation, diagnosis, and treatment are similar in children and adults.
  - Duke's criteria are applicable to the pediatric population.
  - There is about a 5% mortality rate for children with IE.

Co-morbidities

- Important pre-disposing and co-morbid conditions that increase the incidence and complications are detailed as per the incidence and epidemiology section, and include the presence of a prosthetic heart valve, the presence of an intracardiac device, unrepaired cyanotic congenital heart disease, a prior history of infective endocarditis, chronic rheumatic heart disease, age-related degenerative valvular lesions, hemodialysis, diabetes, HIV infections, intravenous drug use, age greater than 65, poor dental hygiene, and dental infection.

Pitfalls in Diagnosis

Critical Steps Not to Miss

- All patients in whom IE is being considered need three sets of correctly drawn blood cultures prior to the administration of antibiotics.
- All patients in whom IE is being considered need to have echocardiography as soon as possible.
- It is important to know that embolic complications (for example, septic pulmonary emboli, cerebrovascular emboli) can occur before the diagnosis of IE is made, and may be a clue to the diagnosis.
- IE associated with injection drug use is limited to the tricuspid valve about half the time, and as such usually has no murmur that can be appreciated by auscultation, and will have no peripheral manifestations of IE. There is a

higher incidence of septic pulmonary emboli in IE among injection drug users, so the diagnosis of pulmonary abscess should lead one to suspect and evaluate for the diagnosis of IE.

Mimics

- Many diseases can present with fever and diffuse/multi-organ symptoms, including many infections, vasculitides, connective tissue diseases, and malignant diseases.
- Many diseases can be associated with bacteremia, such as skin and soft tissue infections, osteomyelitis, pneumonia, meningitis, and others.

Time-Dependent Interventions

- It is important to obtain three sets of appropriately drawn blood cultures prior to the initiation of antibiotics.
- An echocardiogram needs to be performed as soon as possible in any patient in whom the diagnosis of IE is being seriously considered.
- Patients that present acutely with fever and other constitutional symptoms should have empiric antibiotics initiated only after blood cultures are drawn.
- Patients may present with acute complications of IE, such as brain abscess, cerebrovascular accident from emboli/infarct, pulmonary embolism, pulmonary abscess, splenic abscess/infarct, renal abscess/infarct, and vertebral osteomyelitis. These patients need to have the complication treated.
- Patients who develop acute heart failure, or who have significant embolic complications, may require urgent surgical valve replacement or repair.

Overall Principles of Treatment

- The goal of treatment is the eradication of the causative agent of IE, with sterilization of the valve, blood, and all involved organs.
- This usually requires prolonged courses of bactericidal antibiotics.
- Multiple professional societies and organizations have published guidelines for the administration of antibiotics in IE. All are available both in printed and online formats.
- Surgery may be required to aid in removing infected material and draining associated abscesses.
- Patients who present acutely with fever and have a high clinical concern for endocarditis (i.e., a known risk factor or predisposing factor) should have

empiric therapy initiated after three sets of blood cultures are obtained. Empiric therapy should generally cover the most likely etiologic organisms. In developed countries that would be staphylococci, streptococci, and enterococci. For this reason, most empiric regimens should include vancomycin (15-20 mg/kg/dose, every 12 hours, not to exceed 2 grams per dose.).
- Subsequent therapy should be guided by culture results and sensitivity results.
- Therapy usually continues for at least 6-weeks.
- Surgical therapy, either valve repair or replacement, will be necessary in up to 50% of cases. The need for early valve surgery (surgery occurring during the initial course of antibiotics) is indicated by: acutely decompensated heart failure; inability to control infection marked by persistent bacteremia; and the prevention of embolic events.

Disease Course

- In-hospital mortality can range from 10–20%, based upon the predisposing factors (10% for native valve lesions to 40% for prosthetic valve lesions).
- The six-month mortality ranges from 25–30%, and the 5-year mortality approaches 40%.
- Complications of IE can include multiple organ systems (such as cardiovascular, central nervous system, renal, and musculoskeletal), and can occur from multiple pathologic mechanisms (direct extension (abscess), embolization of infected and thrombotic material, and damage and scarring of infected structures (mycotic aneurysm).
- Multiple complications can occur in the same patient.
- Cardiovascular complications include:
    - Heart failure (can be acute or chronic). Heart failure is the most common indication for valve surgery. Heart failure is also the leading cause of death among patients with IE.
    - Abscess around the affected valve.
    - Pericarditis.
    - Intracardiac fistula.
    - Mycotic aneurysm. These can develop in any vessel, including intracerebral vessels, and are most common at areas of weakness such as bifurcations.
- Central Nervous system complications include:
    - Stroke
    - Brain abscess
    - Meningitis

- Renal complications include:
  - Kidney abscess
  - Kidney infarction
  - Immune-mediated glomerulonephritis
- Musculoskeletal complications include:
  - Vertebral osteomyelitis
  - Septic arthritis
- Prolonged antibiotic therapy can also be associated with complications (especially allergic and renal complications).

Related Evidence

Papers of particular importance have been highlighted as:
*** Of key importance*

Practice Guideline

Vogkou CT, Vlachogiannis NI, Palaiodimos L, Kousoulis AA. The causative agents in infective endocarditis: a systematic review comprising 33,214 cases. Eur J Clin Microbiol Infect Dis. 2016 May 11. [Epub ahead of print] Review. PubMed PMID: 27170145. http://www.ncbi.nlm.nih.gov/pubmed/26320109 **

Baltimore RS, Gewitz M, Baddour LM, Beerman LB, Jackson MA, Lockhart PB, Pahl E, Schutze GE, Shulman ST, Willoughby R Jr; American Heart Association Rheumatic Fever, Endocarditis, and Kawasaki Disease Committee of the Council on Cardiovascular Disease in the Young and the Council on Cardiovascular and Stroke Nursing. Infective Endocarditis in Childhood: 2015 Update: A Scientific Statement From the American Heart Association. Circulation. 2015 Oct 13;132(15):1487-515. https://doi.org/10.1161/CIR.0000000000000298. Epub 2015 Sep 15. Review. PubMed PMID: 26373317. http://www.ncbi.nlm.nih.gov/pubmed/26373317

Baddour LM, Wilson WR, Bayer AS, Fowler VG Jr, Tleyjeh IM, Rybak MJ, Barsic B, Lockhart PB, Gewitz MH, Levison ME, Bolger AF, Steckelberg JM, Baltimore RS, Fink AM, O'Gara P, Taubert KA; American Heart Association Committee on Rheumatic Fever, Endocarditis, and Kawasaki Disease of the Council on Cardiovascular Disease in the Young, Council on Clinical Cardiology, Council on Cardiovascular Surgery and Anesthesia, and Stroke Council. Infective Endocarditis in Adults: Diagnosis, Antimicrobial Therapy, and Management of Complications: A Scientific Statement for Healthcare Professionals From the American Heart Association. Circulation. 2015 Oct 13;132(15):1435-86. https://

doi.org/10.1161/CIR.0000000000000296. Epub 2015 Sep 15. Review. Erratum in: Circulation. 2015 Oct 27;132(17):e215. PubMed PMID: 26373316. http://www.ncbi.nlm.nih.gov/pubmed/26373316 **

Meta-Analysis

Anantha Narayanan M, Mahfood Haddad T, Kalil AC, Kanmanthareddy A, Suri RM, Mansour G, Destache CJ, Baskaran J, Mooss AN, Wichman T, Morrow L, Vivekanandan R. Early versus late surgical intervention or medical management for infective endocarditis: a systematic review and meta-analysis. Heart. 2016 Jun 15;102(12):950-7. https://doi.org/10.1136/heartjnl-2015-308589. Epub 2016 Feb 11. PubMed PMID: 26869640. http://www.ncbi.nlm.nih.gov/pubmed/26869640

Chatterjee S, Sardar P. Early surgery reduces mortality in patients with infective endocarditis: insight from a meta-analysis. Int J Cardiol. 2013 Oct 3;168(3):3094-7. https://doi.org/10.1016/j.ijcard.2013.04.078. Epub 2013 May 1. PubMed PMID: 23642830. http://www.ncbi.nlm.nih.gov/pubmed/23642830

Review

Martí-Carvajal AJ, Dayer M, Conterno LO, Gonzalez Garay AG, Martí-Amarista CE, Simancas-Racines D. A comparison of different antibiotic regimens for the treatment of infective endocarditis. Cochrane Database Syst Rev. 2016 Apr 19;4:CD009880. https://doi.org/10.1002/14651858.CD009880.pub2. Review. PubMed PMID: 27092951. http://www.ncbi.nlm.nih.gov/pubmed/27092951 **

Cahill TJ, Prendergast BD. Infective endocarditis. Lancet. 2016 Feb 27;387(10021):882-93. https://doi.org/10.1016/S0140-6736(15)00067-7. Epub 2015 Sep 1. Review. PubMed PMID: 26341945. http://www.ncbi.nlm.nih.gov/pubmed/26341945 **

Tattevin P, Watt G, Revest M, Arvieux C, Fournier PE. Update on blood culture-negative endocarditis. Med Mal Infect. 2015 Jan-Feb;45(1-2):1-8. https://doi.org/10.1016/j.medmal.2014.11.003. Epub 2014 Nov 15. Review. PubMed PMID: 25480453. http://www.ncbi.nlm.nih.gov/pubmed/25480453

Thuny F, Grisoli D, Cautela J, Riberi A, Raoult D, Habib G. Infective endocarditis: prevention, diagnosis, and management. Can J Cardiol. 2014 Sep;30(9):1046-57. https://doi.org/10.1016/j.cjca.2014.03.042. Epub 2014 Apr 3. Review. PubMed PMID: 25151287. http://www.ncbi.nlm.nih.gov/pubmed/25151287

Thanavaro KL, Nixon JV. Endocarditis 2014: an update. Heart Lung. 2014 Jul-Aug;43(4):334-7. https://doi.org/10.1016/j.hrtlng.2014.03.009. Epub 2014 Apr 26. Review. PubMed PMID: 24780242. http://www.ncbi.nlm.nih.gov/pubmed/24780242 **

Pettersson GB, Hussain ST, Shrestha NK, Gordon S, Fraser TG, Ibrahim KS, Blackstone EH. Infective endocarditis: an atlas of disease progression for describing, staging, coding, and understanding the pathology. J Thorac Cardiovasc Surg. 2014 Apr;147(4):1142-1149.e2. https://doi.org/10.1016/j.jtcvs.2013.11.031. Epub 2013 Dec 14. Review. PubMed PMID: 24507402. http://www.ncbi.nlm.nih.gov/pubmed/24507402 **

Al-Omari A, Cameron DW, Lee C, Corrales-Medina VF. Oral antibiotic therapy for the treatment of infective endocarditis: a systematic review. BMC Infect Dis. 2014 Mar 13;14:140. https://doi.org/10.1186/1471-2334-14-140. Review. PubMed PMID: 24624933; PubMed Central PMCID: PMC4007569. http://www.ncbi.nlm.nih.gov/pubmed/24624933 **

Bruun NE, Habib G, Thuny F, Sogaard P. Cardiac imaging in infectious endocarditis. Eur Heart J. 2014 Mar;35(10):624-32. https://doi.org/10.1093/eurheartj/eht274. Epub 2013 Jul 30. Review. Erratum in: Eur Heart J. 2014 Sep 7;35(34):2334. PubMed PMID: 23900698. http://www.ncbi.nlm.nih.gov/pubmed/23900698

Bin Abdulhak AA, Baddour LM, Erwin PJ, Hoen B, Chu VH, Mensah GA, Tleyjeh IM. Global and regional burden of infective endocarditis, 1990-2010: a systematic review of the literature. Glob Heart. 2014 Mar;9(1):131-43. https://doi.org/10.1016/j.gheart.2014.01.002. Review. PubMed PMID: 25432123. http://www.ncbi.nlm.nih.gov/pubmed/25432123

Iung B, Erba PA, Petrosillo N, Lazzeri E. Common diagnostic flowcharts in infective endocarditis. Q J Nucl Med Mol Imaging. 2014 Mar;58(1):55-65. Epub 2013 Nov 14. Review. PubMed PMID: 24231795. http://www.ncbi.nlm.nih.gov/pubmed/24231795 **

Htwe TH, Khardori NM. Cardiac emergencies: infective endocarditis, pericarditis, and myocarditis. Med Clin North Am. 2012 Nov;96(6):1149-69. https://doi.org/10.1016/j.mcna.2012.09.003. Review. PubMed PMID: 23102482. http://www.ncbi.nlm.nih.gov/pubmed/23102482 **

Pierce D, Calkins BC, Thornton K. Infectious endocarditis: diagnosis and treatment. Am Fam Physician. 2012 May 15;85(10):981-6. Review. PubMed PMID: 22612050. http://www.ncbi.nlm.nih.gov/pubmed/22612050

Use PubMed Clinical Queries to find the most recent evidence. Use this search strategy:

("infective endocarditis" OR "Endocarditis"[Majr:NoExp] OR "Endocarditis, Bacterial"[Mesh] OR "bacterial endocarditis")

Chapter 40
Interstitial Lung Disease

Christopher J. Rees, Charles V. Pollack, Jr., and Victoria G. Riese

Name and Synonyms

Interstitial Lung Disease (ILD); Diffuse Parenchymal Lung Disease (DPLD); Diffuse Infiltrative Lung Disease (DILD)

Incidence/Epidemiology

- The interstitial lung diseases encompass more than 200 individual diseases, all with unique incidences and epidemiology.
- The incidence of specific disorders depends upon many factors, including age, sex, smoking status, environmental and occupational exposures, medications used, exposure to radiation, and medical history.
- Most are rare diseases.
- The most common of these disorders, idiopathic pulmonary fibrosis (IPF), accounts for about 55 % of all ILD diagnoses. It has an incidence that ranges from 10–25/100,000 in the population between 40 and 50 years old, to >175/100,000 in those over age 75.
- All of these disorders are associated with considerable morbidity and mortality.

C. J. Rees
Emergency Department, Pennsylvania Hospital, Philadelphia, PA, USA

C. V. Pollack, Jr. (✉)
Department of Emergency Medicine, Thomas Jefferson University, Philadelphia, PA, USA

V. G. Riese
Librarian Consultant, Eldersburg, MD, USA

C. V. Pollack, Jr. (ed.), *Differential Diagnosis of Cardiopulmonary Disease*,
https://doi.org/10.1007/978-3-319-63895-9_40

Differential Diagnosis

- The differential diagnosis is broad and encompasses all diseases that can present primarily with dyspnea and cough, such as asthma, COPD, CHF, and bronchiectasis, among others.
- The differential diagnosis within this class of disorders is also very broad, with over 200 individual diseases to consider.

Pathophysiology and Etiology

- ILD is a broad category of diseases that share pathologic involvement of the lung parenchyma and common clinical, radiologic, and physiologic manifestations.
- These are all non-malignant and non-infectious diseases.
- There are several different classification schemes for these diseases. Some schemes classify based upon whether there is a known cause. Some classify based upon primary underlying histopathology (inflammation with fibrosis versus granulomatous.) Some systems classify based upon a combination of both known cause and underlying histopathology.
- Inflammation and fibrosis. This pathophysiologic process starts with some injury or insult to the epithelial surface of the lung that leads to a diffuse inflammatory response in the air spaces and alveoli. This may remit or become chronic. If the inflammatory becomes chronic, the inflammation spreads to the lung interstitium and vasculature, which can lead to permanent interstitial fibrosis and scarring. This then leads to progressive and permanent impairment in physiologic parameters such as gas exchange and ventilation. Most of these disorders are difficult to treat and resistant to treatment.

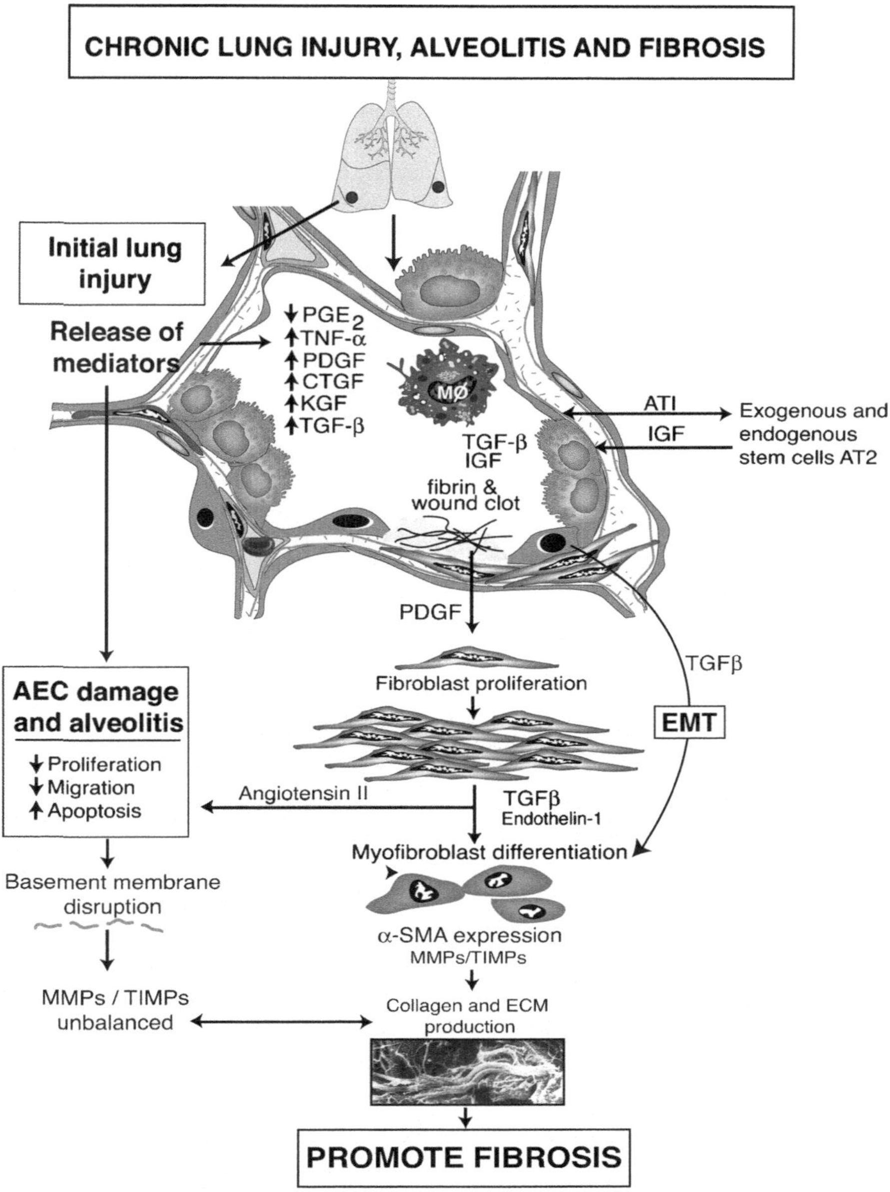

A schematic drawing of pathogenetic mechanism of alveolar epithelial cells (AEC) in lung injury alveolitis and fibrosis. An initial injury of known or unknown etiology provokes an unresolved inflammation or AEC damage and alveolitis. Alveolitis is an initial event in the pathogenesis of lung fibrosis. A fibrin clot forms early and serves as a provisional matrix for the migration and proliferation of endogenous

AEC stem cells. Bone marrow-derived stem cells, HSCs, can also contribute to the populations of AECs. Activated epithelial cells secrete numerous mediators that create a strong profibrotic microenvironment in lung fibrosis inducing AEC injury, alveolitis and apoptosis. Also injured AEC exhibit a defect in the release of some antifibrotic mediators such as prostaglandinE-2 (PGE2). Epithelial cell damage and cell death during alveolitis induce the formation of gaps in the epithelial basement membrane. Progression from the acute phase of lung injury is accompanied by abnormal alveolar reepitalization, tissue repair and remodeling, which may result in progressive fibrosis. AEC produce MMPs that increase basement membrane disruption and allow fibroblast migration, proliferation and differentiation to myofibroblasts. Myofibroblasts secrete extracellular matrix proteins, mainly collagens. An imbalance between MMPs and TIMPs provokes the progressive deposit of the extracellular matrix (ECM) and abnormal collagen accumulation and promotes fibrosis. Alveolar macrophages and AEC secrete TGF-β1, which induces epithelial mesenchymal transition (EMT), and this may contribute to fibroblast/myoflbroblast accumulation in the processes of fibrosis. [Gharaee-Kermani M, Gyetko MR, Hu B, Phan SH. New Insights into the Pathogenesis and Treatment of Idiopathic Pulmonary Fibrosis: A Potential Role for Stem Cells in the Lung Parenchyma and Implications for Therapy. Pharmaceutical Research. 2007 Apr 12;24(5):819–41.] *Caption from original*

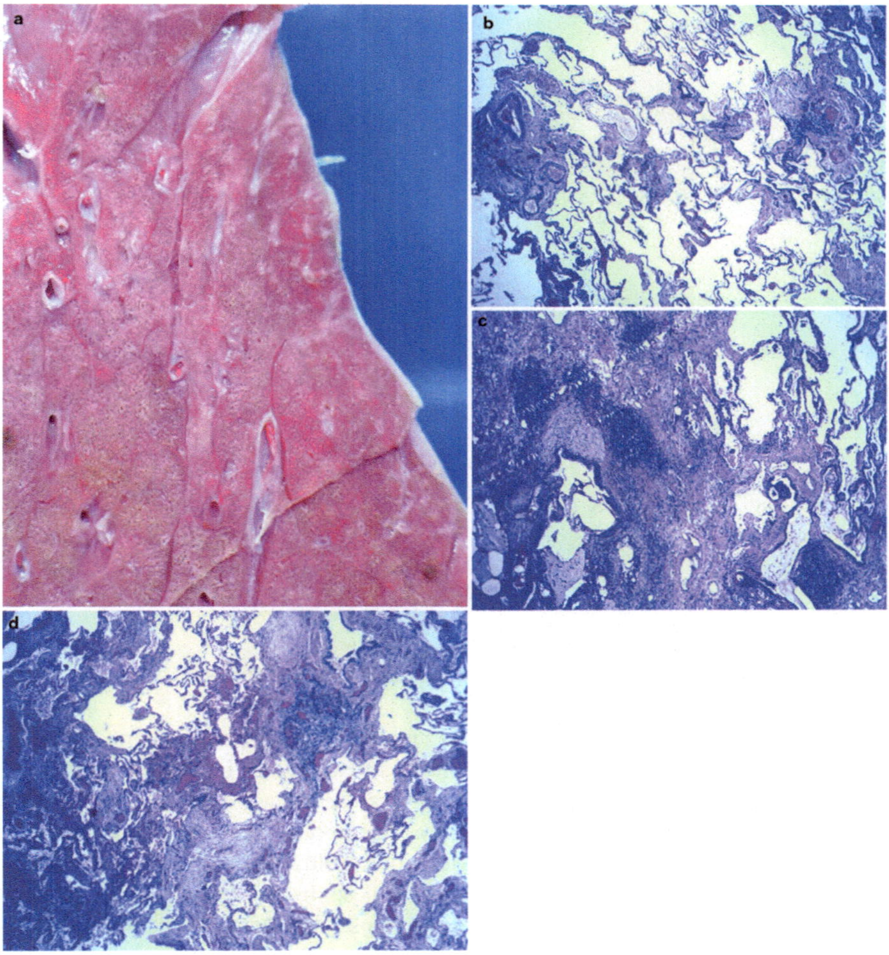
a
b
c
d

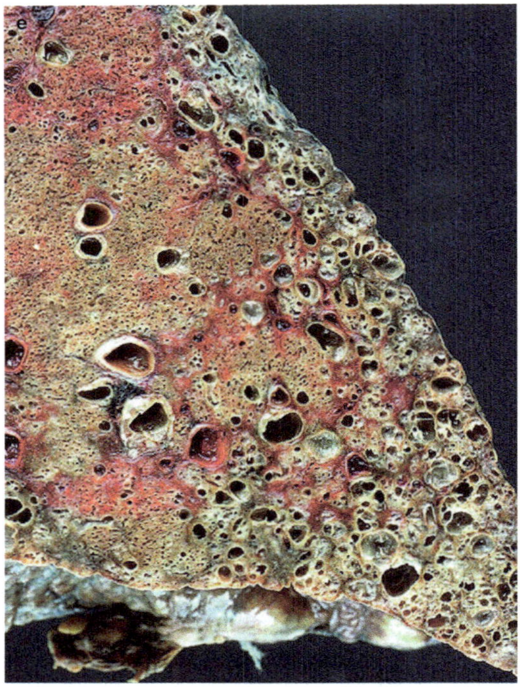

Idiopathic pulmonary fibrosis (interstitial lung disease, idiopathic interstitial pneumonias) with varying alveolar and interstitial inflammatory infiltrates, progressive interstitial fibrosis, secondary hypertensive vascular disease, and a final stage with honeycombing of the lungs. Note the fleshy gross appearance of the lungs in earlier stages (a), with various microscopic interstitial infiltrates (b–d) and gross honeycombing at the end stage (e). The etiology of these diseases is inhomogeneous, as demonstrated by the large variety of terms in use. In many cases, these diseases appear to be autoimmune, either primary or secondary in the course of other systemic autoimmune disorders, but frequently the etiology remains obscure. These disorders are grouped together because of similar clinical manifestations, including severe shortness of breath, diffuse abnormalities of lung mechanics and gas exchange, and diffuse abnormalities in chest radiographs and CT scans, as well as similar clinical outcomes [Krueger GRF, Wagner M, Oldham SAA. Pathology of the Respiratory Tract. In: Krueger GRF, Buja LM, editors. Atlas of Anatomic Pathology with Imaging [Internet]. London: Springer London; 2013 [cited 2015 May 28]. p. 105–89. Available from: http://link.springer.com/10.1007/978-1-4471-2846-5_3] *Caption adapted from original*

- The granulomatous disorders are marked by the pathologic accumulation of inflammatory cells and epithelial cells into granulomas within lung tissue. Many of these patients can remain with mild-to-moderate symptoms, and many may improve with treatment.

- A helpful schema clinically is to group these disorders as to whether the cause is known or unknown.
- Known causes: Inflammatory pathology unless otherwise labeled.
  - Associated with connective-tissue diseases (most commonly rheumatoid arthritis, scleroderma, and polymyositis).
  - Hypersensitivity pneumonitis (e.g., farmer's lung and bird fancier's lung). Granulomatous.
  - Pneumonoconioses (asbestosis, silicosis, coal miner's lung).
  - Drug-induced (chemotherapeutic agents, amiodarone, methotrexate).
  - Smoking-related.
  - Pulmonary Langerhans cell histiocytosis.
  - Respiratory bronchiolitis ILD.
  - Desquamative interstitial pneumonia.
  - Acute eosinophilic pneumonia.
  - Radiation-induced.
  - Toxic-inhalation induced (e.g., cocaine, ammonia, etc.).
- Unknown Causes: Inflammatory pathology unless labeled otherwise.
  - Idiopathic pulmonary fibrosis.
  - Sarcoidosis. Granulomatous.
  - Other idiopathic interstitial pneumonias.
  - Cryptogenic organizing pneumonia (bronchiolitis obliterans organizing pneumonia).
  - Nonspecific interstitial pneumonia.
  - Lymphocytic interstitial pneumonia.
  - Acute interstitial pneumonia.
  - Eosinophilic pneumonias.
  - Pulmonary vasculitides. Mostly granulomatous.
  - Pulmonary lymphangioleiomyomatosis.
  - Pulmonary alveolar proteinosis.
  - Many other rare disorders.

Presentation

Typical/"Classic"

- Dyspnea is the most common and prominent complaint in ILD.
- Classically, patients will have dyspnea with a persistent, non-productive cough associated with diffuse, interstitial infiltrates on chest x-ray.
- Often, patients will have been treated with one or several courses of antibiotics for typical and atypical pneumonia. This non-response to antibiotics should raise suspicion for an ILD.

- The most common time course of presentation is chronic, with symptoms ongoing over months-to-years. A sub-acute presentation over weeks-to-months is also common.
- A detailed history is very important in the evaluation of a patient with a suspected ILD. It can help to narrow the differential to a manageable number of conditions. The history should include detailed questioning as to the pattern and timing of symptoms, smoking history, a detailed environmental and occupational history, and a family history.
- Patients with inflammatory/fibrotic disorders will often have bibasilar "dry" crackles on physical exam. These are often also called "Velcro" crackles as they sound like Velcro being pulled apart.
- Cyanosis and clubbing can occur with advanced disease, and are noted in up to 30% of patients with advanced idiopathic pulmonary fibrosis.

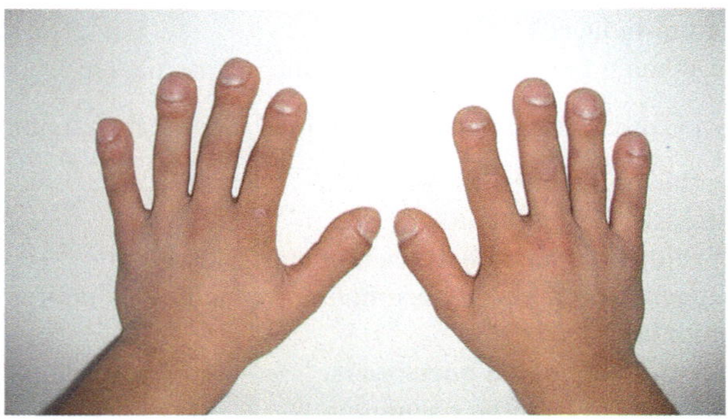

Clubbing of the fingers [Karkucak M, Erturk E, Capkin E, Akyazi H, Ozden G, Tosun M. Primary hypertrophic osteoarthropathy (pachydermoperiostosis): a case report. Rheumatology International. 2007 Jan 11;27(4):403–5.] *Caption from original*

https://www.youtube.com/watch?v=9C5RFb1qWT8
Audio recording of crackles, including late inspiratory crackles.

Atypical

- An acute presentation is unusual, happening mostly in disorders with an allergic basis.
- Some disorders will present in an episodic fashion with acute exacerbations that improve with treatment (sarcoidosis).
- Wheezing and chest pain are not common presenting complaints/findings, except in sarcoidosis.
- Hemoptysis is uncommon, but may be seen in the alveolar hemorrhage syndromes.

Primary Differential Considerations

- Early consideration should be given to
  - ARDS
  - Sarcoidosis
  - Pneumoconiosis
  - Hypersensitivity or drug-induced pneumonitis
  - Pulmonary edema
  - Pneumonia

History and Physical Exam

Findings That Confirm Diagnosis

- There are no historical or physical exam findings that can confirm the diagnosis.
- The diagnosis is confirmed with appropriate findings on high-resolution CT of the lungs, or by specific pathologic findings on lung biopsy.

Factors That Suggest Diagnosis

- A classic presentation as described, with slowly progressive dyspnea, a chronic non-productive cough, and diffuse infiltrates on chest x-ray, with symptoms that don't improve with antibiotic treatment, should clearly raise suspicion for an ILD.
- A careful physical examination can help to identify related systemic processes such as any evidence of a connective-tissue disease.

Factors That Exclude Diagnosis

- There are no historical or physical exam findings that can exclude the diagnosis.
- A normal high-resolution CT scan of the lungs would essentially rule out the diagnosis.

Ancillary Studies

Laboratory

- Most patients will have had routine laboratory studies (CBC, basic chemistries) checked, but they are unlikely to be helpful.
- Specific laboratory evaluation for specific disorders being considered should be performed.
- A raised lactate dehydrogenase (LDH) level is a common, non-specific finding in many ILDs.
- The serum level of angiotensin-converting enzyme (ACE) is commonly elevated in sarcoidosis.
- Anti-nuclear Ab and anti-immunoglobulin Ab (rheumatoid factor) can be found even in patients without an obvious connective-tissue disease.
- If a vasculitis is suspected, it may be helpful to check for the presence of anti-neutrophil cytoplasmic Ab's and anti-basement membrane Ab.

Imaging

- Most evaluations for ILD are initiated and suspected based upon an abnormal chest x-ray But plain CXRs are neither sensitive nor specific for a diagnosis of ILD. In fact, up to 20% of patients with ILD can have a CXR that is read as normal. CXR findings correlate poorly with clinical findings, and also with the histopathologic stage of the disease.
- High-resolution CT (HRCT) of the chest is the imaging study of choice for the diagnosis of any diffuse interstitial process. The classic "honeycombing" of lung tissue is an end-stage finding.
- HRCT can narrow the differential diagnosis, and in some cases can confirm the diagnosis.
- The pattern of abnormalities, distribution of abnormalities, and associated findings (pleural effusions, lymphadenopathy) found on HRCT, used in conjunction with the clinical context, can sometimes confirm the diagnosis. This can obviate the need for a lung biopsy.

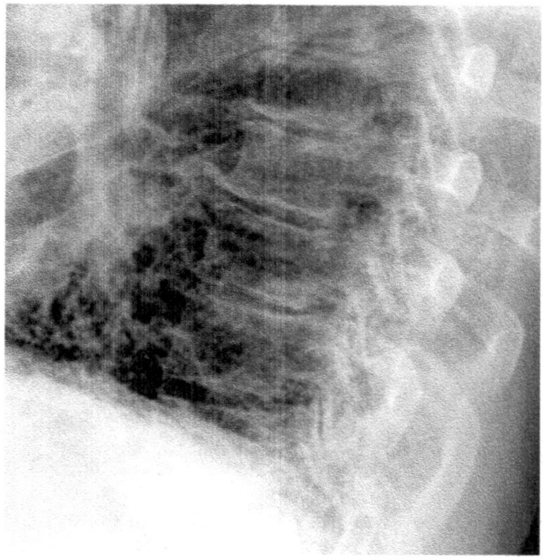

Interstitial lung disease in polymyositis. Magnification lateral-view chest radiograph showing lower zonal reticular interstitial lung disease. [Berney S, Heldmann M. Chapter 14. In: Crapo J, editor. Bone's atlas of pulmonary and critical care medicine. 3rd ed. Philadelphia: Current Medicine; 2005. ISBN: 1-57340-211-7] *Caption from original*

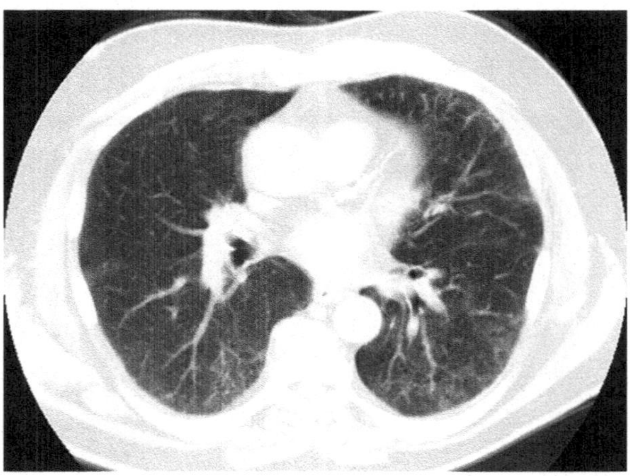

High-resolution computed tomography images from a patient with respiratory bronchiolitis interstitial lung disease demonstrating areas of faint, patchy ground glass opacification and reticular thickening. [Coley CJ, Tolle LB, Hasvold J, Schmidt LA, Flaherty KR. Non-specific, Unclassifiable, and Rare Idiopathic Interstitial Pneumonia: Acute Interstitial Pneumonia, Respiratory Bronchiolitis Interstitial Pneumonia, Desquamative Interstitial Pneumonia, Nonspecific Interstitial Pneumonia. In: Cottin V, Cordier J-F, Richeldi L, editors. Orphan Lung Diseases [Internet]. London: Springer London; 2015 [cited 2015 May 28]. p. 349–62. Available from: http://link.springer.com/10.1007/978-1-4471-2401-6_23] *Caption from original*

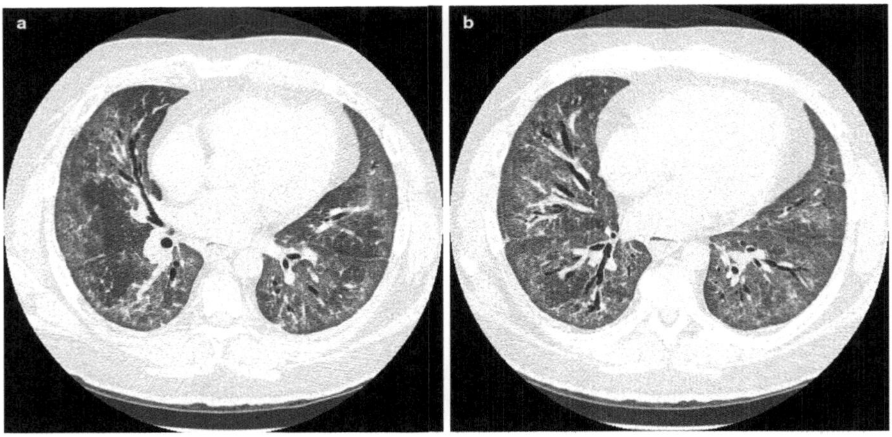

High-resolution computed tomography from the mid (panel a) and lower (panel b) lung fields of patient with nonspecific interstitial pneumonia. The images demonstrate patchy areas of ground glass opacification, reticular thickening and traction bronchiectasis. Some subpleural sparing of disease can be appreciated. Honeycombing is absent. [Coley CJ, Tolle LB, Hasvold J, Schmidt LA, Flaherty KR. Non-specific, Unclassifiable, and Rare Idiopathic Interstitial Pneumonia: Acute Interstitial Pneumonia, Respiratory Bronchiolitis Interstitial Pneumonia, Desquamative Interstitial Pneumonia, Nonspecific Interstitial Pneumonia. In: Cottin V, Cordier J-F, Richeldi L, editors. Orphan Lung Diseases [Internet]. London: Springer London; 2015 [cited 2015 May 28]. p. 349–62. Available from: http://link.springer.com/10.1007/978-1-4471-2401-6_23] *Caption from original*

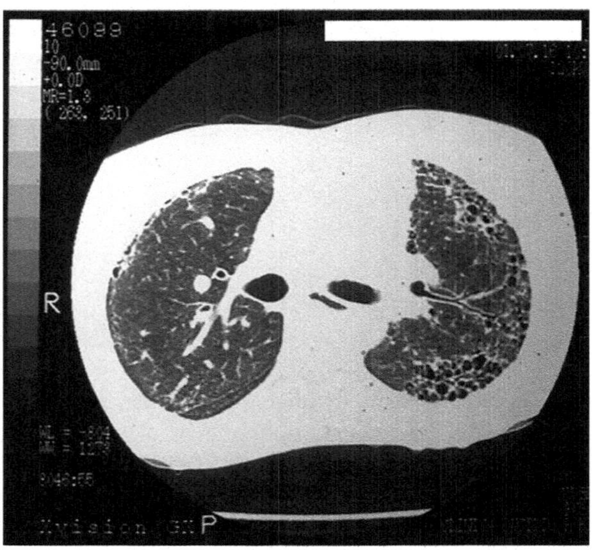

CT diffuse interstitial lung disease with honeycombing. [Teixeira Moreira Almeida M do S, Dias LT, Fernandes SJS, Almeida JVM. Spontaneous pneumomediastinum and subcutaneous emphysema in systemic sclerosis. Rheumatology International. 2007 Apr 10;27(7):675–7.] *Caption from original*

Pulmonary Function Tests

- Spirometry is helpful in evaluating the extent of disease.
- Most forms of ILD will produce a restrictive pattern of PFTs (COPD gives an obstructive pattern). This includes a reduced total lung capacity (TLC), functional residual capacity (FRC), and residual volume (RV).
- Forced expiratory volume in one second (FEV1) and functional vital capacity (FVC) are often reduced, but their ratio is usually normal or increased, as opposed to COPD, where there is a reduced ratio.
- Lung volumes continue to decrease as the disease progresses and lung compliance worsens (the lungs become "stiff").
- The rate of decline of PFTs can have prognostic significance.
- The diffusing capacity to carbon monoxide (DLCO) is reduced in most ILDs, but this is a nonspecific finding and does not correlate with disease stage.
- Arterial blood gases can be normal, but may also show hypoxia from ventilation perfusion mismatch. Ventilation perfusion mismatch occurs because as the fibrosis worsens, lung compliance reduces (the lungs become more stiff). This reduces ventilation in these areas of the lung, but perfusion in these areas remains the same. This leads to blood that has not been adequately oxygenated returning to the heart, which allows this "venous" blood to mix with oxygenated blood in the left heart.
- Carbon dioxide retention is uncommon in ILD (it is more common in COPD), but if present it indicates severe, end-stage disease.
- Exercise pulmonary testing can be used to follow disease progression.

Lung Biopsy

- Lung biopsy may be necessary if the diagnosis is in question after work-up, including HRCT.
- Lung biopsy is the most effective method for diagnosis and assessment of disease severity.
- If possible, a biopsy should be performed prior to the initiation of treatment.
- Bronchoscopy with transbronchial biopsy is usually the first approach to obtaining lung tissue for biopsy. However, this approach gives small tissue samples, and often cannot lead to a definitive diagnosis.
- In these cases it may be necessary to perform a surgical lung biopsy. Surgical lung biopsy has a diagnostic yield of nearly 90%.
- Surgical lung biopsy is usually performed under video-assisted thoracoscopic surgery (VATS). However, this approach can have a mortality of 2% and a complication rate of 5–10%.

- Bronchoalveolar lavage during bronchoscopy is not useful in the diagnosis of ILD, but may help offer alternative diagnoses (cancer or infections), or assess for complications of ILD (also cancer and infections).

Special Populations

Age

Infants and Children

- Interstitial lung disease does occur in infants and children. It is marked by pulmonary symptoms with diffuse pulmonary infiltrates on lung imaging.
- It is very rare in this age group, with a reported incidence between 1.5–3.6 cases per 1 million in those under the age of 16.
- Many of the causes of ILD in children are similar to the causes in adults, but there are syndromes unique to infants and neonates. These include:
  - Diffuse developmental disorders. This includes alveolar capillary dysplasia with misalignment of the pulmonary veins (ACD-MPV), and acinar dysplasia.
  - Disorders of lung growth and development. This group includes pulmonary hypoplasia and chronic neonatal lung disease with bronchopulmonary dysplasia.
  - Neuroendocrine cell hyperplasia of infancy (NEHI). This is a very rare disorder with an unknown etiology.
  - Pulmonary interstitial glycogenolysis (PIG).
  - Genetic disorders of surfactant production and metabolism.
- In neonates and infants, ILD often presents with unexplained respiratory failure.
- In older infants and children the presentation can be non-specific and includes persistent and unexplained tachypnea, chronic cough, hypoxemia, exercise intolerance, and clubbing of the digits. ILD can also present as failure to thrive and unexplained feeding difficulties. Children above age 2 are more likely to present with exercise intolerance and clubbing.
- The work-up should begin with a complete history and physical examination. The evaluation should initially focus on assessing and excluding the more common causes of respiratory symptoms with diffuse infiltrates. These include: infectious causes, congenital heart disease, and cystic fibrosis. Other rare causes can include immunodeficiencies and structural lung and airway abnormalities.
- The evaluation can then follow as described above for adults.
- An important addition to the evaluation of ILD in children, especially in neonates with respiratory failure and children with suspected ILD and another

affected sibling, is genetic testing for mutations of surfactant production and metabolism. Finding one of these mutations can be diagnostic and obviate the need for lung biopsy.

- Treatment is often supportive (avoiding respiratory irritants, nutritional support, oxygen for hypoxemia, appropriate vaccinations, and appropriate treatment of intercurrent infections), and should be guided by the specific syndrome.
- The prognosis greatly depends upon the specific disorder. Some will spontaneously remit.
- The prognosis is generally poor with ACD-MPV, surfactant mutations, and if pulmonary hypertension complicates ILD.
- Lung transplantation can be considered for end-stage disease not responding to therapy.

Adults

- ILD can present across the spectrum of age groups. The age at presentation can be a significant help in narrowing the differential.

Co-morbidities

- The presence of other or multiple co-morbidities can make the diagnosis and management of ILD more challenging. Of particular concern would be the presence of cancer, heart disease, congestive heart failure, diabetes mellitus, and renal failure.

Pitfalls in Diagnosis

Critical Steps Not to Miss

- Consideration of the diagnosis is the first critical step. Strong consideration of the diagnosis should be given when a patient has not responded to several courses of antibiotics for presumed infectious pneumonia when there are diffuse infiltrates on the CXR.
- When considering the diagnosis, it is critical to take an exhaustive history that should include a complete occupational, travel, and hobby/leisure activity history.
- HRCT is a critical test in the evaluation of suspected ILD.

Mimics

- With several hundred different forms of ILD, any of these may mimic another.
- Other diseases that can present with a cough, dyspnea, and diffuse infiltrates include: primary or metastatic cancer, atypical pneumonias, congestive heart failure, and bronchiectasis.

Time-Dependent Interventions

- Most ILDs are insidious and progress slowly.
- Diagnosis often requires months, and symptoms may have been ongoing and worsening for months to years.
- Some of these diseases may present in an acute fashion, developing over days to weeks. These can include allergy, vasculitides, acute interstitial pneumonia, eosinophilic pneumonia, and hypersensitivity pneumonitis.
- In patients with known ILD, acute respiratory worsening, especially if over 4 weeks or less, is usually due to either acute infection or pulmonary edema.

Overall Principles of Treatment

- Treatment should be tailored to the specific disorder if possible.
- The course can be highly variable, but most ILDs are chronic and progressive.
- There is no therapy to reverse fibrosis once present, so the goal of therapy is usually to reduce inflammation to limit any further damage.
- Oxygen should be used if the patient is hypoxemic (resting PaO2 <55 mmHg)
- Pulmonary rehabilitation has been shown to improve quality of life.
- Glucocorticoids are the most commonly used pharmacologic agents in the majority of ILDs. They are commonly started at high doses, up to 1 mg/kg/day, and continued for 1–3 months. If there has been a response, they are slowly tapered over 3–12 months. Too rapid tapering can lead to recurrence. Many patients will require a maintenance dose of steroids. However, the overall response rate is low.
- If patients on glucocorticoids don't improve, or if their condition worsens, second-line agents include cyclophosphamide and azathioprine. These agents can be used alone or in combination with glucocorticoids.

Disease Course

- Most cases are chronic, slowly progressive, and resistant to most treatments.
- Lung transplant can be considered for end-stage disease.

Related Evidence

Papers of particular interest have been highlighted as:
*** Of key importance*

Practice Guideline

Cottin V, Crestani B, Valeyre D, Wallaert B, Cadranel J, Dalphin JC, Delaval P, Israel-Biet D, Kessler R, Reynaud-Gaubert M, Aguilaniu B, Bouquillon B, Carré P, Danel C, Faivre JB, Ferretti G, Just N, Kouzan S, Lebargy F, Marchand-Adam S, Philippe B, Prévot G, Stach B, Thivolet-Béjui F, Cordier JF; French National Reference Centre; Network of Competence Centres for Rare Lung Diseases. Diagnosis and management of idiopathic pulmonary fibrosis: French practical guidelines. Eur Respir Rev. 2014 Jun;23(132):193-214. doi: 10.1183/09059180.00001814. PMID: 24881074. http://www.ncbi.nlm.nih.gov/pubmed/24881074 **

Travis WD, Costabel U, Hansell DM, King TE Jr, Lynch DA, Nicholson AG, Ryerson CJ, Ryu JH, Selman M, Wells AU, Behr J, Bouros D, Brown KK, Colby TV, Collard HR, Cordeiro CR, Cottin V, Crestani B, Drent M, Dudden RF, Egan J, Flaherty K, Hogaboam C, Inoue Y, Johkoh T, Kim DS, Kitaichi M, Loyd J, Martinez FJ, Myers J, Protzko S, Raghu G, Richeldi L, Sverzellati N, Swigris J, Valeyre D; ATS/ERS Committee on Idiopathic Interstitial Pneumonias. An official American Thoracic Society/European Respiratory Society statement: Update of the international multidisciplinary classification of the idiopathic interstitial pneumonias. Am J Respir Crit Care Med. 2013 Sep 15;188(6):733-48. doi: 10.1164/rccm.201308-1483ST. PMID: 24032382. http://www.ncbi.nlm.nih.gov/pubmed/24032382 **

Diagnosis and Management of Suspected Idiopathic Pulmonary Fibrosis: Idiopathic Pulmonary Fibrosis. National Clinical Guideline Centre (UK). London: Royal College of Physicians (UK); 2013 Jun. PMID: 25340234.http://www.ncbi.nlm.nih.gov/pubmed/25340234 **

Meyer KC, Raghu G, Baughman RP, Brown KK, Costabel U, du Bois RM, Drent M, Haslam PL, Kim DS, Nagai S, Rottoli P, Saltini C, Selman M, Strange C, Wood B; American Thoracic Society Committee on BAL in Interstitial Lung Disease. An official American Thoracic Society clinical practice guideline: the clinical utility of bronchoalveolar lavage cellular analysis in interstitial lung disease. Am J Respir Crit Care Med. 2012 May 1;185(9):1004-14. doi: 10.1164/rccm.201202-0320ST. PMID: 22550210. http://www.ncbi.nlm.nih.gov/pubmed/22550210 **

Bradley B, Branley HM, Egan JJ, Greaves MS, Hansell DM, Harrison NK, Hirani N, Hubbard R, Lake F, Millar AB, Wallace WA, Wells AU, Whyte MK, Wilsher ML; British Thoracic Society Interstitial Lung Disease Guideline Group, British Thoracic Society Standards of Care Committee; Thoracic Society of Australia; New Zealand Thoracic Society; Irish Thoracic Society. Interstitial lung disease guideline: the British Thoracic Society in collaboration with the Thoracic Society of Australia and New Zealand and the Irish Thoracic Society. Thorax. 2008 Sep;63 Suppl 5:v1-58. doi: 10.1136/thx.2008.101691. PMID: 18757459. http://www.ncbi.nlm.nih.gov/pubmed/18757459 **

Review

Oldham JM, Noth I. Idiopathic pulmonary fibrosis: early detection and referral. Respir Med. 2014 Jun;108(6):819-29. doi: 10.1016/j.rmed.2014.03.008. PMID: 24746629. http://www.ncbi.nlm.nih.gov/pubmed/24746629 **

Kuo CS, Young LR. Interstitial lung disease in children. Curr Opin Pediatr. 2014 Jun;26(3):320-7. doi: 10.1097/MOP.0000000000000094. PMID: 24752172. http://www.ncbi.nlm.nih.gov/pubmed/24752172 **

Antoniou KM, Margaritopoulos GA, Tomassetti S, Bonella F, Costabel U, Poletti V. Interstitial lung disease. Eur Respir Rev. 2014 Mar 1;23(131):40-54. doi: 10.1183/09059180.00009113. PMID: 24591661. http://www.ncbi.nlm.nih.gov/pubmed/24591661 **

Walsh SL, Hansell DM. High-resolution CT of interstitial lung disease: a continuous evolution. Semin Respir Crit Care Med. 2014 Feb;35(1):129-44. doi: 10.1055/s-0033-1363458. PMID: 24481766. http://www.ncbi.nlm.nih.gov/pubmed/24481766 **

Soares JJ, Deutsch GH, Moore PE, Fazili MF, Austin ED, Brown RF, Sokolow AG, Hilmes MA, Young LR. Childhood interstitial lung diseases: an 18-year retrospective analysis. Pediatrics. 2013 Oct;132(4):684-91. doi: 10.1542/peds.2013-1780. PMID: 24081995. http://www.ncbi.nlm.nih.gov/pubmed/24081995 **

Hilman BC, Amaro-Galvez R. Diagnosis of interstitial lung disease in children. Paediatr Respir Rev. 2004 Jun;5(2):101-7. PMID: 15135119. http://www.ncbi.nlm.nih.gov/pubmed/15135119

Use PubMed Clinical Queries to find the most recent evidence. Use this search strategy:

“Lung Diseases, Interstitial”[Mesh] OR “Interstitial Lung Disease”

Chapter 41
Ischemic Cardiomyopathy

Charles V. Pollack, Jr., Melissa Platt, Richard M. Cantor, and Jaime Friel Blanck

Name and Synonyms

Ischemic cardiomyopathy

- Heart failure; there is some overlap with Dilated Cardiomyopathy (the term *ischemic cardiomyopathy* refers to severe coronary artery disease PLUS global left ventricular dysfunction)

Incidence/Epidemiology

- It is the most common cause of heart failure in developed countries.
- It effects approximately one out of 100 people.
    - Occurs most often middle-aged-to-elderly men.

C. V. Pollack, Jr. (✉)
Department of Emergency Medicine, Thomas Jefferson University, Philadelphia, PA, USA

M. Platt
Department of Emergency Medicine, University of Louisville, Louisville, KY, USA

R. M. Cantor
Department of Emergency Medicine and Pediatrics, State University of New York Upstate Medical University, Syracuse, NY, USA

J. F. Blanck
Welch Medical Library, Johns Hopkins University, Baltimore, MD, USA

C. V. Pollack, Jr. (ed.), *Differential Diagnosis of Cardiopulmonary Disease*, https://doi.org/10.1007/978-3-319-63895-9_41

Differential Diagnosis

- Nonischemic cardiomyopathy
- Dilated cardiomyopathy
- Restrictive cardiomyopathy
- Hypertrophic cardiomyopathy
- Peripartum cardiomyopathy
- Infectious cardiomyopathy

Pathophysiology and Etiology

- Impaired left ventricular function (less than 35–40 %) that results from coronary artery disease
  - may result from irreversible loss of myocardial cells from infarction.
  - may result from contractility deficit that is variable in the setting of ischemic but not frankly infarcted myocardial cells.
  - Ejection fraction less than 35–40 %.

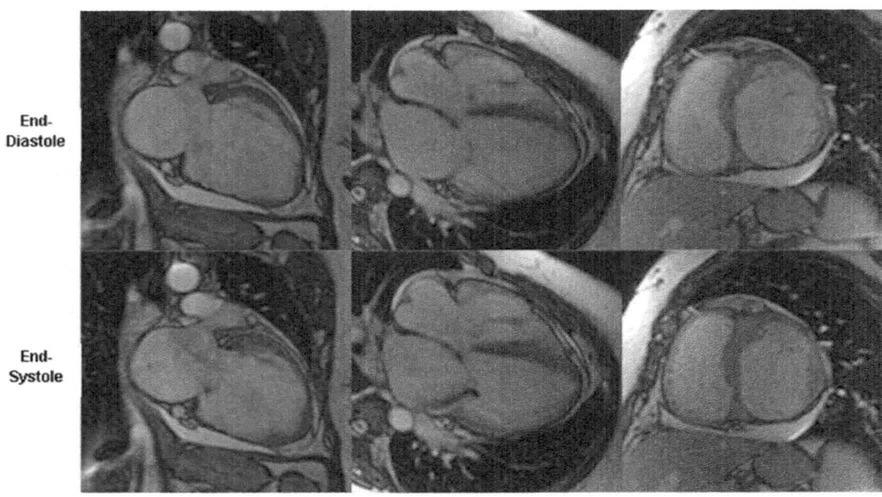

Ischemic cardiomyopathy demonstrating inferior wall thinning and akinesis in the two chamber image (far left). In the four chamber image (middle) there is lateral wall akinesis with RV dilatation and markedly reduced RV free wall shortening and minimal tricuspid annular movement from end-diastole to end-systole. In the short axis images there is RV dilatation with reduced free wall thickening and severe LV systolic dysfunction. The LV inferior wall akinesis is also present in the inferior portion of the interventricular septum [Dell'Italia LJ. The Right Ventricle in Left Heart Failure. In: Voelkel NF, Schranz D, editors. The Right Ventricle in Health and Disease [Internet]. New York, NY: Springer New York; 2015 [cited 2015 Oct 22]. p. 361–90. Available from: http://link.springer.com/10.1007/978-1-4939-1065-6_17] *Caption from original*

Presentation

Typical/"Classic"

- Patients usually have a clear clinical history of coronary heart disease.
- Shortness of breath, with or without chest pain.
- Edema which may cause weight gain.
- Easy fatigability.
- Palpitations.
- Dizziness, lightheadedness, or syncope.

Atypical

- An atypical presentation would manifest as unexplained easy fatigability without the other symptoms noted above.

Primary Differential Considerations

- Consider acute heart failure of other etiologies, acute coronary syndrome, pulmonary embolism, and primary ventricular arrhythmia.

History and Physical Exam

Findings That Confirm Diagnosis

- There are no clinical findings that irrefutably confirm the diagnosis of ischemic cardiomyopathy.

Factors that Suggest Diagnosis

- Fatigue.
- Dyspnea on exertion, shortness of breath.
- Orthopnea, paroxysmal nocturnal dyspnea.
- Increasing edema, weight, or abdominal girth.
- Physical exam may note:
  - Tachypnea
  - Tachycardia
  - Hypertension
  - Hypoxia
  - Jugular venous distension (JVD)
  - Pulmonary crackles and/or wheezes
  - S_3 gallop
  - Peripheral edema
- The level of cardiac compensation determines which signs are present.

Factors That Exclude Diagnosis

- While there are no clinical factors that can exclude ischemic cardiomyopathy in the patient with heart failure symptoms, the finding (on imaging) of no significant coronary artery disease essentially removes the diagnosis from consideration.

Ancillary Studies

Laboratory

- Cardiac biochemical markers
- Brain-type natriuretic peptide (BNP) or NT-pro-BNP
- Coronary risk profile including lipid profile

Electrocardiography

- Left ventricular hypertrophy.
- Left bundle branch block is not uncommon.
- Nonspecific ST-T wave changes and Q waves are common and may reflect past infarction or current ischemia as much as the cardiomyopathy.

Imaging

- Chest x-ray:
  - Cardiomegaly is uniformly present.
  - There may be signs of heart failure, with pulmonary vascular congestion and Kerley B lines.
- Echocardiography is commonly performed to assess pump function.
- Needs evaluation for coronary artery disease, usually including exercise stress testing with myocardial imaging.

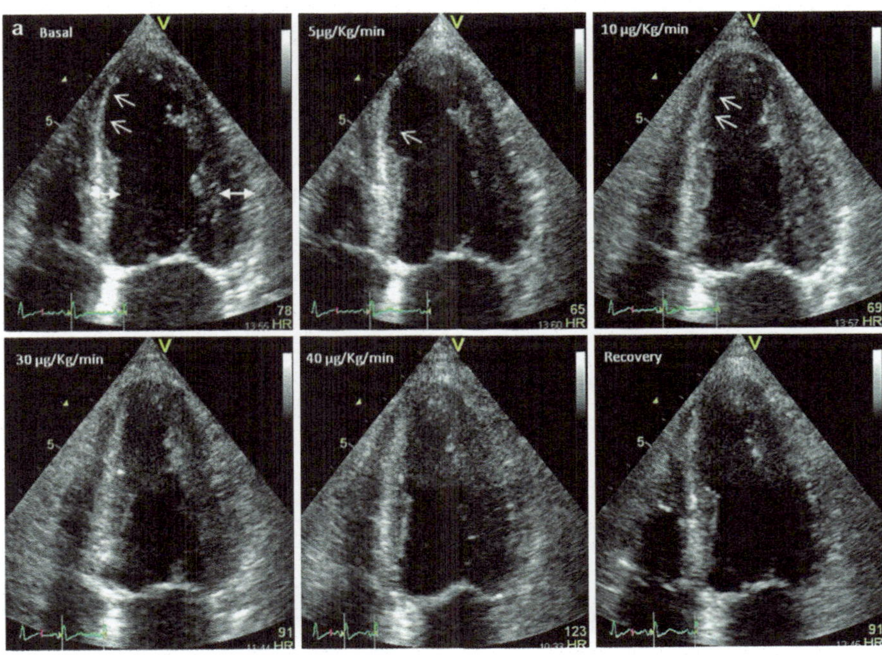

Example of a patient with ischemic cardiomyopathy (left ventricular ejection fraction 35%). At baseline, the resting echocardiography shows areas of thinning (<1 cm markers) in the mid and apical segments of the septal wall (arrows) whereas the lateral wall and the basal segment of the septum show preserved thickness (double arrows). During low-dose and peak-dose dobutamine stress echocardiography, the mid and apical segments of the septal wall show improved thickening (arrows) consistent with myocardial viability. [Delgado V, Schinkel AFL, Yiu K-H, Bax JJ. Nuclear Imaging to Assess Infarction, Reperfusion, No-Reflow, and Viability. In: Kaski JC, Hausenloy DJ, Gersh BJ, Yellon DM, editors. Management of Myocardial Reperfusion Injury [Internet]. London: Springer London; 2012 [cited 2015 Sep 15]. p. 161–89. Available from: http://link.springer.com/10.1007/978-1-84996-019-9_8] *Caption adapted from original*

- Cardiac catheterization with coronary angiography is reasonable for a patient with new-onset heart failure of uncertain cause, who would be eligible for revascularization.
- Noninvasive coronary arteriography including CT or cardiovascular magnetic resonance imaging is also available if the patient does not have angina or is not a candidate for revascularization.

Special Populations

Age

- Most patients with ischemic cardiomyopathy have experienced a transmural myocardial infarction. That means most of these patients are at least 50 years of age.

Co-morbidities

- Coronary artery disease with risk factor:
  - A family history of heart disease
  - Hypertension
  - Smoking
  - Hypercholesterolemia
  - Obesity
  - Diabetes
  - End-stage kidney disease

Pediatric Considerations

- Ischemic cardiomyopathy is generally not a pediatric disease.

Pitfalls in Diagnosis

Critical Steps not to Miss

- Diagnosis consists of 2 steps:
  - 1) The detection of significant coronary artery disease
  - 2) The detection of potentially reversible myocardial function

Mimics

- Chest pain alone is insufficient to make the diagnosis.
  - Nonischemic cardiomyopathy may have chest pain that resembles angina.

Time Dependent Interventions

- The most time-sensitive issue to address is any current ischemia.

Overall Principles of Treatment

- Medical therapy of heart failure:
  - ACE inhibitors.
  - Beta-blockers.
  - Statin as part of secondary prevention of established coronary heart disease.
  - Loop diuretic and dietary salt restriction in patients with fluid volume overload.
  - Removal of drugs that adversely affect systolic dysfunction like nonsteroidal anti-inflammatory drugs, antiarrhythmic drugs, certain calcium channel blockers.

- Device therapy:
  - Implantable cardioverter-defibrillator for prevention of sudden cardiac death.

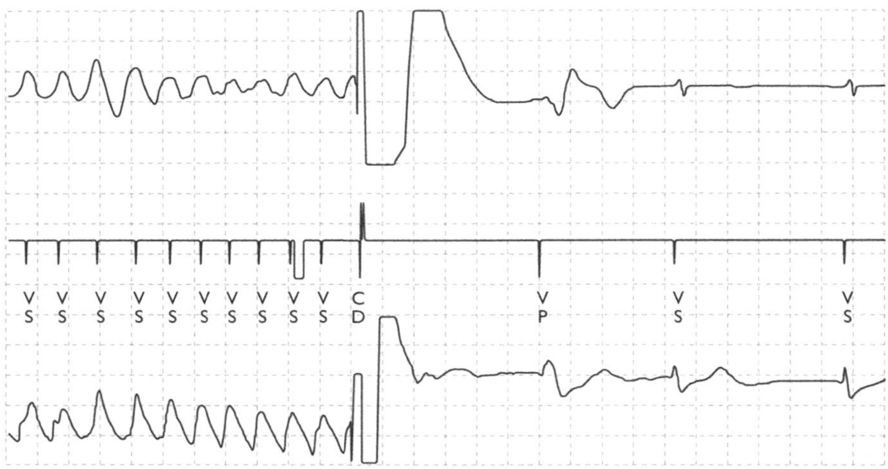

Intracardiac electrogram of implantable cardioverter-defibrillator (ICD) shock terminating ventricular fibrillation in patient with ischemic cardiomyopathy. The ICD is the most effective therapy for prevention of sudden death in patients with heart failure. The use of the ICD for primary prevention of sudden cardiac death has provided the impetus for identification of individuals at highest risk of sudden death. In this example, the ICD accurately recognized ventricular fibrillation and terminated the rhythm with a shock. [Sauer W, Nayak H, Marchlinski F. Chapter 08. In: Shivkumar K, Weiss J, Fonarow G, Narula J, editors. Atlas of electrophysiology in heart failure. Philadelphia: Current Medicine; 2005. (Braunwald E, editor. Atlas of heart diseases; vol. 15); ISBN: 1-57340-225-7] *Caption from original*

- Biventricular pacing for patients in sinus rhythm, LVEF <35 %, prolonged QRS duration and symptoms despite medical therapy.
- Coronary artery bypass graft surgery or angioplasty may improve cardiac blood flow.
- Heart transplant may be tried if other treatments have failed.
- Risk reduction measures for secondary prevention is indicated in patient with ischemic cardiomyopathy includes aspirin, control of hypertension and diabetes, and cessation of smoking.

- Decision to proceed with medical therapy and/or surgical revascularization in patients with ischemic cardiomyopathy should be individualized.

Disease Course

- Ischemic cardiomyopathy is an independent predictor of mortality.
- Prognosis is related primarily to the degree of ventricular dysfunction and the extent of coronary artery disease.

Related Evidence

Papers of particular interest have been highlighted as:
*** Of key importance*

Practice Guideline

Mammen L, Woodard PK, Abbara S, Dorbala S, Javidan-Nejad C, Julsrud PR, Kirsch J, Kramer CM, Krishnamurthy R, Laroia AT, Shah AB, Vogel-Claussen J, White RD; Expert Panel on Cardiac Imaging. ACR appropriateness criteria® nonischemic myocardial disease with clinical manifestations (ischemic cardiomyopathy already excluded). J Thorac Imaging. 2014 Jul;29(4):W44-7. https://doi.org/10.1097/RTI.0000000000000096. PubMed PMID: 24905633. http://www.ncbi.nlm.nih.gov/pubmed/24905633 **

Yancy CW, Jessup M, Bozkurt B, Butler J, Casey DE Jr, Drazner MH, Fonarow GC, Geraci SA, Horwich T, Januzzi JL, Johnson MR, Kasper EK, Levy WC, Masoudi FA, McBride PE, McMurray JJ, Mitchell JE, Peterson PN, Riegel B, Sam F, Stevenson LW, Tang WH, Tsai EJ, Wilkoff BL; American College of Cardiology Foundation; American Heart Association Task Force on Practice Guidelines. 2013 ACCF/AHA guideline for the management of heart failure: a report of the American College of Cardiology Foundation/American Heart Association Task Force on Practice Guidelines. J Am Coll Cardiol. 2013 Oct 15;62(16):e147-239. https://doi.org/10.1016/j.jacc.2013.05.019. Epub 2013 Jun 5. PubMed PMID: 23747642. http://www.ncbi.nlm.nih.gov/pubmed/23747642 **

McMurray JJ, Adamopoulos S, Anker SD, Auricchio A, Böhm M, Dickstein K, Falk V, Filippatos G, Fonseca C, Gomez-Sanchez MA, Jaarsma T, Køber L, Lip GY, Maggioni AP, Parkhomenko A, Pieske BM, Popescu BA, Rønnevik PK, Rutten FH, Schwitter J, Seferovic P, Stepinska J, Trindade PT, Voors AA, Zannad F, Zeiher A; ESC Committee for Practice Guidelines. ESC Guidelines for the diagnosis and treatment of acute and chronic heart failure 2012: The Task Force for the Diagnosis and Treatment of Acute and Chronic Heart Failure 2012 of the European Society of Cardiology. Developed in collaboration with the Heart Failure Association (HFA) of the ESC. Eur Heart J. 2012 Jul;33(14):1787-847. https://doi.org/10.1093/eurheartj/ehs104. Epub 2012 May 19. Erratum in: Eur Heart J. 2013. http://www.ncbi.nlm.nih.gov/pubmed/22611136 Jan;34(2):158. PubMed PMID: 22611136. http://www.ncbi.nlm.nih.gov/pubmed?term=22611136 **

Review

Pfeiffer MP, Biederman RW. Cardiac MRI: A General Overview with Emphasis on Current Use and Indications. Med Clin North Am. 2015 Jul;99(4):849-61. https://doi.org/10.1016/j.mcna.2015.02.011. Review. PubMed PMID: 26042886. http://www.ncbi.nlm.nih.gov/pubmed/26042886

Kramer CM. Role of Cardiac MR Imaging in Cardiomyopathies. J Nucl Med. 2015. Jun;56 Suppl 4:39S-45S. https://doi.org/10.2967/jnumed.114.142729. PubMed PMID: 26033902; PubMed Central PMCID: PMC4465292. http://www.ncbi.nlm.nih.gov/pubmed/26033902 **

Velazquez EJ, Bonow RO. Revascularization in severe left ventricular dysfunction. J Am Coll Cardiol. 2015 Feb 17;65(6):615-24. https://doi.org/10.1016/j.jacc.2014.10.070. Review. PubMed PMID: 25677320. http://www.ncbi.nlm.nih.gov/pubmed/25677320 **

Gracieux J, Sanders GD, Pokorney SD, Lopes RD, Thomas K, Al-Khatib SM. Incidence and predictors of appropriate therapies delivered by the implantable cardioverter defibrillator in patients with ischemic cardiomyopathy: a systematic review. Int J Cardiol. 2014 Dec 20;177(3):990-4. https://doi.org/10.1016/j.ijcard.2014.09.170. Epub 2014 Oct 5. Review. PubMed PMID: 25449512. http://www.ncbi.nlm.nih.gov/pubmed/25449512 **

Satoh H, Sano M, Suwa K, Saitoh T, Nobuhara M, Saotome M, Urushida T, Katoh H, Hayashi H. Distribution of late gadolinium enhancement in various types of cardiomyopathies: Significance in differential diagnosis, clinical features and prognosis. World J Cardiol. 2014 Jul 26;6(7):585-601. https://doi.org/10.4330/wjc.v6.i7.585. Review. PubMed PMID: 25068019; PubMed Central PMCID: PMC4110607. http://www.ncbi.nlm.nih.gov/pubmed/25068019

Shah BN, Senior R. Role of viability imaging in the post-STICH era. Curr Opin Cardiol. 2014 Mar;29(2):145-51. https://doi.org/10.1097/HCO.0000000000000047. Review. PubMed PMID: 24385081. http://www.ncbi.nlm.nih.gov/pubmed/24385081 **

Lipshultz SE, Cochran TR, Briston DA, Brown SR, Sambatakos PJ, Miller TL, Carrillo AA, Corcia L, Sanchez JE, Diamond MB, Freundlich M, Harake D, Gayle T, Harmon WG, Rusconi PG, Sandhu SK, Wilkinson JD. Pediatric cardiomyopathies: causes, epidemiology, clinical course, preventive strategies and therapies. Future Cardiol. 2013 Nov;9(6):817-48. https://doi.org/10.2217/fca.13.66. Review. PubMed PMID: 24180540; PubMed Central PMCID: PMC3903430. http://www.ncbi.nlm.nih.gov/pubmed/24180540

Bui AL, Horwich TB, Fonarow GC. Epidemiology and risk profile of heart failure. Nat Rev Cardiol. 2011 Jan;8(1):30-41. https://doi.org/10.1038/nrcardio.2010.165. Epub 2010 Nov 9. Review. PubMed PMID: 21060326; PubMed Central PMCID: PMC3033496. http://www.ncbi.nlm.nih.gov/pubmed/21060326 **

de Haan S, Knaapen P, Beek AM, de Cock CC, Lammertsma AA, van Rossum AC, Allaart CP. Risk stratification for ventricular arrhythmias in ischaemic cardiomyopathy: the value of non-invasive imaging. Europace. 2010 Apr;12(4):468-74.

https://doi.org/10.1093/europace/euq064. Review. PubMed PMID: 20338987. http://www.ncbi.nlm.nih.gov/pubmed/20338987 **

Weissman G, Asch FM. Myocardial viability in chronic ischemic cardiomyopathy: similarities and discordance of different diagnostic approaches. J Cardiovasc Transl Res. 2009 Mar;2(1):24-9. https://doi.org/10.1007/s12265-008-9083-4. Epub 2008 Dec 31. Review. PubMed PMID: 20559966. http://www.ncbi.nlm.nih.gov/pubmed/20559966 **

Chrysohoou C, Greenberg M, Stefanadis C. Non-invasive methods in differentiating ischaemic from non-ischaemic cardiomyopathy. A review paper. Acta Cardiol. 2006 Aug;61(4):454-62. Review. PubMed PMID: 16970057. http://www.ncbi.nlm.nih.gov/pubmed/16970057 **

Bax JJ. Assessment of myocardial viability in ischemic cardiomyopathy. Heart Lung Circ. 2005;14 Suppl 2:S8-13. Epub 2005 Nov 7. Review. PubMed PMID: 16352289. http://www.ncbi.nlm.nih.gov/pubmed/16352289 **

Allman KC, Shaw LJ, Hachamovitch R, Udelson JE. Myocardial viability testing and impact of revascularization on prognosis in patients with coronary artery disease and left ventricular dysfunction: a meta-analysis. J Am Coll Cardiol. 2002 Apr 3;39(7):1151-8. PubMed PMID: 11923039. http://www.ncbi.nlm.nih.gov/pubmed?term=11923039 **

Felker GM, Shaw LK, O'Connor CM. A standardized definition of ischemic cardiomyopathy for use in clinical research. J Am Coll Cardiol. 2002 Jan 16;39(2):210-8. PubMed PMID: 11788209. http://www.ncbi.nlm.nih.gov/pubmed?term=11788209 **

Clinical Trial

Pecini R, Møller DV, Torp-Pedersen C, Hassager C, Køber L. Heart failure etiology impacts survival of patients with heart failure. Int J Cardiol. 2011 Jun 2;149(2):211-5. https://doi.org/10.1016/j.ijcard.2010.01.011. Epub 2010 Mar 2. PubMed PMID: 20193969. http://www.ncbi.nlm.nih.gov/pubmed/20193969/ **

Carson P, Wertheimer J, Miller A, O'Connor CM, Pina IL, Selzman C, Sueta C, She L, Greene D, Lee KL, Jones RH, Velazquez EJ; STICH Investigators. The STICH trial (Surgical Treatment for Ischemic Heart Failure): mode-of-death results. JACC Heart Fail. 2013 Oct;1(5):400-8. https://doi.org/10.1016/j.jchf.2013.04.012. Epub 2013 Sep 11. PubMed PMID: 24621972; PubMed Central PMCID: PMC3829618. http://www.ncbi.nlm.nih.gov/pubmed/24621972

Fonarow GC, Abraham WT, Albert NM, Stough WG, Gheorghiade M, Greenberg BH, O'Connor CM, Pieper K, Sun JL, Yancy CW, Young JB; OPTIMIZE-HF Investigators and Hospitals. Factors identified as precipitating hospital admissions for heart failure and clinical outcomes: findings from OPTIMIZE-HF. Arch Intern Med. 2008 Apr 28;168(8):847-54. https://doi.org/10.1001/archinte.168.8.847. PubMed PMID: 18443260. http://www.ncbi.nlm.nih.gov/pubmed/18443260?dopt=Abstract&holding=npg **

Cohort Study

He J, Ogden LG, Bazzano LA, Vupputuri S, Loria C, Whelton PK. Risk factors for congestive heart failure in US men and women: NHANES I epidemiologic follow-up study. Arch Intern Med. 2001 Apr 9;161(7):996-1002. PubMed PMID: 11295963. http://www.ncbi.nlm.nih.gov/pubmed/11295963

Velazquez EJ, Williams JB, Yow E, Shaw LK, Lee KL, Phillips HR, O'Connor CM, Smith PK, Jones RH. Long-term survival of patients with ischemic cardiomyopathy treated by coronary artery bypass grafting versus medical therapy. Ann Thorac Surg. 2012 Feb;93(2):523-30. https://doi.org/10.1016/j.athoracsur.2011.10.064. PubMed PMID: 22269720; PubMed Central PMCID: PMC3638256. http://www.ncbi.nlm.nih.gov/pubmed/22269720 **

Comparative Study

Maltais S, Tchantchaleishvili V, Schaff HV, Daly RC, Suri RM, Dearani JA, Topilsky Y, Stulak JM, Joyce LD, Park SJ. Management of severe ischemic cardiomyopathy: left ventricular assist device as destination therapy versus conventional bypass and mitral valve surgery. J Thorac Cardiovasc Surg. 2014 Apr;147(4):1246-50. https://doi.org/10.1016/j.jtcvs.2013.04.012. Epub 2013 Jun 12. PubMed PMID: 23764411. http://www.ncbi.nlm.nih.gov/pubmed/23764411 **

Moran AE, Forouzanfar MH, Roth GA, Mensah GA, Ezzati M, Flaxman A, Murray CJ, Naghavi M. The global burden of ischemic heart disease in 1990 and 2010: the Global Burden of Disease 2010 study. Circulation. 2014 Apr 8;129(14):1493-501. https://doi.org/10.1161/CIRCULATIONAHA.113.004046. Epub 2014 Feb 26. Review. PubMed PMID: 24573351; PubMed Central PMCID: PMC4181601. http://www.ncbi.nlm.nih.gov/pubmed/24573351 **

Kwon DH, Hachamovitch R, Popovic ZB, Starling RC, Desai MY, Flamm SD, Lytle BW, Marwick TH. Survival in patients with severe ischemic cardiomyopathy undergoing revascularization versus medical therapy: association with end-systolic volume and viability. Circulation. 2012 Sep 11;126(11 Suppl 1):S3-8. PubMed PMID: 22965991. http://www.ncbi.nlm.nih.gov/pubmed/22965991 **

Use PubMed Clinical Queries to find the most recent evidence. Use this search strategy:

“Myocardial Ischemia”[Mesh] OR “Ischemic cardiomyopathy”

Chapter 42
Kawasaki Disease

Richard M. Cantor, Charles V. Pollack, Jr., and Jaime Friel Blanck

Name and Synonyms

Kawasaki Disease

- Also known as mucocutaneous lymph node syndrome.

Incidence/Epidemiology

- One of the most common vasculitides of infancy and childhood.
- Its highest incidence is in East Asian children. One in 100 Japanese children will develop KD by age 5.
- Within the US, there is a winter-spring predominance of cases. Incidence estimates vary between ethnic groups in the US, with lowest rates reported amongst Caucasian children.
- Peak incidences occur before the age of one year. Eighty to 90% of cases affect children less than 5 years of age.
- The etiology of KD remains unknown. See legend.

R. M. Cantor
Department of Emergency Medicine and Pediatrics, State University of New York Upstate Medical University, Syracuse, NY, USA

C. V. Pollack, Jr. (✉)
Department of Emergency Medicine, Thomas Jefferson University, Philadelphia, PA, USA

J. F. Blanck
Welch Medical Library, Johns Hopkins University, Baltimore, MD, USA

C. V. Pollack, Jr. (ed.), *Differential Diagnosis of Cardiopulmonary Disease*,
https://doi.org/10.1007/978-3-319-63895-9_42

Single etiologic agent
Uncommon agent that immunologically cross-reacts with, common agent
Common agent with unusual host response
Multiple etiologic agents with final common pathway
Common agents with unusual host response

Paradigms for the cause of Kawasaki disease or syndrome. Debate continues as to whether Kawasaki disease is caused by a single etiologic agent ("disease") or by multiple different agents that result in a stereotyped host response ("syndrome"). [Burns J, Glodé M. Chapter 10. In: Wilfert CM, editor. Pediatric infectious diseases. Philadelphia: Current Medicine; 1999. (Mandell GL, editor. Atlas of infectious diseases; vol. 11). ISBN: 0-443-06526-8] *Caption from original*

Differential Diagnosis

- Kawasaki Disease is accompanied by fever, an exanthema, profound mucous membrane involvement, and lymphadenitis. As such the differential diagnosis includes, but is not limited to:
  - Measles
  - Adenoviral infections
  - Scarlet fever
  - Echoviral infections
  - EBV infections
  - Rocky Mountain Spotted Fever
  - Systemic juvenile rheumatoid arthritis

Pathophysiology and Etiology

- The etiology of KD remains unknown.
- The basic pathology involves a widespread vasculitis, with particular involvement of medium-sized arteries (i.e., the coronaries).
- Coronary involvement will result in the development of aneurysms and generalized dilatation. See legend.

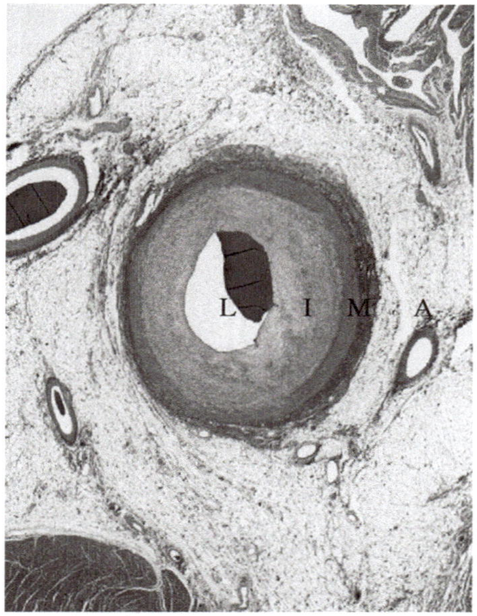

Coronary artery of a patient who died of pachymeningitis 9 months after contracting Kawasaki disease [Takahashi K, Oharaseki T, Yokouchi Y, Naoe S, Saji T. Kawasaki disease: basic and pathological findings. Clinical and Experimental Nephrology. 2013 Oct;17(5):690–3.] *Caption adapted from original*

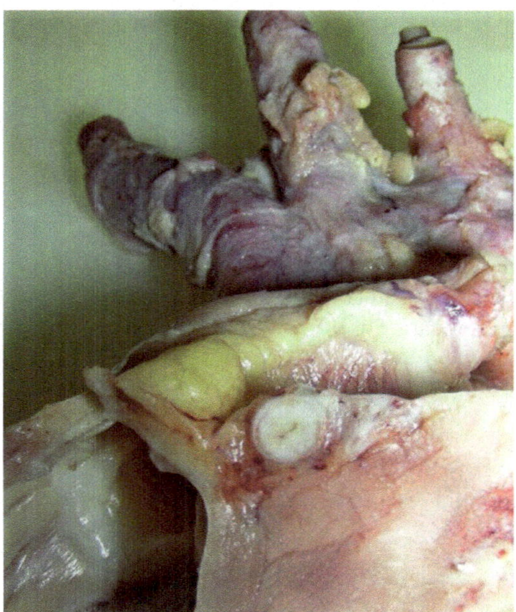

Coronary artery vasculitis in a child with treatment-resistant Kawasaki disease and ischemic cardiomyopathy [Markelj G, Avčin T. Systemic Corticosteroids in Childhood Vasculitides. In: Cimaz R, editor. Systemic Corticosteroids for Inflammatory Disorders in Pediatrics [Internet]. Cham: Springer International Publishing; 2015 [cited 2015 Aug 28]. p. 77–94. Available from: http://link.springer.com/10.1007/978-3-319-16056-6_7] *Caption from original*

Presentation

Typical/"Classic"

- **Fever** is the most common presenting sign. It is usually present for more than 4 days, and generally unresponsive to antipyretic therapy. It is most often greater than 38.5° C.
- **Mucositis** involves the development of red, cracked lips and a strawberry tongue. See figure.

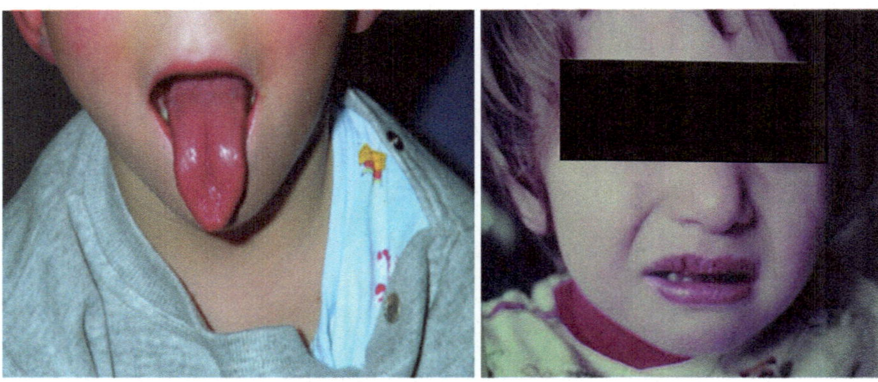

Strawberry tongue, mucosal redness, and cracked lips in a 3-year-old boy [Falcini F. Kawasaki Disease. In: Matucci-Cerinic M, Furst D, Fiorentino D, editors. Skin Manifestations in Rheumatic Disease [Internet]. New York, NY: Springer New York; 2014 [cited 2015 Sep 4]. p. 283–8. Available from: http://link.springer.com/10.1007/978-1-4614-7849-2_34, courtesy of Fernanda Falcini, MD] *Caption from original*

- **Conjunctival** involvement occurs in more than 85 % of patients. Though generally a superficial disease, some cases will go on to develop uveitis. See

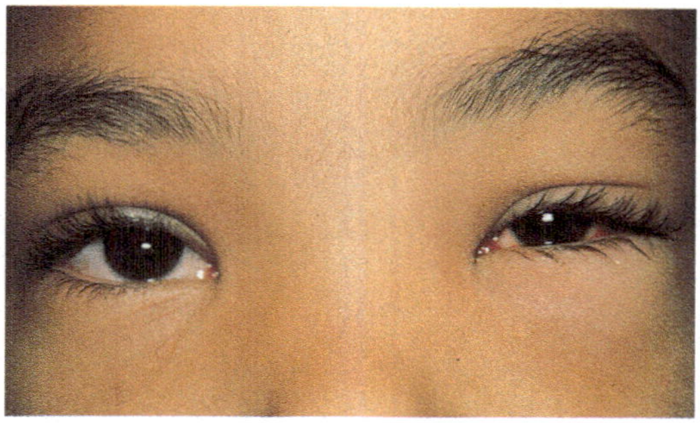

Hemorrhagic conjunctivitis. A, In this case of conjunctivitis, the lids are not thickened and crusted but diffusely swollen. [Wald ER. Eye and Orbit Infections. In: Brook I, editor. Atlas of Upper Respiratory and Head and Neck Infections, 2e. Philadelphia: Current Medicine; 2000. (Mandell GL, editor. Atlas of infectious diseases; vol. 4). ISBN: 1-57340-140-4] *Caption from original*

- The **rash** is polymorphous. It usually involves the development of erythematous papules with variable distribution.
- One of the later findings is **induration** of the hands and feet. During the convalescent phase, distal **desquamation** occurs in 80 % of cases. See figure.

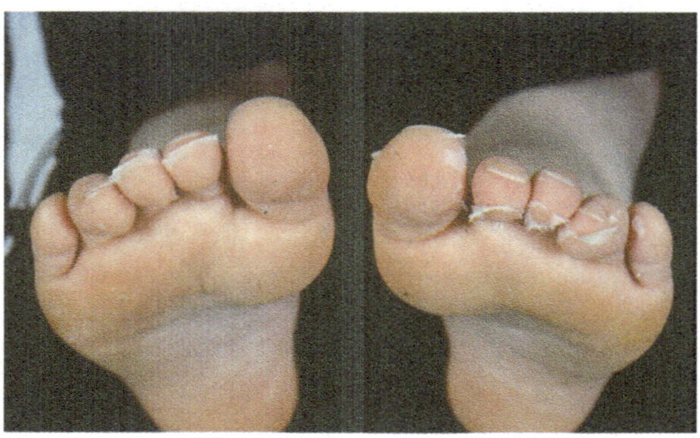

Kawasaki disease. Peeling of the top of the toes [Schneider R, Laxer R. Rheumatology. In: Laxer R, Ford-Jones EL, Friedman J, Gerstle T, editors. The Hospital for Sick Children: atlas of pediatrics. Philadelphia: Current Medicine; 2005. ISBN: 1-57340-188-9] *Caption adapted from original*

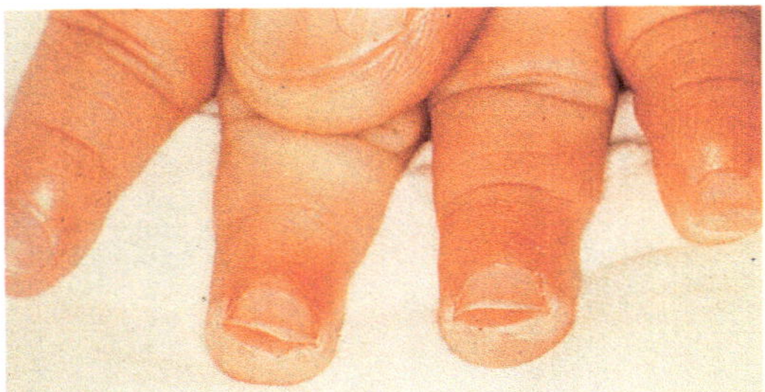

Periungual desquamation during the convalescent phase of Kawasaki disease. The peeling is usually noted after the acute signs and symptoms of inflammation have subsided in the 2nd to 3rd week of the illness. [Burns J, Glodé M. Chapter 10. In: Wilfert CM, editor. Pediatric infectious diseases. Philadelphia: Current Medicine; 1999. (Mandell GL, editor. Atlas of infectious diseases; vol. 11). ISBN: 0-443-06526-8] *Caption from original*

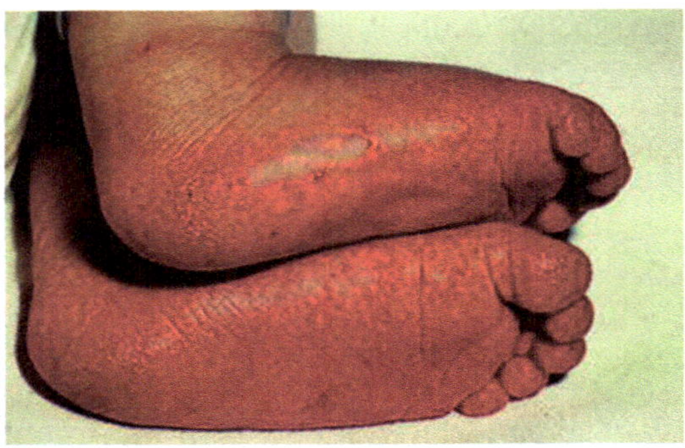

Desquamating rash in child with Kawasaki disease. [Watts RA, Scott DGI. Kawasaki Disease. In: Watts RA, Scott DGI, editors. Vasculitis in Clinical Practice [Internet]. Cham: Springer International Publishing; 2015 [cited 2015 Aug 28]. p. 117–26. Available from: http://link.springer.com/10.1007/978-3-319-14871-7_11] *Caption from original*

- The presence of **lymphadenopathy** is the least consistent finding of KD.

Atypical

- There is a subcategory of KD, namely incomplete, or atypical KD. It is important for the clinician to recognize this entity, since early treatment of KD will prove cardioprotective.

- Studies of children with incomplete KD demonstrate the following variances from the typical findings:
  - Cervical adenopathy was absent in 90 % of infants.
  - Fifty percent have no rash.
  - Peripheral extremity changes were absent in 40 % of patients.
- Consistent findings seen in both typical and atypical KD include fever and mucous membrane involvement.

Primary Differential Considerations

- The most common differential considerations for KD are acute focal infections such as:
  - Orbital cellulitis
  - Lymphangitis
  - Retropharyngeal or peritonsillar abscess
- The rash of KD may look similar to:
  - Measles

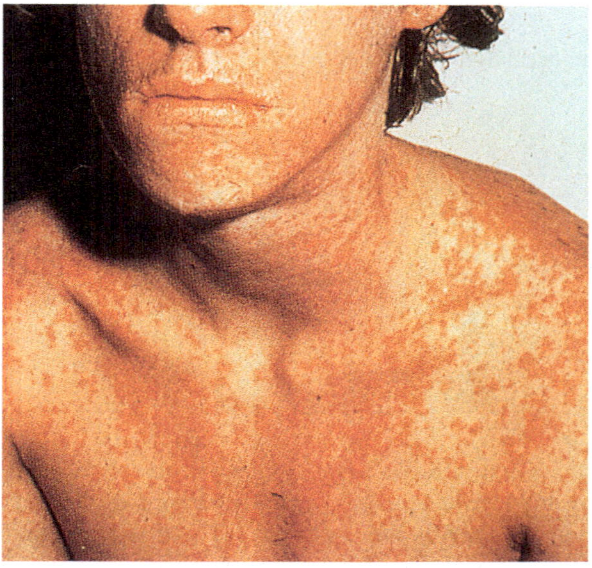

Typical erythematous maculopapular rash of measles. Measles is an acute febrile infection caused by the rubeola virus and characterized by a prodrome of fever and upper respiratory symptoms followed by the characteristic measles exanthem. The rash, which is erythematous and maculopapular, usually begins on the head and spreads downward to involve the trunk and upper and lower extremities. [Gilsdorf J, Shope T. Viral exanthems of childhood. In: Fekety R, editor. External manifestations of systemic infections. Philadelphia: Current Medicine; 1996. 237 p. (Mandell GL, editor. Atlas of infectious diseases; vol. 6.) ISBN:0-443-07760-6] *Caption from original*

- Rocky Mountain Spotted Fever

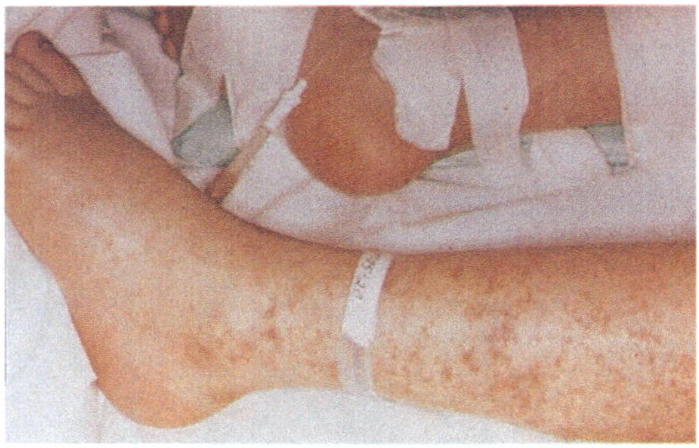

Petechial lesions in Rocky Mountain spotted fever. [Woodward T, Sexton D, Walker D, Bleck T. Chapter 09. In: Stevens DL, editor. Skin, Soft Tissue, Bone and Joint Infections. Philadelphia: Current Medicine; 1995. 250 p. (Mandell GL, editor. Atlas of Infectious Diseases; vol. 2.) ISBN:1-878132-44-X] *Caption adapted from original*

- Staphylococcal Scalded Skin Syndrome

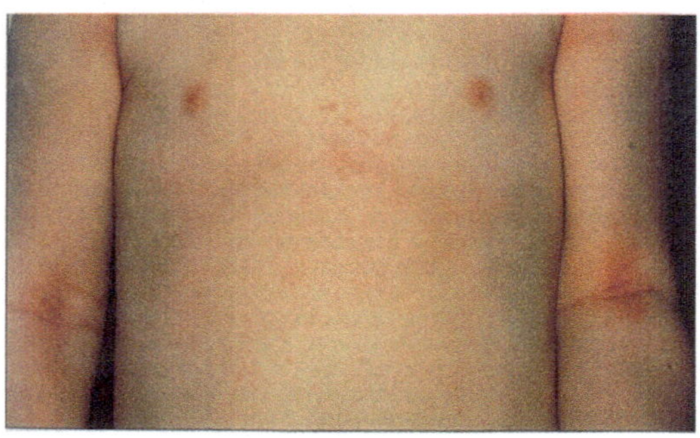

Staphylococcal scalded skin syndrome. A faint macular erythema is present on the trunk and arms of a febrile 4-year-old girl. The redness is accentuated in the skinfolds of the upper arms and the antecubital area. This disease occurs from the effects of epidermolytic toxins produced by some strains of *S. aureus*, most commonly group II phage types. The patients are usually children less than 5 years of age, in whom the staphylococci commonly colonize the mucous membranes of the nasopharynx, vagina, or conjunctivae, from which the toxin is readily absorbed. This disorder is rare in adults, apparently because they can inactivate or eliminate the toxins by immunologic mechanisms or urinary excretion. Affected adults usually have had suppurative infections, rather than just mucosal colonization, and severely compromised renal or immune function. [Hirschmann J, Bleck T. Chapter 02. In: Stevens DL, editor. Skin, Soft Tissue, Bone and Joint Infections. Philadelphia: Current Medicine; 1995. 250 p. (Mandell GL, editor. Atlas of Infectious Diseases; vol. 2.) ISBN: 1-878132-44-X] *Caption from original*

- Toxic Epidermal Necrolysis

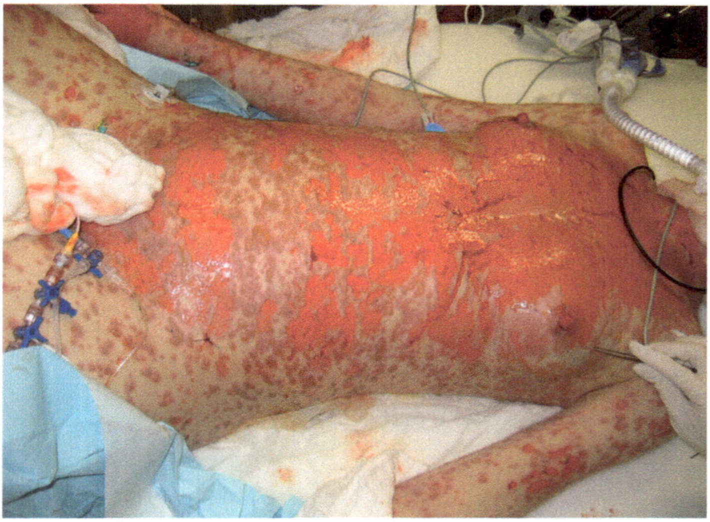

Toxic epidermal necrolysis in a female patient covering more than 30% of the total body surface area. A special critical care infrastructure such as that provided in burn centers with positive pressure units providing a constant environmental temperature of more than 30° C and an adjustable atmospheric humidity of 70% should be considered in the early course of the disease [Struck MF, Hilbert P, Mockenhaupt M, Reichelt B, Steen M. Severe cutaneous adverse reactions: emergency approach to non-burn epidermolytic syndromes. Intensive Care Medicine. 2010 Jan;36(1):22–32.] *Caption from original*

History and Physical Exam

- Most children will seek medical care due to the presence of high fevers. They will be irritable, paradoxically (i.e., not wanting to be touched). There will be a history of a rash, red eyes, and cracked lips. The rash, if present, will often be a chief complaint.

Findings That Confirm Diagnosis

- Commonly accepted diagnostic criteria for Kawasaki disease include the presence of fever for at least 5 days AND at least 4 of the 5 following criteria:
  - Conjunctival injection
  - Oral mucous membrane changes (fissured lips, strawberry tongue)
  - Peripheral extremity changes (erythema of palms/soles, edema of hands and feet, periungual desquamation)
  - Polymorphous rash
  - Cervical lymphadenopathy
- Laboratory findings consistent with a diagnosis of KD include:
  - Elevated ESR or CRP
  - Elevated WBC
  - Anemia (normochromic/normocytic)
  - Thrombocytosis (< 450,000 after 5 days)
  - Pyuria
  - Elevated liver enzymes
- Decreased serum albumin

Factors That Suggest Diagnosis

- In all published reports, the presence of fever for more than 5 days, in any pediatric age group, should raise suspicion for atypical forms of KD.

Factors that Exclude Diagnosis

- The absence of fever essentially rules out KD.

Ancillary studies

Laboratory

- The use of the laboratory is mandatory when evaluating all cases of suspected KD.

- Recommended tests include:
  - ESR or CRP
  - CBC with differential
  - Urinalysis
  - Liver function tests
  - Serum albumin

Electrocardiography

- ECG findings are not helpful.

Cardiac Enzymes

- Not indicated.

Special Populations

Age

- There have been reported cases of KD in adolescents.

Co-morbidities

- Case reports have described associated arthritis in older patients with KD.

Pitfalls in Diagnosis

- One must consider KD (in any form) when evaluating infants and children with prolonged febrile illnesses.
- Early consultation with Pediatric Cardiology is mandatory in suspected cases.

Critical Steps Not to Miss

- When presented with a patient with irritability, fever, and rash, always consider KD in your differential.

Mimics

- Measles
- Adenoviral infections
- Scarlet fever
- Echoviral infections
- EBV infections
- Rocky Mountain Spotted Fever
- Systemic juvenile rheumatoid arthritis

Time-Dependent Interventions

- Obtaining a Pediatric Cardiology consult is always indicated.
- Recommended pharmacologic treatments include:
    - Administration of a single dose of IV immunoglobulin (IVIG) (2 mg/kg) over 8 to 12 hours.
    - Administration of aspirin. The recommended initial dose is 80 to 100 mg/kg/day in 4 divided doses.

Overall Principles of Treatment

- The primary goals of KD management are to prevent the development of coronary lesions and to relieve symptoms.

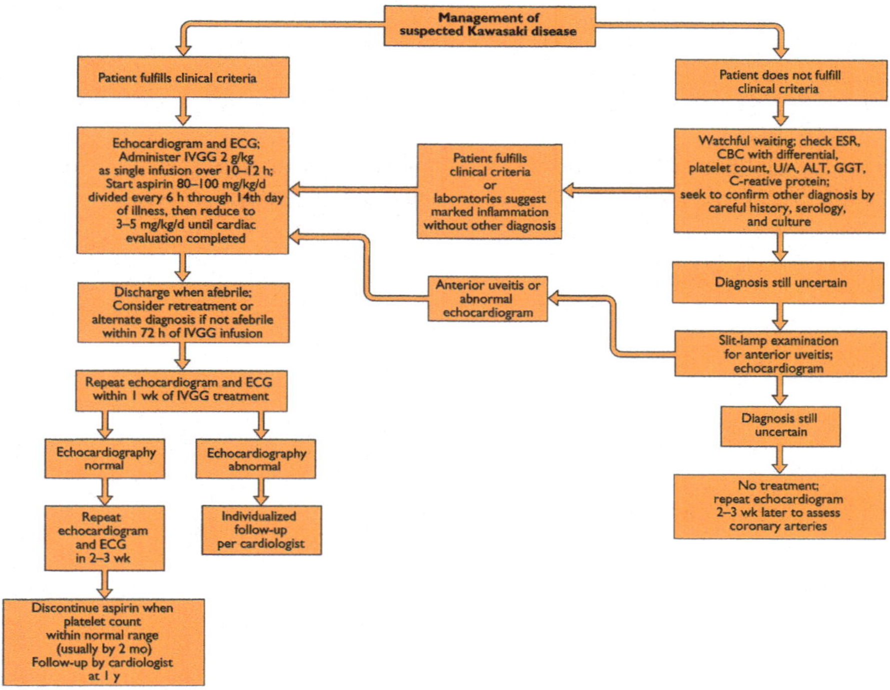

Algorithm for management of patients with suspected Kawasaki disease. The current recommended therapy for patients with Kawasaki disease who present within the first 10 days of illness is intravenous gamma globulin (IVGG), 2 g/kg as a single infusion over 10 to 12 hours, in conjunction with aspirin (80 to 100 mg/kg/d divided into four doses through illness day 14, then 3 to 5 mg/kg/d until cardiac evaluation is completed). The mechanism of action of IVGG has not been elucidated, although downregulation of the inflammatory response after treatment has clearly been demonstrated. ALT—alanine aminotransferase; CBC—complete blood count; ECG—electrocardiogram; ESR—erythrocyte sedimentation rate; GGT—γ-glutamyl transferase; U/A—urinalysis.[Burns J, Glodé M. Chapter 10. In: Wilfert CM, editor. Pediatric infectious diseases. Philadelphia: Current Medicine; 1999. (Mandell GL, editor. Atlas of infectious diseases; vol. 11). ISBN: 0-443-06526-8] *Caption adapted from original*

TARGETS OF THERAPY IN KAWASAKI DISEASE

LIFESTYLE MODIFICATIONS	PHARMACOLOGIC THERAPY	SURGICAL INTERVENTION
Implementation of heart-healthy diet, with specific recommendations guided by serum liqid profile	Goals	CABG
Prevention or cessation of smoking	Decrease overall prevalence and size of coronary artery aneurysms	PTCA
Physical activity guided by status of coronary arteries and use of antithrombolytic therapy (see Figs. 9-29–9-34 for stratified recommendations)	Prevent coronary artery thrombosis in patients with aneurysms	Stents
Maintenance of healthy weight	Treat ischemic heart disease in patients with coronary aneurysms	Cardiac transplantation

Targets of therapy for Kawasaki disease (KD). Children with KD and their parents should receive lifestyle modification counseling. This is especially important because various follow-up studies in children with coronary aneurysms in the acute phase have indicated that even when these aneurysms regress, there is persisting vascular dysfunction. This may put these children at risk for accelerated atherosclerosis in adulthood. [Taubert K, Newburger J. Kawasaki Disease. In: Creager MA, editor. Atlas of Vascular Disease. 2e, Philadelphia: Current Medicine; 2003. (Braunwald E, series editor, vol 07). ISBN: 1-57340-191-9] *Caption adapted from original*

Disease Course

- Long-term outcomes for children treated early with IVIG and salicylates are very favorable.

Related Evidence

Papers of particular interest have been highlighted as:
*** Of key importance*

Practice Guideline

Research Committee of the Japanese Society of Pediatric Cardiology; Cardiac Surgery Committee for Development of Guidelines for Medical Treatment of Acute Kawasaki Disease. Guidelines for medical treatment of acute Kawasaki disease: report of the Research Committee of the Japanese Society of Pediatric Cardiology and Cardiac Surgery (2012 revised version). Pediatr Int. 2014 Apr;56(2):135-58. https://doi.org/10.1111/ped.12317. PubMed PMID: 24730626. http://www.ncbi.nlm.nih.gov/pubmed/24730626 **

JCS Joint Working Group. Guidelines for diagnosis and management of cardiovascular sequelae in Kawasaki disease (JCS 2008)--digest version. Circ J. 2010 Sep;74(9):1989-2020. Epub 2010 Aug 18. PubMed PMID: 20724794. http://www.ncbi.nlm.nih.gov/pubmed/20724794

Japanese Circulation Society Joint Research Group. Guidelines for diagnosis and management of cardiovascular sequelae in Kawasaki disease. Pediatr Int. 2005 Dec;47(6):711-32. PubMed PMID: 16354233. http://www.ncbi.nlm.nih.gov/pubmed/16354233

Ayusawa M, Sonobe T, Uemura S, Ogawa S, Nakamura Y, Kiyosawa N, Ishii M, Harada K; Kawasaki Disease Research Committee. Revision of diagnostic guidelines for Kawasaki disease (the 5th revised edition). Pediatr Int. 2005 Apr;47(2):232-4. PubMed PMID: 15771703. http://www.ncbi.nlm.nih.gov/pubmed/15771703

Newburger JW, Takahashi M, Gerber MA, Gewitz MH, Tani LY, Burns JC, Shulman ST, Bolger AF, Ferrieri P, Baltimore RS, Wilson WR, Baddour LM, Levison ME, Pallasch TJ, Falace DA, Taubert KA; Committee on Rheumatic Fever, Endocarditis, and Kawasaki Disease, Council on Cardiovascular Disease in the Young, American Heart Association. Diagnosis, treatment, and long-term management of Kawasaki disease: a statement for health professionals from the Committee on Rheumatic Fever, Endocarditis, and Kawasaki Disease, Council on Cardiovascular Disease in the Young, American Heart Association. Pediatrics. 2004 Dec;114(6):1708-33. Erratum in: Pediatrics. 2005 Apr;115(4):1118. PubMed PMID: 15574639. http://www.ncbi.nlm.nih.gov/pubmed/15574639 **

Meta-Analysis

Chen S, Dong Y, Yin Y, Krucoff MW. Intravenous immunoglobulin plus corticosteroid to prevent coronary artery abnormalities in Kawasaki disease: a meta-analysis. Heart. 2013 Jan;99(2):76-82. https://doi.org/10.1136/heartjnl-2012-302126. Epub 2012 Aug 6. Review. PubMed PMID: 22869678. http://www.ncbi.nlm.nih.gov/pubmed/22869678 **

Review

Rowley AH. The Complexities of the Diagnosis and Management of Kawasaki Disease. Infect Dis Clin North Am. 2015 Sep;29(3):525-37. https://doi.org/10.1016/j.idc.2015.05.006. Epub 2015 Jul 4. Review. PubMed PMID: 26154665; PubMed Central PMCID: PMC4552602. http://www.ncbi.nlm.nih.gov/pubmed/26154665 **

Greco A, De Virgilio A, Rizzo MI, Tombolini M, Gallo A, Fusconi M, Ruoppolo G, Pagliuca G, Martellucci S, de Vincentiis M. Kawasaki disease: an evolving paradigm. Autoimmun Rev. 2015 Aug;14(8):703-9. https://doi.org/10.1016/j.autrev.2015.04.002. Epub 2015 Apr 13. Review. PubMed PMID: 25882057. **

Shulman ST, Rowley AH. Kawasaki disease: insights into pathogenesis and approaches to treatment. Nat Rev Rheumatol. 2015 Aug;11(8):475-82. https://doi.org/10.1038/nrrheum.2015.54. Epub 2015 Apr 28. Review. PubMed PMID: 25907703. http://www.ncbi.nlm.nih.gov/pubmed/25907703 **

Singh S, Vignesh P, Burgner D. The epidemiology of Kawasaki disease: a global update. Arch Dis Child. 2015 Jun 25. pii: archdischild-2014-307536. https://doi.org/10.1136/archdischild-2014-307536. [Epub ahead of print] Review. PubMed PMID:26111818. http://www.ncbi.nlm.nih.gov/pubmed/26111818

Brown LM, Duffy CE, Mitchell C, Young L. A practical guide to pediatric coronary artery imaging with echocardiography. J Am Soc Echocardiogr. 2015 Apr;28(4):379-91. https://doi.org/10.1016/j.echo.2015.01.008. Epub 2015 Feb 15. Review. PubMed PMID: 25691000. http://www.ncbi.nlm.nih.gov/pubmed/25691000

Seaton KK, Kharbanda A. Evidence-based management of Kawasaki disease in the emergency department. Pediatr Emerg Med Pract. 2015 Jan;12(1):1-20; quiz 21. Review. PubMed PMID: 25693305. http://www.ncbi.nlm.nih.gov/pubmed/25693305

Dimitriades VR, Brown AG, Gedalia A. Kawasaki disease: pathophysiology, clinical manifestations, and management. Curr Rheumatol Rep. 2014 Jun;16(6):423. https://doi.org/10.1007/s11926-014-0423-x. Review. PubMed PMID: 24744086. http://www.ncbi.nlm.nih.gov/pubmed/24744086

Sánchez-Manubens J, Bou R, Anton J. Diagnosis and classification of Kawasaki disease. J Autoimmun. 2014 Feb-Mar;48-49:113-7. https://doi.org/10.1016/j.jaut.2014.01.010. Epub 2014 Jan 28. Review. PubMed PMID: 24485156. http://www.ncbi.nlm.nih.gov/pubmed/24485156 **

Eleftheriou D, Levin M, Shingadia D, Tulloh R, Klein NJ, Brogan PA. Management of Kawasaki disease. Arch Dis Child. 2014 Jan;99(1):74-83. https://doi.org/10.1136/archdischild-2012-302841. Epub 2013 Oct 25. Review. PubMed PMID: 24162006; PubMed Central PMCID: PMC3888612. http://www.ncbi.nlm.nih.gov/pubmed/24162006

Takahashi K, Oharaseki T, Yokouchi Y. Update on etio and immunopathogenesis of Kawasaki disease. Curr Opin Rheumatol. 2014 Jan;26(1):31-6. https://doi.org/10.1097/BOR.0000000000000010. Review. PubMed PMID: 24247115. http://www.ncbi.nlm.nih.gov/pubmed/24247115

Bayers S, Shulman ST, Paller AS. Kawasaki disease: part I. Diagnosis, clinical features, and pathogenesis. J Am Acad Dermatol. 2013 Oct;69(4):501.e1-11; quiz 511-2. https://doi.org/10.1016/j.jaad.2013.07.002. Review. PubMed PMID: 24034379. http://www.ncbi.nlm.nih.gov/pubmed/24034379 **

Jamieson N, Singh-Grewal D. Kawasaki Disease: A Clinician's Update. Int J Pediatr. 2013;2013:645391. https://doi.org/10.1155/2013/645391. Epub 2013 Oct 27. Review. PubMed PMID: 24282419; PubMed Central PMCID: PMC3826559. http://www.ncbi.nlm.nih.gov/pubmed/24282419 **

Yim D, Curtis N, Cheung M, Burgner D. Update on Kawasaki disease: epidemiology, aetiology and pathogenesis. J Paediatr Child Health. 2013 Sep;49(9):704-8. https://doi.org/10.1111/jpc.12172. Epub 2013 Apr 7. Review. PubMed PMID: 23560706. http://www.ncbi.nlm.nih.gov/pubmed/23560706

Yim D, Curtis N, Cheung M, Burgner D. An update on Kawasaki disease II: clinical features, diagnosis, treatment and outcomes. J Paediatr Child Health. 2013 Aug;49(8):614-23. https://doi.org/10.1111/jpc.12221. Epub 2013 May 7. Review. PubMed PMID: 23647873. http://www.ncbi.nlm.nih.gov/pubmed/23647873 **

Golshevsky D, Cheung M, Burgner D. Kawasaki disease--the importance of prompt recognition and early referral. Aust Fam Physician. 2013 Jul;42(7):473-6.

Review. PubMed PMID: 23826599. http://www.ncbi.nlm.nih.gov/pubmed/23826599 **

Son MB, Newburger JW. Kawasaki disease. Pediatr Rev. 2013 Apr;34(4):151-62. https://doi.org/10.1542/pir.34-4-151. Review. PubMed PMID: 23547061. http://www.ncbi.nlm.nih.gov/pubmed/23547061 **

Dominguez SR, Anderson MS. Advances in the treatment of Kawasaki disease. Curr Opin Pediatr. 2013 Feb;25(1):103-9. https://doi.org/10.1097/MOP.0b013e32835c1122. Review. PubMed PMID: 23283289. http://www.ncbi.nlm.nih.gov/pubmed/23283289

Hartopo AB, Setianto BY. Coronary artery sequel of Kawasaki disease in adulthood, a concern for internists and cardiologists. Acta Med Indones. 2013 Jan;45(1):69-75. Review. PubMed PMID: 23585413. http://www.ncbi.nlm.nih.gov/pubmed/23585413

Manlhiot C, Christie E, McCrindle BW, Rosenberg H, Chahal N, Yeung RS. Complete and incomplete Kawasaki disease: two sides of the same coin. Eur J Pediatr. 2012 Apr;171(4):657-62. https://doi.org/10.1007/s00431-011-1631-2. Epub 2011 Dec 3. PubMed PMID: 22134803. http://www.ncbi.nlm.nih.gov/pubmed/22134803

Kuo HC, Yang KD, Chang WC, Ger LP, Hsieh KS. Kawasaki disease: an update on diagnosis and treatment. Pediatr Neonatol. 2012 Feb;53(1):4-11. https://doi.org/10.1016/j.pedneo.2011.11.003. Epub 2012 Jan 17. Review. PubMed PMID: 22348488. http://www.ncbi.nlm.nih.gov/pubmed/22348488 **

Uehara R, Belay ED. Epidemiology of Kawasaki disease in Asia, Europe, and the United States. J Epidemiol. 2012;22(2):79-85. Epub 2012 Feb 4. Review. PubMed PMID: 22307434; PubMed Central PMCID: PMC3798585. http://www.ncbi.nlm.nih.gov/pubmed/22307434

Case Study

Fradin KN, Rhim HJ. An adolescent with fever, jaundice, and abdominal pain: an unusual presentation of Kawasaki disease. J Adolesc Health. 2013 Jan;52(1):131-3 https://doi.org/10.1016/j.jadohealth.2012.06.007. Epub 2012 Aug 11. Review. PubMed PMID:23260847. http://www.ncbi.nlm.nih.gov/pubmed/?term=10.1016%2Fj.jadohealth.2012.06.007

General

Falcini F, Ozen S, Magni-Manzoni S, Candelli M, Ricci L, Martini G, Cuttica RJ, Oliveira S, Calabri GB, Zulian F, Pistorio A, La Torre F, Rigante D. Discrimination between incomplete and atypical Kawasaki syndrome versus other febrile diseases in childhood: results from an international registry-based study. Clin Exp

Rheumatol. 2012 Sep-Oct;30(5):799-804. Epub 2012 Oct 17. PubMed PMID: 23020938. http://www.ncbi.nlm.nih.gov/pubmed/23020938

Perrin L, Letierce A, Guitton C, Tran TA, Lambert V, Koné-Paut I. Comparative study of complete versus incomplete Kawasaki disease in 59 pediatric patients. Joint Bone Spine. 2009 Oct;76(5):481-5. https://doi.org/10.1016/j.jbspin.2008.11.015. Epub 2009 Oct 6. PubMed PMID: 19811939. http://www.ncbi.nlm.nih.gov/pubmed/19811939

Use PubMed Clinical Queries to find the most recent evidence. Use this search strategy:"http://www.ncbi.nlm.nih.gov/pubmed/22634168"

"Mucocutaneous Lymph Node Syndrome"[Mesh] OR "Mucocutaneous Lymph Node Syndrome"[tiab] OR "kawasaki"[tiab]

Chapter 43
Laryngospasm

Charles V. Pollack, Jr., Melissa Platt, Richard M. Cantor, and Victoria G. Riese

Name and Synonyms

Laryngospasm

Incidence/Epidemiology

- Incidence is 8.6/1000 in adults.
- Higher incidence of 27.6/1000 was noted in children perioperatively.
- Overall incidence is just under 1 % in both adult and pediatric anesthesia.
- Increased in infants

C. V. Pollack, Jr. (✉)
Department of Emergency Medicine, Thomas Jefferson University, Philadelphia, PA, USA

M. Platt
Department of Emergency Medicine, University of Louisville, Louisville, KY, USA

R. M. Cantor
Department of Emergency Medicine and Pediatrics, State University of New York Upstate Medical University, Syracuse, NY, USA

V. G. Riese
Librarian Consultant, Eldersburg, MD, USA

C. V. Pollack, Jr. (ed.), *Differential Diagnosis of Cardiopulmonary Disease*,
https://doi.org/10.1007/978-3-319-63895-9_43

Differential Diagnosis

- Epiglottitis
- Croup
- Tracheitis
- Retropharyngeal abscess
- Infectious mononucleosis
- Aspirated foreign body
- Laryngeal trauma
- Anaphylaxis
- Angioedema
- Vocal cord dysfunction
- Congenital anomalies

Pathophysiology and Etiology

- Acute manifestation of vocal cord dysfunction beyond the normal airway protective reflex
- Usually precipitated by irritation of the vocal cords
- May be incomplete or complete
- May occur as a complication of anesthesia, especially with ketamine
- May occur during intubation procedures or post extubation

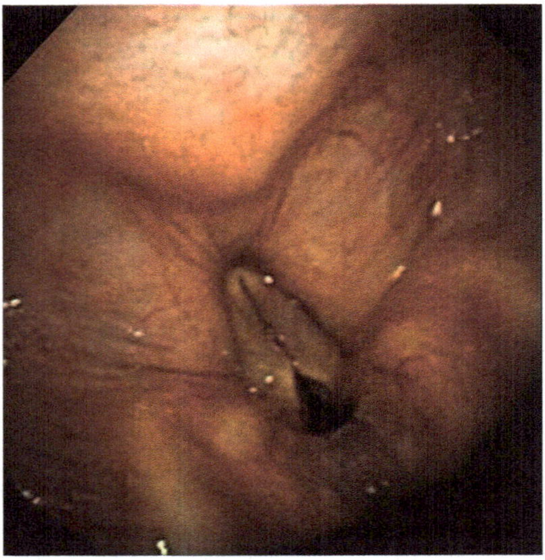

Partial laryngospasm is not uncommon during and at the end of a bronchoscopic procedure [Goudra BG, Singh PM, Borle A, Farid N, Harris K. Anesthesia for

Advanced Bronchoscopic Procedures: State-of-the-Art Review. Lung. 2015 Aug;193(4):453–65.] *Caption from original*

Presentation

Typical/"Classic"

- Patient will describe a choking sensation and be unable to breathe or speak.
- Patient may have stridor.
- Episode may last only minutes.

Atypical

- If prolonged, may lead to hypoxia and hypercapnea
- Vocal cord dysfunction usually is chronic, and worsening of stridor may be a clue to a progressive anatomic problem.

Primary Differential Considerations

- Angioedema
- Asthma
- Epiglottitis
- Croup
- Laryngomalacia
- Tracheal foreign body
- Vocal cord paralysis or tumor

History and Physical Exam

Findings That Confirm Diagnosis

- The diagnosis is made clinically (as below), then attention is turned to the underlying cause.

Factors That Suggest Diagnosis

- Lack of upper airway patency
- Inspiratory stridor if partial obstruction
- Decreased chest wall movement
- Fever suggests an infectious etiology
- Sensation of choking and inability to breathe or speak
- Increased respiratory effort
- Tracheal tug
- Paradoxic respiratory effort
- Oxygen desaturation with or without bradycardia

Factors That Exclude Diagnosis

- A patent trachea with no increased breathing effort excludes significant laryngospasm, but stridor, even in the presence of normal respiratory effort, warrants further evaluation for a fluid or evolving clinical scenario.

Ancillary Studies

Imaging

- Imaging should never interfere with stabilization of a critical obstruction.
- Soft tissue radiographs of the neck may help diagnose epiglottitis/croup/foreign body.

Special Populations

Age

Co-morbidities

- Those with reactive airway disease are more prone to laryngospasm during intubation.

Pediatric Considerations

- Seen mainly in children, especially in infants 1–3 months of age.
- Has been reported in association with ketamine use; however, this is thought to be idiosyncratic in etiology.

Pitfalls in Diagnosis

Critical Steps Not to Miss

- Triggering factors:
  - Painful stimulation
  - Primary vagal hypertonicity
  - Insufficient depth of anesthesia on endotracheal intubation
  - Irritants:
  - Blood
  - Mucus
  - Laryngoscope blade
  - Suction catheter
  - Surgical debris or other foreign body

Mimics

- Other causes of upper airway obstruction, such as a foreign body, may cause a clinical picture similar to that of laryngospasm, but with normal vocal cord action.

Time-Dependent Interventions

- Acute upper airway compromise/obstruction may be a life-threatening emergency.
- Prompt recognition is needed.

Overall Principles of Treatment

- Factors influencing the choice of treatment:
  - Degree of airway compromise
  - Etiology of laryngospasm
  - Presence of fever
  - Acuteness of symptom onset
  - History of injury
  - Age
- Treatment options:
  - Suctioning of foreign material from the oropharynx
  - Removal or avoidance of painful stimuli
  - "Jaw thrust" at the angle of the mandible while applying positive pressure ventilation with oxygen by bag and mask
  - Laryngospasm pressure
  - Lidocaine: 1 to 1.5 mg/kg intravenously (IV)
  - Topical lidocaine: direct administration to vocal cords
  - Succinylcholine: recommended dose varying from 0.25 to 1 mg/kg IV or 4 mg/kg intramuscularly; must be followed by definitive airway and ventilation management

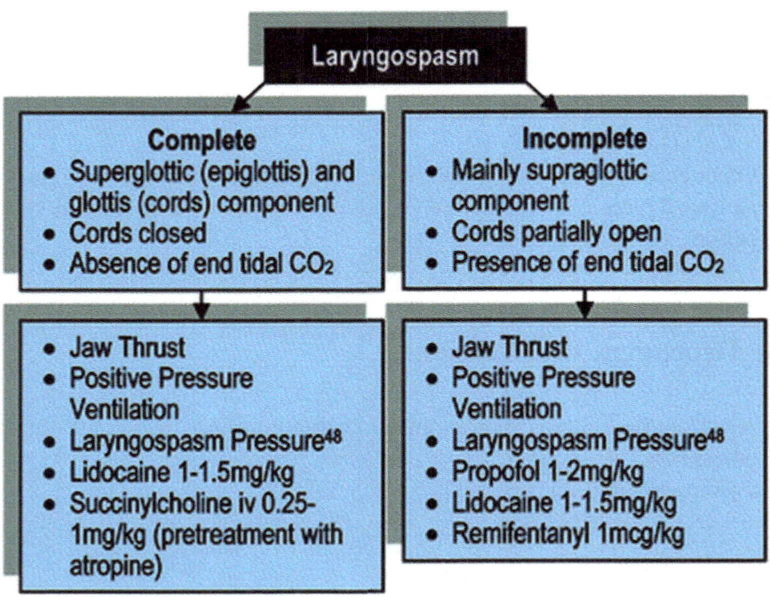

Classification and treatment options of laryngospasm [Finucane BT, Tsui BCH, Santora AH. Principles of airway management [Internet]. New York: Springer;

2010. Chapter 10, Pediatric airway management; [cited 2015 Aug 13]; p. 415–513. Available from: http://link.springer.com/10.1007/978-0-387-09558-5_10] *Caption from original*

1.	Identification and removal of the noxious stimulus (blood, secretions)
2.	Chin lift and jaw thrust
3.	Positive airway pressure with 100 % oxygen
4.	Intravenous succinylcholine (0.5–1 mg/kg) or intramuscular (1–4 mg/kg) if no IV access
5.	Deepen anesthesia with propofol or inhalational agent
6.	Endotracheal intubation if required

Treatment of laryngospasm [Adams MC, Bittner EA. Ear, Nose, and Throat Surgery. In: Sikka PK, Beaman ST, Street JA, editors. Basic Clinical Anesthesia [Internet]. New York, NY: Springer New York; 2015 [cited 2016 May 16]. p. 489–99. Available from: http://link.springer.com/10.1007/978-1-4939-1737-2_37] *Caption from original*

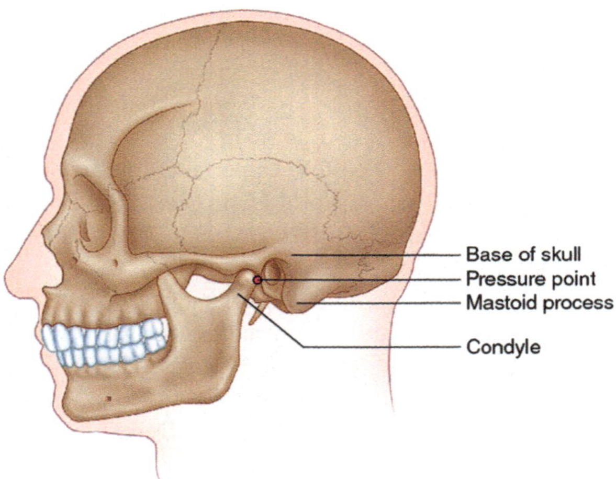

Laryngospasm notch [Gal JS, Yudkowitz FS, Rothschild MA. Pediatric otolaryngology. In: Levine AI, Govindaraj S, DeMaria, S, editors. Anesthesiology and otolaryngology [Internet]. New York: Springer; 2013 [cited 2015 Aug 13]. p. 333–64. Available from: http://link.springer.com/10.1007/978-1-4614-4184-7_20] *Caption from original*

Disease Course

- People experiencing laryngospasm describe a sensation of choking and cannot breathe or speak.
- As the airways slowly open, the person may have stridor.
- The episode may last only a minute or two before breathing returns to normal.
- Some people lose consciousness during these episodes.
- Underlying pathology will determine extended course and risk of recurrence.

Related Evidence

Papers of particular interest have been highlighted as:
** *Of key importance*

Review

Ciorba A, Bianchini C, Zuolo M, Feo CV. Upper aerodigestive tract disorders and gastro-oesophageal reflux disease. World J Clin Cases. 2015 Feb 16;3(2):102-11. https://doi.org/10.12998/wjcc.v3.i2.102. PMID: 25685756. http://www.ncbi.nlm.nih.gov/pubmed/25685756 **

Mihara T, Uchimoto K, Morita S, Goto T. The efficacy of lidocaine to prevent laryngospasm in children: a systematic review and meta-analysis. Anaesthesia. 2014 Dec;69(12):1388-96. https://doi.org/ 10.1111/anae.12788. PMID: 24992191. http://www.ncbi.nlm.nih.gov/pubmed/24992191 **

Green SM, Roback MG, Krauss B; Emergency Department Ketamine Meta-Analysis Study Group. Laryngospasm during emergency department ketamine sedation: a case-control study. Pediatr Emerg Care. 2010 Nov;26(11):798-802. https://doi.org/10.1097/PEC.0b013e3181fa8737. PMID: 20944510. http://www.ncbi.nlm.nih.gov/pubmed/20944510 **

Al-alami AA, Zestos MM, Baraka AS. Pediatric laryngospasm: prevention and treatment. Curr Opin Anaesthesiol. 2009 Jun;22(3):388-95. PMID: 19434787. http://www.ncbi.nlm.nih.gov/pubmed/19434787 **

Gdynia HJ, Kassubek J, Sperfeld AD. Laryngospasm in neurological diseases. Neurocrit Care. 2006;4(2):163-7. PMID: 16627908. http://www.ncbi.nlm.nih.gov/pubmed/16627908 **

Poelmans J, Tack J. Extraoesophageal manifestations of gastro-oesophageal reflux. Gut. 2005 Oct;54(10):1492-9. PMID: 16162955. http://www.ncbi.nlm.nih.gov/pubmed/16162955 **

Ead H. Review of laryngospasm and noncardiogenic pulmonary edema. Dynamics. 2003 Fall;14(3):9-12. PMID: 14725141. http://www.ncbi.nlm.nih.gov/pubmed/14725141 **

Landsman IS. Mechanisms and treatment of laryngospasm. Int Anesthesiol Clin. 1997 Summer;35(3):67-73. PMID: 9361977. http://www.ncbi.nlm.nih.gov/pubmed/9361977 **

Cohort Study

Obholzer RJ, Nouraei SA, Ahmed J, Kadhim MR, Sandhu GS. An approach to the management of paroxysmal laryngospasm. J Laryngol Otol. 2008 Jan;122(1):57-60. PMID: 17319986. http://www.ncbi.nlm.nih.gov/pubmed/17319986 **

Visvanathan T, Kluger MT, Webb RK, Westhorpe RN. Crisis management during anaesthesia: laryngospasm. Qual Saf Health Care. 2005 Jun;14(3):e3. PMID: 15933300. http://www.ncbi.nlm.nih.gov/pubmed/15933300 **

Case Study

Murray RC, Powell D, Curry JM, Sperling MR, Evans JJ, Spiegel JR. Epileptic laryngospasm presenting as a primary sleep disturbance. Arch Otolaryngol Head Neck Surg. 2010 Oct;136(10):1025-7. https://doi.org/10.1001/archoto.2010.174. PMID: 20956752. http://www.ncbi.nlm.nih.gov/pubmed/20956752 **

Use PubMed Clinical Queries to find the most recent evidence. Use this search strategy:
"Laryngismus"[Mesh] OR "Laryngospasm"

Chapter 44
Mallory-Weiss Syndrome

Christopher J. Rees, Richard M. Cantor, Charles V. Pollack, Jr., and Victoria G. Riese

Name and Synonyms

Mallory-Weiss Syndrome

- Mallory-Weiss Tear

Incidence/Epidemiology

- Mallory-Weiss tears are the fourth most common cause of upper gastrointestinal bleeding in adults.
- They account for 5 % of all upper gastrointestinal (UGI) bleeding cases.
- Three percent of deaths from UGI bleeding are the result of Mallory-Weiss tears.
- It is much less common in children.
- Mortality may be up to 3 %, but most mortality is associated with significant co-morbidities, such as portal hypertension, known coagulopathy, or older age.

C. J. Rees
Emergency Department, Pennsylvania Hospital, Philadelphia, PA, USA

R. M. Cantor
Department of Emergency Medicine and Pediatrics, State University of New York Upstate Medical University, Syracuse, NY, USA

C. V. Pollack, Jr. (✉)
Department of Emergency Medicine, Thomas Jefferson University, Philadelphia, PA, USA

V. G. Riese
Librarian Consultant, Eldersburg, MD, USA

C. V. Pollack, Jr. (ed.), *Differential Diagnosis of Cardiopulmonary Disease*,
https://doi.org/10.1007/978-3-319-63895-9_44

Differential Diagnosis

- Chest pain typically occurs with Mallory-Weiss tears, but is usually overshadowed in the presentation by the complaint of hematemesis. Mallory-Weiss tears cause UGI bleeding.
- All the causes of acute UGI bleeding need to be considered, including:
  - peptic ulcer disease (gastric and duodenal ulcers and erosions)
  - esophageal varices
  - esophagitis
  - duodenitis
- Older patients who may have coronary artery disease may develop angina from the exertion of vomiting or from the anemia that results from blood loss.
- Esophageal rupture, which only rarely causes UGI bleeding, may present with chest pain.

Pathophysiology and Etiology

- A Mallory-Weiss tear is a 1- to 4-cm longitudinal tear through the mucosa and submucosa of the esophagus or cardiac region of the stomach. The tear causes pain that may radiate into the chest.
- Bleeding results from extension of the tear into the submucosal arterial or venous plexus.
- It is usually associated with sudden increases in intra-abdominal pressure, especially from forceful vomiting.
- It also may be seen after other events that result in large increases in intra-abdominal pressure, such as straining, coughing, and seizures. It also has been noted after colonoscopy preps containing PEG (polyethylene glycol).
- Most will stop spontaneously and heal within 24–48 hours.

Presentation

Typical/"Classic"

- Acute onset of bright red hematemesis, typically following several episodes of forceful vomiting.
- May be associated with chest pain, epigastric pain, and/or back pain.
- Patient often has a history of recent, heavy alcohol use (40–80 %) or a known history of a hiatal hernia.
- Most often, patients are hemodynamically stable. A minority of cases present with bleeding significant enough to cause hemodynamic instability.

Atypical

- May be found incidentally on endoscopy performed for other reasons.

Primary Differential Considerations

- Upon initial presentation of bright red hematemesis, more serious diagnoses should be considered before attributing the findings to a Mallory-Weiss tear, such as:
  - Esophageal rupture
  - Gastric or peptic ulcer bleeding
  - Consideration should also be given to posterior epistaxis.

History and Physical Exam

Findings That Confirm Diagnosis

- There are no pathognomonic findings on history and physical exam that confirm the diagnosis.
- The diagnosis can be confirmed by upper endoscopy.

Factors That Suggest Diagnosis

- The acute onset of bright red hematemesis after prolonged, forceful vomiting associated with hemodynamic stability will strongly suggest the diagnosis.

Factors That Exclude Diagnosis

- The finding on endoscopy of another cause for UGI bleeding.

Ancillary Studies

Laboratory

- There are no laboratory tests that are specific to the diagnosis.
- Blood loss is often minimal, so the hemoglobin may be mildly reduced.

Imaging

- No specific imaging study helps in making the diagnosis, but imaging may help exclude other causes.
- Upper endoscopy is the study of choice to confirm the diagnosis and also for therapeutic intervention if indicated.

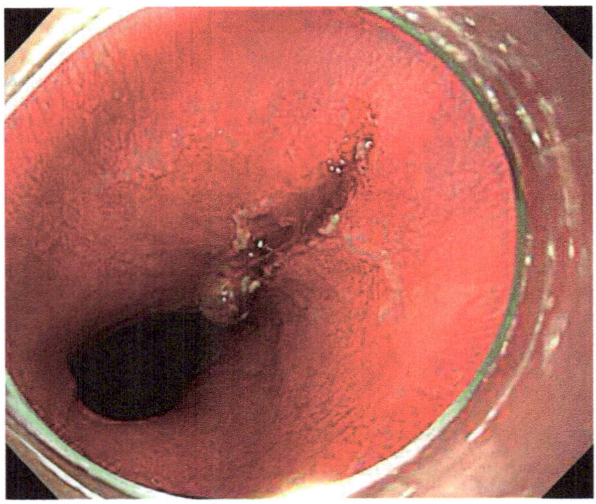

Mallory–Weiss tear. A nonbleeding tear at the gastroesophageal junction extending proximally. [Park JM. Miscellaneous esophageal diseases. In: Chun HJ, Yang S-K, Choi M-G, editors. Clinical gastrointestinal endoscopy. Berlin Heidelberg: Springer; 2014. p. 87–98. Available from: http://link.springer.com/10.1007/978-3-642-35626-1_7] *Caption adapted from original*

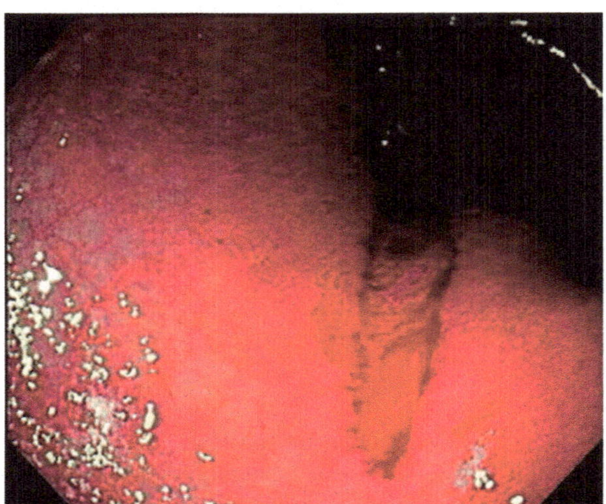

Mallory–Weiss tear in patient with acute bleeding. [Schroder JN, Branch MS. Mallory–Weiss syndrome. In: Pryor AD, Pappas TN, Branch MS, editors. Gastrointestinal bleeding. New York: Springer; 2010. p. 79–84. Available from: http://link.springer.com/10.1007/978-1-4419-1693-8_7] *Caption from original*

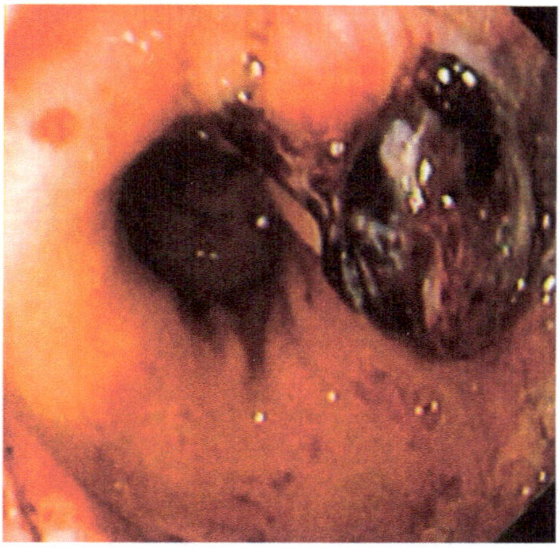

A Mallory-Weiss tear with an adherent clot. [Bozymski E, Kenney C, Orlando R, Feldman M. Gastroenterology and hepatology. In: Orlando RC, Feldman M, editors. Atlas of esophageal diseases. 2nd ed. Philadelphia: Current Medicine; 2002. 248 p. ISBN: 1-57340-181-1] *Caption adapted from original*

Special Populations

Age

- Slightly more common in older individuals.
- Uncommon in children, except perhaps in patients with cyclic vomiting disorders.

Co-morbidities

- Up to 80 % of cases are associated with alcoholism.
- Also associated with hiatal hernia.

Pitfalls in Diagnosis

Critical Steps Not to Miss

- It is important to initially consider the more serious causes of UGI bleeding.

Mimics

- Mallory-Weiss tears can mimic other causes of UGI bleeding, such as peptic ulcers and esophageal variceal bleeding.

Time-Dependent Interventions

- Any patient with hemodynamic instability should be resuscitated, as would any patient in shock.
- Most patients are stable, and there are no time-dependent interventions.

Overall Principles of Treatment

- Most Mallory-Weiss tears stop spontaneously and do not cause physiologically significant bleeding.
- Ninety percent heal spontaneously within 24–48 hours.
- It is most important to distinguish Mallory-Weiss tears from more severe causes of UGI bleeding.
- Treatment is usually supportive, and most patients will be started on acid suppressive therapy.
- Less than 10 % of patients will have significant bleeding. These patients are given treatment similar to that of patients with other causes of UGI bleeding, with resuscitation and stabilization, and transfusions as needed.
- Endoscopic-guided therapies are usually the treatment of choice in patients with more significant bleeding. Endoscopic therapies include thermal coagulation, local injection of epinephrine or vasopressin, or balloon tamponade. In very rare cases, interventional radiologic embolization may be indicated, and even more rarely, surgical management may be indicated.
- Most patients should be admitted or observed for at least 24 hours to document stability and to allow time for endoscopy to confirm the diagnosis.

Disease Course

- The course is usually mild and self-limited.
- Ninety percent will heal spontaneously within 24–48 hours.
- Up to 7 % may re-bleed. Risk factors for re-bleeding include portal hypertension and coagulopathy.

Related Evidence

Papers of particular interest have been highlighted as:
*** Of key importance*

Review

Feinman M, Haut ER. Upper gastrointestinal bleeding. Surg Clin North Am. 2014 Feb;94(1):43-53. https://doi.org/10.1016/j.suc.2013.10.004. PMID: 24267496. http://www.ncbi.nlm.nih.gov/pubmed/24267496 **

Khamaysi I, Gralnek IM. Acute upper gastrointestinal bleeding (UGIB) - initial evaluation and management. Best Pract Res Clin Gastroenterol. 2013 Oct;27(5):633-8. https://doi.org/10.1016/j.bpg.2013.09.002. PMID: 24160923. http://www.ncbi.nlm.nih.gov/pubmed/24160923 **

Schenker MP, Majdalany BS, Funaki BS, Yucel EK, Baum RA, Burke CT, Foley WD, Koss SA, Lorenz JM, Mansour MA, Millward SF, Nemcek AA Jr, Ray CE Jr. ACR Appropriateness Criteria® on upper gastrointestinal bleeding. J Am Coll Radiol. 2010 Nov;7(11):845-53. https://doi.org/10.1016/j.jacr.2010.05.029. PMID: 21040865. http://www.ncbi.nlm.nih.gov/pubmed/21040865 **

Morales P, Baum AE. Therapeutic alternatives for the Mallory-Weiss tear. Curr Treat Options Gastroenterol. 2003 Feb;6(1):75-83. PMID:12521575. http://www.ncbi.nlm.nih.gov/pubmed/12521575 **

Cohort Study

Banerjee S, Bellamkonda S, Gumaste VV. The Blatchford score is an useful index in the management of Mallory-Weiss tear and gastrointestinal bleeding: experience from an urban community hospital. Acta Gastroenterol Belg. 2012 Dec;75(4):432-7. PMID: 23402087. http://www.ncbi.nlm.nih.gov/pubmed/23402087 **

Kortas DY, Haas LS, Simpson WG, Nickl NJ 3rd, Gates LK Jr. Mallory-Weiss tear: predisposing factors and predictors of a complicated course. Am J Gastroenterol. 2001 Oct;96(10):2863-5. PMID: 11693318. http://www.ncbi.nlm.nih.gov/pubmed/11693318 **

Case Study

Bishop PR, Nowicki MJ, Parker PH. Vomiting-induced hematemesis in children: Mallory-Weiss tear or prolapse gastropathy? J Pediatr Gastroenterol Nutr. 2000 Apr;30(4):436-41. PMID: 10776958. http://www.ncbi.nlm.nih.gov/pubmed/10776958 **

Use PubMed Clinical Queries to find the most recent evidence. Use this search strategy:

"Mallory-Weiss Syndrome"[Mesh] OR "Mallory Weiss"

Chapter 45
Mediastinal Masses

Christopher J. Rees, Richard M. Cantor, Charles V. Pollack, Jr., and Victoria G. Riese

Name and Synonyms

Mediastinal masses

- Mediastinal tumors

Incidence/Epidemiology

- Mediastinal masses often are incidental findings of chest imaging performed for other reasons.

Differential Diagnosis

- Many neoplasms may present as mediastinal masses.
- They may be either benign or malignant lesions.
- The differential diagnosis is guided by location (anterior, middle, posterior) within the mediastinum.

C. J. Rees
Emergency Department, Pennsylvania Hospital, Philadelphia, PA, USA

R. M. Cantor
Department of Emergency Medicine and Pediatrics, State University of New York Upstate Medical University, Syracuse, NY, USA

C. V. Pollack, Jr. (✉)
Department of Emergency Medicine, Thomas Jefferson University, Philadelphia, PA, USA

V. G. Riese
Librarian Consultant, Eldersburg, MD, USA

C. V. Pollack, Jr. (ed.), *Differential Diagnosis of Cardiopulmonary Disease*, https://doi.org/10.1007/978-3-319-63895-9_45

Pathophysiology and Etiology

- The anterior mediastinum is the anatomic space that extends from the posterior aspect of the sternum to the anterior aspect of the great vessels and pericardium. Contained within the anterior mediastinum are the thymus, lymph nodes, and internal mammary arteries and veins. It is the most common location for mediastinal masses in adults. The most common masses found within the anterior mediastinum (in decreasing order of prevalence) are thymomas, teratomas (germ-cell tumors), lymphoma, and thyroid masses that extend into the anterior mediastinum.
- The middle mediastinum extends from the anterior pericardium to the posterior pericardium. It contains the heart, great vessels, airway, lymph nodes, and phrenic nerve. The most common cause of a mass within the middle mediastinum is lymphadenopathy from lymphoma, sarcoidosis or other granulomatous diseases, infectious processes, and metastatic lung cancer.
- The posterior mediastinum extends from the posterior aspect of the pericardium and trachea to the spine. It contains the descending thoracic aorta, esophagus, thoracic duct, azygous veins, posterior lymph nodes, spinal ganglia, and sympathetic chain. Neurogenic tumors are the most common posterior mediastinal tumors, especially in children.

Presentation

Typical/"Classic"

- Masses within the mediastinum are often asymptomatic.
- They commonly are found while undergoing diagnostic studies for other reasons.
- Symptoms, if present, usually result from direct compression from tumors or direct infiltration into surrounding structures.
- Compression, obstruction, or infiltration of airway structures may lead to cough, stridor, hemoptysis, shortness of breath, or pain. Hoarseness may result from phrenic nerve compression. Dysphagia may result from compression (either intrinsic or extrinsic) of the esophagus.
- Superior vena cava syndrome is a symptom complex due to compression or infiltration of the superior vena cava by a pathologic process in a contiguous structure. The most common causes are malignancies (either primary or metastatic) within the mediastinum. Dyspnea is the most common symptom, but facial swelling and "fullness" and arm swelling usually are present. The most characteristic exam finding is distension of the veins in the arm and neck.
- Malignant masses are more likely to be symptomatic.
- Many tumors, especially the lymphoproliferative tumors, may cause constitutional symptoms such as fevers, night sweats, and weight loss.

Atypical

- Mediastinal masses are often asymptomatic. More dramatic presentations, such as acute dyspnea, pneumonia with hemoptysis, or severe pain, are less common.

Primary Differential Considerations

- When evaluating a patient suspected of having a mediastinal mass, one also should consider these differential diagnoses:
  - Cysts
  - Enlarged thyroid
  - Aneurysm (aortic arch or proximal great vessels)
  - Loculated pleural effusion
  - Pneumonia

History and Physical Exam

Findings That Confirm Diagnosis

- There are no historical or physical exam findings that can confirm the diagnosis.
- The diagnosis usually is confirmed by imaging studies, most commonly CT scan of the chest. Biopsies may also be needed to confirm specific pathology.

Factors That Suggest Diagnosis

- These are often asymptomatic and found incidentally when performing diagnostic imaging studies for other reasons.
- Symptoms are nonspecific, but any of the symptoms reviewed in the classic presentation section above should suggest the diagnosis. Often, persistence of nonspecific symptoms results in the diagnostic study that leads to the diagnosis.

Factors That Exclude Diagnosis

- If a mediastinal mass is suspected, imaging (CT or magnetic resonance [MR]) with or without biopsy is required to exclude it or establish an alternative diagnosis.

Ancillary Studies

Laboratory

- Laboratory studies are often nonspecific.
- Lymphoproliferative tumors may be associated with anemia and other hematopoietic cell line abnormalities.
- Some specific tumors will have biologic tumor marker abnormalities.

Imaging

- Most mediastinal masses are found incidentally while performing diagnostic imaging of the chest for other reasons.
- They most often are discovered on either plain chest x-ray or CT scan of the chest.
- The diagnostic study of choice is usually a contrast-enhanced CT scan of the chest.

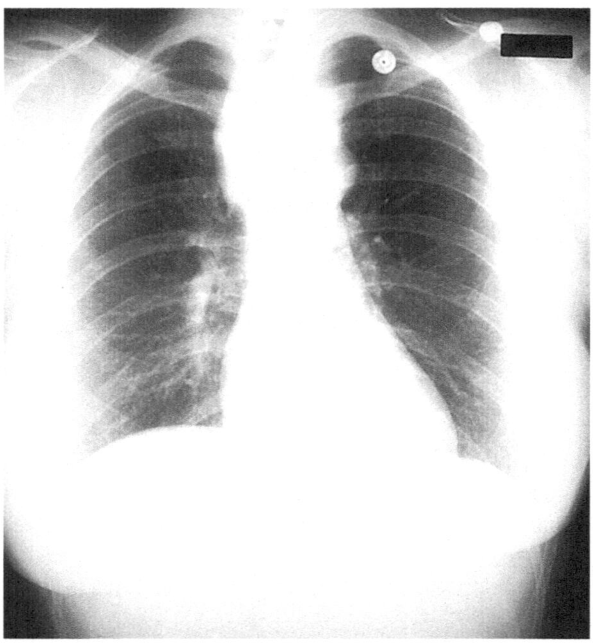

CXR demonstrating an anterior superior mediastinal mass. [Szokol J, Vender J. Respiratory emergencies (pulmonary aspiration of gastric contents, acute epiglottis, anterior mediastinal mass). In: Tremper KK, editor. Principles of anesthetic techniques and anesthetic emergencies. Philadelphia: Current Medicine; 1998. 195 p. (Miller RD, editor. Atlas of anesthesia; vol. 4). ISBN: 0-443-07903-X]

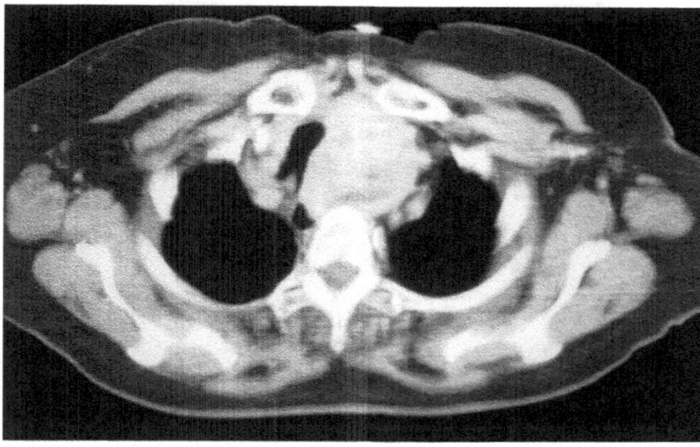

CT scan demonstrating a large anterior mediastinal mass. [Szokol J, Vender J. Respiratory emergencies (pulmonary aspiration of gastric contents, acute epiglottis, anterior mediastinal mass). In: Tremper KK, editor. Principles of anesthetic techniques and anesthetic emergencies. Philadelphia: Current Medicine; 1998. 195 p. (Miller RD, editor. Atlas of anesthesia; vol. 4). ISBN: 0-443-07903-X]

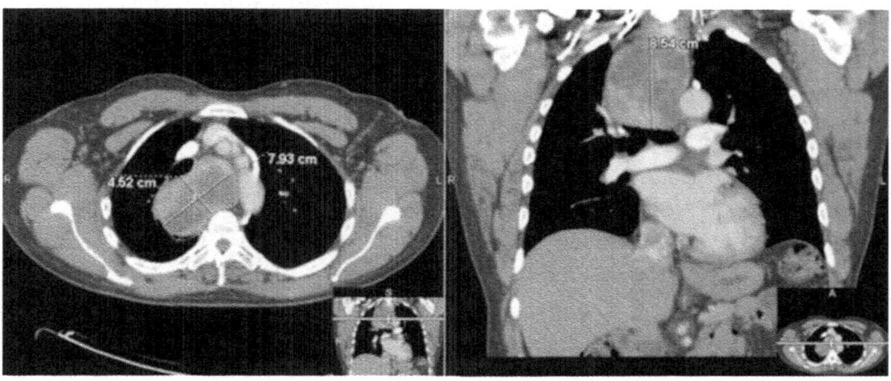

CT of the chest revealing a posterior mediastinal mass that extends all the way down to the aortic arch with tracheal compression and deviation. [From article: Novel thoracoscopic approach to posterior mediastinal goiters: report of two cases. Journal of Cardiothoracic Surgery. 2008;3(1):55. https://doi.org/10.1186/1749-8090-3-55, at http://link.springer.com/article/10.1186%2F1749-8090-3-55/fulltext.html; by Faisal Al-Mufarrej, Marc Margolis, Barbara Tempesta, Eric Strother, Farid Gharagozloo, © Al-Mufarrej et al; licensee BioMed Central Ltd. 2008; licensed under Creative Commons Attribution License BY 2.0 http://creativecommons.org/licenses/by/2.0] *Caption from original*

Special Populations

Age

- The etiologies of mediastinal masses differ in children and adults as per the etiology section above.
- Most mediastinal masses in children are discovered on routine chest radiographs.
- Warning signs in pediatric mediastinal masses are similar to those seen in adults, such as weight loss, cough, shortness of breath, or localized wheezing. Inexperienced readers are often concerned about the normal mediastinal silhouette of the thymus in young patients.

Co-morbidities

- Expected co-morbidities depend on the cell type of the mass.
- The clearest associations are between thymoma and myasthenia gravis and between chronic lung disease and pulmonary tumors.

Pitfalls in Diagnosis

Critical Steps Not to Miss

- Advanced imaging (CT/MR) will guide the diagnostic evaluation.

Mimics

- Thyroid enlargement and pulmonary infections are the diagnoses most likely to initially be confused with a mediastinal mass.

Time-Dependent Interventions

- Patients with respiratory or cardiovascular insufficiency (uncommon at presentation) must be stabilized.

Overall Principles of Treatment

- Treatment depends on the type of neoplasm and whether any symptomatic obstruction or compression exists.
- As with most neoplasms, a tissue diagnosis must be confirmed to guide appropriate treatment. This commonly can be achieved by percutaneous biopsy guided by imaging of the appropriate anatomic area, such as CT scan, endoscopy (both endobronchial and esophageal), and echocardiography. In rare cases, video-assisted mediastinoscopy or thoracoscopy will need to be performed.

Disease Course

- The disease course depends on the specific diagnosis.

Related Evidence

Papers of particular interest have been highlighted as:
*** Of key importance*

Practice Guideline

Ray CE Jr, English B, Funaki BS, Burke CT, Fidelman N, Ginsburg ME, Kinney TB, Kostelic JK, Kouri BE, Lorenz JM, Nair AV, Nemcek AA Jr, Owens CA, Saleh AG, Vatakencherry G, Mohammed TL. ACR appropriateness criteria® radiologic management of thoracic nodules and masses. J Am Coll Radiol. 2012 Jan;9(1):13-9. https://doi.org/10.1016/j.jacr.2011.09.013. PMID: 22221631. http://www.ncbi.nlm.nih.gov/pubmed/22221631 **

Review

Peterson CM, Buckley C, Holley S, Menias CO. Teratomas: a multimodality review. Curr Probl Diagn Radiol. 2012 Nov-Dec;41(6):210-9. https://doi.org/10.1067/j.cpradiol.2012.02.001. PMID: 23009771. http://www.ncbi.nlm.nih.gov/pubmed/23009771 **

Ray CE Jr, Mohammed TL. Review of ACR Appropriateness Criteria® Radiologic Management of Thoracic Nodules and Masses. J Thorac Imaging. 2012 Jul;27(4):W85-6. https://doi.org/10.1097/RTI.0b013e31825420e2. PMID: 22847592. http://www.ncbi.nlm.nih.gov/pubmed/22847592 **

Ranganath SH, Lee EY, Restrepo R, Eisenberg RL. Mediastinal masses in children. AJR Am J Roentgenol. 2012 Mar;198(3):W197-216. https://doi.org/10.2214/AJR.11.7027. PMID: 22358017. http://www.ncbi.nlm.nih.gov/pubmed/22358017 **

Hamid UI, Jones JM. Mediastinal mass. BMJ Case Rep. 2010 Oct 4;2010. pii: bcr1120092471. https://doi.org/10.1136/bcr.11.2009.2471. PMID: 22778081. http://www.ncbi.nlm.nih.gov/pubmed/22778081 **

Domínguez Malagón H, Pérez Montiel D. Mediastinal germ cell tumors. Semin Diagn Pathol. 2005 Aug;22(3):230-40. PMID: 16711404. http://www.ncbi.nlm.nih.gov/pubmed/16711404 **

Jaggers J, Balsara K. Mediastinal masses in children. Semin Thorac Cardiovasc Surg. 2004 Fall;16(3):201-8. PMID: 15619186. http://www.ncbi.nlm.nih.gov/pubmed/15619186 **

Strollo DC, Rosado-de-Christenson ML. Primary mediastinal malignant germ cell neoplasms: imaging features. Chest Surg Clin N Am. 2002 Nov;12(4):645-58. PMID: 12471868. http://www.ncbi.nlm.nih.gov/pubmed/12471868 **

Use PubMed Clinical Queries to find the most recent evidence. Use this search strategy: (“Mediastinal Neoplasms”[Mesh] OR mediastinal mass*)

Chapter 46
Mediastinitis

Christopher J. Rees, Richard M. Cantor, Charles V. Pollack, Jr., and Victoria G. Riese

Name and Synonyms

Mediastinitis

Incidence/Epidemiology

- Acute necrotizing mediastinitis is a life-threatening infection of the mediastinum.
- Historically, it was an uncommon but deadly complication of retropharyngeal space infections that tracked downward from the prevertebral fascia into the posterior mediastinum. Currently, acute mediastinitis occurs most often after cardiovascular or thoracic surgery.
- It also may result from esophageal perforation/rupture.
- The incidence postoperatively ranges from 0.5–5 %, but most large, experienced centers have rates lower than 2 %.

C. J. Rees
Emergency Department, Pennsylvania Hospital, Philadelphia, PA, USA

R. M. Cantor
Department of Emergency Medicine and Pediatrics, State University of New York Upstate Medical University, Syracuse, NY, USA

C. V. Pollack, Jr. (✉)
Department of Emergency Medicine, Thomas Jefferson University, Philadelphia, PA, USA

V. G. Riese
Librarian Consultant, Eldersburg, MD, USA

C. V. Pollack, Jr. (ed.), *Differential Diagnosis of Cardiopulmonary Disease*,
https://doi.org/10.1007/978-3-319-63895-9_46

- The incidence is higher for heart transplant patients and those with cardiac assist devices in place.
- The mortality approaches 25 %, even with appropriate treatment.

Differential Diagnosis

- The differential diagnosis is broad and includes any cause of sepsis syndrome, especially during the postoperative period.

Pathophysiology and Etiology

- The pathophysiology of postoperative mediastinitis is complex, but the final common pathway appears to be intraoperative wound contamination. It may occur even in the presence of meticulous surgical technique and sterile preparation. It seems to be related more to host factors than surgical technique.
- Recognized risk factors for postoperative mediastinitis include:
  - Diabetes or perioperative hyperglycemia
  - Obesity
  - Peripheral vascular disease
  - Tobacco use
  - Prior cardiac surgery
  - Dissection of the internal mammary artery
  - Procedure longer than 5 hours
  - The need to return to the operating room within 4 days
  - Prolonged postoperative ICU stay
- A single organism causes most cases.
- Virtually any organism can cause mediastinitis, but the most commonly reported are:
  - Methacillin-sensitive *Staphylococcus aureus* (MSSA), 45 %
  - Methacillin-resistant *S. aureus* (MRSA), 16 %
  - Gram-negative rods, 17 %
  - Coagulase-negative staphylococci, 13 %
  - Streptococci, 5 %
- Mediastinitis also may result from esophageal rupture, with direct spread of esophageal contents into the mediastinum.
- Other (uncommon) causes include:
  - complication of retropharyngeal space infection
  - rupture of a mediastinal abscess
  - direct extension of empyema into the mediastinum
- Bacteremia is present in more than 50 % of cases.

Presentation

Typical/"Classic"

- Classically, patients with postoperative mediastinitis will have fever, tachycardia, chest pain, sternal instability from a sternal wound infection, and/or purulent wound drainage from the sternal area. Patients with nonoperatively related mediastinitis also often present with a sepsis-like syndrome or frank sepsis.

Atypical

- Patients may present with postoperative fever alone.
- Patients may be found to have asymptomatic postoperative bacteremia.
- Patients may show signs only of superficial wound infection.
- The infection may take a more indolent course, with vague symptoms.

Primary Differential Considerations

- Early in the evaluation of patients with symptoms of mediastinitis, consider the following important differential diagnoses:
    - Acute coronary syndrome
    - Aortic dissection
    - Pulmonary embolism
    - Acute pericarditis
    - Pneumothorax
    - Deep neck infection
    - Pneumonia
    - Esophageal rupture

History and Physical Exam

Findings That Confirm Diagnosis

- Intraoperative findings of purulent discharge with necrotizing infection can confirm the diagnosis.
- Patients who present within two weeks of cardiovascular or thoracic surgery with fever, tachycardia, chest pain, sternal wound instability, and sternal wound infection may be considered to have mediastinitis, and treatment should be initiated immediately.

Factors That Suggest Diagnosis

- Patients presenting postoperatively with sepsis or a sepsis-like syndrome with no other obvious source, especially if there is bacteremia.

Factors That Exclude Diagnosis

- A normal, uncomplicated postoperative course excludes the diagnosis.

Ancillary Studies

Laboratory

- Patients often manifest the laboratory abnormalities associated with sepsis or an acute infectious process, such as leukocytosis with bandemia or leftward shift, acidosis, and an elevated lactate level.
- Bacteremia is present in more than 50 % of cases.

Imaging

- Plain chest radiography is sometimes helpful in suggesting alternative causes for the fever, such as pneumonia or atelectasis. The x-ray also may reveal findings that increase suspicion for mediastinitis in the correct clinical setting, such as pleural or pericardial effusion, empyema, and pneumomediastinum, all of which may result from mediastinitis.

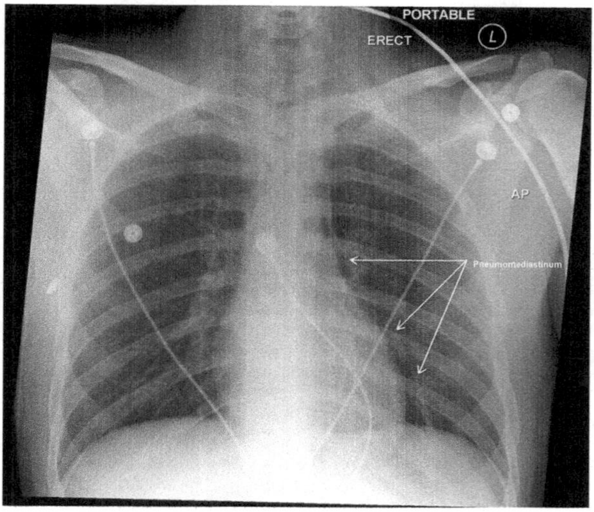

Chest X-ray showing pneumomediastinum. [From article: Pneumomediastinum from nasal insufflation of cocaine. International Journal of Emergency Medicine. 2010 Dec;3(4):435–7. https://doi.org/10.1007/s12245-010-0205-9, at http://link.springer.com/article/10.1007%2Fs12245-010-0205-9; by Brian T. Kloss, Claire E. Broton, Elliot Rodriguez, © Springer-Verlag London Ltd 2010; licensed under Creative Commons Attribution License BY 2.0 http://creativecommons.org/licenses/by/2.0] *Caption adapted from original*

- CT of the chest with intravenous contrast is the study of choice if the diagnosis is in question. CT is most helpful in the following situations:
  - In patients with systemic signs and symptoms (fever, tachycardia, hypotension, chest pain), with or without bacteremia, when there are no signs of a sternal wound infection or instability
  - When there is clinical evidence of a sternal wound infection but no systemic signs or symptoms
  - In the evaluation of asymptomatic, postoperative bacteremia

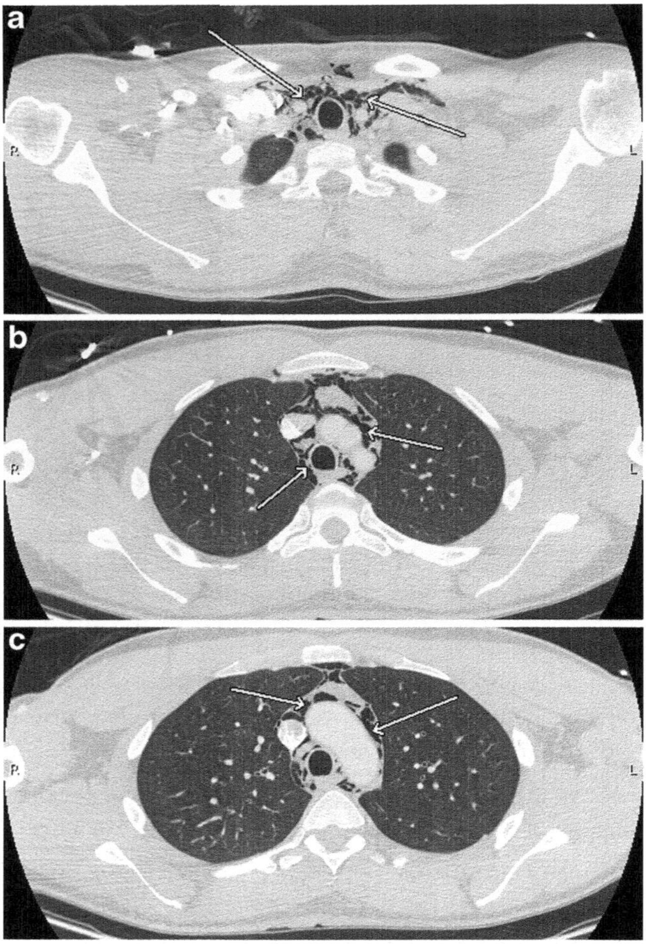

Contrast-enhanced CT with arrows showing pneumomediastinum [From article: Pneumomediastinum from nasal insufflation of cocaine. International Journal of Emergency Medicine. 2010 Dec;3(4):435–7. https://doi.org/10.1007/s12245-010-0205-9, at http://link.springer.com/article/10.1007%2Fs12245-010-0205-9; by Brian T. Kloss, Claire E. Broton, Elliot Rodriguez, © Springer-Verlag London Ltd 2010; licensed under Creative Commons Attribution License BY 2.0 http://creativecommons.org/licenses/by/2.0] *Caption adapted from original*

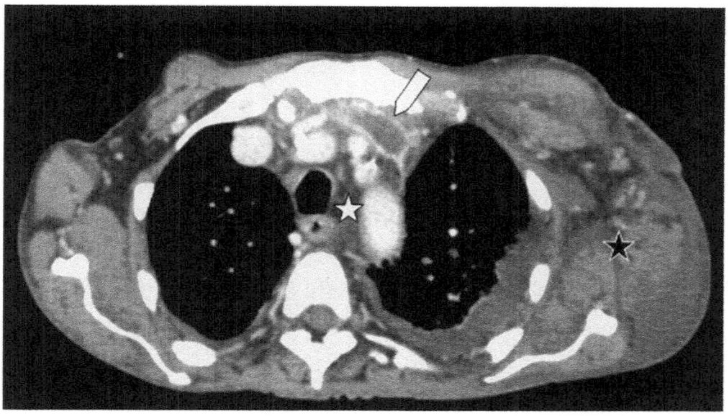

Contrast-enhanced CT scan of descending necrotizing mediastinitis at the lower neck shows brachiocephalic vein thrombosis (arrow), increased density of the middle mediastinal space (white asterisk), and bilateral pleural effusion. In addition, swelling of the left soft tissues of the thorax is evident (black asterisk) [Scaglione M, Pinto A, Romano S, Giovine S, Sparano A, Romano L. Determining optimum management of descending necrotizing mediastinitis with CT; experience with 32 cases. Emerg Radiol. 2005 Jul;11(5):275–80.] *Caption adapted from original*

Special Populations

Age

- Mediastinitis may occur at any age but is most common in older patients after cardiac or thoracic surgery.
- Mediastinitis also may occur in the pediatric population as a complication of cardiovascular or thoracic surgery, or as a complication of retropharyngeal abscess.
- Soft tissue neck infections in children (parapharyngeal abscess, peritonsillar abscess, retropharyngeal abscess, dental abscess, etc.) also contribute to the development of mediastinitis.

Co-morbidities

- Review of the etiologies of acute mediastinitis will indicate co-morbidities of interest. Diabetes, obesity, tobacco use, peripheral arterial disease, and prior cardiac/thoracic surgery are the most concerning.

Pitfalls in Diagnosis

Critical Steps Not to Miss

- Consideration of the diagnosis is the first critical step. Patients who present with sepsis or sepsis-like syndrome postoperatively or those with evidence of a sternal wound infection need urgent resuscitation and institution of broad-spectrum antibiotic coverage while a more definitive diagnosis is pursued.

Mimics

- Many other infectious processes can mimic mediastinitis. Pneumonia and empyema may occur in isolation but also may coexist or be a complication of mediastinitis.
- Superficial sternal wound infection may mimic mediastinitis.

Time-Dependent Interventions

- Consideration of the diagnosis and adequate resuscitation and antibiotic coverage are critical.
- Mortality increases as the infection and necrosis progress.

Overall Principles of Treatment

- Adequate resuscitation and antibiotic coverage are critical.
- Definitive treatment usually involves surgical debridement and continued antibiotics.

Disease Course

- The mortality of postoperative mediastinitis may approach 50 %, even with adequate treatment.
- The occurrence of postoperative mediastinitis is associated with an increased mortality rate that continues for 10 years postoperatively.

Related Evidence

Papers of particular interest have been highlighted as:
*** Of key importance*

Practice Guideline

Edwards FH, Engelman RM, Houck P, Shahian DM, Bridges CR; Society of Thoracic Surgeons. The Society of Thoracic Surgeons Practice Guideline Series: Antibiotic Prophylaxis in Cardiac Surgery, Part I: Duration. Ann Thorac Surg. 2006 Jan;81(1):397-404. PMID: 16368422. http://www.ncbi.nlm.nih.gov/pubmed/16368422 **

Review

Mangukia CV, Agarwal S, Satyarthy S, Datt V, Satsangi D. Mediastinitis following pediatric cardiac surgery. J Card Surg. 2014 Jan;29(1):74-82. https://doi.org/10.1111/jocs.12243. PMID: 24267786. http://www.ncbi.nlm.nih.gov/pubmed/24267786 **

Yu AW, Rippel RA, Smock E, Jarral OA. In patients with post-sternotomy mediastinitis is vacuum-assisted closure superior to conventional therapy? Interact Cardiovasc Thorac Surg. 2013 Nov;17(5):861-5. https://doi.org/10.1093/icvts/ivt326. PMID: 23912622. http://www.ncbi.nlm.nih.gov/pubmed/23912622 **

Lepelletier D, Bourigault C, Roussel JC, Lasserre C, Leclère B, Corvec S, Pattier S, Lepoivre T, Baron O, Despins P. Epidemiology and prevention of surgical site infections after cardiac surgery. Med Mal Infect. 2013 Oct;43(10):403-9. https://doi.org/10.1016/j.medmal.2013.07.003. PMID: 23988675. http://www.ncbi.nlm.nih.gov/pubmed/23988675 **

Kocher GJ, Hoksch B, Caversaccio M, Wiegand J, Schmid RA. Diffuse descending necrotizing mediastinitis: surgical therapy and outcome in a single-centre series. Eur J Cardiothorac Surg. 2012 Oct;42(4):e66-72. https://doi.org/10.1093/ejcts/ezs3 85. PMID: 22761501. http://www.ncbi.nlm.nih.gov/pubmed/22761501 **

Migliario M, Bello L, Greco Lucchina A, Descending necrotizing mediastinitis. Two cases consequent on odontogenic infections and a review of literature. 2010 Oct;59(10):551-60. PMID: 21048547. http://www.ncbi.nlm.nih.gov/pubmed/21048547

Weaver E, Nguyen X, Brooks MA. Descending necrotising mediastinitis: two case reports and review of the literature. Eur Respir Rev. 2010 Jun;19(116):141-9. https://doi.org/10.1183/09059180.00001110. PMID: 20956183. http://www.ncbi.nlm.nih.gov/pubmed/20956183 **

Athanassiadi KA. Infections of the mediastinum. Thorac Surg Clin. 2009 Feb;19(1):37-45, vi. https://doi.org/10.1016/j.thorsurg.2008.09.012. PMID: 19288819. http://www.ncbi.nlm.nih.gov/pubmed/19288819 **

Singhal P, Kejriwal N, Lin Z, Tsutsui R, Ullal R. Optimal surgical management of descending necrotising mediastinitis: our experience and review of literature. Heart Lung Circ. 2008 Apr;17(2):124-8. PMID: 18060838. http://www.ncbi.nlm.nih.gov/pubmed/18060838 **

Keib CN, Pelham JC. Mediastinitis following coronary artery bypass graft surgery: pathogenesis, clinical presentation, risks, and management. J Cardiovasc Nurs. 2006 Nov-Dec;21(6):493-9. PMID: 17293742. http://www.ncbi.nlm.nih.gov/pubmed/17293742 **

Akman C, Kantarci F, Cetinkaya S. Imaging in mediastinitis: a systematic review based on aetiology. Clin Radiol. 2004 Jul;59(7):573-85. PMID: 15208062. http://www.ncbi.nlm.nih.gov/pubmed/15208062 **

Use PubMed Clinical Queries to find the most recent evidence. Use this search strategy: "Mediastinitis"[Mesh] OR "Mediastinitis"

Chapter 47
Mitral Valve Prolapse

Charles V. Pollack, Jr., Richard M. Cantor, and Victoria G. Riese

Name and Synonyms

Mitral Valve Prolapse (MVP); systolic click-murmur syndrome; Barlow's syndrome

Incidence/Epidemiology

- MVP is the most common heart valve abnormality, found in about 3–5% of the US population.
- The clinical syndrome associated with MVP is quite variable, but it is usually benign.

Differential Diagnosis

- The primary differential considerations for chest pain associated with MVP are mitral regurgitation and anxiety/panic attacks.
- Older patients with chest pain and palpitations should be evaluated for possible ACS.

C. V. Pollack, Jr. (✉)
Department of Emergency Medicine, Thomas Jefferson University,
Philadelphia, PA, USA

R. M. Cantor
Department of Emergency Medicine and Pediatrics, State University of New York Upstate
Medical University, Syracuse, NY, USA

V. G. Riese
Librarian Consultant, Eldersburg, MD, USA

C. V. Pollack, Jr. (ed.), *Differential Diagnosis of Cardiopulmonary Disease*,
https://doi.org/10.1007/978-3-319-63895-9_47

Pathophysiology and Etiology

- Mitral valve prolapse is a ballooning of a competent (or minimally incompetent) mitral valve into the left atrium during left ventricular systole. This anatomic defect may result from:
  - Redundant mitral leaflet tissue (myxomatous degeneration)
  - Elongated or redundant chordae tendineae
  - Inherited connective tissue disorders such as Marfan's and Ehler-Danlos syndromes

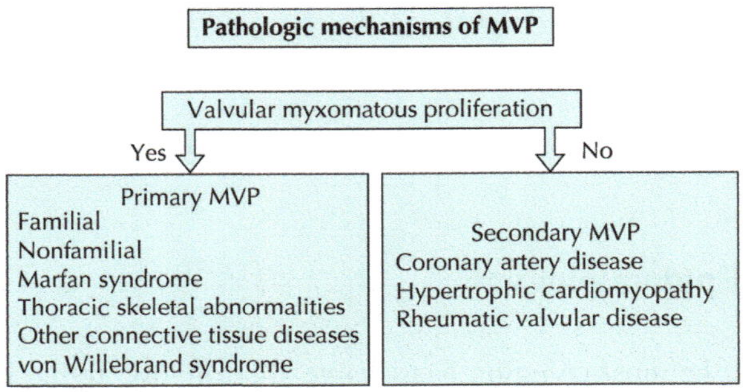

Causes of mitral valve prolapse. A variety of pathologic mechanisms involving any of the functional components of the mitral valve apparatus can result in MVP. Prominent among these is valvular collagen disruption and myxomatous infiltration, termed primary MVP. In most cases, primary MVP is an inherited disorder; it can also occur in a nonfamilial, isolated form. Less commonly, primary MVP is associated with connective tissue diseases. The most important of these is Marfan syndrome, where it can be detected echocardiographically in greater than 90% of affected patients. Thoracic skeletal abnormalities (pectus excavatum, pectus carinatum, straight back syndrome, scoliosis) are also associated with primary MVP. Primary MVP may be a manifestation of a generalized disorder of connective tissue, with a variable range of phenotypic expression within and outside of the cardiovascular system. For example, it can also be associated with myxomatous changes and prolapse of the tricuspid (40%), pulmonic (10%), and aortic valves (2%). The histologic changes are similar to those seen in the mitral valve. Other associated conditions include ostium secundum atrial septal defect and Wolff-Parkinson-White syndrome. Secondary MVP occurs in the absence of myxomatous valvular proliferation and can occur in patients with hypertrophic cardiomyopathy and occasionally as a result of coronary artery disease. Prior rheumatic fever may result in secondary MVP, especially of the anterior leaflet. [Prabhu S, O'Rourke R, Rahimtoola S. Chapter 10. In: Braunwald E, editor. Atlas of Heart Disease: Valvular Heart Disease, Volume 11, 1e. St. Louis, Mo.: Current Medicine; 1997. 200 p. ISBN: 1-878132-30-X] *Caption adapted from original*

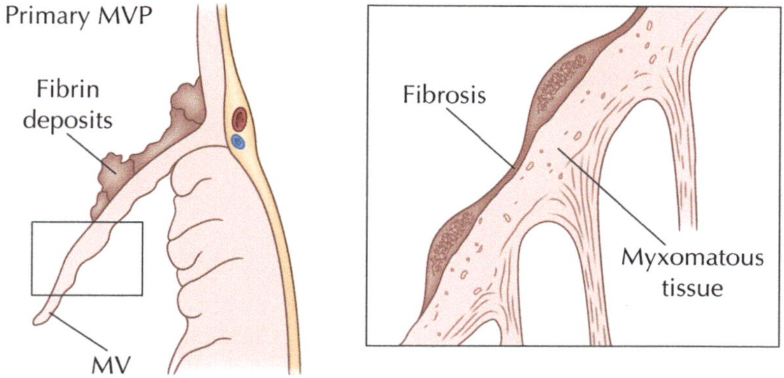

Primary mitral valve prolapse. Histopathology of primary mitral valve prolapse (MVP). A, The normal mitral valve (MV) is composed of three layers: 1) the atrialis, a thin layer of collagen and elastic tissue along the atrial aspect of the leaflet; 2) the fibrosa (ventricularis), a denser layer of collagen along the ventricular aspect; and 3) the spongiosa, the fine myxomatous connective tissue layer between the two. B, In primary MVP, dissolution of collagen bundles occurs primarily with secondary myxomatous proliferation of the spongiosa and interruption of the fibrosa and fibrosis of the atrial and ventricular surfaces of the valve. These secondary effects appear to occur as a response to repeated stress on the valve apparatus. Focal endothelial disruption occurs commonly and may provide a site for thrombus formation. Fibrin deposits often form at the MV–left atrial angle. Similar histologic changes can occur in the chordae tendineae and result in chordal thinning and rupture. Myxomatous degeneration of the annulus can occur as well, especially in patients with connective tissue disorders, resulting in annular dilation and calcification and worsening of mitral regurgitation. [Prabhu S, O'Rourke R, Rahimtoola S. Chapter 10. In: Braunwald E, editor. Atlas of Heart Disease: Valvular Heart Disease, Volume 11, 1e. St. Louis, Mo.: Current Medicine; 1997. 200 p. ISBN: 1-878132-30-X] *Caption adapted from original*

- The ballooning often causes a click that is audible on cardiac auscultation. If there is any incompetence to the overlapping leaflets, a murmur will also result.
- The chest pain associated with MVP, which is typically described as sharp or stabbing, is *not* anginal in origin. MVP is not associated with coronary artery disease nor does it have any other direct relation to myocardial ischemia.
- Chest pain in MVP is often associated with anxiety or panic disorder.
- Besides chest pain and anxiety, MVP is also associated with a variety of symptoms that can prompt acute presentation, including:
  - Autonomic dysfunction
  - Palpitations from both supraventricular and ventricular premature beats
  - Lightheadedness
  - Syncope

- Very rarely, the redundant valve leaflets in MVP can be a nidus for vegetations of endocarditis. This is (relatively) much more common in the frankly regurgitant mitral valve.

Presentation

Typical/"Classic"

- Many patients with MVP are asymptomatic. Chest pain due to MVP is most often described as sharp and stabbing, associated with anxiety, and is occasionally accompanied by palpitations.

Palpitations
Chest pain
Dyspnea
Fatigue
Syncope and lightheadedness
Focal neurologic events
Anxiety

Symptoms in mitral valve prolapse. The most common symptom is palpitations, which often correlates poorly with arrhythmias on ambulatory electrocardiographic monitoring. Chest pain is usually atypical and does not resemble angina pectoris. The etiology is unknown. It has been suggested that the prolapsing mitral valve places undue tension on the papillary muscles and results in subendocardial ischemia. Dyspnea and fatigue may occur without mitral regurgitation or objective impairment of exercise tolerance. Syncope and presyncope may occur in association with postural hypotension and arrhythmias but often are present without any clinical correlates. Transient neurologic events occur with greater frequency in patients with MVP, although the overall incidence is quite low. These may be the result of platelet and fibrin emboli occurring at sites of endothelial disruption and at the mitral valve–left atrial junction. The true association of MVP and neuropsychiatric syndromes remains controversial. [Prabhu S, O'Rourke R, Rahimtoola S. Chapter 10. In: Braunwald E, editor. Atlas of Heart Disease: Valvular Heart Disease, Volume 11, 1e. St. Louis, Mo.: Current Medicine; 1997. 200 p. ISBN: 1-878132-30-X] *Caption adapted from original*

- Patients may or may not report a previously detected click or murmur.

Atypical

- Typical anginal features (pressure-like pain, midsternum perhaps radiating to jaw or left upper extremity, related to exertion) would be very unusual in describing pain caused by MVP.

Primary Differential Considerations

- When evaluating a patient suspected of having MVP, one should also consider the following differential diagnoses:
  - Mitral regurgitation
  - Anxiety

History and Physical Exam

Findings That Confirm Diagnosis

- The diagnosis of MVP is typically made upon cardiac auscultation. There is usually a mid-systolic ejection click thought to be caused either by the tensing of the elongated chordae or by the snapping of the redundant valve leaflet tissue at the peak of systole.

https://www.youtube.com/watch?v=PsmGx2XMxF8
Audio of mid-systolic click

- The murmur, which is less consistently identified than the click, is usually high-pitched, crescendo-decrescendo, and heard best at the apex.

https://www.youtube.com/watch?v=MMJBSd5Z_Uc&list=PL85424CD4340A8D55
Audio of mitral regurgitation murmur

- The click and murmur occur earlier and louder with standing and with Valsalva, and occur later and more quietly (and indeed may disappear) with squatting and isometric exercise.

https://www.youtube.com/watch?v=AHBzu5zhFuA
Video on mitral valve prolapse and mitral regurgitation. Offers animation of blood flow and muscle movement.

Factors That Suggest Diagnosis

- The click and murmur are suggestive of MVP even without chest pain.
- Other body habitus characteristics of connective tissue disease may be helpful.

Thoracic skeletal abnormalities
Arachnodactyly
High-arched palate
Low body weight (< 90% ideal)
Low blood pressure (< 120 mm Hg systolic)
Orthostatic hypotension and tachycardia

Physical findings in mitral valve prolapse. General physical findings in MVP. Thoracic skeletal abnormalities can be seen in association with MVP. Arachnodactyly may be seen without other evidence for Marfan syndrome and these cases may represent formes frustes of this disorder. Patients with MVP tend to have low body weight, low systolic blood pressure, and postural hypotension and tachycardia. These signs may be related to a combination of autonomic dysfunction and reduced intravascular volume in these patients. [Prabhu S, O'Rourke R, Rahimtoola S. Chapter 10. In: Braunwald E, editor. Atlas of Heart Disease: Valvular Heart Disease, Volume 11, 1e. St. Louis, Mo.: Current Medicine; 1997. 200 p. ISBN: 1-878132-30-X] *Caption adapted from original*

Factors That Exclude Diagnosis

- No history or physical findings can definitively exclude MVP; an echocardiogram is required.

Ancillary Studies

Laboratory

- There are no diagnostic laboratory studies for MVP.

Imaging

- Echocardiography can confirm or refute the diagnosis of MVP and can differentiate it from mitral regurgitation.

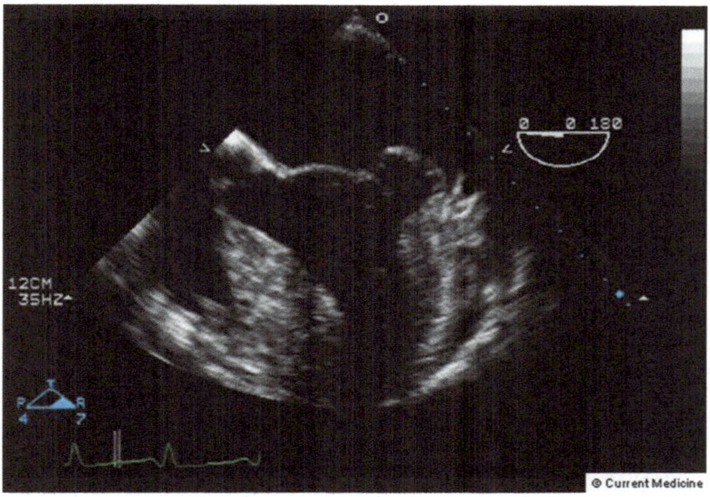

Mitral valve prolapse: transesophageal echocardiogram. Transesophageal echocardiogram showing prolapse of the mitral valve. [Greer DM, Kamalian S, Silverman SB, Mitha AP, Kinnecom CE, Sanborn DY, Greenberg SM, Ogilvy CS, Lev MH, Kistler JP, Furie KL, Camargo ECS de. Cerebrovascular Disease. In: Rosenberg RN, editor. Atlas of Clinical Neurology [Internet]. Current Medicine Group; 2009 [cited 2015 May 20]. p. 133–214. Available from: http://link.springer.com/chapter/10.1007/978-1-57340-359-7_5] *Caption adapted from original*

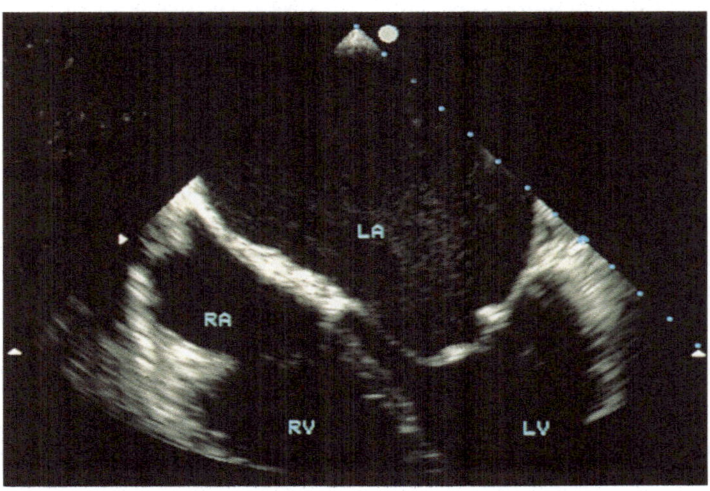

Mitral valve prolapse. Two-dimensional image transesophageal echocardiographic image of mitral valve with severe prolapse of the posterior leaflet due to chordal rupture. B, Doppler color flow image of the same valve with a large regurgitant jet (arrow) directed away from the prolapsed leaflet. LA—left atrium; LV—left ventricle; RA—right atrium; RV—right ventricle. [Clements F, de Bruijn N,

Bennett-Guerrero E, Newman M, Reves JG. Chapter 1. In: Miller RD, Muravchick S, editors. Atlas of Anesthesia: Subspecialty Care, Volume 5, 1e. Philadelphia: Current Medicine; 1998. 236 p. ISBN: 0-443-07905-6] *Caption from original*

https://www.youtube.com/watch?v=h6aJSuUTVb0
Video depicting echocardiography of mitral valve prolapse.

- It has been thought in the past that echocardiographic studies "overdiagnosed" MVP. This concern can be alleviated at least in part by relying on the parasternal long-axis view.
- Other imaging or tests are sometimes helpful.

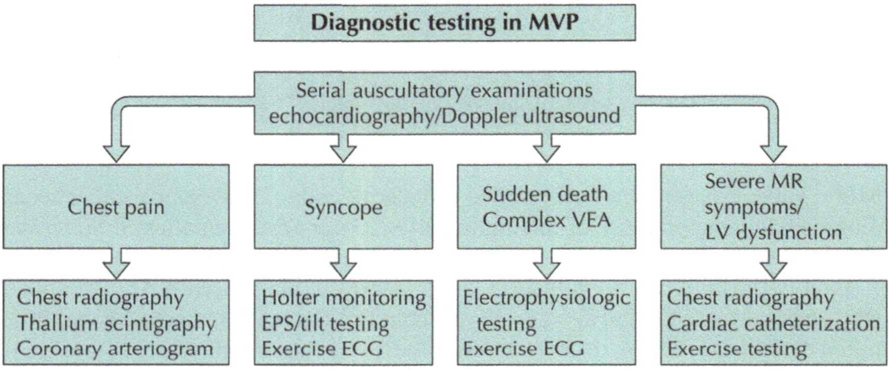

Diagnostic testing in mitral valve prolapse (MVP). The diagnosis of MVP is based on the presence of typical auscultatory findings detected during carefully performed serial examinations. Echocardiography (M-mode, two-dimensional, and Doppler) is the single most useful test in the definition of MVP. It is used to assess natural history and prognosis, the presence of associated conditions (e.g., atrial septal defect, hypertrophic cardiomyopathy), the need for antibiotic prophylaxis, and the degree of mitral regurgitation (MR). Echocardiography should not supplant the physical examination in the diagnosis of MVP; up to 10% of patients diagnosed with MVP by typical auscultatory findings will have a non-diagnostic two-dimensional echocardiogram. Electrocardiography (ECG) is routinely performed to assess for ventricular preexcitation and resting ST- and T-wave abnormalities. The tests listed in the lowest level of the flow diagram are not required for the diagnosis of MVP, but they are useful in assessing certain symptoms and complications that can occur in this disorder. EPS—electrophysiology; LV—left ventricular; MR—mitral regurgitation; VEA—ventricular ectopic arrhythmia. [Prabhu S, O'Rourke R, Rahimtoola S. Chapter 10. In: Braunwald E, editor. Atlas of Heart Disease: Valvular Heart Disease, Volume 11, 1e. St. Louis, Mo.: Current Medicine; 1997. 200 p. ISBN: 1-878132-30-X] *Caption from original*

Special Populations

Age and Gender

- MVP is more common in females than males.
- It is most commonly diagnosed in the second or third decade of life.
- MVP in children most often presents with palpitations.
- Children will often describe a "butterfly" in their chest.

Co-morbidities

- Connective tissue diseases such as Marfan's are often associated with MVP.

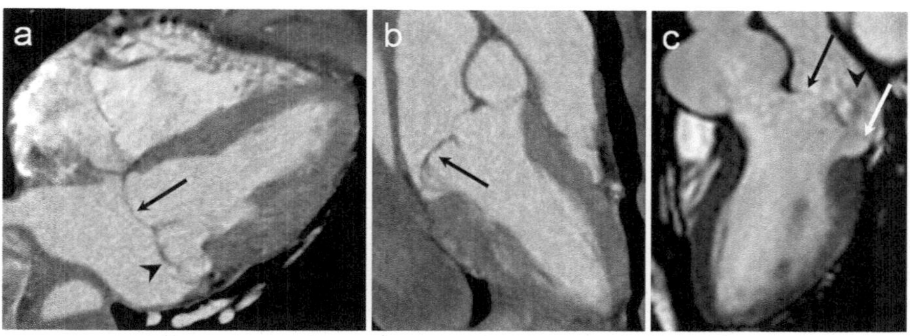

A 33-year-old woman with Marfan syndrome and mitral valve prolapse. a, b Four- (a) and two-chamber (b) CT images in systole show entire anterior mitral leaflet prolapse (arrows) and P2 prolapse in the posterior mitral leaflet (arrowheads). c Three-chamber balanced-steady state precession cine cardiac MRI in systole demonstrates bileaflet mitral prolapse (arrows) and a dephasing jet from mitral regurgitation (arrowhead) [Ko SM, Song MG, Hwang HK. Evaluation of the aortic and mitral valves with cardiac computed tomography and cardiac magnetic resonance imaging. Int J Cardiovasc Imaging. 2012 Nov 9;28(2):109–27.] *Caption from original*

Pitfalls in Diagnosis

Critical Steps Not to Miss

- There are no critical steps in diagnosing MVP. The clinical situation is more important if mitral regurgitation has developed. Either way, an echocardiogram is diagnostic.

Mimics

- Acute anxiety or panic disorder can mimic MVP, especially if there is a coincident heart murmur or history thereof.
- It is unlikely that chest pain associated with MVP will be confused with anginal pain.

Time-Dependent Interventions

- There are no time-dependent interventions in the diagnosis and management of MVP.

Overall Principles of Treatment

- For most cases of MVP, reassurance of the benign nature of the valve abnormality is sufficient.

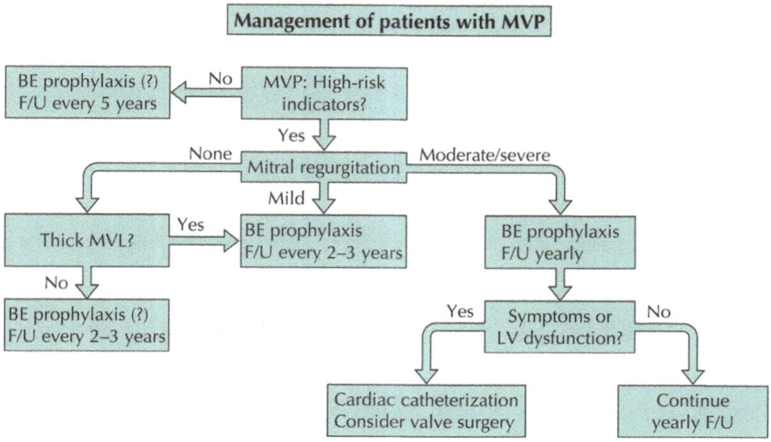

Management of mitral valve prolapse. Management of patients with mitral valve prolapse (MVP). High-risk characteristics in MVP patients are additive, that is, the more indicators present, the greater the total risk. The majority of patients with MVP are asymptomatic and have no or minimal high-risk indicators. They are treated with reassurance and can lead a normal life. Clinical and echocardiographic assessment every 5 years is reasonable to determine passage into a higher risk group. If any high-risk indicators are present, patients can be further stratified based on the presence of mitral regurgitation (MR). Some authorities advocate prophylaxis for bacterial endocarditis (BE) only if MVP is associated with MR or thickened mitral valve leaflets (MVL). However, given the variability of physical findings and the dynamic nature of MR in MVP, prophylaxis may be reasonable in all patients with MVP. Patients with MVP and severe MR should be managed in the same manner as patients with severe MR due to other causes. The decision to proceed with valve surgery is based on the presence of symptoms or impairment of left ventricular (LV) systolic function. Mitral valve reconstructive surgery can often be used in lieu of valve replacement to correct regurgitant floppy valves. Compared with valve replacement, valve repair is associated with a lower operative and late mortality, lower long-term thromboembolic risk, and lower BE risk. F/U—follow-up. [Prabhu S, O'Rourke R, Rahimtoola S. Chapter 10. In: Braunwald E, editor. Atlas of Heart Disease: Valvular Heart Disease, Volume 11, 1e. St. Louis, Mo.: Current Medicine; 1997. 200 p. ISBN: 1-878132-30-X] *Caption adapted from original*

- For patients with frequent chest pain, palpitations, or other autonomic manifestations, beta-adrenergic blockage may provide symptomatic relief.
- An echocardiogram will provide a basis for deciding whether or not patients with MVP should receive antibiotic prophylaxis prior to dental procedures or other procedures that could result in transient bacteremia.
- Patients with mitral regurgitation should be managed by a cardiologist.

Disease Course

- MVP generally runs a benign course.

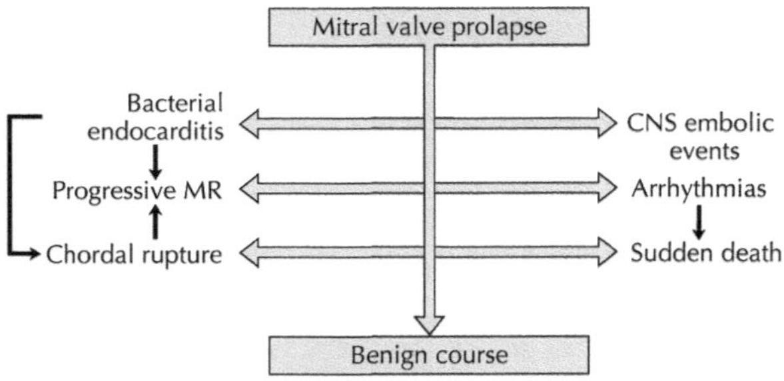

Clinical course in mitral valve prolapse. Overview of the clinical course in MVP. The majority of patients with MVP follow a benign course and their age-adjusted survival is similar to persons without MVP. However, serious complications can occur in 10% to 20% of patients. These include infective endocarditis, chordal rupture, progressive mitral regurgitation (MR), life-threatening arrhythmias, neurologic and embolic events, and sudden death. The risk of infective endocarditis is five to eight times greater in patients with MVP than in the general population and MVP is the leading underlying diagnosis in patients with endocarditis. Progressive MR is often accelerated by infective endocarditis or chordal rupture. The overall incidence of ophthalmologic and central nervous system (CNS) embolic events is generally low. An increase in risk for CNS events associated with MVP is detectable in patients who do not have other cerebrovascular risk factors, especially young women. Sudden death is the least common complication of MVP and occurs mainly in patients with significant MR, reduced ventricular function, and malignant ventricular arrhythmias. [Prabhu S, O'Rourke R, Rahimtoola S. Chapter 10. In: Braunwald E, editor. Atlas of Heart Disease: Valvular Heart Disease, Volume 11, 1e. St. Louis, Mo.: Current Medicine; 1997. 200 p. ISBN: 1-878132-30-X] *Caption adapted from original*

- Patients should be evaluated intermittently to assess for progression to mitral regurgitation.

Related Evidence

Papers of particular interest have been highlighted as:
*** Of key importance*

Practice Guideline

Joint Task Force on the Management of Valvular Heart Disease of the European Society of Cardiology (ESC); European Association for Cardio-Thoracic Surgery (EACTS), Vahanian A, Alfieri O, Andreotti F, Antunes MJ, Barón-Esquivias G, Baumgartner H, Borger MA, Carrel TP, De Bonis M, Evangelista A, Falk V, Iung B, Lancellotti P, Pierard L, Price S, Schäfers HJ, Schuler G, Stepinska J, Swedberg K, Takkenberg J, Von Oppell UO, Windecker S, Zamorano JL, Zembala M. Guidelines on the management of valvular heart disease (version 2012). Eur Heart J. 2012 Oct;33(19):2451-96. https://doi.org/10.1093/eurheartj/ehs109. PMID: 22922415. http://www.ncbi.nlm.nih.gov/pubmed/22922415 **

Lang RM, Badano LP, Tsang W, Adams DH, Agricola E, Buck T, Faletra FF, Franke A, Hung J, de Isla LP, Kamp O, Kasprzak JD, Lancellotti P, Marwick TH, McCulloch ML, Monaghan MJ, Nihoyannopoulos P, Pandian NG, Pellikka PA, Pepi M, Roberson DA, Shernan SK, Shirali GS, Sugeng L, Ten Cate FJ, Vannan MA, Zamorano JL, Zoghbi WA; American Society of Echocardiography; European Association of Echocardiography. EAE/ASE recommendations for image acquisition and display using three-dimensional echocardiography. J Am Soc Echocardiogr. 2012 Jan;25(1):3-46. https://doi.org/10.1016/j.echo.2011.11.010.. PMID: 22183020. http://www.ncbi.nlm.nih.gov/pubmed/22183020 **

Review

Benenstein R, Saric M. Mitral valve prolapse: role of 3D echocardiography in diagnosis. Curr Opin Cardiol. 2012 Sep;27(5):465-76. https://doi.org/10.1097/HCO.0b013e328356afe9. PMID: 22874124. http://www.ncbi.nlm.nih.gov/pubmed/22874124

Loardi C, Alamanni F, Trezzi M, Kassem S, Cavallotti L, Tremoli E, Pacini D, Parolari A. Biology of mitral valve prolapse: the harvest is big, but the workers are few. Int J Cardiol. 2011 Sep 1;151(2):129-35. https://doi.org/10.1016/j.ijcard.2010.11.004. PMID: 21168228. http://www.ncbi.nlm.nih.gov/pubmed/21168228

Shah PM. Current concepts in mitral valve prolapse--diagnosis and management. J Cardiol. 2010 Sep;56(2):125-33. https://doi.org/10.1016/j.jjcc.2010.06.004. PMID: 20702064. http://www.ncbi.nlm.nih.gov/pubmed/20702064 **

Hayek E, Gring CN, Griffin BP. Mitral valve prolapse. Lancet. 2005 Feb 5-11;365(9458):507-18. PMID: 15705461. http://www.ncbi.nlm.nih.gov/pubmed/15705461 **

Cohort Study

Guven B, Eroglu AG, Babaoglu K, Demir T, Güzeltas A, Oztunc F, Saltik L. QT dispersion and diastolic functions in differential diagnosis of primary mitral valve prolapse and rheumatic mitral valve prolapse. Pediatr Cardiol. 2008 Mar;29(2):352-8. PMID: 17917767. http://www.ncbi.nlm.nih.gov/pubmed/17917767 **

Case Study

Tagarakis GI, Karantzis I, Tsolaki F, Stylianakis GE, Daskalopoulos ME, Tsilimingas NB. Classic and non-classic forms of mitral valve prolapse. Anadolu Kardiyol Derg. 2012 Feb;12(1):2-4. https://doi.org/10.5152/akd.2012.001. PMID: 22214735. http://www.ncbi.nlm.nih.gov/pubmed/22214735 **

Use PubMed Clinical Queries to find the most recent evidence. Use this search strategy:
"Mitral Valve Prolapse"[Mesh] OR "mitral valve prolapse"

Chapter 48
Mitral Valve Regurgitation

Charles V. Pollack, Jr. and Jaime Friel Blanck

Name and Synonyms

Mitral valve regurgitation
Mitral valve incompetence
Mitral valve insufficiency

Incidence/Epidemiology

- Mitral valve disorders are the second-most common valvulopathies (aortic valve is most common).
- Mitral regurgitation (MR) may be acute or chronic. The chronic form is most often related to prior rheumatic fever, the incidence of which is decreasing in the industrialized world. The acute form is most often a complication of acute inferior wall myocardial infarction, and is rare but potentially catastrophic.
- MR is more common in females.

Differential Diagnosis

- The differential diagnosis of MR includes
  - Endocarditis
  - Aortic regurgitation/insufficiency
  - Ventricular septal defect

C. V. Pollack, Jr. (✉)
Department of Emergency Medicine, Thomas Jefferson University, Philadelphia, PA, USA

J. F. Blanck
Welch Medical Library, Johns Hopkins University, Baltimore, MD, USA

C. V. Pollack, Jr. (ed.), *Differential Diagnosis of Cardiopulmonary Disease*,
https://doi.org/10.1007/978-3-319-63895-9_48

Pathophysiology and Etiology

- The explicit pathophysiology of MR is reduced resistance to emptying of the left ventricle (LV), with regurgitant return of LV blood to the left atrium (LA).

Primary mitral regurgitation:
Mitral valve prolapse: the most common cause of mitral regurgitation in developed countries
Rheumatic disease: more common in underdeveloped countries. Usually manifests as mitral stenosis or double mitral lesion
Annular calcification: associated with aging. Does not cause severe mitral regurgitation
Infective or marantic endocarditis (associated with connective tissue disease)
Trauma that may produce rupture of the *chordae tendinae* and acute mitral regurgitation
Congenital anomalies, principally mitral cleft
Secondary to drugs: anorexigens, carbergoline, pergolide or ergotamine
Secondary mitral regurgitation:
Dilation and dysfunction of the left ventricle that causes stretching and distortion on the mitral valve annulus leading to centrally directed mitral regurgitation
Ischaemic heart disease, usually as a result of ischaemia or necrosis of the posterior papillary muscle, which can lead to acute mitral regurgitation
Hypertrophic obstructive cardiomyopathy, caused by the movement of the mitral valve anterior leaflet due to the "Venturi effect" caused by outflow tract obstruction

Causes of mitral regurgitation. [Suárez-Mier MP, Morentin B, Cobo M, Castedo E, García-Pavía P. Pathology of the Heart Valves. In: Lucena JS, García-Pavía P, Suarez-Mier MP, Alonso-Pulpon LA, editors. Clinico-Pathological Atlas of Cardiovascular Diseases [Internet]. Cham: Springer International Publishing; 2015 [cited 2016 Apr 4]. p. 171–200. Available from: http://link.springer.com/10.1007/978-3-319-11146-9_7] *Caption from original*

- In acute MR, this typically results from rupture of the papillary muscles that connect the chordae tendinae to the cardiac wall. Loss of papillary muscle function leads to incompetence of one or more of the valve leaflets. When the LV contracts, its contents flow both ante- and retrograde, significantly reducing forward cardiac output and disrupting LA function.

	Primary ("Organic")	Secondary ("Functional")
Acute	Papillary muscle ischemia	Acute ischemic LV dilatation
	Ruptured papillary muscle (trauma, infarction)	
	Flail mitral valve leaflet	
	Ruptured chordae tendinae	
	Endocarditis (leaflet perforation)	
Chronic	Flail mitral valve leaflet	Chronic ischemic mitral regurgitation (CIMR)
	Mitral valve prolapse	Non-ischemic LV dilatation (failure of leaflets to coapt)
	Ruptured chordae tendinae	Non-ischemic LV systolic dysfunction
	Degeneration (myxomatous, endocarditis, calcification)	Hypertrophic cardiomyopathy
	Rheumatic	Right ventricular pacing
	Congenital	Aortic insufficiency [1]

Classification of mitral regurgitation by mechanism and acuity [From article: Echocardiographic assessment of ischemic mitral regurgitation. Cardiovasc Ultrasound. 2014 Dec 1;12(1):46. https://doi.org/10.1186/1476-7120-12-46, at https://link.springer.com/article/10.1186%2F1476-7120-12-46; by David M Dudzinski, Judy Hung, © Dudzinski and Hung 2014; licensee BioMed Central Ltd.; licensed under Creative Commons Attribution License BY 4.0 http://creativecommons.org/licenses/by/4.0] *Caption from original*

- In chronic MR, damage to the valve apparatus (as in rheumatic heart disease) leads gradually to LA and LV enlargement and the patient remains largely asymptomatic until LV systolic dysfunction develops. Fatigue, dyspnea, and diminished exercise tolerance ensue. Frank heart failure may follow over time. With LV dilatation, the risk of atrial fibrillation and its attendant risk of thromboembolic complications rises.

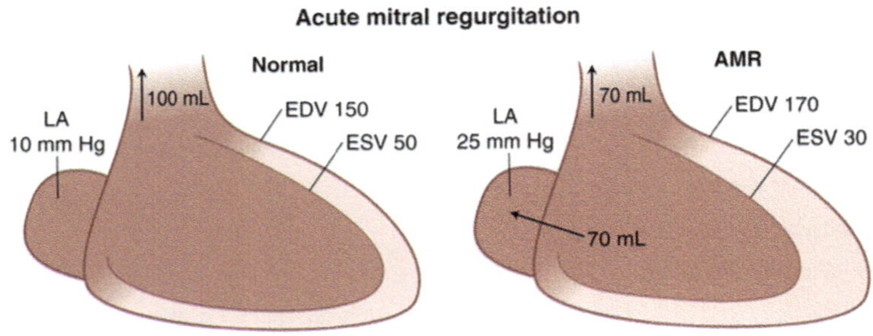

	Preload SL, μ	Afterload ESS, *Kdyne/cm²*	CF	EF	RF	FSV, *mL*
N	2.07	90	N	0.67	0.0	100
AMR	2.25	60	N	0.82	0.50	70

A

Pathophysiology of acute mitral regurgitation (AMR). A, AMR. Left ventricular (LV) sarcomere length (SL) is increased, but afterload (as estimated by end-systolic stress [ESS]) is initially reduced, as the LV ejects into the low impedance left atrium (LA). Contractile function (CF) is unchanged, but ejection fraction (EF) increases. The regurgitant fraction (RF) in this example is 50%. Forward stroke volume (FSV) is reduced from 100 to 70 mL. Pressure in the unprepared and relatively noncompliant LA rises abruptly to 25 mm Hg. [O'Gara P. Chapter 9. In: Libby P, editor. Essential Atlas of Cardiovascular Disease. 4th ed. Philadelphia: Current Medicine Group; 2009.] *Caption adapted from original*

- Chronic MR can also be caused by a host of other diseases, especially connective tissue disorders such as lupus and scleroderma.
- MR is distinct from mitral valve prolapse (MVP), in which there is ballooning of the mitral valve leaflets during LV systole, but there is no valve incompetence

Presentation

Typical/"Classic"

- The presentation of MR depends on whether it is acute or chronic. Acute MR, which often occurs proximal to an inferior wall myocardial infarction (MI) or as a complication of infective endocarditis, classically presents with
  - Shortness of breath
  - Chest pain
  - Orthopnea
  - Pulmonary edema
- Chronic MR may be asymptomatic for years, prior to presenting with decreased exercise tolerance and orthopnea.

Atypical

- Patients with acute MR may present hemodynamically unstable, requiring immediate intervention including use of a balloon pump.
- The damaged valve leaflets in MR are at risk for bacterial vegetations and endocarditis.
- MR may present with thromboembolism, from thrombi that form as a result of concomitant atrial fibrillation.

Primary Differential Considerations

- Consider the following diagnoses:
  - Aortic stenosis
  - Aortic insufficiency
  - Ventricular septal defect

History and Physical Examination

- Check for a thrill at the cardiac apex.
- Check for a brisk carotid upstroke.
- On cardiac auscultation, check for
  - Wide splitting of S2
  - Presence of an S3
  - Holosystolic, high-pitch, blowing murmur best heard over the apex

https://www.med.ucla.edu/wilkes/MRmain.htm

Mitral Regurgitation. [Systolic Murmurs - Mitral Regurgitation; The Auscultation Assistant; Christopher Cable, MD, https://www.med.ucla.edu/wilkes/]
Listen for rales in the lower lung fields

http://www.easyauscultation.com/rales

Rales. [Rales Lung Sounds; Easy Auscultation; www.easyauscultation.com; copyright 2015, MedEdu LLC]

- Peripheral findings of heart failure, including a hypoperfused state, may be apparent in acute MR.

Findings That Confirm Diagnosis

- The echocardiogram confirms the diagnosis. The MR murmur in the context of MR symptoms (starting with exertional dyspnea), should prompt the imaging study.

Factors That Suggest Diagnosis

- Prior to diagnostic confirmation with echo, presence of two or more of the symptoms cited above suggests MR.
- The lack of a history of rheumatic fever does not exclude the diagnosis.
- Signs of pulmonary hypertension or right heart failure in the presence of a holosystolic murmur are suggestive of MR.

Factors That Exclude Diagnosis

- MR is definitively excluded only by an echocardiogram showing competence of the mitral valve.

Ancillary Studies

Laboratory

- It is helpful to send routine laboratory studies such as basic chemistries and a complete blood count to evaluate for other causes of the patient's symptoms.
- There may be value to checking a brain-type natriuretic peptide (BNP) level, especially if the patient has heart failure symptoms.

Electrocardiography

- The ECG should be obtained and interpreted promptly. Findings on electrocardiography may include the following:
  - Ischemic changes or new Q-waves in the inferior leads.
  - Left ventricular hypertrophy.
  - Left atrial enlargement as manifest by wide P-waves in II, III, and aVF.

Imaging

- The chest x-ray may be helpful in the evaluation of possible MR. Look for straightening of the left border of the cardiac silhouette or a double shadow in the right cardiac silhouette. Frank cardiomegaly and signs of pulmonary edema may be evident in acute MR or in late stages of chromic MR, but usually does not occur until fairly late in the disease progression.
- Echocardiography is the most sensitive and specific noninvasive test for MR. Transthoracic 2-D echo can usually confirm the diagnosis, and with Doppler echo and color jet imaging the degree of incompetence can be clearly delineated.

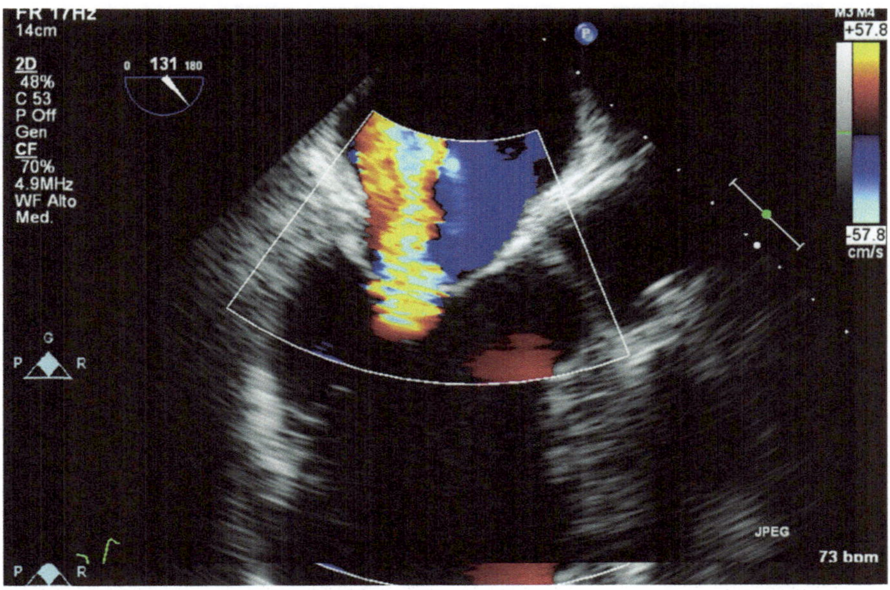

Transesophageal echocardiography (TEE) long-axis view. The picture shows severe ischemic mitral regurgitation (vena contracta 0.67 cm) [Colombo A, Godino C, Agricola E. The Degree and Type of Mitral Regurgitation Present at the Baseline Is Not Always a Good Predictor of the Procedural Technical Needs or of the Final Result. In: Feldman T, Franzen O, Low R, Rogers J, Yeo KK, editors. Atlas of Percutaneous Edge-to-Edge Mitral Valve Repair [Internet]. Springer London; 2013 [cited 2017 May 3]. p. 521–3. Available from: http://link.springer.com/chapter/10.1007/978-1-4471-4294-2_41] *Caption from original*

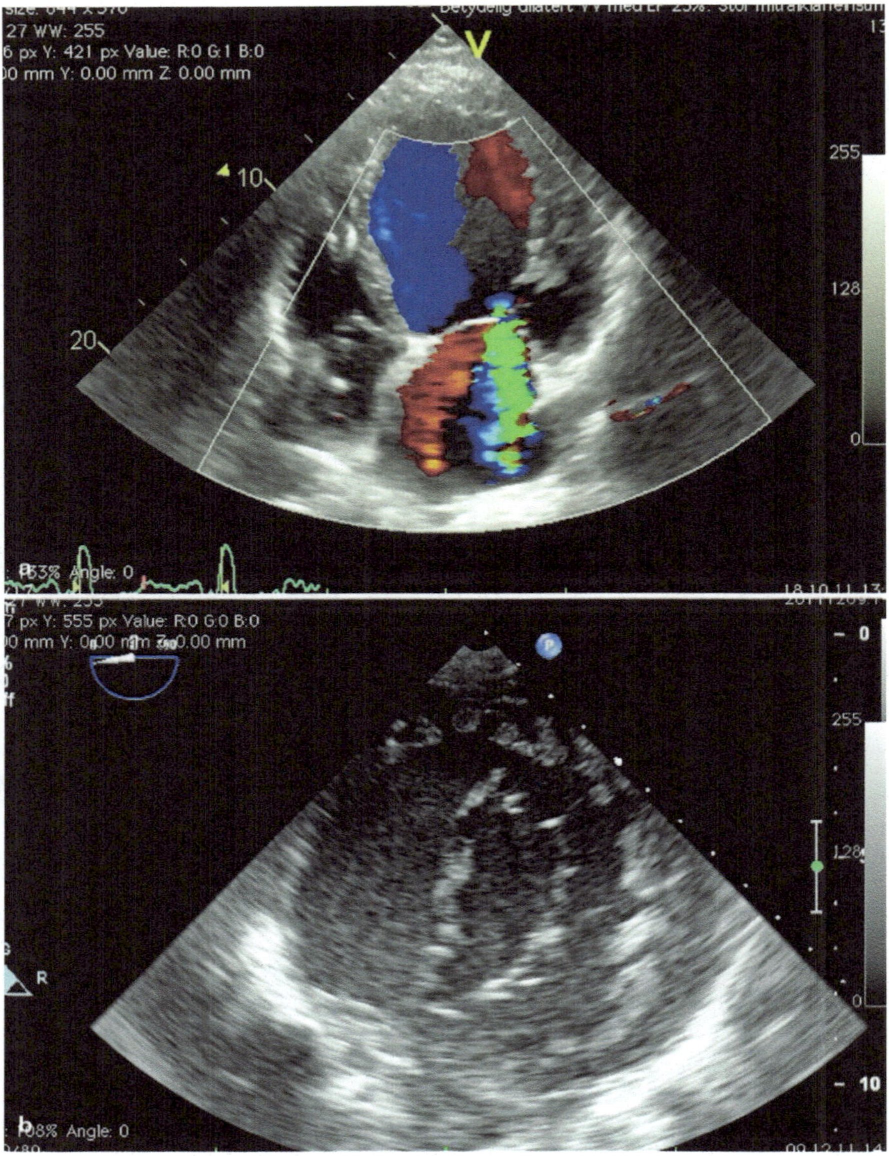

Transesophageal echo demonstrated very extensive mitral regurgitation located centrally between A2 and P2, dilated mitral annulus (4.4 × 4.8 cm) with malcoaptation of leaflets due to tenting of the leaflets. Coaptation depth 13 mm, coaptation length 2 mm. Four-chamber view (a) showing a very large, central mitral regurgitation reaching the roof of the left atrium. In the transgastric, short axis view (b) we measured the opening area of the mitral orifice to be more than 4 cm2. [Dahle G, Andersen KA, Brekke M, Rein KA. Functional Mitral Regurgitation with a Wide Extension of the Central Regurgitant Jet. In: Feldman T, Franzen O, Low R, Rogers

J, Yeo KK, editors. Atlas of Percutaneous Edge-to-Edge Mitral Valve Repair [Internet]. Springer London; 2013 [cited 2017 May 3]. p. 525–32. Available from: http://link.springer.com/chapter/10.1007/978-1-4471-4294-2_42] *Caption adapted from original*

Special Populations

Age

- Acute onset MR follows the age distribution for myocardial infarction, although infective endocarditis may cause MR at younger ages.
- Chronic MR usually becomes symptomatic later in life.

Co-morbidities

- The most important co-morbidities are underlying cardiopulmonary disease, including coronary artery disease and heart failure. Atrial fibrillation increases the risk of thromboembolic complications in MS.

Pitfalls in Diagnosis

Critical Steps Not to Miss

- An echocardiogram should be obtained early in the evaluation of patients with signs and symptoms suggestive of MR.
- Stabilize patients who present with hemodynamic compromise and poor oxygenation.

Mimics

- The echocardiogram will resolve differential considerations.

Time-Dependent Interventions

- The most important intervention is to stabilize patients with hemodynamic instability.
- Recognition of acute MR and heart failure may require life-saving intervention, including resuscitation and placement of a balloon pump.

Overall Principles of Treatment

- Afterload reduction is key in acute resuscitation.
- Biventricular pacing and an aortic balloon pump may be required.

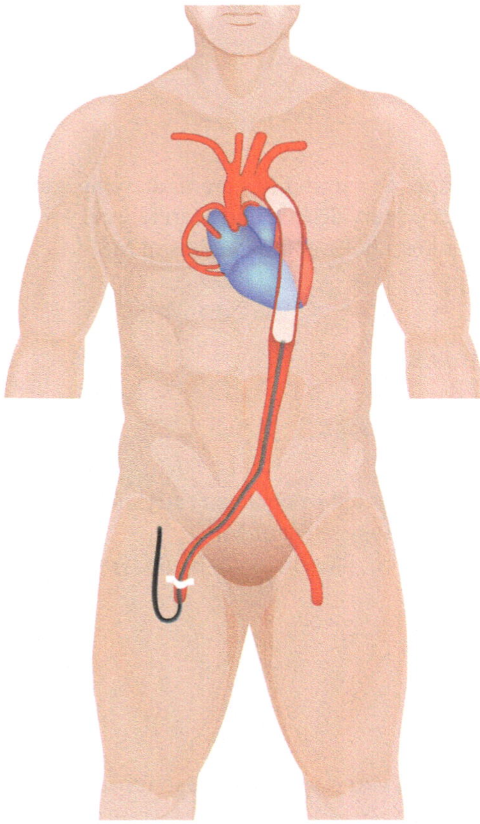

Illustration of an intra-aortic balloon pump [Baker ZP, Keenan JB, Khalpey Z. Difficult Decisions in Cardiothoracic Surgery: Acute Cardiogenic Shock. In: Surgical Decision Making [Internet]. Springer International Publishing; 2016 [cited

2017 May 3]. p. 165–75. Available from: http://link.springer.com/chapter/10.1007/978-3-319-29824-5_16] *Caption from original*

- In chromic MR, nitrates, diuretics, and beta-blockers may be helpful in controlling MR symptoms.
- Sodium restriction with or without diuretic therapy can help ease symptoms of pulmonary vascular congestion.
- Rate control and thromboembolic protection should be provided to MS patients with atrial fibrillation.
- Surgical repair or mitral valve replacement may be required in severe cases.

Disease Course

- Prognosis is dependent on the severity of the MR and underlying co-morbidities.
- Co-morbid heart failure or atrial fibrillation worsens the course.

Related Evidence

Papers of particular interest have been highlighted as:
*** Of key importance*

Practice Guideline

American Association for Thoracic Surgery Ischemic Mitral Regurgitation Consensus Guidelines Writing Committee., Kron IL, Acker MA, Adams DH, Ailawadi G, Bolling SF, Hung JW, Lim DS, LaPar DJ, Mack MJ, O'Gara PT, Parides MK, Puskas JD. 2015 The American Association for Thoracic Surgery Consensus Guidelines: Ischemic mitral valve regurgitation. J Thorac Cardiovasc Surg. 2016 Apr;151(4):940-56. https://doi.org/10.1016/j.jtcvs.2015.08.127. Epub 2016 Feb 4. Review. PubMed PMID: 26995621. https://www.ncbi.nlm.nih.gov/pubmed/26995621 **

Nishimura RA, Otto CM, Bonow RO, Carabello BA, Erwin JP 3rd, Guyton RA, O'Gara PT, Ruiz CE, Skubas NJ, Sorajja P, Sundt TM 3rd, Thomas JD; ACC/AHA Task Force Members. 2014 AHA/ACC Guideline for the Management of Patients With Valvular Heart Disease: a report of the American College of Cardiology/American Heart Association Task Force on Practice Guidelines. Circulation. 2014 Jun 10;129(23):e521-643. https://doi.org/10.1161/CIR.0000000000000031. Erratum in: Circulation. 2014 Sep 23;130(13):e120. Dosage error in article text. Circulation. 2014 Jun 10;129(23):e651. PubMed PMID: 24589853. https://www.ncbi.nlm.nih.gov/pubmed/24589853 **

O'Gara PT, Calhoon JH, Moon MR, Tommaso CL; American College of Cardiology.; American Association for Thoracic Surgery.; Society for Cardiovascular Angiography and Interventions.; Society of Thoracic Surgeons. Transcatheter therapies for mitral regurgitation: a professional society overview from the american college of cardiology, the american association for thoracic surgery, society for cardiovascular angiography and interventions foundation, and the society of thoracic surgeons. Catheter Cardiovasc Interv. 2014 May 1;83(6):849-63. https://doi.org/10.1002/ccd.25306. Review. PubMed PMID: 24867626. https://www.ncbi.nlm.nih.gov/pubmed/24867626 **

Lancellotti P, Moura L, Pierard LA, Agricola E, Popescu BA, Tribouilloy C, Hagendorff A, Monin JL, Badano L, Zamorano JL; European Association of Echocardiography. European Association of Echocardiography recommendations for the assessment of valvular regurgitation. Part 2: mitral and tricuspid regurgitation (native valve disease). Eur J Echocardiogr. 2010 May;11(4):307-32. https://doi.org/10.1093/ejechocard/jeq031. PubMed PMID: 20435783. https://www.ncbi.nlm.nih.gov/pubmed/20435783 **

Meta-Analysis

Teng Z, Ma X, Zhang Q, Yun Y, Ma C, Hu S, Zou C. Additional mitral valve procedure and coronary artery bypass grafting versus isolated coronary artery bypass grafting in the management of significant functional ischemic mitral regurgitation: a meta-analysis. J Cardiovasc Surg (Torino). 2017 Feb;58(1):121-130. https://doi.org/10.23736/S0021-9509.16.08852-2. Epub 2015 Jun 18. Review. PubMed PMID: 26086215. https://www.ncbi.nlm.nih.gov/pubmed/26086215

Salmasi MY, Acharya M, Humayun N, Baskaran D, Hubbard S, Vohra H. Is valve repair preferable to valve replacement in ischaemic mitral regurgitation? A systematic review and meta-analysis. Eur J Cardiothorac Surg. 2016 Jul;50(1):17-28. https://doi.org/10.1093/ejcts/ezw053. Epub 2016 Mar 23. Review. PubMed PMID: 27009102. https://www.ncbi.nlm.nih.gov/pubmed/27009102

Zhang H, Liu Y, Qiu S, Liang W, Jiang L. Short-Term and Long-Term Survival After Revascularization with or without Mitral Valve Surgery of Patients with Ischemic Mitral Valve Regurgitation: A Meta-Analysis. Med Sci Monit. 2015 Dec 4;21:3784-91. PubMed PMID: 26635041; PubMed Central PMCID: PMC4672719. https://www.ncbi.nlm.nih.gov/pubmed/26635041

Sündermann SH, Czerny M, Falk V. Open vs. Minimally Invasive Mitral Valve Surgery: Surgical Technique, Indications and Results. Cardiovasc Eng Technol. 2015 Jun;6(2):160-6. https://doi.org/10.1007/s13239-015-0210-5. Epub 2015 Jan 21. Review. PubMed PMID: 26577232. https://www.ncbi.nlm.nih.gov/pubmed/26577232

Dayan V, Soca G, Cura L, Mestres CA. Similar survival after mitral valve replacement or repair for ischemic mitral regurgitation: a meta-analysis. Ann Thorac

Surg. 2014 Mar;97(3):758-65. https://doi.org/10.1016/j.athoracsur.2013.10.044. Epub 2013 Dec 25. PubMed PMID: 24370200. https://www.ncbi.nlm.nih.gov/pubmed/24370200

Review

Poelaert JI, Bouchez S. Perioperative echocardiographic assessment of mitral valve regurgitation: a comprehensive review. Eur J Cardiothorac Surg. 2016 Nov;50(5):801-812. Epub 2016 Jun 3. Review. PubMed PMID: 27261073. https://www.ncbi.nlm.nih.gov/pubmed/27261073 **

Argulian E, Borer JS, Messerli FH. Misconceptions and Facts About Mitral Regurgitation. Am J Med. 2016 Sep;129(9):919-23. https://doi.org/10.1016/j.amjmed.2016.03.010. Epub 2016 Apr 5. Review. PubMed PMID: 27059381. https://www.ncbi.nlm.nih.gov/pubmed/27059381 **

Nishimura RA, Vahanian A, Eleid MF, Mack MJ. Mitral valve disease—current management and future challenges. Lancet. 2016 Mar 26;387(10025):1324-34. https://doi.org/10.1016/S0140-6736(16)00558-4. Review. PubMed PMID: 27025438. https://www.ncbi.nlm.nih.gov/pubmed/27025438 **

Badhwar V, Smith AJ, Cavalcante JL. A pathoanatomic approach to the management of mitral regurgitation. Trends Cardiovasc Med. 2016 Feb;26(2):126-34. https://doi.org/10.1016/j.tcm.2015.05.007. Epub 2015 Jun 29. Review. PubMed PMID: 26139247. https://www.ncbi.nlm.nih.gov/pubmed/26139247 **

Paulsen JM, Smith TW. Echocardiographic Imaging of the Mitral Valve for Transcatheter Edge-to-Edge Repair. Interv Cardiol Clin. 2016 Jan;5(1):17-31. https://doi.org/10.1016/j.iccl.2015.08.002. Epub 2015 Oct 17. Review. PubMed PMID: 27852479. https://www.ncbi.nlm.nih.gov/pubmed/27852479 **

McClung JA. Native and Prosthetic Valve Emergencies. Cardiol Rev. 2016 Jan-Feb;24(1):14-8. https://doi.org/10.1097/CRD.0000000000000079. Review. PubMed PMID: 26147306. https://www.ncbi.nlm.nih.gov/pubmed/26147306

Asgar AW, Mack MJ, Stone GW. Secondary mitral regurgitation in heart failure: pathophysiology, prognosis, and therapeutic considerations. J Am Coll Cardiol. 2015 Mar 31;65(12):1231-48. https://doi.org/10.1016/j.jacc.2015.02.009. Review. Erratum in: J Am Coll Cardiol. 2015 May 26;65(20):2265. PubMed PMID: 25814231. https://www.ncbi.nlm.nih.gov/pubmed/25814231

Zeng X, Tan TC, Dudzinski DM, Hung J. Echocardiography of the mitral valve. Prog Cardiovasc Dis. 2014 Jul-Aug;57(1):55-73. https://doi.org/10.1016/j.pcad.2014.05.010. Review. PubMed PMID: 25081402. https://www.ncbi.nlm.nih.gov/pubmed/25081402 **

Suri RM, Schaff HV, Enriquez-Sarano M. Mitral valve repair in asymptomatic patients with severe mitral regurgitation: pushing past the tipping point. Semin Thorac Cardiovasc Surg. 2014 Summer;26(2):95-101. https://doi.org/10.1053/j.semtcvs.2014.07.004. Epub 2014 Jul 30. Review. PubMed PMID: 25441000. https://www.ncbi.nlm.nih.gov/pubmed/25441000

Ducas RA, White CW, Wassef AW, Farag A, Bhagirath KM, Freed DH, Tam JW. Functional mitral regurgitation: current understanding and approach to management. Can J Cardiol. 2014 Feb;30(2):173-80. https://doi.org/10.1016/j.cjca.2013.11.022. Epub 2013 Nov 23. Review. PubMed PMID: 24461918. https://www.ncbi.nlm.nih.gov/pubmed/24461918 **

de Marchena E, Badiye A, Robalino G, Junttila J, Atapattu S, Nakamura M, De Canniere D, Salerno T. Respective prevalence of the different carpentier classes of mitral regurgitation: a stepping stone for future therapeutic research and development. J Card Surg. 2011 Jul;26(4):385-92. https://doi.org/10.1111/j.1540-8191.2011.01274.x. Review. PubMed PMID: 21793928. https://www.ncbi.nlm.nih.gov/pubmed/21793928

Use PubMed Clinical Queries to find the most recent evidence. Use this search strategy: "Mitral Valve Insufficiency"[Mesh] OR "Mitral Valve Regurgitation"[tiab] OR "Mitral Regurgitation"[tiab] OR "Mitral Valve Incompetence"[tiab] OR "Mitral Incompetence"[tiab] OR "Mitral Insufficiency"[tiab] OR "Mitral Valve Insufficiency"[tiab]

Chapter 49
Mitral Valve Stenosis

Charles V. Pollack, Jr. and Jaime Friel Blanck

Name and Synonyms

Mitral valve stenosis

Incidence/Epidemiology

- Mitral stenosis (MS), a narrowing of the channel between the left atrium and left ventricle, is most often a late sequela of acute rheumatic fever; it is occasionally congenital.
- The incidence of rheumatic fever is steadily diminishing in the US and the developed world.
- About two-thirds of patients with rheumatic MS are female.
- Symptoms usually manifest during the third or fourth decade of life and most patients are unaware that they ever had rheumatic fever.

Differential Diagnosis

- MS can be diagnosed definitively with echocardiography, so it can therefore be confirmed expeditiously if suspected. The symptoms associated with MS can overlap with those of a handful of other syndromes, such as:
  - Endocarditis
  - Left atrial myxoma
  - Atrial septal defect

C. V. Pollack, Jr. (✉)
Department of Emergency Medicine, Thomas Jefferson University, Philadelphia, PA, USA

J. F. Blanck
Welch Medical Library, Johns Hopkins University, Baltimore, MD, USA

C. V. Pollack, Jr. (ed.), *Differential Diagnosis of Cardiopulmonary Disease*,
https://doi.org/10.1007/978-3-319-63895-9_49

Pathophysiology and Etiology

- In MS, the valve leaflets are thickened and coarsened by fibrous tissue and/or calcific deposits. The mitral commissures eventually fuse and the valve cusps become rigid. The chordae tendineae also fuse and shorten, and eventually the aperture of the funnel-shaped valve narrows.

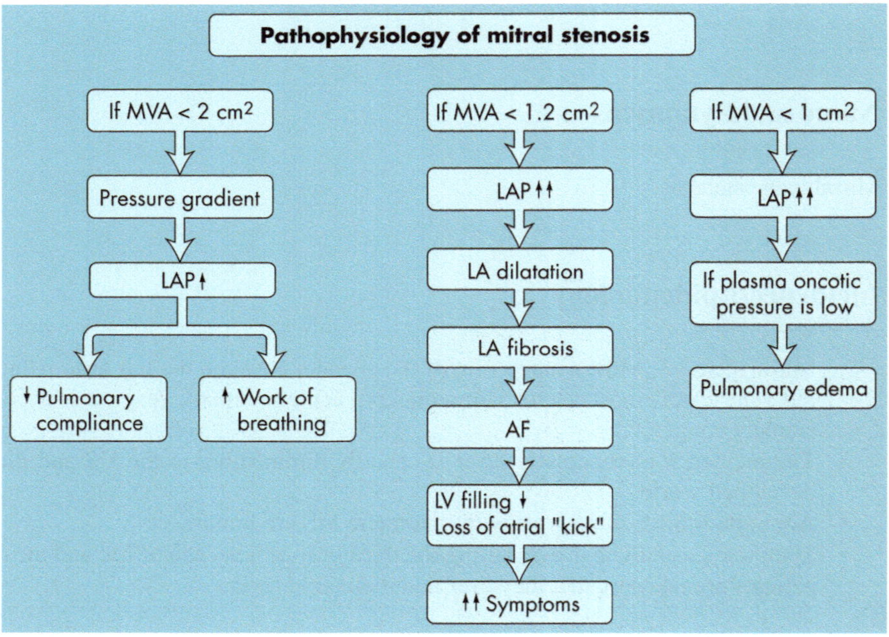

Pathophysiology of mitral valve stenosis. AF—atrial fibrillation; LA—left atrial; LAP—left atrial pressure; MVA—mitral valve area. [Clements F, de Bruijn N, Bennett-Guerrero E, Newman M, Reves JG. Chapter 1. In: Miller RD, Muravchick S, editors. Atlas of Anesthesia: Subspecialty Care, Volume 5, 1e. Philadelphia: Current Medicine; 1998. 236 p. ISBN: 0-443-07905-6] *Caption from original*

- The damage to the valve caused by the initial rheumatic insult is exacerbated over years by inflammatory and traumatic changes that occur because of altered flow patterns across the leaflets.
- MS eventually becomes symptomatic as the left atrium must generate higher and higher pressures to empty into the left ventricle across the narrower and narrower valve. In adults, the normal valve diameter is 4–6 cm^2. Symptoms usually are not apparent until the diameter is 2–2.5 cm^2. The left atrial pressure required to pump blood across that opening begins to increase dramatically at

that point, and patients may experience dyspnea and/or tachycardia on exertion. With severe MS, marked by a valve diameter of 1 cm^2 or less, a left atrial pressure of 25 mm Hg or more is required to maintain a normal cardiac output. This level of pressure in turn increases pulmonary venous and capillary pressures and further reduces pulmonary compliance, resulting in worsening dyspnea. Symptoms are worse with physical stress or exertion that increases heart rate because in tachycardia, diastole is shortened disproportionately compared to systole, leaving less time available for flow across the mitral valve.
- As left atrial, pulmonary capillary, and pulmonary arterial pressures rise, it becomes more difficult for the right ventricle to empty its full volume into the lungs for oxygenation, ultimately reducing cardiac output.
- When severe, pulmonary hypertension results in tricuspid and pulmonic valve incompetence and right-sided heart failure, or "cor pulmonale." With pulmonary hypertension there is also an increased risk of atrial fibrillation and its attendant thromboembolic complications.

Presentation

Typical/"Classic"

- The presentation of MS varies along a continuum, determined by the extent of valve narrowing and presence of pulmonary hypertension. Patients are usually asymptomatic for decades, but then symptoms typically progress continuously over a period of 2–3 years once dyspnea or cough with exertion begins to occur. The symptoms that suggest MS include:
  - Shortness of breath
  - Chest pain
  - Palpitations
  - Hemoptysis
  - Decreased exercise tolerance

Atypical

- Patients with advanced MS may have signs of right heart failure, such as severe dependent edema, liver congestion, and ascites.
- Hoarseness may develop from compression of the left recurrent laryngeal nerve by the enlarged left atrium as it hypertrophies to overcome the pressure gradient in the stenotic mitral valve.

- The damaged valve leaflets in MS are at risk for bacterial vegetations and endocarditis.
- MS may present with thromboembolism, from thrombi that form in the enlarged atrial appendages of patients with advanced MS.

Primary Differential Considerations

- Mitral stenosis, once symptomatic, may prompt searches for primary pulmonary causes of dyspnea, such as bronchitis, pneumonia, pulmonary edema, or pulmonary hypertension of other etiology.
- Other cardiac diagnoses to be considered are limited to atrial myxoma, atrial septal defect, heart failure, and arrhythmia. Early echocardiography can establish the culprit.

History and Physical Examination

- "Mitral facies"—purplish patches on the cheeks—has been described as being commonly seen in these patients.
- Ask about dyspnea, chest pain, or palpitations with exertion; ask about previous echocardiograms or a history of heart murmur.
- Ask about hemoptysis.
- Inquire about a history of rheumatic fever.
- Listen carefully over the heart for a low-pitched, rumbling, diastolic murmur, accentuated by exercise and diminished by Valsalva. Other suggestive findings on cardiac auscultation include:
    - Loud, snapping first heart sound.
    - Opening snap of the mitral valve, heard best in exhalation at or just medial to the cardiac apex.
- A diastolic thrill may be palpable at the cardiac apex. Check with the patient in the left lateral recumbent position.
- Look for pedal edema, jugular venous distension, or ascites as indications of right heart involvement.

Findings That Confirm Diagnosis

- The echocardiogram confirms the diagnosis. The MS murmur, opening snap, and diastolic thrill noted above, particularly in the context of MS symptoms (starting with exertional dyspnea), should prompt the imaging study.

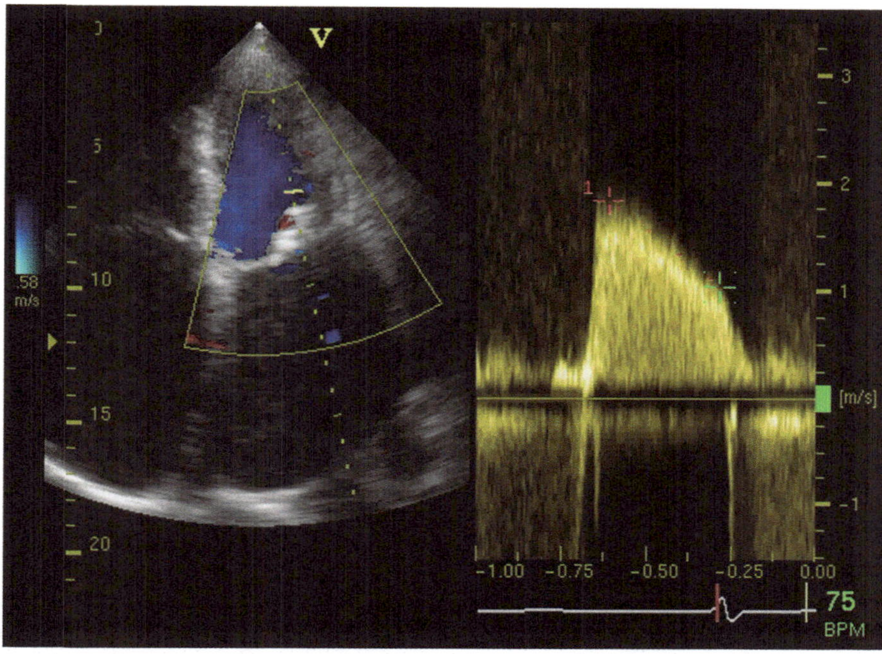

Rheumatic mitral stenosis. Continuous-wave Doppler flow recording demonstrates a pressure half-time of 220 μsec yielding an estimated orifice area of 1 cm^2. [Garcia M, Liu Z. Chapter; In: Vannan MA, Lang RM, Rakowski H, Tajik AJ, Braunwald E, editors. Atlas of Echocardiography. 1e. Philadelphia, PA: Current Medicine Group; 2005. 312 p. ISBN: 1-57340-217-6] *Caption from original*

https://www.easyauscultation.com/cases?coursecaseorder=14&courseid=31
Mitral stenosis murmur. [Mitral Stenosis (Diastolic Murmur); Easy Auscultation; www.easyauscultation.com; copyright 2015, MedEdu LLC]

Factors That Suggest Diagnosis

- Prior to diagnostic confirmation with echo, presence of two or more of the symptoms cited above suggests MS.
- The lack of a history of rheumatic fever does not exclude the diagnosis.
- Signs of pulmonary hypertension or right heart failure in the presence of a diastolic murmur are suggestive of MS.

Factors That Exclude Diagnosis

- MS is definitively excluded only by an echocardiogram showing unimpeded flow across the mitral valve.

Ancillary Studies

Laboratory

- It is helpful to send routine laboratory studies, such as basic chemistries and a complete blood count, to evaluate for other causes for the patient's symptoms.
- There may be value to checking a brain-type natriuretic peptide (BNP) level, especially if the patient has heart failure symptoms.
- Liver and renal function should be evaluated.

Electrocardiography

- The ECG should be obtained and interpreted promptly. If MS is suspected, look for a tall and peaked P-wave in lead II and an upright P-wave in lead V_1. These findings are more prominent with more advanced MS.

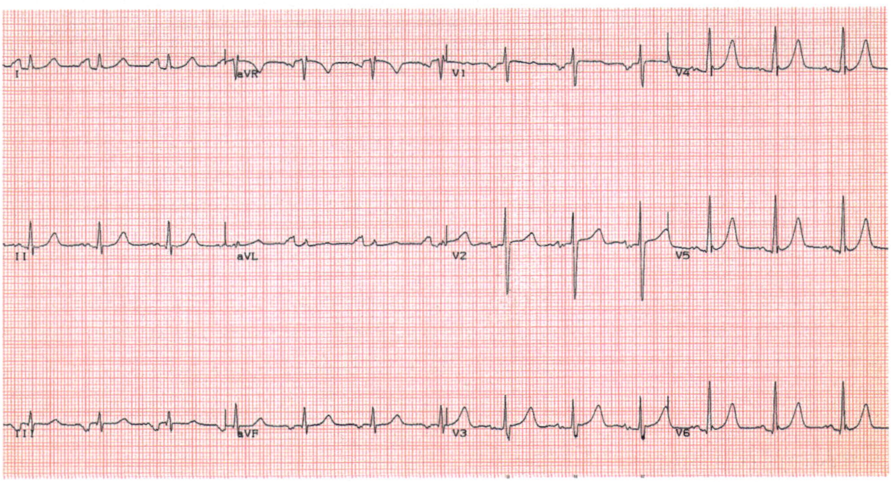

Electrocardiographic (ECG) signs in MS. A, The ECG findings from a patient with MS and regular sinus rhythm is normal except for signs of left atrial (LA) enlargement, that is, a P wave widened to 0.12 second or more. In lead II, the P wave has a double peak often characterized by an M-shaped configuration. In lead V1, the late negative portion of the P wave is characteristically increased in both width and depth. The P-wave changes are also called "P mitrale." [Kawanishi D, Rahimtoola S. Chapter; In: Braunwald E, editor. Atlas of Heart Disease: Valvular Heart Disease, Volume 11, 1e. St. Louis, Mo.: Current Medicine; 1997. 200 p. ISBN: 1-878132-30-X] *Caption adapted from original*

Imaging

- The chest x-ray may be helpful in the evaluation of possible MS. Look for straightening of the left border of the cardiac silhouette and prominence of the main pulmonary arteries. Prominence of the upper lobe pulmonary vasculature may be seen. In rare cases, a calcified mitral valve may be seen. Frank cardiomegaly usually does not occur until fairly late in the disease progression.
- Echocardiography is the most sensitive and specific noninvasive test for MS. Transthoracic 2-D echo can usually confirm the diagnosis, and with Doppler echo and color flow imaging the actual size and function of the valve can be assessed. In the past, cardiac catheterization was used to determine a therapeutic plan—i.e., whether surgery is required—but latest-generation echo now usually suffices.

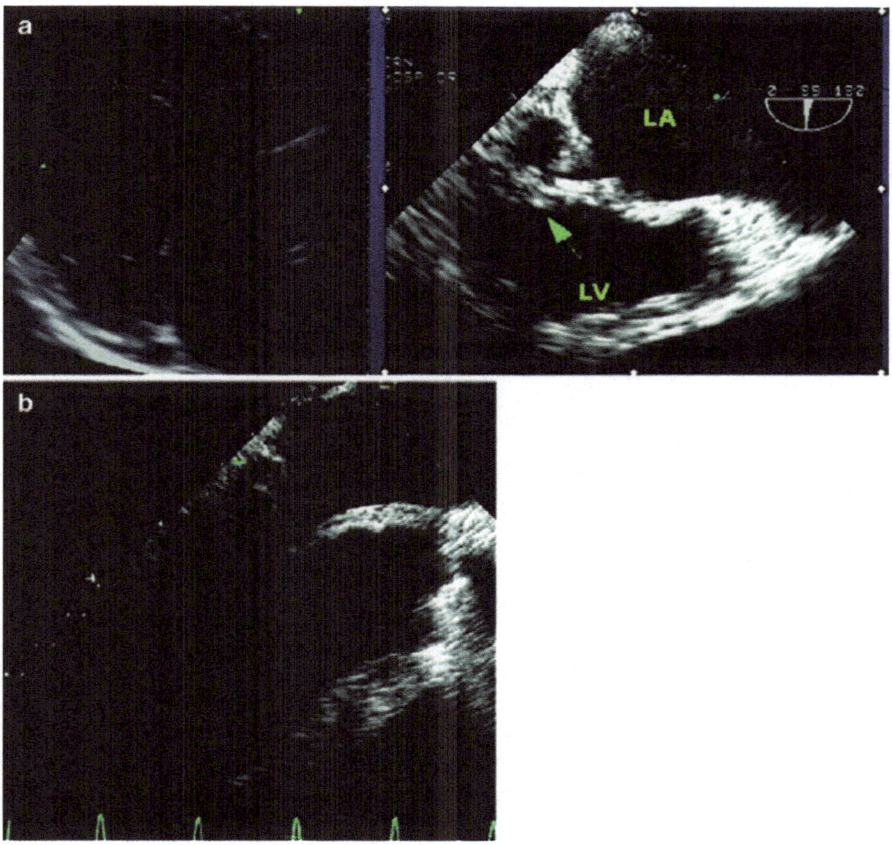

Echocardiographic features of mitral stenosis. (a) Rheumatic mitral stenosis. This figure demonstrates typical findings of rheumatic mitral stenosis (MS). The left panel shows hockey stick deformity of the anterior leaflet of the mitral valve in diastole. This appearance is a manifestation of the preferential involvement of the tips of the leaflets with the inflammatory/fibrosis process. This leads to relatively preserved mobility of the body with restricted mobility of the tip and the typical appearance. The right panel is a TEE from a different patient. The green arrow shows severe thickening and shortening of the chordae tendinae. Another common feature of rheumatic mitral stenosis is commissural fusion. The presence of commissural fusion may be a good predictor of who will respond to balloon valvuloplasty. (b) Other etiologies of mitral stenosis. Other etiologies of mitral stenosis include radiation and connective tissue disorders. Systemic lupus erythematosus causes diffuse thickening of the body of the valve leaflet as opposed to the tips in rheumatic heart disease [Akhter N, Mikati IA. Mitral Prolapse Regurgitation and Mitral Stenosis. In: Abraham T, editor. Case Based Echocardiography [Internet]. Springer London; 2010 [cited 2017 May 4]. p. 195–218. Available from: http://link.springer.com/chapter/10.1007/978-1-84996-151-6_17] *Caption adapted from original*

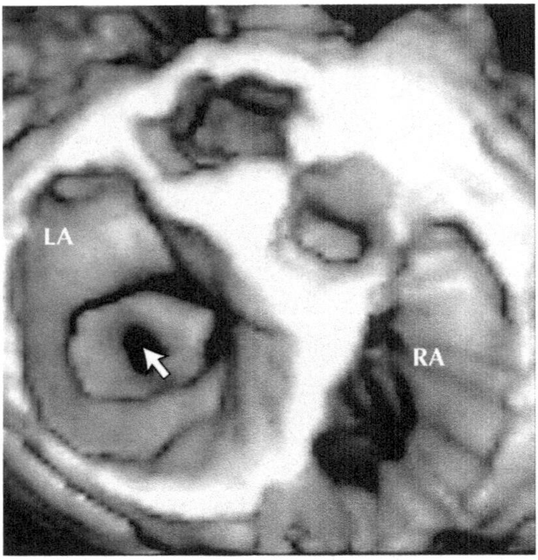

Three-dimensional echocardiographic (3DE) images of mitral valve (MV) from a patient with mitral stenosis. A, The MV as seen from above the left atrium (LA). The right atrium (RA) is seen to the right of LA and aorta anteriorly adjoining both atria. This type of 3DE sections displays MV and the narrowed MV orifice (arrow) in a view that stimulates intraoperative visualization [Hsu T, Yao J, De Castro S, Pandian N. Chapter; In: Lee RT, Braunwald E, editors. Atlas of Cardiac Imaging. Philadelphia: Current Medicine; 1998. ISBN: 0-443-07567-0] *Caption adapted from original*

Special Populations

Age

- Onset of MS symptoms is usually in the third or fourth decades of life.

Co-morbidities

- The most important co-morbidities are underlying cardiopulmonary disease, including heart failure and pulmonary hypertension. Atrial fibrillation increases the risk of thromboembolic complications in MS.

Pitfalls in Diagnosis

Critical Steps Not to Miss

- An echocardiogram should be obtained early in the evaluation of patients with signs and symptoms suggestive of MS.
- Stabilize patients who present with hemodynamic compromise and poor oxygenation.

Mimics

- The echocardiogram will resolve differential considerations.

Time-Dependent Interventions

- The most important intervention is to stabilize patients with hemodynamic instability.
- Recognition of pulmonary hypertension and right heart failure will prompt immediate therapy.

Overall Principles of Treatment

- The goals of medical treatment for MS are to:
    - Protect against recurrent rheumatic fever.
    - Protect against infective endocarditis.
    - Provide symptomatic relief.

- Sodium restriction with or without diuretic therapy can help ease symptoms of pulmonary vascular congestion.
- Beta-blockers may also provide some symptomatic relief for patients in sinus rhythm by prolonging diastolic filling time.
- Rate control and thromboembolic protection should be provided to MS patients with atrial fibrillation.
- Rheumatic fever prophylaxis with antibiotics providing Group A beta-hemolytic strep protection should be considered, as should antibiotic prophylaxis for infective endocarditis in association with interventions that may seed the bloodstream with bacteria, such as some dental procedures.
- Percutaneous balloon commissurotomy is the procedure of choice when medical therapy is insufficient to provide symptom relief.
- Surgical repair or mitral valve replacement may be required in severe cases or those in which commissurotomy does not provide relief.

Disease Course

- Prognosis is dependent on the severity of the MS.
- Co-morbid heart failure or atrial fibrillation worsens the course.
- The availability of percutaneous commissurotomy has improved the course of symptomatic MS.

Related Evidence

Papers of particular interest have been highlighted as:
*** Of key importance*

Practice Guideline

Nishimura RA, Otto CM, Bonow RO, Carabello BA, Erwin JP 3rd, Guyton RA, O'Gara PT, Ruiz CE, Skubas NJ, Sorajja P, Sundt TM 3rd, Thomas JD; ACC/AHA Task Force Members. 2014 AHA/ACC Guideline for the Management of Patients With Valvular Heart Disease: a report of the American College of Cardiology/American Heart Association Task Force on Practice Guidelines. Circulation. 2014 Jun 10;129(23):e521-643. https://doi.org/10.1161/CIR.0000000000000031. Erratum in: Circulation. 2014 Sep 23;130(13):e120. Dosage error in article text. Circulation. 2014 Jun 10;129(23):e651. PubMed PMID: 24589853. https://www.ncbi.nlm.nih.gov/pubmed/24589853 **

Nishimura RA, Otto CM, Bonow RO, Carabello BA, Erwin JP 3rd, Guyton RA, O'Gara

PT, Ruiz CE, Skubas NJ, Sorajja P, Sundt TM 3rd, Thomas JD; American College of Cardiology/American Heart Association Task Force on Practice Guidelines. 2014 AHA/ACC guideline for the management of patients with valvular heart disease: a report of the American College of Cardiology/American Heart Association Task Force on Practice Guidelines. J Am Coll Cardiol. 2014 Jun 10;63(22):e57-185. https://doi.org/10.1016/j.jacc.2014.02.536. Epub 2014 Mar 3. Erratum in: J Am Coll Cardiol. 2014 Jun 10;63(22):2489. Dosage error in article text. PubMed PMID: 24603191. https://www.ncbi.nlm.nih.gov/pubmed/24603191

Zamorano J, de Agustín JA. Three-dimensional echocardiography for assessment of mitral valve stenosis. Curr Opin Cardiol. 2009 Sep;24(5):415-9. https://doi.org/10.1097/HCO.0b013e32832e165b. Review. PubMed PMID: 19550310. https://www.ncbi.nlm.nih.gov/pubmed/19130998 **

Baumgartner H, Hung J, Bermejo J, Chambers JB, Evangelista A, Griffin BP, Iung B, Otto CM, Pellikka PA, Quiñones M; EAE/ASE.. Echocardiographic assessment of valve stenosis: EAE/ASE recommendations for clinical practice. Eur J Echocardiogr. 2009 Jan;10(1):1-25. https://doi.org/10.1093/ejechocard/jen303. Epub 2008 Dec 8. Review. Erratum in: Eur J Echocardiogr. 2009 May;10(3):479. PubMed PMID: 19065003. https://www.ncbi.nlm.nih.gov/pubmed/19065003 **

Review

Oktay AA, Gilliland YE, Lavie CJ, Ramee SJ, Parrino PE, Bates M, Shah S, Cash ME, Dinshaw H, Qamruddin S. Echocardiographic Assessment of Degenerative Mitral Stenosis: A Diagnostic Challenge of an Emerging Cardiac Disease. Curr Probl Cardiol. 2017 Mar;42(3):71-100. https://doi.org/10.1016/j.cpcardiol.2017.01.002. Epub 2017 Jan 10. Review. PubMed PMID: 28232004. https://www.ncbi.nlm.nih.gov/pubmed/28232004

Nunes MC, Nascimento BR, Lodi-Junqueira L, Tan TC, Athayde GR, Hung J. Update on percutaneous mitral commissurotomy. Heart. 2016 Apr;102(7):500-7. https://doi.org/10.1136/heartjnl-2015-308091. Review. PubMed PMID: 26743926. https://www.ncbi.nlm.nih.gov/pubmed/26743926 **

Nishimura RA, Vahanian A, Eleid MF, Mack MJ. Mitral valve disease—current management and future challenges. Lancet. 2016 Mar 26;387(10025):1324-34. https://doi.org/10.1016/S0140-6736(16)00558-4. Review. PubMed PMID: 27025438. https://www.ncbi.nlm.nih.gov/pubmed/27025438 **

Baird CW, Marx GR, Borisuk M, Emani S, del Nido PJ. Review of Congenital Mitral Valve Stenosis: Analysis, Repair Techniques and Outcomes. Cardiovasc Eng Technol. 2015 Jun;6(2):167-73. https://doi.org/10.1007/s13239-015-0223-0. Review. PubMed PMID: 26577233. https://www.ncbi.nlm.nih.gov/pubmed/26577233 **

Zeng X, Tan TC, Dudzinski DM, Hung J. Echocardiography of the mitral valve. Prog Cardiovasc Dis. 2014 Jul-Aug;57(1):55-73. https://doi.org/10.1016/j.

pcad.2014.05.010. Review. PubMed PMID: 25081402. https://www.ncbi.nlm.nih.gov/pubmed/25081402 **

Wunderlich NC, Beigel R, Siegel RJ. Management of mitral stenosis using 2D and 3D echo-Doppler imaging. JACC Cardiovasc Imaging. 2013 Nov;6(11):1191-205. https://doi.org/10.1016/j.jcmg.2013.07.008. Review. PubMed PMID: 24229772. https://www.ncbi.nlm.nih.gov/pubmed/24229772 **

Magne J, Lancellotti P, Pierard LA. Stress echocardiography and mitral valvular heart disease. Cardiol Clin. 2013 May;31(2):311-21. https://doi.org/10.1016/j.ccl.2013.03.008. Review. PubMed PMID: 23743079. https://www.ncbi.nlm.nih.gov/pubmed/23743079

Krapf L, Dreyfus J, Cueff C, Lepage L, Brochet E, Vahanian A, Messika-Zeitoun D. Anatomical features of rheumatic and non-rheumatic mitral stenosis: potential additional value of three-dimensional echocardiography. Arch Cardiovasc Dis. 2013 Feb;106(2):111-5. https://doi.org/10.1016/j.acvd.2012.11.004. Review. PubMed PMID: 23527915. https://www.ncbi.nlm.nih.gov/pubmed/23527915 **

andrashekhar Y, Westaby S, Narula J. Mitral stenosis. Lancet. 2009 Oct 10;374(9697):1271-83. https://doi.org/10.1016/S0140-6736(09)60994-6. Review. PubMed PMID: 19747723. https://www.ncbi.nlm.nih.gov/pubmed/19747723 **

Messika-Zeitoun D, Iung B, Brochet E, Himbert D, Serfaty JM, Laissy JP, Vahanian A. Evaluation of mitral stenosis in 2008. Arch Cardiovasc Dis. 2008 Oct;101(10):653-63. https://doi.org/10.1016/j.acvd.2008.06.016. Review. PubMed PMID: 19056072. https://www.ncbi.nlm.nih.gov/pubmed/19056072

Cohort Study

Gerede DM, Ongun A, Tulunay Kaya C, Acıbuca A, Özyüncü N, Erol Ç. Use of strain and strain rate echocardiographic imaging to predict the progression of mitral stenosis: a 5-year follow-up study the progression of mitral stenosis: a 5-year follow-up study. Anatol J Cardiol. 2016 Oct;16(10):772-777. https://doi.org/10.14744/AnatolJCardiol.2015.6590. PubMed PMID: 27182618. https://www.ncbi.nlm.nih.gov/pubmed/27182618

Pasca I, Dang P, Tyagi G, Pai RG. Survival in Patients with Degenerative Mitral Stenosis: Results from a Large Retrospective Cohort Study. J Am Soc Echocardiogr. 2016 May;29(5):461-9. https://doi.org/10.1016/j.echo.2015.12.012. PubMed PMID:

26936152. https://www.ncbi.nlm.nih.gov/pubmed/26936152

Use PubMed Clinical Queries to find the most recent evidence. Use this search strategy: (“Mitral Valve Stenosis”[Mesh] OR “mitral valve stenosis”[tiab] OR “mitral stenosis”[tiab] OR “mitral stenoses”[tiab] OR “mitral valve stenoses”[tiab])

Chapter 50
Myocarditis

Charles V. Pollack, Jr., Richard M. Cantor, and Victoria G. Riese

Name and Synonyms

Myocarditis

- Carditis, cardiac inflammation

Incidence/Epidemiology

- There are many diverse causes of myocarditis, and disease severity varies widely; therefore, the overall incidence of the disease is unknown.
- It is estimated that as many as 1–3 % of patients with acute viral infections may develop at least subclinical viral myocarditis.
- Overall, myocarditis is an unusual cause of acute chest pain. Although usually benign and self-limited, severe myocardial injury may occur.

Differential Diagnosis

- The differential considerations for myocarditis include all other causes of acute chest pain. These include, in particular, the potentially life-threatening diagnoses of acute coronary syndrome (ACS; unstable angina, NSTEMI, STEMI), pulmonary embolism, and aortic dissection.

C. V. Pollack, Jr. (✉)
Department of Emergency Medicine, Thomas Jefferson University, Philadelphia, PA, USA

R. M. Cantor
Department of Emergency Medicine and Pediatrics, State University of New York Upstate Medical University, Syracuse, NY, USA

V. G. Riese
Librarian Consultant, Eldersburg, MD, USA

C. V. Pollack, Jr. (ed.), *Differential Diagnosis of Cardiopulmonary Disease*,
https://doi.org/10.1007/978-3-319-63895-9_50

- Pneumonia, pleurisy, and pneumothorax should also be considered.
- Some patients with myocarditis have transient (or persistent) myocardial dysfunction, which brings heart failure, arrhythmias, and pericarditis into the differential.

Pathophysiology and Etiology

- Myocarditis is inflammation of the cardiac muscle. It may result from infection, secondary reaction, autoimmune problems, or exposures as follows:

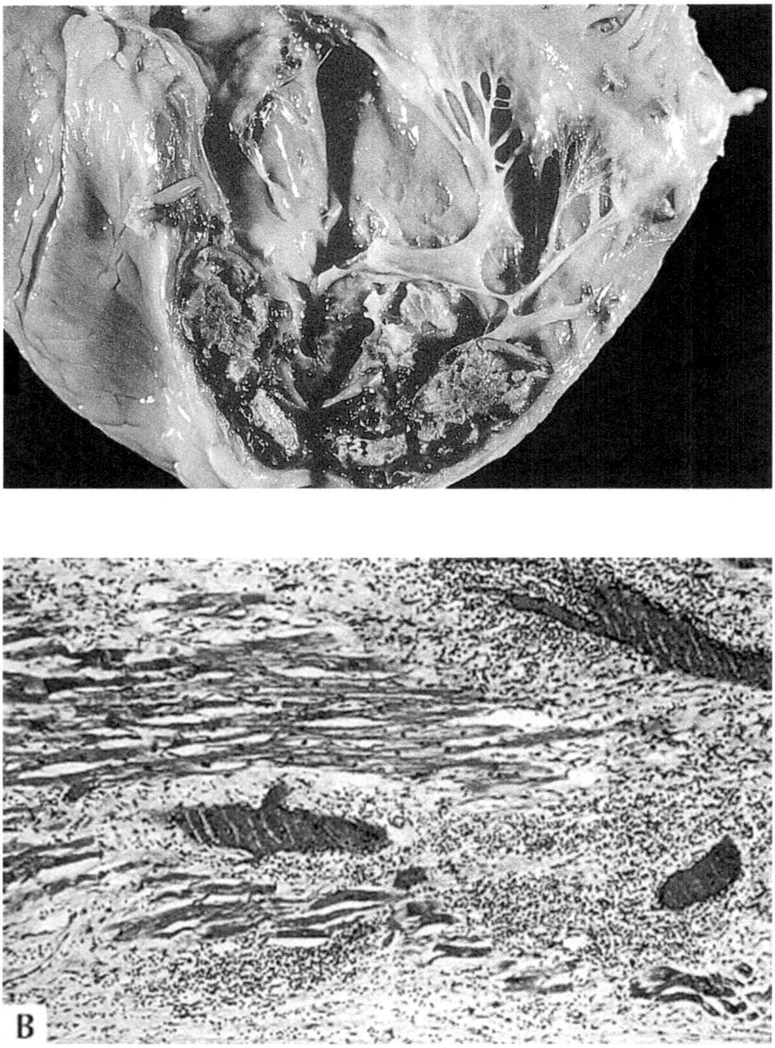

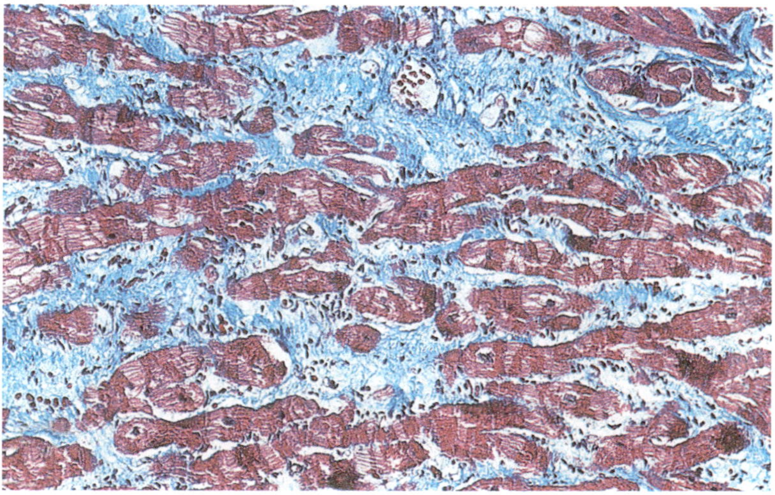

c

Gross autopsy specimen and photomicrographs of myocarditis. A, Gross autopsy specimen of a heart with fulminant myocarditis. The right ventricle is cut along the long axis to demonstrate an apical mural thrombus. B, Low-power photomicrograph of the myocardium revealing extensive mononuclear inflammation, which has replaced large clusters of myocytes that have undergone necrosis. Fulminant myocarditis is characterized by a nonspecific, severe influenza-like illness and the distinct onset of cardiac involvement. The patient's condition deteriorates rapidly, and the disorder frequently results in profound hemodynamic compromise and multisystem failure. Endomyocardial biopsies from fulminant myocarditis patients demonstrate unequivocal active myocarditis and are particularly notable for very extensive inflammatory infiltrates and numerous foci of myocyte necrosis. Within 1 month, the patients usually recover left ventricular function completely or die [045]. In contrast, acute myocarditis describes the clinical spectrum of the largest group of patients with active or borderline myocarditis. These patients have minimally dilated, hypokinetic left ventricles on presentation. The onset of cardiac symptoms is frequently indistinct, and some patients provide a vague history consistent with (but not diagnostic of) an antecedent viral illness. Active or borderline myocarditis is present on initial (but not subsequent) endomyocardial biopsies. Some patients in this group appear to respond to immunosuppressive therapy [046], while others experience either partial recovery of ventricular function or continue to deteriorate to end-stage dilated cardiomyopathy. (045. Rockman HA, Adamson RM, Dembitsky WP, et al. Acute fulminant myocarditis: long-term follow-up after circulatory support with left ventricular assist device. Am Heart J. 1991; 121:922 -926.) (046. Jones SR, Herskowitz A, Hutchins GM, et al. Effects of immunosuppressive therapy in biopsy-proved myocarditis and borderline myocarditis on left ventricular function. Am J Cardiol. 1991; 68:370 -376). C, Masson's trichrome (which stains collagen blue) of an endomyocardial biopsy of a patient with chronic active myocarditis. Note the extensive collagen deposition characteristically seen in end-stage dilated cardiomyopathy. Patients with chronic active myocarditis usually have a vague clinical presentation. Such patients have a slowly progressive course that inevitably deteriorates but may be punctuated by brief, often-dramatic but unsustained responses to immunosuppressive therapy. Serial endomyocardial biopsies demonstrate ongoing myocarditis with the development of extensive interstitial fibrosis. Inflammatory infiltrates in this subgroup of myocarditis patients may contain multinucleated giant cells. [Herskowitz A, Ansari A, Abelmann W. Myocarditis. In: Lee RT, Braunwald E, editors. Atlas of cardiac imaging. Philadelphia: Current Medicine; 1998. Chapter 9. (Braunwald E, editor. Atlas of heart diseases; vol. 2). ISBN: 0-443-07567-0; 2002-01-23] *Caption from original*

Etiologies of Human Myocarditis: Infectious

Viral	Protozoal and metazoal
Coxsackievirus (A and B)	Trypanosomiasis
Parvovirus	Toxoplasmosis
Echovirus	Malaria
Influenza	Schistosomiasis
Cytomegalovirus	Trichinosis
Hepatitis	Bacterial
Mumps	Diphtheria
Herpes simplex	Tuberculosis
Rabies	Legionella
EBV	Brucella
HIV	Clostridium
Rickettsial	Salmonella/shigella
Q fever	Meningococcus
Rocky Mountain spotted fever	Yersinia
Scrub typhus	Spirochetal
Fungal	Borrelia (Lyme)
Cryptococcus	
Candidiasis	
Histoplasmosis	
Aspergillus	

Infectious causes of human myocarditis. Most cases of myocarditis are clinically idiopathic and likely represent the largest subgroup of cases of human myocarditis (Liu PP, Mason JW. Advances in the understanding of myocarditis. Circulation. 2001; 104:1076 -1082.). EBV—Epstein-Barr virus. [Baughman K. Etiologies of human myocarditis: infectious, viral, protozoal, and metazoal. In: Libby P, editor.

Essential atlas of cardiovascular disease. Philadelphia: Current Medicine; 2009. Chapter 6. ISBN: 978-1-57340-309-2; 2009-05-21;] *Caption adapted from original*

Infectious	Immune-mediated	Toxic	Other/unknown
All types of microorganisms	Post-infectious	Drugs	Sarcoidosis
1. Virus	Systemic disorders	Toxins	Giant cell myocarditis
2. Fungus	Drug hypersensitivity		
3. Bacteria	Transplant rejection		
4. Protozoa			
5. Parasite			

How myocarditis can be sub-typed/grouped [Baandrup U. Myocarditis/inflammatory cardiomyopathy. In: Suvarna SK, editor. Cardiac pathology. London: Springer; 2013. p. 133-46. Book https://doi.org/10.1007/978-1-4471-2407-8; Chapter: 8; Chapter https://doi.org/10.1007/978-1-4471-2407-8_8; 2013-01-01] *Caption from original*

- Viral infection, including but not limited to
  - Coxsackie B virus (most common)
  - Enterovirus
  - Adenovirus
  - Influenza
  - HIV
  - Mumps
  - Rubeola
- Bacterial infection, including but not limited to
  - Diphtheria
  - *Streptococcus*
  - *Mycoplasma*
  - Tuberculosis
- Acute rheumatic fever
- Protozoal infection, including but not limited to
  - Chagas disease

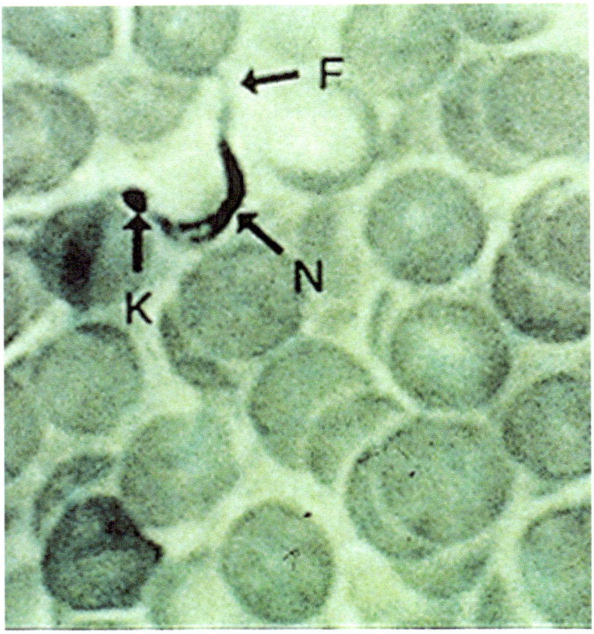

American trypanosomiasis (Chagas' disease): myocarditis. The most common infection of the heart worldwide is Chagas' disease, caused by the protozoan parasite Trypanosoma cruzi, which is spread by reduviid insects (Kirchhoff LV. American trypanosomiasis (Chagas' disease): a tropical disease now in the United States. N Engl J Med. 1993; 329:639 -644.). Infection with T. cruzi is endemic in Latin America and is now increasingly observed in the United States. Acute Chagas' disease is characterized by the systemic spread of the parasites to muscle, including myocardium. A, T. cruzi isolated from the blood of a patient with Chagas' disease. The trypomastigote is shown in mouse blood (Giemsa stain, × 2000). B, Histopathology of acute Chagas' myocarditis with a mononuclear infiltration. The arrows denote myocytes containing amastigote forms of the parasites (hematoxylin and eosin, × 360). C, High magnification of an infected myocyte (hematoxylin and eosin, × 900). F—flagellum; K—kinetoplast of amastigotes; N—nucleus. American trypanosomiasis (Chagas' disease): myocarditis [Hare J. Pathologic etiologies of heart failure. In: Colucci WS, editor. Atlas of heart failure. 5th ed. Philadelphia: Current Medicine; 2008. Chapter 3. (Braunwald E, editor. Atlas of heart diseases; vol. 4). ISBN: 1-57340-261-3; 2008-04-23] *Caption from original*

- toxoplasmosis
- Spirochetal infection, including but not limited to
  - Syphilis
  - Lyme disease

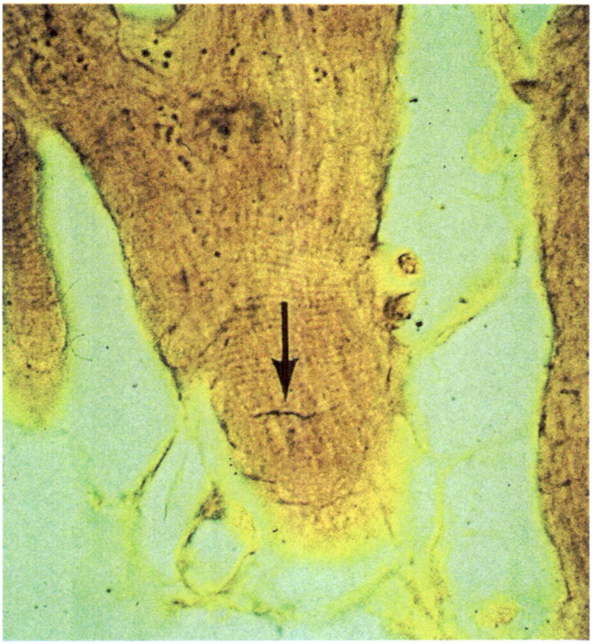

Borrelia burgdorferi in human myocardium: Lyme myocarditis. Detection of the spirochete Borrelia burgdorferi (arrow) in human myocardium (modified Steiner's silver stain). Lyme disease, a multisystem disorder caused by infection with B. burgdorferi, produces cardiac disease, notably arrhythmias and myocarditis, as a tertiary manifestation [045]. Here the spirochete is demonstrated in myocardium from a patient with a 4-year history of dilated cardiomyopathy and a serologic profile consistent with chronic Lyme disease. [Hare J. Pathologic etiologies of heart failure. In: Colucci WS, editor. Atlas of heart failure. 5th ed. Philadelphia: Current Medicine; 2008. Chapter 3. (Braunwald E, editor. Atlas of heart diseases; vol. 4). ISBN: 1-57340-261-3; 2008-04-23] *Caption from original*

- Rickettsial infection, including but not limited to
  - Rocky Mountain spotted fever

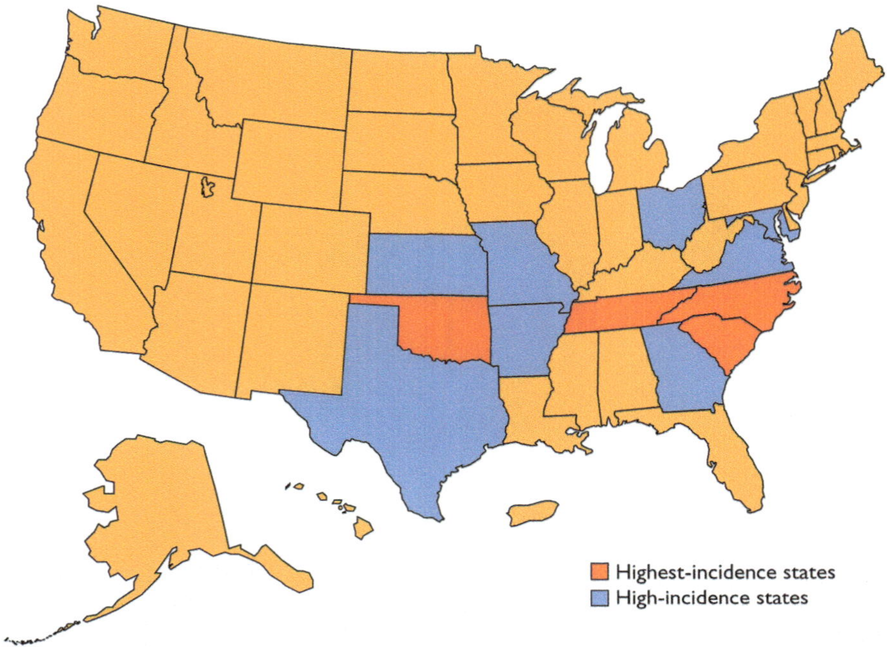

Incidence of Rocky Mountain spotted fever in the United States. High and medium incidence rates of Rocky Mountain spotted fever (RMSF) in the United States. Although RMSF has now been reported in almost every state, four states (North Carolina, South Carolina, Tennessee, and Oklahoma) have reported the highest number of cases in recent years. Other high incidence states in recent years include Maryland, Virginia, Georgia, Tennessee, Ohio, Missouri, Arkansas, Texas, and Kansas. Certain focal regions, such as Cowan and Rowan counties in North Carolina, are considered hyperendemic. [Spach D. Chapter 14. In: Wilfert S, editor. Pediatric infectious diseases. Philadelphia: Current Medicine; 1998. (Mandell GL, editor. Atlas of infectious diseases; vol. 11). ISBN: 0-443-06526-8; 2002-01-23] *Caption from original*

- Fungal infection, including but not limited to
  - Candidiasis
  - Histoplasmosis
- Systemic inflammatory disease, including but not limited to
  - Giant cell myocarditis
  - Sarcoidosis

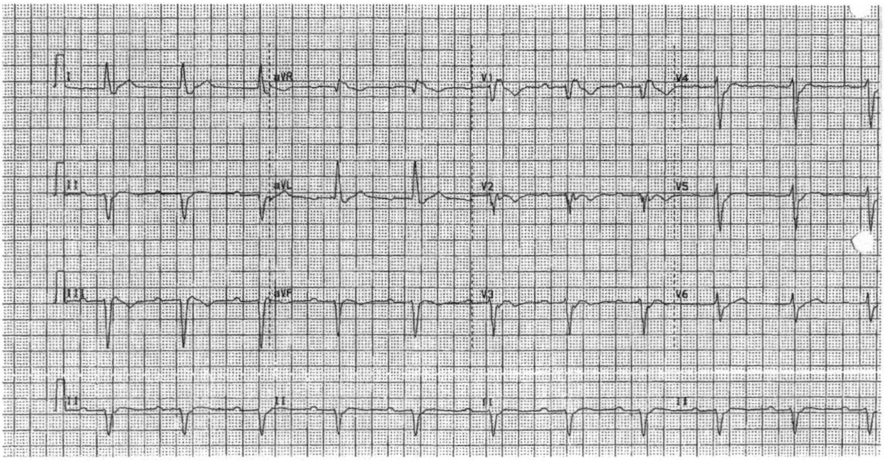

Sarcoidosis of the heart. Resting ECG in a patient with advanced sarcoidosis. The tracing shows evidence of first-degree atrioventricular block as well as a right bundle branch block pattern. Echocardiography showed no evidence of regional wall motion abnormality and an estimated left ventricular ejection fraction of 40%. The patient underwent cardiac catheterization, which demonstrated no evidence of coronary artery disease. Based on the prior history of pulmonary sarcoidosis and the presence of conduction system abnormalities and cardiomyopathy in the absence of coronary artery disease, the patient was felt to have cardiac sarcoidosis. The patient underwent electrophysiologic study, which demonstrated inducible sustained ventricular tachycardia. An implantable cardio-defibrillator device was placed. [Tanoue L, Elias J. Sarcoidosis. In: Crapo J, editor. Bone's atlas of pulmonary medicine. 3rd ed. Philadelphia: Current Medicine; 2005. Chapter 12; ISBN: 1-57340-211-7; 2005-01-14] *Caption adapted from original*

- Kawasaki's disease
- Crohn's disease
- Radiation exposure
- Chemical or drug toxicity, including but not limited to
  - Chemotherapeutic agents such as doxorubicin and anthracyclines
  - Antiseizure drugs such as phenytoin and carbamazepine
  - Antibiotics such as penicillin and chloramphenicol
- Envenomations, including but not limited to
  - Black widow spider bites

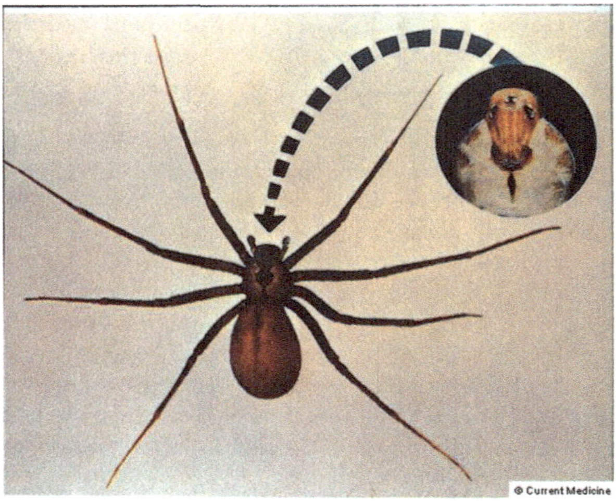

Neurotoxic black widow spider. The black widow spider (Latrodectus mactans) elaborates a venom that can cause severe neurologic dysfunction. The female (shown here) contains a red hourglass mark on the abdomen and is one of the most aggressive and most dangerous of the American spiders. (From US Government Printing Office [9].) 009. Venomous Arthropod Handbook. USAF School of Aerospace Medicine, Brooks Air Force Base, Texas 78235. Stock no. 008-070-00397-0, catalog no. D 301-35:161/43. Washington, DC: US Government Printing Office; 1977 [Prockop L, Brock C, Spencer P. Neurotoxic disorders. In: Rosenberg RN, editor. Atlas of clinical neurology. 3rd ed. Philadelphia: Current Medicine; 2009. p. 543-64. ISBN: 978-1-57340-283-5; 2009-01-28;] *Caption adapted from original*

- Scorpion stings

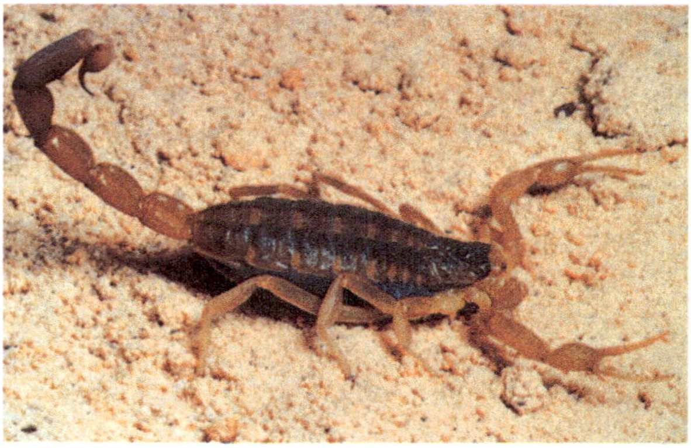

Scorpion envenomation. Scorpions secrete a complex mixture of substances, including an array of proteins with neuropharmacologic and enzymatic activity. The venom is delivered from a tail stinger. (From Anon [008].) 008. Anon: Venomous

Arthropod Handbook. USAF School of Aerospace Medicine, Brooks Air Force Base, Texas 78235. Stock No. 008–070–00397–0, catalog no. D 301.35: 161/43. Washington, DC: US Government Printing Office; 1977 [Gold B, Schnell J, Spencer P. Neurotoxic disorders. In: Rosenberg RN, editor. Atlas of clinical neurology. 2nd ed. Philadelphia: Current Medicine; 2003. Chapter 14. ISBN: 1-57340-175-7; 2002-01-24] *Caption adapted from original*

- Snake venom

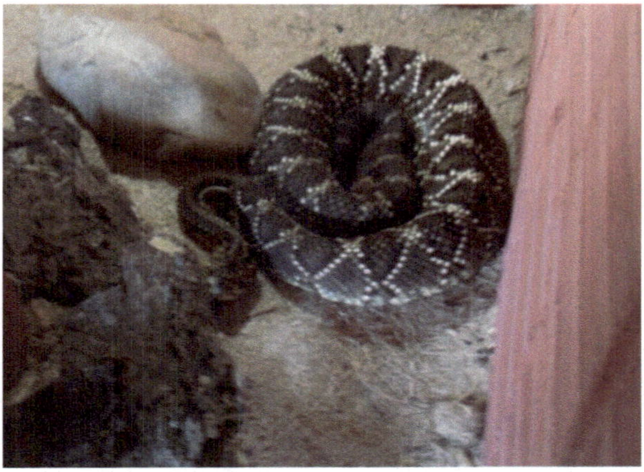

Rattlesnake (*Crotalus durissus*). [From article: The use of zootherapeutics in folk veterinary medicine in the district of Cubati, Paraíba State, Brazil. J Ethnobiol Ethnomed. 2007 Sep;3(1):32. https://doi.org/10.1186/1746-4269-3-32, at http://link.springer.com/article/10.1186%2F1746-4269-3-32/fulltext.html; by Raynner RD Barboza, Wedson de MS Souto, José da S Mourão, © Barboza et al; licensee BioMed Central Ltd. 2007; licensed under Creative Commons Attribution License BY 2.0 http://creativecommons.org/licenses/by/2.0] *Caption from original*

- Postpartum
- Idiopathic
- The common denominator of all these diverse causes is inflammation and potential dysfunction of myocardial cells, the consequences of which may range from subclinical to life threatening. Damage to the adjacent cardiac conduction system is common, with arrhythmias the potential result. Exploration of possible underlying causes is important to determine specific treatments beyond basic support of heart function.

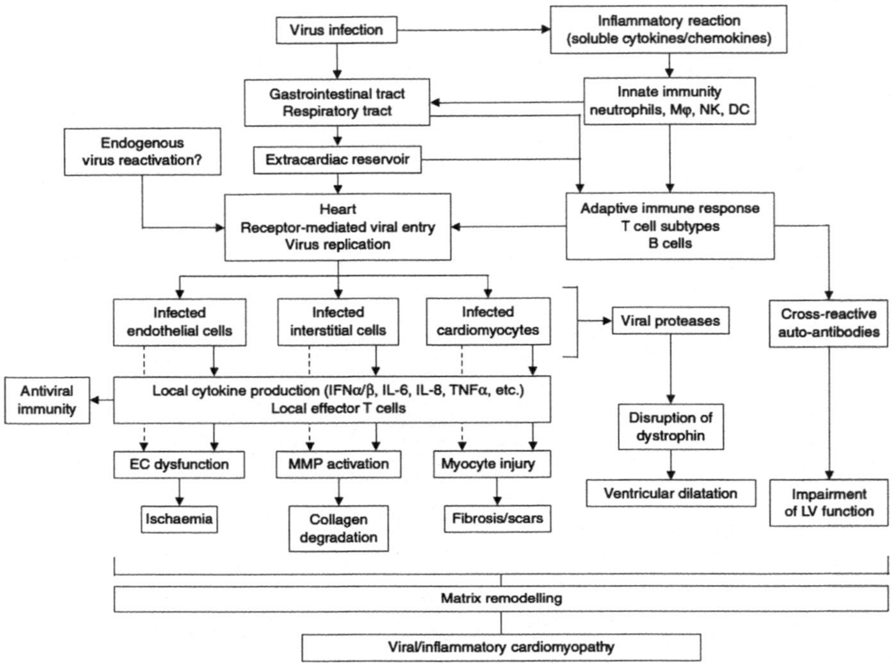

Causes of myocardial injury in viral and post-infectious heart disease. Myocardial tissue injury emerges during different phases of infectious myocarditis from direct virus-associated and/or immune-mediated tissue injury. DC = dendritic cells; EC = endothelial cells; IFN = interferon; IL = interleukin; LV = left ventricular; Mφ = monocytes; MMP = matrix metalloproteinase; NK = natural killer cells; TNFα = tumour necrosis factor-α. [Kühl U, Schultheiss HP. Viral myocarditis. Drugs. 2009 Jul;69(10):1287-302. https://doi.org/10.2165/00003495-200969100-00001; Published: 2009-07-01] *Caption from original*

Presentation

Typical/"Classic"

- Because of the broad range of etiologies, there is no "classic" presentation of myocarditis. Common features that may prompt presentation for care include:
  - Acute or chronic heart failure
  - Chest pain
  - Arrhythmias
  - Exercise intolerance
  - Fever, chills, and other signs and symptoms of systemic illness
- Signs and symptoms range from quite mild to life threatening.

Aspecific	1. Gastrointestinal: nausea and vomiting, cramp, diarrhea, appetite loss, abdominal and epigastric pain 2. Respiratory: cough, pharyngeal pain 3. General: increased fever, general fatigue, arthralgia and myalgia, headache, and back pain
Cardiac	1. Chest pain or discomfort (particularly common in young patients with coronary vasospasm), concomitant pericarditis, syncope, palpitations, dyspnea 2. Heart failure: generalized fatigue, intolerance to exercise and dyspnea. Subsequently acute or fulminant cardiogenic shock 3. Sinus tachycardia (most common, especially out of proportion with concomitant fever), premature atrial and ventricular contraction, atrial fibrillation, and ventricular tachycardia. I and II degree, up to complete AV block (more common with infiltrative and GCM), RBBB, and LBBB

Clinical presentation of myocarditis. [Cortinovis B, Scanziani M, Celotti S. ECMO in myocarditis and rare cardiomyopathies. In: Sangalli F, Patroniti N, Pesenti A, editors. ECMO-extracorporeal life support in adults. Milan: Springer; 2014. p. 137-49; Book https://doi.org/10.1007/978-88-470-5427-1; Chapter: 12; Chapter https://doi.org/10.1007/978-88-470-5427-1_12; Published: 2014-01-01] *Caption from original*

Atypical

- Because of the broad range of etiologies and co-morbidities, atypical or distracting presentations of myocarditis are common.

Primary Differential Considerations

- Prompt consideration also should be given to the possible diagnosis of ACS, pulmonary edema, cardiac tamponade, and cardiomyopathy.

History and Physical Exam

Findings That Confirm Diagnosis

- The diagnosis of myocarditis is usually presumptive, based on recognition of the combination of suggestive symptoms, a potential exposure, and clinical suspicion.

Diagnostic test	Common features
Chest radiography	Cardiomegaly, pulmonary vascular congestion, and/or pleural effusion (depending on right ventricular and tricuspid valve dysfunction). No specific abnormalities
ECG	Completely normal or with minor, aspecific abnormalities to markedly abnormal Brady- and tachyarrhythmias, conduction abnormalities, ST and T wave alterations, abnormal Q wave, low voltage, and poor R wave progression. Patterns of infarction or pericarditis. Presence of Q wave associated with a severe course, higher early cardiac enzymes, worse LV function, and higher incidence of cardiogenic shock, but not necessarily with a worse long-term outcome (31)
Cardiac enzymes	CPK MB, TnT, and TnI may be elevated (reflecting the extent of myocardial injury). TnI probably superior to CPK MB early in the disease, TnT levels correlating with more extensive damage
Echocardiography	Highly variable, from a completely normal to a markedly abnormal Various degrees of hypokinesis most commonly (mild hypokinesis limited to areas of focal infiltration, segmental wall motion abnormalities or diffuse involvement, with severe hypokinesis) LVEF or FS reduced, not necessarily with LV dilatation
Magnetic resonance imaging	Areas of inflammation and infiltration, mostly focal within the first 2 weeks, more diffuse within 4 weeks. Extent of the lesion correlates with LV dysfunction
Endomyocardial biopsy	5–10 samples from RV septum. Submit 4–5 to light microscopic examination. Transmission electron microscopy may be useful but reserved to infiltrative disorders Routine viral genome testing only for referral centers Several patterns of infiltration (histiocytic and mononuclear), varying in severity and structural abnormalities of myocardium

Diagnostic test results in myocarditis. [Cortinovis B, Scanziani M, Celotti S. ECMO in myocarditis and rare cardiomyopathies. In: Sangalli F, Patroniti N, Pesenti A, editors. ECMO-extracorporeal life support in adults. Milan: Springer; 2014. p. 137-49; Book https://doi.org/10.1007/978-88-470-5427-1; Chapter: 12; Chapter https://doi.org/10.1007/978-88-470-5427-1_12; Published: 2014-01-01] *Caption adapted from original*

- The diagnosis cannot be fully confirmed without endomyocardial biopsy.

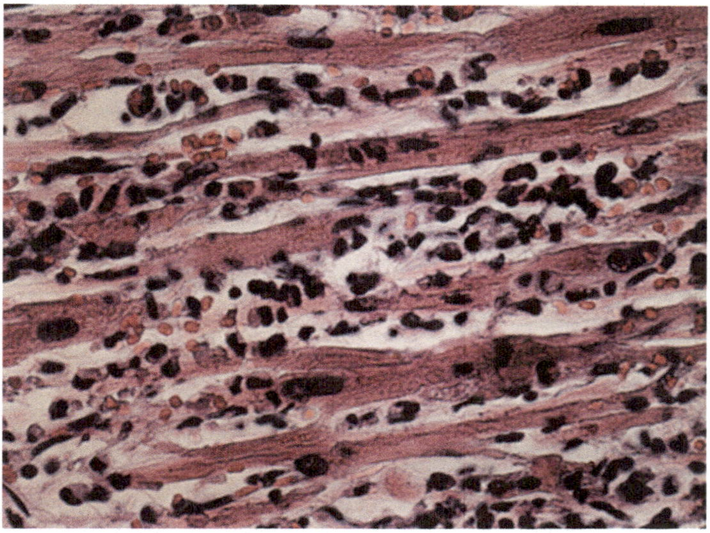

Severe myocarditis. Infiltrative disorders. A, Histologic section of myocardium showing severe myocarditis (hematoxylin-eosin stain ×50). Panel A shows the histology of the heart of a college student who came home for the winter holidays and died suddenly during Christmas dinner with her family. She was apparently asymptomatic in spite of the presence of severe myocarditis. B, Endomyocardial biopsy of a young woman who was successfully resuscitated from an episode of sudden death. At the time of electrophysiologic studies, an endomyocardial biopsy was obtained that showed non-necrotizing granulomas (arrow), leading to the diagnosis of isolated cardiac sarcoidosis. [Fishbein M, Chen PS. Structural substrates for arrhythmias in heart failure. In: Shivkumar K, Weiss J, Fonarow G, Narula J, editors. Atlas of electrophysiology in heart failure. Philadelphia: Current Medicine; 2005. Chapter 2. (Braunwald E, editor. Atlas of heart diseases; vol. 15); ISBN: 1-57340-225-7; Published: 2005-07-18; Braunwald, Eugene] *Caption adapted from original*

Factors That Suggest Diagnosis

- Systemic illness, chest pain, and exposure to an etiologic concern are suggestive and should prompt consideration of the diagnosis. Detection of arrhythmia in this setting is more suggestive.
- Associated pericarditis may result in an audible friction rub.

http://www.easyauscultation.com/myocarditis
Myocarditis heart sounds. [Myocarditis Page; Easy Auscultation; www.easyauscultation.com; copyright 2015, MedEdu LLC]

- Patients with more significant or advanced disease may have an audible S3 heart sound.
- One might arrive at the diagnosis by first recognizing the underlying cause (such as toxic drug exposure, viral infection, or systemic inflammatory disease) and then attributing cardiac symptoms to the myocarditis.

Factors That Exclude Diagnosis

- No history or physical findings can definitively exclude myocarditis.

Ancillary Studies

Laboratory

- There are no diagnostic laboratory studies for myocarditis other than endomyocardial biopsy, which demonstrates inflammation of the myocardial cells.
- Some laboratory studies may be helpful in raising suspicion of myocarditis, evaluating causative/co-morbid conditions, or both. These may include:
  - Complete blood count
  - Erythrocyte sedimentation rate (ESR) or C-reactive protein (CRP)
  - Cardiac enzymes (CPK-MB and/or troponin)
  - Viral antibody titers
  - Rheumatologic studies

Imaging

- Echocardiography may be used to evaluate the extent of heart failure.

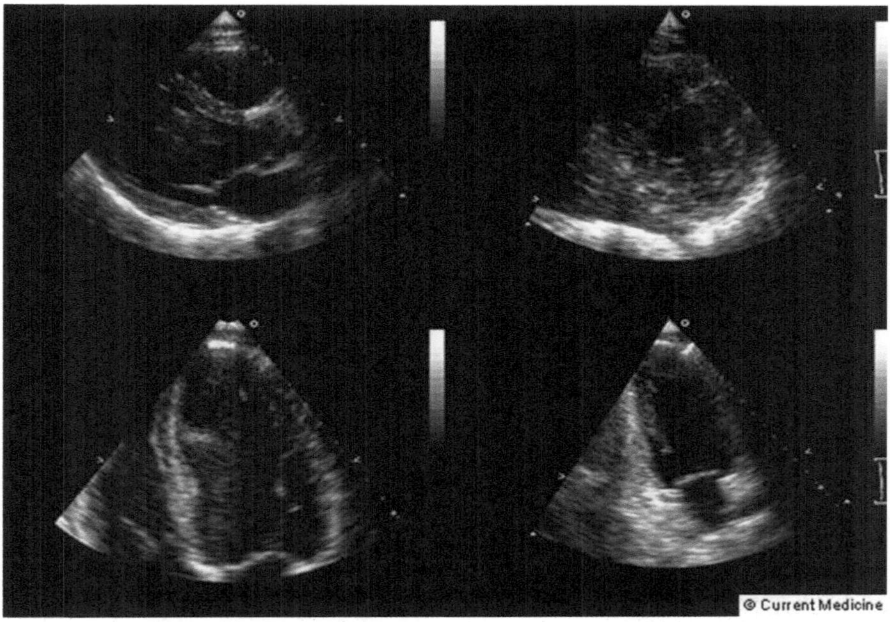

Transthoracic echocardiography in suspected acute myocarditis. Transthoracic echocardiography: Three long axis views (upper left and lower panels) and one short axis view (upper right panel) are shown. Severely reduced ejection fraction with preserved left ventricular size is demonstrated; valvular function was normal, as was the right ventricular size and function. [Strohm O, Friedrich M. Chapter 12. In: Manning WJ, editor. Atlas of cardiovascular magnetic resonance. Philadelphia: Current Medicine; 2009; ISBN: 978-1-57340-299-6; Published: 2009-01-16] *Caption from original*

- Magnetic resonance scanning with gadolinium may identify areas of myocardial inflammation.

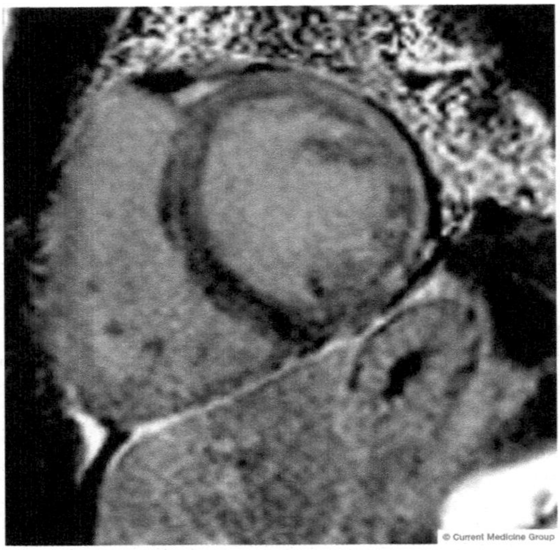

Acute myocarditis. A 20-year-old male student who was previously healthy developed an influenza-like illness while visiting Mexico. He developed worsened dyspnea and was found to have severe depression of left ventricular (LV) global systolic function and moderate LV dilatation. At hospital admission, he had frequent nonsustained ventricular tachycardia, physical findings consistent with cardiogenic shock, with an LV ejection fraction (LVEF) quantified by volumetric cine cardiac magnetic resonance (CMR) to be 25% (A). Serial blood and urine cultures revealed no bacterial pathogens. Endomyocardial biopsy revealed moderate interstitial fibrosis only. Contrast-enhanced late gadolinium enhancement (LGE) imaging demonstrated diffuse and patchy enhancement of the anterolateral and inferolateral wall (B). These CMR findings are consistent with diffuse acute myocardial inflammation and edema presumably from acute viral myocarditis. The patient fortunately followed a stable and then progressively improving clinical course in the months following initial presentation. [Kwong R. Cardiac magnetic resonance imaging. In: Libby P, editor. Essential atlas of cardiovascular disease. Philadelphia: Current Medicine; 2009. Chapter 16. ISBN: 978-1-57340-309-2; Published: 2009-05-21;] *Caption from original*

- Electrocardiographic findings are usually nonspecific but may suggest ACS.

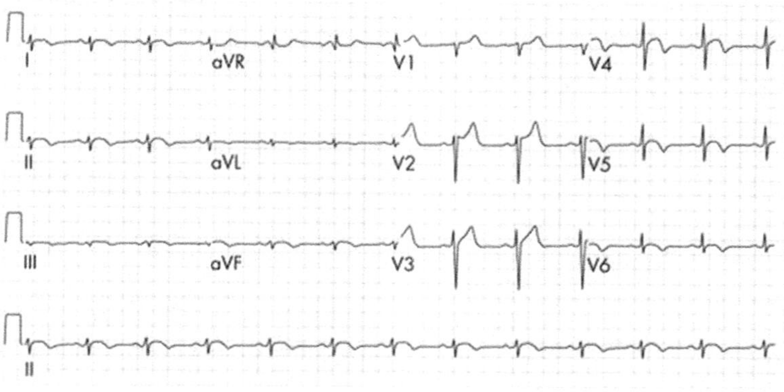

ECG in suspected acute myocarditis. 12-Lead electrocardiogram at presentation, demonstrating nonischemic changes in the ST and T segments. Physical examination revealed severe chest pain and shortness of breath (New York Heart Association III), blood pressure 98/58 mm Hg, and heart rate 97 bpm. aVF—augmented voltage, unipolar left leg lead; aVL—augmented voltage, unipolar left arm lead; aVR—augmented voltage, unipolar right arm lead. [Strohm O, Friedrich M. Chapter 12. In: Manning WJ, editor. Atlas of cardiovascular magnetic resonance. Philadelphia: Current Medicine; 2009; ISBN: 978-1-57340-299-6; Published: 2009-01-16] *Caption from original*

Special Populations

Age and Gender

- Perhaps owing to the diverse etiologies of the disease, there is no age or gender predilection for myocarditis in general. Obviously, some causes affect specific groups, such as postpartum myocarditis in women and viral myocarditis in younger patients.
- In the pediatric population, viral etiologies predominate, specifically enteroviral (Coxsackie B), parvovirus B19, adenovirus, and human herpes 6.
- In children, the mean age at diagnosis is 9 years, with bimodal peaks at 9 months of age and 16 years.
- Affected infants will manifest signs of congestive heart failure, including tachypnea, tachycardia, and increased work of breathing and diaphoresis when feeding.

Co-morbidities

- The list of etiologies provided above signifies the major co-morbidities of interest.
- Of particular note are HIV disease—in which myocarditis may be caused by direct viral infection; associated opportunistic infections, such as toxoplasmosis; or related disorders, such as Kaposi's sarcoma—and malignancies treated with doxorubicin or anthracyclines, which are particularly cardiotoxic.
- Lyme disease is complicated by myocarditis in about 10 % of cases.
- Chagas' disease bears mention because it is one of the most common forms of heart disease in Central and South America. Most patients with this infection (cased by the protozoan *Trypanosoma cruzi*) develop chronic cardiomyopathy and heart failure without an acute phase of myocarditis, but it should still be considered in migrants from or visitors to endemic areas.
- Because viral etiologies of myocarditis are common, it should be remembered that patients may give a history of a recent febrile illness, either upper respiratory or gastrointestinal.

Pitfalls in Diagnosis

Critical Steps Not to Miss

- Failing to consider the diagnosis of myocarditis, especially in patients with more severe presentations, may be costly. The disease may be mistaken for ACS, viral syndrome, pneumonia, and fatigue associated with co-morbid conditions.

Mimics

- Many of the mimics and causes of myocarditis are themselves treatable. Preoccupation with such management may lead the clinician to overlook the specific myocardial involvement.

Time-Dependent Interventions

- Patients who present with fulminant heart failure, symptoms consistent with ACS, a pneumonia-like syndrome, or significant arrhythmias must be quickly evaluated and stabilized as the work-up proceeds.

Overall Principles of Treatment

- Treatment of myocarditis is in large part dependent on the cause. Usually—but not always—treating the etiology improves the patient's myocardial function.
- Treat infections if possible (with viral myocarditis, only supportive therapy may be feasible)
- Remove the offending agent/drug if it can be identified
- Treat heart failure, if present, with diuretics, nitrates, and inotropes as needed.

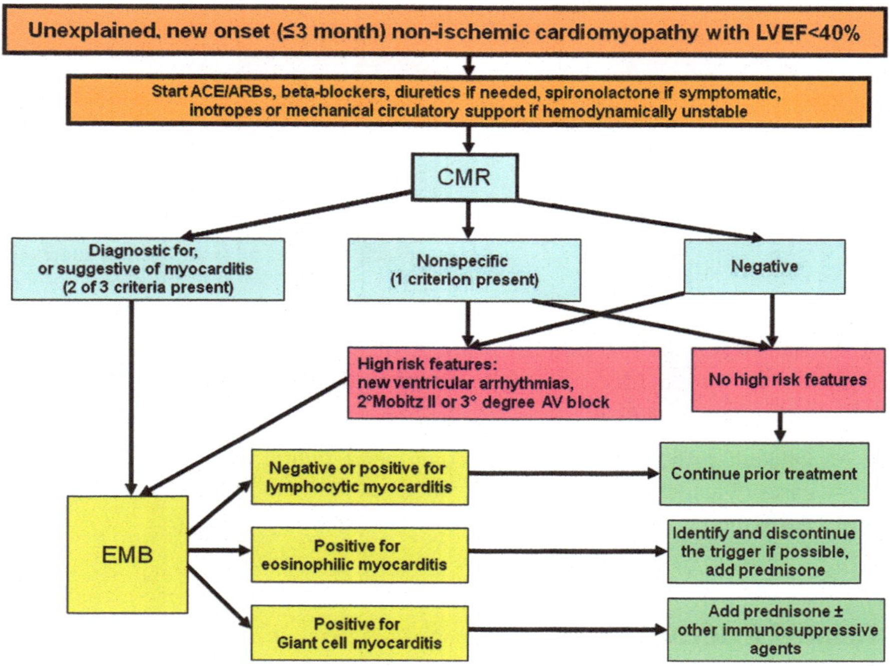

Algorithm for diagnostic work-up and treatment of myocarditis. CMR cardiac magnetic resonance, LVEF left ventricular ejection fraction, EMB endomyocardial biopsy. [Guglin M, Nallamshetty L. Myocarditis: diagnosis and treatment. Curr Treat Options Cardiovasc Med. 2012 Dec;14(6): 637-51; https://doi.org/10.1007/s11936-012-0204-7; Published: 2012-12-01] *Caption adapted from original*

- Specific antiarrhythmic therapy is usually not helpful, but if arrhythmias persist after correction of any oxygenation and electrolyte derangements, antiarrhythmics may be used. Digoxin is not recommended in the treatment of myocarditis.

Disease Course

- Myocarditis is a self-limited disease in most cases.

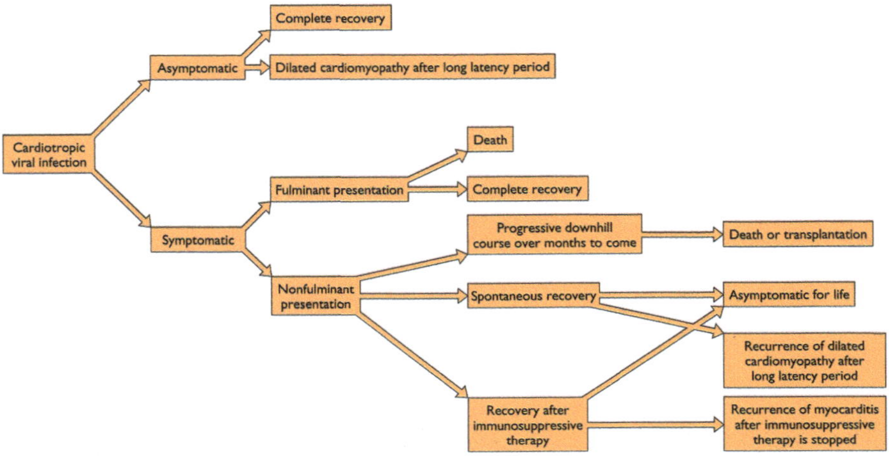

Natural history of human myocarditis [Herskowitz A, Ansari A. Myocarditis. In: Abelmann WH, editor. Cardiomyopathies, myocarditis, and pericardial disease. Philadelphia: Current Medicine; 1996. (Braunwald E, editor. Atlas of heart diseases; vol. 2).] *Caption from original*

- Dilated cardiomyopathy and chronic heart failure may result from severe cases of acute myocarditis.
- Arrhythmias associated with myocarditis can rarely be fatal.

Related Evidence

Papers of particular interest have been highlighted as:
*** Of key importance*

Practice Guidelines

CS Joint Working Group. Guidelines for diagnosis and treatment of myocarditis (JCS 2009): digest version. Circ J. 2011;75(3):734-43. PMID: 21304213. http://www.ncbi.nlm.nih.gov/pubmed/21304213 **

Review

Thiene G, Bruneval P, Veinot J, Leone O. Diagnostic use of the endomyocardial biopsy: a consensus statement. Virchows Arch. 2013 Jul;463(1):1-5. https://doi.org/10.1007/s00428-013-1430-4. PMID: 23748875. http://www.ncbi.nlm.nih.gov/pubmed/23748875

Elamm C, Fairweather D, Cooper LT. Pathogenesis and diagnosis of myocarditis. Heart. 2012 Jun;98(11):835-40. https://doi.org/10.1136/heartjnl-2012-301686. PMID: 22442199. http://www.ncbi.nlm.nih.gov/pubmed/22442199 **

Kühl U, Schultheiss HP. Myocarditis: early biopsy allows for tailored regenerative treatment. Dtsch Arztebl Int. 2012 May;109(20):361-8. https://doi.org/10.3238/arztebl.2012.0361. PMID: 22685492. http://www.ncbi.nlm.nih.gov/pubmed/22685492

Kindermann I, Barth C, Mahfoud F, Ukena C, Lenski M, Yilmaz A, Klingel K, Kandolf R, Sechtem U, Cooper LT, Böhm M. Update on myocarditis. J Am Coll Cardiol. 2012 Feb 28;59(9):779-92. https://doi.org/10.1016/j.jacc.2011.09.074. PMID: 22361396. http://www.ncbi.nlm.nih.gov/pubmed/22361396 **

Sagar S, Liu PP, Cooper LT Jr. Myocarditis. Lancet. 2012 Feb 25;379(9817):738-47. https://doi.org/10.1016/S0140-6736(11)60648-X. PMID: 22185868. http://www.ncbi.nlm.nih.gov/pubmed/22185868

Simpson KE, Canter CE. Acute myocarditis in children. Expert Rev Cardiovasc Ther. 2011 Jun;9(6):771-83. https://doi.org/10.1586/erc.11.70. PMID: 21714608. http://www.ncbi.nlm.nih.gov/pubmed/21714608 **

Kühl U, Schultheiss HP. Myocarditis in children. Heart Fail Clin. 2010 Oct;6(4):483-96, viii-ix. https://doi.org/10.1016/j.hfc.2010.05.009. PMID: 20869648. http://www.ncbi.nlm.nih.gov/pubmed/20869648 **

Blauwet LA, Cooper LT. Myocarditis. Prog Cardiovasc Dis. 2010 Jan-Feb;52(4):274-88. https://doi.org/10.1016/j.pcad.2009.11.006. PMID: 20109598. http://www.ncbi.nlm.nih.gov/pubmed/20109598 **

Magnani JW, Dec GW. Myocarditis: current trends in diagnosis and treatment. Circulation. 2006 Feb 14;113(6):876-90. PMID: 16476862. http://www.ncbi.nlm.nih.gov/pubmed/16476862 **

Use PubMed Clinical Queries to find the most recent evidence. Use this search strategy:

"Myocarditis"[Mesh] OR "myocarditis"

Chapter 51
Neuromuscular Disease: Myasthenia Gravis, Guillain-Barré, Amyotrophic Lateral Sclerosis

Charles V. Pollack, Jr. and Jaime Friel Blanck

Name and Synonyms

Neuromuscular Disease, inclusive of:

- myasthenia gravis (MG)
- Guillain-Barre syndrome (GBS)
- amyotrophic lateral sclerosis (ALS) or Lou Gehrig's Disease

This diverse group of neurologic diseases can, through different mechanisms, cause disordered breathing. MG is a disease of the neuromuscular junction, GBS is a demyelinating neuropathy, and ALS is a motor-neuron degenerative disorder.

Incidence/Epidemiology

- MG has an incidence of around 20/100,000 patients. Women are affected more commonly than men, with the typical MG patients being females in their 20s and 30s and males in their 50s and 60s.
- GBS is rare, with an incidence of about 1/100,000 patients. Males are more commonly affected than females, and the incidence increases with age. There have also been occasional transient increases in incidence attributable to the use of specific influenza vaccines.
- ALS is rare, with an incidence of fewer than 3/100,000 patients. Males are somewhat more frequently affected than females.

C. V. Pollack, Jr. (✉)
Department of Emergency Medicine, Thomas Jefferson University, Philadelphia, PA, USA

J. F. Blanck
Welch Medical Library, Johns Hopkins University, Baltimore, MD, USA

C. V. Pollack, Jr. (ed.), *Differential Diagnosis of Cardiopulmonary Disease*,
https://doi.org/10.1007/978-3-319-63895-9_51

Differential Diagnosis

- The differential diagnosis for MG includes
  - Botulism
  - Multiple sclerosis (MS)
  - Lambert-Eaton Syndrome

Feature	Myasthenia gravis	Eaton–Lambert syndrome
Most commonly associated malignancy	Thymoma (40%)	Small cell lung cancer (1–3%)
Antibody target	Acetylcholine receptor	Voltage-gated calcium channel
Area of NMJ affected	Postsynaptic membrane	Presynaptic membrane
Common presenting feature	Ocular and bulbar weakness	Limb weakness, oculomotor sparing
Ocular and bulbar muscle involvement	Common	Rare
Autonomic dysfunction	None	Common
Deep tendon reflexes	Normal	Reduced
Strength improved by	Rest, sleep	Exercise

Myasthenia gravis vs. Lambert–Eaton syndrome. [Chelico L, McRae K. Thymic Surgery and Paraendocrine Syndromes. In: Slinger, MD, FRCPC P, editor. Principles and Practice of Anesthesia for Thoracic Surgery [Internet]. New York, NY: Springer New York; 2011 [cited 2016 Mar 29]. p. 211–23. Available from: http://link.springer.com/10.1007/978-1-4419-0184-2_15] *Caption from original*

- The differential diagnosis for GBS includes
  - Botulism
  - MG
  - MS
  - Spinal cord tumor
  - Lyme disease
- The differential diagnosis for ALS includes
  - Spinal cord disease/tumor/compression
  - Myopathy
  - Lead or mercury poisoning

Pathophysiology and Etiology

- MG is characterized by weakness and rapid fatigability of skeletal muscle. It is a result of ineffective nerve firing activity at the neuromuscular junction (NMJ), which in turn is caused by a decrease in the number of available acetylcholine (ACh) receptors. ACh is the neurotransmitter at the NMJ, and the receptors are decreased in number because of an antibody-mediated autoimmune disorder.

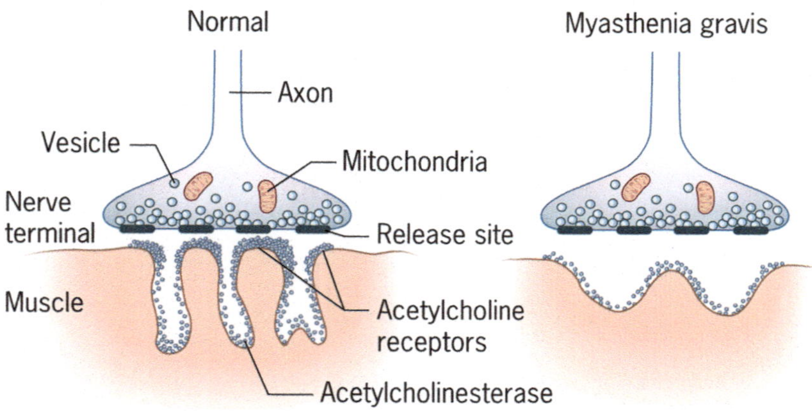

Myasthenia gravis. Myasthenia gravis affects approximately 25,000 patients or 50 to 125 cases per million. Features of myasthenia gravis are weakness (focal or generalized) and skeletal and muscle fatigability, which generally increases with repeated activity and improves with rest. An example is ptosis, which is improved with 3 minutes of eye closure (rest). Approximately three quarters of patients with myasthenia gravis have abnormalities of the thymus (thymic lymphoid hyperplasia [85%] or thymoma [15%]). A thymectomy frequently improves the symptoms of myasthenia gravis, but this has been more common in patients with hyperplasia than with thymoma. [Loehrer Sr, P. Henley, J. Johnson, D. Chapter 30. In: Markman, M, editor: Volume 3: Atlas of Cancer. 1 edition. Philadelphia: Current Medicine Group; 2002. ISBN: 0-7817-4280-3] *Caption adapted from original*

- GBS is a demyelinating neuropathy. Myelin is a protein that covers nerve sheaths and greatly increases nerve conduction velocities. GBS is a "polyneuropathy," meaning that many peripheral nerves in the body are affected. The muscles at the periphery—in the hands and feet—are affected first, because the nerve sheaths supplying them are the longest, and therefore the problems with "insulation" are more pronounced there. This is probably an autoimmune process, but the specific etiology remains obscure.
- ALS is the most common form of progressive and likely the most devastating of the motor neuron diseases. ALS gradually affects both upper motor neurons (motor cortex and corticospinal cells) and lower motor neurons (anterior

horn cells in the spinal cord and brainstem motor cells that innervate the bulbar muscles). As these nerve cells die, the innervated muscle fibers atrophy and lose function.

Presentation

Typical/"Classic"

- MG typically presents with:
  - Extraocular muscle weakness leading to ptosis.

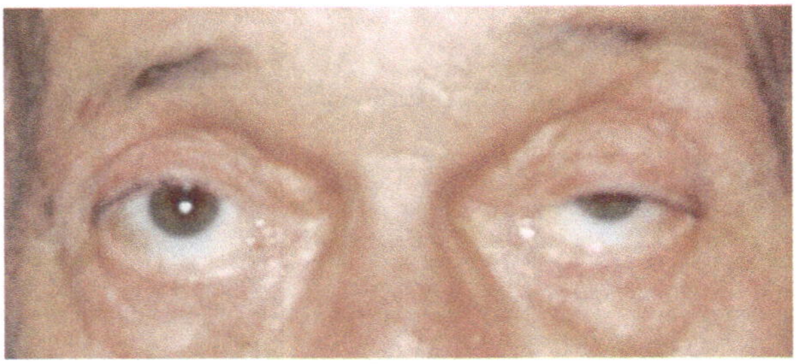

Left-sided ptosis in a patient with myasthenia gravis before initiation of therapy with cholinergic drugs and immunosuppressants. [Finsterer J. Ptosis: Causes, Presentation, and Management. Aesthetic Plastic Surgery. 2003 Jun 1;27(3):193–204.] *Caption from original*

- Bulbar and facial muscle weakness.
- Inability to hold head up.
- Easy fatigability of routine and repetitive tasks.
- Exacerbations of this chronic disease may be prompted by such diverse stimuli as:
  - Acute illness
  - Medications
  - Emotional stress
  - Menstruation
  - Immunization
- GBS typically presents with the following characteristics:
  - "Ascending weakness"; that is, feet before hands, and then extremities toward trunk. The cranial nerves are usually affected later in the course, leading to double vision and difficulties speaking and swallowing.

  - Ultimately, in severe cases, patients are quadriplegic and have ventilatory failure.
  - Most patients complain of numbness or burning paresthesias prior to the onset of weakness.
  - More than half of patients with GBS complain of severe pain, especially in proximal muscle groups.
  - Autonomic nerves are often involved as GBS progresses, leading to orthostatic hypotension, tachy- or bradycardia, and facial flushing.
  - Cardiac arrhythmias may develop.
  - There is usually a benign viral prodrome 2–4 weeks before the onset of weakness.

- ALS typically presents with:

  - Progressive loss of strength and function.
  - Limb involvement first, then with bulbar involvement (the latter manifests as difficulty swallowing and voice changes).
  - "Pseudobulbar" manifestations—exaggerated emotions, sometimes inappropriate emotional responses.

Atypical Presentations

- MG may sometimes present with:

  - Isolated muscle weakness and no extraocular or bulbar involvement.
  - Acute respiratory failure without preceding ocular or bulbar worsening.

- GBS may sometimes present with:

  - Weakness in the cranial nerves *prior to* the extremities. This is called the Miller-Fisher variant of GBS.
  - Asymmetric or incomplete weakness, which may delay consideration of the diagnosis.
  - No history of viral prodrome or influenza vaccination.

- ALS may sometimes present with:

  - Bulbar involvement preceding limb involvement.
  - Numbness and paresthesias (sensory function is ordinarily preserved in ALS).

Primary Differential Considerations

- These are unusual diseases. The differential diagnosis for each is usually limited to other neural or neuromuscular diseases as described above. These patients do not ordinarily present with primary cardiorespiratory symptoms.

History and Physical Exam

Findings That Confirm Diagnosis

- The diagnosis of MG is confirmed with laboratory demonstration of antibodies to acetylcholine receptors. Electromyography (EMG) and nerve conduction studies (NCS) are also used to confirm the diagnosis.
- The edrophonium test can be performed at the bedside and has reasonably high sensitivity.

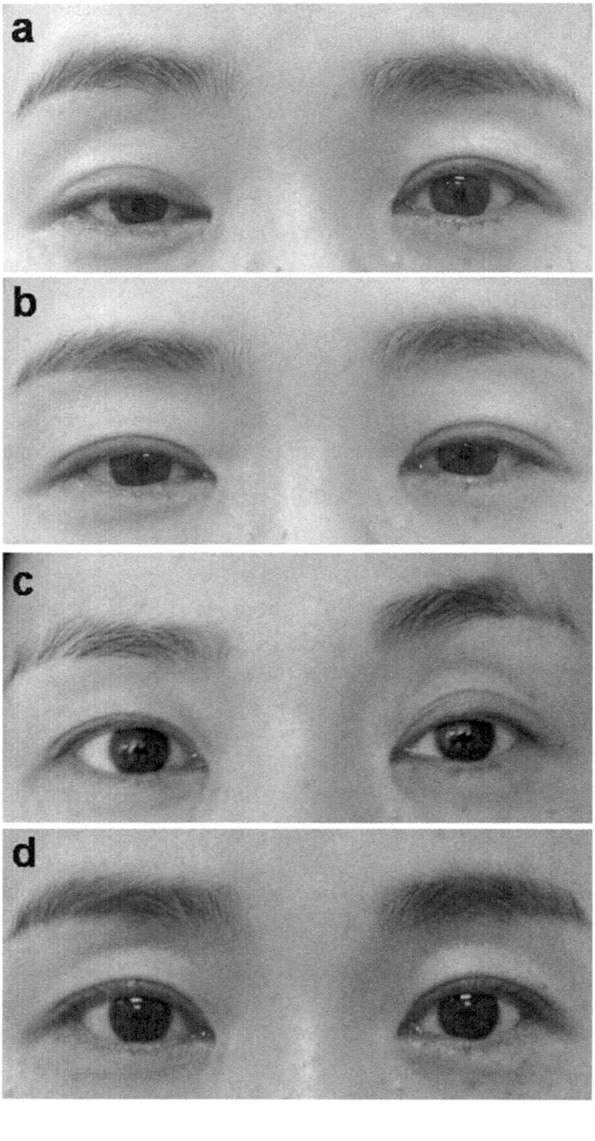

Ptosis in a patient with ocular myasthenia gravis. The patient showed right ptosis when referred to our hospital (a). Edrophonium injection improved right ptosis and induced minor left ptosis (b). After intravenous methylprednisolone therapy, right ptosis was satisfactorily relieved, however, left ptosis got appeared (c). Left ptosis was resolved after 1-month observation without additional immunosuppressive therapy (d)[Nishijima H, Ueno T, Suzuki C, Baba M, Tomiyama M. Eyelid ptosis enhanced after steroid pulse therapy in ocular myasthenia gravis: a case report. Neurological Sciences. 2015 Jun;36(6):1055–6.] *Caption from original*

- On physical exam the disease is characterized by weakness in repetitive activities that improves with rest.
- The “ice bag test” for ptosis may be used to evaluate for MG.
- The diagnosis of GBS cannot be confirmed at the bedside. EMG and NCS are helpful, as is evaluation of the cerebrospinal fluid.
- The diagnosis of ALS is often challenging. EMG and NCS are useful. There are no confirmatory bedside tests.

Factors That Suggest Diagnosis

- MG:
  - Positive edrophonium test
  - Positive ice-bag test
  - Ptosis in the absence of thyroid disease
  - Ventilator capacity can be assessed by testing negative inspiratory force (NIF)
- GBS:
  - Symmetric ascending weakness
  - Viral-like prodrome or immunization 2-4 weeks prior to onset of weakness

Viral infections	
	Cytomegalovirus
	Influenza
	Parainfluenza
	Epstein-Barr virus
	Cocksackie
	Echo
	Measles
	Mumps
	Rubella
	Herpes simplex virus
	Herpes Zoster virus
	Hepatitis A and B virus
	Human immunodeficiency virus
Bacterial and other infections	
	Campylobacter jejuni
	Mycoplasma pneumoniae
	Typhoid
	Shigella
	Legionella pneumonia
	Cyclospora
Systemic illnesses	
	Hodgkin's lymphoma
	Thyroid disease
	Addison's disease
	Leukemia
	Paraproteinemia
	Solid tumors (lung cancer)
	Sarcoidosis
	Systemic lupus erythematosus
	Surgery
	Trauma
	Vaccination
	Pregnancy

Antecedent illnesses associated with Guillain-Barré syndrome. [Piccione EA, Salame K, Katirji B. Guillain-Barré Syndrome and Related Disorders. In: Katirji B, Kaminski HJ, Ruff RL, editors. Neuromuscular Disorders in Clinical Practice [Internet]. New York, NY: Springer New York; 2014 [cited 2016 Mar 29]. p. 573–603. Available from: http://link.springer.com/10.1007/978-1-4614-6567-6_28] *Caption from original*

- ALS:
  - "slapping gait"
  - Involuntary emotional exaggerations

	Tongue strength				p
	Abnormal (n = 20) median (range)/ n (%)		Normal (n = 34) median (range)/ n (%)		
Sex (male)	7	(35)	18	(51)	0.26*
Onset site (bulbar)	13	(65)	6	(18)	<0.00*
Bulbar symptoms (presence)	17	(85)	9	(32)	<0.00*
Bulbar signs (presence)	15	(75)	5	(15)	<0.00*
Gastrostomy (presence)	12	(60)	14	(41)	0.09*
MPT (<10 sec)[a]	6	(35)	5	(17)	0.28*
Age at diagnosis (year)	66.0	(20.0–80.0)	63.5	(40.0–79.0)	0.52**
Time from symptoms to diagnosis (month)	12.0	(6.0–60.0)	10.0	(4.0–60.0)	0.70**

Clinical and demographic characteristics of the 54 patients with amyotrophic lateral sclerosis [From article: Prognostic value of decreased tongue strength on survival time in patients with amyotrophic lateral sclerosis. Journal of Neurology. 2012 Nov;259(11):2360–5. https://doi.org/10.1007/s00415-012-6503-9, at http://link.springer.com/article/10.1007%2Fs00415-012-6503-9; by J. G. Weikamp, H. J. Schelhaas, J. C. M. Hendriks, B. J. M. de Swart, A. C. H. Geurts, © The Author(s) 2012; licensed under Creative Commons Attribution License BY 2.0 http://creativecommons.org/licenses/by/2.0] *Caption from original*

Factors That Exclude Diagnosis

- In patients with weakness, no historical or physical examination factors can completely exclude these diagnoses at all stages.

Ancillary Studies

Laboratory

- For MG:
  - Ordinary baseline lab studies are not helpful.
  - Serologic testing for antibodies to ACh receptors should be performed.

- For GBS:
  - Ordinary baseline lab studies are not helpful.
  - Evaluate cerebrospinal fluid (from lumbar puncture) for protein levels, which are ordinarily high (unless patient has HIV) in GBS.
  - Liver function tests are abnormal in one-third to one-half of GBS patients.
- For ALS:
  - Ordinary baseline lab studies are not helpful.

Imaging

- MG:
  - Chest radiography or CT chest may show a thymoma. A normal chest radiograph does not exclude MG.
- GBS:
  - MRI with gadolinium contrast may show enhancement at the nerve root, but this is not a consistent finding in patients diagnosed with GBS.
- ALS:
  - Imaging studies are needed only to exclude other etiologies of weakness.

Other

- MG:
  - As above, the following tests are potentially useful:
  - Ice-pack test
  - EMG
  - NCS
  - serology
- GBS:
  - Serology
  - Lumbar puncture
  - EMG
  - NCS
- ALS:
  - Genetic testing (familial in a small number of cases)
  - EMG
  - NCS

Special Populations

Age

- MG:
  - MG can occur at any age.
  - It typically occurs earlier in females than males.
- GBS:
  - Incidence increases with increasing age
- ALS:
  - Slightly more common in men than in women.

Co-morbidities

- MG:
  - The most common co-morbidities are thyroid disease, lupus, and rheumatoid arthritis.
- GBS:
  - The most common co-morbidities are COPD, diabetes, and obesity.
- ALS:
  - The most common co-morbidity is cardiovascular disease.

Pitfalls in Diagnosis

Critical Steps Not to Miss

- These are unusual diseases. Early consideration to the diagnosis should be given or it may be missed on multiple presentations.

Mimics

- Other neuropathies
- Other neuromuscular disorders
- Botulism

Time-Dependent Interventions

- Time-dependent interventions are present only in the rare case of presentation with ventilator failure.

C	Conduction block, bradycardia, asystole
R	Rapid progression of motor weakness
I	Infection
T	Tachyarrhythmias
I	Intensive care monitoring of respiratory and autonomic dysfunction
C	Complications of critical illness: pulmonary embolism, myocardial infarction
A	Airway: ventilatory failure, bulbar weakness
L	Labile blood pressure: hypertension/hypotension

The word "critical" is used as a mnemonic for the different indications

Clinical Indications for admission to the ICU in patients with Guillain-Barré Syndrome [Cordova FC, Lim MRC, Criner GJ. Neuromyopathies in the Critically Ill. In: Criner GJ, Barnette RE, D'Alonzo GE, editors. Critical Care Study Guide [Internet]. New York, NY: Springer New York; 2010 [cited 2016 Mar 29]. p. 541–70. Available from: http://link.springer.com/10.1007/978-0-387-77452-7_29] *Caption from original*

Overall Principles of Treatment

- MG:
  - MG is a chronic disease.
  - Symptoms can be generally managed with anticholinesterase medications and immunosuppressants.
  - Plasmapherseis can be used in severe or recurrent exacerbations.
  - Thymectomy may be considered.
  - Intravenous immunoglobulin is generally beneficial
- GBS:
  - GBS is generally managed with support only, although this may entail prolonged mechanical ventilation.
- ALS:
  - Treatment of ALS is supportive.

Disease Course

- MG:
  - With close medical management, MG can generally be well tolerated by patients.
- GBS:
  - The course of GBS may be prolonged, but patients usually substantially recover.
- ALS:
  - ALS is an inexorably fatal disease.

Related Evidence

Papers of particular interest have been highlighted as:
*** Of key importance*

Review

Ansar V, Valadi N. Guillain-Barré syndrome. Prim Care. 2015 Jun;42(2):189-93. https://doi.org/10.1016/j.pop.2015.01.001. Epub 2015 Mar 20. Review. PubMed PMID: 25979580. http://www.ncbi.nlm.nih.gov/pubmed/25979580 **

Sussman J, Farrugia ME, Maddison P, Hill M, Leite MI, Hilton-Jones D. Myasthenia gravis: Association of British Neurologists' management guidelines. Pract Neurol. 2015 Jun;15(3):199-206. https://doi.org/10.1136/practneurol-2015-001126. Review. PubMed PMID: 25977271. http://www.ncbi.nlm.nih.gov/pubmed/25977271

Valadi N. Evaluation and management of amyotrophic lateral sclerosis. Prim Care. 2015 Jun;42(2):177-87. https://doi.org/10.1016/j.pop.2015.01.009. Epub 2015 Apr 7. Review. PubMed PMID: 25979579. http://www.ncbi.nlm.nih.gov/pubmed/25979579 **

Verstraete E, Foerster BR. Neuroimaging as a New Diagnostic Modality in Amyotrophic Lateral Sclerosis. Neurotherapeutics. 2015 Apr;12(2):403-16. https://doi.org/10.1007/s13311-015-0347-9. Review. PubMed PMID: 25791072; PubMed Central PMCID: PMC4404464. http://www.ncbi.nlm.nih.gov/pubmed/25791072

Wakerley BR, Yuki N. Mimics and chameleons in Guillain-Barré and Miller Fisher syndromes. Pract Neurol. 2015 Apr;15(2):90-9. https://doi.org/10.1136/practneurol-2014-000937. Epub 2014 Sep 19. Review. PubMed PMID: 25239628. http://www.ncbi.nlm.nih.gov/pubmed/25239628

Bucchia M, Ramirez A, Parente V, Simone C, Nizzardo M, Magri F, Dametti S, Corti S. Therapeutic development in amyotrophic lateral sclerosis. Clin Ther. 2015 Mar 1;37(3):668-80. https://doi.org/10.1016/j.clinthera.2014.12.020. Epub 2015 Feb 7. Review. PubMed PMID: 25666449. http://www.ncbi.nlm.nih.gov/pubmed/25666449

Turner MR, Swash M. The expanding syndrome of amyotrophic lateral sclerosis: a gclinical and molecular odyssey. J Neurol Neurosurg Psychiatry. 2015 Jun;86(6):667-73. https://doi.org/10.1136/jnnp-2014-308946. Epub 2015 Feb 2. Review. PubMed PMID: 25644224; PubMed Central PMCID: PMC4453495. http://www.ncbi.nlm.nih.gov/pubmed/25635517

Malik R, Lui A, Lomen-Hoerth C. Amyotrophic lateral sclerosis. Semin Neurol. 2014 Nov;34(5):534-41. https://doi.org/10.1055/s-0034-1396007. Epub 2014 Dec 17. Review. PubMed PMID: 25520025. http://www.ncbi.nlm.nih.gov/pubmed/25520025 **

Gilhus NE, Nacu A, Andersen JB, Owe JF. Myasthenia gravis and risks for comorbidity. Eur J Neurol. 2015 Jan;22(1):17-23. https://doi.org/10.1111/ene.12599. Epub 2014 Oct 30. Review. PubMed PMID: 25354676. http://www.ncbi.nlm.nih.gov/pubmed/25354676

Tiryaki E, Horak HA. ALS and other motor neuron diseases. Continuum (Minneap Minn). 2014 Oct;20(5 Peripheral Nervous System Disorders):1185-207. https://doi.org/10.1212/01.CON.0000455886.14298.a4. Review. PubMed PMID: 25299277. http://www.ncbi.nlm.nih.gov/pubmed/25299277 **

van den Berg B, Walgaard C, Drenthen J, Fokke C, Jacobs BC, van Doorn PA. Guillain-Barré syndrome: pathogenesis, diagnosis, treatment and prognosis. Nat Rev Neurol. 2014 Aug;10(8):469-82. https://doi.org/10.1038/nrneurol.2014.121. Epub 2014 Jul 15. Review. PubMed PMID: 25023340. http://www.ncbi.nlm.nih.gov/pubmed/25023340 **

Eldar AH, Chapman J. Guillain Barré syndrome and other immune mediated neuropathies: diagnosis and classification. Autoimmun Rev. 2014 Apr-May;13(4-5):525-30. https://doi.org/10.1016/j.autrev.2014.01.033. Epub 2014 Jan 13. Review. PubMed PMID: 24434363. http://www.ncbi.nlm.nih.gov/pubmed/24434363

Berrih-Aknin S, Frenkian-Cuvelier M, Eymard B. Diagnostic and clinical classification of autoimmune myasthenia gravis. J Autoimmun. 2014 Feb-Mar;48-49:143-8. https://doi.org/10.1016/j.jaut.2014.01.003. Epub 2014 Feb 13. Review. PubMed PMID: 24530233. http://www.ncbi.nlm.nih.gov/pubmed/24530233 **

Sieb JP. Myasthenia gravis: an update for the clinician. Clin Exp Immunol. 2014 Mar;175(3):408-18. https://doi.org/10.1111/cei.12217. Review. PubMed PMID: 24117026; PubMed Central PMCID: PMC3927901. http://www.ncbi.nlm.nih.gov/pubmed/24117026 **

Xiao J, Simard AR, Shi FD, Hao J. New strategies in the management of Guillain-Barré syndrome. Clin Rev Allergy Immunol. 2014 Dec;47(3):274-88. https://doi.

org/10.1007/s12016-013-8388-5. Review. PubMed PMID: 24057598. http://www.ncbi.nlm.nih.gov/pubmed/24057598

Al-Chalabi A, Hardiman O. The epidemiology of ALS: a conspiracy of genes, environment and time. Nat Rev Neurol. 2013 Nov;9(11):617-28. https://doi.org/10.1038/nrneurol.2013.203. Epub 2013 Oct 15. Review. PubMed PMID: 24126629. http://www.ncbi.nlm.nih.gov/pubmed/24126629

Le Panse R, Berrih-Aknin S. Autoimmune myasthenia gravis: autoantibody mechanisms and new developments on immune regulation. Curr Opin Neurol. 2013 Oct;26(5):569-76. https://doi.org/10.1097/WCO.0b013e328364d6cd. Review. PubMed PMID: 23995274. http://www.ncbi.nlm.nih.gov/pubmed/23995274 **

Godoy DA, Mello LJ, Masotti L, Di Napoli M. The myasthenic patient in crisis: an update of the management in Neurointensive Care Unit. Arq Neuropsiquiatr. 2013 Sep;71(9A):627-39. https://doi.org/10.1590/0004-282X20130108. Review. PubMed PMID: 24141444. http://www.ncbi.nlm.nih.gov/pubmed/24141444 **

Walling AD, Dickson G. Guillain-Barré syndrome. Am Fam Physician. 2013 Feb 1;87(3):191-7. Review. PubMed PMID: 23418763. http://www.ncbi.nlm.nih.gov/pubmed/23418763 **

Kiernan MC, Vucic S, Cheah BC, Turner MR, Eisen A, Hardiman O, Burrell JR, Zoing MC. Amyotrophic lateral sclerosis. Lancet. 2011 Mar 12;377(9769):942-55. https://doi.org/10.1016/S0140-6736(10)61156-7. Epub 2011 Feb 4. Review. PubMed PMID: 21296405. http://www.ncbi.nlm.nih.gov/pubmed/21296405 **

Mao ZF, Mo XA, Qin C, Lai YR, Olde Hartman TC. Course and prognosis of myasthenia gravis: a systematic review. Eur J Neurol. 2010 Jul;17(7):913-21. https://doi.org/10.1111/j.1468-1331.2010.03017.x. Epub 2010 Apr 12. Review. PubMed PMID: 20402761. http://www.ncbi.nlm.nih.gov/pubmed/20402761

Use PubMed Clinical Queries to find the most recent evidence. Use this search strategy: “Neuromuscular Diseases”[tiab] OR “neuromuscular disease”[tiab] “Myasthenia Gravis”[Mesh] OR “Amyotrophic Lateral Sclerosis”[Mesh] OR “Guillain-Barre Syndrome”[Mesh] OR “Myasthenia Gravis” OR “Amyotrophic Lateral Sclerosis” OR “Guillain-Barre Syndrome”

Chapter 52
Noncardiogenic Pulmonary Edema

Charles V. Pollack, Jr., Melissa Platt, Richard M. Cantor, and Victoria G. Riese

Name and Synonyms

Noncardiogenic Pulmonary Edema (NCPE)

- Acute respiratory distress syndrome (ARDS), high-altitude pulmonary edema, neurogenic pulmonary edema, reperfusion pulmonary edema, re-expansion pulmonary edema

Incidence/Epidemiology

- Less common than cardiogenic pulmonary edema
- ARDS incidence is uncertain but has been on the decline.
- Overall mortality is 50–75 % and prognosis varies with the patient's age, the cause of ARDS, and the number of organs involved.
- No single variable has been found to predict patient outcome.
- Even the degree of hypoxemia has not been valuable in this regard.

C. V. Pollack, Jr. (✉)
Department of Emergency Medicine, Thomas Jefferson University, Philadelphia, PA, USA

M. Platt
Department of Emergency Medicine, University of Louisville, Louisville, KY, USA

R. M. Cantor
Department of Emergency Medicine and Pediatrics, State University of New York Upstate Medical University, Syracuse, NY, USA

V. G. Riese
Librarian Consultant, Eldersburg, MD, USA

C. V. Pollack, Jr. (ed.), *Differential Diagnosis of Cardiopulmonary Disease*,
https://doi.org/10.1007/978-3-319-63895-9_52

Differential Diagnosis

- Cardiogenic pulmonary edema
- High-altitude pulmonary edema
- Neurogenic pulmonary edema
- Reperfusion pulmonary edema
- Re-expansion pulmonary edema
- Opioid overdose
- Salicylate toxicity
- Pulmonary embolism
- Viral infections
- Pulmonary veno-occlusive disease
- Eclampsia
- Inhaled toxins
- Aspiration
- Disseminated intravascular coagulation
- Acute hemorrhagic pancreatitis
- Sepsis
- Smoke inhalation
- Oxygen toxicity

Pathophysiology and Etiology

- The clinical coincidence of bilateral alveolar infiltrates causing hypoxemia in the absence of pneumonia or congestive heart failure
- It is caused by various disorders responsible for protein and fluid accumulation in the alveoli.
- Unlike cardiogenic pulmonary edema, it is not caused by high pulmonary capillary pressure.
- Most common mechanism is an increase in pulmonary capillary permeability and elevated intravascular pressure.
- The major cause of NCPE is ARDS, followed by high-altitude and neurogenic pulmonary edema.
- A subset of NCPE, neurogenic pulmonary edema, may occur after seizure or stroke and is thought to be centrally mediated.

Presentation

Typical/"Classic"

- Patients classically present with profound dyspnea and diaphoresis.
- Onset often is sudden.

- Anxiety due to hypoxemia.
- Cough is common.
- Tachypnea and tachycardia.

Atypical

- Gradual onset (over 24 hours) is less common.
- Patients may complain only of paroxysmal nocturnal dyspnea or orthopnea.
- Chest pain more predominant than dyspnea would be atypical but has been reported.

Primary Differential Considerations

- Myocardial ischemia
- Pneumothorax
- Pulmonary edema of other causes (cardiogenic, neurogenic)
- Pulmonary embolism
- ARDS

History and Physical Exam

Findings That Confirm Diagnosis

- There are no clinical findings that confirm NCPE specifically; it is a combined clinical and radiographic diagnosis.

Factors That Suggest Diagnosis

- Earliest sign is increased respiratory rate.
- Shortness of breath is the most common symptom.
- A pulmonary artery wedge pressure less than 18 mm Hg favors NCPE over cardiogenic pulmonary edema.
- NCPE usually has bounding pulses, no gallop, and no jugular venous distention.
- Fine inspiratory rales are noted.
- Cough with frothy sputum may be present.

Factors That Exclude Diagnosis

- No clinical findings can exclude NCPE, but clear lung fields on auscultation make it unlikely.

Ancillary Studies

Laboratory

- B-type natriuretic peptide (BNP) has been used to distinguish heart failure from lung disease.
  - Intermediate values are not helpful.
  - Role of biomarker in pulmonary edema has limited utility.
- In NCPE, the ratio of pulmonary edema fluid protein to plasma protein concentration is 0.7 or greater.

Electrocardiography

- Usually does not show signs of ischemia

Imaging

- Chest x-ray:
  - Usually a normal cardiac silhouette.
  - Bilateral pulmonary edema, frequently in a "butterfly" pattern, is a consistent finding.
  - Air bronchograms often are seen, but Kerley lines are not.

Cardiogenic	Noncardiogenic
Lower lobes	Peripheral
Perihilar	Patchy
No air bronchograms	Air bronchograms
Large heart and vascular pedicle	No cardiovascular enlargement
May be asymmetric in COPD	May be asymmetric in COPD*

*chronic obstructive pulmonary disease

Chest radiograph in cardiogenic versus noncardiogenic pulmonary edema. [Vilar J, Andreu J. The lung parenchyma: radiological presentation of alveolar pattern. In: Coche EE, Ghaye B, de Mey J, Duyck P, editors. Comparative interpretation of CT and standard radiography of the chest [Internet]. Berlin Heidelberg: Springer; 2011 [cited 2015 Aug 13]. p. 221–45. Available from: http://link.springer.com/10.1007/978-3-540-79942-9_9] *Caption from original*

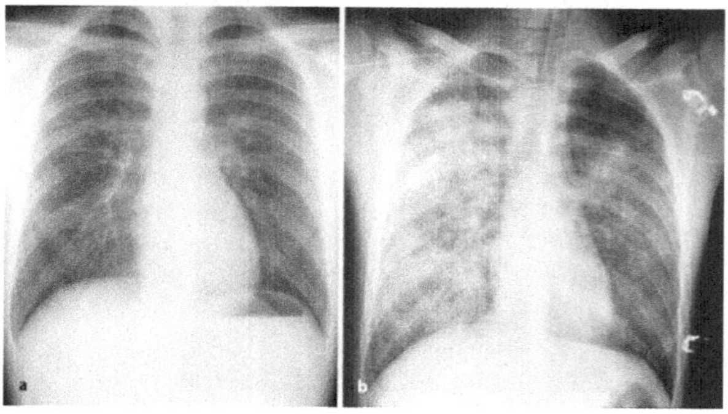

a. ARDS stage I. b. ARDS stage II. [Häuser H, Wohlgemuth WA. Bildgebende diagnostik des thorax bei intensivpatienten. Der Anaesthesist. 2005 Aug;54(8):827–48.]

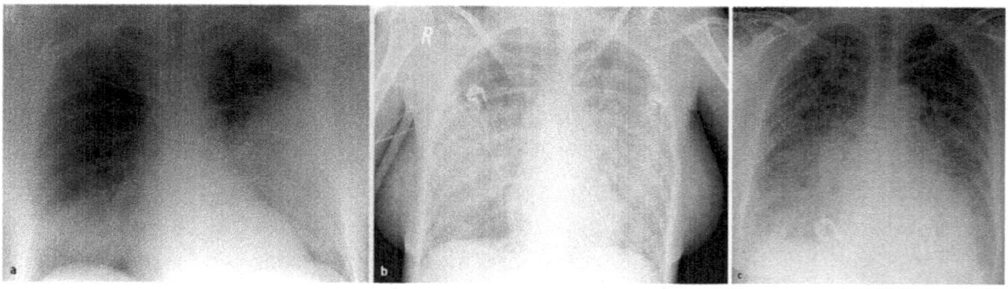

The most common causes of hypoxemic ARI: a severe, community-acquired pneumonia; b ARDS during sepsis; c cardiogenic pulmonary edema [Westhoff M, Rosseau S. Nichtinvasive beatmung bei akuter respiratorischer insuffizienz: indikationen und grenzen. Der Pneumologe. 2010 Mar;7(2):89–99.] *Caption translated from original*

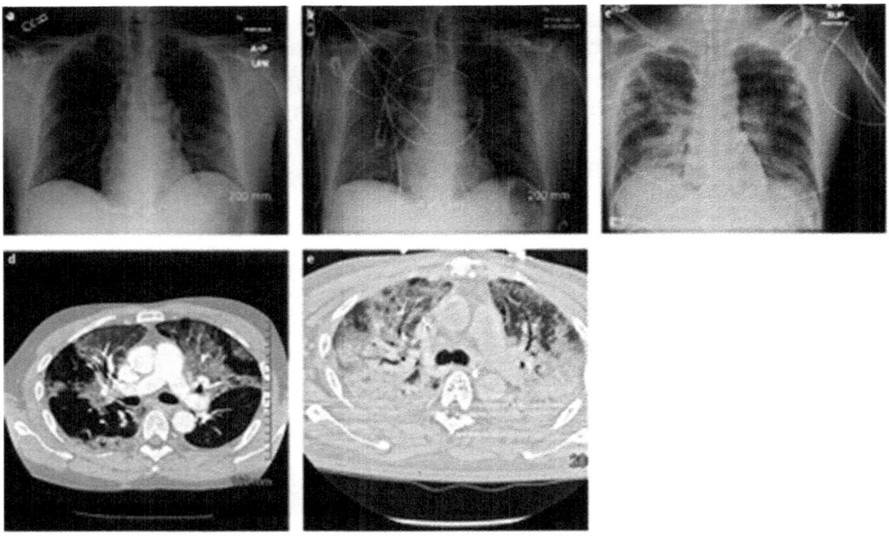

Acute respiratory distress syndrome (ARDS) following abdominal infection: imaging progression. a Relatively normal chest X-ray 12 h after abdominal surgery for sepsis. The patient was starting to experience dyspnea and some hypoxia. A normal chest X-ray is frequent in the early symptomatic stages of ARDS. b Four hours later, there is mild but definite interstitial thickening. c Thirty hours later, there is a dense bat's-wing consolidation in the perihilar areas. A Swan-Ganz catheter was inserted to rule out heart failure as a cause of the edema. d A computed tomography scan on day 3 shows the antigravity distribution of the ground-glass opacification that appeared to be perihilar on the chest X-ray. e In a different patient, 5 days after onset of ARDS, the edema is visible ventrally, whereas there is atelectasis, dorsally, in the gravity-dependent areas [Goodman LR. Imaging the intensive care patient. In: Hodler J, von Schulthess GK, Zollikofer CL, editors. Diseases of the heart, chest and breast 2011–2014 [Internet]. Milan: Springer; 2011 [cited 2015 Aug 13]. p. 66–9. Available from: http://link.springer.com/10.1007/978-88-470-1938-6_10] *Caption from original*

- CT:
  - CT scan is not required to make the diagnosis of NCPE.
  - When CT is performed, the scan looks similar to that of ARDS.

Special Populations

Age

- Because NCPE is a secondary event, it may occur across the age spectrum, but in general, it is more likely in elderly patients.

- In the pediatric patient, NCPE has been associated with any form of upper airway disease, including croup and epiglottitis, and choking episodes.

Co-morbidities

- Eclampsia in pregnancy may cause pulmonary edema.

Pitfalls in Diagnosis

- At times, both cardiogenic and NCPE may occur simultaneously.

Critical Steps Not to Miss

- Although pulmonary edema is the most prominent feature of ARDS, the two terms should not be used interchangeably.
- Hypoalbuminemia alone is not a cause of pulmonary edema.

Mimics

- The primary mimic of NCPE is cardiogenic pulmonary edema. Initial management of the two illnesses is similar and focuses on supporting oxygenation and reducing preload.

Time-Dependent Interventions

- Try to maintain a $Pa0_2$ of 60 mm Hg through use of oxygen and mechanical ventilation.

Overall Principles of Treatment

- Treatment varies depending on the underlying pathophysiology.
  - For example, descent to a lower altitude is the mainstay of treatment for high-altitude pulmonary edema.

- Currently, no known measures exist to correct the permeability abnormality in ARDS.
- Treatment is largely supportive and aimed at ensuring adequate ventilation and oxygenation.
    - Goal of treatment is to keep the $Pa0_2$ >60 mm Hg without injuring lungs with excessive O_2 or volutrauma/barotrauma.
- Lowering the pulmonary artery wedge pressure with diuretics and fluid restriction may improve pulmonary function in ARDS.
- Positive pressure ventilation is useful in severe NCPE.

Disease Course

- NCPE commonly develops within 24 hours of onset of the initial insult.
    - Presentation may be delayed 5 days.
- Begins with mild signs and symptoms that may progress rapidly to hypoxic respiratory failure
- Most patients require a high FiO_2 and will require mechanical ventilation.
- Ventilator-associated pneumonia is a frequent complication of ARDS.
- In severe cases, pulmonary scarring and diffuse alveolar damage may occur, especially if mechanical ventilation is used.

Related Evidence

Papers of particular interest have been highlighted as:
*** Of key importance*

Review

Mann A, Early GL. Acute respiratory distress syndrome. Mo Med. 2012 Sep-Oct;109(5):371-5. PMID: 23097941. http://www.ncbi.nlm.nih.gov/pubmed/23097941 **

Bajwa SS, Kulshrestha A. Diagnosis, prevention and management of postoperative pulmonary edema. Ann Med Health Sci Res. 2012 Jul;2(2):180-5. https://doi.org/10.4103/2141-9248.105668. PMID: 23439791. http://www.ncbi.nlm.nih.gov/pubmed/23439791 **

Mac Sweeney R, McAuley DF, Matthay MA. Acute lung failure. Semin Respir Crit Care Med. 2011 Oct;32(5):607-25. https://doi.org/10.1055/s-0031-1287870. PMID: 21989697. http://www.ncbi.nlm.nih.gov/pubmed/21989697 **

Matuschak GM, Lechner AJ. Acute lung injury and the acute respiratory distress syndrome: pathophysiology and treatment. Mo Med. 2010 Jul-Aug;107(4):252-8. PMID: 20806836. http://www.ncbi.nlm.nih.gov/pubmed/20806836 **

Ead H. Review of laryngospasm and noncardiogenic pulmonary edema. Dynamics. 2003 Fall;14(3):9-12. PMID: 14725141. http://www.ncbi.nlm.nih.gov/pubmed/14725141 **

Perina DG. Noncardiogenic pulmonary edema. Emerg Med Clin North Am. 2003 May;21(2):385-93. PMID: 12793620. http://www.ncbi.nlm.nih.gov/pubmed/12793620 **

Mortelliti MP, Manning HL. Acute respiratory distress syndrome. Am Fam Physician. 2002 May 1;65(9):1823-30. PMID: 12018805. http://www.ncbi.nlm.nih.gov/pubmed/12018805 **

Briasoulis E, Pavlidis N. Noncardiogenic pulmonary edema: an unusual and serious complication of anticancer therapy. Oncologist. 2001;6(2):153-61. PMID: 11306727. http://www.ncbi.nlm.nih.gov/pubmed/11306727 **

Fulkerson WJ, MacIntyre N, Stamler J, Crapo JD. Pathogenesis and treatment of the adult respiratory distress syndrome. Arch Intern Med. 1996 Jan 8;156(1):29-38. PMID: 8526694. http://www.ncbi.nlm.nih.gov/pubmed/8526694 **

Use PubMed Clinical Queries to find the most recent evidence. Use this search strategy: "Noncardiogenic pulmonary edema" OR "NCPE" OR "Non cardiogenic pulmonary edema"

Chapter 53
Peptic Ulcer Disease

Christopher J. Rees, Charles V. Pollack, Jr., and Victoria G. Riese

Name and Synonyms

Peptic Ulcer Disease (PUD)

- Gastric or Duodenal Ulcers

Incidence/Epidemiology

- Peptic ulcer disease (PUD) affects about 4 million adults in the United States, with an incidence of 0.09–0.3 % per patient year.
- Estimated annual cost to the health care system is around $15 billion, with an overall economic effect on the economy for health care, lost work, etc. of $50 billion.
- People who are infected with *Helicobacter pylori* have a lifetime prevalence of up to 20 %. Those who are uninfected have a lifetime prevalence of 5–10 %.
- The incidence of PUD has been falling steadily in the United States and all other developed nations.
- At one time, there was a decided male predominance; now, the rate is about equal in both genders.

C. J. Rees
Emergency Department, Pennsylvania Hospital, Philadelphia, PA, USA

C. V. Pollack, Jr. (✉)
Department of Emergency Medicine, Thomas Jefferson University, Philadelphia, PA, USA

V. G. Riese
Librarian Consultant, Eldersburg, MD, USA

C. V. Pollack, Jr. (ed.), *Differential Diagnosis of Cardiopulmonary Disease*,
https://doi.org/10.1007/978-3-319-63895-9_53

Differential Diagnosis

- The differential diagnosis of PUD is broad and includes all causes of chest and upper abdominal pain. All the causes of acute chest and abdominal pain, especially those that are immediately life threatening (e.g., acute myocardial infarction, pulmonary embolism, aortic dissection, perforated ulcer, perforated esophagus, acute cholecystitis, acute pancreatitis) must be considered first.
- In addition, there is a syndrome called non-ulcer dyspepsia that presents very similarly to PUD, but in which no ulcer or gastritis is found. The official criteria for diagnosis of non-ulcer dyspepsia is a chronic, recurrent upper abdominal pain or discomfort for at least 1 month that is present at least 25 % of the time and in which there is no evidence of organic disease. It is thought this condition may result from ulcers that are too small to be seen, acid hypersecretion, bile reflux, malabsorption, motility disorders, or sphincter of Oddi dysfunction, or that it may be functional.
- Gastritis (gastric mucosal inflammation without ulcer formation) also may have a presentation identical to that of PUD.
- *Peptic ulcer disease* refers to ulcers that develop within either the stomach (gastric) or duodenum. Although there may be subtle differences in presentation, risk factors, and natural history, the treatment remains very similar for both. Therefore, it often is not immediately necessary to refine the diagnosis to one or the other before beginning empiric treatment.

Pathophysiology and Etiology

- The upper gastrointestinal (GI) tract is regularly bathed in acid. Injury to the mucosal lining allows damage to underlying cells, which may result in ulceration and bleeding. There are a limited number of causes of PUD, including:
  - Infection with *H. pylori*, a bacterium whose growth disrupts the acid-protective barrier of the gastric mucosa:
    - *H. pylori* is more common in lower socioeconomic strata.
    - It is spread by the fecal–oral route.
    - It increases the risk of gastric carcinoma.
  - Use and abuse of nonsteroidal anti-inflammatory drugs (NSAIDs), which reduces mucosal protection from acid via interference with prostaglandin production in the upper GI mucosa.
  - Toxins such as cigarette smoke exposure and regular alcohol ingestion.
  - Hyperacidic states such as chronic anxiety.
  - Gastrin-producing tumor (Zollinger–Ellison syndrome) is a rare cause.

Presentation

Typical/"Classic"

- Chest or upper abdominal pain is typical, with the pain often described as burning or gnawing.
  - Pain may radiate to the back.
  - Pain usually occurs 2 to 3 hours after eating, at bedtime, or in the early morning hours, when gastric acid production levels are high.
  - Pain usually is relieved by eating.
  - Antacids often relieve the pain, but neither relief nor the absence of relief is pathognomonic.

Atypical

- Patients may describe only back pain; some duodenal ulcers may present with right scapular or shoulder pain.
- Patients may describe increased belching, but this is more typical of biliary tract disease.
- Vomiting is an atypical symptom of PUD. The presence of vomiting should raise concern for another diagnosis.
- Other symptoms that occasionally may be attributed to PUD but that should raise concerns for other conditions, especially malignancy, include weight loss, early satiety, dysphagia, unexplained anemia, and occult GI bleeding. Patients with any of these symptoms and those older than 55 years at first diagnosis should undergo endoscopy to exclude malignancy as the cause.

Primary Differential Considerations

- Patients with signs and symptoms of PUD may warrant an evaluation for:
  - Acute coronary syndrome
  - Esophagitis
  - Cholelithiasis and cholecystitis

History and Physical Exam

Findings That Confirm Diagnosis

- There are no historical or physical examination features that confirm the diagnosis.
- The diagnosis can be confirmed only by direct visualization through endoscopy.

Factors That Suggest Diagnosis

- A history as discussed in the presentation section may suggest the diagnosis.
- The absence of another cause of chest or abdominal pain may suggest the diagnosis.
- The initial diagnosis usually is clinical and treatment is started empirically, unless any of the "red flag" symptoms discussed under the atypical presentation section are present.

Factors That Exclude Diagnosis

- There are no historical or physical examination factors that exclude the diagnosis.
- Patients diagnosed with another cause of the initial symptoms may be acutely ill, which in and of itself is a risk factor for PUD.
- PUD may coexist with any other diagnosis.
- The only factor that excludes the diagnosis is a normal endoscopy that fully visualizes the stomach and duodenum.

Ancillary Studies

Laboratory

- Lab tests should include a complete blood count to look for anemia; measurement of serum electrolyte, blood urea nitrogen, and creatinine levels; liver function tests; and lipase testing to help evaluate for other diagnoses. In patients presenting with chest pain, cardiac biomarker testing may be indicated.
- Patients with a presumptive diagnosis of PUD should be tested for *H. pylori* infection.
    - The method for *H. pylori* testing depends on whether empiric treatment is to be initiated or the patient is proceeding to endoscopy.
    - Noninvasive tests for *H. pylori* include serologic testing for IgG. These tests have a low sensitivity and specificity; therefore, the positive predictive value of a positive test in a low-prevalence population (e.g., most of the United States) is low, limiting the usefulness of these tests. Urea breath tests have sensitivity and specificity above 95 %, so they are used frequently.

Stool antigen (Ag) tests to look for *H. pylori* have sensitivity and specificity above 90 %; these tests commonly are used to confirm cure 4 weeks after treatment completion.

- Invasive, endoscopically based tests include the rapid urease test, direct histologic examination, polymerase chain reaction tests, and culture. The only one of these tests routinely used in clinical practice is the rapid urease test. The others are expensive, as well as time and resource intensive; therefore they usually are used only used in research settings.
- If the clinical suspicion for infection is high, one positive test confirms infection. However, one negative test does not exclude infection, and a second test should be performed.
- In cases of acute bleeding, the biopsy rapid urease and stool Ag tests lack specificity; therefore, if testing must be done in this setting, the urea breath test should be used.

Imaging

- There are no diagnostic imaging findings of PUD
- Upper GI endoscopy is the diagnostic study of choice.

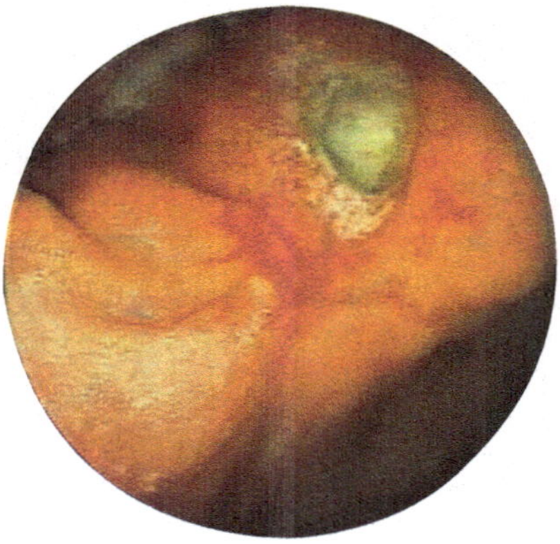

Gastric ulcer with greenish adherent exudate. [Graham D, Genta R. Helicobacter pylori. In: Lorber B, editor. Intra-abdominal infections, hepatitis and gastroenteritis. Philadelphia: Current Medicine; 1996. (Mandell GL, editor. Atlas of infectious diseases; vol. 7). ISBN 0-443-07730-4]

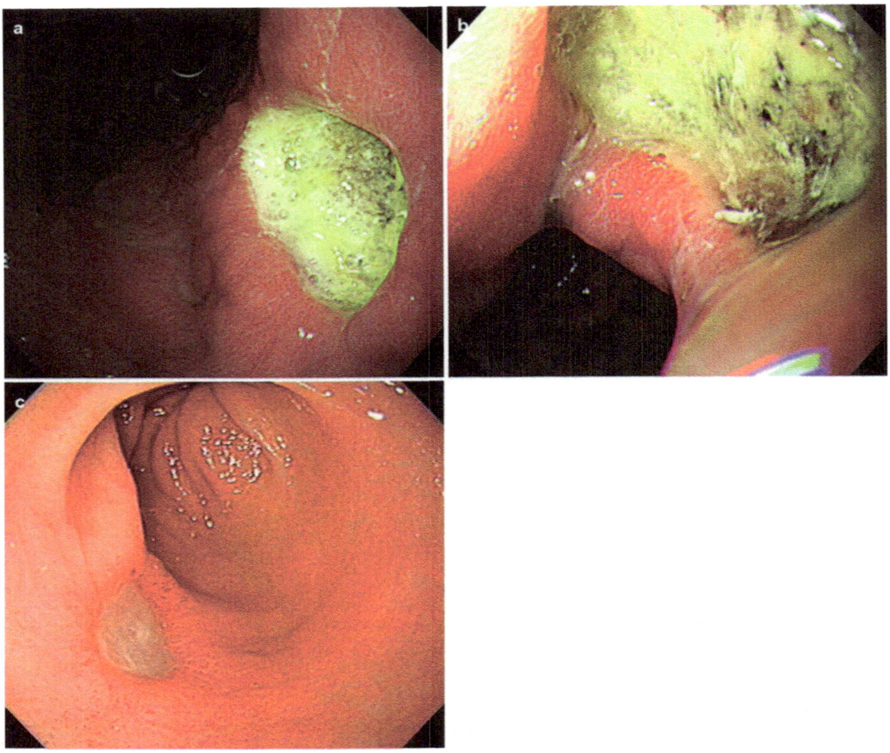

Endoscopic features of active gastric ulcers. (a) well-circumscribed and deeply penetrating active ulcer (b) Black pigmented area shown on close observation (c) clean ulcer base and a regular shape ulceration without exudate. [Lee SK. Gastritis and gastric ulcers. In: Chun HJ, Yang S-K, Choi M-G, editors. Clinical gastrointestinal endoscopy [Internet]. Berlin, Heidelberg: Springer; 2014 [cited 2015 Aug 28]. p. 99–122. Available from: http://link.springer.com/10.1007/978-3-642-35626-1_8] *Caption from original*

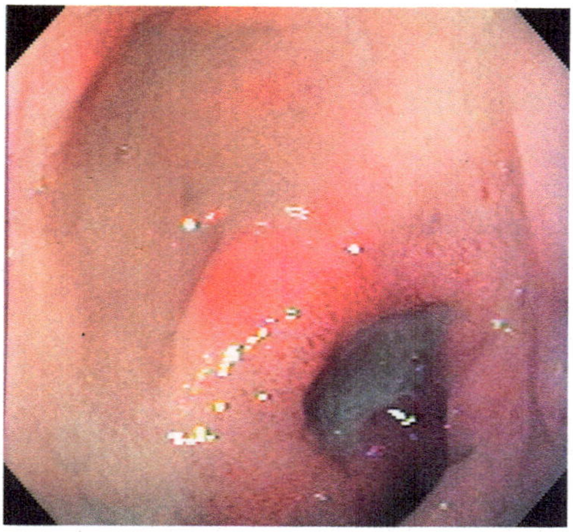

Duodenal ulcer. A deep duodenal ulcer is seen. There is surrounding inflammation with hyperemia of the mucosa. [Wilcox MC. Helicobacter pylori. In Feldman M, editor. Stomach and duodenum. Philadelphia: Current Medicine; 1996. Chapter 7. (Feldman M, editor. Gastroenterology and hepatology; vol. 3). ISBN: 0-443-07843-2]

Special Populations

Age

- The incidence of PUD increases with age.
- The incidence of upper GI bleeding from PUD increases with age.
- PUD rarely is encountered in the pediatric population.
- Younger children often present with emesis, hemorrhage, and perforation.
- *H. pylori* rarely is seen in pediatric patients; in this age range, most PUD is idiopathic.

Co-morbidities

- Patients who are acutely ill, such as those in intensive care units, have higher rates of PUD.
- Patients who smoke, abuse alcohol, use NSAIDs daily, or are maintained on glucocorticoids also are at higher risk for PUD.

Pitfalls in Diagnosis

Critical Steps Not to Miss

- It is important not to ascribe symptoms to PUD prematurely, before evaluating for the more immediately life-threatening conditions that may present similarly.

Mimics

- The pain from PUD may mimic the pain of cardiac ischemia.
- Non-ulcer dyspepsia
- Gastritis
- Esophageal disorders

Time-Dependent Interventions

- If patients present with upper GI bleeding, they must be resuscitated and stabilized urgently.

Overall Principles of Treatment

- Most patients can be started empirically on a trial of acid suppression based on the history and normal physical examination findings. Most patients will be started on proton-pump inhibitors (PPIs), as these provide much greater acid suppression than H2-blockers.
- Patients with any of the red-flag symptoms discussed in the atypical presentation section, as well as those over 55 years old, should be referred to a gastroenterologist for endoscopy to confirm the diagnosis and rule out malignancy.
- Patients who test positive for *H. pylori* must be given appropriate antibiotic treatment to eradicate the infection. The recurrence rate of *H. pylori*–associated ulcers is 65–95 % if the infection is not eradicated and <10 % if it is. Generally, patients are started on a combination of antibiotics (most commonly, clarithromycin and amoxicillin) with a PPI. The antibiotics are given for 2 weeks; there is controversy over whether to discontinue the PPI at 2 weeks as well.
- All patients should be counseled on lifestyle modifications as appropriate. Patients who smoke cigarettes should try to quit, alcohol intake should be limited, and NSAIDs, including aspirin, should be avoided.

Disease Course

- Ulcers that are not treated, those that are poorly treated, and, rarely, even those that are adequately treated may develop many complications. Some may be life threatening.
- In order of prevalence, the most common complications of PUD are:
  - Bleeding, typically from inflamed mucosa, but sometimes from ulcer erosion into a submucosal vessel.
    - Hemorrhage is more common in older patients.
  - Perforation of the ulcer through the gastric or duodenal wall, most often posteriorly and causing severe back pain from leakage of gastric contents.
  - Gastric outlet obstruction from chronic inflammation and swelling around an ulcer in or near the gastroduodenal junction.

Related Evidence

Papers of particular interest have been highlighted as:
*** Of key importance*

Practice Guideline

Koletzko S, Jones NL, Goodman KJ, Gold B, Rowland M, Cadranel S, Chong S, Colletti RB, Casswall T, Elitsur Y, Guarner J, Kalach N, Madrazo A, Megraud F, Oderda G; H pylori Working Groups of ESPGHAN and NASPGHAN. Evidence-based guidelines from ESPGHAN and NASPGHAN for Helicobacter pylori infection in children. J Pediatr Gastroenterol Nutr. 2011 Aug;53(2):230-43. https://doi.org/10.1097/MPG.0b013e3182227e90. PMID: 21558964. http://www.ncbi.nlm.nih.gov/pubmed/21558964 **

ASGE Standards of Practice Committee, Banerjee S, Cash BD, Dominitz JA, Baron TH, Anderson MA, Ben-Menachem T, Fisher L, Fukami N, Harrison ME, Ikenberry SO, Khan K, Krinsky ML, Maple J, Fanelli RD, Strohmeyer L. The role of endoscopy in the management of patients with peptic ulcer disease. Gastrointest Endosc. 2010 Apr;71(4):663-8. https://doi.org/10.1016/j.gie.2009.11.026. PMID: 20363407. http://www.ncbi.nlm.nih.gov/pubmed/20363407 **

Meta-Analysis

Leontiadis GI, Sharma VK, Howden CW. Proton pump inhibitor therapy for peptic ulcer bleeding: Cochrane collaboration meta-analysis of randomized controlled trials. Mayo Clin Proc. 2007 Mar;82(3):286-96. PMID: 17352364. http://www.ncbi.nlm.nih.gov/pubmed/17352364

Review

Leontiadis GI, Molloy-Bland M, Moayyedi P, Howden CW. Effect of comorbidity on mortality in patients with peptic ulcer bleeding: systematic review and meta-analysis. Am J Gastroenterol. 2013 Mar;108(3):331-45; quiz 346. https://doi.org/10.1038/ajg.2012.451. PMID: 23381016. http://www.ncbi.nlm.nih.gov/pubmed/23381016

Wilkins T, Khan N, Nabh A, Schade RR. Diagnosis and management of upper gastrointestinal bleeding. Am Fam Physician. 2012 Mar 1;85(5):469-76. PMID: 22534226. http://www.ncbi.nlm.nih.gov/pubmed/22534226 **

Yeomans ND. The ulcer sleuths: The search for the cause of peptic ulcers. J Gastroenterol Hepatol. 2011 Jan;26 Suppl 1:35-41. https://doi.org/10.1111/j.1440-1746.2010.06537.x. PMID: 21199512. http://www.ncbi.nlm.nih.gov/pubmed/21199512

Najm WI. Peptic ulcer disease. Prim Care. 2011 Sep;38(3):383-94, vii. https://doi.org/10.1016/j.pop.2011.05.001. PMID 21872087. http://www.ncbi.nlm.nih.gov/pubmed/21872087 **

Holle GE. Pathophysiology and modern treatment of ulcer disease. Int J Mol Med. 2010 Apr;25(4):483-91. PMID: 20198295. http://www.ncbi.nlm.nih.gov/pubmed/20198295

Malfertheiner P, Chan FK, McColl KE. Peptic ulcer disease. Lancet. 2009 Oct 24;374(9699):1449-61. https://doi.org/10.1016/S0140-6736(09)60938-7. PMID 19683340. http://www.ncbi.nlm.nih.gov/pubmed/19683340 **

Ramakrishnan K, Salinas RC. Peptic ulcer disease. Am Fam Physician. 2007 Oct 1;76(7):1005-12. Review. PMID: 17956071. http://www.ncbi.nlm.nih.gov/pubmed/17956071 **

Louw JA. Peptic ulcer disease. Curr Opin Gastroenterol. 2006 Nov;22(6):607-11. PMID: 17053437. http://www.ncbi.nlm.nih.gov/pubmed/17053437 **

Chelimsky G, Czinn S. Peptic ulcer disease in children. Pediatr Rev. 2001 Oct;22(10):349-55. PMID: 11581488. http://www.ncbi.nlm.nih.gov/pubmed/11581488 **

Use PubMed Clinical Queries to find the most recent evidence. Use this search strategy:

"Peptic Ulcer"[Mesh] OR "Peptic ulcer"

Chapter 54
Pericardial Effusion

Charles V. Pollack, Jr., Melissa Platt, Richard M. Cantor, and Jaime Friel

Name and Synonyms

Pericardial effusion; tamponade

Incidence/Epidemiology

- 60 % of cases are related to a known or suspected underlying process.
- Malignancies with the highest prevalence of pericardial effusion include lung, breast, and leukemia/lymphoma.

C. V. Pollack, Jr. (✉)
Department of Emergency Medicine, Thomas Jefferson University, Philadelphia, PA, USA

M. Platt
Department of Emergency Medicine, University of Louisville, Louisville, KY, USA

R. M. Cantor
Department of Emergency Medicine and Pediatrics, State University of New York Upstate Medical University, Syracuse, NY, USA

J. Friel
Welch Medical Library, Johns Hopkins University, Baltimore, MD, USA

C. V. Pollack, Jr. (ed.), *Differential Diagnosis of Cardiopulmonary Disease*,
https://doi.org/10.1007/978-3-319-63895-9_54

Differential Diagnosis

- Acute pericarditis
- Autoimmune disease
- Postmyocardial infarction or cardiac surgery
- Sharp or blunt chest trauma
- Malignancy
- Mediastinal radiation
- Renal failure with uremia
- Myxedema
- Aortic dissection extending into pericardium
- Dilated cardiomyopathy
- Pulmonary edema
- Pulmonary embolism
- Myocarditis

Pathophysiology and Etiology

- Accumulated fluid within the pericardial sac exceeds the small amount that is normally present.
  - 25–50 ml may be physiologic
- May develop rapidly or slowly.
- Accumulation of pericardial fluid into a closed space increases intrapericardial pressure.
- Cardiac tamponade is present when intrapericardial pressure becomes high enough to impede cardiac filling and function.
  - May occur with small amounts of fluid (~80 cc) when the pericardial cavity fills quickly; effusions may accumulate slowly to much higher volumes (up to 2 L) without symptoms.
  - Occurs when diastolic filling pressures equalize and prohibit effective pump function

Malignancy
Postoperative (postpericardiotomy)
Cardiac puncture from invasive procedures (electrophysiology studies, cardiac catheterization, pacemaker/ICD implantation)
Ischemic heart disease related (postinfarct as in Dressler's Syndrome; myocardial rupture)
Infectious
Immune/connective tissue diseases (lupus; rheumatoid arthritis; vasculitides)
Idiopathic
Renal failure
Drug-related and anticoagulants
Postradiation
Chest trauma
Hypothyroidism
Amyloidosis

Etiologies of pericardial effusion [Tsang TSM, Sinak LJ, Oh JK. Pericardial Effusion, Tamponade, and Constriction. In: Nihoyannopoulos P, Kisslo J, editors. Echocardiography [Internet]. London: Springer London; 2009 [cited 2015 Sep 2]. p. 297–310. Available from: http://link.springer.com/10.1007/978-1-84882-293-1_14] *Caption from original*

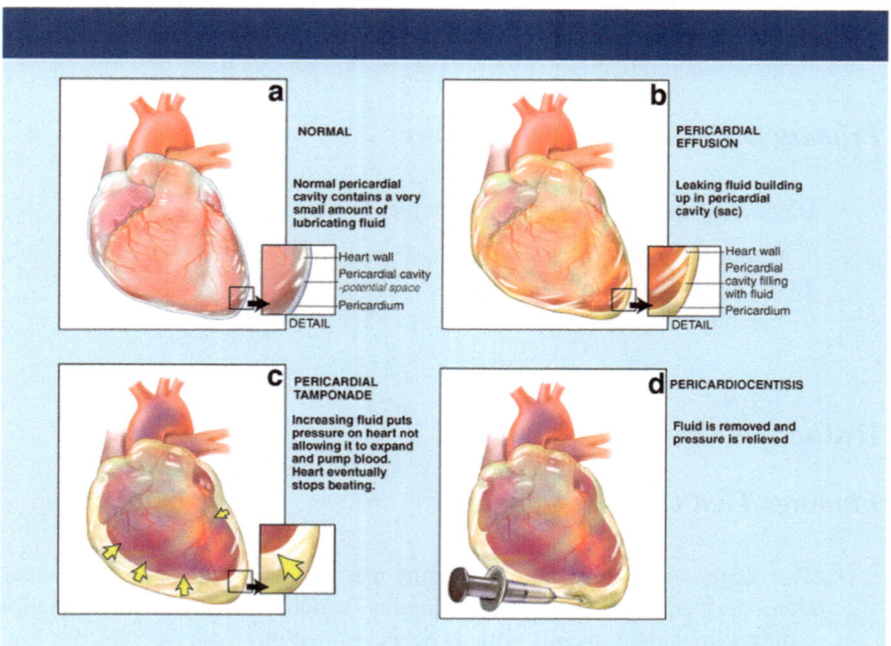

Illustrations demonstrate the progressive effects of a large pericardial effusion on the heart (a–c). If the effusion is large enough to compress the cardiac chambers it will ultimately limit cardiac output. In this setting, an emergency pericardiocentesis is necessary (d) [Towbin R. The bowed catheter sign: a risk for pericardial tamponade. Pediatric Radiology. 2008 Mar;38(3):331–5.] *Caption from original*

Presentation

Typical/"Classic"

- Many patients with pericardial effusion have no symptoms.
- Signs and symptoms may not occur until a large amount of fluid has collected over time.
- Beck triad of pericardial **tamponade**: Hypotension, muffled heart sounds, jugular venous distention.

Atypical

- Atypical presentations might include primary complaints of syncope, shortness of breath (especially on exertion), and chest pain.

Primary Differential Considerations

- Diagnostic approach consists of 3 steps:
  1. Confirm the presences of a pericardial effusion
  2. Assess its hemodynamic impact
  3. Establish the cause of the effusion

History and Physical Exam

Findings That Confirm Diagnosis

- The diagnosis is strongly suggested by the finding of concomitant hypotension, muffled heart sounds, and jugular venous distention. Confirmation requires imaging, typically with an echocardiogram.

Factors That Suggest Diagnosis

- Chest pain
- Syncope
- Cough
- Ewart's sign (triangular area of dullness at the tip of the left scapula along with tubular breath sounds and egophony at the same location)
- May have fever in the setting of pericarditis
- Elevated jugular venous pressure
- Edema
- Pulsus paradoxus
- Pericardial friction rub
- Tachycardia
- Hepatojugular reflux
- Tachypnea
- Hepatosplenomegaly

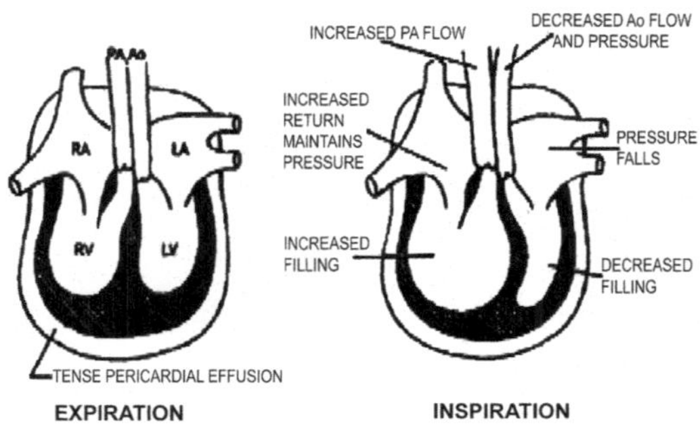

Pulsus paradoxus expiration and inspiration. [Reprinted from Curr Probl Cardiol., Vol. 29, Iss. 9, Goldstein JA. Cardiac tamponade, constrictive pericarditis, and restrictive cardiomyopathy. Pages 503-567, Copyright 2004, with permission from Elsevier].

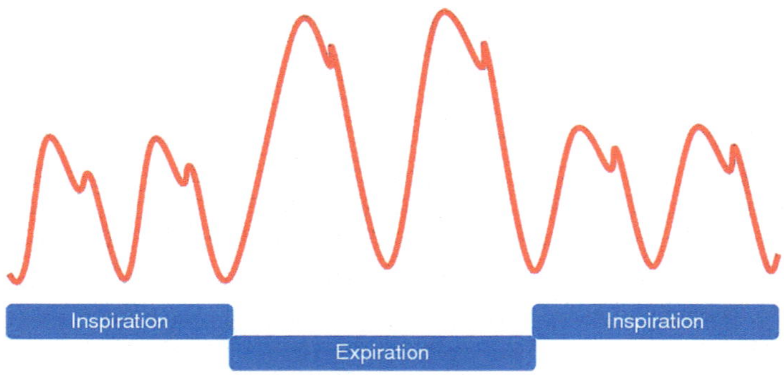

Pulsus paradoxus demonstrating an exaggerated decline in systolic blood pressure during inspiration, resulting from an increase in negative intrathoracic pressure [Patel S, Kronzon I. History and Physical Examination of a Patient with Pericardial Disease. In: Herzog E, editor. Management of Pericardial Disease [Internet]. Cham: Springer International Publishing; 2014 [cited 2015 Sep 2]. p. 27–35. Available from: http://link.springer.com/10.1007/978-3-319-06124-5_3] *Caption from original*

Factors That Exclude Diagnosis

- The absence of a pericardial effusion on echocardiogram is the only way to exclude the diagnosis with certainty.

Ancillary Studies

Laboratory

- Cardiac biomarkers may be elevated with acute myopericarditis or myocardial infarction.
- Moderate or large effusions etiology may be established with fluid and/or pericardial tissue analysis.
  - Fluid analysis may be obtained if clinical suspicion of purulent, tuberculous, or neoplastic pericarditis.
- CBC.
- Chemistry profile with renal function.
- Thyroid function.
- ANA testing.

ECG

- Sinus tachycardia.
- Low QRS voltage.
- Electrical Alternans.
- The combination of low voltage with sinus tachycardia should raise concern about pericardial effusion with tamponade.
- Electrical alternans with sinus tachycardia is highly specific of pericardial effusion.
    - Its absence does not exclude cardiac tamponade.

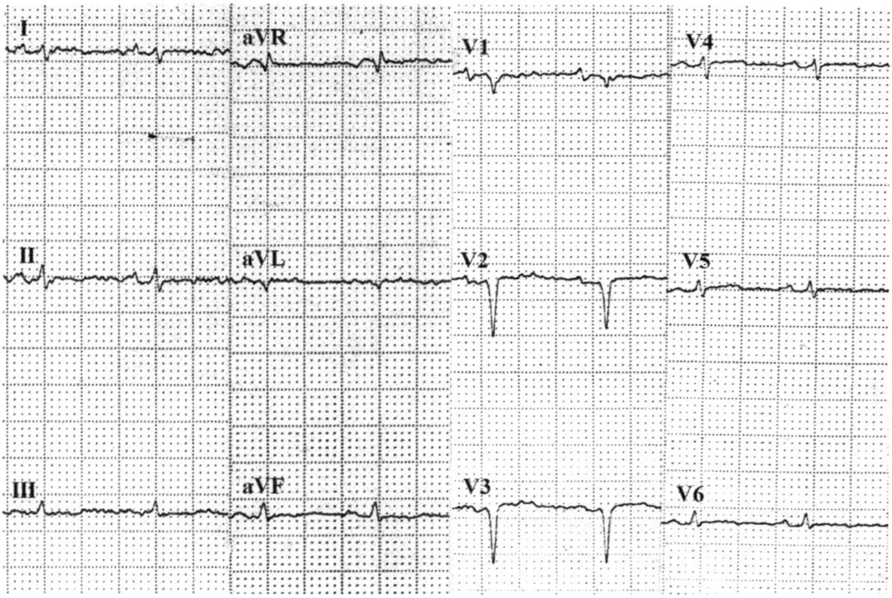

ECG in a patient with massive pericardial effusion causing pericardial tamponade. The key feature is a significant decrease in the QRS voltage in all leads [Romanò M. The Electrocardiogram in Diseases of the Pericardium and Myocardium. Text Atlas of Practical Electrocardiography [Internet]. Milano: Springer Milan; 2015 [cited 2015 Sep 2]. p. 209–12. Available from: http://link.springer.com/10.1007/978-88-470-5741-8_13] *Caption from original*

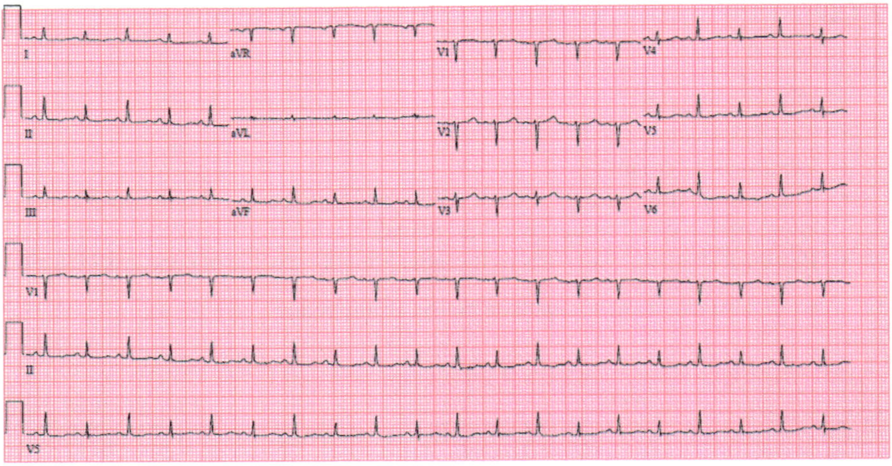

EKG demonstrating electrical alternans [Aksoy O, Rodriguez L. Tamponade. In: Anwaruddin S, Martin JM, Stephens JC, Askari AT, editors. Cardiovascular Hemodynamics [Internet]. Totowa, NJ: Humana Press; 2013 [cited 2015 Sep 2]. p. 181–96. Available from: http://link.springer.com/10.1007/978-1-60761-195-0_9] *Caption from original*

Imaging

- Chest x-ray
  - Variable.
  - Depends on etiology and size of effusion.
    - Small-to-moderate effusions (less than 200–300 ml) may not be apparent on CXR.
  - Enlarged cardiac silhouette "water bottle heart" is not specific and cannot be considered diagnostic.

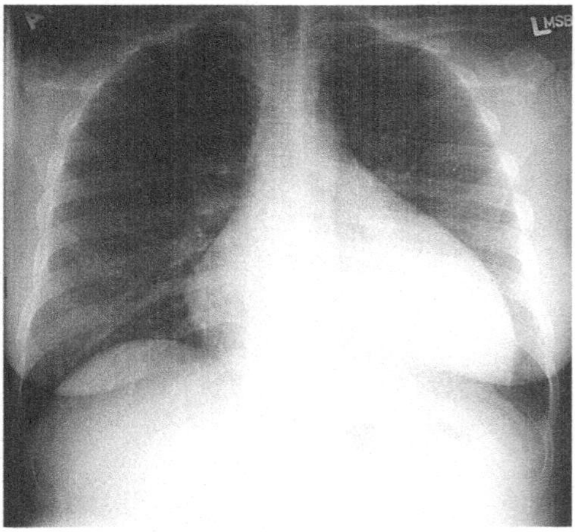

Chest radiograph of a large pericardial effusion. The cardiac diameter is markedly enlarged and the cardiac silhouette has a characteristic globular shape. This picture is seen in slowly developing chronic effusions when there is time for the pericardium to stretch. In an acute cardiac tamponade caused by bleeding into the pericardium the chest radiograph may show little or no cardiac enlargement. [Woodcock B. Hemodynamic Emergencies. In: Miller RD, Tremper KK, editors. Atlas of Anesthesia: Principles of Anesthetic Techniques and Anesthetic Emergencies, Volume 4, 1e. Vol. IV. Philadelphia: Current Medicine; 1998. 195 p.] *Caption from original*

Echocardiography

- Sensitive and specific for pericardial effusion.
- Can provide information regarding the hemodynamic significance of the effusion.
- Small effusions (50–100 mL) can be seen posterior to the left ventricle.
- Most sensitive and specific view is the accumulation of pericardial fluid above the right atrium in the apical four chamber view with the patient in the left lateral decubitus.
- Plays important role in diagnosis of cardiac tamponade.
    - Collapse of the right atrium at end diastole and the right ventricle in early diastole.
    - Reciprocal changes in left and right ventricular volumes with respiration.
    - Dilation of IVC and less than a 50 % reduction in its diameter during inspiration.

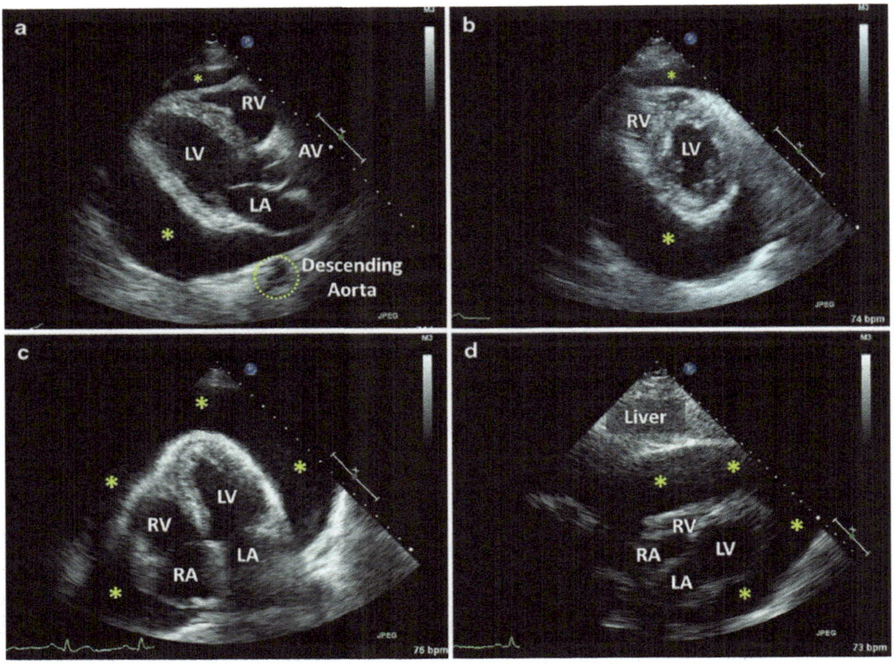

Pericardial effusion. Transthoracic echocardiogram demonstrates a large pericardial effusion (asterisks) in a 47-year-old woman with breast cancer. Panel a: Parasternal long axis view demonstrates typical interposition of the pericardial effusion (asterisks) between the heart and the descending thoracic aorta. This finding differentiates a pericardial effusion from a left pleural effusion in which there is no such interposition between the heart and the descending thoracic aorta. Panel b: Parasternal short axis at the level of the papillary muscles demonstrates that the pericardial effusion (asterisks) is larger posterior to the left ventricle that anterior to the right ventricle. This is due to gravity in this supine patient. Panel c: In the apical 4-chamber view, note that the pericardial effusion (asterisks) surrounds the cardiac apex. This feature helps distinguish a pericardial effusion from a pleural effusion. Panel d: Subcostal view demonstrates a large pericardial effusion (asterisks). Abbreviations: AV aortic valve, LA left atrium, LV left ventricle, RA right atrium, RV right ventricle [Saric M. Echocardiography in Pericardial Disease. In: Herzog E, editor. Management of Pericardial Disease [Internet]. Cham: Springer International Publishing; 2014 [cited 2015 Sep 2]. p. 49–70. Available from: http://link.springer.com/10.1007/978-3-319-06124-5_5] *Caption from original*

CT and MRI

- May be used after non-diagnostic echocardiography.

- May be useful when quantification and localization of pericardial fluid is important, when complex effusions are present, or when epicardial fat and pleural effusions need to be excluded.

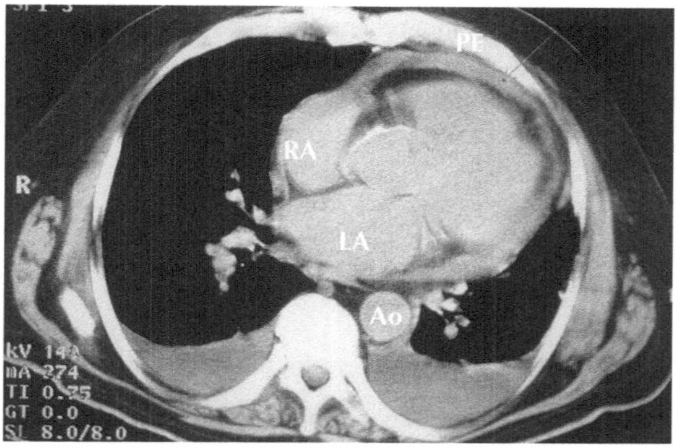

Pericardial effusion (PE). PEs are usually well shown by echocardiography. However, they are often a finding on conventional computed tomography (CT) scan or ultrafast CT (UFCT; Imatron, South San Francisco, CA). CT may show loculated pericardial fluid that cannot be shown by echocardiography. A, On unenhanced scans, a PE often has attenuation similar to soft tissue and therefore has the same density as do myocardium and blood pool. PE is usually visible as a layer of abnormal thickening separated from the heart by a line of low-attenuation epicardial fat, as shown in this example. Sometimes the epicardial fat is very thin; however, it still should be visible. Ao—aorta; LA—left atrium; RA—right atrium. [Hartnell G. Chapter 7. In: Lee RT, Braunwald E, editors. Atlas of Cardiac Imaging. Atlas of Heart Diseases, Volume 01, Philadelphia: Current Medicine; 1998. ISBN: 0-443-07567-0] *Caption adapted from original*

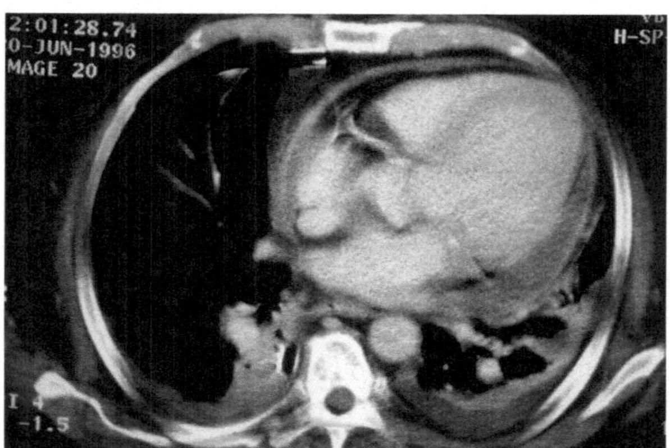

B, If there is doubt whether there is a PE or if there is no epicardial fat, intravenous contrast medium will enhance the myocardium but not the pericardial fluid. The attenuation of the myocardium will increase, as shown in this patient with lymphoma invading the pericardium, whereas the attenuation of the pericardial fluid (here mostly loculated posteriorly) is unchanged, enhancing the difference between the two. Although CT is not recommended as the first line method for detecting PEs, it frequently shows underlying conditions such as tumor, which may lead to pericardial effusion. In addition, in patients who are poor subjects for echocardiography, CT will show PEs, including effusions loculated in areas difficult to examine by echocardiography. [Hartnell G. Chapter 7. In: Lee RT, Braunwald E, editors. Atlas of Cardiac Imaging. Atlas of Heart Diseases, Volume 01, Philadelphia: Current Medicine; 1998. ISBN: 0-443-07567-0] *Caption adapted from original*

Special Populations

- Populations at particular risk for development of a pericardial effusion include patients with
  - Malignancy
  - Renal failure
  - Autoimmune diseases, such as lupus
  - Certain unusual systemic infections, such as tuberculosis
  - Some viral infections, incluing HIV
  - Very recent myocardial infarction
  - Very recent heart surgery

Age

- Most common in the fourth and fifth decades of life.
- Within the pediatric population, reported cases of pericardial effusion are most likely due to enteroviral infections, specifically Coxsackie viral infections. Other pediatric specific etiologies include malignancies, specifically the leukemias.
- In addition, cases of pediatric myocarditis may involve the pericardium as well.

Co-morbidities

- Patients with heart disease, renal failure, or malignancy are at risk of developing pericardial effusion.

Pitfalls in Diagnosis

Critical Steps Not to Miss

- Rapid diagnosis of cardiac tamponade is needed for urgent treatment.
- No positive-pressure ventilation because of its adverse effects on venous return and cardiac output.

Mimics

- Cardiomyopathy, which also causes diminished cardiac output and an enlarged cardiac silhouette on chest radograph.

Time-Dependent Interventions

- Drainage of a pericardial effusion is often performed for therapeutic benefit, as in cardiac tamponade.
- Patients with a pericardial effusion and evidence of hemodynamic compromise should undergo urgent drainage.
- Cardiac tamponade is initially treated with expansion of intravascular volume and urgent pericardial drainage.

Overall Principles of Treatment

- Development of pericardial effusion may have implications for prognosis and diagnosis.
- Patient with effusion who are hemodynamically stable do not require immediate drainage.
- Manage underlying cause:
  - NSAIDs or prednisone for inflammatory effusions
  - Diuretics for heart failure-associated effusions
  - Antibiotic if infection is suspected
  - Malignant effusions may respond as the underlying cancer is treated with chemotherapy or radiation
- The choice between pericardiocentesis and open surgical drainage is multifactorial and institution specific:
  - Both techniques allow for rapid relief of cardiac tamponade
  - Both allow for fluid analysis if needed

- A percutaneous continuous catheter drain may be placed for intermittent or continuous removal until the rate of fluid return is negligible.

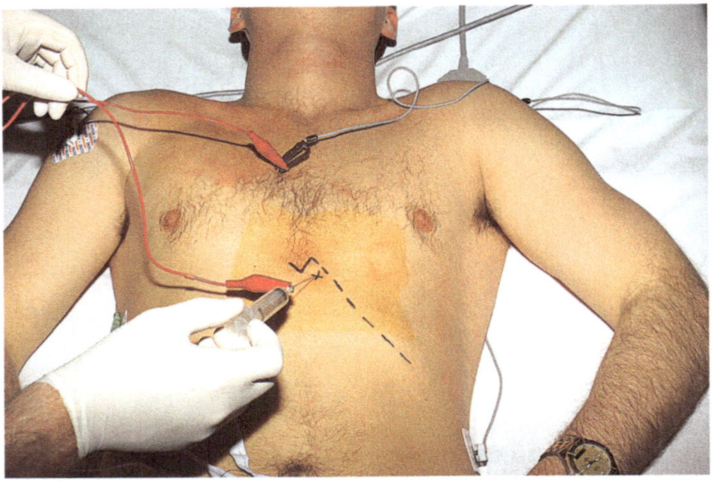

Pericardiocentesis [Woodcock B. Hemodynamic Emergencies. In: Miller RD, Tremper KK, editors. Atlas of Anesthesia: Principles of Anesthetic Techniques and Anesthetic Emergencies, Volume 4, 1e. Vol. IV. Philadelphia: Current Medicine; 1998. 195 p.]

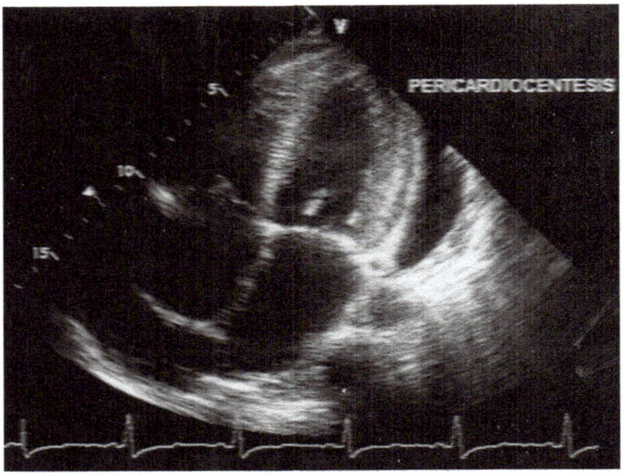

Echocardiographically guided pericardiocentesis. In addition to confirming the presence, location, and distribution of pericardial effusion, two-dimensional echocardiography can enhance the safety of percutaneous pericardiocentesis by identifying the optimal entry site (the point at which the distance from skin to prominent fluid accumulation is minimized, with no intervening vital organ). Once the needle has entered the pericardial space and a sheath or catheter is inserted, confirmation and documentation of intrapericardial location can be achieved by injecting a small amount of agitated saline. A moderate-to-large size pericardial effusion is present as shown in the modified apical four-chamber view (A). [Goldstein S, Pita F. Chapter 9. In: Vannan MA, Lang RM, Rakowski H, Tajik AJ, Braunwald E, editors. Atlas of Echocardiography. 1e. Philadelphia, PA: Current Medicine Group; 2005. 312 p. ISBN: 1-57340-217-6] *Caption adapted from original*

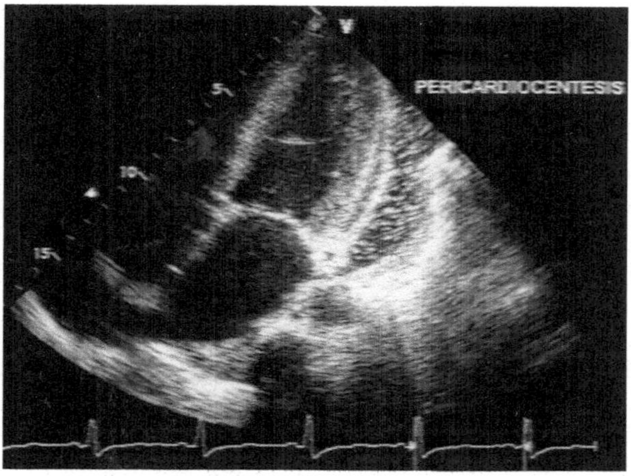

Proper catheter location is confirmed by the echogenic microbubbles observed within the pericardial space (B). This technique should be used routinely to minimize complications. [Goldstein S, Pita F. Chapter 9. In: Vannan MA, Lang RM, Rakowski H, Tajik AJ, Braunwald E, editors. Atlas of Echocardiography. 1e. Philadelphia, PA: Current Medicine Group; 2005. 312 p. ISBN: 1-57340-217-6] *Caption adapted from original*

Disease Course

- Often self-limited or responsive to NSAIDs or corticosteroids.
- Many secondary cases are responsive to better management of underlying disease.
- Perform follow-up echocardiography to rule out accumulation and constrictive physiology.

Related Evidence

Papers of particular interest have been highlighted as:
*** Of key importance*

Review

Virk SA, Chandrakumar D, Villanueva C, Wolfenden H, Liou K, Cao C. Systematic review of percutaneous interventions for malignant pericardial effusion. Heart. 2015 Oct 15;101(20):1619-26. https://doi.org/10.1136/heartjnl-2015-307907. Epub 2015 Jul 15. Review. PubMed PMID: 26180077. http://www.ncbi.nlm.nih.gov/pubmed/26180077

Chandraratna PA, Mohar DS, Sidarous PF. Role of echocardiography in the treatment of cardiac tamponade. Echocardiography. 2014 Aug;31(7):899-910. https://doi.org/10.1111/echo.12605. Epub 2014 Apr 4. Review. PubMed PMID: 24697811. http://www.ncbi.nlm.nih.gov/pubmed/24697811 **

Perera P, Lobo V, Williams SR, Gharahbaghian L. Cardiac echocardiography. Crit Care Clin. 2014 Jan;30(1):47-92, v. https://doi.org/10.1016/j.ccc.2013.08.003. Review.

PubMed PMID: 24295841. http://www.ncbi.nlm.nih.gov/pubmed/24295841

Argulian E, Messerli F. Misconceptions and facts about pericardial effusion and tamponade. Am J Med. 2013 Oct;126(10):858-61. https://doi.org/10.1016/j.amjmed.2013.03.022. Epub 2013 Jul 24. Review. PubMed PMID: 23891285. http://www.ncbi.nlm.nih.gov/pubmed/23891285

Seferović PM, Ristić AD, Maksimović R, Simeunović DS, Milinković I, Seferović Mitrović JP, Kanjuh V, Pankuweit S, Maisch B. Pericardial syndromes: an update after the ESC guidelines 2004. Heart Fail Rev. 2013 May;18(3):255-66. https://doi.org/10.1007/s10741-012-9335-x. Review. PubMed PMID: 22855353. http://www.ncbi.nlm.nih.gov/pubmed/22855353

Imazio M, Adler Y. Management of pericardial effusion. Eur Heart J. 2013 Apr;34(16):1186-97. https://doi.org/10.1093/eurheartj/ehs372. Epub 2012 Nov 2. Review. PubMed PMID: 23125278. http://www.ncbi.nlm.nih.gov/pubmed/23125278 **

Burazor I, Imazio M, Markel G, Adler Y. Malignant pericardial effusion. Cardiology. 2013;124(4):224-32. https://doi.org/10.1159/000348559. Epub 2013 Apr 5. Review. PubMed PMID: 23571453. http://www.ncbi.nlm.nih.gov/pubmed/23571453

Loukas M, Walters A, Boon JM, Welch TP, Meiring JH, Abrahams PH. Pericardiocentesis: a clinical anatomy review. Clin Anat. 2012 Oct;25(7):872-81. https://doi.org/10.1002/ca.22032. Epub 2012 Jan 31. Review. PubMed PMID: 22294431. http://www.ncbi.nlm.nih.gov/pubmed/22294431

Sykes JA, Verma R, Peshkovsky C, O'Connor B, Malik F, Lubega J, Malhotra S, McQueen D, Mikkilineni S, Kalyanaraman M. Early repair of large infant ventricular septal defect despite respiratory syncytial virus-induced respiratory failure with postrepair chylous pericardial effusion requiring pleuropericardial window: a case report and review of the literature. Pediatr Emerg Care. 2012 Oct;28(10):1072-7. https://doi.org/10.1097/PEC.0b013e31826cedc6. Review. PubMed PMID: 23034497. http://www.ncbi.nlm.nih.gov/pubmed/23034497

Imazio M. Contemporary management of pericardial diseases. Curr Opin Cardiol. 2012 May;27(3):308-17. https://doi.org/10.1097/HCO.0b013e3283524fbe. Review. PubMed PMID: 22450720. http://www.ncbi.nlm.nih.gov/pubmed/22450720

Dudzinski DM, Mak GS, Hung JW. Pericardial diseases. Curr Probl Cardiol. 2012 Mar;37(3):75-118. https://doi.org/10.1016/j.cpcardiol.2011.10.002. Review. PubMed PMID:22289657. http://www.ncbi.nlm.nih.gov/pubmed/22289657

Grecu L. Cardiac tamponade. Int Anesthesiol Clin. 2012 Spring;50(2):59-77. https://doi.org/10.1097/AIA.0b013e318254053e. Review. PubMed PMID: 22481556. http://www.ncbi.nlm.nih.gov/pubmed/22481556 **

Bodson L, Bouferrache K, Vieillard-Baron A. Cardiac tamponade. Curr Opin Crit Care. 2011 Oct;17(5):416-24. https://doi.org/10.1097/MCC.0b013e3283491f27. Review. PubMed PMID: 21716107. http://www.ncbi.nlm.nih.gov/pubmed/21716107 **

Schairer JR, Biswas S, Keteyian SJ, Ananthasubramaniam K. A systematic approach to evaluation of pericardial effusion and cardiac tamponade. Cardiol Rev. 2011 Sep-Oct;19(5):233-8. https://doi.org/10.1097/CRD.0b013e31821e202c. Review. PubMed PMID: 21808166. http://www.ncbi.nlm.nih.gov/pubmed/21808166

Imazio M, Mayosi BM, Brucato A, Markel G, Trinchero R, Spodick DH, Adler Y. Triage and management of pericardial effusion. J Cardiovasc Med (Hagerstown). 2010 Dec;11(12):928-35. https://doi.org/10.2459/JCM.0b013e32833e5788. Review. PubMed PMID:20814314. http://www.ncbi.nlm.nih.gov/pubmed/20814314 **

Imazio M, Brucato A, Mayosi BM, Derosa FG, Lestuzzi C, Macor A, Trinchero R, Spodick DH, Adler Y. Medical therapy of pericardial diseases: part II: Noninfectious pericarditis, pericardial effusion and constrictive pericarditis. J Cardiovasc Med (Hagerstown). 2010 Nov;11(11):785-94. Review. PubMed PMID: 20925146. http://www.ncbi.nlm.nih.gov/pubmed/20925146

O'Connor CJ, Tuman KJ. The intraoperative management of patients with pericardial tamponade. Anesthesiol Clin. 2010 Mar;28(1):87-96. https://doi.org/10.1016/j.anclin.2010.01.011. Review. PubMed PMID: 20400042. http://www.ncbi.nlm.nih.gov/pubmed/20400042 **

Imazio M, Brucato A, Trinchero R, Adler Y. Diagnosis and management of pericardial diseases. Nat Rev Cardiol. 2009 Dec;6(12):743-51. doi:10.1038/nrcardio.2009.185. Epub 2009 Oct 27. Review. PubMed PMID: 19859068. http://www.ncbi.nlm.nih.gov/pubmed/19859068

Dib C, Tajik AJ, Park S, Kheir ME, Khandieria B, Mookadam F. Chylopericardium in adults: a literature review over the past decade (1996-2006). J Thorac Cardiovasc Surg. 2008 Sep;136(3):650-6. https://doi.org/10.1016/j.jtcvs.2008.03.033. Epub 2008 Jun 2. Review. PubMed PMID: 18805268. http://www.ncbi.nlm.nih.gov/pubmed/18805268

Restrepo CS, Lemos DF, Lemos JA, Velasquez E, Diethelm L, Ovella TA, Martinez S, Carrillo J, Moncada R, Klein JS. Imaging findings in cardiac tamponade with emphasis on CT. Radiographics. 2007 Nov-Dec;27(6):1595-610. Review. PubMed PMID: 18025505. http://www.ncbi.nlm.nih.gov/pubmed/18025505 **

Ojeda W, Martínez-Toro JA. Diagnosis and management of pericardial effusions. P R Health Sci J. 2006 Sep;25(3):255-8. Review. PubMed PMID: 17203796. http://www.ncbi.nlm.nih.gov/pubmed/17203796 **

Levy PY, Habib G, Collart F, Lepidi H, Raoult D. Etiological diagnosis of pericardial effusion. Future Microbiol. 2006 Aug;1(2):229-39. Review. PubMed PMID: 17661668. http://www.ncbi.nlm.nih.gov/pubmed/17661668

Clinical Trial

Imazio M, Belli R, Beqaraj F, Giammaria M, Lestuzzi C, Hoit B, LeWinter M, Spodick DH, Adler Y; DROP Investigators. DRainage Or Pericardiocentesis alone for recurrent nonmalignant, nonbacterial pericardial effusions requiring intervention: rationale and design of the DROP trial, a randomized, open-label, multicenter study. J Cardiovasc Med (Hagerstown). 2014 Jun;15(6):510-4. https://doi.org/10.2459/JCM.0b013e3283621d26. PubMed PMID: 23867908. http://www.ncbi.nlm.nih.gov/pubmed/23867908 **

General

Labovitz AJ, Noble VE, Bierig M, Goldstein SA, Jones R, Kort S, Porter TR, Spencer KT, Tayal VS, Wei K. Focused cardiac ultrasound in the emergent setting: a consensus statement of the American Society of Echocardiography and American College of Emergency Physicians. J Am Soc Echocardiogr. 2010 Dec;23(12):1225-30. https://doi.org/10.1016/j.echo.2010.10.005. PubMed PMID: 21111923. http://www.ncbi.nlm.nih.gov/pubmed/21111923

Use PubMed Clinical Queries to find the most recent evidence. Use this search strategy: "Pericardial Effusion"[Mesh] OR "Cardiac Tamponade"[Mesh] OR "pericardial effusion" OR "Pericardial effusions" OR "cardiac tamponade" OR "pericardial tamponade"

Chapter 55
Pleural Effusion

Charles V. Pollack, Jr., Melissa Platt, Richard M. Cantor, and Victoria G. Riese

Name and Synonyms

Pleural Effusion

- Hydrothorax, chylothorax, malignant effusion, parapneumonic effusion

Incidence/Epidemiology

- Pleural effusions may develop as a result of more than 50 different disorders.
  - The most common causes are congestive heart failure, malignancy, severe pneumonia, and thromboembolism.
  - A particularly worrisome, potentially infectious cause is tuberculosis.
  - In pediatrics, the incidence of parapneumonic effusions is increasing.

C. V. Pollack, Jr. (✉)
Department of Emergency Medicine, Thomas Jefferson University, Philadelphia, PA, USA

M. Platt
Department of Emergency Medicine, University of Louisville, Louisville, KY, USA

R. M. Cantor
Department of Emergency Medicine and Pediatrics, State University of New York Upstate Medical University, Syracuse, NY, USA

V. G. Riese
Librarian Consultant, Eldersburg, MD, USA

C. V. Pollack, Jr. (ed.), *Differential Diagnosis of Cardiopulmonary Disease*,
https://doi.org/10.1007/978-3-319-63895-9_55

Differential Diagnosis

- The differential diagnosis of pleural effusion is quite broad and includes the following:
  - Congestive heart failure
  - Hepatic hydrothorax
  - Nephrotic syndrome
  - Hypoproteinemia
  - Glomerulonephritis
  - Superior vena cava obstruction
  - Malignancy
  - Pneumonia
  - Tuberculosis
  - Pulmonary embolism
  - Fungal infection
  - Pancreatic pseudocyst
  - Intra-abdominal abscess
  - Post coronary artery bypass graft surgery
  - Post–cardiac injury syndrome
  - Pericardial disease
  - Meigs syndrome
  - Ovarian hyperstimulation syndrome
  - Rheumatoid pleuritis
  - Lupus
  - Drug-induced pleural disease
  - Asbestos pleural effusion
  - Uremia
  - Chylothorax
  - Acute respiratory distress syndrome
  - Chronic pleural thickening
  - Malignant mesothelioma

Pathophysiology and Etiology

- The pleural space (which lies between the parietal pleura and visceral pleura) is a potential anatomic space which normally holds only a small amount of sterile fluid. Fluid is filtered by the parietal pleura and absorbed by the visceral pleura. Governed by Starling's equation, blood and pleural fluid are in hydrostatic and oncotic balance. When an imbalance exists between the blood and pleural hydrostatic and oncotic pressure, fluid accumulates in the pleural space. Pleural effusions develop whenever influx of fluid into the pleural space exceeds lymphatic efflux.

- There are two types of pleural effusions: transudative and exudative.
  - The fluid in a transudative effusion contains very little protein but is otherwise similar to plasma.
    - Most transudates result from heart failure, but sometimes they are seen in advanced liver disease, nephrotic syndrome, and hypoalbuminemia.
  - The fluid in an exudative effusion is protein rich and is generally associated with pneumonia ("parapneumonic effusion") or cancer ("malignant effusion").

Presentation

Typical/"Classic"

- Small pleural effusions may be entirely asymptomatic.
- Large pleural effusions may present with significant respiratory distress that usually is insidious in onset.
- In pediatrics, the most common presenting symptoms are fever, cough, malaise, anorexia, chest pain, and dyspnea.

Atypical

- Chest pain in isolation is unusual; a viral-type prodrome with low-grade fever preceding chest pain is more common.

Primary Differential Considerations

- The underlying disease process may dominate or obscure the signs and symptoms of the pleural effusion.

History and Physical Exam

Findings That Confirm Diagnosis

- The diagnosis cannot be confirmed without imaging.

Factors That Suggest Diagnosis

- Localized reduced breath sounds on auscultation and dullness to percussion in the same area suggest pleural fluid collection.
- A history of typical predisposing diagnoses, such as heart failure, pneumonia, nephrotic syndrome, liver disease, or malignancy, in a patient with the aforementioned physical findings should prompt imaging. Pleural friction rub is sometimes appreciated and may suggest the diagnosis.

http://www.easyauscultation.com/cases?coursecaseorder=7&courseid=201
Pleural friction rub. [Pleural Rubs; Easy Auscultation; www.easyauscultation.com; copyright 2015, MedEdu LLC]

Factors That Exclude Diagnosis

- The absence of effusion on radiographic study is the only way to exclude the diagnosis with certainty.
- Symmetric breath sounds on auscultation and the absence of dullness to percussion in the lower lung fields make the diagnosis of pleural effusion unlikely. Small loculated effusions may still be present, however, and must be excluded by imaging.

Ancillary Studies

Laboratory

- Usual laboratory studies for evaluating co-morbidities should be obtained.
- If pleural tap is performed, fluid should be sent for Gram stain, cytology, cell count, cultures, protein, lactate dehydrogenase (LDH), and glucose.
  - As menti.oned earlier, transudative fluid has little protein (pleural protein to serum protein < 0.5).

Infection
Bacterial
Mycobacterial
Fungal
Parasitic
Mixed
Gastrointestinal disease
Esophageal perforation
Mediastinitis
Subdiaphragmatic infection
Other
Collagen-vascular disease
Malignancy
Uremia
Drug-induced disease
Pulmonary embolism
Abestosis
Sarcoidosis
Radiation injury
Trauma
Hemothorax
Chylothorax

Differential diagnosis of exudative pleural effusion. Once an effusion is classified as exudative, diagnostic considerations include many infectious and noninfectious diseases. [Salmon C, Bryant R. Pleural effusion and empyema. In: Simberkoff MS, editor. Pleuropulmonary and bronchial infections. Philadelphia: Current Medicine; 1996. Chapter 10. (Mandell GL, editor. Atlas of infectious diseases; vol. 6). ISBN: 0-443-07740-1] *Caption from original*

- The measurement of pleural cholesterol, triglycerides, and amylase also may provide useful information in selected patients.
  - Blood cultures should be performed in all children with parapneumonic effusions. Blood cultures are positive in 10–22 % of children with complicated parapneumonic effusions.
  - In certain instances, tuberculosis testing may be warranted.

Imaging

- Chest radiography (posteroanterior [PA] or anteroposterior upright and lateral decubitus radiographs) confirms the following:
  - Blunting or obliteration of the costophrenic angle on an upright chest radiograph
  - A “meniscus sign” (rim of fluid ascending the lateral chest wall) may be seen.
  - On a PA view, opacification of more than half the thorax suggests a large effusion.
  - On a PA view, opacification of more than one quarter but less than half of the thorax suggests a moderate-sized effusion.
  - A decubitus permits free fluid to layer out on the dependent chest wall and may help distinguish the meniscus from pleural thickening.

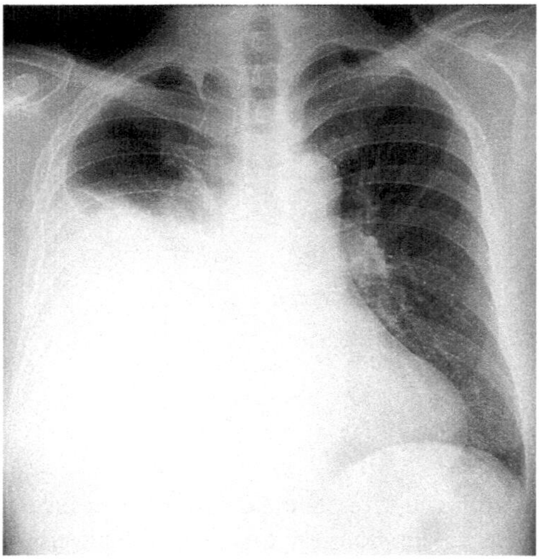

Pleural effusion. Pleural effusion is present in about 6% of patients with ascites, and more often it is on the right side. This is the result of a defect in the diaphragm that allows the ascitic fluid to pass up into the pleural cavity. In contrast, a left-sided pleural effusion in an ascitic patient may indicate pulmonary pathology. Occasionally, a pleural effusion can be seen in the absence of ascites caused by the negative intrathoracic pressure drawing up the ascitic fluid through the diaphragmatic defect into the pleural cavity. Thoracocentesis is followed by rapid refilling of the pleural cavity because of the negative intrathoracic pressure. Control of the pleural effusion can only be achieved with the control of ascites. Insertion of a permanent chest tube can lead to the development of a fistula and is not recommended. /Wong F. Cirrhosis: ascites and spontaneous bacterial peritonitis. In: Maddrey WC, series editor. Atlas of the liver, 4e. Philadelphia: Current Medicine; 2007 (Feldman M, editor. Atlas of gastroenterology and hepatology) ISBN: 1-57340-241-9] *Caption from original*

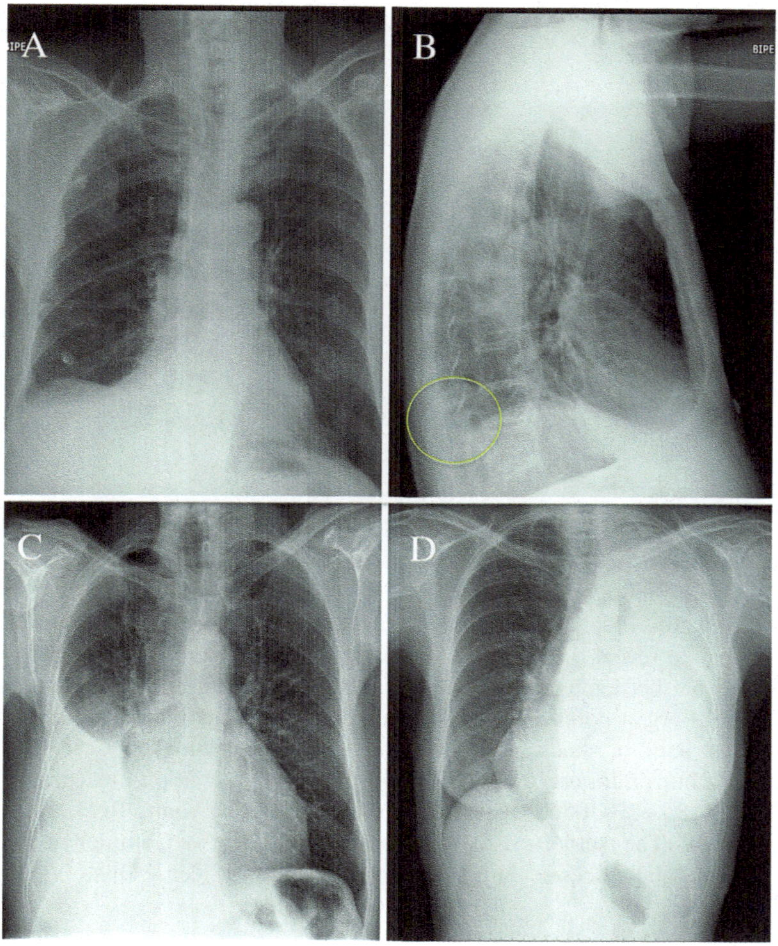

Different chest x-ray images in patients with pleural effusion. (a) Postero-anterior (PA) chest x-ray of a patient with minimal pleural effusion impossible to be detected in this projection. (b) Lateral chest x-ray of the same patient. The circle shows a detectable posterior costo-phrenic angle blunting confirming the presence of minimal pleural effusion. (c) PA chest x-ray of a patient with a moderate right pleural effusion. (d) PA chest x-ray of a patient with a massive left pleural effusion with contralateral mediastinal shift *[*Call S, Sánchez D, Rami-Porta R. Diagnosis and treatment of malignant pleural effusion. In: Kiselevsky MV, editor. Malignant effusions [Internet]. Dordrecht, Netherlands: Springer; 2012 [cited 2015 Aug 28]. p. 23–55. Available from: http://link.springer.com/10.1007/978-94-007-4783-8_3*]* *Caption from original*

- Ultrasound is particularly helpful in guiding thoracentesis.
  - Preferred modality in pediatrics
  - Superior to CT because of better accuracy in detecting early loculations and septations

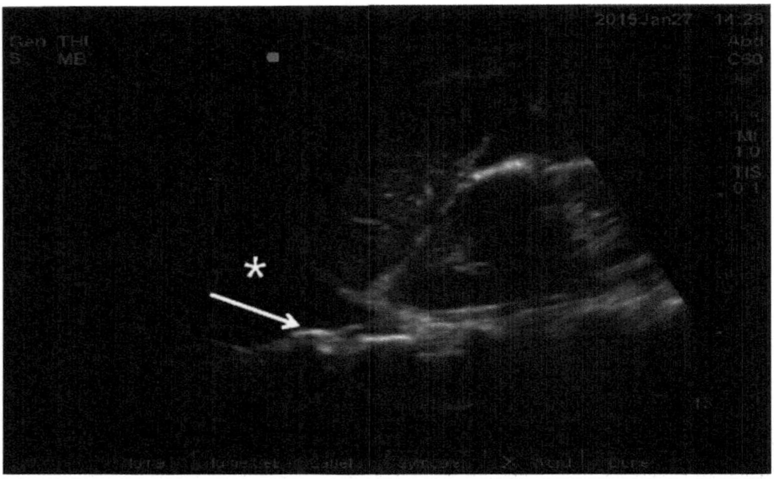

Pleural effusion. Pleural effusion (*asterisk*) permits the ultrasound beam to penetrate deeply to reveal the vertebral stripe (*arrow*). The vertebral stripe will not be visible above the diaphragm if the lung is aerated [From article: Clinically integrated multi-organ point-of-care ultrasound for undifferentiated respiratory difficulty, chest pain, or shock: a critical analytic review. J Intensive Care. 2016 Aug 15;4(1):54. https://doi.org/10.1186/s40560-016-0172-1, at http://link.springer.com/article/10.1186%2Fs40560-016-0172-1/fulltext.html; by Young-Rock Ha, Hong-Chuen Toh, © The Author(s). 2016; licensed under Creative Commons Attribution 4.0 International License http://creativecommons.org/licenses/by/4.0/] *Caption from original*

- Chest CT
  - Can identify small effusions and determine whether larger effusions are loculated, and may identify underlying disease

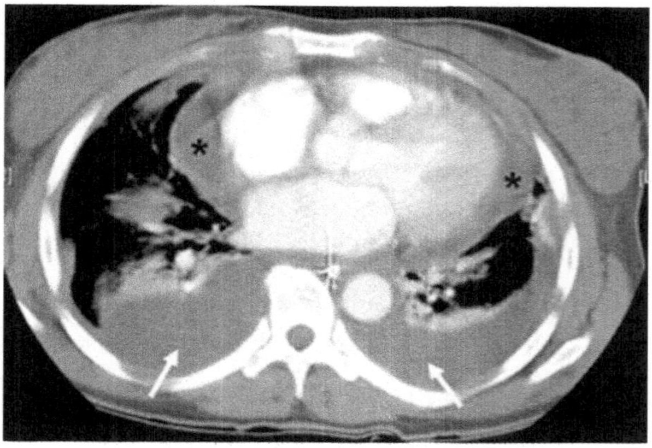

Pleural effusion in systemic lupus erythematosus. Enhanced CT scan at systemic lupus erythematosus (SLE) presentation. Bilateral pleural (arrows) and pericardial (asterisk) effusions resolved promptly with therapy. [Berney S, Heldmann M. Chapter 14. In: Crapo J, editor. Bone's atlas of pulmonary and critical care medicine. 3rd ed. Philadelphia: Current Medicine; 2005. ISBN: 1-57340-211-7] *Caption adapted from original*

Special Populations

Age

- Pleural effusion may occur at any age, although owing to the greater number of underlying disease processes (heart failure, cirrhosis, uremia, malignancy), the incidence increases with age.
- The most common cause of pleural effusion in the pediatric population is lung infection (parapneumonic effusion).
  - Within the pediatric population, reported cases of pleural effusion are on the rise, usually as a result of resistant organisms causing the primary infectious process.
  - Many emergency departments are using ultrasound to accurately diagnose pleural effusions in infants and children.

Co-morbidities

- Because pleural effusion likely is the result of an underlying disease process, those with a history of congestive heart failure, cirrhosis, nephrotic syndrome, mesothelioma, esophageal rupture, certain rheumatologic diseases, or drug-induced lupus, to name a few, also are at risk for pleural effusions.

Pitfalls in Diagnosis

Critical Steps Not to Miss

- Any child who remains febrile or unwell 48 hours after initiation of antibiotic therapy for pneumonia should be reevaluated for possible pleural effusion.
- Always consider pulmonary embolism as a potential underlying cause of effusion.

Time-Dependent Interventions

- Emergency thoracentesis may be warranted for severe respiratory distress.

Overall Principles of Treatment

- Empyema mandates chest tube insertion.
- If effusion does not have a clear etiology, pleural fluid analysis is required.
- Heart failure–associated effusions usually improve with diuresis for the underlying disease.
- Many small effusions are not clinically important and resolve spontaneously.

Disease Course

- Malignant pleural effusions seldom resolve spontaneously.
- Effusions that do not clear with management of underlying disease are more worrisome.
- Effusions may recur, especially in patients with chronic underlying disease, such as heart failure, cirrhosis, or nephrotic syndrome.
- Effusions associated with acute disease, such as pneumonia, usually do not recur.

Related Evidence

Papers of particular interest have been highlighted as:
*** Of key importance*

Practice Guideline

Hooper C, Lee YC, Maskell N; BTS Pleural Guideline Group. Investigation of a unilateral pleural effusion in adults: British Thoracic Society Pleural Disease Guideline 2010. Thorax. 2010 Aug;65 Suppl 2:ii4-17. https://doi.org/10.1136/thx.2010.136978. PMID: 20696692. http://www.ncbi.nlm.nih.gov/pubmed/20696692 **

Roberts ME, Neville E, Berrisford RG, Antunes G, Ali NJ; BTS Pleural Disease Guideline Group. Management of a malignant pleural effusion: British Thoracic Society Pleural Disease Guideline 2010. Thorax. 2010 Aug;65 Suppl 2:ii32-40. https://doi.org/10.1136/thx.2010.136994. PMID: 20696691. http://www.ncbi.nlm.nih.gov/pubmed/20696691 **

Havelock T, Teoh R, Laws D, Gleeson F; BTS Pleural Disease Guideline Group. Pleural procedures and thoracic ultrasound: British Thoracic Society Pleural Disease Guideline 2010. Thorax. 2010 Aug;65 Suppl 2:ii61-76. https://doi.org/10.1136/thx.2010.137026. PMID: 20696688. http://www.ncbi.nlm.nih.gov/pubmed/20696688 **

Review

Wilcox ME, Chong CA, Stanbrook MB, Tricco AC, Wong C, Straus SE. Does this patient have an exudative pleural effusion? The Rational Clinical Examination systematic review. JAMA. 2014 Jun 18;311(23):2422-31. https://doi.org/10.1001/jama.2014.5552. PMID: 24938565. http://www.ncbi.nlm.nih.gov/pubmed/24938565 **

Villena Garrido V, Cases Viedma E, Fernández Villar A, de Pablo Gafas A, Pérez Rodríguez E, Porcel Pérez JM, Rodríguez Panadero F, Ruiz Martínez C, Salvatierra Velázquez A, Valdés Cuadrado L. Recommendations of diagnosis and treatment of pleural effusion. Update. Arch Bronconeumol. 2014 Jun;50(6):235-49. https://doi.org/10.1016/j.arbres.2014.01.016. PMID: 24698396. http://www.ncbi.nlm.nih.gov/pubmed/24698396 **

Corcoran JP, Hallifax R, Rahman NM. Advances in the management of pleural disease. Expert Rev Respir Med. 2013 Oct;7(5):499-513. https://doi.org/10.1586/17476348.2013.838016. PMID: 24138694 http://www.ncbi.nlm.nih.gov/pubmed/24138694 **

Thomas JM, Musani AI. Malignant pleural effusions: a review. Clin Chest Med. 2013 Sep;34(3):459-71. https://doi.org/10.1016/j.ccm.2013.05.004. PMID: 23993817. http://www.ncbi.nlm.nih.gov/pubmed/23993817 **

Light RW. Pleural effusions. Med Clin North Am. 2011 Nov;95(6):1055-70. https://doi.org/10.1016/j.mcna.2011.08.005. PMID: 22032427. http://www.ncbi.nlm.nih.gov/pubmed/22032427 **

McGrath EE, Anderson PB. Diagnosis of pleural effusion: a systematic approach. Am J Crit Care. 2011 Mar;20(2):119-27; quiz 128. https://doi.org/10.4037/ajcc2011685. PMID: 21362716. http://www.ncbi.nlm.nih.gov/pubmed/21362716 **
McGrath EE, Anderson PB. Diagnostic tests for tuberculous pleural effusion. Eur J Clin Microbiol Infect Dis. 2010 Oct;29(10):1187-93. https://doi.org/10.1007/s10096-010-0986-z. PMID: 20556468. http://www.ncbi.nlm.nih.gov/pubmed/20556468 **

Use PubMed Clinical Queries to find the most recent evidence. Use this search strategy:

"Pleural Effusion"[Mesh] OR "Pleural Effusion" OR "Pleural Effusions"

Chapter 56
Pleurisy

Charles V. Pollack, Jr., Richard M. Cantor, and Victoria G. Riese

Name and Synonyms

Pleurisy

- Pleuritic, pleuritic pain

Incidence/Epidemiology

- Pleurisy or pleuritic pain is common and nonspecific.
- There are no clear incidence data, as many patients with pleurisy do not seek medical attention. Others may have significant chest pain as a result of pleurisy.

Differential Diagnosis

- The differential considerations for chest pain due to pleurisy include immediate life threats such as pulmonary embolism, acute coronary syndrome, and aortic dissection.

C. V. Pollack, Jr. (✉)
Department of Emergency Medicine, Thomas Jefferson University,
Philadelphia, PA, USA

R. M. Cantor
Department of Emergency Medicine and Pediatrics, State University of New York Medical University, Syracuse, NY, USA

V. G. Riese
Librarian Consultant, Eldersburg, MD, USA

C. V. Pollack, Jr. (ed.), *Differential Diagnosis of Cardiopulmonary Disease*,
https://doi.org/10.1007/978-3-319-63895-9_56

- Less severe differential considerations include pneumonia and pneumothorax, which may cause pleuritic pain, as well as chest wall pain and anxiety.
- Pericarditis may present similarly.
- Acute chest syndrome in sickle cell disease is a differential consideration in at-risk patients.

Pathophysiology and Etiology

- The pleura is a two-layer membrane in the thorax. The outer, or parietal, layer lines the chest cavity, whereas the inner, or visceral, layer adheres tightly to the lungs. Between these layers is a tiny space that normally contains a small amount of lubricating fluid. In pneumothorax, this space contains air, and in pleural effusion, this space contains larger amounts of fluid.

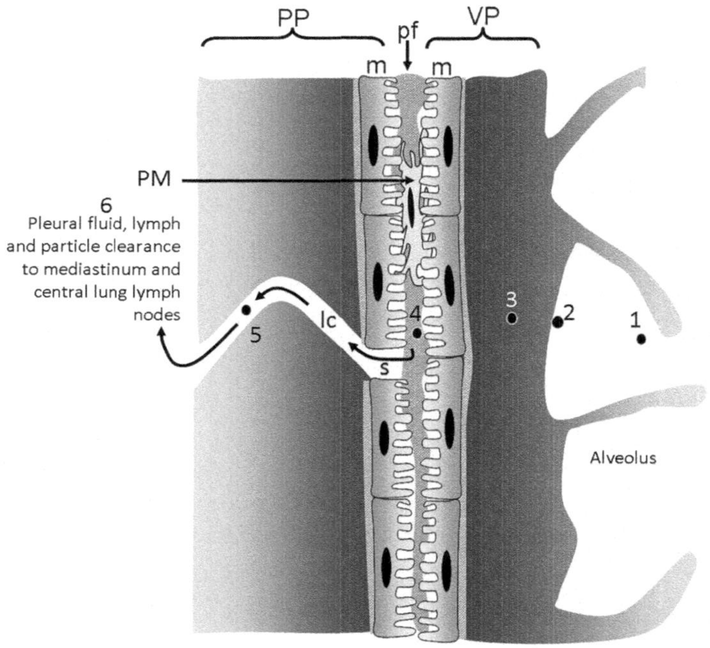

Diagrammatic representation of the relationship between the visceral and parietal pleurae. The visceral pleura (VP) and the parietal pleura (PP) are seen in close apposition separated by a pleural space that contains a small volume of pleural fluid (pf). Contact between the 2 pleurae is made via the mesothelial cell layers (m) on the surface of the parietal and visceral pleurae. Pleural macrophages (PM) are present in the pleural space. The rigid chest wall is tightly locked to the lungs by the adherence of the visceral pleura to the parietal pleura allowing movements of the chest wall caused by the action of the diaphragmatic muscle and intercostal muscle (IM) to expand and relax the lungs, allowing pulmonary inspiration and expiration. The pathway for particles to reach the pleural space is unknown but the path for an airborne particle (1) that deposits in the distal alveoli (2) is shown as it passes into the interstitium (3) enters the pleural space (4) and exits through a stoma in the parietal pleura (s) into a lymphatic capillary (lc, 5) to enter the lymph flow to the lymph nodes in the mediastinum and central lung. [From article: Asbestos, carbon nanotubes and the pleural mesothelium: a review of the hypothesis regarding the role of long fibre retention in the parietal pleura, inflammation and mesothelioma. Part Fibre Toxicol. 2010 Mar;7:5. https://doi.org/10.1186/1743-8977-7-5, at http://link.springer.com/article/10.1186/1743-8977-7-5; by Ken Donaldson, Fiona A Murphy, Rodger Duffin, Craig A Poland, © Donaldson et al; licensee BioMed Central Ltd. 2010; licensed under Creative Commons Attribution License BY 2.0 http://creativecommons.org/licenses/by/2.0] *Caption from original*

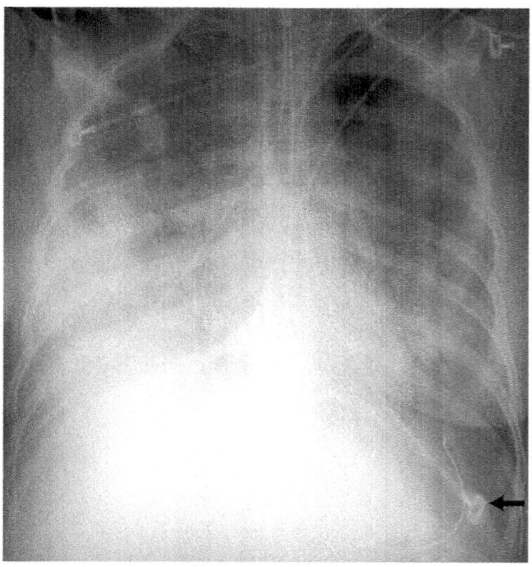

Pneumothorax . A, Chest radiograph of a critically ill patient with a deep sulcus sign on the left (arrow), consistent with the diagnosis of a pneumothorax. B. Chest radiograph of a critically ill patient on mechanical ventilation with the presence of a right loculated tension pneumothorax (arrow). Note the increase in volume of the right hemithorax, depression of the right hemidiaphragm, and contralateral mediastinal shift. [Huggins J, Sahn S. Pleural disease. In: Crapo J, editor. Bone's atlas of pulmonary and critical care medicine. Philadelphia: Current Medicine; 2005. Chapter 25. ISBN: 1-57340-211-7; 2005-01-14] *Caption from original*

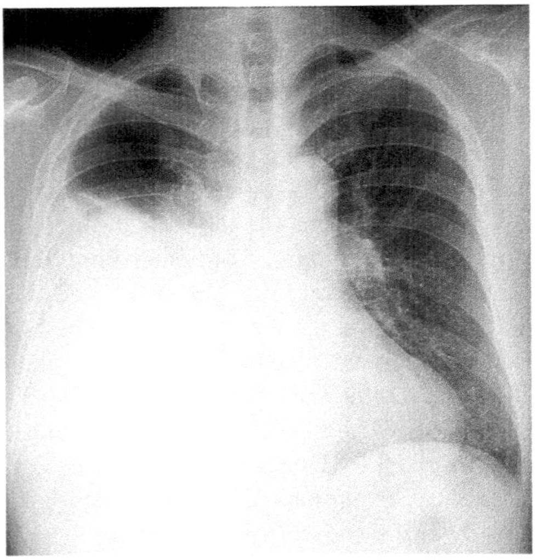

Pleural effusion in ascites. Pleural effusion. [Wong W. Cirrhosis: ascitis and spontaneous bacterial peritonitis. In: Maddrey W, editor. Atlas of the liver. 4th ed. Philadelphia: Current Medicine; 2006. Chapter 10 (Feldman M, editor. Gastroenterology and hepatology; vol. 1; ISBN: 1-57340-241-9; 2006-06-27] *Caption adapted from original*

- Inflammation of the pleura causes the two layers to rub together and results in pain and dyspnea. Although the underlying problem may be the actual cause of dyspnea (pneumonia, pneumothorax), pleurisy itself does not actually *cause* shortness of breath or ventilatory compromise. Instead, the patient perceives dyspnea because of pain on inspiration, which may involuntarily limit inspiratory effort.

Presentation

Typical/"Classic"

- The classic presentation of pleuritic pain is:
  - Acute or relatively acute onset
  - One-sided
  - Exacerbated by inspiration, cough, sneeze, or sudden movement
  - Worse when lying down than when sitting up
  - May extend to shoulder (raising concern of acute coronary syndrome) or abdomen

- A pleural friction rub may be heard.

https://www.youtube.com/watch?v=t2QE0O_exAQ
Audio of pleural friction rub.

http://www.easyauscultation.com/cases?coursecaseorder=7&courseid=201
Pleural Friction Rub [Pleural Rubs; Easy Auscultation; www.easyauscultation.com; copyright 2015, MedEdu LLC]

Atypical

- Because of underlying pathology, pleurisy may present with dyspnea that is more concerning to the patient than the chest pain.
- With pneumonia, fever may be a dominant symptom.

Primary Differential Considerations

- Keeping in mind that pleurisy may be either an independent diagnosis or a symptom of many other thoracic illnesses, the differential diagnosis is broad.
- The most worrisome primary differential considerations are pulmonary embolism and pneumonia.
- Myocardial ischemia and pleural effusion with pleuritis also should be considered early on.

History and Physical Exam

Findings That Confirm Diagnosis

- History and physical examination are not diagnostic for pleurisy.

Factors That Suggest Diagnosis

- Typical pain description (see earlier) with exacerbations from deep breathing or coughing. A change in position is suggestive.
- A pleural friction rub in patients with chest pain indicates pleural involvement.

https://www.youtube.com/watch?v=t2QE0O_exAQ
Audio of pleural friction rub.

Factors That Exclude Diagnosis

- There are no history or physical findings that conclusively exclude pleurisy.

Ancillary Studies

Laboratory

- There are no diagnostic laboratory studies for pleurisy.
- Laboratory tests target suspected underlying disease.
- If measured, erythrocyte sedimentation rate and C-reactive protein may be elevated in patients with pleurisy, but these tests are not essential for the diagnosis or treatment.

Imaging

- Chest radiography does not reveal pleurisy itself, but may reveal the underlying cause.
- Chest radiography or CT scanning may exclude pneumothorax and pulmonary embolism as causes of pleurisy.

Special Populations

Age and Gender

- The epidemiology of pleurisy follows that of the underlying cause. Therefore, it may occur at any age from childhood to old age. Some diseases (e.g., lung cancer) have a gender predilection, and secondary pleurisy therefore will follow that.
- Pleurisy in children is synonymous with any atraumatic cause of chest pain.
- Texidor's twinge, or precordial catch, is a benign cause of musculoskeletal chest pain in children. It is associated with brief, sharp, painful episodes near the left sternal border.
- Pleurodynia, or Bornholm disease, is an infrequent complication of Coxsackie B infections
  - It is characterized by sudden, severe episodes of unilateral chest pain, restricting air entry (hence the name "devil's grip").
  - It resolves spontaneously.

Co-morbidities

- Typical co-morbidities (and underlying causes) of pleurisy include:
  - Viral and bacterial lower respiratory tract infections
  - Chest wall trauma
  - Recent thoracic surgery
  - Sickle cell disease
  - Pulmonary embolism
  - Autoimmune disease (lupus, rheumatoid arthritis)
  - Pneumothorax
  - Pericarditis
  - Tuberculosis

Pitfalls in Diagnosis

Critical Steps Not to Miss

- Pleurisy is a symptom, not a disease. Therefore, there are no critical steps in the evaluation of pleurisy.
- Because there are underlying causes of pleurisy that are immediate life threats, evaluation for acute coronary syndrome, pulmonary embolism, and pneumonia should be considered early.

Mimics

- The entire constellation of diagnoses underlying chest pain syndrome, especially those often accompanied by dyspnea, can mimic the pain and overall presentation of pleurisy.
- Pericarditis may mimic pleurisy in presentation. Listen for a pericardial friction rub.

http://www.easyauscultation.com/acute-pericarditis

Acute Pericarditis Audio Recordings. [Acute Pericarditis; Easy Auscultation; www.easyauscultation.com; copyright 2015, MedEdu LLC]

Time-Dependent Interventions

- Underlying disease may be rapidly fatal, but therapy is targeted at the cause of the pleurisy not the pleurisy itself.

Overall Principles of Treatment

- Treatment of the symptoms of pleurisy usually is successful with nonsteroidal anti-inflammatory drugs.
- Treatment of the underlying disease usually will diminish pleurisy symptoms.

Disease Course

- Pleurisy will resolve as the underlying condition clears. There typically is no anatomic damage to the pleura, with the possible exception of tube thoracostomy for pneumothorax. Rarely, patients develop chronic pleuritic pain after chest tube placement.

Related Evidence

Papers of particular interest have been highlighted as:
*** Of key importance*

Review

Jeon D. Tuberculous pleurisy: an update. Tuberc Respir Dis (Seoul). 2014 Apr;76(4):153-9. https://doi.org/10.4046/trd.2014.76.4.153. PMID: 24851127. http://www.ncbi.nlm.nih.gov/pubmed/24851127 **

Cagle PT, Allen TC. Pathology of the pleura: what the pulmonologists need to know. Respirology. 2011 Apr;16(3):430-8. https://doi.org/10.1111/j.1440-1843.2011.01957.x. PMID: 21362105. http://www.ncbi.nlm.nih.gov/pubmed/21362105 **

Kass SM, Williams PM, Reamy BV. Pleurisy. Am Fam Physician. 2007 May 1;75(9):1357-64. PMID: 17508531. http://www.ncbi.nlm.nih.gov/pubmed/17508531 **

English JC, Leslie KO. Pathology of the pleura. Clin Chest Med. 2006 Jun;27(2): 157-80. PMID: 16716811. http://www.ncbi.nlm.nih.gov/pubmed/16716811 **

Segura RM. Useful clinical biological markers in diagnosis of pleural effusions in children. Paediatr Respir Rev. 2004;5 Suppl A:S205-12. PMID: 14980272. http://www.ncbi.nlm.nih.gov/pubmed/14980272 **

Cohort Study

Valdés L, Alvarez D, San José E, Penela P, Valle JM, García-Pazos JM, Suárez J, Pose A. Tuberculous pleurisy: a study of 254 patients. Arch Intern Med. 1998 Oct 12;158(18):2017-21. PMID: 9778201. http://www.ncbi.nlm.nih.gov/pubmed/9778201

Comparative Study

Bösner S, Haasenritter J, Hani MA, Keller H, Sönnichsen AC, Karatolios K, Schaefer JR, Baum E, Donner-Banzhoff N. Gender differences in presentation and diagnosis of chest pain in primary care. BMC Fam Pract. 2009 Dec 14;10:79. https://doi.org/10.1186/1471-2296-10-79. PMID: 20003406. http://www.ncbi.nlm.nih.gov/pubmed/20003406

Use PubMed Clinical Queries to find the most recent evidence. Use this search strategy:

("Pleurisy"[Mesh] OR "Pleurisy")

Chapter 57
Pneumoconiosis

Christopher J. Rees, Charles V. Pollack, Jr., and Victoria G. Riese

Name and Synonyms

Pneumoconiosis
Black Lung Disease (Coal Worker's Pneumoconiosis)
Asbestosis
Silicosis

Incidence/Epidemiology

- The incidence of pneumoconiosis in Western nations has been declining for the past 20 years. However, in developing nations, where regulatory oversight is not as consistent, the incidence of these disorders continues to increase.
- From 1968 through 1992 in the United States, there were 100,800 death certificates listing pneumoconiosis as a contributing or primary cause of death.
- In 2013, there reportedly were about 250,000 deaths worldwide from pneumoconiosis.
- The most common pneumoconioses are the result of exposure to coal dust, silica, and asbestos.

C. J. Rees
Emergency Department, Pennsylvania Hospital, Philadelphia, PA, USA

C. V. Pollack, Jr. (✉)
Department of Emergency Medicine, Thomas Jefferson University, Philadelphia, PA, USA

V. G. Riese
Librarian Consultant, Eldersburg, MD, USA

C. V. Pollack, Jr. (ed.), *Differential Diagnosis of Cardiopulmonary Disease*,
https://doi.org/10.1007/978-3-319-63895-9_57

Differential Diagnosis

- The differential diagnosis of pneumoconiosis is broad and includes the entire spectrum of diseases that may present with cough and dyspnea, such as asthma, chronic obstructive pulmonary disease (COPD), congestive heart failure (CHF), pneumonia, lung cancer, and all the other interstitial lung diseases (ILDs).

Pathophysiology and Etiology

- Pneumoconioses are a group of ILDs caused by the chronic inhalation of inorganic dusts.
- *Pneumoconiosis* classically refers only to dusts that cause a fibrotic, restrictive pattern of lung disease.
- Exposure to organic dusts tends to cause reactive airway disease that may mimic asthma or, more chronically, obstructive diseases such as COPD.

Table Some types of pneumoconiosis according to dust and lung reaction

Inorganic Dust	**Type of Disease**	**Lung Reaction**
Asbestos	Asbestosis	Fibrosis
Silica (Quartz)	Silicosis	Fibrosis
Coal	Coal Pneumoconiosis	Fibrosis
Beryllium	Beryllium Disease	Fibrosis
Tungsten Carbide	Hard Metal Disease	Fibrosis
Iron	Siderosis	No Fibrosis
Tin	Stannosis	No Fibrosis
Barium	Baritosis	No Fibrosis
Organic Dust		
Mouldy hay, straw and grain	Farmer's lung	Fibrosis
Droppings and feathers	Bird fancier's lung	Fibrosis
Mouldy sugar cane	Bagassosis	Fibrosis
Compost dust	Mushroom worker's lung	No Fibrosis
Dust or mist	Humidifier fever	No Fibrosis
Dust of heat-treated sludge	Sewage sludge disease	No Fibrosis
Mould dust	Cheese washers' lung	No Fibrosis
Dust of dander, hair particles, and dried urine of rats	Animal handlers' lung	No Fibrosis

Some types of pneumoconiosis according to dust and lung reaction [*What are the Effects of Dust on the Lungs?, http://www.ccohs.ca/oshanswers/chemicals/lungs_dust.html, OSH Answers Fact Sheets,* Canadian Centre for Occupational Health and Safety (CCOHS), *October 1, 2012.* Reproduced with the permission of CCOHS, *2016.*]

- Exposure to organic dusts also may cause a distinct syndrome: hypersensitivity pneumonitis.
- This discussion is limited to the classic pneumoconioses.
- The etiology of these diseases usually is multifactorial, with occupational and environmental factors (such as exposure to cigarette smoke) interacting with genetic risk to produce a spectrum of disease activity in affected individuals.
- Many different industries and metals may be associated with the development of pneumoconiosis. This discussion centers on the three most common: coal dust, silica, and asbestos.
- The exact pathophysiologic mechanisms by which these substances produce fibrosis are not well elucidated. In general, it involves chronic immune activation due to direct exposure, phagocytosis of the inorganic particles by macrophages, and the generation of reactive oxygen species with subsequent oxidative injury to the lung tissue.

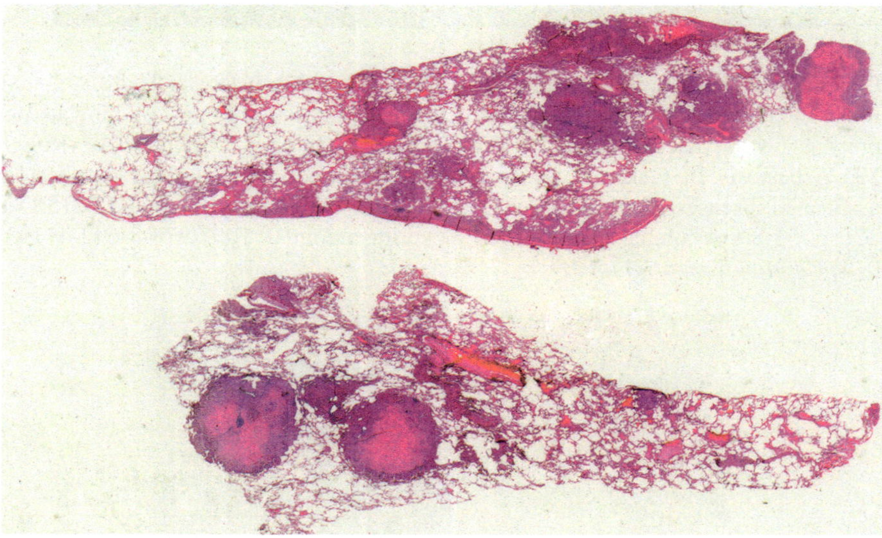

Silicosis. "Dirty" macrophages in a subpleural perilymphatic and peribronchovascular distribution associated with bronchiolocentric fibrotic nodules (haematoxylin–eosin, ×20. Courtesy Dr Alberto Cavazza Reggio Emilia, Italy). [Spagnolo P, Sverzellati N, Wells AU, Hansell DM. Imaging aspects of the diagnosis of sarcoidosis. Eur Radiol. 2014 Apr;24(4):807-16.] *Caption from original*

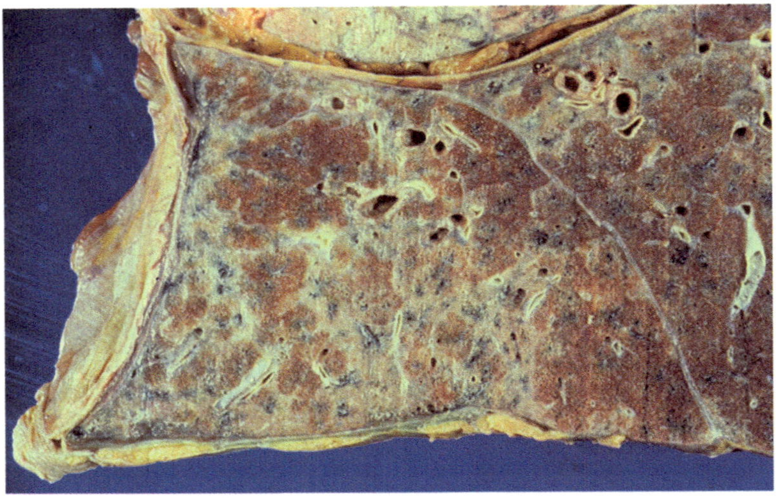

Coronal section of the lower lobe in an insulator with asbestosis. There is coarse linear interstitial fibrosis, but changes of advanced fibrosis or honeycombing are not present. Note accompanying visceral pleural fibrosis [Sporn TA, Roggli VL. Asbestosis. In: Oury TD, Sporn TA, Roggli VL, editors. Pathology of asbestos-associated diseases [Internet]. Berlin, Heidelberg: Springer; 2014 [cited 2015 Dec 22]. p. 53-80. Available from: http://link.springer.com/10.1007/978-3-642-41193-9_4] *Caption from original*

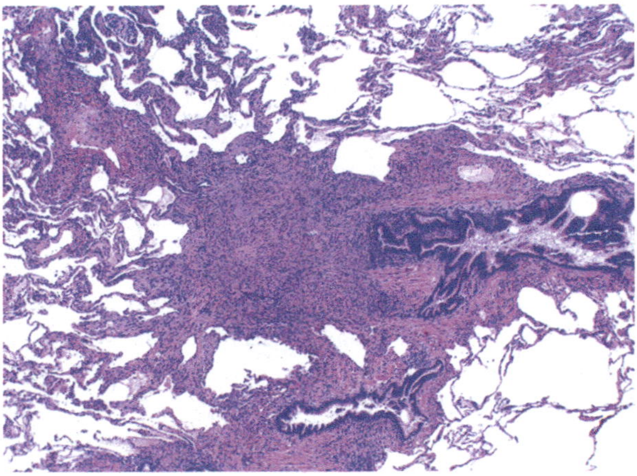

Silicosis. There is a cuff of dust-filled histiocytes around a small bronchiole [Colby TV, Leslie KO. Pathology of diffuse lung disease. In: Baughman RP, du Bois RM, editors. Diffuse lung disease [Internet]. New York: Springer; 2012 [cited 2016 Jan 14]. p. 49-70. Available from: http://link.springer.com/10.1007/978-1-4419-9771-5_4] *Caption from original*

- Coal dust: Coal is a combustible rock formed over eons by the biologic and geologic processing of dead plant matter. Coal is considered a fossil fuel, and the burning of coal is the largest source of energy for electricity generation worldwide. Long-term exposure (>10–20 years) to coal dust in coal mines may cause coal worker's pneumoconiosis (CWP). Inhaled coal dust appears to become phagocytized by macrophages, which tend to group together and develop into "coal macules" within the lung tissue. CWP may be classified radiographically and clinically into simple or complicated CWP. Cigarette smoking does not appear to increase the incidence of CWP.
  - Simple CWP is diagnosed when coal macules grow to about 2–5 mm and become visible on plain chest x-ray (CXR; within upper lung zones). These patients usually are asymptomatic. Simple CWP may be seen in about 10–15 % of coal miners who have worked in the mines for 20 years or more.

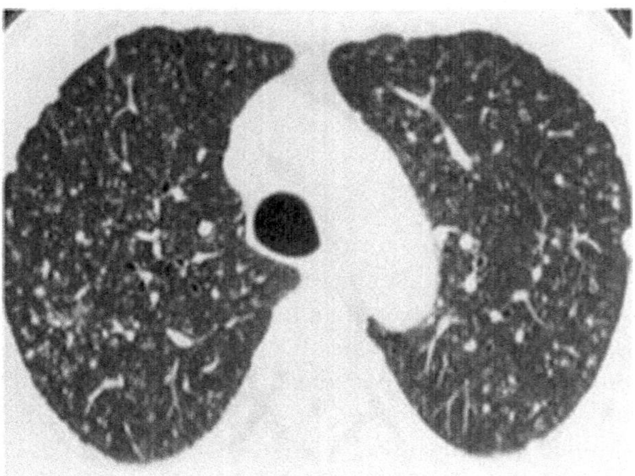

Coal workers pneumoconiosis. HRCT at the level of the upper lobes exhibits a "nodular without tree-in-bud pattern" characterized by ill-defined centrilobular nodules of slightly variable size that have an upper lobe and posterior predominance. A distinctive characteristic occasionally observed is that the micronodules of CWP tend to be less sharply defined and of more granular density than those of silicosis. [From article: Mimics in chest disease: interstitial opacities. Insights Imaging. 2013 Feb;4(1):9-27. https://doi.org/10.1007/s13244-012-0207-7, at http://link.springer.com/article/10.1007%2Fs13244-012-0207-7; by Anastasia Oikonomou, Panos Prassopoulos, © The Author(s) 2012; licensed under Creative Commons Attribution License http://creativecommons.org/licenses/by/2.0] *Caption and text from original*

- Complicated CWP is diagnosed when these macules coalesce into nodules 1 cm or larger. These nodules may take up an entire lobe. These patients usually have symptoms of dyspnea and chronic cough with a restrictive physiology. When the macules become very large and associated with fibrosis, the term *progressive massive fibrosis* (PMF) may be applied. This also is often referred to as "black lung". These patients have severe symptoms associated with hypoxia and a high mortality rate.

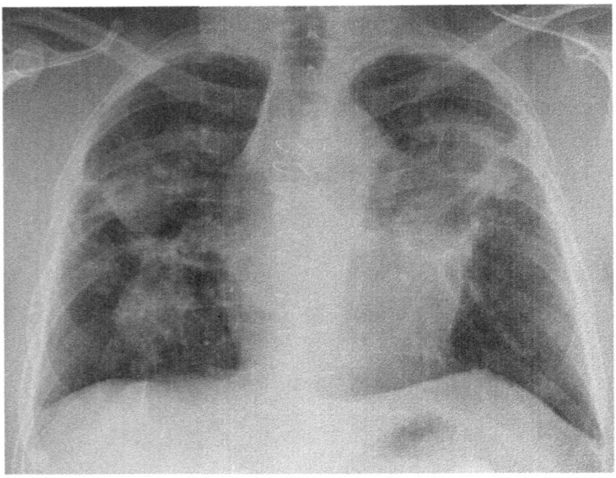

Coal worker's pneumoconiosis. PA chest film: This study demonstrates progressive massive fibrosis, which is usually seen in the upper lobes and posterior to midline on lateral view. Peripheral to the masses is lucency, also very characteristic as the masses "migrate" toward the hila [Goodman PC. Radiography and CT of occupational and environmental lung diseases. In: Huang Y-CT, Ghio AJ, Maier LA, editors. A clinical guide to occupational and environmental lung diseases [Internet]. Totowa, NJ: Humana Press; 2012 [cited 2015 Dec 22]. p. 59-92. Available from: http://link.springer.com/10.1007/978-1-62703-149-3_4] *Caption from original*

- Silica: Free silica (silicon dioxide, SiO_2, crystalline quartz) is commonly encountered by employees in the mining, stonecutting, cement manufacturing, and other stone-related industries. In general, many years of exposure are required to develop pulmonary fibrosis. Silicosis also may be classified as simple or complicated. There also is a much less common syndrome from acute, high-intensity exposure: acute silicosis. Silica is taken up by alveolar macrophages, to which it is toxic. Patients with silicosis therefore have an increased risk for atypical lung infections associated with decreased macrophage function, such as tuberculosis, atypical mycobacteria, and fungi.
  - Simple silicosis, like simple CWP, is marked by the appearance on CXR of small (0.3–5-mm) round opacities in the upper lobes. These patients are mostly asymptomatic. About 20 % of patients will have associated calcification of their hilar lymph nodes, which gives a characteristic "eggshell" appearance on CXR and high-resolution CT (HRCT).

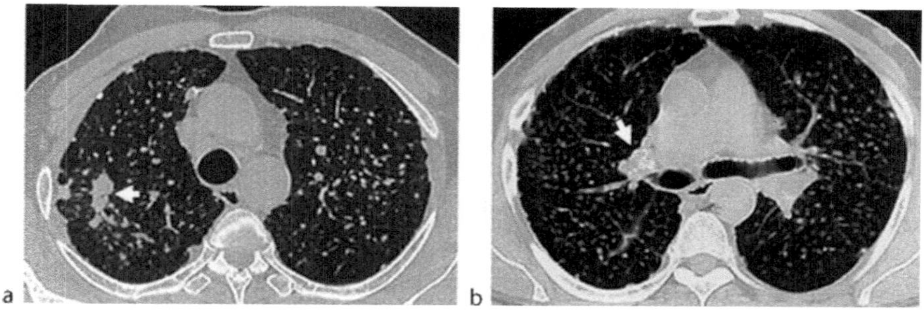

Silicotic nodules. (a) Centrilobular and randomly distributed pleural nodules and large opacity (arrow) due to complicated silicosis (progressive massive fibrosis). (b) Egg-shell calcification (arrow) in lymph nodes. [Hering KG. Pneumoconioses. In: Baert AL, editor. Encyclopedia of diagnostic imaging [Internet]. Berlin, Heidelberg: Springer; 2008 [cited 2015 Dec 22]. p. 1509-12. Available from: http://www.springerlink.com/index/10.1007/978-3-540-35280-8_1976] *Caption from original*

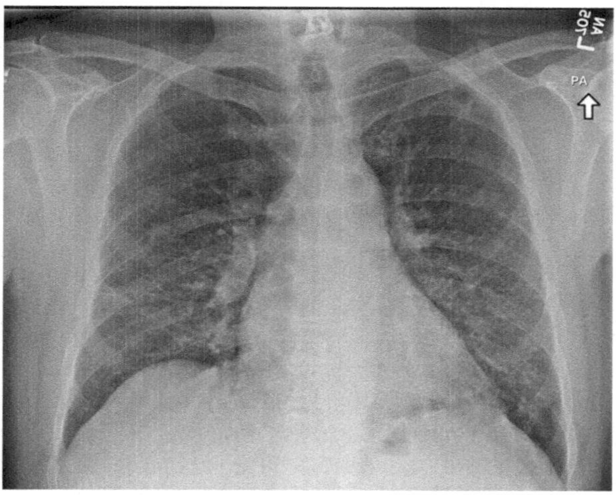

Silicosis. PA chest film demonstrates bilateral small nodules seen best over the lingual. [Goodman PC. Radiography and CT of occupational and environmental lung diseases. In: Huang Y-CT, Ghio AJ, Maier LA, editors. A clinical guide to occupational and environmental lung diseases [Internet]. Totowa, NJ: Humana Press; 2012 [cited 2015 Dec 22]. p. 59-92. Available from: http://link.springer.com/10.1007/978-1-62703-149-3_4] *Caption from original*

- Complicated silicosis occurs when the nodules grow or coalesce to greater than 1 cm in diameter. This usually is associated with significant fibrosis and usually leads to symptoms. As in CWP, these fibrotic nodules may become quite large and also lead to PMF and significant functional impairment and mortality. Once the process of fibrosis starts, it may continue even in the absence of continued exposure.

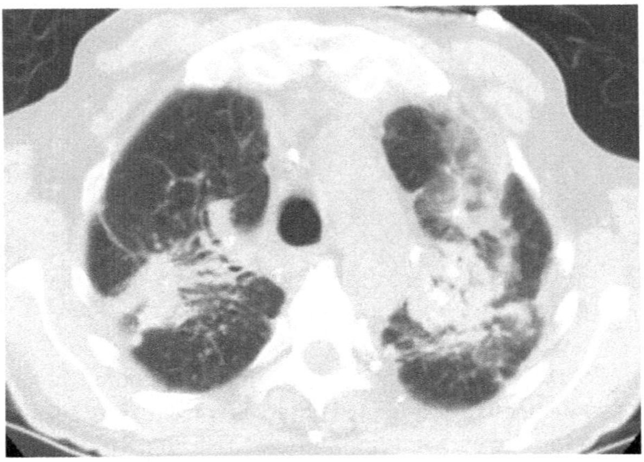

Silicosis. Single slice from a CT scan in lung windows demonstrates the typical upper posterior location of conglomerate opacities or progressive massive fibrosis in a patient with silicosis. Note the small clustered nodules posterior to the right-sided PMF as well as the bilateral hilar and mediastinal calcified lymph nodes. Also note that some calcified parenchymal nodules are incorporated in the PMF. [Goodman PC. Radiography and CT of occupational and environmental lung diseases. In: Huang Y-CT, Ghio AJ, Maier LA, editors. A clinical guide to occupational and environmental lung diseases [Internet]. Totowa, NJ: Humana Press; 2012 [cited 2015 Dec 22]. p. 59-92. Available from: http://link.springer.com/10.1007/978-1-62703-149-3_4] *Caption from original*

  - Acute silicosis is an uncommon syndrome that occurs after short-term exposure (about 1 year) to high concentrations of silica in confined spaces (e.g., from sandblasting or tunneling through rock with a high quartz content). It is manifest with progressive dyspnea and a chronic, usually nonproductive cough, although the patient occasionally may have gelatinous sputum, with low-grade fever and constitutional symptoms. CXR usually reveals a diffuse miliary pattern but may show diffuse alveolar opacities. HRCT shows a characteristic "crazy paving" pattern.

- Asbestos: *Asbestos* is a general term that refers to several mineral silicates. Silicate minerals are the predominant minerals in rock and make up 90 % of the earth's crust. These silicates differ from silica, which is silicon dioxide; rather, silicates have many different ratios of silicon to oxygen. Asbestos is characterized by being made up of long, thin, fiber-like crystals. Each visible fiber is composed of millions of microscopic "fibrils" that may be released by abrasion and other processes. Asbestos has been mined and used for millennia. It has excellent thermal, electrical, and acoustic insulating properties and is markedly fire resistant. Although synthetic materials largely have replaced asbestos use in developed nations, asbestos continues to be mined and used widely in developing countries. Asbestos predominantly affects the respiratory tract and causes pleural fibrosis, pulmonary fibrosis, cancers of the respiratory tract, and pleural and pulmonary mesothelioma. The development of asbestos-related diseases is directly related to the extent and duration of exposure. In general, more than 10 years of exposure is necessary for any of these diseases to develop.

- *Asbestosis* is the term given to the pneumoconiosis associated with asbestos exposure. It is a diffuse, nodular, interstitial fibrosing disease of the lung. CXR usually shows the typical progression of disease, usually with pleural plaques as the initial finding. These plaques are observed as thickening or calcification of the parietal pleura, usually along the diaphragmatic border. Pleural plaques are a clue to significant asbestos exposure; they generally are asymptomatic and in isolation do not signify underlying pulmonary disease. Benign pleural effusions also may occur. As the disease progresses, CXR will show linear opacities in the lung bases that may become irregularly shaped and spread into the middle and upper lung zones. Severe disease may be associated with a diffuse ground-glass appearance and/or honeycombing on CXR. Once patients become symptomatic, they demonstrate restrictive pulmonary disease with decreased lung volumes and decreased diffusing capacity.

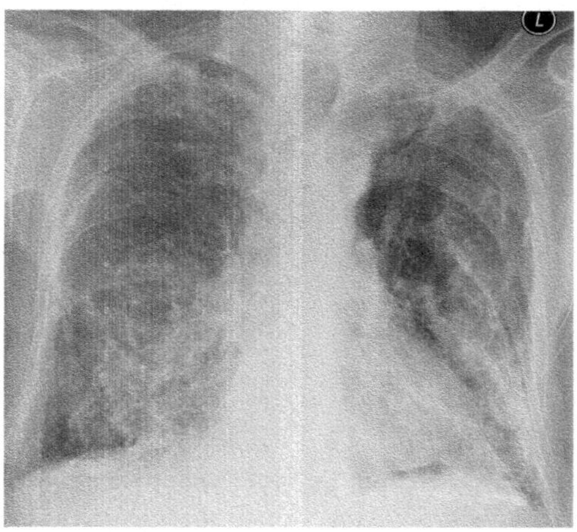

Asbestosis and asbestos-related pleural plaques. PA chest film demonstrates bibasilar heterogeneous irregular lung opacities (look at lung overlying both costophrenic angles) as well as calcified bilateral pleural plaques, many seen en face, which makes assessment of underlying lung disease difficult [Goodman PC. Radiography and CT of occupational and environmental lung diseases. In: Huang Y-CT, Ghio AJ, Maier LA, editors. A clinical guide to occupational and environmental lung diseases [Internet]. Totowa, NJ: Humana Press; 2012 [cited 2015 Dec 22]. p. 59-92. Available from: http://link.springer.com/10.1007/978-1-62703-149-3_4] *Caption from original*

- Other asbestos-related pulmonary disease:
  - Lung cancer is the most common cancer associated with asbestos exposure. It is directly related to the extent and duration of the exposure.

Smoking dramatically increases the risk of lung cancer in those exposed to asbestos. The risk is beyond what would be expected from just adding each risk (asbestos exposure and smoking) individually.

- Mesothelioma. Pleural and peritoneal mesothelioma is associated with asbestos exposure. It may occur with much less exposure and with prolonged latent periods (up to 40 years). Smoking does not appear to increase the risk of mesothelioma. Mesothelioma is much less common than lung cancer.

Presentation

Typical/"Classic"

- Pneumoconiosis may range from asymptomatic findings on imaging to severe, life-threatening restrictive pulmonary disease.
- Patients who develop symptoms usually will have slowly progressive shortness of breath and a dry cough.
- It usually is possible to obtain a history of occupational exposure to a known cause of pneumoconiosis.
- On examination, symptomatic patients usually have fine, inspiratory crackles.
- CXR and/or HRCT of the lungs usually show the typical changes of the inciting pneumoconiosis (see "Imaging").

Atypical

- Silicosis rarely may present more acutely, in patients who have been exposed to large amounts of silica dust in a small space (such as in tunneling and sandblasting). Acute silicosis may occur with short-term exposure (1 year or less). The presentation of acute silicosis is unlike that of usual silicosis (or other pneumoconioses), as it is not a restrictive disease. Although patients with acute silicosis have shortness of breath and cough, the cough may produce a copious amount of thick, white sputum. CXR may show diffuse, miliary nodules that subsequently develop into lobar consolidations. HRCT reveals the characteristic crazy-paving appearance of the lung parenchyma.

Primary Differential Considerations

- Pneumonia
- Acute exacerbation of COPD
- Pulmonary edema
- Acute exacerbation of asthma
- Lung cancer

History and Physical Exam

Findings That Confirm Diagnosis

- The diagnosis often may be nearly confirmed by a history of prolonged occupational exposure to a known inciting agent.
- There are no pathognomic physical examination findings for pneumoconiosis. Patients often demonstrate the signs of restrictive lung disease, such as diffuse, fine inspiratory crackles. Later findings with more advanced disease may include digital clubbing and hypoxia.
- The aforementioned findings together with a confirmatory imaging study confirm the diagnosis.

Factors That Suggest Diagnosis

- A history of occupational exposure to a known inciting agent should suggest the diagnosis.
- Symptoms that occur, or worsen, only while the patient is at work strongly suggest an occupational cause.

Factors That Exclude Diagnosis

- The complete lack of any occupational/environmental/hobby exposure to any of the known inciting agents for pneumoconiosis should lead to evaluation for an alternative diagnosis.

Ancillary Studies

Pulmonary Function Studies

- Pulmonary function tests (PFTs) may be very helpful in the diagnosis of pneumoconiosis. PFTs should show a restrictive pattern, with diffusely decreased lung volumes (total lung capacity [TLC], functional residual capacity [FRC], residual volume [RV], and forced vital capacity [FVC]) and a decreased diffusing capacity for carbon monoxide (DLCO). As opposed to obstructive lung disease (asthma, COPD), airway resistance in restrictive lung disease is normal.

Laboratory

- There are no laboratory studies particularly helpful for the diagnosis or management of pneumoconiosis.

Imaging

- CXR:
    - The plain CXR may be extremely useful in the diagnosis of pneumoconiosis.
    - In general, small round opacities in the upper lung zones are characteristic of both simple silicosis and simple CWP.
    - In both silicosis and CWP, the nodules may coalesce and grow to 1 cm or greater. Both diseases also progress to significant pulmonary fibrosis with larger areas of opacity as well as lung volume loss, usually noted in the upper lung zones. Sometimes these changes involve an entire lobe or even multiple lobes; this situation is termed progressive massive fibrosis.
    - About 20 % of patients with silicosis will develop calcification of the hilar lymph nodes, as seen on CXR; this is termed eggshell calcification and is characteristic of silicosis.
    - Asbestosis is characterized by pleural plaques (usually diaphragmatic) and small linear opacities in the lung bases. These opacities may spread to include all lung fields.
- HRCT of the lungs:

- HRCT is very helpful in the diagnosis and evaluation of all the ILDs.
- The changes associated with these diseases may be appreciated earlier and be more characteristic on HRCT as compared with CXR.
- HCRT has been shown to improve the detection and diagnosis of asbestosis compared with plain CXR.

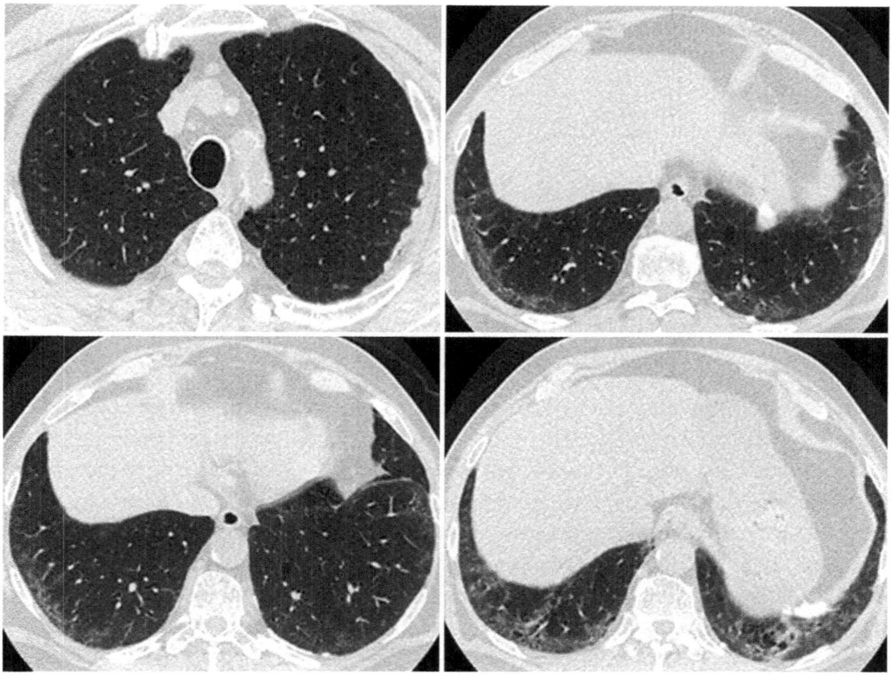

HRCT scan of a 62 year old plumber with asbestosis showing linear opacities and subpleural nodular opacities (upper left), ground-glass attenuation, subpleural honeycombing, and calcified plaques [Müller-Quernheim J, Zissel G, Kayser G, Prasse A. Chronic beryllium disease and other interstitial lung diseases of occupational origin. In: Cottin V, Cordier J-F, Richeldi L, editors. Orphan lung diseases [Internet]. London: Springer; 2015 [cited 2015 Dec 22]. p. 473-91. Available from: http://link.springer.com/10.1007/978-1-4471-2401-6_30] *Caption from original*

- HRCT may lead to consideration of alternative ILDs in the differential diagnosis.
- HRCT may demonstrate the crazy-paving pattern typical of acute silicosis.

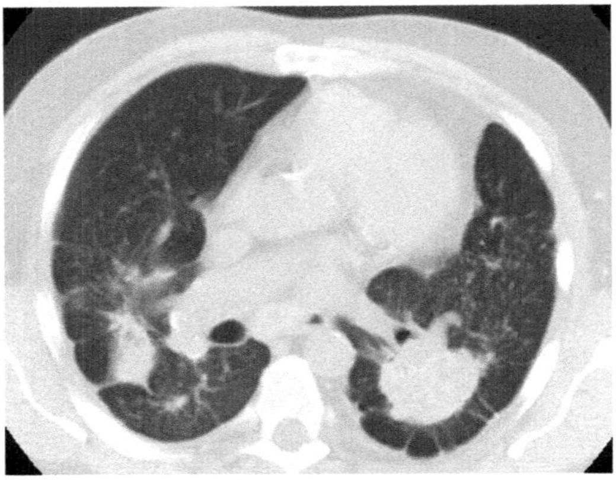

Coal worker's pneumoconiosis. Single slice of a CT scan demonstrates progressive massive fibrosis as represented by the larger opacities posterior to midline in the upper lobes. Just adjacent to the masses are very small nodular opacities which represent the earlier changes of coal worker's pneumoconiosis. As these small nodules coalesce, the large opacities are formed. As the masses migrate centrally, areas of emphysema are formed in the lung periphery as seen here bilaterally [Goodman PC. Radiography and CT of occupational and environmental lung diseases. In: Huang Y-CT, Ghio AJ, Maier LA, editors. A clinical guide to occupational and environmental lung diseases [Internet]. Totowa, NJ: Humana Press; 2012 [cited 2015 Dec 22]. p. 59-92. Available from: http://link.springer.com/10.1007/978-1-62703-149-3_4] *Caption adapted from original*

Special Populations

Age

- Given the decades-long latency between exposure and disease, these are diseases of middle-aged to older adults.

Co-morbidities

- There are multiple comorbidities of importance. Many of these patients also have risk factors for other pulmonary diseases, such as COPD, from other exposures and smoking, making the diagnosis and management more difficult.

- In many patients, the etiology of their pulmonary disease is multifactorial and includes occupational, environmental (smoking, air pollution), and genetic factors.
- Any cause of chronic dyspnea and cough (COPD, CHF, another ILD) may coexist with a pneumoconiosis.
- Patients with silicosis have decreased alveolar macrophage numbers and function, because silica is cytotoxic to these macrophages. These patients then have an increased risk and incidence of pulmonary infections associated with decreased macrophage function, primarily tuberculosis, atypical mycobacterial pneumonia, and fungal pneumonia.
- Silicosis (and to a lesser extent, CWP) also is associated with an increased incidence of autoimmune connective tissue diseases, such as rheumatoid arthritis (both silicosis and CWP) and scleroderma (silicosis only). Seropositive rheumatoid arthritis associated with findings of simple silicosis or simple CWP on CXR has been called Caplan's syndrome.

Pitfalls in Diagnosis

Critical Steps Not to Miss

- It is critical to obtain a complete occupational, environmental, and hobby history to be able to ascertain any significant exposures the patient may have sustained.
- If supported by the history, and the diagnosis is being considered, it is critical to perform appropriate imaging (CXR, HRCT) and PFTs to secure the diagnosis.

Mimics

- Many different diseases may present similarly to pneumoconiosis (with dyspnea and cough), including all the ILDs, COPD, asthma, and CHF.
- With an appropriate history, examination, imaging, and PFTs, the mimics include other restrictive lung diseases, such as other ILDs.

Time-Dependent Interventions

- These disorders tend to be chronic and slowly progressive, so there are no significant time-dependent interventions.

- If a patient presents with hypoxia, oxygen should be administered.
- If a patient is having ventilatory difficulty, ventilation should be supported. Patients with ventilatory difficulty generally have advanced disease, and the approach to managing ventilatory emergencies would ideally have been discussed with the patient and family and decisions made before the acute event.

Overall Principles of Treatment

- There is no specific treatment for any pneumoconiosis.
- Treatment tends to be supportive and should proceed as for most restrictive lung diseases.
- Patients with hypoxia require oxygen.
- Patients with silicosis should be monitored for atypical lung infections, such as tuberculosis.
- All patients should receive routine care as appropriate for any patient with chronic lung disease, including appropriate vaccinations (influenza, pneumococcus).
- Patients who smoke tobacco should be offered all assistance needed to stop.
- Patients still working in an occupation with risk for continued exposure should stop or be moved to a position with no exposure risk.
- These patients may be at increased risk for lung cancer and may need periodic monitoring.

Disease Course

- These diseases are slowly progressive.
- The diseases may continue to progress even after the exposure has stopped.
- There is a large individual variation in the severity of disease. Although development of a pneumoconiosis is related to the extent and duration of exposure, severity of disease is less so.
- Many patients will remain asymptomatic, with only CXR findings, throughout their lives. Some patients may develop only minor symptoms; others may progress to life-altering and -shortening disease.

Related Evidence

Papers of particular interest have been highlighted as:
*** Of key importance*

Review

Prazakova S, Thomas PS, Sandrini A, Yates DH. Asbestos and the lung in the 21st century: an update. Clin Respir J. 2014 Jan;8(1):1-10. https://doi.org/10.1111/crj.12028. PMID: 23711077. http://www.ncbi.nlm.nih.gov/pubmed/23711077 **

Jun JS, Jung JI, Kim HR, Ahn MI, Han DH, Ko JM, Park SH, Lee HG, Arakawa H, Koo JW. Complications of pneumoconiosis: radiologic overview. Eur J Radiol. 2013 Oct;82(10):1819-30. https://doi.org/10.1016/j.ejrad.2013.05.026. PMID: 23791520. http://www.ncbi.nlm.nih.gov/pubmed/23791520 **

Cullinan P, Reid P. Pneumoconiosis. Prim Care Respir J. 2013 Jun;22(2):249-52. https://doi.org/10.4104/pcrj.2013.00055. PMID: 23708110. http://www.ncbi.nlm.nih.gov/pubmed/23708110 **

Karkhanis VS, Joshi JM. Pneumoconioses. Indian J Chest Dis Allied Sci. 2013 Jan-Mar;55(1):25-34. PMID: 23798087. http://www.ncbi.nlm.nih.gov/pubmed/23798087 **

Laney AS, Weissman DN. The classic pneumoconioses: new epidemiological and laboratory observations. Clin Chest Med. 2012 Dec;33(4):745-58. https://doi.org/10.1016/j.ccm.2012.08.005. PMID: 23153613. http://www.ncbi.nlm.nih.gov/pubmed/23153613 **

Leung CC, Yu IT, Chen W. Silicosis. Lancet. 2012 May 26;379(9830):2008-18. https://doi.org/10.1016/S0140-6736(12)60235-9. PMID: 22534002. http://www.ncbi.nlm.nih.gov/pubmed/22534002 **

Review. Yucesoy B, Luster MI. Genetic susceptibility in pneumoconiosis. Toxicol Lett. 2007 Feb 5;168(3):249-54. PMID: 17161563. http://www.ncbi.nlm.nih.gov/pubmed/17161563 **

Use PubMed Clinical Queries to find the most recent evidence. Use this search strategy:

“Pneumoconiosis”[Mesh] OR “Pneumoconiosis”

Chapter 58
Pneumonia

Charles V. Pollack, Jr., Richard M. Cantor, and Victoria G. Riese

Name and Synonyms

Pneumonia

Incidence/Epidemiology

- Pneumonia is an infection of the lung parenchyma.

C. V. Pollack, Jr. (✉)
Department of Emergency Medicine, Thomas Jefferson University,
Philadelphia, PA, USA

R. M. Cantor
Department of Emergency Medicine and Pediatrics, State University of New York Upstate
Medical University, Syracuse, NY, USA

V. G. Riese
Librarian Consultant, Eldersburg, MD, USA

C. V. Pollack, Jr. (ed.), *Differential Diagnosis of Cardiopulmonary Disease*,
https://doi.org/10.1007/978-3-319-63895-9_58

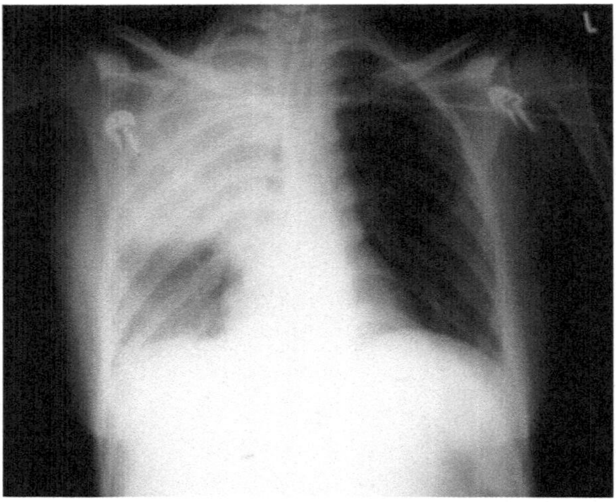

Pneumococcal pneumonia, Chest radiograph of a black African man aged 19 years who presented with a 1-week history of cough, fever, and chest pain. Radiograph shows dense consolidation of the right upper lobe. Differential diagnosis included Klebsiella pneumonia. Sputum Gram stain and blood culture confirmed Streptococcus pneumoniae. The patient also had marked weight loss and oropharyngeal candidiasis. [Lalloo UG, Ambaram A, Vawda F. Pulmonary Complications. In: Mildvan D, editor. International Atlas of AIDS. 4e.: Current Medicine; 2008. 366 p. ISBN: 1-57340-270-2] *Caption adapted from original*

- Chest pain due to pneumonia tends to be pleuritic in nature.
- Pneumonia may be caused by any of a broad variety of infectious agents, including viruses, bacteria, fungi, rickettsiae, and parasites.
- Pneumonia is typically classed as community-acquired (community-acquired pneumonia or "CAP"), healthcare- (or hospital-) associated (HCAP or HAP), or ventilator-associated (VAP). Each of these classifications carries a largely predictable etiologic profile. Classification does not usually affect the chest pain presentation of pneumonia, although pneumococcal pneumonia and infections that cause pleural effusions or lung abscesses typically present with more severe pain.
- The bacterial pathogens that cause pneumonia may be "typical" (such as pneumococcal, *Hemophilus*, or staphylococcal) or "atypical" (such as *Mycoplasma* or *Chlamydophila*). Pathogen does not usually affect the chest pain presentation of pneumonia.

Pathogen	CAP	HAP/HCAP	Adults	Children
Bacteria				
S. pneumoniae	+++	+++	+++	+++
H. influenzae	++	++	++	++
M. pneumoniae	+++	+	++	+++
Chlamydia spp.	+		(+)	++
Klebsiella spp.	+	++		
Legionella spp.	++	+++		
S. aureus	++	+++	+++	+
P. aerugenosa	+	+++	+	
Acinetobacter spp.		++		
Viruses				
RSV	++		+	+++
Rhinovirus	++		(+)	++
Influenza virus	++	+	+	++
Parainfluenza virus	++		+	++
Fungi				
Candida spp.		++1		
Aspergillus spp.		++1		
P. jirovecii		+2		

+ indicates the relative importance of the pathogen and the frequency of isolation in adults or children. 1 of importance in immunocompromised hosts. 2 important opportunistic pathogen in HIV/AIDS patients. CAP, community-acquired pneumonia; HAP, hospital-acquired pneumonia; HCAP, health-care associated pneumonia. Based on collective data [2,5,6,15-18,23,252,253].

Important pathogens causing pneumonia. (See article for data sources.) [From article: Lung epithelium as a sentinel and effector system in pneumonia – molecular mechanisms of pathogen recognition and signal transduction. Respiratory Research. 2006 Jul 8;7(1):97. https://doi.org/10.1186/1465-9921-7-97, at http://link.springer.com/article/10.1186/1465-9921-7-97; by Stefan Hippenstiel, Bastian Opitz, Bernd Schmeck, Norbert Suttorp, © Hippenstiel et al. 2006; licensee BioMed Central Ltd.; licensed under Creative Commons Attribution License BY 2.0 http://creativecommons.org/licenses/by/2.0] *Caption adapted from original*

Differential Diagnosis

- The differential considerations for chest pain due to pneumonia are for the most part other primary lung diagnoses such as pulmonary embolism and pleurisy.
- As in all chest pain presentations, immediate life threats such as acute coronary syndrome and aortic dissection should always be considered.
- Less severe differential considerations include pneumothorax, which can cause pleuritic pain, as well as chest wall pain/costochondritis, and anxiety.
- Pericarditis may present similarly to pneumonia and may also be accompanied by fever.
- Acute chest syndrome in sickle cell disease is a differential consideration in at-risk patients.

Pathophysiology and Etiology

- The clinical manifestations of pneumonia result from a variable combination of actual infection, as well as the host's inflammatory response to the infection.
- The actual etiologic agents behind pneumonia would require an exceedingly long list. For purposes of considering pneumonia in the differential diagnosis of chest pain syndrome, pain is typically caused by inflammation of the pleura. Chest pain in pneumonia can also result from lung abscess, pleural effusion or empyema, myalgias associated with a more systemic infection, or chest wall pain from coughing.

Presentation

Typical/"Classic"

- The classic presentation of pneumonia includes:
  - Cough, which may or may not be productive.
  - Fever, which may be mild or high.
  - Shortness of breath, typically more evident with exertion.
  - Chills.

Atypical

- Especially with "atypical" etiologies, pneumonia may present with more prominent extrapulmonary symptoms, such as headache, myalgias, sore throat, gastroenteritis-type symptoms, or fatigue. Chest pain may or may not be a prominent feature at presentation.
- Elderly patients with pneumonia may present with altered mental status. Chest pain may or may not be a prominent feature at presentation.

Extra-pulmonary symptoms	Chills, nausea, vomiting, altered sensorium, diarrhea, delirium, worsening of a chronic confusion, fall to the ground
Pulmonary symptoms	Dyspnea, pleuritic chest pain
Signs of pneumonia	Fever, crackles, cough
Clinical features suggestive of aspiration pneumonia	Evident macroaspiration
	Reduced level of consciousness
	Dysphagia
	Mechanical or neurological dysfunction of the high gastrointestinal tract

Signs and symptoms most commonly associated with pneumonia in elderly patients. [Falcone M, Blasi F, Menichetti F, Pea F, Violi F. Pneumonia in frail older patients: an up to date. Internal and Emergency Medicine. 2012 Oct;7(5):415–24.] *Caption from original*

- *Mycoplasma* pneumonia may present with ear pain (from bullous myringitis) or with rashes (such as erythema multiforme). Chest pain may or may not be a prominent feature at presentation.

Characteristics	*M. pneumoniae*	*S. pneumoniae*	*p* value
Number	64	68	
Mean age (range), years	36.6 (18–69)	61.8 (19–86)	<0.0001
Male: Female	34: 30	42: 26	0.3791
Co-morbid illness	15 (23)	33 (48)	<0.0001
PSI risk classes**			
I – III	41 (64)	29 (43)	0.0154
IV	23 (36)	39 (57)	
V	0	0	
WBC mean (/μL)	7,400	13,800	<0.0001

*Data represent the numbers of patients, and numbers in parentheses are percentages.
**PSI, pneumonia severity index.

Clinical characteristics in patients with *Mycoplasma pneumoniae* pneumonia and *Streptococcus pneumoniae* pneumonia on admission* [From article: Radiographic features of *Mycoplasma pneumoniae* pneumonia: differential diagnosis and performance timing. BMC Medical Imaging. 2009;9(1):7. https://doi.org/10.1186/1471-2342-9-7, at http://link.springer.com/article/10.1186/1471-2342-9-7; by Naoyuki Miyashita, Tadaaki Sugiu, Yasuhiro Kawai, Keiko Oda, Tetsuya Yamaguchi, Kazunobu Ouchi, Yoshihiro Kobashi, Mikio Oka, © Miyashita et al; licensee BioMed Central Ltd. 2009; licensed under Creative Commons Attribution License BY 2.0 http://creativecommons.org/licenses/by/2.0] *Caption from original*

- *Chlamydophila* pneumonia may present with bronchospasm and wheezing even in nonasthmatics, but it should be noted that patients with underlying asthma or COPD who present with pneumonia are likely to be wheezing. Chest pain may or may not be a prominent feature at presentation.
- Patients with pneumonia may present with overwhelming sepsis, but chest pain is typically not the most prominent feature.

Primary Differential Considerations

- Early consideration should be given to bronchitis, acute exacerbation of COPD, foreign body aspiration, asthma, and ARDS.

History and Physical Exam

Findings That Confirm Diagnosis

- History and physical examination cannot confirm the presence of pneumonia.

Factors That Suggest Diagnosis

- A history of fever, chills, and/or sputum production—especially hemoptysis—is suggestive of pneumonia in the patient with chest pain.
- Findings of consolidation of pulmonary exam—such as egophony and percussion dullness—are suggestive of pneumonia.

http://www.easyauscultation.com/egophony
Egophony. [Egophony Page; Easy Auscultation; www.easyauscultation.com; copyright 2015, MedEdu LLC]

https://www.youtube.com/watch?v=48nzLXnEHvg
Percussion of the Chest (Stanford Medicine 25 video): Demonstrates percussion technique and surface anatomy

- Tachycardia and reduced pulse oximetry readings are suggestive of pneumonia in the patient with chest pain.
- Wheezing, rales, and pleural friction rub may all suggest pneumonia in the patient with chest pain.

http://www.easyauscultation.com/wheezing
Wheezing. [Wheezing; *Easy Auscultation; www.easyauscultation.com; copyright 2015, MedEdu LLC]*

http://www.easyauscultation.com/rales
Rales. [Rales Lung Sounds; Easy Auscultation; www.easyauscultation.com; copyright 2015, MedEdu LLC]

https://www.youtube.com/watch?v=t2QE0O_exAQ
Pleural Friction Rub

Factors That Exclude Diagnosis

- There are no history or physical findings that conclusively exclude pneumonia in the patient with chest pain.

Ancillary Studies

Laboratory

- Bacterial pneumonia is confirmed, not in real time, by the presence of a positive bacterial culture from sputum or blood.
- Various diagnostic tests performed on sputum, blood, or urine can provide confirmation of the etiology of a clinical pneumonia.
- Sputum Gram stain is a notoriously unreliable test for evaluating possible pneumonia.

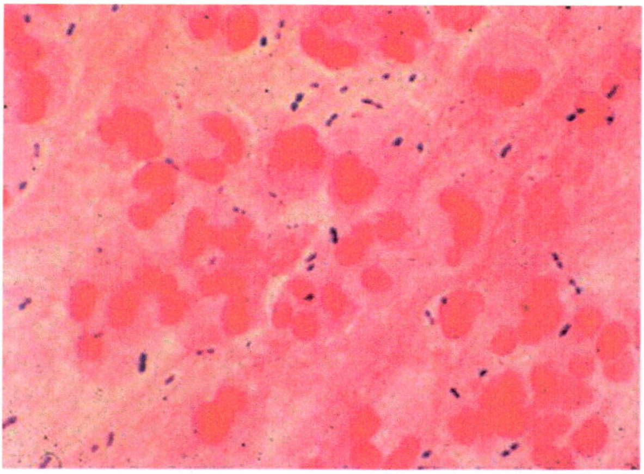

Gram stain of sputum sample from patient with pneumococcal pneumonia. Note diploid organisms surrounded by polymorphonuclear cell infiltrate [Shelburne S, Musher DM. Management of Gram-Positive Bacterial Disease: Staphylococcus aureus, Streptococcal, Pneumococcal and Enterococcal Infections. In: Safdar A, editor. Principles and Practice of Cancer Infectious Diseases [Internet]. Totowa, NJ: Humana Press; 2011 [cited 2015 Jun 2]. p. 409–21. Available from: http://link.springer.com/10.1007/978-1-60761-644-3_35] *Caption from original*

- A CBC in pneumonia will typically show an elevated WBC count except in severely immunocompromised patients. This is also less likely in viral pneumonias.
- *Legionella* pneumonia is often associated with hyponatremia.

	Patients with Legionella that met IDSA/ ATS criteria for Legionella testing	Patients with Legionella that did not meet IDSA/ATS criteria for Legionella testing	All patients with Legionella pneumonia
Male	15	9	24 (65%)
Recent travel	1	0	1 (3%)
History of alcohol abuse	6	0	6 (16%)
Anti-TNF therapy	1	1	2 (5%)
Daily steroid use	0	1	1 (3%)
Cancer	4	4	8 (22%)
Diabetes	5	6	11 (29%)
COPD	5	4	9 (24%)
Solid-organ transplant recipient	0	1	1 (3%)
HIV infection	1	0	1 (3%)
Receipt of antibiotics prior to hospitalization	4	0	4 (11%)
Pleural effusion present at hospital admission	7	0	7 (19%)
ICU admission	14	0	14 (38%)
Abnormal liver function tests	15	5	20 (54%)
Hyponatremia (Sodium < 130 mEq/L)	9	4	13 (35%)
Crude mortality	6	0	6 (16%)

SD, standard deviation; TNF, tumor necrosis factor; COPD, chronic obstructive pulmonary disease; abnormal liver function test defined as above reference range; Crude mortality defined as in-hospital death or discharge to hospice care with impending death.

Characteristics of Adult Patients with *Legionella* Pneumonia, 2005-2009 [From article: How often is a work-up for *Legionella* pursued in patients with pneumonia? A retrospective study. BMC Infectious Diseases. 2011; 11(1):237. https://doi.org/10.1186/1471-2334-11-237, at http://link.springer.com/article/10.1186/1471-2334-11-237; by Brian Hollenbeck, Irene Dupont, Leonard A Mermel, © Hollenbeck et al; licensee BioMed Central Ltd. 2011; licensed under Creative Commons Attribution License BY 2.0 http://creativecommons.org/licenses/by/2.0] *Caption from original*

- Normal laboratory studies do not exclude pneumonia as a cause of chest pain.

Imaging

- Chest radiography can confirm the presence and location of pneumonia.

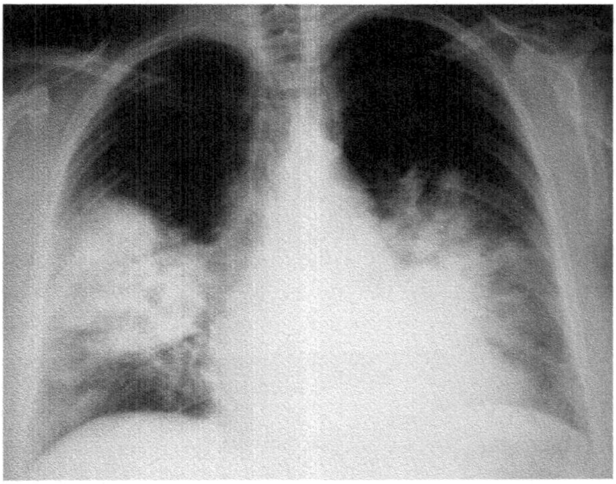

Hospital-acquired pneumonia. Chest radiograph of a patient with hospital-acquired pneumonia. This patient developed bilateral infiltrates after aspirating postoperatively. [Rumbak MJ. Nosocomial infections including pneumonia. In: Crapo JD, editor. Bone's Atlas of Pulmonary Medicine. 3rd edition. Philadelphia, PA: Current Medicine Group; 2005. 338 p. ISBN: 1-57340-211-7] *Caption adapted from original*

- Chest radiography can identify abscesses, cavities, and pleural involvement.

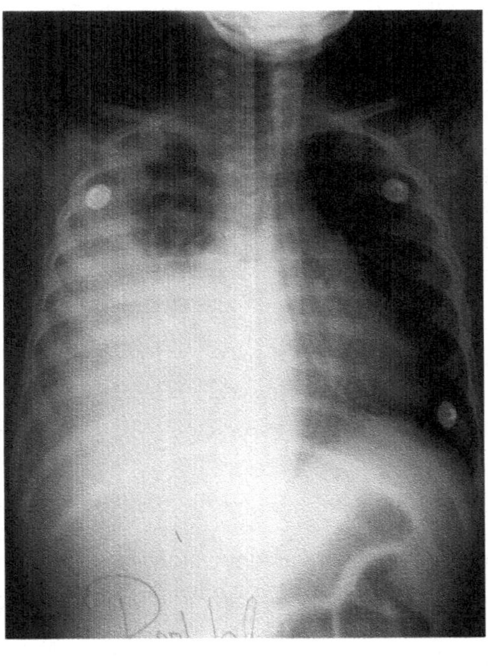

Chest radiograph of a patient with complicated lung abscess. [Ayed AK, Al-Rowayeh A. Lung resection in children for infectious pulmonary diseases. Pediatric Surgery International. 2005 Aug;21(8):604–8.] *Caption from original*

- Chest radiography can be used to follow the treatment success (or lack thereof) of pneumonia management.
- A normal chest radiograph does not exclude pneumonia, as patients who are immunocompromised, dehydrated, or very early in the disease process may not show an infiltrate. Chest CT may be helpful in patients suspected of having pneumonia but lacking diagnostic certainty on plain chest radiography.

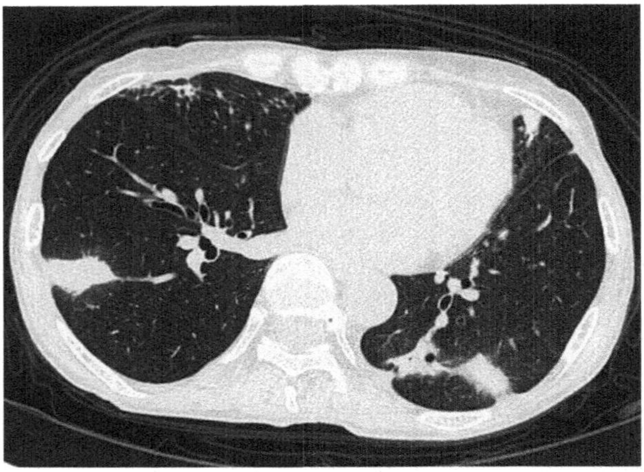

Computed tomography (CT) findings of organizing pneumonia on admission. Multiple consolidations with sub-pleural distribution were detected in both lungs by CT scan. The lesions were accompanied by ground glass opacities. [Nakamura H, Kita J, Kawakami A, Yamasaki S, Ida H, Sakamoto N, Furusu A, Eguchi K. Multiple bone fracture due to Fanconi's syndrome in primary Sjögren's syndrome complicated with organizing pneumonia. Rheumatology International. 2009 Dec;30(2):265–7.] *Caption from original*

Special Populations

Age and Gender

- Pneumonia occurs in all age, ethnic, and socioeconomic groups. It occurs in both males and females.
- Pneumonia often has poorer outcomes at the extremes of age.
- In children, atypical pathogens predominate.
- In newborns and infants, viruses (including RSV), pneumococcus, and aspiration are important etiologic ocnsiderations.

- Current recommendations for the management of community-acquired pneumonia in children include:
    - Viral testing for infants less than 1 year.
    - Avoidance of routine chest radiographs.
    - Omission of blood work, including CBC's and blood cultures.
    - Use of amoxicillin in pre-school children.
    - Use of a macrolide in school-age children.

Co-morbidities

- Co-morbidities associated with the various types of pneumonia include but are not limited to:
    - congestive heart failure
    - cancer
    - chronic renal failure
    - COPD and chronic respiratory failure
    - chronic hepatic disease
    - alcoholism
    - diabetes mellitus
    - neurologic disease
    - immunosuppression, including HIV infection

Pitfalls in Diagnosis

Critical Steps Not to Miss

- Except in significantly compromised patients, pneumonia is most often not a life-threatening diagnosis. Still, it is a cause of significant morbidity, loss of productivity, and cost. Even in immunocompetent patients, pneumonia can cause sepsis and death. It is therefore critical to at least consider the diagnosis in the patient with chest pain, and a chest radiograph often gives useful information.

Mimics

- The entire constellation of diagnoses that underlies chest pain syndrome, especially those often accompanied by dyspnea, can mimic the pain and overall presentation of pneumonia. Be especially cognizant of pulmonary embolism as a mimic, as PE has a higher case-mortality rate than pneumonia.
- Pericarditis may mimic pneumonia in presentation. Listen for a pericardial friction rub.

http://www.easyauscultation.com/acute-pericarditis

Acute Pericarditis Audio Recordings. [Acute Pericarditis; Easy Auscultation; www.easyauscultation.com; copyright 2015, MedEdu LLC]

Time-Dependent Interventions

- Anti-infective therapy, usually at first with empiric antibiotic therapy, should be initiated when the diagnosis of pneumonia is strongly considered or confirmed. Consult your local antibiogram for guidance on choosing a specific agent.
- Choice of antimicrobial is also driven by the classification of the pneumonia (CAP vs HAP vs VAP).

Overall Principles of Treatment

- Anti-infective therapy is the mainstay of pneumonia treatment. Unfortunately, treatment is not always guided by positive microbiologic or virologic results.

Patient status	Treatment
Outpatient (previously healthy without history of antimicrobials in the last 3 months)	Macrolide or Doxycycline
Outpatient (comorbidities such as chronic heart, lung, liver or renal disease, diabetes, alcoholism, malignancy, asplenia, immunosuppressed, or history of antimicrobials in the last 3 months)	Respiratory fluoroquinolone or Beta lactam plus macrolide
Inpatient (non-ICU)	Respiratory fluoroquinolone or Beta lactam plus macrolide
Inpatient (ICU)	Beta lactam plus Either azithromycin or respiratory fluoroquinolone
Inpatient (with concern of *Pseudomonas*)	Antipneumococcal, antipseudomonal beta lactam (piperacillin–tazobactam, cefepime, imipenem, or meropenem) plus ciprofloxacin or levofloxacin or Above beta lactam plus either aminoglycoside or azithromycin or Above beta lactam plus azithromycin and aminoglycoside
Inpatient (with concern of methicillin-resistant *Staphylococcus aureus*)	Add vancomycin or linezolid to regimen

Recommendations for empiric treatment of community-acquired pneumonia. [Nguyen HH. Pneumonia. In: Mainous III AG, Pomeroy C, editors. Management of Antimicrobials in Infectious Diseases [Internet]. Totowa, NJ: Humana Press; 2010 [cited 2015 Jun 3]. p. 169–82. Available from: http://link.springer.com/10.1007/978-1-60327-239-1_9] *Caption from original*

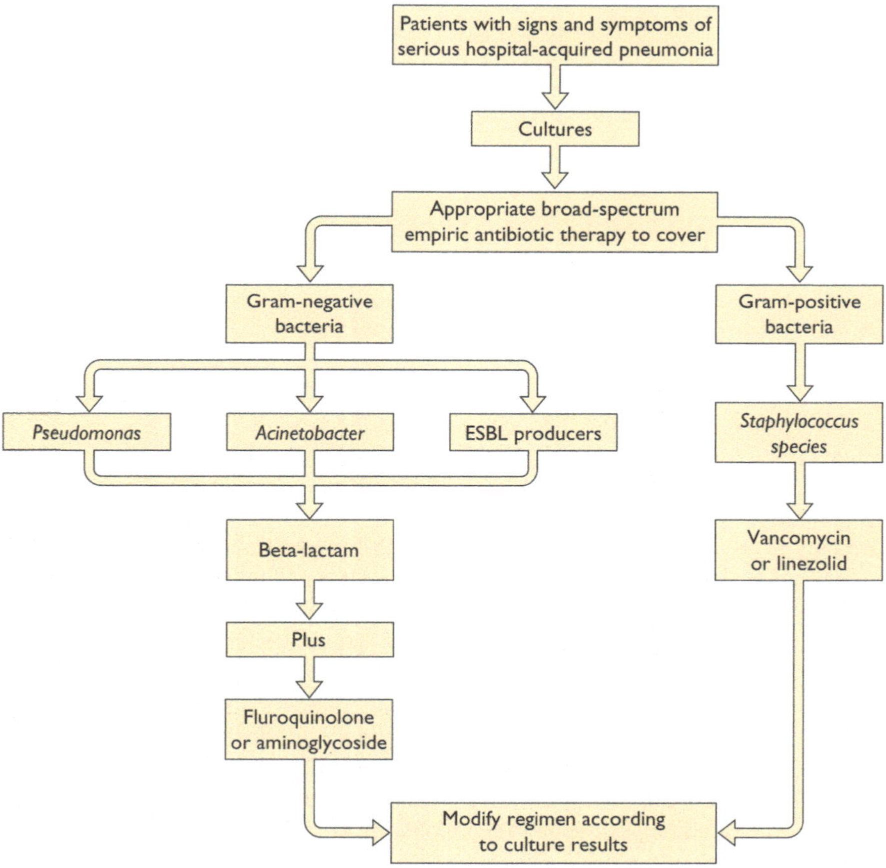

Treatment of patients with ventilator-associated pneumonia (VAP). This algorithm suggests initial broad-spectrum antibiotics to cover gram- negative and gram-positive bacteria. Once the cultures are back from the laboratory, the antibiotics are tailored to the bacteria. “Beta-lactams” here include carbapenems and monolactems. ESBLS and *Acinetobacter* may respond best to carbapenems. ESBL—extended-spectrum β-lactams [Rumbak MJ.Nosocomial infections including pneumonia. In: Crapo JD, editor. Bone's Atlas of Pulmonary Medicine. 3rd edition. Philadelphia, PA: Current Medicine Group; 2005. 338 p. ISBN: 1-57340-211-7] *Caption from original*

- Chest pain associated with pneumonia usually improves quickly as the infection resolves. Non-steroidal anti-inflammatory drugs or narcotics can be given to patients with persistent or severe pain.

Disease Course

- The course pneumonia varies widely with mortality rates as high as 50% in some severely compromised patients, and as low as less than 1% in immunocompetent, nonsmoking adults with CAP.

Related Evidence

Papers of particular interest have been highlighted as:
*** Of key importance*

Practice Guideline

Bradley JS, Byington CL, Shah SS, Alverson B, Carter ER, Harrison C, Kaplan SL, Mace SE, McCracken GH Jr, Moore MR, St Peter SD, Stockwell JA, Swanson JT, Pediatric Infectious Diseases Society and the Infectious Diseases Society of America. The management of community-acquired pneumonia in infants and children older than 3 months of age: clinical practice guidelines by the Pediatric Infectious Diseases Society and the Infectious Diseases Society of America. Clin Infect Dis. 2011 Oct;53(7):e25-76. https://doi.org/10.1093/cid/cir531. PMID: 21880587. http://www.ncbi.nlm.nih.gov/pubmed/21880587 **

Levy ML, Le Jeune I, Woodhead MA, Macfarlaned JT, Lim WS; British Thoracic Society Community Acquired Pneumonia in Adults Guideline Group. Primary care summary of the British Thoracic Society Guidelines for the management of community acquired pneumonia in adults: 2009 update. Endorsed by the Royal College of General Practitioners and the Primary Care Respiratory Society UK. Prim Care Respir J. 2010 Mar;19(1):21-7. https://doi.org/10.4104/pcrj.2010.00014. Erratum in: Prim Care Respir J. 2010 Jun;19(2):108. PMID: 20157684. http://www.ncbi.nlm.nih.gov/pubmed/20157684 **

Lim WS, Baudouin SV, George RC, Hill AT, Jamieson C, Le Jeune I, Macfarlane JT, Read RC, Roberts HJ, Levy ML, Wani M, Woodhead MA; Pneumonia Guidelines Committee of the BTS Standards of Care Committee. BTS guidelines for the management of community acquired pneumonia in adults: update 2009. Thorax. 2009 Oct;64 Suppl 3:iii1-55. https://doi.org/10.1136/thx.2009.121434. PMID: 19783532. http://www.ncbi.nlm.nih.gov/pubmed/19783532 **

Muscedere J, Dodek P, Keenan S, Fowler R, Cook D, Heyland D; VAP Guidelines Committee and the Canadian Critical Care Trials Group. Comprehensive evidence-based clinical practice guidelines for ventilator-associated pneumonia: diagnosis and treatment. J Crit Care. 2008 Mar;23(1):138-47. https://doi.org/10.1016/j.jcrc.2007.12.008. PMID: 1835943. http://www.ncbi.nlm.nih.gov/pubmed/18359431 **

American Thoracic Society; Infectious Diseases Society of America. Guidelines for the management of adults with hospital-acquired, ventilator-associated, and health-care-associated pneumonia. Am J Respir Crit Care Med. 2005 Feb 15;171(4):388-416. PMID: 15699079. http://www.ncbi.nlm.nih.gov/pubmed/15699079 **

Review

Song JY, Eun BW, Nahm MH. Diagnosis of pneumococcal pneumonia: current pitfalls and the way forward. Infect Chemother. 2013 Dec;45(4):351-66. https://doi.org/10.3947/ic.2013.45.4.351. PMID: 24475349. http://www.ncbi.nlm.nih.gov/pubmed/24475349 **

Asrar Khan W, Woodhead M. Major advances in managing community-acquired pneumonia. F1000Prime Rep. 2013 Oct 1;5:43. https://doi.org/10.12703/P5-43. PMID: 24167724. http://www.ncbi.nlm.nih.gov/pubmed/24167724

Ricard JD. New therapies for pneumonia. Curr Opin Pulm Med. 2012 May;18(3):181-6. https://doi.org/10.1097/MCP.0b013e3283520fec. PMID: 22388584. http://www.ncbi.nlm.nih.gov/pubmed/22388584

Lippi G, Meschi T, Cervellin G. Inflammatory biomarkers for the diagnosis, monitoring and follow-up of community-acquired pneumonia: clinical evidence and perspectives. Eur J Intern Med. 2011 Oct;22(5):460-5. https://doi.org/10.1016/j.ejim.2011.02.023. PMID: 21925053. http://www.ncbi.nlm.nih.gov/pubmed/21925053

Watkins RR, Lemonovich TL. Diagnosis and management of community-acquired pneumonia in adults. Am Fam Physician. 2011 Jun 1;83(11):1299-306. PMID: 21661712. http://www.ncbi.nlm.nih.gov/pubmed/21661712 **

Attridge RT, Frei CR. Health care-associated pneumonia: an evidence-based review. Am J Med. 2011 Aug;124(8):689-97. https://doi.org/10.1016/j.amjmed.2011.01.023. PMID: 21663884. http://www.ncbi.nlm.nih.gov/pubmed/21663884 **

Cohort Study

Medford AR, Husain SA, Turki HM, Millar AB. Diagnosis of ventilator-associated pneumonia. J Crit Care. 2009 Sep;24(3):473.e1-6. https://doi.org/10.1016/j.jcrc.2008.06.012. PMID: 19327300. http://www.ncbi.nlm.nih.gov/pubmed/19327300

Comparative Study

van Vugt SF, Verheij TJ, de Jong PA, Butler CC, Hood K, Coenen S, Goossens H, Little P, Broekhuizen BD; GRACE Project Group. Diagnosing pneumonia in patients with acute cough: clinical judgment compared to chest radiography. Eur Respir J. 2013 Oct;42(4):1076-82. https://doi.org/10.1183/09031936.00111012. PMID: 23349450. http://www.ncbi.nlm.nih.gov/pubmed/23349450

Use PubMed Clinical Queries to find the most recent evidence. Use this search strategy:

"Pneumonia"[Mesh] OR "Pneumonia"

Chapter 59
Pneumothorax (Simple)

Charles V. Pollack, Jr., Richard M. Cantor, and Victoria G. Riese

Name and Synonyms

Simple pneumothorax; dropped lung; ruptured lung; ruptured bleb

Incidence/Epidemiology

- Because simple pneumothorax may be largely or completely asymptomatic, the incidence is clearly underestimated. It ranges from 2–60 per 100,000 people per year, depending on gender and associated lung disease.
- Primary spontaneous pneumothorax is more common in men than in women, and is more common in smokers than in nonsmokers.
- Primary spontaneous pneumothorax occurs most commonly in the third decade of life and is rare after the fifth decade.
- Secondary spontaneous pneumothorax tends to occur in older patients because of the prevalence of underlying lung disease in those patients.
- Traumatic pneumothorax can occur at any age and may result from accidental or iatrogenic trauma.

C. V. Pollack, Jr. (✉)
Department of Emergency Medicine, Thomas Jefferson University, Philadelphia, PA, USA

R. M. Cantor
Department of Emergency Medicine and Pediatrics, State University of New York Upstate Medical University, Syracuse, NY, USA

V. G. Riese
Librarian Consultant, Eldersburg, MD, USA

C. V. Pollack, Jr. (ed.), *Differential Diagnosis of Cardiopulmonary Disease*,
https://doi.org/10.1007/978-3-319-63895-9_59

Differential Diagnosis

- The differential considerations for pneumothorax are primarily driven by the size of the pneumothorax and the extent of any underlying lung disease. Exacerbations of asthma and COPD may both precipitate and present similarly to simple pneumothorax. Other causes of dyspnea and pleuritic chest pain, alone or together, should also be considered, including pulmonary embolism, pneumonia, pleurisy, mediastinal disorders, and anxiety.

Pathophysiology and Etiology

- Pneumothorax is defined by the presence of air in the pleural space, which is the ordinarily tiny space between the visceral and parietal layers of the pleura.

Primary spontaneous (simple) pneumothorax
Secondary spontaneous (complicated) pneumothorax
Catamenial pneumothorax
Pneumothorax associated with drug abuse
Iatrogenic pneumothorax
Pneumothorax associated with mechanical ventilation
Traumatic pneumothorax
Tension pneumothorax

Types of pneumothorax. Primary spontaneous pneumothorax occurs in patients without underlying lung disease. It usually occurs in young, tall, slender male patients. Secondary pneumothoraces occur in those patients with underlying lung disease. Pneumothorax has also been associated with drug abuse and is believed to be related to the inhalational route of drug abuse, in which the abuser performs a Valsalva maneuver with generation of pressures greater than 200 cm H2O. Iatrogenic pneumothorax occurs most commonly during attempted central line placement, with the risk between 3% and 6% for subclavian placement and about 1% to 2% with internal jugular catheterization. Traumatic pneumothorax may be caused by blunt or penetrating trauma and may have associated hemopneumothorax and other vascular injuries. [Szokol J, Vender J. Respiratory emergencies (pulmonary aspiration of gastric contents, acute epiglottis, anterior mediastinal mass). In: Tremper KK, editor. Principles of anesthetic techniques and anesthetic emergencies. Philadelphia: Current Medicine; 1998. 195 p. (Miller RD, editor. Atlas of anesthesia; vol. 4). ISBN: 0-443-07903-X] *Caption from original*

- Simple pneumothorax may be small and asymptomatic or larger, resulting in dyspnea. Depending on the size of the pneumothorax, the adjacent lung may be deformed or compressed, or totally collapsed. Simple pneumothorax is differentiated from the more obvious, more symptomatic, and life-threatening "tension pneumothorax" by the fact that in the latter, the pressure in the pleural space is positive throughout the respiratory cycle, resulting in forced deviation of the mediastinum to the contralateral side.

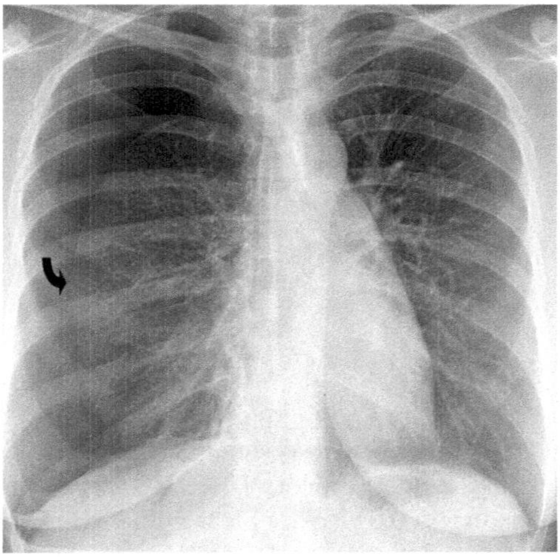

Tension pneumothorax. Portable chest radiograph demonstrates large right-sided tension pneumothorax (curved arrow) with mediastinal shift to the left side [Carter BW, Muse VV. Imaging of Nontraumatic Mediastinal and Pulmonary Processes. In: Singh A, editor. Emergency Radiology [Internet]. New York, NY: Springer New York; 2013 [cited 2015 Aug 31]. p. 321–32. Available from: http://link.springer.com/10.1007/978-1-4419-9592-6_23] *Caption from original*

- Simple pneumothorax may be spontaneous (primary or secondary) or traumatic:
  - Primary spontaneous pneumothorax is usually the result of rupture of an apical pleural bleb or bulla, a small cystic space lying just under the visceral pleura. The designation "primary" is meant to imply the absence of underlying lung disease, but primary spontaneous pneumothorax occurs more commonly in smokers than in nonsmokers, indicating the likely presence of subclinical lung pathology. The "primary" also signifies the absence of a known inciting event, such as trauma. A special case is so-called "catamenial" pneumothorax, which typically occurs in women age 30–40, presents within 48 hours of menses onset, and may be recurrent.

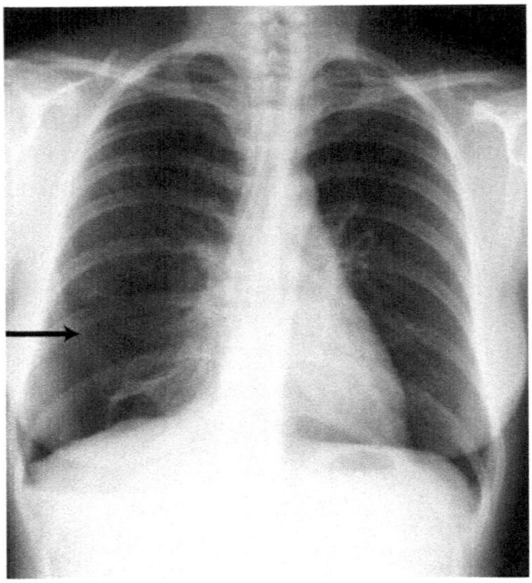

Catamenial pneumothorax. Chest radiograph of a 31-year-old nonsmoking woman with multiple spontaneous right-sided pneumothoraces who presented with acute onset of pleuritic chest pain and dyspnea. There is a large right-sided pneumothorax; the arrow signifies the 1 mm visceral pleural line. [Huggins J, Sahn S. Pleural disease. In: Crapo J, editor. Bone's atlas of pulmonary and critical care medicine. Philadelphia: Current Medicine; 2005. Chapter 25. ISBN: 1-57340-211-7] *Caption adapted from original*

  - Secondary spontaneous pneumothorax has been reported with virtually all lung diseases, but is most common with COPD. Air enters the pleural space through distended or damaged alveoli.
  - Traumatic pneumothorax occurs as a result of physical disruption of the pleura, either from blunt force pressure or from puncture. Puncture may be accidental, as in blunt trauma with rib fracture, or iatrogenic, as in puncture of the pleura during placement of a central venous catheter.

- Primary spontaneous pneumothorax is more likely to occur in tall, thin individuals. There is an association with Marfan's syndrome. It is much more common in smokers than in nonsmokers. There seems to be a familial tendency to develop primary spontaneous pneumothorax. It is also more common during pregnancy.

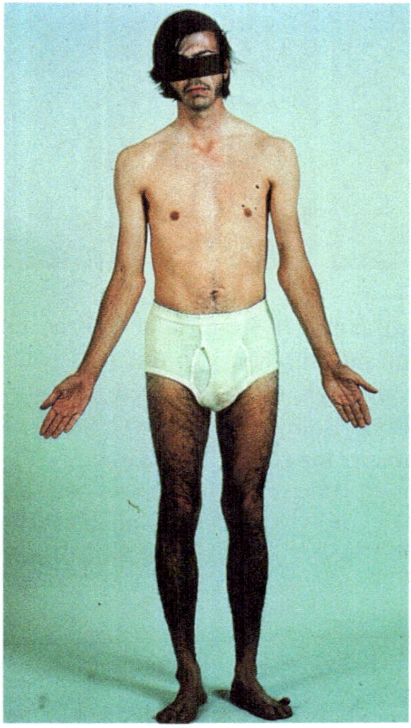

Clinical features. Many of the typical features of Marfan's syndrome are seen in this patient, including arm length greater than height, increased lower to upper extremity ratio, pectus excavatum, and pes planus. [Maricic M, Ko M. Diseases of bone and connective tissue. In: Hunder G, editor. Atlas of rheumatology. Philadelphia: Current Medicine; 2005. Chapter 6. ISBN: 1-57340-210-9] *Caption adapted from original*

- Secondary spontaneous pneumothorax is most common in patients with obstructive lung disease, such as COPD or asthma, in which intrathoracic pressures are higher. It is also more common in pneumonia (including necrotizing pneumonia, *Pneumocystis* pneumonia in AIDS, and tuberculosis), sarcoidosis and other connective tissue diseases, and lung neoplasms.
- Accidental traumatic pneumothorax may result from penetrating or nonpenetrating (blunt) injury. Iatrogenic traumatic pneumothorax has been reported with:
  - Central venous catheter insertion (subclavian or internal jugular)
  - Lung, pleural, or mediastinal biopsy
  - Intercostal nerve block
  - Chest compressions for CPR
  - Positive-end-expiratory pressure (PEEP) ventilation

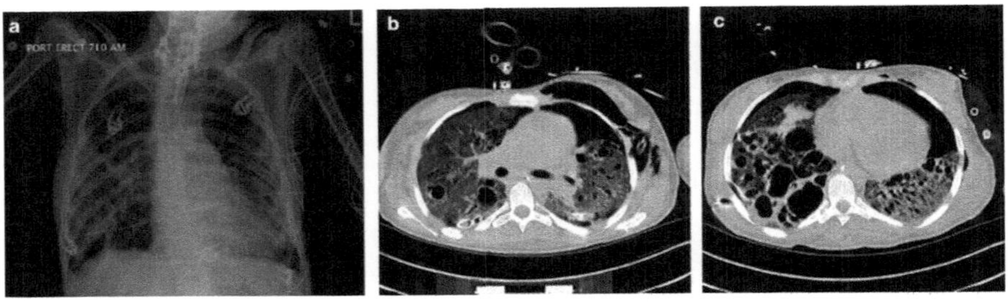

AP chest radiograph (a) axial CT (b, c) confirms the presence of subcutaneous emphysema and bilateral pneumothorax in this ICU patient who developed barotrauma secondary to high levels of PEEP. There is evidence of acute respiratory distress syndrome (ARDS). [Boiselle PM, Dass C, Steiner RM. Radiologic Imaging in the Critically Ill Patient. In: Criner GJ, Barnette RE, D'Alonzo GE, editors. Critical Care Study Guide [Internet]. New York, NY: Springer New York; 2010 [cited 2015 Aug 31]. p. 181–207. Available from: http://link.springer.com/10.1007/978-0-387-77452-7_11] *Caption from original*

Presentation

Typical/"Classic"

- Pleuritic chest pain and shortness of breath are the most common findings in simple pneumothorax at presentation. Pain is often of sudden onset. With larger pneumothorax volumes, patients may manifest hypoxemia and have hemodynamic instability or mental status changes.
- The diagnosis of simple pneumothorax is made on chest radiography—typically a plain CSR, sometimes computed tomography. Ultrasound is occasionally used.
- Patients with traumatic pneumothorax usually offer a pertinent history.
- Patients with primary spontaneous pneumothorax are typically tall and thin and are often smokers.
- Patients presenting with secondary spontaneous pneumothorax often manifest signs and symptoms of their underlying lung disease.

Atypical

- Patients with pneumothorax of sufficient size to be diagnosed will have some dyspnea. Chest pain may not be the presenting complaint.
- There may be distractions to the presentation, as in catamenial pneumothorax, which occurs within 48 hours on onset of menses.

Primary Differential Considerations

- When evaluating a patient suspected of having a pneumothorax, early consideration should be given to these differential diagnoses:
  - Acute coronary syndrome
  - Asthma
  - Pneumonia
  - Pulmonary embolism
  - Rib fracture

History and Physical Exam

Findings That Confirm Diagnosis

- History and physical examination are key to diagnosing simple pneumothorax, but the magnitude of those findings is dependent almost wholly on the side of the pneumothorax. With larger lesions, patients are quite dyspneic. With smaller lesions, the diagnosis may prove elusive. Chest radiography is diagnostic.

Factors That Suggest Diagnosis

- Pleuritic chest pain and dyspnea on history are suggestive but not confirmatory.
- Those same findings in smokers, asthmatics, Marfanoid body habitus, women within 48 hours of menses onset, recent sharp procedure above the diaphragm, or recent thoracic trauma should be suspected of having pneumothorax.
- Patients with larger pneumothoraces are likely to show signs of frank respiratory distress, including tachycardia, tachypnea, diaphoresis, and pallor or cyanosis. These patients are also more likely to manifest asymmetric breath sounds upon careful lung auscultation.
- The larger the pneumothorax, the more likely it is that the patient will have tracheal shift (classic for tension pneumothorax), hyperresonance upon percussion of the affected lung, or jugular venous distention.

Factors That Exclude Diagnosis

- There are no history or physical findings that conclusively exclude simple pneumothorax.

Ancillary Studies

Laboratory

- There are no diagnostic laboratory studies for pneumothorax. Patients with secondary spontaneous pneumothorax should undergo laboratory screening pertinent to their underlying diagnosis.

Imaging

- The diagnosis of simple pneumothorax is confirmed on chest radiography. Small pneumothoraces may only be visible on computed tomography of the chest. Look for a thin line representing the pleura separate from the chest wall. The upright, inspiratory posteroanterior film offers the best opportunity of demonstrating a simple pneumothorax.

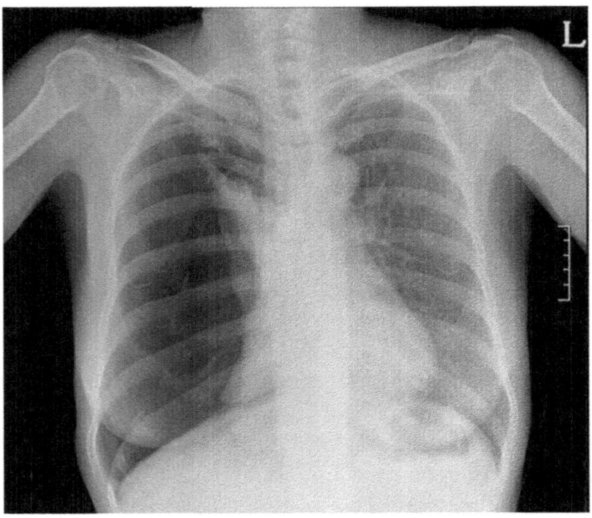

Poteroanterior upright chest X-ray shows large pneumothorax of the right lung [Kim S-H, Yoo W-H. Recurrent pneumothorax associated with pulmonary nodules after leflunomide therapy in rheumatoid arthritis: a case report and review of the literature. Rheumatology International. 2011 Jul;31(7):919–22.] *Caption from original*

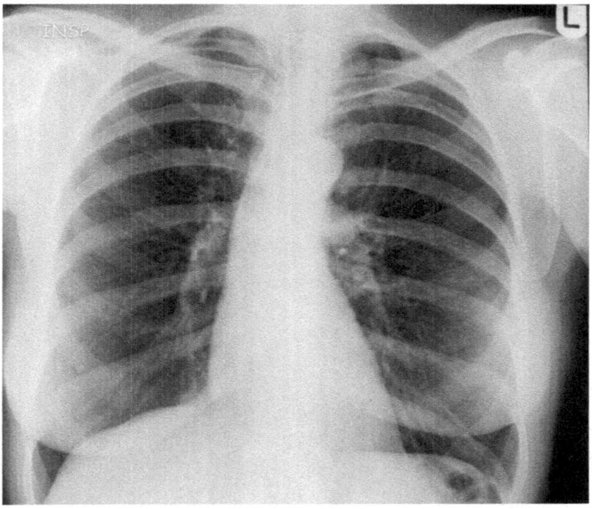

CXR in inspiration showing left sided small pneumothorax [From article: Pneumothorax after a clinical breast fine-needle aspiration of a lump in a patient with Poland syndrome. International Seminars in Surgical Oncology. 2005 Aug 19;2(1):14. https://doi.org/10.1186/1477-7800-2-14, at http://link.springer.com/article/10.1186/1477-7800-2-14; by M Salhab, W Al Sarakbi, N Perry, K Mokbel, © Salhab et al; licensee BioMed Central Ltd. 2005; licensed under Creative Commons Attribution License BY 2.0 http://creativecommons.org/licenses/by/2.0] *Caption from original*

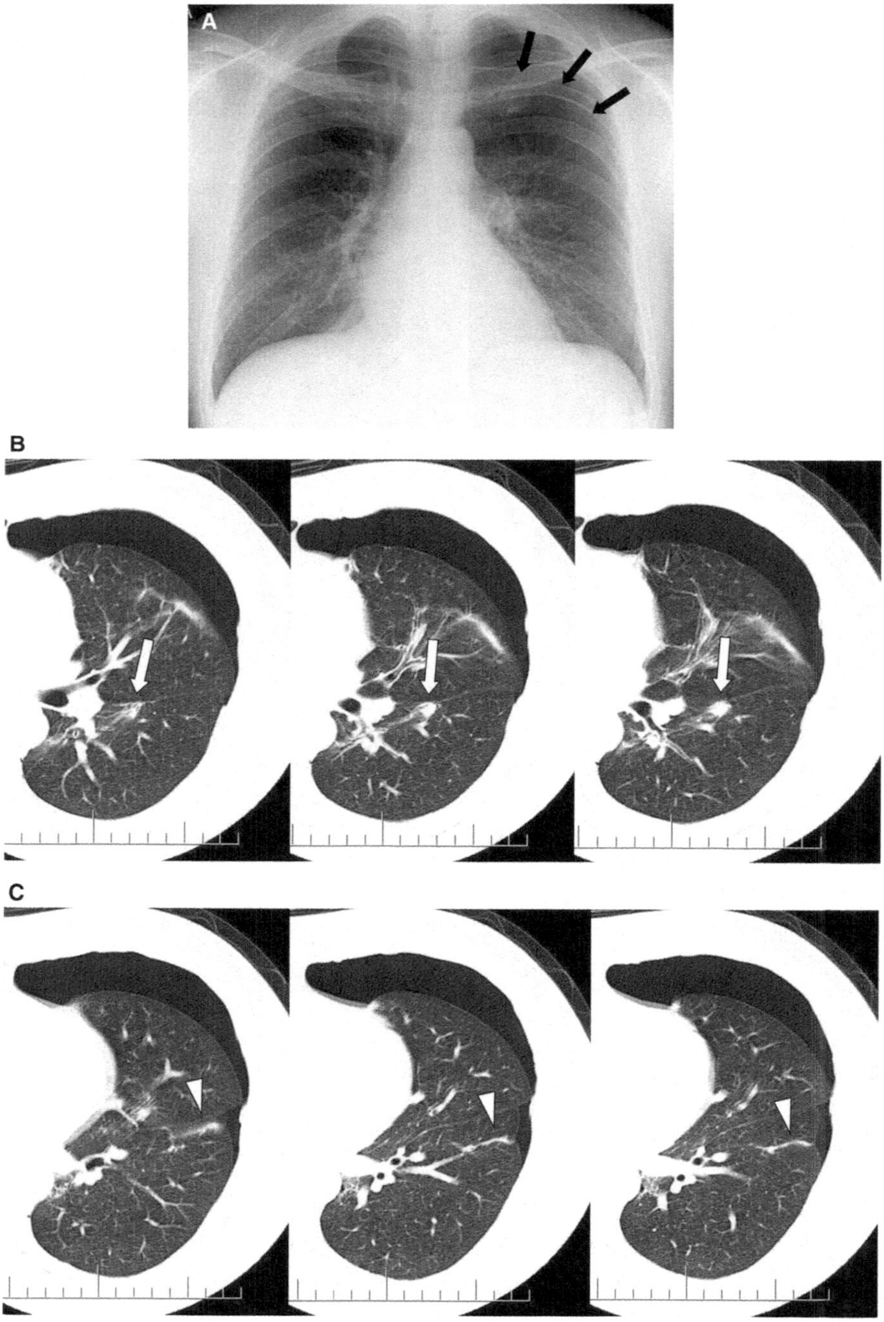
A
B
C

a A radiograph demonstrating pneumothorax of the left lung. The arrow indicates the line of the lung apex. b A computed tomography (CT) scan showing the pneumothorax and an irregular dense nodular shadow (white arrows) beneath the interlobular surface. c A CT scan showing linear-reticular shadows (white arrowheads) in the lung parenchyma within the left lower lobe [Kato T, Ishikawa K, Kadoya M, Okamoto K, Kaji M. Spontaneous pneumothorax in a patient with dendriform pulmonary ossification: report of a case. Surgery Today. 2012 Sep;42(9):903–8.] *Caption from original*

  - The lateral film may be especially helpful.
  - The lateral decubitus film (affected side up) may better demonstrate a simple pneumothorax.
- Ultrasound may be useful in some cases. Look for the "sliding lung sign."

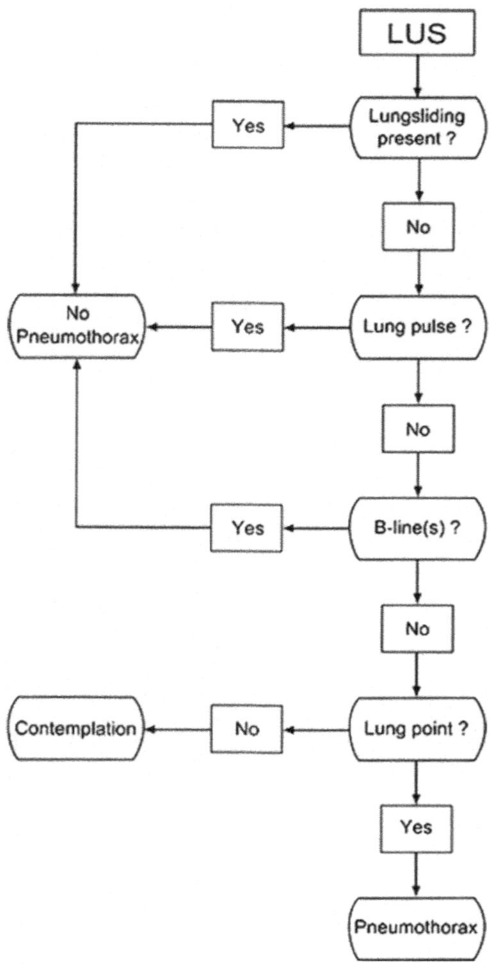

Algorithm for the diagnosis and exclusion of pneumothorax using LUS. Initially one should look for signs which rule out the presence of pneumothorax [lung sliding, lung pulse, B-line(s)] at the anterior surface of the chest. If none of these are present, then one should gradually move the transducer laterally and posterior on the surface of the chest and look for lung point in order to establish the diagnosis of pneumothorax. If neither sign is present, contemplation is needed since pneumothorax can neither be ruled in nor out. In young, previously healthy patients, such as most trauma patients, the absence of lung sliding alone is sufficient to diagnose pneumothorax. In such patients the absence of all signs will be consistent with pneumothorax. In comparison, patients with known lung diseases or previous chest surgery may have a variety of causes for the absence of lung sliding. In such patients the absence of all signs can neither be used to rule in nor to rule out a pneumothorax and further imaging should be performed in order to establish whether pneumothorax is present or absent [From article: Ultrasonography for clinical decision-making and intervention in airway management: from the mouth to the lungs and pleurae. Insights into Imaging. 2014 Apr;5(2):253–79. https://doi.org/10.1007/s13244-014-0309-5, at http://link.springer.com/article/10.1007/s13244-014-0309-5; by Michael S. Kristensen, Wendy H. Teoh, Ole Graumann, Christian B. Laursen, © The Author(s) 2014; licensed under Creative Commons Attribution License https://creativecommons.org/licenses/by/2.0/] *Caption from original*

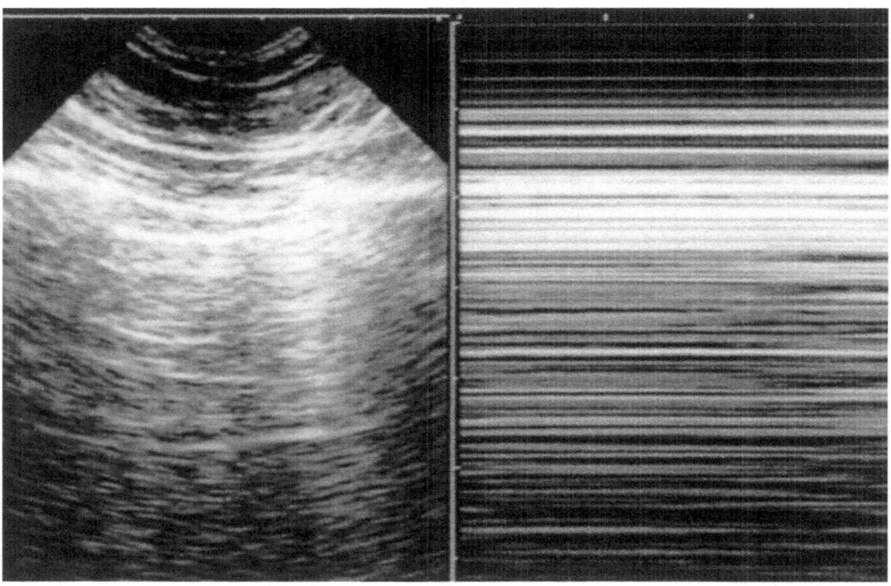

Pneumothorax. *Left* Real-time. Lung sliding or pathological comet-tail artifacts are absent. In real time the pleural line appears completely motionless. *Right* Time motion. This mode objectifies the complete disappearance of lung sliding, without any visible "lung pulse" [Lichtenstein DA, Lascols N, Prin S, Mezière G. The"lung pulse": an early ultrasound sign of complete atelectasis. Intensive Care Medicine. 2003 Dec 1;29(12):2187–92.] *Caption from original*

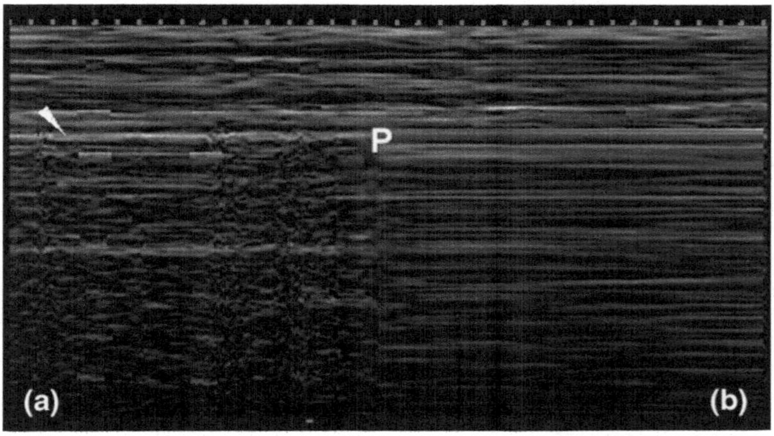

Time-motion mode lung ultrasound. (a) Normal lung and (b) pneumothorax patterns using time-motion mode lung ultrasound. In time motion mode, one must first locate the pleural line (white arrow) and, above it, the motionless parietal structures. Below the pleural line, lung sliding appears as a homogenous granular pattern (a). In the case of pneumothorax and absent lung sliding, horizontal lines only are visualised (b). In a patient examined in the supine position with partial pneumothorax, normal lung sliding and absence of lung sliding may coexist in lateral regions of the chest wall. In this boundary region, called the 'lung point' (P), lung sliding appears (granular pattern) and disappears (strictly horizontal lines) with inspiration when using the time-motion mode. [From article: Clinical review: Bedside lung ultrasound in critical care practice. Crit Care. 2007 Feb 16;11(1):1–9. https://doi.org/10.1186/cc5668, at http://link.springer.com/article/10.1186/cc5668; by Bélaïd Bouhemad, Mao Zhang, Qin Lu, Jean-Jacques Rouby, © BioMed Central Ltd 2007; licensed under Creative Commons Attribution License https://creativecommons.org/licenses/by/2.0/] *Caption from original*

Special Populations

Age and Gender

- Primary spontaneous simple pneumothorax occurs most often in tall, thin adults between the ages of 18 and 40 and is more common in smokers. It is more common in men than in women.
- Secondary spontaneous simple pneumothorax occurs in older patients, often with COPD. It is more common in men than in women.
- Catemenial pneumothorax occurs in menstruating females, most often in the fourth decade of life.
- In the pediatric population, the highest incidence of simple pneumothoraces occurs in the newborn period. In some studies, the incidence approaches 2 in 10,000 live births.

- In adolescents, the development of both pneumothorax and pneumomediastinum has been associated with smoking marijuana and crack cocaine.

Co-morbidities

- Asthma and COPD are common comorbidities.
- Marfan's syndrome and other connective tissue disorders predispose to simple pneumothorax.
- Tobacco use increases the incidence of simple pneumothorax.

Pitfalls in Diagnosis

Critical Steps Not to Miss

- Consideration of the diagnosis is the first critical step. Chest radiography is required to confirm the diagnosis.

Mimics

- The entire constellation of diagnoses that underlies chest pain syndrome, especially those often accompanied by dyspnea, can mimic the pain and overall presentation of simple pneumothorax.

Time-Dependent Interventions

- There are usually no time-dependent interventions in the management of simple pneumothorax. In this way the diagnosis differs sharply from tension pneumothorax, which is immediately life-threatening.
- Patients with significant underlying pulmonary disease may be intolerant of the hypoxemia that may result from simple pneumothorax, even without tension. For those patients, decompression of the pneumothorax (with needle, catheter, or tube thoracostomy) should be performed immediately.

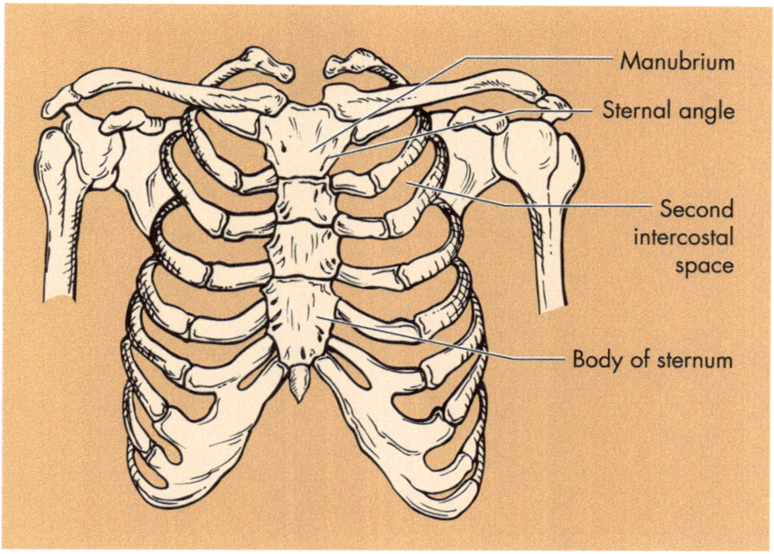

Needle thoracostomy. The occurrence of a pneumothorax in the patient receiving positive pressure ventilation necessitates the placement of a chest tube. If the patient has evidence of a tension pneumothorax and exhibits hemodynamic or respiratory instability, a needle thoracostomy should be undertaken immediately. The procedure involves using a 14-gauge angiocatheter and inserting it into the second intercostal space in the midclavicular line of the side of the pneumothorax. The needle is "walked off" the superior portion of the third rib into the second intercostal space. This is done to prevent laceration of the intercostal vessels. If the tension is not released then a tube thoracostomy should be done in the same location. Once a tension pneumothorax is decompressed, a chest tube must be inserted to prevent reaccumulation of air. The angiocatheter, once it has released the tension in the chest, should not be removed until a chest tube is in place.[Szokol J, Vender J. Respiratory emergencies (pulmonary aspiration of gastric contents, acute epiglottis, anterior mediastinal mass). In: Tremper KK, editor. Principles of anesthetic techniques and anesthetic emergencies. Philadelphia: Current Medicine; 1998. 195 p. (Miller RD, editor. Atlas of anesthesia; vol. 4). ISBN: 0-443-07903-X] *Caption from original*

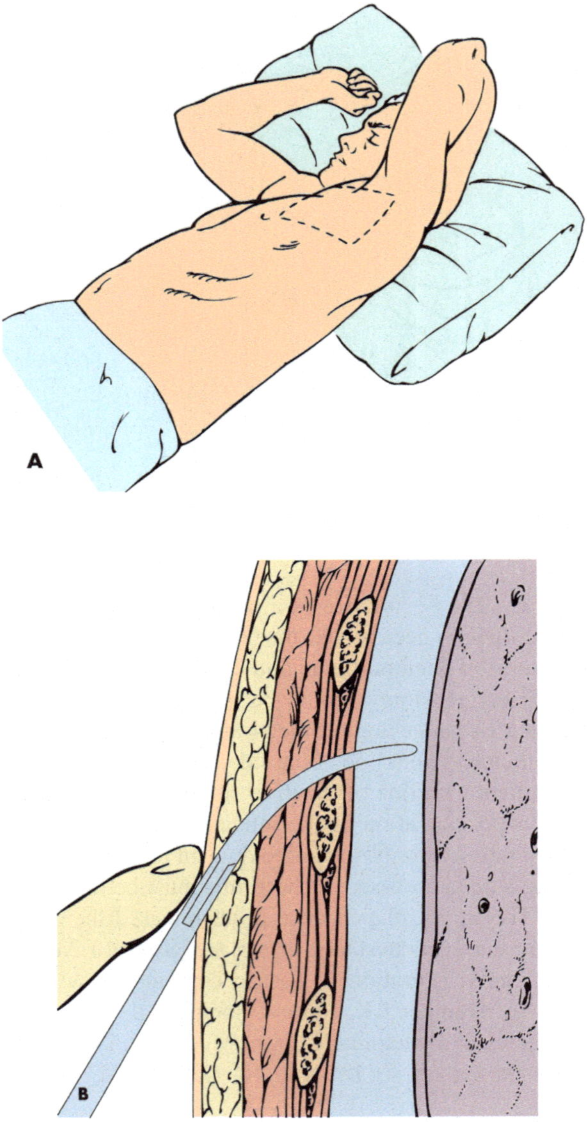
A
B

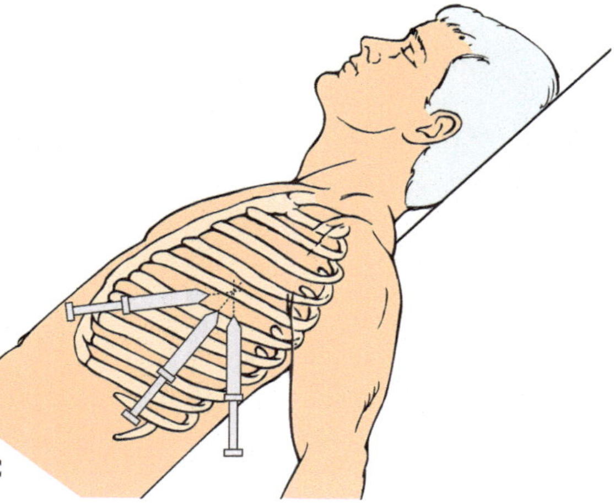

C

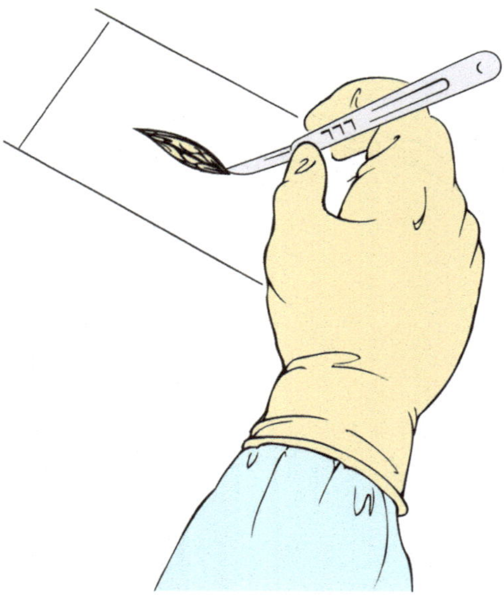

D

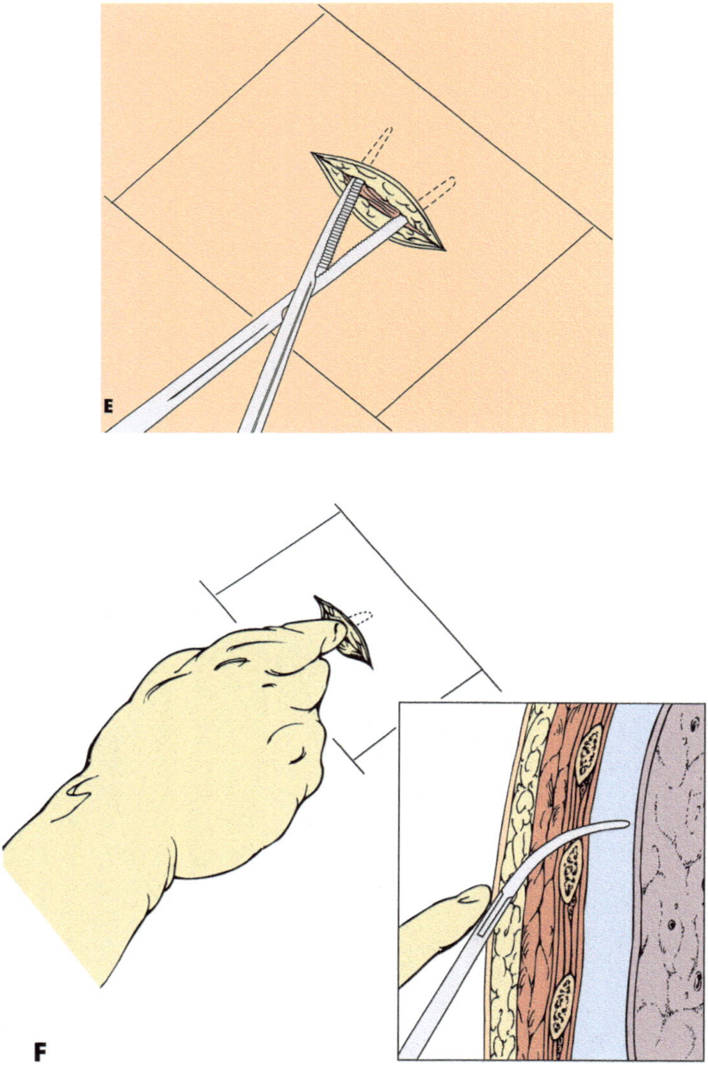
E
F

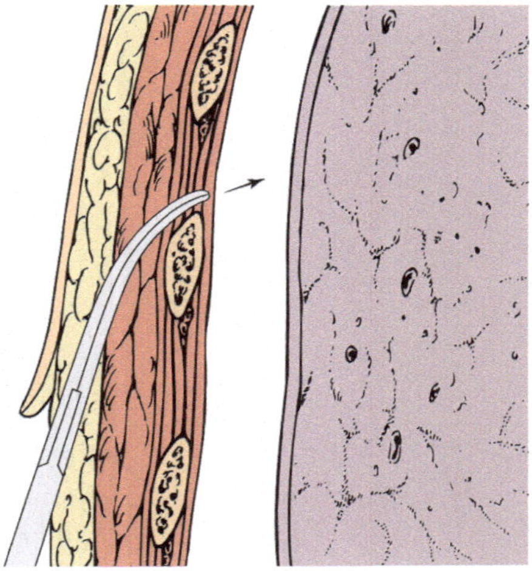

G

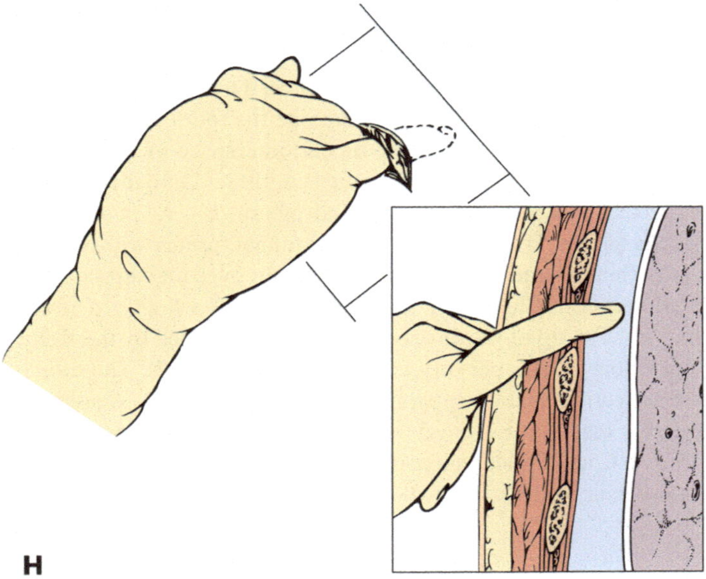

H

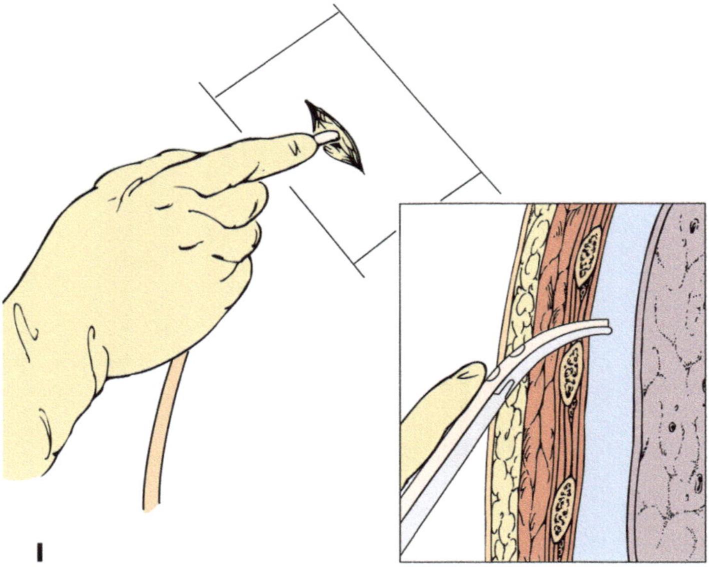

Tube thoracostomy. Tube thoracostomy is indicated to remove air or fluid (including blood) from the pleural space. Preferred sites are the fourth or fifth intercostal space in the anterior axillary line (A) or the second interspace in the midclavicular line (pneumothorax alone) (B). Local anesthetic is infiltrated into the skin, subcutaneous tissue, intercostal muscles, periosteum, and pleura (C). A 2-cm incision is made below the selected rib (D) and a subcutaneous tunnel formed with a Kelly clamp (E). The clamp is then inserted into the pleural space over the superior margin of the upper rib (F and G), followed by insertion of a gloved finger to confirm thoracic penetration (H). The tip of the thoracostomy tube is grasped by the Kelly clamp and inserted posteriorly and superiorly into the pleural space (I). The tube is then connected to a collection-suction apparatus with high-volume flow, adjustable suction, and underwater seal and is sutured to the skin. [Yeston N. Chapter 12. In: Kirby R, editor. Critical Care. Philadelphia: Current Medicine; 1997. (Miller RD, editor. Atlas of anesthesia; vol. 1). ISBN: 0-443-07906-4] *Caption from original*

Overall Principles of Treatment

- Treatment of simple pneumothorax involves evacuation of the air collection between the pleural layers. This should be done for all cases of simple pneumothorax except those that are shown to be very small on chest radiograph and are not causing symptoms; such lesions may be treated with supplemental oxygen and observation. Percutaneous management options include simple aspiration, chest tube placement, one-way valve insertion, and tube thoracostomy with continuous suction.

- Intensity of treatment is driven by size of the pneumothorax, degree of respiratory distress, severity of underlying lung disease, and risk of recurrence. Sometimes pharmacologic agents are instilled into the pleural space in an effort to prevent recurrence.

Disease Course

- It typically takes about 10 days for a simple pneumothorax to completely resolve, although symptoms typically improve much more quickly. Recurrence rates are 25–35 % for primary spontaneous simple pneumothorax and 40–50 % for patients with severe underlying lung disease.

Related Evidence

Papers of particular interest have been highlighted as:
*** Of key importance*

Practice Guideline

MacDuff A, Arnold A, Harvey J, BTS Pleural Disease Guideline Group. Management of spontaneous pneumothorax: British Thoracic Society pleural disease guideline 2010. Thorax. 2010 Aug;65(Suppl 2):ii18-31. PMID: 20696690. http://www.ncbi.nlm.nih.gov/pubmed/20696690 **

Review

Kaneda H, Nakano T, Taniguchi Y, Saito T, Konobu T, Saito Y. Three-step management of pneumothorax: time for a re-think on initial management. Interact Cardiovasc Thorac Surg. 2013 Feb;16(2):186-92. https://doi.org/10.1093/icvts/ivs445. PMID: 23117233. http://www.ncbi.nlm.nih.gov/pubmed/23117233

Ding W, Shen Y, Yang J, He X, Zhang M. Diagnosis of pneumothorax by radiography and ultrasonography: a meta-analysis. Chest. 2011 Oct;140(4):859-66. https://doi.org/10.1378/chest.10-2946. PMID: 21546439. http://www.ncbi.nlm.nih.gov/pubmed/21546439

Wakai AP. Spontaneous pneumothorax. Clin Evid (Online). 2011 Jan 17;2011. pii: 1505. PMID: 21477390. http://www.ncbi.nlm.nih.gov/pubmed/21477390 **

Noppen M. Spontaneous pneumothorax: epidemiology, pathophysiology and cause. Eur Respir Rev. 2010 Sep;19(117):217-9. https://doi.org/10.1183/09059180.00005310. PMID: 20956196. http://www.ncbi.nlm.nih.gov/pubmed/20956196

Tschopp JM, Rami-Porta R, Noppen M, Astoul P. Management of spontaneous pneumothorax: state of the art. Eur Respir J. 2006 Sep;28(3):637-50. PMID: 16946095. http://www.ncbi.nlm.nih.gov/pubmed/16946095 **

Ryan B. Pneumothorax: assessment and diagnostic testing. J Cardiovasc Nurs. 2005 Jul-Aug;20(4):251-3. PMID:16000911. http://www.ncbi.nlm.nih.gov/pubmed/16000911

Cohort Study

Belchis DA, Shekitka K, Gocke CD. Multi-institutional retrospective cohort study of spontaneous pneumothorax. Pathol Res Pract. 2013 Aug;209(8):486-9. https://doi.org/10.1016/j.prp.2013.05.002. PMID: 23778154. http://www.ncbi.nlm.nih.gov/pubmed/23778154

Jalli R, Sefidbakht S, Jafari SH. Value of ultrasound in diagnosis of pneumothorax: a prospective study. Emerg Radiol. 2013 Apr;20(2):131-4. https://doi.org/10.1007/s10140-012-1091-7. PMID: 23179505. http://www.ncbi.nlm.nih.gov/pubmed/23179505

Use PubMed Clinical Queries to find the most recent evidence. Use this search strategy: "Pneumothorax"[Mesh] OR "Pneumothorax"

Chapter 60
Pneumothorax (Tension)

Charles V. Pollack, Jr., Richard M. Cantor, and Victoria G. Riese

Name and Synonyms

Tension Pneumothorax, Dropped Lung

Incidence/Epidemiology

- The incidence of tension pneumothorax is clearly underestimated. Because it results in such dramatic ventilatory and hemodynamic compromise, it often is treated rapidly, before the diagnosis is confirmed. Needle thoracostomy, for example, may relieve tension pneumothorax, but if the presumed diagnosis is incorrect, it creates a simple pneumothorax.
- Tension pneumothorax is a rare complication of primary spontaneous pneumothorax. In the 1800s, the most common underlying cause of tension pneumothorax was pulmonary tuberculosis.

C. V. Pollack, Jr. (✉)
Department of Emergency Medicine, Thomas Jefferson University,
Philadelphia, PA, USA

R. M. Cantor
Department of Emergency Medicine and Pediatrics, State University of New York Upstate
Medical University, Syracuse, NY, USA

V. G. Riese
Librarian Consultant, Eldersburg, MD, USA

C. V. Pollack, Jr. (ed.), *Differential Diagnosis of Cardiopulmonary Disease*,
https://doi.org/10.1007/978-3-319-63895-9_60

- Probably the most common cause of tension pneumothorax in the community is blunt chest trauma. It may occur in the hospital as a complication of mechanical ventilation with positive end-expiratory pressure (PEEP), which may or may not be associated with a sharp procedure (such as central line placement). Rupture of blebs during PEEP ventilation is an important cause of significant pneumothorax.

Differential Diagnosis

- The differential considerations for tension pneumothorax are quite limited. Given the dramatic presentation with tracheal shift and extraordinary hemodynamic and ventilatory compromise, the diagnosis is usually straightforward. This is important because emergency treatment is required.
- If the tracheal deviation and unilateral hyperresonance described below are not readily apparent, other dramatic diagnoses, such as overwhelming pulmonary embolism or cardiac rupture, may be considered.

Pathophysiology and Etiology

- Pneumothorax is defined by the presence of air in the pleural space, which is the usually tiny space between the visceral and parietal layers of the pleura.
- Tension pneumothorax occurs when the abnormal gas-filled space become so large that the ipsilateral lung completely collapses and the pressure in the pleural space is positive throughout the respiratory cycle. The expanding gas eventually extends across the mediastinum and affects the volume and function of the contralateral lung.

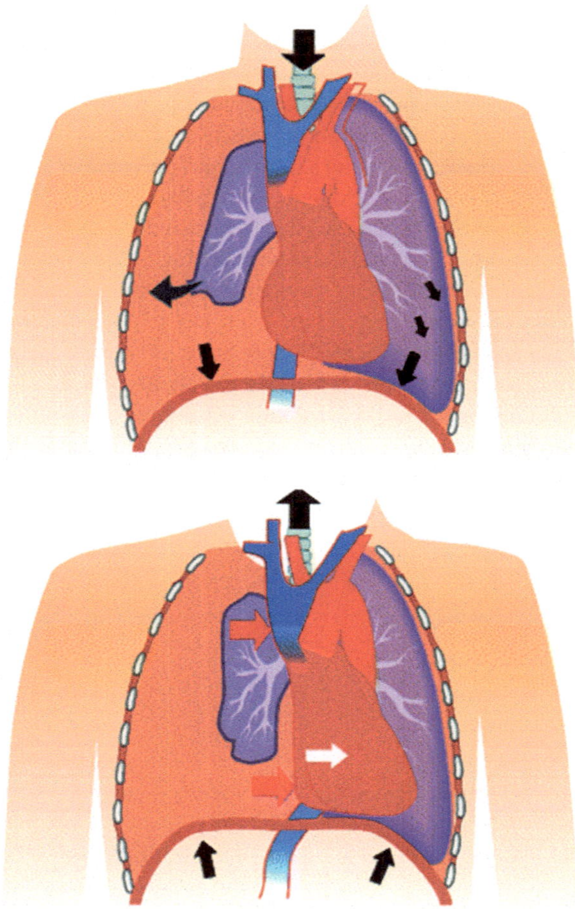

Tension pneumothorax, a feared and immediately life-threatening complication of pneumothorax. At the site of the lung injury, a valve mechanism occurs so that air leaks out but not back in. In a closed pneumothorax (intact chest wall) this leads to an increase of intrapleural pressure. The mediastinum is pushed toward the unaffected side, leading to ventilatory insufficiency on that side. The most threatening consequence of this condition is the pressure on the large chest veins with impairment of the refilling of the heart, which can lead to a rapidly progressing circulatory collapse. Immediate normalization of the pressure with needle thoracotomy is a prerequisite for survival [Lennquist S. Medical response to major incidents and disasters. Berlin Heidelberg: Springer; 2012. Chapter 7, Incidents caused by physical trauma; p. 111–96. Book https://doi.org/10.1007/978-3-642-21895-8; Chapter: 7; Chapter https://doi.org/10.1007/978-3-642-21895-8_7; Published: 2012-01-01] *Caption from original*

- The ventilatory compromise associated with tension pneumothorax results from the burden of trying to overcome consistent positive intrathoracic pressure combined with the loss of functional lung volume.
- The circulatory compromise associated with tension pneumothorax results in part from the impact of continuous positive pressure on the mediastinum, which reduces both venous return to the heart and cardiac output.
- Tension pneumothorax may be diagnosed as a complication in patients in whom simple pneumothorax has already been recognized, or it may present *de novo*.
- Tension pneumothorax in the outpatient setting is often the result of trauma, which is more commonly blunt (nonpenetrating) than penetrating. In the hospital, iatrogenic trauma may result from sharp procedures that violate the pleura (central line placement, lymph node or lung biopsy, etc.) or from positive-pressure ventilation, especially in patients with blebs.
- Tension pneumothorax in nontraumatic settings is most often the result of a severe infection process, such as necrotizing pneumonia. Pneumothorax is more common in smokers than nonsmokers, and is more common in patients with Marfan's syndrome and other connective tissue disorders associated with a tall, thin body type.

Presentation

Typical/"Classic"

- Tension pneumothorax presents dramatically—with a hypotensive patient who cannot ventilate effectively.
- Classically, the trachea is deviated out of the midline away from the collapsed lung.
- The ipsilateral hemithorax is hyperresonant (because it is filled with gas and the lung is collapsed) and may be visibly distended. Breath sounds are absent on that side.
- If the patient is on mechanical ventilation, airway pressure alarms will sound.
- The patient is hypotensive and tachycardic.

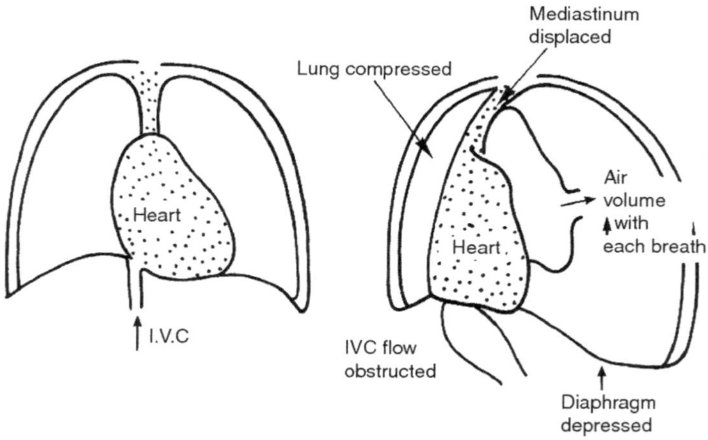

The effect of tension pneumothorax on ventilation and venous return [Hutson JM, Beasley SW. The Surgical Examination of Children, 2e. Berlin Heidelberg: Springer; 2013. Chapter 12, Trauma; p. 151–83. Book https://doi.org/10.1007/978-3-642-29814-1] *Caption from original*

- Jugular venous distension is present.
- Although chest radiography is diagnostic, it is often said that tension pneumothorax should never be diagnosed by x-ray, because delays in obtaining imaging may lead to further deterioration and death of the patient. If the diagnosis is suspected, treatment with decompressive needle thoracostomy should begin immediately.

Atypical

- Given the underlying pathophysiology of tension pneuomothorax, presentation is almost always "typical" (see above). The presentation may be slightly less dramatic very early and slightly obscured in the ICU when the patient is on a ventilator.
- Bilateral pneumothoraces with tension may present without tracheal deviation, but other cardinal features, especially hemodynamic collapse, will be present.

Primary Differential Considerations

- Because the clinical presentation of tension pneumothorax is so dramatic, there are few immediate differential considerations. In fact, pausing to consider other possibilities is dangerous to the patient. The only other immediate considerations might be severe shock or acute respiratory distress syndrome.

History and Physical Exam

Findings That Confirm Diagnosis

- Tension pneumothorax is a clinical diagnosis. Whether or not the patient has been injured, whether in the hospital or in the community, the findings of severe cardiopulmonary distress and volume/pressure shift in the chest are suggestive enough of the diagnosis that treatment should be empirically undertaken.

Factors That Suggest Diagnosis

- Each of the cardinal findings—respiratory distress, cardiovascular compromise, tracheal shift, asymmetry of sound and appearance in the two sides of the chest—points to the diagnosis.
- Appreciation of trauma or the presence and extent of underlying pulmonary disease may be helpful.

Factors That Exclude Diagnosis

- Tension pneumothorax results from the impact of persistently positive intrapleural pressure. Even finding a concomitant diagnosis (pulmonary embolism, pneumonia) not associated with this pressure shift does not exclude tension pneumothorax.

Ancillary Studies

Laboratory

- There are no diagnostic laboratory studies for tension pneumothorax. Obtaining "resuscitation labs" is appropriate but must not delay treatment with decompressive needle thoracostomy.

Imaging

- Tension pneumothorax is readily identified on chest radiograph. However, it is often said that tension pneumothorax should never be diagnosed by x-ray, because delays in obtaining imaging may lead to further deterioration and death of the patient. If the diagnosis is suspected, treatment with decompressive needle thoracostomy should begin immediately.

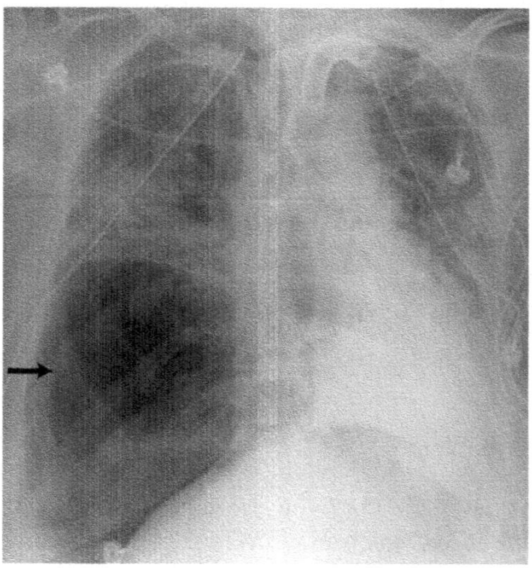

Tension pneumothorax. A, Chest radiograph of a critically ill patient with a deep sulcus sign on the left (arrow), consistent with the diagnosis of a pneumothorax. B. Chest radiograph of a critically ill patient on mechanical ventilation with the presence of a right loculated tension pneumothorax (arrow). Note the increase in volume of the right hemithorax, depression of the right hemidiaphragm, and contralateral mediastinal shift. [Huggins J, Sahn S. Pleural disease. In: Crapo J, editor. Bone's atlas of pulmonary and critical care medicine. Philadelphia: Current Medicine; 2005. Chapter 25. ISBN: 1-57340-211-7; Published: 2005-01-14] *Caption from original*

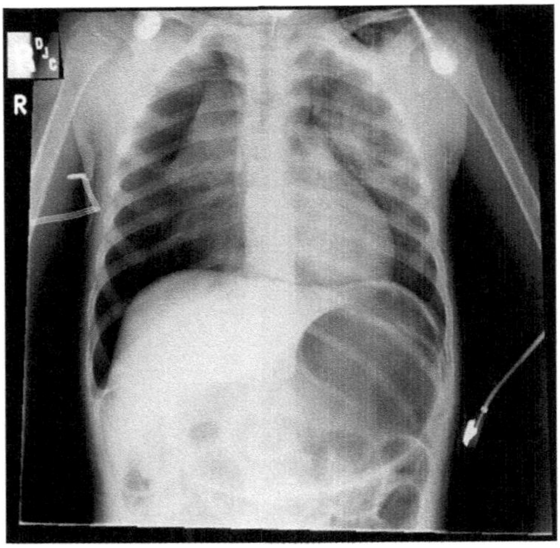

Chest radiograph of the chest showing tension pneumothorax on the right side [Parray T, Siddiqui SM, Hughes M, Shah S. Tension pneumothorax and subcutaneous emphysema during retrieval of an ingested lithium button battery. J Anesth. 2010 Jun;24(3):469–71. https://doi.org/10.1007/s00540-010-0908-3; Published: 2010-06-10] *Caption from original*

- There is no role for CT or ultrasound imaging in patients with tension pneumothorax.

Special Populations

Age and Gender

- Because the potential etiologies of tension pneumothorax are so varied, there are limited age and gender predilections. Patients with chronic obstructive pulmonary disease (COPD; who are more likely older males) have more blebs, the rupture of which may eventually lead to tension pneumothorax, especially in the setting of positive pressure ventilation.
- Because tension pneumothorax may be a complication of untreated or extensive simple pneumothorax, the age and gender considerations discussed for the former may be applicable.
- It cannot be stressed enough that consideration of differential diagnoses, special populations, etc. must not result in delay in recognition and immediate treatment of tension pneumothorax.
- Within the pediatric population, both simple and tension pneumothoraces are rarely encountered.

- There are, however, well recognized associated pediatric conditions that may present with pneumothoraces, such as cystic fibrosis, reactive airway disease, Marfan's syndrome, and Ehlers-Danlos syndrome.

Co-morbidities

- Asthma and COPD are common comorbidities. Pneumonia may be associated with either simple or tension pneumothorax.
- Marfan's syndrome and other connective tissue disorders predispose to pneumothorax.

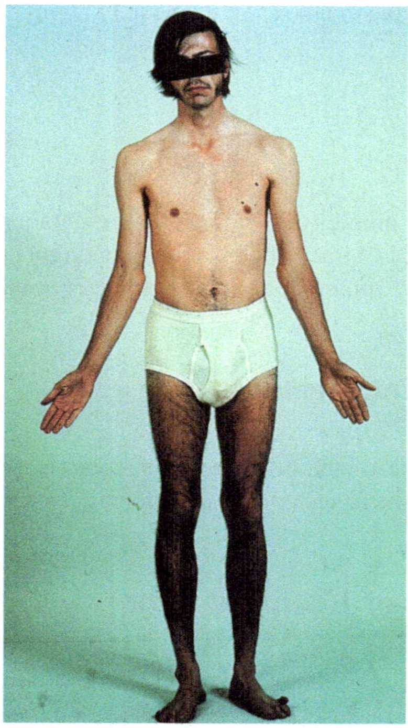

Clinical features of Marfan syndrome. Clinical features. Many of the typical features of Marfan's syndrome are seen in this patient, including arm length greater than height, increased lower to upper extremity ratio, pectus excavatum, and pes planus. Marfan's syndrome is characterized by autosomal dominant inheritance and has a prevalence of one in 20,000. A disorder of fibrillin, a glycoprotein abundant in the aortic media, skin, and ciliary zones, has recently been implicated as the most likely cause of this disorder. Musculoskeletal features include limbs disproportionately long for trunk size (dolichostenomelia), arachnodactyly, pectus excavatum or carinatum, scoliosis, pes planus, and joint hypermobility. Serious extraskeletal features include dilation of the aortic root (leading to aortic dissection) and upward subluxation of the lens. [Maricic M, Ko M. Diseases of bone and connective tissue. In: Hunder G, editor. Atlas of rheumatology. Philadelphia: Current Medicine; 2005. Chapter 6. ISBN: 1-57340-210-9; Published: 2005-01-18] *Caption from original*

- Tobacco use increases the incidence of pneumothorax.

Pitfalls in Diagnosis

Critical Steps Not to Miss

- Consideration of the diagnosis in the acutely compromised patient is the first critical step.

Mimics

- There are no real mimics of the dramatic presentation of tension pneumothorax. In the absence of tracheal deviation, one might consider large pulmonary embolism, cardiac rupture, or other intrathoracic catastrophe.

Time-Dependent Interventions

- Immediate release of the positive intrapleural pressure is required. Needle thoracostomy is the fastest means of relieving the tension.

Overall Principles of Treatment

- Treatment of tension pneumothorax is best provided by simple needle thoracostomy. The needle is usually inserted into the second or third intercostal space, in the midclavicular line, of the ipsilateral side. A rush of air through the needle confirms the diagnosis. The patient should then undergo formal tube thoracostomy while other hemodynamic support measures, as needed, are taken.

Video that describes the pathophysiology, diagnosis, and technique for decompressing a tension pneumothorax.
https://www.youtube.com/watch?v=ZZO5EEILnAA

Video covering the indications, instruments, and approach for performing a needle decompression of the chest
https://www.youtube.com/watch?v=UvHJ4pjNh2Q

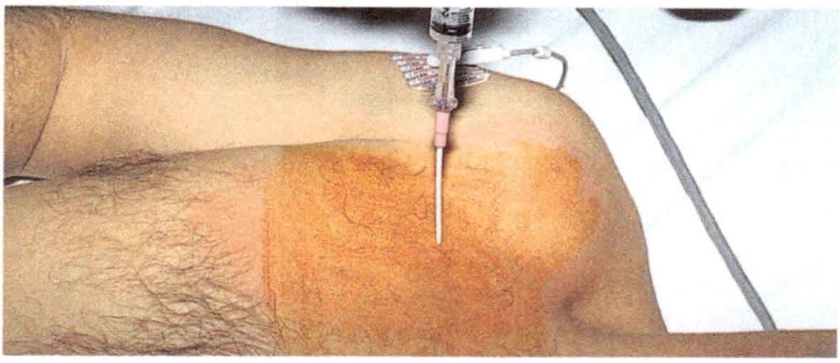

Needling the chest for tension pneumothorax. This procedure is performed with readily available equipment and can be accomplished rapidly before a chest tube is obtained and inserted. A, A 12- or 14-gauge intravenous cannula is inserted in the second intercostal space in the midclavicular line. The cannula is inserted on the side of the pneumothorax, if known, or it can be inserted bilaterally, if the side is not evident clinically or if bilateral pneumothoraxes are suspected. [Woodcock B. Hemodynamic emergencies. In: Tremper K, Miller R, editors. Atlas of anesthesia. Philadelphia: Current Medicine; 1998. Chapter 11. ISBN: 0-443-07903-X; Published: 2002-01-22] *Caption from original*

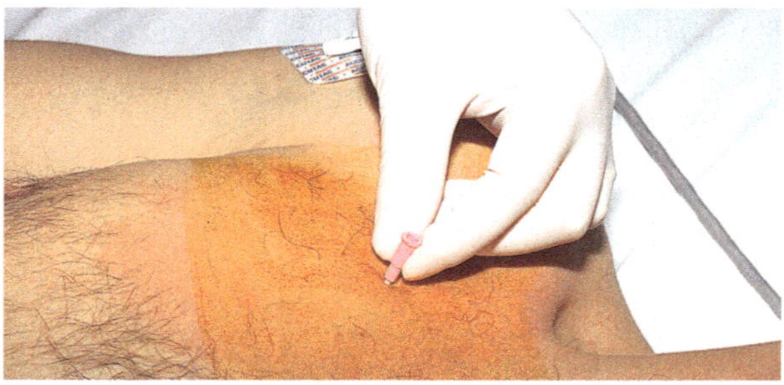

B, Entry into a tension pneumothorax is confirmed by air rushing rapidly through the needle. There is risk of causing pulmonary damage with needle insertion if a pneumothorax is not present, and this technique should be reserved for the patient who is rapidly deteriorating and cannot tolerate any delay for chest radiography. [Woodcock B. Hemodynamic emergencies. In: Tremper K, Miller R, editors. Atlas of anesthesia. Philadelphia: Current Medicine; 1998. Chapter 11. ISBN: 0-443-07903-X; Published: 2002-01-22] *Caption from original*

Video that demonstrates how to insert a chest tube for trauma.
https://www.youtube.com/watch?v=qyJkh-ghl70

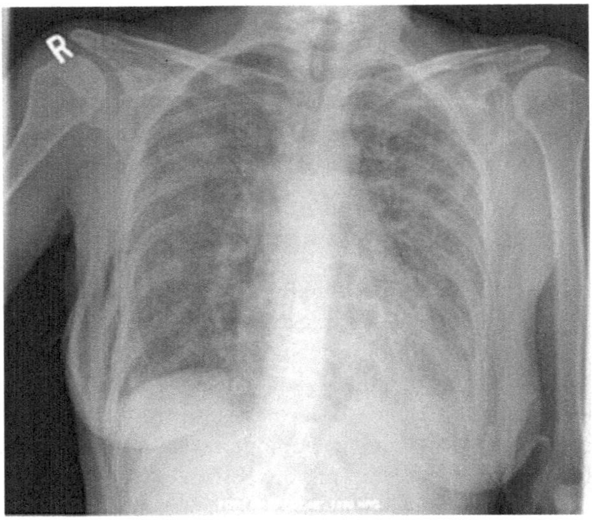

Chest radiograph obtained after decompression showing resolution of tension pneumothorax with a small apical crescent of residual right pneumothorax. [Wachsman AM, Hoffer EK, Forauer AR, Silas AM, Gemery JM. Tension pneumothorax after placement of a tunneled pleural drainage catheter in a patient with recurrent malignant pleural effusions. Cardiovasc Intervent Radiol. 2007 May;30(3):531–3. https://doi.org/10.1007/s00270-006-0073-0; Published: 2007-06-01] *Caption from original*

Disease Course

- Tension pneumothorax is fatal if untreated. Ultimate recovery after initial treatment depends on a variety of factors, including comorbidity burden and extent of other injuries.

Related Evidence

Papers of particular interest have been highlighted as:
*** Of key importance*

Practice Guideline

MacDuff A, Arnold A, Harvey J, BTS Pleural Disease Guideline Group. Management of spontaneous pneumothorax: British Thoracic Society pleural disease guideline 2010. Thorax. 2010 Aug;65(Suppl 2):ii18-31. PMID: 20696690. http://www.ncbi.nlm.nih.gov/pubmed/20696690 **

Review

Leigh-Smith S, Harris T. Tension pneumothorax–time for a re-think? Emerg Med J. 2005 Jan;22(1):8-16. PMID: 15611534. http://www.ncbi.nlm.nih.gov/pubmed/15611534 **

Barton ED. Tension pneumothorax. Curr Opin Pulm Med. 1999 Jul;5(4):269-74. PMID: 10407699. http://www.ncbi.nlm.nih.gov/pubmed/10407699 **

Clinical Trial

Notrica DM, Garcia-Filion P, Moore FO, Goslar PW, Coimbra R, Velmahos G, Stevens LR, Petersen SR, Brown CV, Foulkrod KH, Coopwood TB Jr, Lottenberg L, Phelan HA, Bruns B, Sherck JP, Norwood SH, Barnes SL, Matthews MR, Hoff WS, Demoya MA, Bansal V, Hu CK, Karmy-Jones RC, Vinces F, Hill J, Pembaur K, Haan JM. Management of pediatric occult pneumothorax in blunt trauma: a subgroup analysis of the American Association for the Surgery of Trauma multicenter prospective observational study. J Pediatr Surg. 2012 Mar;47(3):467-72. https://doi.org/10.1016/j.jpedsurg.2011.09.037. PMID: 22424339. http://www.ncbi.nlm.nih.gov/pubmed/22424339 **

Cohort Study

Yoon JS, Choi SY, Suh JH, Jeong JY, Lee BY, Park YG, Kim CK, Park CB. Tension pneumothorax, is it a really life-threatening condition? J Cardiothorac Surg. 2013 Oct 15;8:197. https://doi.org/10.1186/1749-8090-8-197. PMID: 24128176. http://www.ncbi.nlm.nih.gov/pubmed/24128176

Case Study

Mayordomo-Colunga J, Rey C, Medina A, Concha A. Iatrogenic tension pneumothorax in children: two case reports. J Med Case Rep. 2009 Jun 30;3:7390. https://doi.org/10.4076/1752-1947-3-7390. PMID: 19830199. http://www.ncbi.nlm.nih.gov/pubmed/19830199 **

Watts BL, Howell MA. Tension pneumothorax: a difficult diagnosis. Emerg Med J. 2001 Jul;18(4):319-20. PMID: 11435384. http://www.ncbi.nlm.nih.gov/pubmed/11435384

Use PubMed Clinical Queries to find the most recent evidence. Use this search strategy:

"Tension Pneumothorax"

Chapter 61
Pulmonary Embolism

Charles V. Pollack, Jr., Richard M. Cantor, and Victoria G. Riese

Name and Synonyms

Pulmonary embolism (PE); venous thromboembolism

Incidence/Epidemiology

- Pulmonary embolism is relatively common and is clearly underreported, as it is the most common cause of in-hospital death, and autopsies are not always performed on these patients.

C. V. Pollack, Jr. (✉)
Department of Emergency Medicine, Thomas Jefferson University,
Philadelphia, PA, USA

R. M. Cantor
Department of Emergency Medicine and Pediatrics, State University of New York Upstate
Medical University, Syracuse, NY, USA

V. G. Riese
Librarian Consultant, Eldersburg, MD, USA

C. V. Pollack, Jr. (ed.), *Differential Diagnosis of Cardiopulmonary Disease*,
https://doi.org/10.1007/978-3-319-63895-9_61

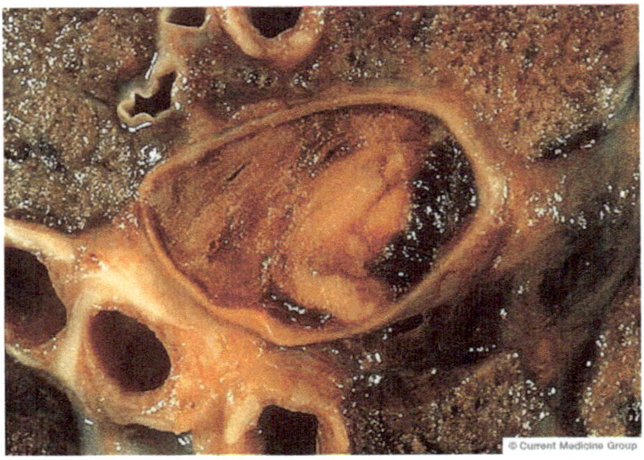

Autopsy specimen demonstrating pulmonary embolism. The patient subsequently suffered a cardiac arrest and died 3 days later despite maximal resuscitative efforts. At autopsy, the right main pulmonary artery, seen in cross-section, was filled with thrombus of varying age. [Goldhaber SZ, Piazza G. Interventional cardiology. In: Libby P, editor. Essential Atlas of Cardiovascular Disease. 4th ed. Philadelphia: Current Medicine Group; 2009. 432 p. ISBN: 978-1-57340-309-2] *Caption adapted from original*

- On the other hand, PE is likely diagnosed now more than in previous times because of the ubiquitous availability of computed tomographic (CT) pulmonary angiography.
- The estimated incidence of PE in the US is about 1 case per 1,000 persons per year.
- The incidence of venous thromboembolism (PE plus deep venous thrombosis, or DVT) is increasing as the population ages and as obesity, cancer, and longer lifespans with debilitating disease all become more common.

Differential Diagnosis

- The differential considerations for chest pain due to PE includes acute coronary syndrome and aortic dissection, both of which—like PE—are potentially life-threatening.
- Less severe differential considerations include pleurisy, pneumonia, pneumothorax, chest wall pain, and anxiety.
- With significant hypoxemia patients may present with syncope, near-syncope, or seizure, so the differential considerations for those entities also must be entertained.
- Acute chest syndrome in sickle cell disease is a differential consideration in at-risk patients.

Pathophysiology and Etiology

- As the name implies, PE is an embolic phenomenon. The usual embolus is a thrombus that originates in a deep vein, typically in the lower extremities or pelvis, or occasionally from the upper extremities or other sources.

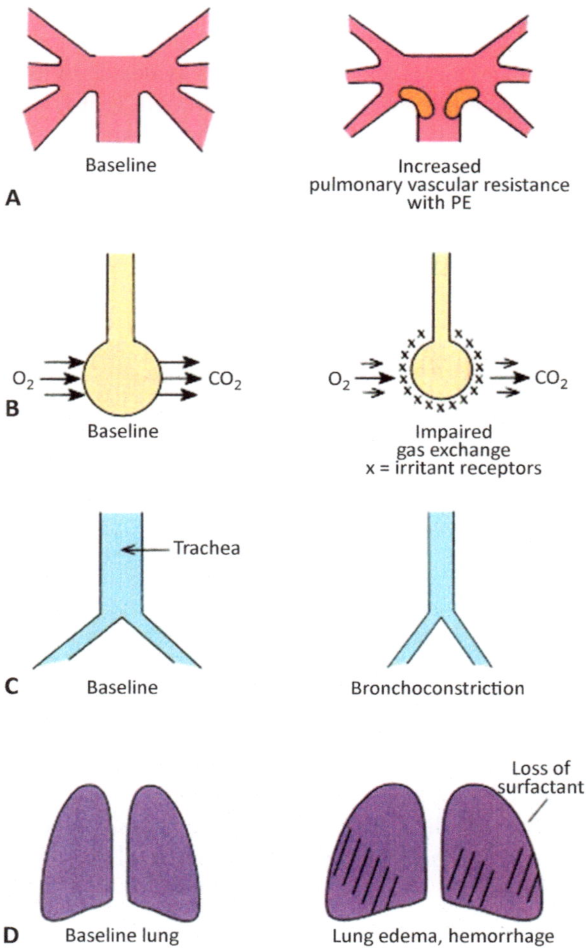

Pathophysiology of pulmonary embolism (PE). A, Increased pulmonary vascular resistance due to vascular obstruction, vasoconstriction by neurohumoral agents, vasoconstriction because of baroreceptors in the pulmonary arteries (which sense pressure exerted against the wall of the pulmonary artery by blood flowing past an obstructing blood clot), or increased pulmonary artery pressure. Baroreceptors may induce reflex pulmonary vasoconstriction. B, Impaired gas exchange due to irritant receptors, increased alveolar dead space (from vascular obstruction), hypoxemia (from alveolar hypoventilation), and right-to-left shunting; impaired carbon monoxide transfer due to loss of gas exchange surface also occurs. C, Increased airway resistance due to bronchoconstriction. D, Decreased pulmonary compliance due to lung edema and hemorrhage as well as loss of surfactant. [Chapter 3 in: Braunwald E, Goldhaber S, editors. Cardiopulmonary Diseases and Cardiac Tumors. Atlas of Heart Diseases. 1st edition. Philadelphia: Current Medicine; 1995. ISBN: 1-878132-23-7.] *Caption from original*

- The thrombus fragments and detaches (or may detach in its entirety), passes through the right atrium, tricuspid valve, and right ventricle, and into the pulmonary vasculature. It lodges in a vessel either proximally or distally, depending on its size and pulmonary flow dynamics. Infarction of pulmonary tissue occurs when obstruction is complete and there is no collateral blood flow to that tissue.
- The result of pulmonary infarction is pain and hypoxemia (the extent of which relates to the volume of tissue infarcted). In some cases, the infarction will cause bleeding or sloughing of bloody tissue into the alveolar space, and hemoptysis may ensue.
- Even in the absence of frank infarction, PE results in pain, dyspnea, increased alveolar dead space and ventilation : perfusion (V:Q) mismatch.

Presentation

Typical/"Classic"

- The classic PE presentation is characterized by the combination of dyspnea, pleuritic chest pain, hypoxemia, and hemoptysis. Of these, hemoptysis is the least consistent.
- An even more "classic" presentation would include a known history of, or evidence of, DVT. Recall, however, that pelvic vein DVTs do not always cause significant findings on physical examination, and also that DVT from any source may *completely* embolize, leaving no clinical or ultrasonographic evidence behind.

Atypical

- The classic presentation is not typical. The most consistent finding in acute PE is dyspnea. The presentation of dyspnea and tachycardia together should always prompt consideration of PE.
- Patients with PE may present with syncope, seizure, or with sudden death.
- Patients with massive PE may present with hemodynamic collapse.

- Depending on the area of lung involved, presenting pain in PE may be in the flank or abdomen.
- Patients with PE may present with wheezing and may be confused with asthma or COPD.
- The coincidence of fever and chest pain in PE may mimic pneumonia.

Primary Differential Considerations

- Pulmonary embolism carries an immediate life threat and as such should be considered at the top of the list of differential considerations that present with the signs and symptoms described above. Other diagnostic considerations that are potentially immediately life-threatening include:
  - acute coronary syndrome
  - aortic dissection
  - tension pneumothorax
  - shock
- Other less acute but important differential diagnoses to consider include:
  - simple pneumothorax
  - pneumonia
  - pleurisy

History and Physical Exam

Findings That Confirm Diagnosis

- History and physical examination are not diagnostic for PE.

Factors That Suggest Diagnosis

- History and physical findings are dependent upon the size of the PE. PE is typically classed as:
  - Massive, implying hemodynamic compromise, or
  - Submassive, implying clear symptoms but with intact hemodynamics
- Known DVT, risk for DVT, or swollen extremity suggestive of DVT is suggestive. A prior history of PE puts the patient at increased life-long risk for another episode.

- Findings of two or more of the cardinal symptoms (dyspnea, pleuritic chest pain, hypoxemia, and hemoptysis) should prompt serious consideration of PE.
- Local wheezes in the affected area are commonly heard.

- There are predictive scores, such as that published by Wells, which may be useful.

Criteria			**Points**
1. Suspected PE			3.0
2. An alternative diagnosis is less likely than PE			3.0
3. Heart rate > 100 beats/min			1.5
4. Immobilization or surgery in previous 4 weeks			1.5
5. Previous DVT/PE			1.5
6. Hemoptysis			1.0
7. Malignancy (on treatment or treated within past 6 months)			1.0
Score	**Mean probability of PE**	**% of Patients with this score**	**Risk**
<2	3.6	40	low
2–6	20.5%	53	medium
>6	66.7%	7	high

Wells criteria for assessment of pre-test probability of pulmonary embolism (Data from Wells et al., 2000)[McIntyre LK, Langdale LA. Pulmonary Embolism. In: Bland, KI, Sarr, MG, Büchler, MW, Csendes, A, Garden, OJ, Wong, J (Eds.), editors. General Surgery [Internet]. Springer London; 2009 [cited 2016 May 27]. p. 263–72. Available from: http://link.springer.com/referenceworkentry/10.1007/978-1-84628-833-3_25] *Caption from original*

- The Geneva Score is another such predictive tool. Many authorities hold, however, that clinical gestalt (that is, the evaluator's clinical impression) is superior—or at least noninferior—to any validated scoring systems.

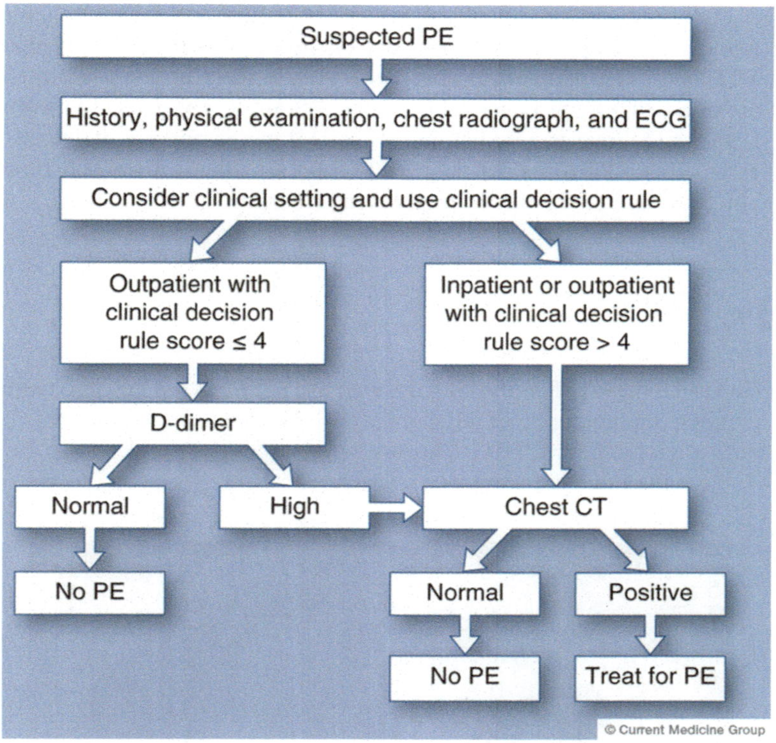

Algorithm for diagnosis of pulmonary embolism. An integrated approach. [Goldhaber SZ, Piazza G. Interventional cardiology. In: Libby P, editor. Essential Atlas of Cardiovascular Disease. 4th ed. Philadelphia: Current Medicine Group; 2009. 432 p. ISBN: 978-1-57340-309-2] *Caption adapted from original*

Factors That Exclude Diagnosis

- There are no history or physical findings that conclusively exclude PE.

Ancillary Studies

Laboratory

- There are no diagnostic laboratory studies for PE.
- Arterial blood gases may be used to calculate an arterial-alveolar oxygen gradient or to quantify hypoxemia, although in most cases transcutaneous pulse oximetry is sufficient.

- A D-dimer assay (D-dimer is a byproduct of fibrin degradation, and can be found in the body when there is active or chronic clotting) is very sensitive for VTE but is not particularly specific. It should therefore be used to reassure providers that there is *not* a PE. In the setting of low clinical probability, a negative D-dimer is very helpful. If the D-dimer is positive, it should not be assumed that PE (or underlying DVT) is present, but further evaluation (usually by imaging) should ordinarily then be performed.

Imaging

- The usual means of confirming the diagnosis of PE is with contrast-enhanced computed tomography of the thorax (called a computed tomographic pulmonary angiogram, or CTPA). This test is very sensitive for detecting PE down to the subsegmental pulmonary artery level.

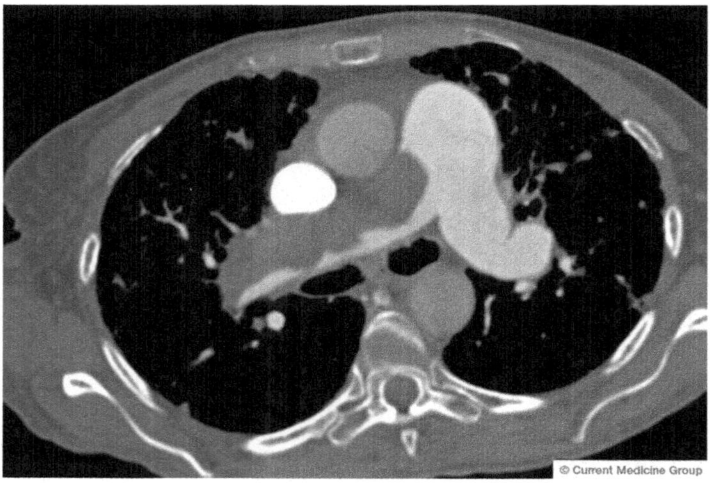

Chest computed tomography in pulmonary embolism. Diagnosis of acute pulmonary embolism (PE) by CT of the chest. This image is from a 59-year-old woman with advanced sarcoidosis who underwent chest CT as part of an evaluation before lung transplantation. The CT demonstrated a previously unsuspected PE indicated by the large filling defect in the right main pulmonary artery. [Goldhaber SZ, Piazza G. Interventional cardiology. In: Libby P, editor. Essential Atlas of Cardiovascular Disease. 4th ed. Philadelphia: Current Medicine Group; 2009. 432 p. ISBN: 978-1-57340-309-2] *Caption from original*

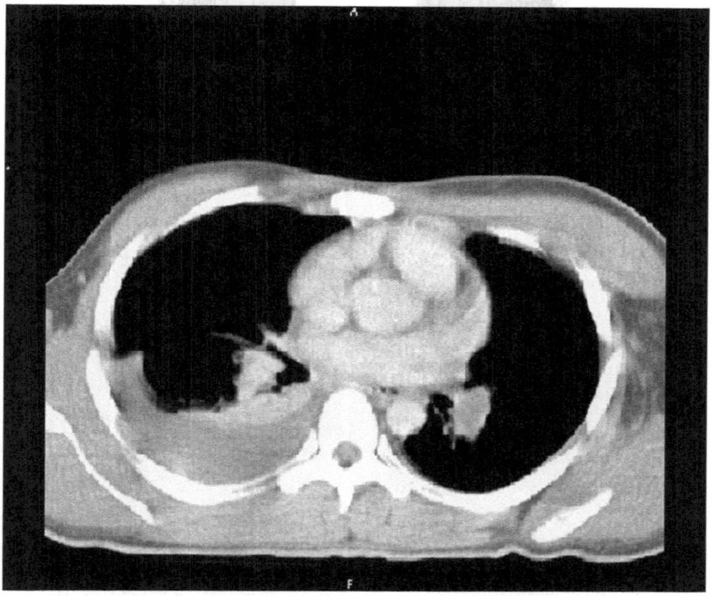

Acute pulmonary embolism. CECT chest showing thrombus in left pulmonary artery with right pleural effusion. [Vikram S, Jacob P, Nair CG, Vaidyanathan S. Gastric Carcinoma—A Rare Presentation. Indian Journal of Surgical Oncology. 2010 Dec;1(4):346–8.] *Caption from original*

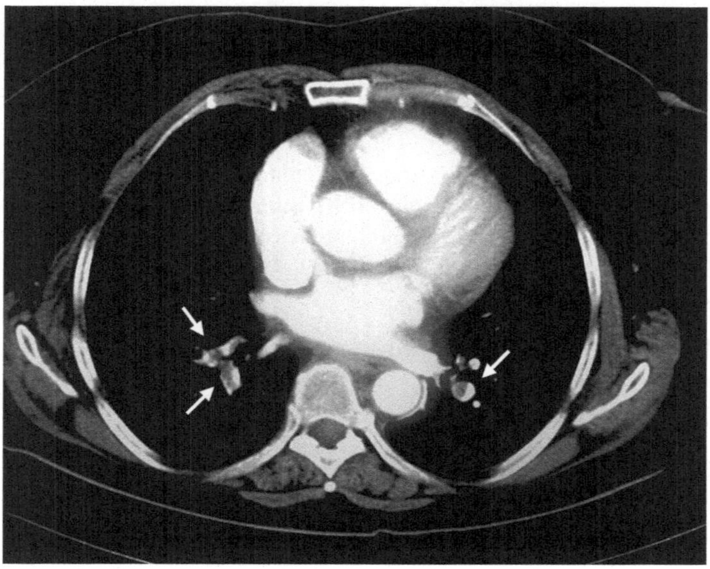

Visualization of a filling defect in the lumen of a vessel. *Arrows* indicate multiple filling defects in segmental branches of both pulmonary arteries diagnostic of bilateral pulmonary embolism. [Garcia-Bolado A, Del Cura JL. CT venography vs ultrasound in the diagnosis of thromboembolic disease in patients with clinical suspicion of pulmonary embolism. Emergency Radiology. 2007 Nov;14(6):403–9.] *Caption adapted from original*

- Because contrast material is required, CTPA may not be feasible in patients with renal insufficiency and should not be performed in pregnant patients.
- CT may also reveal suggestive right ventricular enlargement in PE.

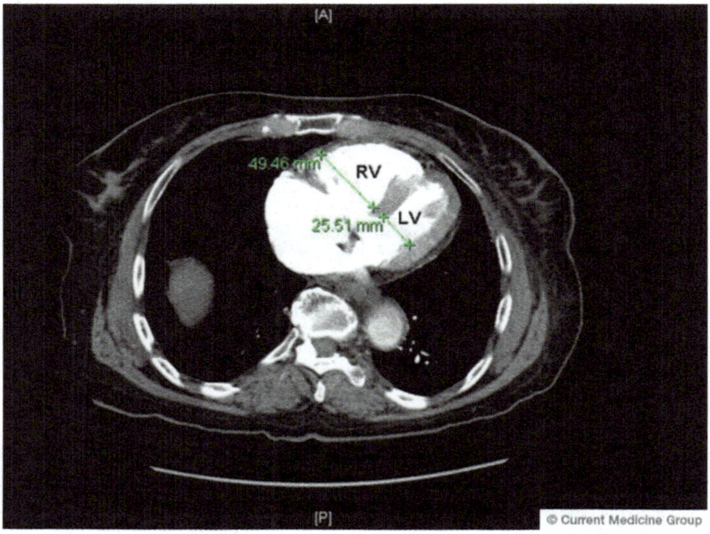

Chest computed tomography (CT) demonstrating right ventricular (RV) enlargement. This chest CT image demonstrates RV enlargement with a ratio of RV dimension to left ventricular (LV) dimension of 1.9. [Goldhaber SZ, Piazza G. Interventional cardiology. In: Libby P, editor. Essential Atlas of Cardiovascular Disease. 4th ed. Philadelphia: Current Medicine Group; 2009. 432 p. ISBN: 978-1-57340-309-2] *Caption adapted from original*

- MRI of the chest can be used to evaluate for PE in patients who cannot undergo CT imaging.

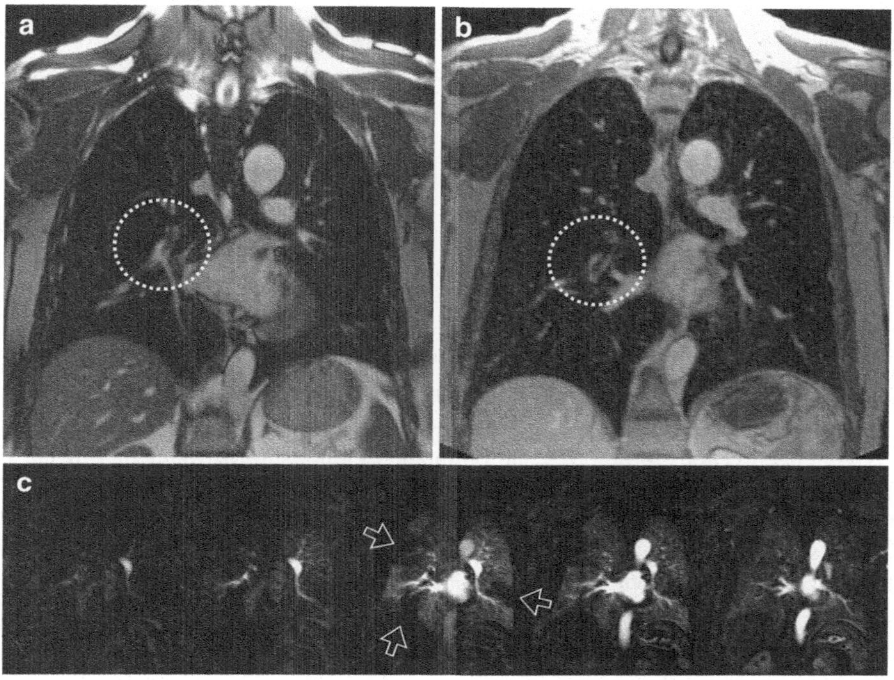

MRI of acute pulmonary embolism. A 55-year-old patient with acute pulmonary embolism. Coronal steady-state free precession images acquired during free breathing (a) and contrast-enhanced coronal 3d flash angiogram acquired in breathhold (b; embolus inside the right lower lobe artery circled); c series of subtracted images from the first pass perfusion study, perfusion deficits marked with open arrows at the image obtained at peak lung enhancement; 1.5-T MRI scanner [Biederer J, Mirsadraee S, Beer M, Molinari F, Hintze C, Bauman G, Both M, Van Beek EJR, Wild J, Puderbach M. MRI of the lung (3/3)—current applications and future perspectives. Insights into Imaging. 2012 Aug;3(4):373–86.] *Caption adapted from original*

- Ventilation-perfusion imaging (V/Q scan) is a nuclear medicine study that can demonstrate mismatches between ventilation and perfusion of the lungs and therefore indirectly identify PE. The test is more difficult to interpret than CT or MRI and is notably compromised in patients with existing lung disease such as COPD. It is still sometimes used when patients cannot receive contrast for CTPA.

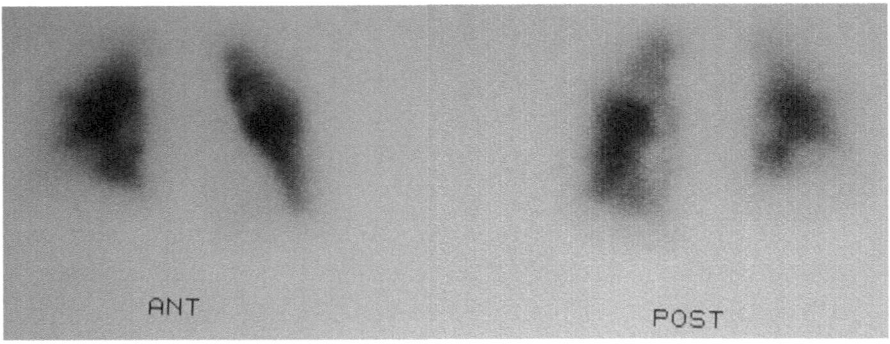

Ventilation-perfusion scan was interpreted as a high probability for pulmonary embolism involving the right lung and left upper lung. Patient was diagnosed as having deep venous thrombosis and pulmonary embolism. [Kawaguchi Y, Mine T, Kawana I, Umemura S. Protein-losing enteropathy, deep venous thrombosis and pulmonary embolism in a patient with generalized inflammatory polyposis in remission stage of ulcerative colitis. Clinical Journal of Gastroenterology. 2009 Jun;2(3):156–60.] *Caption adapted from original*

- An echocardiogram will typically demonstrate right ventricular strain with larger PEs and may occasionally show the thrombus.

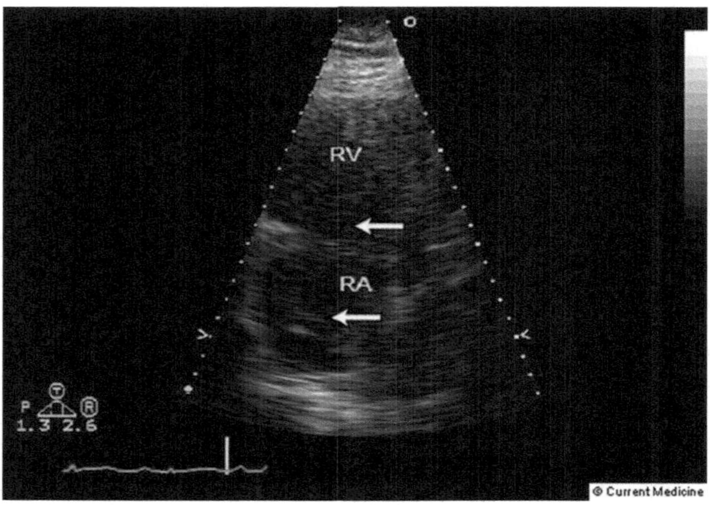

Echocardiogram of pulmonary embolism with thrombus in transit. Pulmonary embolism, thrombus in transit. Apical four-chamber view, demonstrating large mobile thrombi (arrows) within a dilated and hypokinetic RA and RV, which is consistent with acute pulmonary emboli. The appearance of thrombus in transit has been described as similar to "sausage links." Because most pulmonary emboli originate from the deep veins in the legs, it is hypothesized that the valves within the deep veins create indentations in the thrombus, which contribute to the "sausage link" appearance. [Mangion J, Solomon S. Chapter 15. In: Vannan MA, Lang RM, Rakowski H, Tajik AJ, Braunwald E, editors. Atlas of Echocardiography. 1e. Philadelphia, PA: Current Medicine Group; 2005. 312 p. ISBN: 1-57340-217-6] *Caption from original*

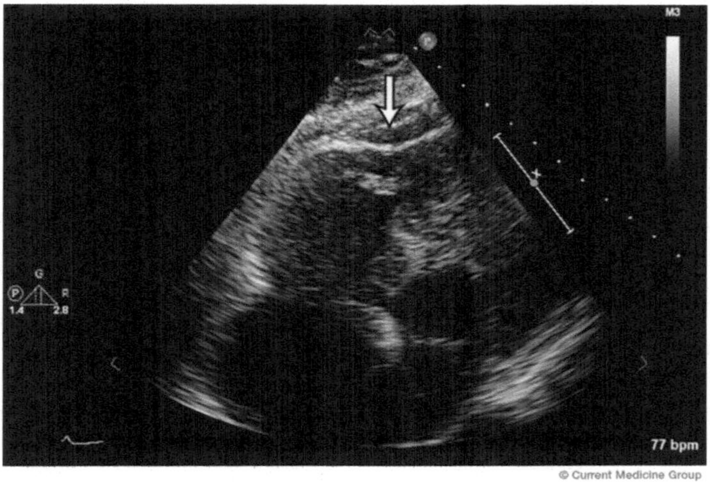

Echocardiographic assessment of pulmonary embolism. Pulmonary embolism. Apical four-chamber view, demonstrating right ventricular (RV) dilatation, hypokinesis, as well as McConnell's sign (arrow), which are markers of acute pulmonary embolism. [Mangion J, Solomon S. Echocardiography. In: Libby P, editor. Essential Atlas of Cardiovascular Disease. 4th ed. Philadelphia: Current Medicine Group; 2009. 432 p. ISBN: 978-1-57340-309-2] *Caption adapted from original*

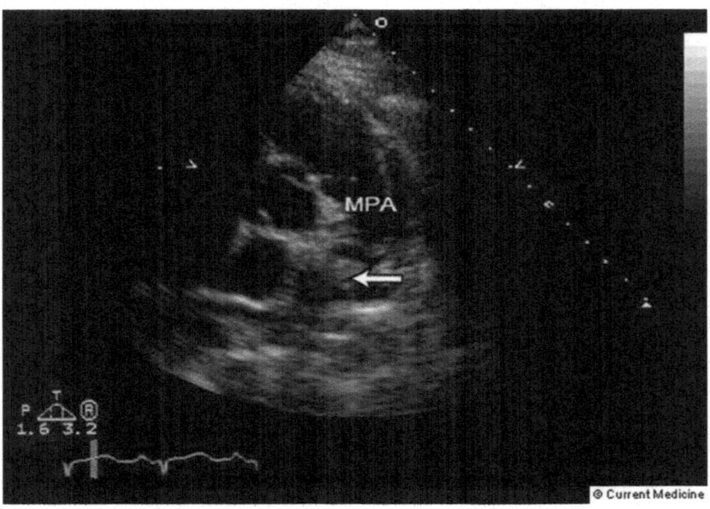

Echocardiogram of pulmonary embolism with right pulmonary artery thrombus Pulmonary embolism, thrombus within the right pulmonary artery (*arrow*). Main pulmonary artery and bifurcation view. Although echocardiography is often used in the setting of pulmonary embolism, it is not recommended as a routine imaging test for the diagnosis of pulmonary embolism because most patients with pulmonary embolism will have a "normal" echo. In patients with known pulmonary emboli, or with strong clinical suspicion for pulmonary emboli, it is important to visualize the pulmonary artery and branches, as in this case example. MPA—main pulmonary artery. [Mangion J, Solomon S. Echocardiography. In: Libby P, editor. Essential Atlas of Cardiovascular Disease. 4th ed. Philadelphia: Current Medicine Group; 2009. 432 p. ISBN: 978-1-57340-309-2] *Caption from original*

- Ultrasound of the extremities can identify DVT as a potential source of PE. Keep in mind that an entire DVT focus can embolize, creating PE and leaving behind no clot to be detected in the extremities.
- Electrocardiographic manifestations of PE are inconsistent, but the "classic" S1Q3T3 pattern is occasionally seen. Tachycardia is the most common finding on ECG in PE patients.

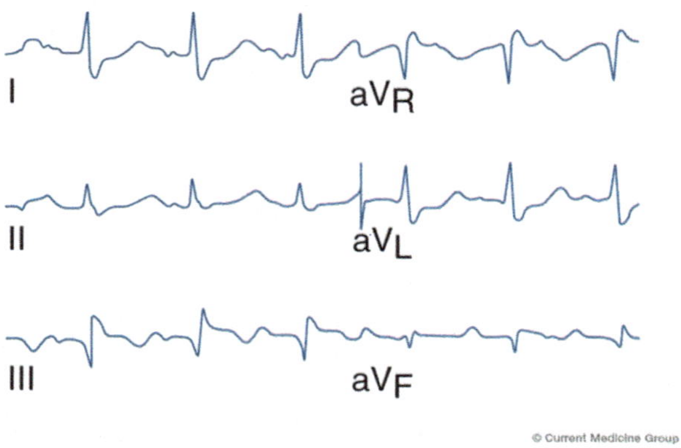

Electrocardiogram in pulmonary embolism. Electrocardiogram of a 64-year-old woman who was hospitalized with "atypical chest pain" and subsequently diagnosed with pulmonary embolism (PE). This patient's electrocardiogram shows sinus tachycardia, incomplete right bundle branch block, an S wave in lead I, Q wave in lead III, and T-wave inversion in lead III. This so-called S1Q3T3 pattern along with the new incomplete right bundle branch block is indicative of right ventricular strain in the setting of pressure overload from PE. [Goldhaber SZ, Piazza G. Interventional cardiology. In: Libby P, editor. Essential Atlas of Cardiovascular Disease. 4th ed. Philadelphia: Current Medicine Group; 2009. 432 p. ISBN: 978-1-57340-309-2] *Caption adapted from original*

Special Populations

Age and Gender

- The risk of PE increases with age.
- In general, the risk of PE is higher in men (perhaps owing to higher rates of cigarette smoking, cancer, and obesity), but women have higher risk when pregnant, in the post-partum period, and when taking hormone therapy (both oral contraceptives and replacement therapy).
- Blacks have higher rates of PE than whites in the US, and also have higher mortality with PE.
- The incidence of PE in children has risen sharply during the past decade, as a result of either more sensitive testing methods or greater survival from serious diseases (e.g., malignancies).
- The vast majority of PE in children is associated with the presence of central venous catheters, usually for the provision of chemotherapy or total parenteral nutrition (TPN).
- Within the adolescent population, adult risk factors apply.

Co-morbidities

- Hereditary thrombophilia (such as Protein C deficiency, antithrombin deficiency, Factor V Leiden) increases the risk of thromboembolism.
- Any state associated with increased levels of female hormones (including both pregnancy and prescribed therapy) increases the risk of thromboembolism.
- COPD is associated with PE, but that may derive from tobacco exposure more than from structural lung disease.
- Post-operative DVT and PE are common, owing primarily to post-op immobility, especially without prophylaxis such as low-molecular weight heparins.
- Prior VTE is a life-long risk factor for recurrent disease.
- Both malignancy and most forms of cancer treatment (surgery, chemotherapy, hormonal therapy) increase the risk of thromboembolism.
- Obesity increases the risk of thromboembolism.

Pitfalls in Diagnosis

Critical Steps Not to Miss

- Consideration of the diagnosis is the first critical step. Therapeutic anticoagulation may be initiated while awaiting formal confirmation of the diagnosis.

Mimics

- The entire constellation of diagnoses that underlies chest pain syndrome, especially those often accompanied by dyspnea, can mimic the pain and overall presentation of PE.
- Sudden cardiac death may mimic or be a presentation of PE.
- Syncope or near-syncope may mimic or be a presentation of PE.

Time-Dependent Interventions

- Pulmonary embolism can be rapidly fatal.
- Parenteral anticoagulation therapy should be initiated upon high suspicion or confirmation of PE.
- Patients with PE and hemodynamic compromise (inability to support blood pressure or oxygenation) should be immediately evaluated for suitability for thrombolytic therapy.

PRINCIPAL INCLUSION CRITERIA	MAJOR EXCLUSION CRITERIA
Massive pulmonary embolism	Intracranial disease
Anatomically small or moderate size pulmonary embolism with hemodynamic instability (*eg*, prior cardiopulmonary disease)	Recent major trauma or surgery
Hemodynamically stable, but right ventricular dysfunction detected on baseline echocardiogram	Active bleeding, known bleeding diathesis, or unexplained anemia
Normal echocardiogram and moderate size pulmonary embolism associated with massive pelvic or leg vein thrombosis	Uncontrolled hypertension

Inclusion and exclusion criteria for thrombolysis. The greatest challenge of thrombolysis for pulmonary embolism is gaining a thorough familiarity of when it should be utilized and, conversely, when it should be withheld. [Chapter 3 in: Braunwald E, Goldhaber S, editors. Cardiopulmonary Diseases and Cardiac Tumors. Atlas of Heart Diseases. 1st edition. Philadelphia: Current Medicine; 1995. ISBN: 1-878132-23-7.] *Caption from original*

Overall Principles of Treatment

- Treatment of PE is with anticoagulation. Anticoagulants prevent clot progression while the body's native thrombolytic defenses gradually break down the clot and while collateral perfusion channels develop around the occluded vessel.

- Anticoagulation is recommended for at least 3 months after PE, but may be extended to 6 or 12 months or even longer based on the patient's thrombotic risk and the bleeding risk while on anticoagulants.

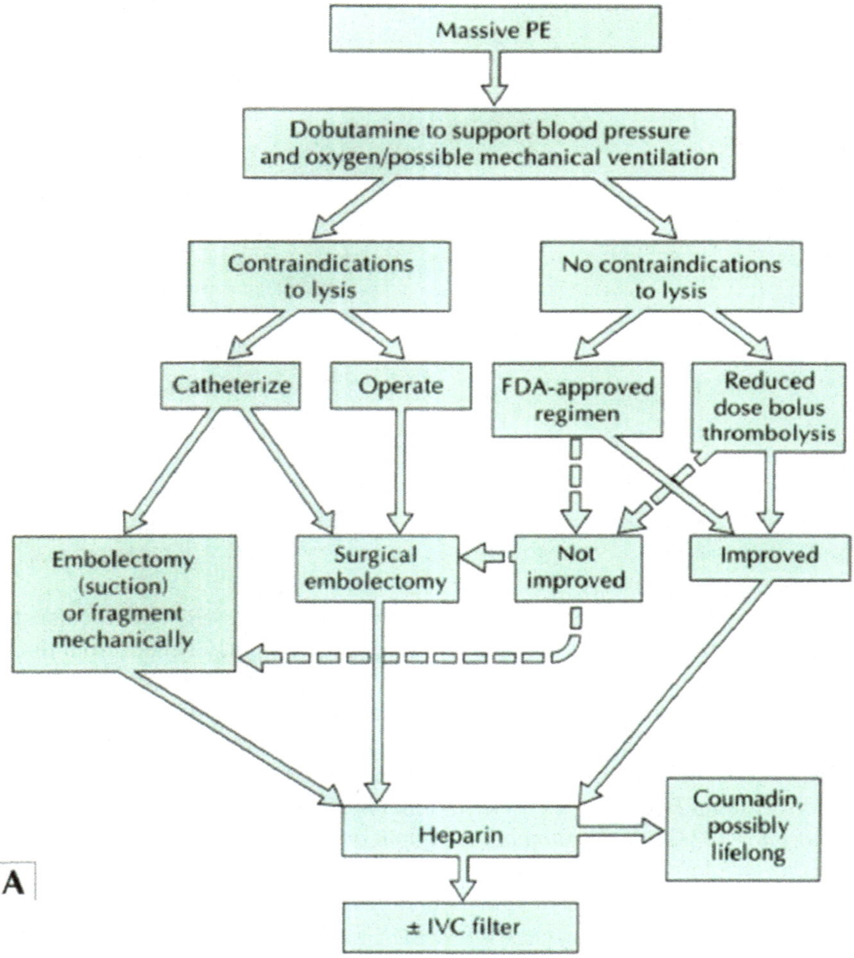

A

Protocols for treating different types of pulmonary embolism (PE). The optimal duration of Coumadin has not been studied in patients with pulmonary embolism. A, The patient who is hemodynamically compromised can receive an array of pharmacologic or mechanical interventions designed to lyse, remove, and dissipate the embolism while maintaining adequate right ventricular function. Consideration should be given to placement of a filter in the inferior vena cava (IVC) to prevent recurrent embolism that may be fatal in a patient with persistently compromised cardiopulmonary status. [Chapter 3 in: Braunwald E, Goldhaber S, editors. Cardiopulmonary Diseases and Cardiac Tumors. Atlas of Heart Diseases. 1st edition. Philadelphia: Current Medicine; 1995. ISBN: 1-878132-23-7.] *Caption from original*

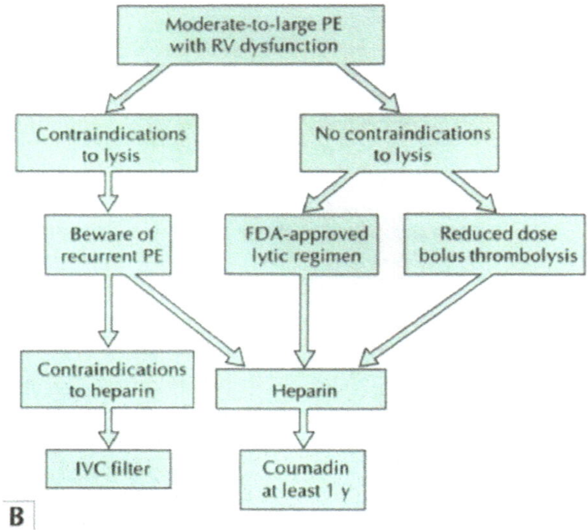

B, Moderate to large pulmonary embolism with associated right ventricular dysfunction. Although they are normotensive, these patients may benefit from thrombolytic therapy or suction catheter embolectomy not only to reverse right ventricular dysfunction rapidly and hasten pulmonary reperfusion but also to reduce the frequency of such adverse clinical events as recurrent embolism [Chapter 3 in: Braunwald E, Goldhaber S, editors. Cardiopulmonary Diseases and Cardiac Tumors. Atlas of Heart Diseases. 1st edition. Philadelphia: Current Medicine; 1995. ISBN: 1-878132-23-7.] *Caption adapted from original*

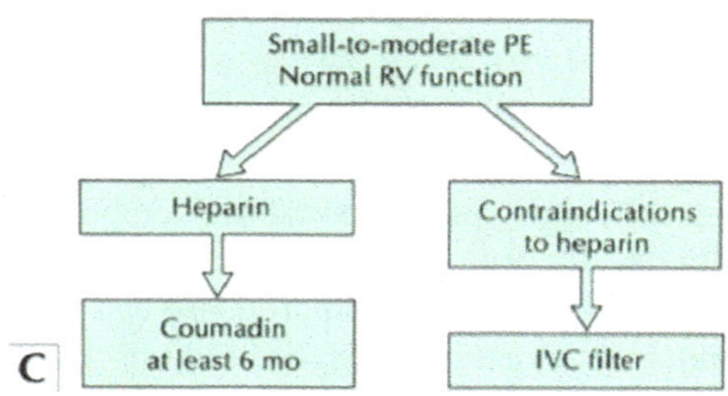

C, Small to moderate pulmonary embolism with normal right ventricular function. The prognosis of these patients is usually good with anticoagulation therapy alone. [Chapter 3 in: Braunwald E, Goldhaber S, editors. Cardiopulmonary Diseases and

Cardiac Tumors. Atlas of Heart Diseases. 1st edition. Philadelphia: Current Medicine; 1995. ISBN: 1-878132-23-7.] *Caption from original*

- Hemodynamically unstable PE is likely to benefit from thrombolytic therapy if contraindications do not exist.
- Remove or ameliorate risk as possible (e.g., stop smoking, lose weight if obese, discontinue birth control pills, etc).

Disease Course

- PE can be fatal. The true case mortality rate is not known owing to minor PEs that may not even be diagnosed on one end of the disease spectrum, and lack of autopsy data on the other end.
- Repeated PE may result in a serious disease called chronic thromboembolic pulmonary hypertension, or CTEPH.

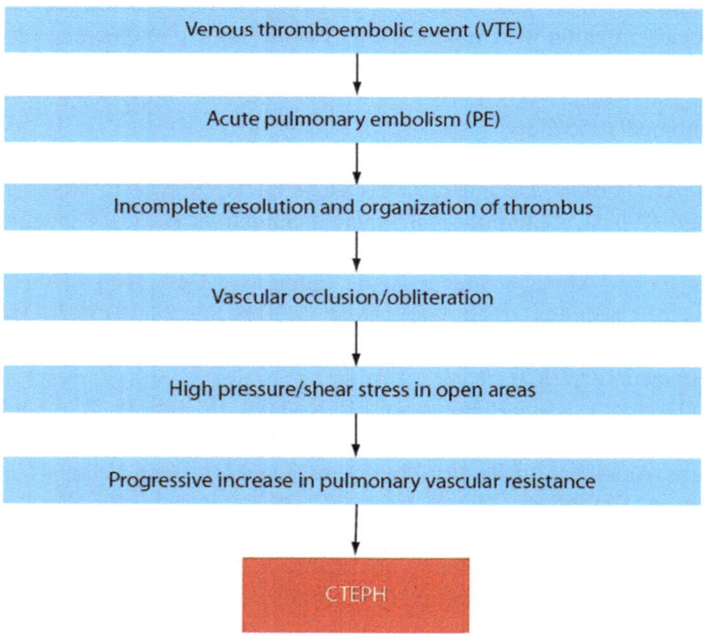

Embolic hypothesis of CTEPH. [Humbert M, Lang IM, Mayer E. Chronic thromboembolic pulmonary hypertension (CTEPH): specific disease characteristics and similarities to idiopathic pulmonary arterial hypertension. Clinical Research in Cardiology Supplements. 2010 Sep;5(S2):12–5.] *Caption from original*

- Most patients with first submassive PE, treated with early anticoagulation, have full recovery.

Related Evidence

Papers of particular interest have been highlighted as:
*** Of key importance*

Practice Guideline

Kearon C, Akl EA, Comerota AJ, Prandoni P, Bounameaux H, Goldhaber SZ, Nelson ME, Wells PS, Gould MK, Dentali F, Crowther M, Kahn SR; American College of Chest Physicians. Antithrombotic therapy for VTE disease: Antithrombotic Therapy and Prevention of Thrombosis, 9th ed: American College of Chest Physicians Evidence-Based Clinical Practice Guidelines. Chest. 2012 Feb;141(2 Suppl):e419S-94S. https://doi.org/10.1378/chest.11-2301. PMID: 22315268. http://www.ncbi.nlm.nih.gov/pubmed/22315268 **

Bajc M, Neilly JB, Miniati M, Schuemichen C, Meignan M, Jonson B; EANM Committee. EANM guidelines for ventilation/perfusion scintigraphy : Part 1. Pulmonary imaging with ventilation/perfusion single photon emission tomography. Eur J Nucl Med Mol Imaging. 2009 Aug;36(8):1356-70. https://doi.org/10.1007/s00259-009-1170-5. PMID:19562336. http://www.ncbi.nlm.nih.gov/pubmed/19562336 **

Torbicki A, Perrier A, Konstantinides S, Agnelli G, Galiè N, Pruszczyk P, Bengel F, Brady AJ, Ferreira D, Janssens U, Klepetko W, Mayer E, Remy-Jardin M, Bassand JP; ESC Committee for Practice Guidelines (CPG). Guidelines on the diagnosis and management of acute pulmonary embolism: the Task Force for the Diagnosis and Management of Acute Pulmonary Embolism of the European Society of Cardiology (ESC). Eur Heart J. 2008 Sep;29(18):2276-315. https://doi.org/10.1093/eurheartj/ehn310. PMID: 18757870. http://www.ncbi.nlm.nih.gov/pubmed/18757870 **

Snow V, Qaseem A, Barry P, Hornbake ER, Rodnick JE, Tobolic T, Ireland B, Segal J, Bass E, Weiss KB, Green L, Owens DK; Joint American College Of Physicians/american Academy Of Family Physicians Panel On Deep Venous Thrombosis/pulmonary Embolism. Management of venous thromboembolism: a clinical practice guideline from the American College of Physicians and the American Academy of Family Physicians. Ann Fam Med. 2007 Jan-Feb;5(1):74-80. PMID: 17261867. http://www.ncbi.nlm.nih.gov/pubmed/17261867

Meta-Analysis

Singh B, Parsaik AK, Agarwal D, Surana A, Mascarenhas SS, Chandra S. Diagnostic accuracy of pulmonary embolism rule-out criteria: a systematic review and meta-analysis. Ann Emerg Med. 2012 Jun;59(6):517-20.e1-4. https://doi.org/10.1016/j.annemergmed.2011.10.022. PMID: 22177109. http://www.ncbi.nlm.nih.gov/pubmed/22177109

Pasha SM, Klok FA, Snoep JD, Mos IC, Goekoop RJ, Rodger MA, Huisman MV. Safety of excluding acute pulmonary embolism based on an unlikely clinical probability by the Wells rule and normal D-dimer concentration: a meta-analysis. Thromb Res. 2010 Apr;125(4):e123-7. https://doi.org/10.1016/j.thromres.2009.11.009. PMID: 19942258. http://www.ncbi.nlm.nih.gov/pubmed/19942258

Review

Lapner ST, Kearon C. Diagnosis and management of pulmonary embolism. BMJ. 2013 Feb 20;346:f757. https://doi.org/10.1136/bmj.f757. PMID: 23427133. http://www.ncbi.nlm.nih.gov/pubmed/23427133 **

Dijk FN, Curtin J, Lord D, Fitzgerald DA. Pulmonary embolism in children. Paediatr Respir Rev. 2012 Jun;13(2):112-22. https://doi.org/10.1016/j.prrv.2011.09.002. PMID: 22475258. http://www.ncbi.nlm.nih.gov/pubmed/22475258 **

Bettmann MA, Baginski SG, White RD, Woodard PK, Abbara S, Atalay MK, Dorbala S, Haramati LB, Hendel RC, Martin ET 3rd, Ryan T, Steiner RM. ACR Appropriateness Criteria® acute chest pain–suspected pulmonary embolism. J Thorac Imaging. 2012 Mar;27(2):W28-31. https://doi.org/10.1097/RTI.0b013e31823efeb6. PMID: 22343403. http://www.ncbi.nlm.nih.gov/pubmed/22343403 **

Use PubMed Clinical Queries to find the most recent evidence. Use this search strategy:

"Pulmonary Embolism"[Mesh] OR "pulmonary embolism"

Chapter 62
Pulmonary Fibrosis

Charles V. Pollack, Jr., Melissa Platt, Richard M. Cantor, Victoria G. Riese, and Jaime Friel Blanck

Name and Synonyms

Pulmonary Fibrosis

- Synonyms:
    - Chronic interstitial pneumonitis
    - Hamman–Rich syndrome
    - Diffuse fibrosing alveolitis

Incidence/Epidemiology

- Idiopathic pulmonary fibrosis affects about 128,100 people in the United States
    - 48,000 new cases diagnosed annually
    - 40,000 people die each year

C. V. Pollack, Jr. (✉)
Department of Emergency Medicine, Thomas Jefferson University, Philadelphia, PA, USA

M. Platt
Department of Emergency Medicine, University of Louisville, Louisville, KY, USA

R. M. Cantor
Department of Emergency Medicine and Pediatrics, State University of New York Upstate Medical University, Syracuse, NY, USA

V. G. Riese
Librarian Consultant, Eldersburg, MD, USA

J. F. Blanck
Welch Medical Library, Johns Hopkins University, Baltimore, MD, USA

C. V. Pollack, Jr. (ed.), *Differential Diagnosis of Cardiopulmonary Disease*,
https://doi.org/10.1007/978-3-319-63895-9_62

Differential Diagnosis

- The differential diagnosis is broad and includes acute and chronic lung infections, pneumoconioses, collagen vascular diseases, and hypersensitivity syndromes.
  - Usually a diagnosis of exclusion
  - Sarcoidosis
  - Histiocytosis X
  - Collagen vascular disease
  - Drug-induced pulmonary toxicity
  - Eosinophilic pneumonia
  - Farmer's lung
  - Histoplasmosis
  - Pneumonia (aspiration, bacterial, fungal, viral)
  - Pneumonitis (interstitial)
  - Pulmonary edema
  - Restrictive lung disease
  - Silicosis
  - Tobacco worker's lung

Pathophysiology and Etiology

- Scarring throughout the lungs results in impaired gas exchange.

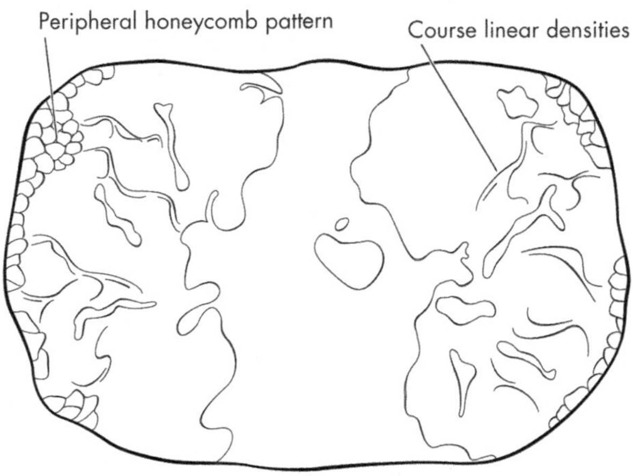

Pathophysiology of idiopathic pulmonary fibrosis. Schematic representation of chest computed tomography in IPF, showing coarse linear densities and a peripheral honeycomb pattern. [Smith M, Grichnik K. Anesthetic considerations for lung transplant and thoracic aortic surgery. In: Reves JG, editor. Cardiothoracic anesthesia. Philadelphia: Current Medicine; 1999. (Miller RD, editor. Atlas of anesthesia; vol. 8). ISBN: 0-443-07974-9] *Caption adapted from original*

- Associated with many conditions, including:
  - Infection
  - Pneumoconiosis (asbestos, silica)
  - Radiation exposure
  - Lupus, rheumatoid arthritis
  - Certain medications, including amiodarone
  - Granulomatous processes such as pulmonary sarcoidosis and Wegener's granulomatosis
  - Idiopathic: fibrosis develops without an identifiable cause
    - Most common form

Presentation

Typical/"Classic"

- Onset usually is gradual as symptoms worsen from a dry cough through dyspnea on exertion to dyspnea at rest.

Shortness of breath, exercise limitation
Cough
Age > 50 years
Crackles on physical examination (>80%)
Clubbing on physical examination (>20–50%)
Restrictive defect (reduced lung volumes) on pulmonary function tests
Hypoxemia (at rest or with exercise)
Characteristic HRCT scan

Clinical features of idiopathic pulmonary fibrosis [Lynch JP, Belperio JA. Idiopathic pulmonary fibrosis. In: Baughman RP, du Bois RM, editors. Diffuse lung disease [Internet]. New York, NY: Springer; 2012 [cited 2015 Sep 9]. p. 171–94. Available from: http://link.springer.com/10.1007/978-1-4419-9771-5_10] Caption from original

Atypical

- Occasionally seen as Hamman–Rich syndrome, in which symptoms and deterioration progress rapidly.

Primary Differential Considerations

Patients with signs and symptoms consistent with pulmonary fibrosis also may need to be evaluated for other lung and cardiopulmonary diseases, including:

- Pneumoconiosis
- Pneumonia
- Congestive heart failure
- Drug-induced lung toxicity
- Radiation pneumonitis
- Sarcoidosis
- Restrictive lung disease

History and Physical Exam

Findings That Confirm Diagnosis

Imaging (and often lung biopsy) is required to confirm the diagnosis of pulmonary fibrosis

Factors That Suggest Diagnosis

- History of occupational exposure
- History of connective tissue disease, inflammatory bowel disease, or malignancy
- Medication history
- Smoking history
- Prior irradiation
- Physical exam findings are nonspecific
  - Crackles may be present
  - Clubbing of the digits may occur

Factors That Exclude Diagnosis

- A productive cough is unusual.
- Wheezing and chest pain are uncommon signs.

Ancillary Studies

Imaging

- Plain chest radiography typically shows reticulonodular opacities and sometimes a "ground glass" appearance of the lung fields.
  - This is nonspecific, and advanced imaging is required in the evaluation.
- Chest CT reveals "honeycomb lung" with cysts that grow larger as the disease advances.

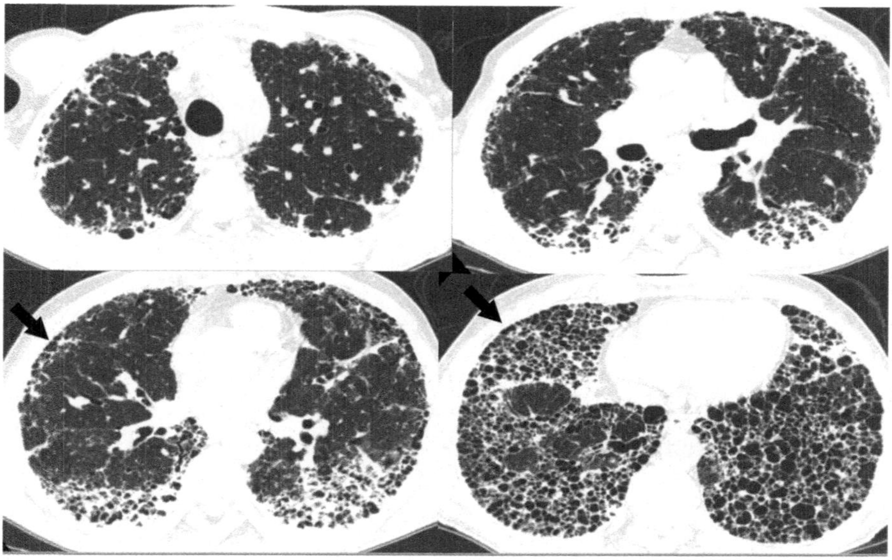

Multiple axial HRCT images show basilar- and peripheral-predominant pulmonary fibrosis characterized by reticulation, traction bronchiolectasis, and subpleural honeycombing (arrows), diagnostic of UIP [Chung JH, Kanne JP. Imaging of idiopathic pulmonary fibrosis. In: Meyer KC, Nathan SD, editors. Idiopathic pulmonary fibrosis [Internet]. Totowa, NJ: Humana Press; 2014 [cited 2015 Sep 9]. p. 55–75. Available from: http://link.springer.com/10.1007/978-1-62703-682-5_4] *Caption from original*

Special Populations

- Those with certain occupational, medication, or tobacco exposure are at increased risk.

Pediatric Considerations

- Pulmonary fibrosis generally is not a pediatric disease.
- As in the adult, it may be associated with certain medications, if taken by the child.
- At the extremes of chronicity (i.e. bronchopulmonary dysplasia, bronchiolitis, cystic fibrosis), it may develop.

Pitfalls in Diagnosis

Critical Steps Not to Miss

- Diagnosis needs a complete, thorough history and physical including occupation, drug exposures, and family history to exclude other diagnoses.

Mimics

- Many symptoms may be shared with a variety of pulmonary and cardiac diseases.

Time-Dependent Interventions

- Fibrosis is a chronic disease; unless the patient presents with acute ventilatory failure, there are no time-critical interventions.

Overall Principles of Treatment

- The course typically is inexorably downhill, with no consistently effective pharmacotherapy.
  - In some cases, corticosteroid therapy may be beneficial.
- Lung transplantation is reserved for very advanced cases.

Disease Course

- Scarring is permanent once it has developed.
- As the disease progresses, it may lead to pulmonary hypertension, cor pulmonale, respiratory failure, and increased risk of lung cancer.

Related Evidence

Papers of particular interest have been highlighted as:
*** Of key importance*

Practice Guideline

Travis WD, Costabel U, Hansell DM, King TE Jr, Lynch DA, Nicholson AG, Ryerson CJ, Ryu JH, Selman M, Wells AU, Behr J, Bouros D, Brown KK, Colby TV, Collard HR, Cordeiro CR, Cottin V, Crestani B, Drent M, Dudden RF, Egan J, Flaherty K, Hogaboam C, Inoue Y, Johkoh T, Kim DS, Kitaichi M, Loyd J, Martinez FJ, Myers J, Protzko S, Raghu G, Richeldi L, Sverzellati N, Swigris J, Valeyre D; ATS/ERS Committee on Idiopathic Interstitial Pneumonias. An official American Thoracic Society/European Respiratory Society statement: update of the international multidisciplinary classification of the idiopathic interstitial pneumonias. Am J Respir Crit Care Med. 2013 Sep 15;188(6):733-48. https://doi.org/10.1164/rccm.201308-1483ST. PMID: 24032382. http://www.ncbi.nlm.nih.gov/pubmed/24032382 **

National Clinical Guideline Centre (UK). Diagnosis and management of suspected idiopathic pulmonary fibrosis: idiopathic pulmonary fibrosis. London: Royal College of Physicians (UK); 2013 Jun. PMID: 25340234. http://www.ncbi.nlm.nih.gov/pubmed/25340234 **

Raghu G, Collard HR, Egan JJ, Martinez FJ, Behr J, Brown KK, Colby TV, Cordier JF, Flaherty KR, Lasky JA, Lynch DA, Ryu JH, Swigris JJ, Wells AU, Ancochea J, Bouros D, Carvalho C, Costabel U, Ebina M, Hansell DM, Johkoh T, Kim DS, King TE Jr, Kondoh Y, Myers J, Müller NL, Nicholson AG, Richeldi L, Selman M, Dudden RF, Griss BS, Protzko SL, Schünemann HJ; ATS/ERS/JRS/ALAT Committee on Idiopathic Pulmonary Fibrosis. An official ATS/ERS/JRS/ALAT statement: idiopathic pulmonary fibrosis: evidence-based guidelines for diagnosis and management. Am J Respir Crit Care Med. 2011 Mar 15;183(6):788-824. https://doi.org/10.1164/rccm.2009-040GL. PMID: 21471066. http://www.ncbi.nlm.nih.gov/pubmed/21471066 **

Review

Dowman L, Hill CJ, Holland AE. Pulmonary rehabilitation for interstitial lung disease. Cochrane Database Syst Rev. 2014 Oct 6;10:CD006322. https://doi.org/10.1002/14651858.CD006322.pub3. PMID: 25284270. http://www.ncbi.nlm.nih.gov/pubmed/25284270

Covvey JR, Mancl EE. Recent evidence for pharmacological treatment of idiopathic pulmonary fibrosis. Ann Pharmacother. 2014 Sep 8. pii: 1060028014551015. PMID: 25202034. http://www.ncbi.nlm.nih.gov/pubmed/25202034 **

Ryu JH, Moua T, Daniels CE, Hartman TE, Yi ES, Utz JP, Limper AH. Idiopathic pulmonary fibrosis: evolving concepts. Mayo Clin Proc. 2014 Aug;89(8):1130-42. https://doi.org/10.1016/j.mayocp.2014.03.016. PMID: 24867394. http://www.ncbi.nlm.nih.gov/pubmed/24867394 **

Kistler KD, Nalysnyk L, Rotella P, Esser D. Lung transplantation in idiopathic pulmonary fibrosis: a systematic review of the literature. BMC Pulm Med. 2014 Aug 16;14:139. https://doi.org/10.1186/1471-2466-14-139. PMID: 25127540. http://www.ncbi.nlm.nih.gov/pubmed/25127540

Renzoni E, Srihari V, Sestini P. Pathogenesis of idiopathic pulmonary fibrosis: review of recent findings. F1000Prime Rep. 2014 Aug 1;6:69. https://doi.org/10.12703/P6-69. PMID: 25165568. http://www.ncbi.nlm.nih.gov/pubmed/25165568 **

Kekevian A, Gershwin ME, Chang C. Diagnosis and classification of idiopathic pulmonary fibrosis. Autoimmun Rev. 2014 Apr-May;13(4-5):508-12. https://doi.org/10.1016/j.autrev.2014.01.037. PMID: 24424167. http://www.ncbi.nlm.nih.gov/pubmed/24424167 **

Woodcock HV, Maher TM. The treatment of idiopathic pulmonary fibrosis. F1000Prime Rep. 2014 Mar 3;6:16. https://doi.org/10.12703/P6-16. PMID: 24669297. http://www.ncbi.nlm.nih.gov/pubmed/24669297 **

Atkins CP, Loke YK, Wilson AM. Outcomes in idiopathic pulmonary fibrosis: a meta-analysis from placebo controlled trials. Respir Med. 2014 Feb;108(2):376-87. https://doi.org/10.1016/j.rmed.2013.11.007. PMID: 24440032. http://www.ncbi.nlm.nih.gov/pubmed/24440032 **

Ley B, Collard HR. Epidemiology of idiopathic pulmonary fibrosis. Clin Epidemiol. 2013 Nov 25;5:483-92. https://doi.org/10.2147/CLEP.S54815. PMID: 24348069. http://www.ncbi.nlm.nih.gov/pubmed/24348069 **

King C, Nathan SD. Identification and treatment of comorbidities in idiopathic pulmonary fibrosis and other fibrotic lung diseases. Curr Opin Pulm Med. 2013 Sep;19(5):466-73. https://doi.org/10.1097/MCP.0b013e328363f460. PMID: 23912191. http://www.ncbi.nlm.nih.gov/pubmed/23912191

Archontogeorgis K, Steiropoulos P, Tzouvelekis A, Nena E, Bouros D. Lung cancer and interstitial lung diseases: a systematic review. Pulm Med. 2012;2012:315918. https://doi.org/10.1155/2012/315918. PMID: 22900168. http://www.ncbi.nlm.nih.gov/pubmed/22900168

Chua F, Sly PD, Laurent GJ. Pediatric lung disease: from proteinases topulmonary fibrosis. Pediatr Pulmonol. 2005 May;39(5):392-401. PubMedPMID: 15786437.

Rigante D, Stabile A. Diagnostic clues in the idiopathic pulmonary fibrosis of children. Minerva Pediatr. 2004 Apr;56(2):157-60. PubMed PMID: 15249899.

Use PubMed Clinical Queries to find the most recent evidence. Use this search strategy:

"Pulmonary Fibrosis"[Mesh] OR "Pulmonary Fibrosis"

Chapter 63
Pulmonary Hypertension

Christopher J. Rees, Charles V. Pollack, Jr., and Jaime Friel Blanck

Name and Synonyms

Pulmonary Hypertension; Idiopathic Pulmonary Hypertension; Pulmonary Arterial Hypertension; Primary Pulmonary Hypertension

Incidence/Epidemiology

- The incidence and prevalence of pulmonary hypertension is difficult to ascertain, as the disease has 5 general classes as defined by The World Health Organization (see Pathophysiology and Etiology section below), all with multiple etiologies.
- Pulmonary hypertension affects all age groups, races, and both sexes.
- The incidence varies among the different groups and etiologies.
- Group 1 (pulmonary arterial hypertension) is rare, with an estimated incidence of about 10 cases per one million adults. Group 1 affects adults younger than those in the other groups.

C. J. Rees
Emergency Department, Pennsylvania Hospital, Philadelphia, PA, USA

C. V. Pollack, Jr. (✉)
Department of Emergency Medicine, Thomas Jefferson University, Philadelphia, PA, USA

J. F. Blanck
Welch Medical Library, Johns Hopkins University, Baltimore, MD, USA

C. V. Pollack, Jr. (ed.), *Differential Diagnosis of Cardiopulmonary Disease*,
https://doi.org/10.1007/978-3-319-63895-9_63

Differential Diagnosis

- The differential diagnosis of pulmonary hypertension is broad, as the presenting symptoms of pulmonary hypertension are nonspecific.
- The most common initial symptom is dyspnea on exertion, and the differential diagnosis of this complaint is broad and includes a large spectrum of pulmonary, cardiac, and metabolic diseases.
- Initial symptoms often include dyspnea on exertion (the most common initial symptom), atypical chest pain, and exertional syncope. These symptoms are slowly progressive and often long-standing when the patient presents for care.
- It is important to consider pulmonary hypertension in the differential of patients being evaluated for any of these complaints.
- As the presenting symptoms are nonspecific, the diagnosis of pulmonary hypertension is often delayed for months to years after symptoms begin.

Pathophysiology and Etiology

- Pulmonary hypertension refers to elevated pulmonary arterial pressure. It is defined as a mean pulmonary arterial pressure of greater than or equal to 25 mm Hg at rest, usually measured during right heart catheterization.
- It can occur as a primary condition, with hypertension only within the pulmonary system; or, it can occur has a secondary condition in the context of pressure elevation within the pulmonary venous system. Primary pulmonary hypertension (outdated term) is now referred to as idiopathic pulmonary arterial hypertension (IPAH), and secondary pulmonary hypertension is referred to as pulmonary hypertension (PH). When referring to the group of disorders collectively, pulmonary hypertension is the appropriate term.
- IPAH has no identifiable cause, whereas PH generally has an identifiable cause, such as heart disease, thromboembolic pulmonary disease, and chronic lung disease.
- The World Health Organization has recently re-classified pulmonary hypertension into five broad groups based upon etiology.
    - Group 1: Pulmonary arterial hypertension (PAH). This group includes idiopathic PH (IPAH), familial (heritable) PAH, and PAH due to diseases that share the common pathologic basis of involvement of the small pulmonary muscular arterioles. This includes PAH caused by drugs and toxins, PAH secondary to connective tissue diseases, HIV infection, portal hypertension, congenital heart disease, and schistosomiasis.
    - Group 2: This is PH due to left heart disease.
    - Group 3: PH secondary to chronic lung disease and/or hypoxemia.
    - Group 4: PH secondary to chronic thromboembolic pulmonary disease. Often referred to as chronic thromboembolic pulmonary hypertension (CTEPH).

  - Group 5: PH due to unclear multifactorial mechanisms.

- Group 1. Patients with idiopathic and familial PAH are pathologically and clinically nearly identical. The distinction can only be made when and if a patient with PAH is found to have a genetic defect known to cause PAH. It is estimated that up to 10 % of patients in Group 1 have familial PAH. The mutation BMPR2 is the most common mutation to cause familial PAH. It may account for up to 80 % of all cases of familial PAH. Other causes of Group 1 PAH include:
  - Drugs and toxins. Several drugs are known to induce PAH. These include appetite suppressants (fenfluramine, dexfenfluramine, aminorex, and diethylpropion), toxic rapeseed oil, and benfluorex. Other drugs that are considered to be possible causes of PAH include: amphetamines, L-tryptophan, methamphetamines, cocaine, phenylpropolamine, St. John's Wort, dasatinib, and interferon.
  - Connective tissue diseases. Systemic sclerosis (scleroderma), Rheumatoid arthritis, and systemic lupus erythematous (SLE) can cause PAH. The mechanism is unknown.
  - HIV. PAH occurs in about 0.5 % of patients with HIV. The cause is unknown.
  - Portal hypertension associated with chronic liver disease can lead to PAH. When portal hypertension and pulmonary hypertension are present together it is called portopulmonary hypertension.
  - Congenital heart disease. PAH can develop in patients with large left-to-right intracardiac shunts due to congenital heart disease such as atrial septal defects and ventricular septal defects. PAH can also develop in patients with left-to-right shunts from great artery defects. PAH develops due to increased pulmonary blood volume and subsequent pressure overload.
  - Schistosomiasis. Schistosomiasis is rare in the United States and other developed nations, but it is the most prevalent cause of PAH worldwide.

- Group 2. Pulmonary hypertension from left heart disease. Characterized by elevated left atrial and pulmonary venous pressures. Left atrial hypertension is most commonly caused by left ventricular systolic or diastolic dysfunction and mitral or aortic valvular disease. Other, less common, causes include: restrictive cardiomyopathies, constrictive pericarditis, left atrial myxoma, and congenital cardiomyopathies.
- Group 3. Group 3 PH is PH caused by underlying lung diseases and/or hypoxemia. This includes: chronic obstructive pulmonary disease (COPD), interstitial lung diseases (ILD), and obstructive sleep apnea (OSA), especially in the presence of obesity hypoventilation syndrome and hypoxemia.
- Group 4. Group 4 PH is PH caused by thromboembolic disease. Chronic thromboembolic pulmonary hypertension (CTEPH) occurs from chronic, small pulmonary emboli with occlusion of the pulmonary vasculature. This leads to pulmonary hypertension and vascular remodeling.
- Group 5. Pulmonary hypertension from unclear and multifactorial mechanisms. Examples include PH due to sickle cell anemia and other hemolytic anemias.

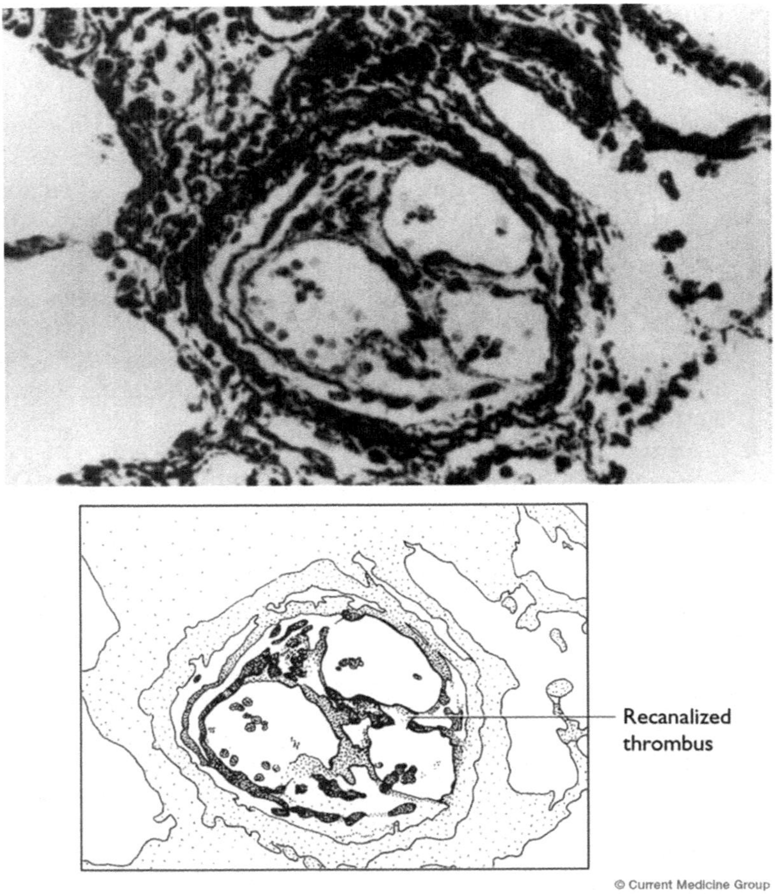

Vascular pathology in idiopathic pulmonary arterial hypertension. Thrombotic arteriopathy in a pathologic specimen from a patient with idiopathic pulmonary arterial hypertension. Evidence of thrombosis with recanalization can be observed in pathologic specimens from patients with idiopathic pulmonary arterial hypertension. [Goldhaber SZ, Piazza G. Interventional cardiology. In: Libby P, editor. Essential Atlas of Cardiovascular Disease. 4th ed. Philadelphia: Current Medicine Group; 2009. 432 p. ISBN: 978-1-57340-309-2] *Caption from original*

Presentation

Typical/"Classic"

- The symptoms of pulmonary hypertension are non-specific. In retrospect, patients are often found to have complained of dyspnea on exertion and fatigue. These are not uncommonly attributed to other causes, such as age, deconditioning, or a coexisting and/or alternative medical condition.

- These early symptoms are caused by the inability to adequately increase cardiac output to match demand during exertion.
- Because the initial symptoms of PH can be very vague and nonspecific, patients are often not correctly diagnosed for several years after the development of symptoms.
- As PH is a chronic and progressive disease, the diagnosis is often not considered until the patient develops severe symptoms. These include exertional chest pain, exertional syncope, and signs of right heart failure such as peripheral edema.
- PH is frequently only considered and identified during the evaluation and work-up for an alternative diagnostic consideration.

Atypical

- It is difficult to define an atypical presentation of a process with such vague symptoms and signs.
- Ortner's Syndrome is one such defined atypical presentation of PH. It is marked by cough, hoarseness, and hemoptysis secondary to compression of the recurrent laryngeal nerve by a dilated main pulmonary artery.

Primary Differential Considerations

- Patients with signs and symptoms referable to pulmonary hypertension should also be evaluated early on for other potentially accurate diagnoses, such as:
  - dilated cardiomyopathy
  - pulmonic valve stenosis
  - mitral valve stenosis

History and Physical Exam

Findings That Confirm Diagnosis

- There are no historical or physical examination findings that are pathognomic for pulmonary hypertension.
- The diagnosis is only confirmed by diagnostic testing. Right heart catheterization is currently the standard test for confirmation of the diagnosis.

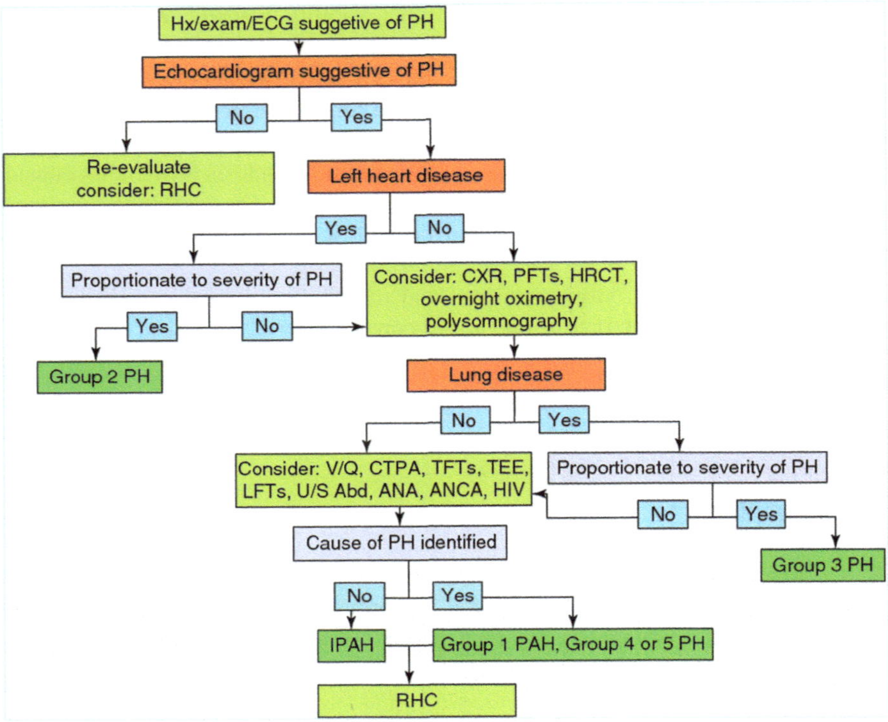

Suggested algorithm for evaluation of suspected pulmonary hypertension. Hx clinical history, Exam clinical examination, ECG electrocardiogram, PH pulmonary hypertension, CXR chest radiograph, PFTs pulmonary function tests, V/Q ventilation/perfusion scintigraphy, CTPA computed tomography pulmonary angiography, TFTs thyroid function tests, TEE transesophageal echocardiogram, LFTs liver function tests, U/S abd ultrasound of the abdomen, ANA antinuclear antibody, ANCA anti-neutrophil cytoplasmic antibody, HIV human immunodeficiency virus serology, IPAH idiopathic pulmonary arterial hypertension, RHC right heart catheterization [Judge EP, O'Callaghan D, Gaine SP. Pulmonary Vascular Disease. In: Rosendorff C, editor. Essential Cardiology [Internet]. New York, NY: Springer New York; 2013 [cited 2015 Sep 29]. p. 603–25. Available from: http://link.springer.com/10.1007/978-1-4614-6705-2_35] *Caption from original*

Factors That Suggest Diagnosis

- The diagnosis should be considered in any patient (especially a patient with any of the associated diseases and exposures as detailed in the Etiology section) with complaints of progressive dyspnea on exertion.

- The work-up and evaluation of a patient with dyspnea on exertion is broad, and should include studies (such as a chest x-ray, echocardiogram, or CT chest) that may give clues to the presence of PH.
- Physical exam findings in PH are also nonspecific, especially early in the disease course.
- Early in the course of PH, before right heart failure develops, patients may have a loud pulmonic component to the second heart sound, and the second heart sound may be narrowly split or single.
- As right heart failure develops, patients may develop the physical signs as described in the section on cor pulmonale.

Findings	Patients, %
Increase in P_2	93
Tricuspid regurgitation murmur	40
Right-sided S_4	38
Peripheral edema	32
Right-sided S_3	23
Cyanosis	20
Pulmonic insufficiency murmur	13

Physical findings in patients with idiopathic pulmonary arterial hypertension. The physical examination is nonspecific, revealing signs of pulmonary hypertension and right ventricular failure. In the NIH study, the presence of an S3 gallop and tricuspid regurgitation were associated with an increase in right atrial pressure and a decrease in cardiac index; the finding of pulmonic valve insufficiency was associated with a higher mean pulmonary artery pressure. The physical examination helps exclude secondary causes of pulmonary hypertension by an absence of crackles, wheezes, and clubbing. (Data from Rich S, Dantzker DR, Ayres SM, et al. Primary pulmonary hypertension: a national prospective study. Ann Intern Med. 1987; 107:216 -223.) [Singh J, Tapson V, Markewitz B, Elliott GC, Michael J. Chapter 18. In: Crapo J, editor. Bone's atlas of pulmonary and critical care medicine. Philadelphia: Current Medicine; 2005. ISBN: 1-57340-211-7] Caption adapted from original

Factors That Exclude Diagnosis

- There are no reliable historical or physical findings that exclude PH from the differential.

Ancillary Studies

- Extensive diagnostic testing is usually performed on patients thought to have PH, with three common goals:
    - to confirm the diagnosis
    - to attempt to identify an underlying cause
    - to evaluate the severity of the physiologic derangement
- Evaluation often begins with an echocardiogram, and includes multiple other tests as determined by the clinical scenario and symptoms. The diagnosis is usually confirmed by right heart catheterization.

Echocardiography

- Transthoracic echocardiography (TTE) is often the first step in the evaluation and diagnosis of pulmonary hypertension. TTE is used to estimate the pulmonary artery pressure, right ventricular size thickness and function, and right atrial size and function.
- TTE can also be used to assess left heart function, valve function, and any congenital heart anomalies, all three of which are necessary steps in the evaluation of PH.
- As PH progresses, patients will develop findings of right ventricular pressure overload, such as:
    - Paradoxical bulging of the septum into the left ventricle during systole
    - Hypertrophy of the right ventricle
- Echocardiographic findings of right ventricular failure/cor pulmonale are described in the chapter on cor pulmonale.

https://www.youtube.com/watch?v=jpEXFf2tRL4
Video demonstrating Echocardiogram in PH.

https://www.youtube.com/watch?v=3yOdNyTH07g
Video of Echocardiographic findings in PH.

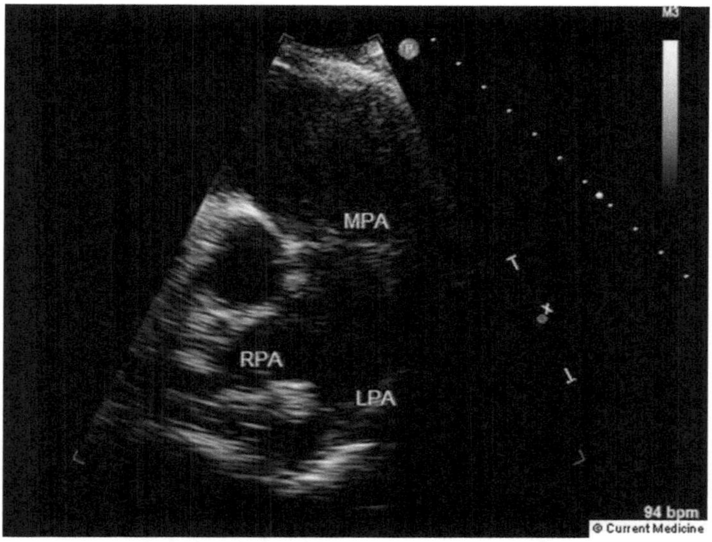

Echocardiogram of severely dilated main pulmonary artery in pulmonary hypertension. Main pulmonary artery (MPA) and bifurcation view, demonstrating severely dilated MPA and branches in a patient with severe pulmonary hypertension. LPA: left pulmonary artery; RPA: right pulmonary artery. [Mangion J, Solomon S. Chapter 15. In: Vannan MA, Lang RM, Rakowski H, Tajik AJ, Braunwald E, editors. Atlas of Echocardiography. 1e. Philadelphia, PA: Current Medicine Group; 2005. 312 p. ISBN: 1-57340-217-6] *Caption from original*

Laboratory

- Typical laboratory tests performed in the evaluation include evaluation for anemia with a complete blood count, and a complete metabolic panel to evaluate electrolytes, renal function, and liver function.
- In the appropriate clinical setting, HIV serology should be checked to screen for HIV-associated PH.
- An antinuclear antibody (ANA) should be sent to evaluate for connective tissue as the cause for PH. Further, more specific connective tissue disease testing can be performed as indicated.
- In areas of increased prevalence, screening for hemolytic anemia such as sickle cell anemia, and screening for Schistosomiasis should be considered.
- Brain natriuretic peptide (BNP) and its precursor, N-terminal pro-brain natriuretic peptide (NT-proBNP), are peptides that are released by myocardial cells when stretched. They are elevated in both right and left heart failure, and are not helpful in distinguishing between the two. Patients with known PH who have elevated levels of either have a worse prognosis than those with normal levels.

Electrocardiography

- The ECG in PH can show a right axis deviation, right ventricular hypertrophy (an R wave/S wave ratio greater than one in lead V1), right atrial enlargement (p pulmonale, an increase P wave amplitude in lead II), and an incomplete or complete right bundle branch block. These ECG changes are almost always present in pulmonary hypertension especially as the disease progresses, but can also be present in many other disease states (they are specific but not sensitive).

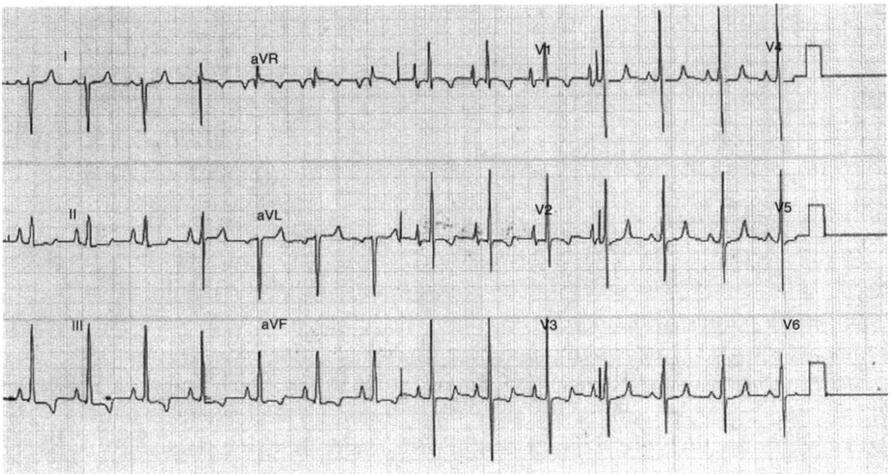

A 12-lead ECG strip of a 31-year-old male patient with pulmonary hypertension (p-pulmonale, right-axis deviation, and right ventricular hypertophy) [Stübgen J-P. Rigid Spine Syndrome: A Noninvasive Cardiac Evaluation. Pediatric Cardiology. 2008 Jan;29(1):45–9.] *Caption from original*

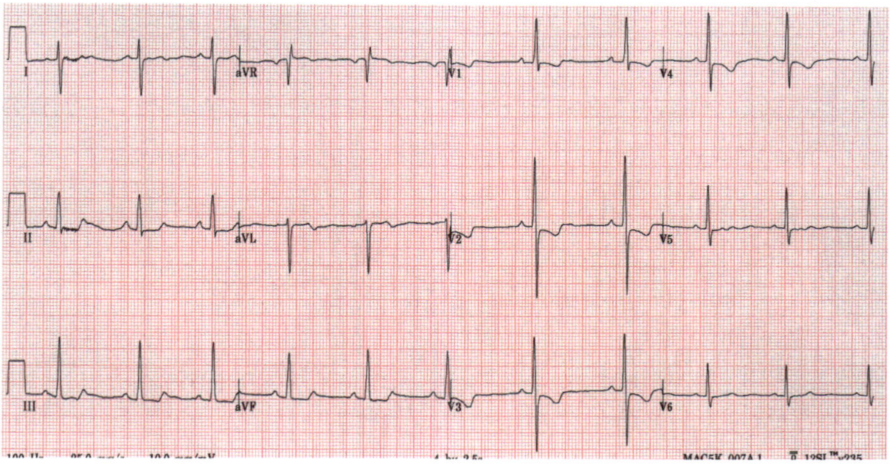

An ECG taken in a patient with idiopathic pulmonary arterial hypertension. Note the signs of right ventricular hypertrophy with a rightward mean frontal QRS axis. [Simon J, Gibbs R, Stefanidis A, Li W. Pulmonary Hypertension Clinical Echocardiography. In: Nihoyannopoulos P, Kisslo J, editors. Echocardiography [Internet]. London: Springer London; 2009 [cited 2015 Sep 3]. p. 229–49. Available from: http://link.springer.com/10.1007/978-1-84882-293-1_10] *Caption from original*

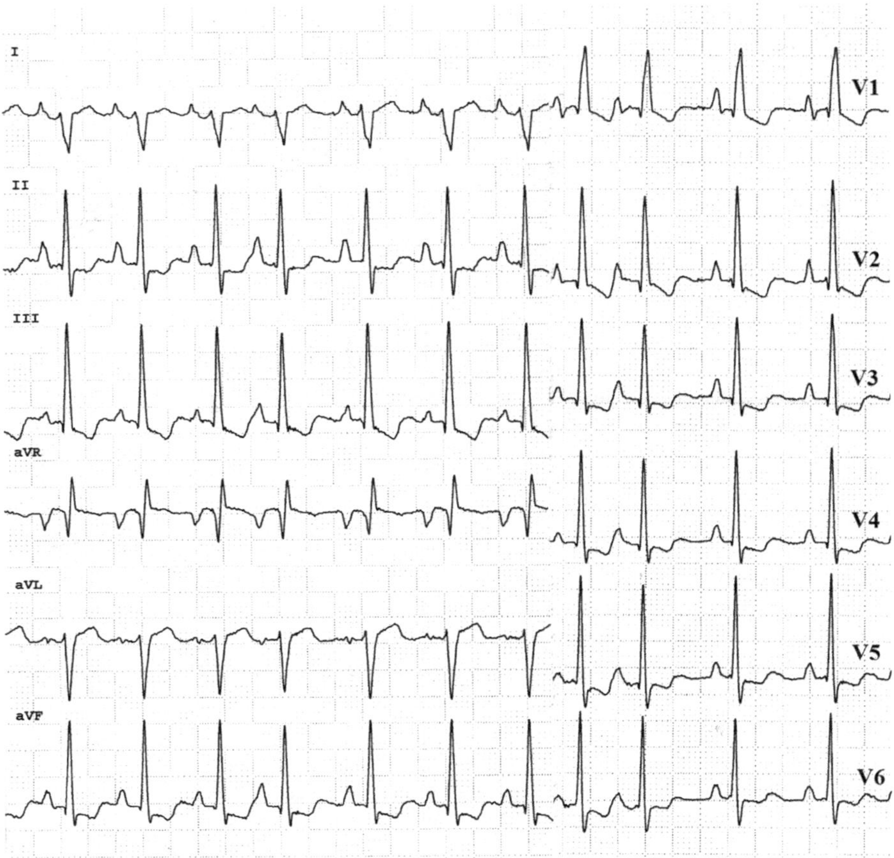

Pulmonary hypertension with severe right atrial and ventricular overload in a young woman. The ECG shows signs of right atrial and ventricular enlargement, the latter manifested by qR complexes in V1-V3 and ST-segment depression. The electrical axis is also deviated to the right. [Romanò M. The Electrocardiogram in Disorders of the Pulmonary Circulation. Text Atlas of Practical Electrocardiography [Internet]. Milano: Springer Milan; 2015 [cited 2015 Sep 3]. p. 213–5. Available from: http://link.springer.com/10.1007/978-88-470-5741-8_14] *Caption from original*

Imaging

Chest X-ray

- Pulmonary hypertension often leads to enlargement of the central pulmonary arteries, i.e., the main pulmonary artery, the hilar vessels, and the descending right pulmonary artery, associated with gradual diminution in the peripheral vessels, leading to hyperlucent peripheral lung fields (oligemia). Other findings on CXR can include:
  - right ventricular enlargement (noted as loss of the retrosternal airspace on a lateral view)
  - right atrial dilatation (noted as a prominent right heart border)
- The chest x-ray can also occasionally help in giving clues to any underlying diseases that may be complicating PA, such as COPD, interstitial lung disease, and congestive heart failure.

https://www.youtube.com/watch?v=9y-PDoJoL2M
Video explaining radiographic findings in PH.

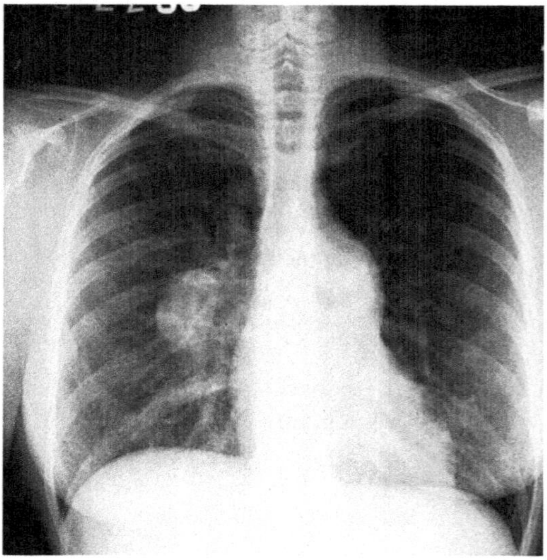

Pulmonary hypertension. A, An injection drug user aged 32 years presented with progressive shortness of breath. Marked dilatation of both pulmonary arteries is shown. For unknown reasons, the incidence of primary pulmonary hypertension is increased in patients with HIV infection. [Lalloo UG, Ambaram A, Vawda F. Pulmonary Complications. In: Mildvan D, editor. International Atlas of AIDS. 4e.: Current Medicine; 2008. 366 p. ISBN: 1-57340-270-2] *Caption adapted from original*

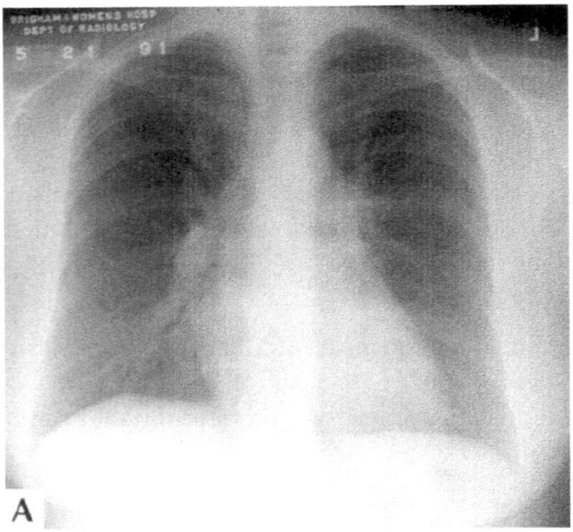

Typical radiograph of a patient with primary pulmonary hypertension and cor pulmonale. Note the peripheral oligemia of the pulmonary vessels with mild bilateral enlargement of the main pulmonary arteries. [Loh E. Chapter 01. In: Goldhaber S, editor. Cardiopulmonary Diseases and Cardiac Tumors. Philadelphia: Current Medicine; 1995 (Braunwald E, editor. Atlas of heart diseases; vol. 3.)] *Caption adapted from original*

Ventilation/Perfusion Scanning (V/Q scan)

- V/Q scan is the imaging of choice in the evaluation of patients for CTEPH (Group 4 PH).
- A normal V/Q scan can nearly exclude chronic thromboembolic disease as the cause for PAH.
- If the V/Q suggests the presence of chronic thromboembolic disease, an angiogram or a CT angiogram should be performed to confirm the diagnosis.

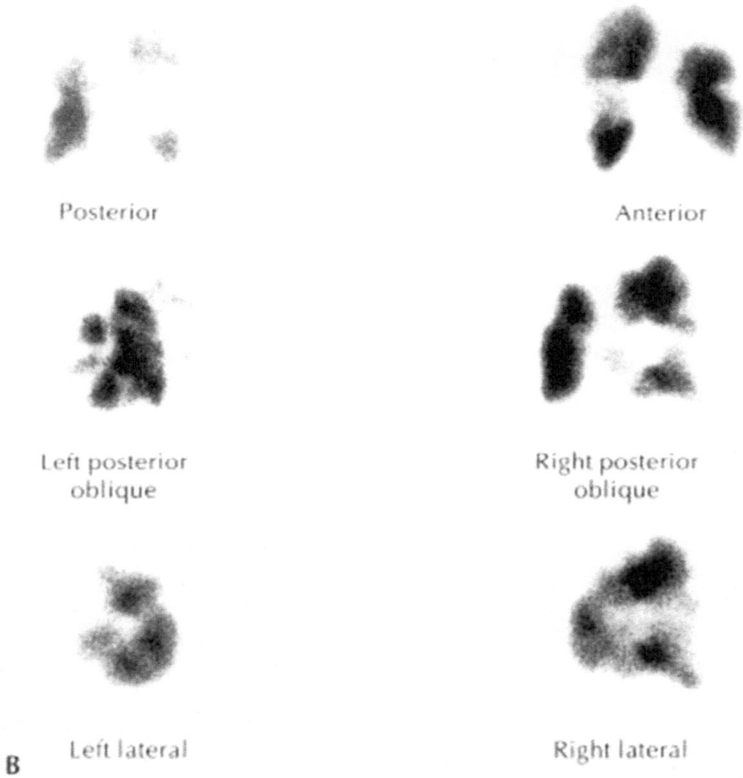

Perfusion lung scan in chronic thromboembolic pulmonary hypertension. B, Perfusion lung scan in a patient with CTEPH. Ventilation scan was normal. [Fedullo P, Auger W, Channick R, Jamieson S, Moser K. Chapter 07. In: Goldhaber S, editor. Cardiopulmonary Diseases and Cardiac Tumors. Philadelphia: Current Medicine; 1995 (Braunwald E, editor. Atlas of heart diseases; vol. 3.)] *Caption adapted from original*

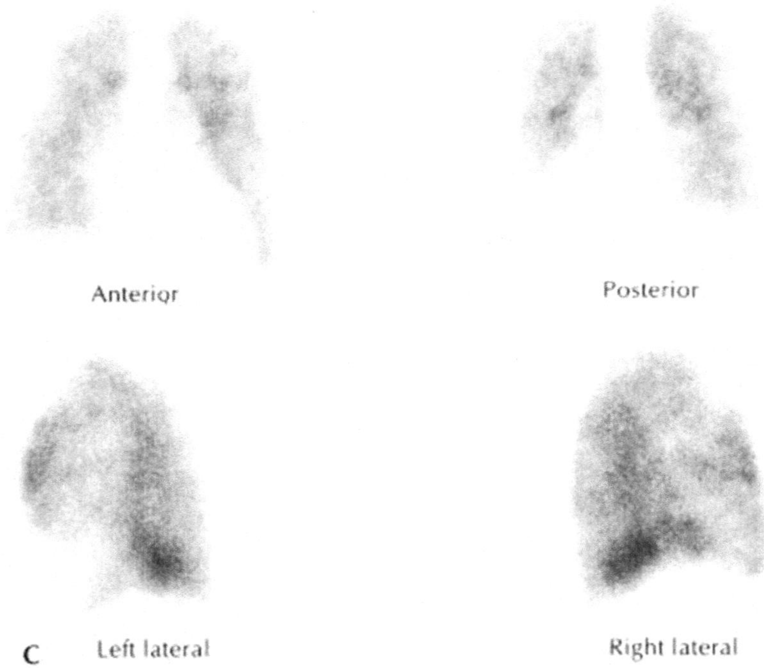

C, Perfusion lung scan in primary pulmonary hypertension. Ventilation-perfusion lung scanning provides an excellent, low-risk, noninvasive means of distinguishing between pulmonary hypertension due to potentially operable CTEPH and obliterative, small-vessel pulmonary hypertension. In chronic thromboembolic disease, at least one (and, more commonly, several) segmental or larger mismatched defect is present. In primary pulmonary hypertension, the perfusion scan is either normal or has a mottled appearance consisting of patchy, subsegmental abnormalities. Although the ventilation-perfusion lung scan can suggest the diagnosis of CTEPH, it is incapable of confirming the diagnosis or establishing surgical feasibility. Any process that occludes major pulmonary arteries, either through external compression (fibrosing mediastinitis, mediastinal tumors) or intraluminal obstruction (thrombus, tumor), will result in similar defects. [Fedullo P, Auger W, Channick R, Jamieson S, Moser K. Chapter 07. In: Goldhaber S, editor. Cardiopulmonary Diseases and Cardiac Tumors. Philadelphia: Current Medicine; 1995 (Braunwald E, editor. Atlas of heart diseases; vol. 3.)] *Caption adapted from original*

CT Scan/MRI

- CT scans of the lungs can be helpful in the evaluation and diagnosis of causes of PH, such as ILD, COPD, CTEPH.

- Cardiac magnetic resonance imaging (MRI), if available, is superior to transthoracic echocardiography in the evaluation of right ventricular structure and function.

Other

- Right heart catheterization is considered the best diagnostic test for confirming the diagnosis of pulmonary hypertension and evaluating the severity of the disease. Pulmonary hypertension is defined as a pulmonary artery (PA) pressure greater than 25 mmHg, and no evidence of left heart disease, as evidenced by either a normal (less than 15 mmHg) left ventricular end-diastolic pressure. All chamber dimensions and pressures can be directly measured.
  - Measuring *only* the pulmonary capillary wedge pressure (PCWP) is insufficient to distinguish PH alone from PH due to left heart disease, as the PCWP may be falsely elevated in all cases of PH due to dilatation of the main pulmonary artery, which prevents accurate measurement of the PCWP.
- Vasoreactivity test. Patients with Group 1 PAH should have a vasoreactivity performed prior to the initiation of any PAH-specific therapy. A small subset of patients with IPAH, hereditable PAH, and drug-induced PAH will have significant hemodynamic and symptomatic improvement with the use of calcium channel blockers. Vasoreactivity testing involves administering a short-acting vasodilator (such as inhaled nitric oxide, or infusions of adenosine or epoprostenol) during right heart catheterization and then measuring the response of the mean pulmonary artery pressure. Patients with a positive vasoreactivity test (decrease in mean PA pressure of at least 10 mm Hg to at least 40 mmHg, an increased or unchanged cardiac output, and insignificant change in systemic blood pressure) should have therapy with a calcium channel blocker started.
- Pulmonary function tests are used to evaluate for underlying lung disease such as interstitial lung disease (ILD) and chronic obstructive pulmonary disease (COPD) as the underlying causes for PH.
- Sleep studies (polysomnography) are used to diagnose obstructive sleep apnea as the underlying cause for PH when the clinical suspicion is high.
- Exercise testing (most commonly the 6-minute walk test) is often performed during the evaluation of or after the diagnosis of PH is established. Exercise testing helps to establish a clinical baseline to guide therapy and measure the response to therapy.

Special Populations

Age

- Pulmonary hypertension is mostly a disease of middle-aged to older adults.
- Group one PAH typically affects younger adults, and is slightly more common in women.
- There is a subset of Group 1 PH (Group 1″) known as persistent pulmonary hypertension of the newborn (PPHN). This is a rare disease of late preterm or term infants with abnormal development of the pulmonary vasculature.
- PH may complicate and be caused by diseases of childhood, congenital heart disease, sickle cell anemia, and cystic fibrosis. However, the development of PH in patients with these disorders is usually a late complication, developing in young adulthood.

Co-morbidities

- Many co-morbid conditions can worsen the prognosis and make the diagnosis of PH difficult. These include but are not limited to, cardiac diseases, other pulmonary diseases, liver disease, and kidney disease.

Pitfalls in Diagnosis

Critical Steps Not to Miss

- It is important to keep PH on your differential diagnosis in the evaluation of patients with exertional dyspnea and fatigue, as the symptoms and exam findings are nonspecific. It is important to diagnose this disorder as early into the clinical course as possible, as this improves the ability to treat the disease and improves the overall prognosis.
- It is important to perform a detailed and specific evaluation for alternative diagnoses and causative factors for PH.
- It is also important to consider all alternative diagnoses that may cause worsening or acute dyspnea in patients with chronic pulmonary and heart disease. This list includes, but is not limited to, pneumonia, CHF, pulmonary embolism, pneumothorax, significant pleural effusion, and acute metabolic issues that can cause dyspnea.

Mimics

- Many diseases can present with exertional dyspnea and fatigue. This includes, but is not limited to, lung diseases such as COPD and ILD, coronary artery disease, valvular heart disease, congenital heart disease, chronic anemia, metabolic diseases, neuromuscular diseases, etc.

Time-Dependent Interventions

- It is important to make the diagnosis as early as possible into the disease course to improve treatments and outcomes.

Overall Principles of Treatment

- Early diagnosis and treatment is important, as less advanced disease responds better to treatment, and outcomes are better.
- Treatment is generally classified as primary therapy, which is treatment directed at the underlying cause of the PH, and advanced therapy, which is therapy directed at PH.
- Certain treatments need to be considered in all patients with PH. These include:
    - Anticoagulation. PH increases the risk for pulmonary thromboembolism through multiple mechanisms. As such, chronic anticoagulation is indicated in all patients with PH, but especially those with Groups 1 (especially IPAH, hereditary PAH, and drug-induced PAH) and 4 PH.
    - Diuretics. Diuretics are useful to reduce fluid retention and associated edema.
    - Oxygen. All patients with hypoxemia should be given oxygen.
    - Pulmonary rehab/exercise therapy. Pulmonary rehabilitation improves patients' exercise tolerance, daily function, and quality of life.
    - Digoxin. Digoxin is positively inotropic, meaning that it can increase the mechanical contractile strength of the heart. Digoxin's therapeutic window is narrow, however, and it has significant toxicities associated with its use. Patients receiving digoxin need to be closely monitored.
- Primary therapy.
    - Group 1 PAH. There are limited therapeutic options for Group 1 PAH patients. Management of the primary disease should be maximized for patients with an identified underlying cause (such as HIV, congenital heart disease, Schistosomiasis). However, this often does not improve symptoms of PAH once they develop and these patients often require advanced therapy for PAH.
    - Group 2. Therapy for the underlying heart disease must be maximized for patients with Group 2 PH.

  - Group 3. These patients need to have their underlying lung disease treated, and they require oxygen therapy if hypoxemic.
  - Group 4. Anticoagulation is the most important treatment for patients with group 4 PH. Some selected patients may benefit from surgical thromboendarterectomy.
  - Group 5. Patients with group 5 PH should have their underlying diseases treated.

- Advanced Therapy. Patients requiring advanced therapy for PH should be referred to and managed by a center with significant experience managing these disorders. All patients should have a complete diagnostic evaluation (which includes right heart catheterization and vasoreactivity test) and functional class staging WHO functional class) prior to initiating advanced therapies.
- WHO Functional Classes for PH.

  - Group 1. Advanced therapy for PH by a specialized center is the treatment of choice for most patients with Group 1 PAH. Patients with a positive vasoreactivitiy test should have a trial of treatment with a either a dihydropyridine calcium channel blocker (e.g., amlodipine and others that end in *–ipine*) or diltiazem. If patients have a negative vasoreactivity test or are non-responders they need to have an alternative advanced therapy agent started. The choice of agent is complex and multifactorial, and best managed by a specialized center.

- Treatment with advanced agents is often guided by WHO functional class, and includes:

  - WHO functional class II or III (oral therapy preferred):

    - Oral endothelin receptor antagonists (ambrisentan, bosentan, macitentan)
    - Oral phosphodiesterase inhibitors (sildenafil, tadalafil)
    - Oral guanylate cyclase stimulants (riociguat)

  - Some patients with WHO functional class III disease may benefit from other parenteral agents such as intravenous epoprostenol, inhaled iloprost, or intravenous trepostinil.
  - WHO functional class IV. Intravenous epoprostenol.

- Patients with refractory disease may be considered for combination drug therapy or surgical therapy.

  - Surgical therapy includes: creation of a right-to-left intracardiac shunt (atrial septostomy, or a Potts shunt, a shunt between the left pulmonary artery and the descending aorta); and bilateral lung or bilateral lung and heart-lung transplantation. These therapies are reserved for refractory cases and should be considered only at highly specialized centers.

Disease Course

- Patients on therapy should be seen at least every three months. Patients on no therapy should also be followed at least every three-to-six months for reevaluation.
- PH is a chronic, progressive, and frequently fatal disease, especially if untreated.
- The course of disease progression and mortality is highly variable and dependent upon the type of PH and the disease severity at diagnosis.
- In general, Group 1 PAH tends to have a more rapid course and worse survival than the other types of PH. Recently reported data from the REVEAL registry (Registry to Evaluate Early and Long-term PAH Disease Management) shows survival rates one, three, five, and seven years from the time of right heart catheterization of 85, 68, 57, and 49 percent, respectively, for Group 1 PAH.
- There is early data that advanced therapy can improve survival in Group 1 PAH.
- The following factors are associated with a poorer prognosis in Group 1 PAH.
    - Age > 45
    - Male
    - WHO functional class III or IV
    - Failure to improve clinically with advanced therapy
    - Evidence of right heart failure on echocardiogram (large right atrial size, elevated right atrial pressure, septal shift during diastole, presence of a pericardial effusion, low right ventricular ejection fraction)
    - Increased NT-pro-BNP or BNP levels
    - Prolonged QRS duration
    - Hypocapnia
    - Certain comorbid conditions (especially interstitial lung disease, COPD, diabetes)
    - Persistent supraventricular arrhythmias (atrial fibrillation or flutter)
    - Long-term use of selective serotonin reuptake inhibitors
- The overall course and prognosis in other types of PH varies greatly and is mostly related to the course of the underlying disease.
- Patients with PH (especially those with PAH) are at increased risk for complications and death from any surgical procedure, use of general anesthesia, or mechanical ventilation.

Related Evidence

Papers of particular interest have been highlighted as:
*** Of key importance*

Practice Guideline

Hayes MM, Vedamurthy A, George G, Dweik R, Klings ES, Machado RF, Gladwin MT, Wilson KC, Thomson CC; American Thoracic Society Implementation Task Force. Pulmonary hypertension in sickle cell disease. Ann Am Thorac Soc. 2014 Nov;11(9):1488-9. https://doi.org/10.1513/AnnalsATS.201408-405CME. PubMed PMID: 25423000. http://www.ncbi.nlm.nih.gov/pubmed/25423000

Klings ES, Machado RF, Barst RJ, Morris CR, Mubarak KK, Gordeuk VR, Kato GJ, Ataga KI, Gibbs JS, Castro O, Rosenzweig EB, Sood N, Hsu L, Wilson KC, Telen MJ, Decastro LM, Krishnamurti L, Steinberg MH, Badesch DB, Gladwin MT; American Thoracic Society Ad Hoc Committee on Pulmonary Hypertension of Sickle Cell Disease. An official American Thoracic Society clinical practice guideline: diagnosis, risk stratification, and management of pulmonary hypertension of sickle cell disease. Am J Respir Crit Care Med. 2014 Mar 15;189(6):727-40. https://doi.org/10.1164/rccm.201401-0065ST. PubMed PMID: 24628312; PubMed Central PMCID: PMC3983842. http://www.ncbi.nlm.nih.gov/pubmed/24628312

Dweik RA, Rounds S, Erzurum SC, Archer S, Fagan K, Hassoun PM, Hill NS, Humbert M, Kawut SM, Krowka M, Michelakis E, Morrell NW, Stenmark K, Tuder RM, Newman J; ATS Committee on Pulmonary Hypertension Phenotypes. An official American Thoracic Society Statement: pulmonary hypertension phenotypes. Am J Respir Crit Care Med. 2014 Feb 1;189(3):345-55. https://doi.org/10.1164/rccm.201311-1954ST. PubMed PMID: 24484330; PubMed Central PMCID: PMC4291177. http://www.ncbi.nlm.nih.gov/pubmed/24484330 **

Khanna D, Gladue H, Channick R, Chung L, Distler O, Furst DE, Hachulla E, Humbert M, Langleben D, Mathai SC, Saggar R, Visovatti S, Altorok N, Townsend W, FitzGerald J, McLaughlin VV; Scleroderma Foundation and Pulmonary Hypertension Association. Recommendations for screening and detection of connective tissue disease-associated pulmonary arterial hypertension. Arthritis Rheum. 2013 Dec;65(12):3194-201. https://doi.org/10.1002/art.38172. PubMed PMID: 24022584; PubMed Central PMCID: PMC3883571. http://www.ncbi.nlm.nih.gov/pubmed/24022584

Task Force for Diagnosis and Treatment of Pulmonary Hypertension of European Society of Cardiology (ESC); European Respiratory Society (ERS); International Society of Heart and Lung Transplantation (ISHLT), Galiè N, Hoeper MM, Humbert M, Torbicki A, Vachiery JL, Barbera JA, Beghetti M, Corris P, Gaine S, Gibbs JS, Gomez-Sanchez MA, Jondeau G, Klepetko W, Opitz C, Peacock A, Rubin L, Zellweger M, Simonneau G. Guidelines for the diagnosis and treatment of pulmonary hypertension. Eur Respir J. 2009 Dec;34(6):1219-63. https://doi.org/10.1183/09031936.00139009. Epub 2009 Sep 12. PubMed PMID: 19749199. http://www.ncbi.nlm.nih.gov/pubmed/19749199 **

McLaughlin VV, Archer SL, Badesch DB, Barst RJ, Farber HW, Lindner JR, Mathier MA, McGoon MD, Park MH, Rosenson RS, Rubin LJ, Tapson VF, Varga J; American College of Cardiology Foundation Task Force on Expert

Consensus Documents; American Heart Association; American College of Chest Physicians; American Thoracic Society, Inc; Pulmonary Hypertension Association. ACCF/AHA 2009 expert consensus document on pulmonary hypertension a report of the American College of Cardiology Foundation Task Force on Expert Consensus Documents and the American Heart Association developed in collaboration with the American College of Chest Physicians; American Thoracic Society, Inc.; and the Pulmonary Hypertension Association. J Am Coll Cardiol. 2009 Apr 28;53(17):1573-619. https://doi.org/10.1016/j.jacc.2009.01.004. PubMed PMID: 19389575. http://www.ncbi.nlm.nih.gov/pubmed/19389575 **

McLaughlin VV, Presberg KW, Doyle RL, Abman SH, McCrory DC, Fortin T, Ahearn G; American College of Chest Physicians. Prognosis of pulmonary arterial hypertension: ACCP evidence-based clinical practice guidelines. Chest. 2004 Jul;126(1 Suppl):78S-92S. Review. PubMed PMID: 15249497. http://www.ncbi.nlm.nih.gov/pubmed/15249497

Review

Lewis G, Hoey ET, Reynolds JH, Ganeshan A, Ment J. Multi-detector CT assessment in pulmonary hypertension: techniques, systematic approach to interpretation and key findings. Quant Imaging Med Surg. 2015 Jun;5(3):423-32. https://doi.org/10.3978/j.issn.2223-4292.2015.01.05. Review. PubMed PMID: 26029645; PubMed Central PMCID: PMC4426108. http://www.ncbi.nlm.nih.gov/pubmed/26029645

Bossone E, Dellegrottaglie S, Patel S, Grunig E, D'Andrea A, Ferrara F, Gargiulo P, D'Alto M, Soricelli A, Cittadini A, Sanz J, Perrone-Filardi P, Rubenfire M. Multimodality imaging in pulmonary hypertension. Can J Cardiol. 2015 Apr;31(4):440-59. https://doi.org/10.1016/j.cjca.2015.02.012. Epub 2015 Feb 18. Review. PubMed PMID: 25840095. http://www.ncbi.nlm.nih.gov/pubmed/25840095

Haddad RN, Mielniczuk LM. An evidence-based approach to screening and diagnosis of pulmonary hypertension. Can J Cardiol. 2015 Apr;31(4):382-90. https://doi.org/10.1016/j.cjca.2015.01.018. Epub 2015 Jan 28. Review. PubMed PMID: 25840091. http://www.ncbi.nlm.nih.gov/pubmed/25840091 **

Mocumbi AO, Thienemann F, Sliwa K. A global perspective on the epidemiology of pulmonary hypertension. Can J Cardiol. 2015 Apr;31(4):375-81. https://doi.org/10.1016/j.cjca.2015.01.030. Epub 2015 Jan 29. Review. PubMed PMID: 25840090. http://www.ncbi.nlm.nih.gov/pubmed/25840090

Lau EM, Humbert M, Celermajer DS. Early detection of pulmonary arterial hypertension. Nat Rev Cardiol. 2015 Mar;12(3):143-55. https://doi.org/10.1038/nrcardio.2014.191. Epub 2014 Nov 25. Review. PubMed PMID: 25421168. http://www.ncbi.nlm.nih.gov/pubmed/25421168

Haeck ML, Vliegen HW. Diagnosis and treatment of pulmonary hypertension. Heart. 2015 Feb;101(4):311-9. https://doi.org/10.1136/heartjnl-2011-301386. Epub 2014 May 22. Review. PubMed PMID: 24855320. http://www.ncbi.nlm.nih.gov/pubmed/24855320 **

Gatzoulis MA, Beghetti M, Landzberg MJ, Galiè N. Pulmonary arterial hypertension associated with congenital heart disease: recent advances and future directions. Int J Cardiol. 2014 Dec 15;177(2):340-7. https://doi.org/10.1016/j.ijcard.2014.09.024. Epub 2014 Sep 28. Review. PubMed PMID: 25443244.http://www.ncbi.nlm.nih.gov/pubmed/25443244

Rich JD, Rich S. Clinical diagnosis of pulmonary hypertension. Circulation. 2014 Nov 11;130(20):1820-30. https://doi.org/10.1161/CIRCULATIONAHA.114.006971. Review. PubMed PMID: 25385937. http://www.ncbi.nlm.nih.gov/pubmed/25385937 **

Baldi F, Fuso L, Arrighi E, Valente S. Optimal management of pulmonary arterial hypertension: prognostic indicators to determine treatment course. Ther Clin Risk Manag. 2014 Oct 7;10:825-39. https://doi.org/10.2147/TCRM.S48920. eCollection 2014. Review. PubMed PMID: 25328398; PubMed Central PMCID: PMC4199557. http://www.ncbi.nlm.nih.gov/pubmed/25328398 **

Nicolarsen J, Ivy D. Progress in the diagnosis and management of pulmonary hypertension in children. Curr Opin Pediatr. 2014 Oct;26(5):527-35. https://doi.org/10.1097/MOP.0000000000000135. Review. PubMed PMID: 25136947; PubMed Central PMCID: PMC4225814. http://www.ncbi.nlm.nih.gov/pubmed/25136947

Taichman DB, Ornelas J, Chung L, Klinger JR, Lewis S, Mandel J, Palevsky HI, Rich S, Sood N, Rosenzweig EB, Trow TK, Yung R, Elliott CG, Badesch DB. Pharmacologic therapy for pulmonary arterial hypertension in adults: CHEST guideline and expert panel report. Chest. 2014 Aug;146(2):449-75. https://doi.org/10.1378/chest.14-0793. Review. PubMed PMID: 24937180; PubMed Central PMCID: PMC4137591. http://www.ncbi.nlm.nih.gov/pubmed/24937180 **

Zamanian RT, Kudelko KT, Sung YK, de Jesus Perez V, Liu J, Spiekerkoetter E. Current clinical management of pulmonary arterial hypertension. Circ Res. 2014 Jun 20;115(1):131-47. https://doi.org/10.1161/CIRCRESAHA.115.303827. Review. PubMed PMID: 24951763; PubMed Central PMCID: PMC4452016. http://www.ncbi.nlm.nih.gov/pubmed/24951763

Lai YC, Potoka KC, Champion HC, Mora AL, Gladwin MT. Pulmonary arterial hypertension: the clinical syndrome. Circ Res. 2014 Jun 20;115(1):115-30. https://doi.org/10.1161/CIRCRESAHA.115.301146. Review. PubMed PMID: 24951762; PubMed Central PMCID: PMC4096686. http://www.ncbi.nlm.nih.gov/pubmed/24951762 **

Moceri P, Baudouy D, Chiche O, Cerboni P, Bouvier P, Chaussade C, Ferrari E. Imaging in pulmonary hypertension: Focus on the role of echocardiography. Arch Cardiovasc Dis. 2014 Apr;107(4):261-71. https://doi.org/10.1016/j.acvd.2014.02.005. Epub 2014 Apr 18. Review. PubMed PMID: 24746538. http://www.ncbi.nlm.nih.gov/pubmed/24746538 **

Alassas K, Mergo P, Ibrahim el-S, Burger C, Safford R, Parikh P, Shapiro B. Cardiac MRI as a diagnostic tool in pulmonary hypertension. Future Cardiol. 2014 Jan;10(1):117-30. https://doi.org/10.2217/fca.13.97. Review. PubMed PMID: 24344668. http://www.ncbi.nlm.nih.gov/pubmed/24344668

Galiè N, Corris PA, Frost A, Girgis RE, Granton J, Jing ZC, Klepetko W, McGoon MD, McLaughlin VV, Preston IR, Rubin LJ, Sandoval J, Seeger W, Keogh A. Updated treatment algorithm of pulmonary arterial hypertension. J Am Coll Cardiol. 2013 Dec 24;62(25 Suppl):D60-72. https://doi.org/10.1016/j.jacc.2013.10.031. Review. PubMed PMID: 24355643. http://www.ncbi.nlm.nih.gov/pubmed/24355643 **

Simonneau G, Gatzoulis MA, Adatia I, Celermajer D, Denton C, Ghofrani A, Gomez Sanchez MA, Krishna Kumar R, Landzberg M, Machado RF, Olschewski H, Robbins IM, Souza R. Updated clinical classification of pulmonary hypertension. J Am Coll Cardiol. 2013 Dec 24;62(25 Suppl):D34-41. https://doi.org/10.1016/j.jacc.2013.10.029. Review. Erratum in: J Am Coll Cardiol. 2014 Feb 25;63(7):746. PubMed PMID: 24355639. http://www.ncbi.nlm.nih.gov/pubmed/24355639

McGoon MD, Benza RL, Escribano-Subias P, Jiang X, Miller DP, Peacock AJ, Pepke-Zaba J, Pulido T, Rich S, Rosenkranz S, Suissa S, Humbert M. Pulmonary arterial hypertension: epidemiology and registries. J Am Coll Cardiol. 2013 Dec 24;62(25 Suppl):D51-9. https://doi.org/10.1016/j.jacc.2013.10.023. Review. PubMed PMID: 24355642. http://www.ncbi.nlm.nih.gov/pubmed/24355642

McLaughlin VV, Gaine SP, Howard LS, Leuchte HH, Mathier MA, Mehta S, Palazzini M, Park MH, Tapson VF, Sitbon O. Treatment goals of pulmonary hypertension. J Am Coll Cardiol. 2013 Dec 24;62(25 Suppl):D73-81. https://doi.org/10.1016/j.jacc.2013.10.034. Review. PubMed PMID: 24355644. http://www.ncbi.nlm.nih.gov/pubmed/24355644

Ivy DD, Abman SH, Barst RJ, Berger RM, Bonnet D, Fleming TR, Haworth SG, Raj JU, Rosenzweig EB, Schulze Neick I, Steinhorn RH, Beghetti M. Pediatric pulmonary hypertension. J Am Coll Cardiol. 2013 Dec 24;62(25 Suppl):D117-26. https://doi.org/10.1016/j.jacc.2013.10.028. Review. PubMed PMID: 24355636. http://www.ncbi.nlm.nih.gov/pubmed/24355636

Lahm T, Chakinala MM. World Health Organization group 5 pulmonary hypertension. Clin Chest Med. 2013 Dec;34(4):753-78. https://doi.org/10.1016/j.ccm.2013.08.005. Epub 2013 Oct 18. Review. PubMed PMID: 24267303. http://www.ncbi.nlm.nih.gov/pubmed/24267303 **

Forfia PR, Trow TK. Diagnosis of pulmonary arterial hypertension. Clin Chest Med. 2013 Dec;34(4):665-81. https://doi.org/10.1016/j.ccm.2013.09.001. Epub 2013 Oct 17. Review. PubMed PMID: 24267297. http://www.ncbi.nlm.nih.gov/pubmed/24267297 **

Taichman DB, Mandel J. Epidemiology of pulmonary arterial hypertension. Clin Chest Med. 2013 Dec;34(4):619-37. https://doi.org/10.1016/j.ccm.2013.08.010. Epub 2013 Oct 18. Review. PubMed PMID: 24267294. http://www.ncbi.nlm.nih.gov/pubmed/24267294

Montani D, Günther S, Dorfmüller P, Perros F, Girerd B, Garcia G, Jaïs X, Savale L, Artaud-Macari E, Price LC, Humbert M, Simonneau G, Sitbon O. Pulmonary arterial hypertension. Orphanet J Rare Dis. 2013 Jul 6;8:97. https://doi.org/10.1186/1750-1172-8-97. Review. PubMed PMID: 23829793; PubMed Central PMCID: PMC3750932. http://www.ncbi.nlm.nih.gov/pubmed/23829793 **

Frazier AA, Burke AP. The imaging of pulmonary hypertension. Semin Ultrasound CT MR. 2012 Dec;33(6):535-51. https://doi.org/10.1053/j.sult.2012.06.002. Review. PubMed PMID: 23168063. http://www.ncbi.nlm.nih.gov/pubmed/23168063

McCann C, Gopalan D, Sheares K, Screaton N. Imaging in pulmonary hypertension, part 1: clinical perspectives, classification, imaging techniques and imaging algorithm. Postgrad Med J. 2012 May;88(1039):271-9. https://doi.org/10.1136/postgradmedj-2011-130292. Epub 2012 Jan 21. Review. PubMed PMID: 22267542. http://www.ncbi.nlm.nih.gov/pubmed/22267542

Heresi GA, Dweik RA. Pulmonary hypertension: evaluation and management. Compr Ther. 2007 Fall;33(3):150-61. Review. PubMed PMID: 18004030. http://www.ncbi.nlm.nih.gov/pubmed/18004030

Edelman JD. Clinical presentation, differential diagnosis, and vasodilator testing of pulmonary hypertension. Semin Cardiothorac Vasc Anesth. 2007 Jun;11(2):110-8. Review. PubMed PMID: 17536115. http://www.ncbi.nlm.nih.gov/pubmed/17536115

Barst RJ, McGoon M, Torbicki A, Sitbon O, Krowka MJ, Olschewski H, Gaine S. Diagnosis and differential assessment of pulmonary arterial hypertension. J Am Coll Cardiol. 2004 Jun 16;43(12 Suppl S):40S-47S. Review. PubMed PMID: 15194177. http://www.ncbi.nlm.nih.gov/pubmed/15194177

General

Colman R, Whittingham H, Tomlinson G, Granton J. Utility of the physical examination in detecting pulmonary hypertension. A mixed methods study. PLoS One. 2014 Oct 24;9(10):e108499. https://doi.org/10.1371/journal.pone.0108499. eCollection 2014. PubMed PMID: 25343585; PubMed Central PMCID: PMC4208756. http://www.ncbi.nlm.nih.gov/pubmed/25343585

Hoeper MM. Definition, classification, and epidemiology of pulmonary arterial hypertension. Semin Respir Crit Care Med. 2009 Aug;30(4):369-75. https://doi.org/10.1055/s-0029-1233306. Epub 2009 Jul 24. PubMed PMID: 19634076. http://www.ncbi.nlm.nih.gov/pubmed/19634076 **

Use PubMed Clinical Queries to find the most recent evidence. Use this search strategy:

"Hypertension, Pulmonary"[Majr:NoExp] OR "Idiopathic pulmonary hypertension"[tiab] OR "pulmonary arterial hypertension"[tiab] OR "pulmonary hypertension"[tiab] OR "idiopathic pulmonary arterial hypertension"[tiab]

Chapter 64
Radiation Pneumonitis

Christopher J. Rees, Charles V. Pollack, Jr., and Jaime Friel Blanck

Name and Synonyms

Radiation Pneumonitis; Radiation-induced Lung Injury (RILI); Radiation Fibrosis

Incidence/Epidemiology

- The incidence of radiation pneumonitis varies widely depending upon the regimen/modality of radiation used, and the size/volume of tissue treated.
- Radiographic changes of pneumonitis are much more common than symptomatic disease.
- Across all cancers, about 50% of patients who receive radiation therapy to the chest, lungs, or mediastinum will develop some radiographic findings of pneumonitis, but only about 10–15 % will develop symptoms.
- About 65 % of all patients with cancer will undergo therapeutic radiation therapy at some point during their cancer treatment. This leads to a large number of people being "at risk" for the development of radiation pneumonitis.

C. J. Rees
Emergency Department, Pennsylvania Hospital, Philadelphia, PA, USA

C. V. Pollack, Jr. (✉)
Department of Emergency Medicine, Thomas Jefferson University, Philadelphia, PA, USA

J. F. Blanck
Welch Medical Library, Johns Hopkins University, Baltimore, MD, USA

C. V. Pollack, Jr. (ed.), *Differential Diagnosis of Cardiopulmonary Disease*,
https://doi.org/10.1007/978-3-319-63895-9_64

Differential Diagnosis

- The differential diagnosis can be broad, and includes all causes of dyspnea and cough, especially in a cancer patient.
- The differential can often be focused to include those processes that have a similar radiographic appearance to radiation pneumonitis. These include:
  - Infection, such as pneumonia, tracheobronchitis, and empyema. Infections can be bacterial, viral, atypical, or fungal.
  - Lymphangitic spread of tumor.
  - Pulmonary embolism (especially if dyspnea is the prominent complaint).
  - Drug reaction.
  - Congestive heart failure (especially in patients who have received chemotherapeutic agents such as doxorubicin).
  - Hypersensitivity pneumonitis-like reaction. This is a less common reaction to radiation that is distinguished from radiation pneumonitis by including areas of the lung outside those that received radiation. It is often bilateral, even if the radiation was only delivered to one lung. It follows a similar time course to early radiation pneumonitis.

Pathophysiology and Etiology

- Ionizing radiation passing through tissue causes the release of large amounts of energy, which can lead to the production of reactive free radicals in the tissue. As water is plentiful, the majority of free radicals include reactive oxygen and hydrogen ions. Other important free radical species include reactive nitrogen species. These free radicals react with and damage other cellular molecules such as DNA, RNA, peptides, and lipids. This can lead to direct cytotoxicity and death to normal lung cells and tissue, especially high turnover cells such as surfactant-producing cells.
- Radiation energy, cell damage, and cell death lead to the activation of inflammatory pathways and the release of a large number of cytokines that can cause inflammatory reactions in lung tissue. Pro-inflammatory cytokines up-regulated after exposure to radiation include, transforming growth factor beta, tumor necrosis factor alpha, interleukin 1-alpha, interleukin-6, platelet-derived growth factor, and basic fibroblast growth factor.
- There are several factors that affect the incidence and risk of the development of radiation pneumonitis.
  - Genetics. In patients with small cell and non-small cell lung cancer, the presence of a mutation in the methylene tetrahydrofolate reductase gene has been shown to be associated with an increased risk for the development

  of radiation pneumonitis. There are other, less well-defined, genetic associations in both breast and lung cancer.
  - The risk of developing radiation pneumonitis is directly related to the volume of lung tissue exposed to radiation.
  - Using the modality of radiation delivery that most limits the dose to the affected tissue helps to prevent the development of radiation-induced lung injury.
  - The risk also increases directly with increasing doses of radiation.
  - Some chemotherapeutic agents are known to increase tissue sensitivity to radiation. These include doxorubicin, gemcitabine, taxanes, dactinomycin, bleomycin, cyclophosphamide, vincristine, mitomicin, recombinant interferon-alpha, and bevacizumab.
  - Concurrent chemotherapy and radiotherapy also appears to increase the risk of radiation pneumonitis, especially in the treatment of breast cancer.
  - Current tobacco-smoking and chronic obstructive pulmonary disease have been associated with a lowered risk of developing radiation pneumonitis in some studies.

- The pathologic changes within the lung after exposure to radiation can be divided into five phases.

  - Immediate phase. These changes occur within hours to days after radiation exposure. It consists of mucosal inflammation, increased capillary permeability, mucous hypersecretion, with subsequent sloughing of alveolar epithelial cells. This is usually asymptomatic.
  - Latent phase. During this phase, goblet cells start to proliferate, leading to an increase in secretions. Radiation has also induced ciliary dysfunction, leading to an inability to clear these increased secretions, which then pool in alveoli.
  - Acute exudative phase. This phase occurs anywhere from 3 to 12 weeks after exposure to radiation. It is during this phase that the clinical syndrome of radiation pneumonitis usually occurs. It is characterized by increased sloughing of epithelial and endothelial cells, microvascular thrombosis, alveolar exudate, with subsequent hyaline membrane formation with narrowing of small airways and pulmonary capillaries.
  - Intermediate phase. During this phase, many patients will have resolution of all changes. Some patients, however, will continue to progress with increased collagen deposition by fibroblasts, resulting in thickening and distortion of the interstitial tissues.
  - Fibrosis. In some cases, fibroblasts can continue to migrate into lung tissue and continue to produce collagen, which leads to disruption of alveolar and vascular tissue. These changes can become clinically apparent in anywhere from 6 months to several years after radiation exposure.

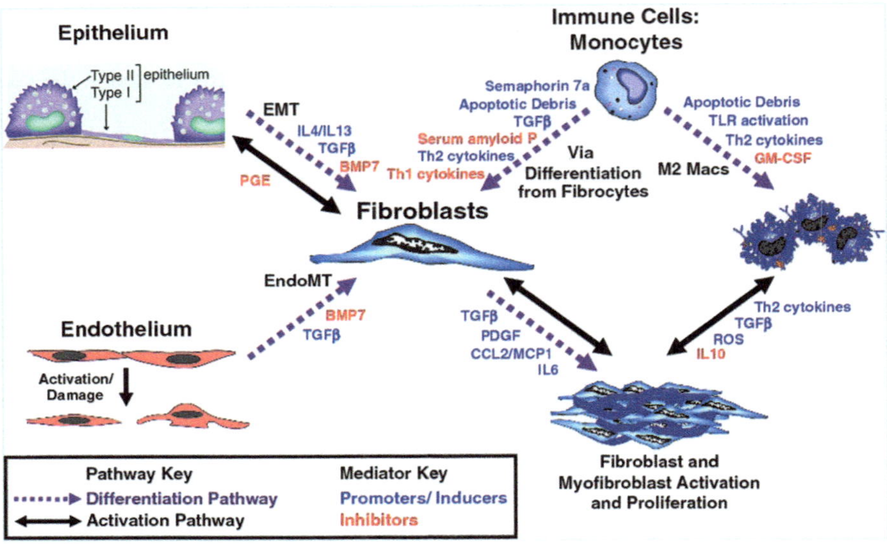

Key cell types associated with fibrosis and the differentiation pathways and mediators that promote and inhibit these pathways. Fibrosis is characterized by excess extracellular matrix deposition from collagen-producing cells including fibroblasts and myofibroblasts. These cells are resident within tissues, generating matrix to support tissue function and homeostasis. However, during fibrosis, fibroblasts become activated, proliferate at greater rates than unactivated cells and are resistant to apoptosis. There is also an increased number of myofibroblasts, which are normally at low levels in non-fibrotic tissue. Monocytes activate fibroblasts through either differentiating to fibrocytes or alternatively activated M2 macrophages. Both of these monocyte-derived cells are found at elevated numbers in the circulation of patients with chronic lung fibrosis and at sites of tissue remodeling. Both epithelial cell and endothelial cell injury is observed at sites of fibrotic tissue remodeling. Moreover, the transition of epithelial cells to mesenchymal cells and endothelial cells to mesenchymal cells has been hypothesized as sources for increased mesenchymal cell numbers in fibrosis. Multiple mediators, especially radiation exposure, have been shown to promote fibrosis and to direct cells to a pro-fibrotic or anti-fibrotic phenotype, with the cellular environment also helping to direct cell phenotype. Many of the mediators shown to induce pro-fibrotic responses are pleiotropic, directing more than cellular response on multiple cell types [Murray LA, Sleeman MA. Fibrosis. In: Sonis ST, Keefe DM, editors. Pathobiology of Cancer Regimen-Related Toxicities [Internet]. New York, NY: Springer New York; 2013 [cited 2015 Dec 22]. p. 167–86. Available from: http://link.springer.com/10.1007/978-1-4614-5438-0_9] *Caption adapted from original*

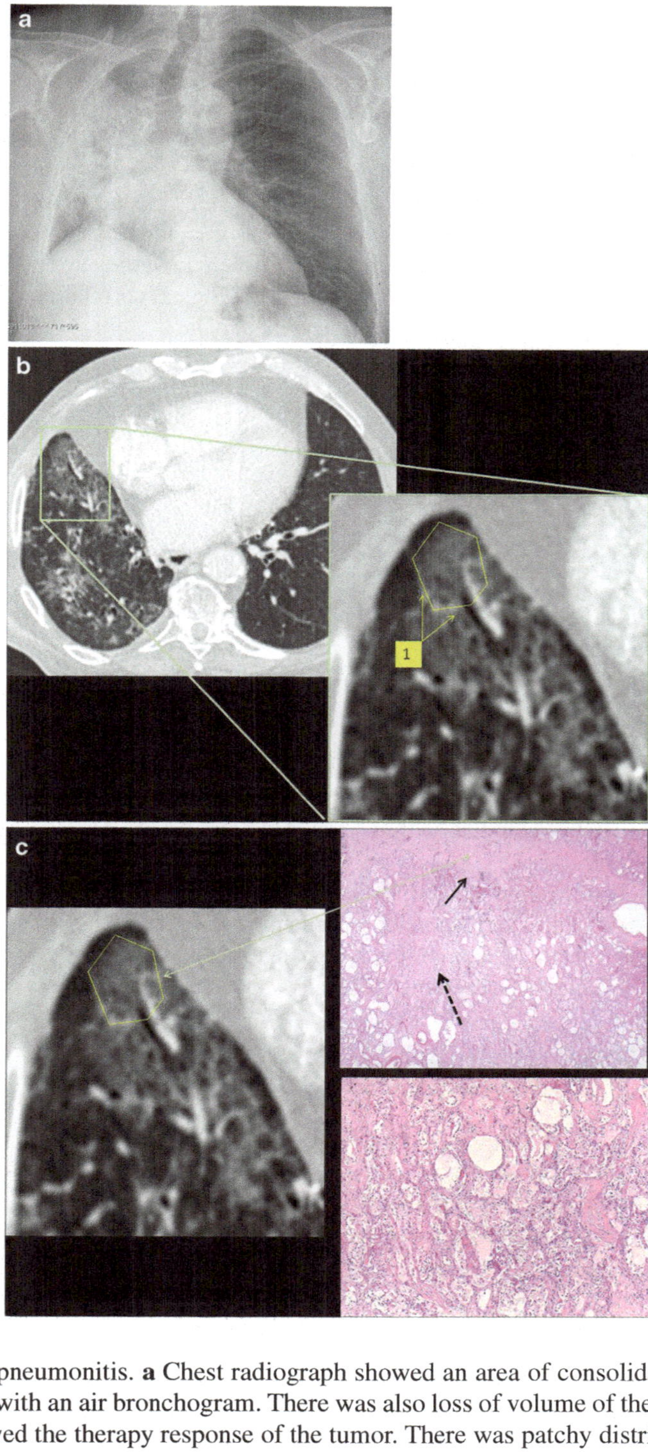

Radiation pneumonitis. **a** Chest radiograph showed an area of consolidation in the right lung with an air bronchogram. There was also loss of volume of the right lung. **b** CT showed the therapy response of the tumor. There was patchy distribution of a crazy-paving pattern with increased lung attenuation (ground-glass opacity) and thickening of the interlobular septa in the right lung (1). **c** Radiological-histopathological correlation. Histological examination after autopsy showed air-space filling with an exudate in combination with thickening of the interlobular septa (arrow), thickening of the interstitium surrounding the airspaces and also the presence of irregular fibrosis (dotted arrow). Alveolar spaces filled with an exudate of proteinaceous material were responsible for the ground-glass opacities on CT. The reticular pattern was due to congestion of capillaries and oedema of the interstitium [De Wever W, Meersschaert J, Coolen J, Verbeken E, Verschakelen JA. The crazy-paving pattern: a radiological-pathological correlation. Insights into Imaging. 2011 Apr;2(2):117–32.] *Caption from original*

Presentation

Typical/"Classic"

- There are two distinct clinical syndromes associated with radiation damage to the lungs: an acute clinical syndrome due to pneumonitis, and a later syndrome caused by fibrosis.
  - Acute radiation pneumonitis. This develops anywhere from 2 weeks to 3 months after exposure to radiation.
    - Most patients remain asymptomatic throughout this period.
    - Most patients will develop radiographic evidence of pneumonitis (patchy opacities within irradiated areas), but only about 50 % have symptoms.
    - As noted in the Pathophysiology section, the pathologic changes during this period include mucosal inflammation with increased and thickened secretions. These pathologic changes lead to the classic symptoms.
    - The classic symptoms include:
      - Dry cough
      - Shortness of breath
      - Fever
    - Physical examination may be normal, but crackles in the area of consolidation may be noted. Patients may also be tachypneic. In about 10 % of cases a small pleural effusion may be present and decreased breath sounds and dullness to percussion over the effusion may be noted. Pleural inflammation may be noted with a pleural rub.
    - The majority of patients who develop symptoms improve spontaneously over 2 – 4 weeks.

- Late radiation pneumonitis/radiation fibrosis. Although the pathologic process leading to fibrosis can start within 2 weeks of radiation exposure, symptoms (if present) don't usually start until 6 months to even years later.
    - Up to 50 % of patients with radiographic abnormalities will remain asymptomatic.
    - The most common symptoms are dry cough and shortness of breath. Fever can occur but is less common than in acute radiation pneumonitis.
    - In advanced cases of radiation fibrosis, patients may develop signs of pulmonary hypertension and cor pulmonale.

Atypical

- Atypically, patients may present with chest pain. The pain is often pleuritic, and often due to pleural inflammation.
- Chest pain may also occur secondary to esophageal irritation or inflammation. Chest pain in this setting in often worsened by swallowing.

Primary Differential Considerations

- Patients with radiation pneumonitis may present with symptoms that prompt consideration of:
    - Other causes of pulmonary fibrosis
    - Acute pneumonia
    - Pulmonary embolism

History and Physical Exam

Findings That Confirm Diagnosis

- There are no historical or physical examination findings that can completely confirm the diagnosis.

Factors That Suggest Diagnosis

- The diagnosis is suggested when a patient presents with the typical symptoms or radiographic changes in the appropriate time frame after receiving radiation, especially when the radiographic changes are confined to the areas irradiated.

Factors That Exclude Diagnosis

- There are no historical or physical examination findings that can completely exclude the diagnosis, except for an absence of exposure to radiation.

Ancillary Studies

Laboratory

- There are no laboratory studies specific to the diagnosis of radiation pneumonitis.
- Routine laboratory studies are often performed in the evaluation to seek other possible causes of symptoms and radiographic changes.
  - For example, a complete blood count (CBC) showing a leukocytosis with a bandemia or leftward shift may help increase the suspicion for an infectious cause. Patients with radiation pneumonitis may have a slight leukocytosis, but without a bandemia or left shift.
  - An elevated brain natriuretic peptide (BNP) may suggest a diagnosis of congestive heart failure.

Imaging

- Chest x-ray. The classic CXR pattern is one of patchy alveolar densities in the areas treated with radiation. Patients who progress to radiation fibrosis may exhibit lung-volume loss with dense opacities. Again, these are within the areas that received radiation. Some patients may have small pleural effusions.
  - Historically, the CXR in radiation pneumonitis would often show a "straight-line" effect. This straight line of radiographic changes did not conform to anatomic boundaries but to the area that was irradiated. Modern methods of radiation administration allow mostly three-dimensional therapy that can closely conform to the tissue needing treatment, so the straight-line effect is no longer a common finding.

Features of alveolar pattern
Lesions in radiation field
Airspace 1–3 months
Fibrosis 6–12 months
Organizing pneumonia may appear

Imaging findings in radiation pneumonitis. The diagnosis of radiation pneumonitis should be made when focal pulmonary disease coincides with the areas of the radiation field [Vilar J, Andreu J. The Lung Parenchyma: Radiological Presentation of Alveolar Pattern. In: Coche EE, Ghaye B, de Mey J, Duyck P, editors. Comparative Interpretation of CT and Standard Radiography of the Chest [Internet]. Berlin, Heidelberg: Springer Berlin Heidelberg; 2011 [cited 2015 Dec 21]. p. 221–45. Available from: http://link.springer.com/10.1007/978-3-540-79942-9_9] *Caption and text from original*

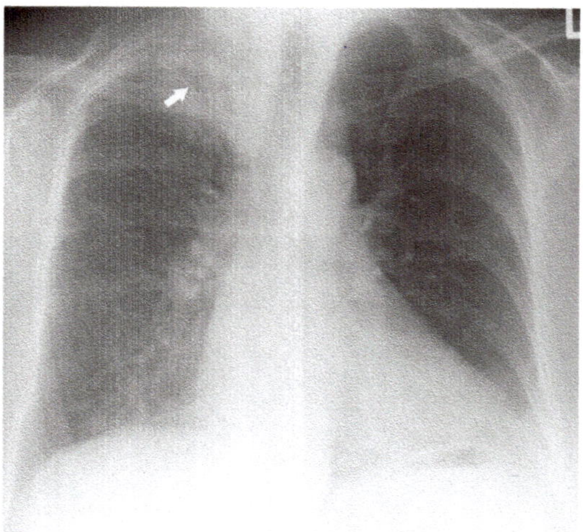

Radiation pneumonitis. PA radiograph shows consolidation (arrow) in the right upper lobe. [Kanne JP, Godwin JD. Imaging the Chest Following Radiation Therapy. In: Ravenel JG, editor. Lung Cancer Imaging [Internet]. New York, NY: Springer New York; 2013 [cited 2015 Dec 21]. p. 153–68. Available from: http://link.springer.com/10.1007/978-1-60761-620-7_13] *Caption from original*

- Computed tomography (CT) of the chest. A CT scan of the chest is frequently performed during the evaluation of these patients. CT is more sensitive than CXR for the diagnosis of radiation pneumonitis. However, a CT scan is more frequently performed to help exclude other causes of the patient's symptoms (as per the Differential Diagnosis section). As with the CXR, lung involvement should follow the irradiated areas.

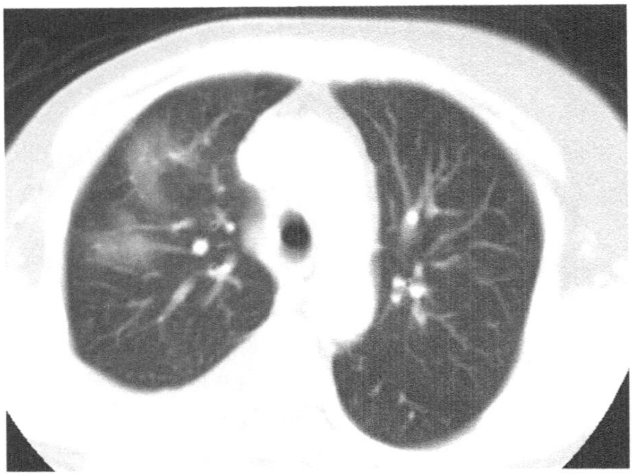

Early radiation pneumonitis changes with ground-glass attenuation in the radiation field 6 weeks after radiotherapy for a localized right side breast cancer.[Murchison JT, van Beek EJR. Complications and Toxicity of Radiotherapy for the Breast, Lung and Heart. In: Kauczor H-U, Bäuerle T, editors. Imaging of Complications and Toxicity following Tumor Therapy [Internet]. Cham: Springer International Publishing; 2015 [cited 2015 Dec 21]. p. 115–28. Available from: http://link.springer.com/10.1007/174_2015_1083] *Caption from original*

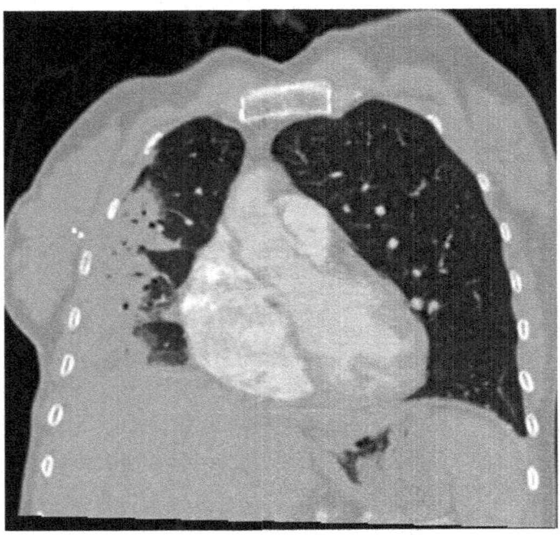

Subacute radiation pneumonitis in a patient treated with radiotherapy for breast cancer 10 weeks earlier. There is consolidation with air bronchograms which is largely limited by the radiation field and is not bounded by fissures [Murchison JT, van Beek EJR. Complications and Toxicity of Radiotherapy for the Breast, Lung and Heart. In: Kauczor H-U, Bäuerle T, editors. Imaging of Complications and Toxicity following Tumor Therapy [Internet]. Cham: Springer International Publishing; 2015 [cited 2015 Dec 21]. p. 115–28. Available from: http://link.springer.com/10.1007/174_2015_1083] *Caption from original*

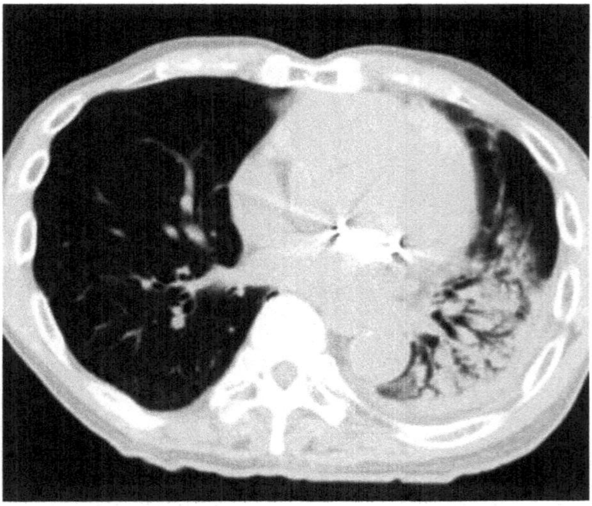

Computed tomography (CT) image of radiation pneumonitis (RP). [From article: Exceptionally high incidence of symptomatic grade 2–5 radiation pneumonitis after stereotactic radiation therapy for lung tumors. Radiation Oncology. 2007;2(1):21. https://doi.org/10.1186/1748-717X-2-21, at http://link.springer.com/article/10.1186/1748-717X-2-21/fulltext.html; by Hideomi Yamashita, Keiichi Nakagawa, Naoki Nakamura, Hiroki Koyanagi, Masao Tago, Hiroshi Igaki, Kenshiro Shiraishi, Nakashi Sasano, Kuni Ohtomo, © Yamashita et al; licensee BioMed Central Ltd. 2007; licensed under Creative Commons Attribution License BY 2.0 http://creativecommons.org/licenses/by/2.0] *Caption adapted from original*

Other

- Pulmonary Function Tests (PFTs). If performed, PFTs will often show diffusely reduced lung volumes, a decreased diffusing capacity for carbon monoxide (DLCO), and an increased alveolar-arterial oxygen gradient. In advanced fibrosis, patients may be hypoxic.
- Bronchoscopy. Bronchoscopy is useful to exclude other diagnoses (as per the differential diagnosis section).

Special Populations

Age

- Age is not a factor in developing radiation pneumonitis. It can occur in any patient who has received radiation to the chest.

Co-morbidities

- Patients with radiation pneumonitis often have multiple co-morbid conditions that can make the diagnosis and management of radiation pneumonitis challenging. Such conditions include chronic obstructive pulmonary disease (COPD), congestive heart failure (CHF), cardiomyopathies, and interstitial lung diseases (ILD).

Pitfalls in Diagnosis

Critical Steps Not to Miss

- It is critical to carefully consider and evaluate for all diagnoses in the differential.

Mimics

- As the symptoms of radiation pneumonitis are non-specific and also occur with many other conditions, many diseases can present identically to radiation pneumonitis (as per the differential diagnosis section).

Time-Dependent Interventions

- Patients with a known cancer, and who present with shortness of breath, cough, and fever, need to be urgently evaluated for either an infectious or thrombotic (pulmonary embolism) etiology as cause of their symptoms. It may be necessary to treat for infection empirically until this can be adequately ruled out. A CT scan of the chest (or suitable alternative) may be necessary to exclude pulmonary embolism.
- Any patient with hypoxia should receive supplemental oxygen.

Overall Principles of Treatment

- Asymptomatic (or minimally symptomatic) patients who are found to have radiographic abnormalities consistent with radiation pneumonitis can be followed without treatment, as many (up to 50 %) will have a spontaneous recovery.
- All symptomatic patients should be offered supportive, symptomatic treatments such as oxygen for hypoxia, anti-tussives for cough, and anti-pyretics for fever.
- Patients who are symptomatic and have had or are in the process of having alternative diagnoses evaluated can be started on glucocorticoids, specifically prednisone starting at 0.5–1 mg/kg/day in divided doses. This treatment recommendation is based upon consensus, expert opinion, as there are no randomized, controlled trials of glucocorticoids in the treatment or radiation pneumonitis.
- When initiated, steroids should be tapered gradually (over 1–3 months) to prevent a recurrence of symptoms.
- Patients who fail to respond to steroids often have rapid disease progression.
- There is no indication for the treatment of radiation fibrosis with steroids.
- Prophylactic administration of glucocorticoids has not been shown to prevent the development of radiation pneumonitis.

Disease Course

- Many patients with radiation pneumonitis (especially if asymptomatic or minimally symptomatic) will improve spontaneously.
- Patients who progress to fibrosis have less likelihood of spontaneous improvement.
- Fibrosis can continue to progress, but many patients will have both clinical and pathologic stabilization after about 18 months.

Related Evidence

Papers of particular interest have been highlighted as:
*** Of key importance*

Meta-Analysis

Baker R, Han G, Sarangkasiri S, DeMarco M, Turke C, Stevens CW, Dilling TJ. Clinical and dosimetric predictors of radiation pneumonitis in a large series of patients treated with stereotactic body radiation therapy to the lung. Int J Radiat Oncol Biol Phys. 2013 Jan 1;85(1):190-5. https://doi.org/10.1016/j.ijrobp.2012.03.041. Epub 2012 Aug 25. PubMed PMID: 22929858. http://www.ncbi.nlm.nih.gov/pubmed/22950387 **

Zhang XJ, Sun JG, Sun J, Ming H, Wang XX, Wu L, Chen ZT. Prediction of radiation pneumonitis in lung cancer patients: a systematic review. J Cancer Res Clin Oncol. 2012 Dec;138(12):2103-16. https://doi.org/10.1007/s00432-012-1284-1. Epub 2012 Jul 29. Review. PubMed PMID: 22842662. http://www.ncbi.nlm.nih.gov/pubmed/22842662 **

Vogelius IR, Bentzen SM. A literature-based meta-analysis of clinical risk factors for development of radiation induced pneumonitis. Acta Oncol. 2012 Nov;51(8):975-83. https://doi.org/10.3109/0284186X.2012.718093. Epub 2012 Sep 5. Review. PubMed PMID: 22950387; PubMed Central PMCID: PMC3557496. http://www.ncbi.nlm.nih.gov/pubmed/22950387 **

Marks LB, Bentzen SM, Deasy JO, Kong FM, Bradley JD, Vogelius IS, El Naqa I, Hubbs JL, Lebesque JV, Timmerman RD, Martel MK, Jackson A. Radiation dose-volume effects in the lung. Int J Radiat Oncol Biol Phys. 2010 Mar 1;76(3 Suppl):S70-6. https://doi.org/10.1016/j.ijrobp.2009.06.091. Review. PubMed PMID: 20171521; PubMed Central PMCID: PMC3576042. http://www.ncbi.nlm.nih.gov/pubmed/20171521

Review

Straub JM, New J, Hamilton CD, Lominska C, Shnayder Y, Thomas SM. Radiation-induced fibrosis: mechanisms and implications for therapy. J Cancer Res Clin Oncol. 2015 Nov;141(11):1985-94. https://doi.org/10.1007/s00432-015-1974-6. Epub 2015 Apr 25. Review. PubMed PMID: 25910988; PubMed Central PMCID: PMC4573901. http://www.ncbi.nlm.nih.gov/pubmed/25910988 **

Ding NH, Li JJ, Sun LQ. Molecular mechanisms and treatment of radiation-induced lung fibrosis. Curr Drug Targets. 2013 Oct;14(11):1347-56. Review. PubMed PMID: 23909719; PubMed Central PMCID: PMC4156316. http://www.ncbi.nlm.nih.gov/pmc/articles/PMC4156316/ **

Benveniste MF, Welsh J, Godoy MC, Betancourt SL, Mawlawi OR, Munden RF. New era of radiotherapy: an update in radiation-induced lung disease. Clin Radiol. 2013 Jun;68(6):e275-90. https://doi.org/10.1016/j.crad.2013.01.013. Epub 2013 Mar 6. Review. PubMed PMID: 23473474; PubMed Central PMCID: PMC3941603. http://www.ncbi.nlm.nih.gov/pubmed/23473474 **

Inoue T, Oh RJ, Shiomi H, Masai N, Miura H. Stereotactic body radiotherapy for pulmonary metastases. Prognostic factors and adverse respiratory events. Strahlenther Onkol. 2013 Apr;189(4):285-92. https://doi.org/10.1007/s00066-012-0290-1. Epub 2013 Feb 20. PubMed PMID: 23420546. http://www.ncbi.nlm.nih.gov/pubmed/23276463 **

Westbury CB, Yarnold JR. Radiation fibrosis–current clinical and therapeutic perspectives. Clin Oncol (R Coll Radiol). 2012 Dec;24(10):657-72. https://doi.org/10.1016/j.clon.2012.04.001. Epub 2012 May 18. Review. PubMed PMID: 22608361. http://www.ncbi.nlm.nih.gov/pubmed/22608361 **

Robbins ME, Brunso-Bechtold JK, Peiffer AM, Tsien CI, Bailey JE, Marks LB. Imaging radiation-induced normal tissue injury. Radiat Res. 2012 Apr;177(4):449-66. Epub 2012 Feb 21. Review. PubMed PMID: 22348250; PubMed Central PMCID: PMC3733443. http://www.ncbi.nlm.nih.gov/pubmed/22348250

Linda A, Trovo M, Bradley JD. Radiation injury of the lung after stereotactic body radiation therapy (SBRT) for lung cancer: a timeline and pattern of CT changes. Eur J Radiol. 2011 Jul;79(1):147-54. https://doi.org/1016/j.ejrad.2009.10.029. Epub 2009 Dec 1. Review. PubMed PMID: 19954913. http://www.ncbi.nlm.nih.gov/pubmed/19954913

Larici AR, del Ciello A, Maggi F, Santoro SI, Meduri B, Valentini V, Giordano A, Bonomo L. Lung abnormalities at multimodality imaging after radiation therapy for non-small cell lung cancer. Radiographics. 2011 May-Jun;31(3):771-89. https://doi.org/10.1148/rg.313105096. Review. PubMed PMID: 21571656. http://www.ncbi.nlm.nih.gov/pubmed/21571656

Williams JP, Johnston CJ, Finkelstein JN. Treatment for radiation-induced pulmonary late effects: spoiled for choice or looking in the wrong direction? Curr Drug Targets. 2010 Nov;11(11):1386-94. Review. PubMed PMID: 20583979; PubMed Central PMCID: PMC2948640. http://www.ncbi.nlm.nih.gov/pubmed/20583979

Krasin MJ, Constine LS, Friedman DL, Marks LB. Radiation-related treatment effects across the age spectrum: differences and similarities or what the old and young can learn from each other. Semin Radiat Oncol. 2010 Jan;20(1):21-9. https://doi.org/10.1016/j.semradonc.2009.09.001. Review. PubMed PMID: 19959028; PubMed Central PMCID: PMC2843498. http://www.ncbi.nlm.nih.gov/pubmed/19959028

Graves PR, Siddiqui F, Anscher MS, Movsas B. Radiation pulmonary toxicity: from mechanisms to management. Semin Radiat Oncol. 2010 Jul;20(3):201-7. https://doi.org/10.1016/j.semradonc.2010.01.010. Review. PubMed PMID: 20685583. http://www.ncbi.nlm.nih.gov/pubmed/20685583 **

Vargas HA, Hampson FA, Babar JL, Shaw AS. Imaging the lungs in patients treated for lymphoma. Clin Radiol. 2009 Nov;64(11):1048-55. https://doi.org/10.1016/j.crad.2009.04.006. Epub 2009 Jun 5. Review. PubMed PMID: 19822237. http://www.ncbi.nlm.nih.gov/pubmed/19822237

Ghafoori P, Marks LB, Vujaskovic Z, Kelsey CR. Radiation-induced lung injury. Assessment, management, and prevention. Oncology (Williston Park). 2008

Jan;22(1):37-47; discussion 52-3. Review. PubMed PMID: 18251282. http://www.ncbi.nlm.nih.gov/pubmed/18251282

Choi YW, Munden RF, Erasmus JJ, Park KJ, Chung WK, Jeon SC, Park CK. Effects of radiation therapy on the lung: radiologic appearances and differential diagnosis. Radiographics. 2004 Jul-Aug;24(4):985-97; discussion 998. Review. PubMed PMID: 15256622. http://www.ncbi.nlm.nih.gov/pubmed/15256622

Comparative Study

Takeda A, Ohashi T, Kunieda E, Sanuki N, Enomoto T, Takeda T, Oku Y, Shigematsu N. Comparison of clinical, tumour-related and dosimetric factors in grade 0-1, grade 2 and grade 3 radiation pneumonitis after stereotactic body radiotherapy for lung tumours. Br J Radiol. 2012 May;85(1013):636–42. https://doi.org/10.1259/bjr/71635286. Epub 2012 Jan 17. PubMed PMID: 22253343; PubMed Central PMCID: PMC3479872. http://www.ncbi.nlm.nih.gov/pubmed/22253343

General

Rutkowska ES, Syndikus I, Baker CR, Nahum AE. Mechanistic modelling of radiotherapy-induced lung toxicity. Br J Radiol. 2012 Dec;85(1020):e1242-8. https://doi.org/10.1259/bjr/28365782. PubMed PMID: 23175489; PubMed Central PMCID: PMC3611730. http://www.ncbi.nlm.nih.gov/pubmed/22929858

Matsuo Y, Shibuya K, Nakamura M, Narabayashi M, Sakanaka K, Ueki N, Miyagi K, Norihisa Y, Mizowaki T, Nagata Y, Hiraoka M. Dose–volume metrics associated with radiation pneumonitis after stereotactic body radiation therapy for lung cancer. Int J Radiat Oncol Biol Phys. 2012 Jul 15;83(4):e545-9. https://doi.org/10.1016/j.ijrobp.2012.01.018. Epub 2012 Mar 19. PubMed PMID: 22436782.

Yirmibesoglu E, Higginson DS, Fayda M, Rivera MP, Halle J, Rosenman J, Xie L, Marks LB. Challenges scoring radiation pneumonitis in patients irradiated for lung cancer. Lung Cancer. 2012 Jun;76(3):350-3. https://doi.org/10.1016/j.lungcan.2011.11.025. Epub 2012 Jan 9. PubMed PMID: 22230037; PubMed Central PMCID: PMC4287383. http://www.ncbi.nlm.nih.gov/pubmed/22230037

Takeda A, Kunieda E, Ohashi T, Aoki Y, Oku Y, Enomoto T, Nomura K, Sugiura M.Severe COPD is correlated with mild radiation pneumonitis following stereotactic body radiotherapy. Chest. 2012 Apr;141(4):858-66. https://doi.org/10.1378/chest.11-1193. Epub 2011 Sep 1. PubMed PMID: 21885726. http://www.ncbi.nlm.nih.gov/pubmed/21885726

Parashar B, Edwards A, Mehta R, Pasmantier M, Wernicke AG, Sabbas A, Kerestez RS, Nori D, Chao KS. Chemotherapy significantly increases the risk of radiation pneumonitis in radiation therapy of advanced lung cancer. Am J Clin Oncol. 2011 Apr;34(2):160-4. https://doi.org/10.1097/COC.0b013e3181d6b40f. PubMed PMID: 20498591.

Use PubMed Clinical Queries to find the most recent evidence. Use this search strategy: "Radiation Pneumonitis"[Mesh] OR "radiation induced lung injury" OR "radiation fibrosis"

Chapter 65
Retropharyngeal Abscess

Christopher J. Rees, Richard M. Cantor, Charles V. Pollack, Jr., and Victoria G. Riese

Name and Synonyms

Retropharyngeal Abscess; Retropharyngeal Cellulitis

Incidence/Epidemiology

- The incidence of retropharyngeal abscess has decreased as the use of antibiotics for pharyngeal and dental infections has increased.
- In children, it is most prevalent between the ages of 2 and 4 years.
- Retropharyngeal abscesses are among the most serious of the cervical deep space infections, as they may spread directly into the mediastinum.

C. J. Rees
Emergency Department, Pennsylvania Hospital, Philadelphia, PA, USA

R. M. Cantor
Department of Emergency Medicine and Pediatrics, State University of New York Upstate Medical University, Syracuse, NY, USA

C. V. Pollack, Jr. (✉)
Department of Emergency Medicine, Thomas Jefferson University, Philadelphia, PA, USA

V. G. Riese
Librarian Consultant, Eldersburg, MD, USA

C. V. Pollack, Jr. (ed.), *Differential Diagnosis of Cardiopulmonary Disease*,
https://doi.org/10.1007/978-3-319-63895-9_65

Differential Diagnosis

- The differential diagnosis of retropharyngeal abscess includes all the other deep neck space infections, pharyngitis, epiglottitis, cervical osteomyelitis, meningitis, angioedema, tumors, and other space-occupying lesions.

Pathophysiology and Etiology

- About half of pediatric cases are preceded by an upper respiratory tract infection. Another quarter are the result of penetrating trauma (e.g., from swallowing chicken bones, iatrogenic trauma after procedures); the remainder are secondary to pharyngitis, dental infections, and, rarely, vertebral osteomyelitis.
- In adults, it now is seen most commonly as an iatrogenic complication of oropharyngeal procedures, a direct extension from other contiguous infectious foci, or a result of penetrating trauma (swallowing of chicken bones, stab wounds, gunshot wounds).
- The retropharyngeal space is a potential space between the posterior prevertebral fascia and the alar fascia. It extends from the base of the skull to the posterior mediastinum at the tracheal bifurcation. It is fused in the midline (so infections usually stay localized to one side) and contains two chains of lymph nodes that drain the nasopharynx, adenoids, and posterior nasal sinuses.
- Children usually have an antecedent infection that is drained by one of the lymph node chains in the retropharyngeal space. The lymph nodes become infected, suppurate, and develop into an abscess. Adults tend to develop infection in the space by direct contamination from penetrating trauma or by contiguous spread from other infections.
- The retropharyngeal space communicates directly with the mediastinum and the lateral pharyngeal space, both of which communicate with the carotid sheath. Infection may spread within all these spaces.
- The infections typically are polymicrobial and include normal flora of the oropharynx.
- The infection often includes oral anaerobes.
- The most commonly found organisms include *Streptococcus viridans*, *Streptococcus pyogenes*, *Staphylococcus aureus*, *Pseudomonas aeruginosa*, *Enterobacter*, *Peptostreptococcus*, and *Fusobacterium*.

Presentation

Typical/"Classic"

- Children more commonly present classically than do adults.
- Commonly presents with fever (65 %), sore throat (76 %), pain or difficulty with swallowing (35 %), and neck spasms with the patient's unwillingness or inability to move (especially extend) the neck (37 %)
- Neck swelling or a discreet neck mass may be present.
- Cervical lymphadenopathy often is present.
- Children often drool and cannot handle oral secretions appropriately.
- Vocal quality may change, with hoarseness or a muted quality to the voice.
- The patient may have respiratory distress and stridor.
- Trismus (difficulty or inability to open the jaw) is present in 20 %.
- Affected patients usually appear ill and toxic, and the onset generally is acute.
- The nonconstitutional symptoms manifested by the patient usually are related to whatever structures are being obstructed or compressed by the abscess cavity.

Atypical

- Onset may be more insidious and less dramatic, especially if the patient has been on antibiotics.
- Early in the course of illness, the symptoms may be identical to those of pharyngitis.

Primary Differential Considerations

- When evaluating a patient in whom retropharyngeal abscess is suspected, early consideration also should be given to the following differential diagnoses:
  - Angioedema
  - Epiglottitis
  - Meningitis
  - Pharyngitis
  - Peritonsillar abscess
  - Caustic ingestion

History and Physical Exam

Findings That Confirm Diagnosis

- There are no confirmatory findings on history and physical examination. The other diagnoses in the differential may present with remarkable similarity.

Factors That Suggest Diagnosis

- The index of suspicion should be high for any child who presents febrile with any combination of the symptoms reviewed in the classic presentation.
- Adults may give a history of a recent procedure or trauma, leading to consideration of the diagnosis.

Factors That Exclude Diagnosis

- There are no historical or physical findings that exclude the diagnosis.
- The diagnosis is excluded only by the absence of an abscess on advanced imaging.

Ancillary Studies

Laboratory

- Lab studies should include the typical tests for any patient who presents febrile with an acute illness. These include (but are not limited to) a complete blood count with differential, electrolyte and renal function tests, serum lactate measurement, blood cultures, and pharynx culture if possible.

Imaging

- Contrast-enhanced CT of the neck is the diagnostic test of choice. A CT scan can differentiate among the different cervical deep space infections, epiglottitis, and other diseases in the differential. CT also may help the otolaryngologist plan appropriate operative intervention.
- Contrast-enhanced MRI also may be performed, but it takes longer and is more difficult for children.

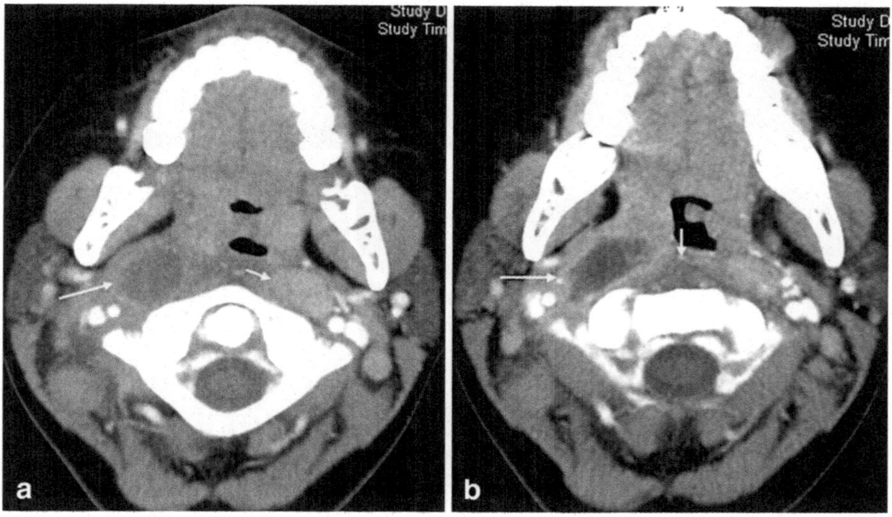

Retropharyngeal abscess. CT scans of the neck of a child at early and later stages of suppurative adenitis evolving into a retropharyngeal abscess. a At an earlier stage, CT image shows right parapharyngeal adenopathy with central necrosis (long arrow). Note the prominent hyperdense adenopathy on the contralateral side (short arrow). b There was no clinical improvement after antibiotic administration. A repeat examination at the same level shows abscess formation on the right (long arrow) causing a mass effect upon the airway and improvement of the adenopathy on the left. The hypodense area in the prevertebral space indicates edema/exudate (short arrow). [Restrepo R, Oneto J, Lopez K, Kukreja K. Head and neck lymph nodes in children: the spectrum from normal to abnormal. Pediatr Radiol. 2009 Aug;39(8):836–46.] *Caption from original*

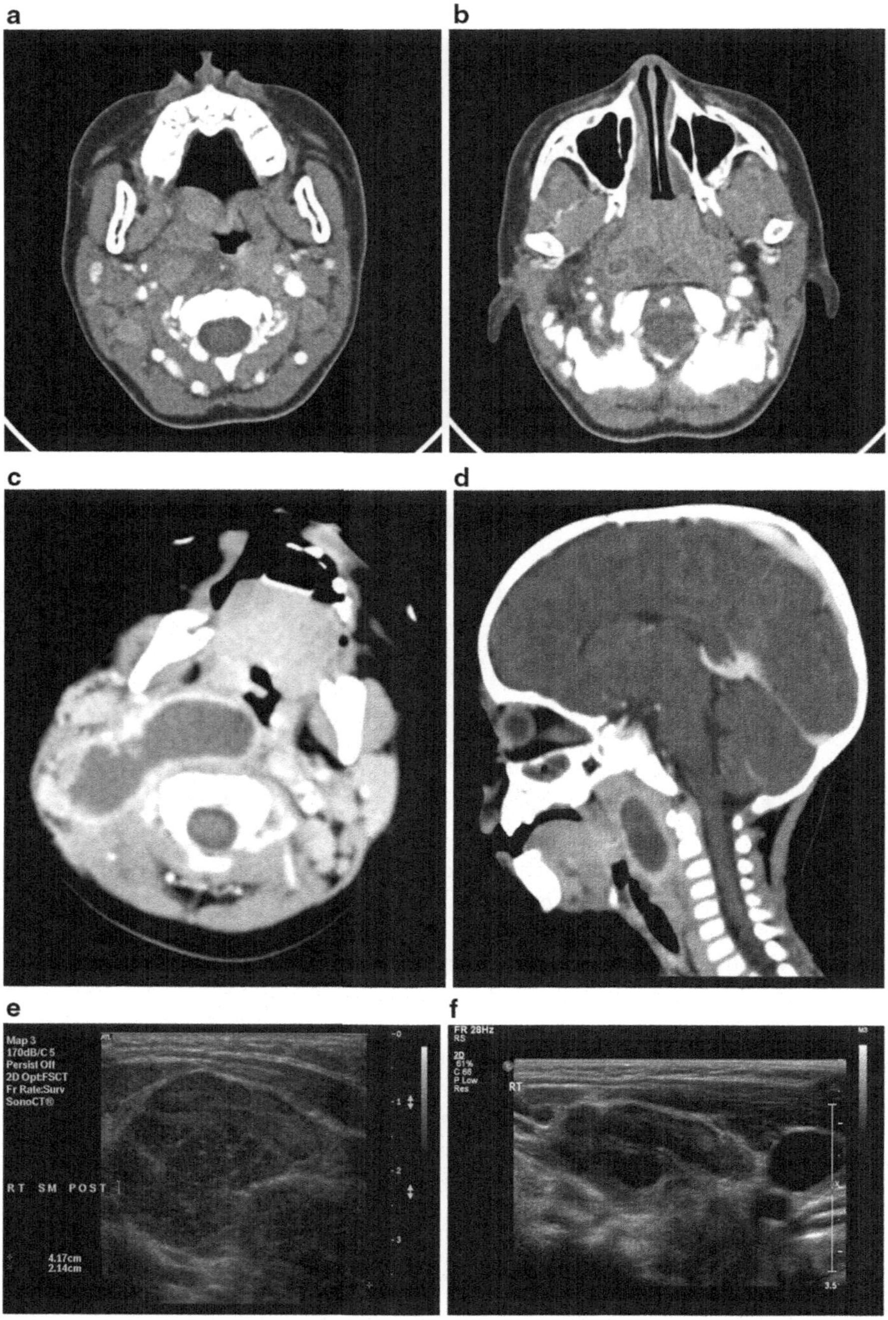

Retropharyngeal infection in two different patients. First patient is an infant with acute pharyngitis and tonsillitis. Axial image of contrast-enhanced CT at the level of the tonsils (a) demonstrates enlarged enhancing retropharyngeal lymph nodes with associated inflammatory phlegmon displacing the right tonsil anteriorly; in the same patient, an axial image at the level of the nasopharynx demonstrates a right-sided suppurated retropharyngeal lymph node (b). Second patient is a 1-year-old girl with complicated ear infection, and axial (c) and sagittal reformat (d) images from contrast-enhanced neck CT demonstrate a large retropharyngeal fluid density rim-enhancing collection consistent with an abscess, which involves the posterior triangle of the neck. An US study before (e) and after (f) surgical drainage of the abscess demonstrated a more complex appearance of the abscess content with thick pus as opposed to the relative simple fluid-like appearance on the CT; the US allows follow-up after drainage and demonstrates collapse of the abscess cavity. [Shiran SI. Imaging of pediatric neck and airway. In: Kountakis SE, editor. Encyclopedia of otolaryngology, head and neck surgery [Internet]. Berlin, Heidelberg: Springer; 2013 [cited 2015 Aug 24]. p. 1277–307. Available from: http://link.springer.com/10.1007/978-3-642-23499-6_414] *Caption from original*

Special Populations

Age

- Retropharyngeal abscess is more common in children, especially those between the ages of 2 and 4 years.
- The child appears ill, sometimes toxic, and febrile.
- Associated signs and symptoms include dysphagia, drooling, neck stiffness, torticollis, change in vocal tone, and trismus.
- In the young child or infant, CT scanning may be necessary to define the extent of the problem.

Co-morbidities

- There are no specific co-morbidities associated with retropharyngeal abscess.

Pitfalls in Diagnosis

Critical Steps Not to Miss

- Consideration of the diagnosis is the first critical step.
- Ensuring that the patient has a secure airway, especially if undergoing diagnostic testing, is critically important.

Mimics

- Retropharyngeal abscess can mimic and be mimicked by all the other cervical deep space infections, pharyngitis and pharyngeal cellulitis, epiglottitis, and the other diagnoses in the differential.

Time-Dependent Interventions

- Retropharyngeal abscesses may progress rapidly. Appropriate resuscitation, cultures, antibiotic treatment, and confirmatory imaging should proceed as quickly as possibly once the diagnosis is considered.

Overall Principles of Treatment

- When the diagnosis of retropharyngeal abscess is seriously considered, patients should undergo rapid resuscitation and receive antibiotic therapy even before confirmatory imaging.
- It is critical to ensure that the patient has a secure airway, especially when going "off unit" for any diagnostic testing.
- Broad-spectrum antibiotic coverage should be initiated to cover the usual oropharyngeal pathogens, including anaerobes.
- Urgent otolaryngologic consultation should be obtained.
- Definitive care often is guided by imaging. If the patient presents early in the course and there is no discrete collection, antibiotic therapy without surgery may arrest further abscess development and be curative. If collection is present, definitive treatment is operative drainage along with continued antibiotic therapy.

Disease Course

- With early and appropriate treatment, most patients will recover fully with few sequela.
- Delays in presentation and treatment may lead to serious complications, including death. Airway compromise may occur; the abscess may rupture spontaneously, with direct spread to contiguous structures, most ominously the mediastinum and carotid sheath.

Related Evidence

Papers of particular interest have been highlighted as:
*** Of key importance*

Review

Debnam JM, Guha-Thakurta N. Retropharyngeal and prevertebral spaces: anatomic imaging and diagnosis. Otolaryngol Clin North Am. 2012 Dec;45(6):1293-310. https://doi.org/10.1016/j.otc.2012.08.004. PMID: 23153750. http://www.ncbi.nlm.nih.gov/pubmed/23153750 **

Reilly BK, Reilly JS. Retropharyngeal abscess: diagnosis and treatment update. Infect Disord Drug Targets. 2012 Aug;12(4):291-6. PMID: 22338591. http://www.ncbi.nlm.nih.gov/pubmed/22338591 **

Caccamese JF Jr, Coletti DP. Deep neck infections: clinical considerations in aggressive disease. Oral Maxillofac Surg Clin North Am. 2008 Aug;20(3):367-80. https://doi.org/10.1016/j.coms.2008.03.001. PMID: 18603197. http://www.ncbi.nlm.nih.gov/pubmed/18603197 **

Osborn TM, Assael LA, Bell RB. Deep space neck infection: principles of surgical management. Oral Maxillofac Surg Clin North Am. 2008 Aug;20(3):353-65. https://doi.org/10.1016/j.coms.2008.04.002. PMID: 18603196. http://www.ncbi.nlm.nih.gov/pubmed/18603196 **

Vieira F, Allen SM, Stocks RM, Thompson JW. Deep neck infection. Otolaryngol Clin North Am. 2008 Jun;41(3):459-83, vii. https://doi.org/10.1016/j.otc.2008.01.002. PMID: 18435993. http://www.ncbi.nlm.nih.gov/pubmed/18435993 **

Chong VF, Fan YF. Radiology of the retropharyngeal space. Clin Radiol. 2000 Oct;55(10):740-8. PMID: 11052873. http://www.ncbi.nlm.nih.gov/pubmed/11052873 **

Tannebaum RD. Adult retropharyngeal abscess: a case report and review of the literature. J Emerg Med. 1996 Mar-Apr;14(2):147-58. PMID: 8740744. http://www.ncbi.nlm.nih.gov/pubmed/8740744 **

Comparative Study

Benmansour N, Benali A, Poirrier AL, Cherkaoui A, Oudidi A, Elalami MN. Retropharyngeal abscess in adults. Rev Laryngol Otol Rhinol (Bord). 2012;133(3):137-9. PMID: 23590102. http://www.ncbi.nlm.nih.gov/pubmed/23590102 **

Case Study

Schott CK, Counselman FL, Ashe AR. A pain in the neck: non-traumatic adult retropharyngeal abscess. J Emerg Med. 2013 Feb;44(2):329-31. https://doi.org/10.1016/j.jemermed.2011.09.028. PMID: 22284974. http://www.ncbi.nlm.nih.gov/pubmed/22284974

Use PubMed Clinical Queries to find the most recent evidence. Use this search strategy:

"Retropharyngeal Abscess"[Mesh] OR "Retropharyngeal Abscess"

Chapter 66
Sarcoidosis

Christopher J. Rees, Richard M. Cantor, Charles V. Pollack, Jr., and Victoria G. Riese

Name and Synonyms

Sarcoidosis; Sarcoid

Incidence/Epidemiology

- Sarcoidosis occurs throughout the world, but its prevalence and racial mix varies from country to country. For example, in the United States sarcoidosis is 3–4 times more common in blacks than whites, but in Ireland and Northern Europe (especially the Nordic countries), it is more prevalent among whites.
- The estimated worldwide prevalence of sarcoidosis is 20–60 cases per 100,000 people per year.
- The disease is usually diagnosed in young, otherwise healthy adults between the ages of 20 and 40, but there is also a second peak at about age 60. There is a slight female predominance. It is rare in children.

C. J. Rees
Emergency Department, Pennsylvania Hospital, Philadelphia, PA, USA

R. M. Cantor
Department of Emergency Medicine and Pediatrics, State University of New York Upstate Medical University, Syracuse, NY, USA

C. V. Pollack, Jr. (✉)
Department of Emergency Medicine, Thomas Jefferson University, Philadelphia, PA, USA

V. G. Riese
Librarian Consultant, Eldersburg, MD, USA

C. V. Pollack, Jr. (ed.), *Differential Diagnosis of Cardiopulmonary Disease*,
https://doi.org/10.1007/978-3-319-63895-9_66

- In the United Stavtes, the lifetime risk among the black population is about 2.5 %. The lifetime risk in the white population is only about 0.85 %.
- Blacks are more likely to present younger and with more acute and severe disease.
- In Ireland, and among African Americans in the United States, there can be a familial predisposition to the disease. This is thought to be due to linkage to the major histocompability complex (MHC). Increased susceptibility to the disease is noted in the presence of certain human leukocyte antigen (HLA) alleles (DRB1, 11, 12, 14, 15, and 17).

Differential Diagnosis

- The differential diagnosis of sarcoidosis is broad, and includes all the diseases that can cause shortness of breath and cough, such as asthma, COPD, interstitial lung disease, pneumonia, and congestive heart failure.
- Sarcoidosis can also present with hilar adenopathy on chest x-ray, so the differential must also include all the diseases associated with mediastinal and hilar adenopathy. This includes tuberculosis (both tuberculosis and atypical mycobacterial infections), fungal infections (such as histoplasmosis, blastomycosis, and Pneumocystis), and cancer (especially lymphoma).
- Other granulomatous diseases of the lungs that need to be considered include: hypersensitivitiy pneumonitis, pneumoconioses (beryllium), drug-induced hypersensitivity (causative agents include methotrexate, etanercept, infliximab, adalimumab, amoxicillin, sirolimus, and fluoxetine, among others), Pulmonary Langerhans cell histiocytosis, foreign body granulomatosis, vasculitides (Wegener's, Churg-Strauss, primary lymphomatoid granulomatosis), and primary immunodeficiencies.
- It is important in the evaluation of someone for presumed sarcoidosis that all these diseases be considered.

Pathophysiology and Etiology

- Sarcoidosis is a multi-system, inflammatory, granulomatous disease of unknown cause.
- The characteristic pathologic finding of sarcoidosis is the presence of noncaseating granulomas in affected tissues. The granulomas contain a mixture of multiple different inflammatory cells, epithelial cells, multi-nucleated giant cells, and fibroblasts. The majority of these granulomas gradually resolve without scarring or fibrosis. Large amounts of scarring, fibrosis, or necrosis should make one consider an alternative diagnosis.

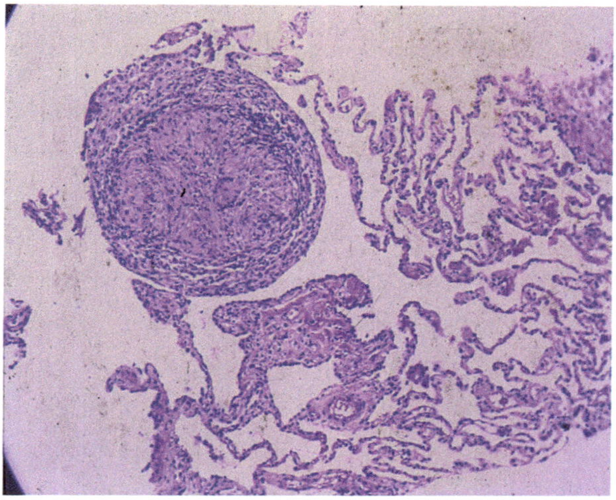

Sarcoidosis: a non-caseating granuloma. [Mahmoudi M, Sharma OP. Sarcoidosis. In: Mahmoudi M, editor. Challenging Cases in Pulmonology [Internet]. New York, NY: Springer New York; 2012 [cited 2015 Jun 9]. p. 253–74. Available from: http://link.springer.com/10.1007/978-1-4419-7098-5_15] *Caption from original*

- Sarcoidosis is thought to result from an exaggerated cell-mediated immune response to an as yet unidentified antigen.
- The etiology remains unknown, despite extensive investigations. An NIH-funded case-control study, Access, that included 700 patients with known sarcoidosis, and nearly 30,000 relatives, could not identify a single etiologic agent.
- Population studies have identified two possible associations: exposure to beryllium and beryllium salts, which can produce granulomas very similar to sarcoidosis. There has also been an increased incidence of sarcoid-like granulomatous disease in people exposed to the dust from the collapse of the World Trade Centers.

Presentation

Typical/"Classic"

- The most common presenting symptoms of sarcoidosis are cough, dyspnea, and chest pain. They are often associated with more constitutional symptoms such as fatigue, fever, and weight loss.
- Nearly one-third of patients are asymptomatic on presentation, and only present with an abnormal CXR.
- Sarcoidosis can affect virtually all organs of the body, but the lung, impacted in over 95 % of cases, is the most frequently affected. The next most fre-

quently involved organ is the skin, which is affected in about 25 % of cases at presentation, but will be involved in nearly one-third of all cases throughout the course of the disease.

- Ninety-five percent of patients eventually diagnosed with sarcoidosis will have pulmonary involvement at presentation. This may manifest as pulmonary symptoms or chest x-ray findings.
- The classic CXR findings of sarcoidosis are hilar adenopathy with associated reticular opacities.
- Patient will often also note eye problems (uveitis) and skin and/or joint lesions on presentation.

Atypical

- Thirty percent of patients will present with predominantly extra-thoracic manifestations of sarcoidosis.
- Löfgren Syndrome is an uncommon, acute, systemic presentation of sarcoidosis. Patients will have fever, erythema nodosum, polyarthralgia, uveitis, and bilateral hilar adenopathy on the CXR.
- Sarcoidosis can affect virtually any organ system in the body. Most of the pathologic and clinical manifestations are due to granulomatous infiltration of the relevant tissues. Some of the more common extra-pulmonary manifestations of sarcoidosis are reviewed below.
    - Skin. Overall, about one-third of patients will develop skin involvement. There are many different skin lesions associated with sarcoidosis, including:
        - Erythema nodosum

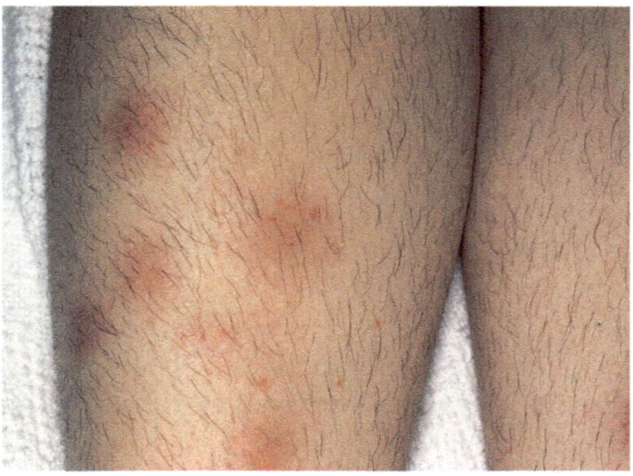

Erythema nodosum. Red nodules of erythema nodosum in the pretibial area. Lesions are usually tender, poorly circumscribed, and located deep within the subcutaneous fat. Their appearance is usually accompanied by an exacerbation in the underlying inflammatory bowel disease. Erythema nodosum occurs in about 4% of patients with ulcerative colitis and in 2% of patients with Crohn's disease. Treatment includes bed rest, systemic or intralesional steroids, nonsteroidal anti-inflammatory agents, potassium iodide, colchicine, and dapsone. [Pandya A. Chapter 12. In Feldman, M, editor. Gastroenterology and Hepatology, Volume 03. Philadelphia: Current Medicine; 1996. ISBN: 0-443-07843-2] *Caption from original*

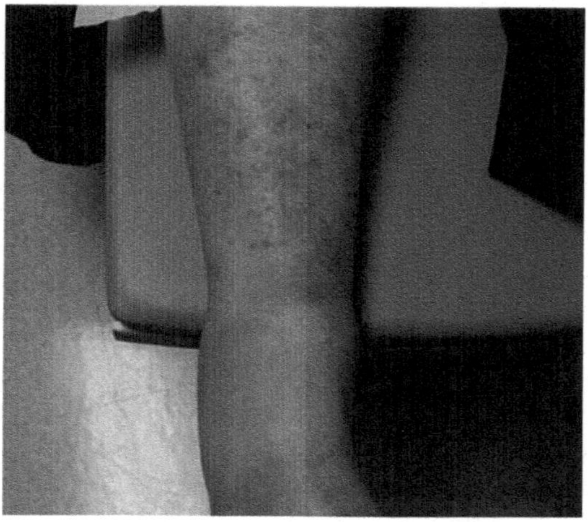

Erythema nodosum on the leg of a sarcoidosis patient [Baughman RP, Lower EE. Sarcoidosis. In: Stone JH, editor. A Clinician's Pearls and Myths in Rheumatology [Internet]. London: Springer London; 2009 [cited 2015 Jun 17]. p. 409–20. Available from: http://link.springer.com/10.1007/978-1-84800-934-9_42] *Caption from original*

- Maculopapular lesions. These are the most common form of skin involvement, and the most common form of chronic disease. They are often asymptomatic and overlooked by patients.

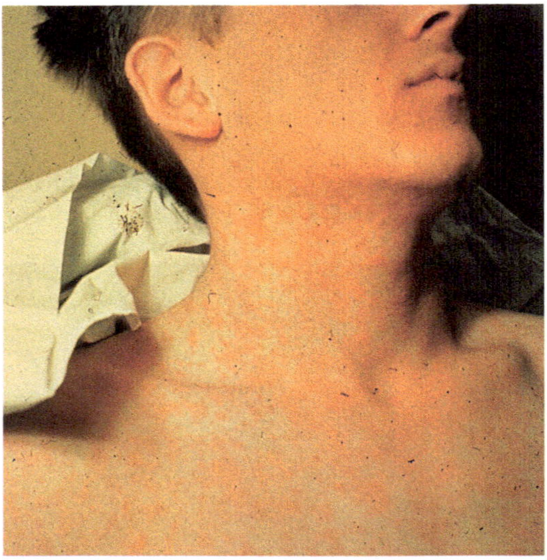

Rash of acquired rubella. The rash of acquired rubella is usually maculopapular, which may eventually coalesce. The rash is usually mild. [Maldonado Y. Chapter 01. In: Wilfert CM, editor. Pediatric infectious diseases. Philadelphia: Current Medicine; 1999. (Mandell GL, editor. Atlas of infectious diseases; vol. 11). ISBN: 0-443-06526-8] *Caption from original*

- Hyper and hypo-pigmentation.

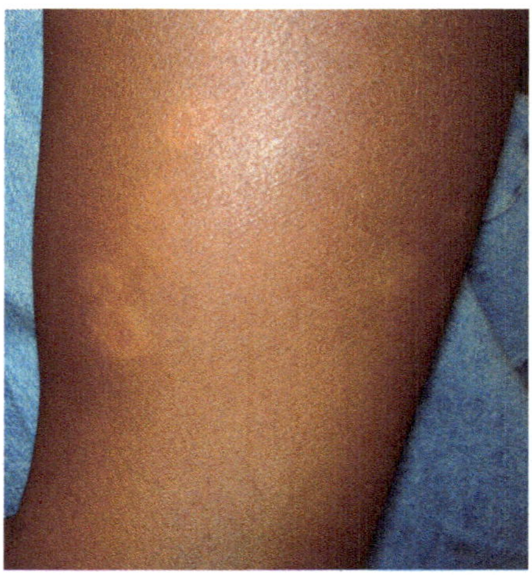

Sarcoidosis on the arm of an African American female demonstrating hypopigmentation. [Goldman S, Pandya AG. Post-inflammatory Hypopigmentation. In: Jackson-Richards D, Pandya AG, editors. Dermatology Atlas for Skin of Color [Internet]. Berlin, Heidelberg: Springer Berlin Heidelberg; 2014 [cited 2015 Jun 17]. p. 9–12.

Available from: http://link.springer.com/10.1007/978-3-642-54446-0_2] *Caption adapted from original*

- Keloid formation.
- Subcutaneous nodules (these are actual granulomas).

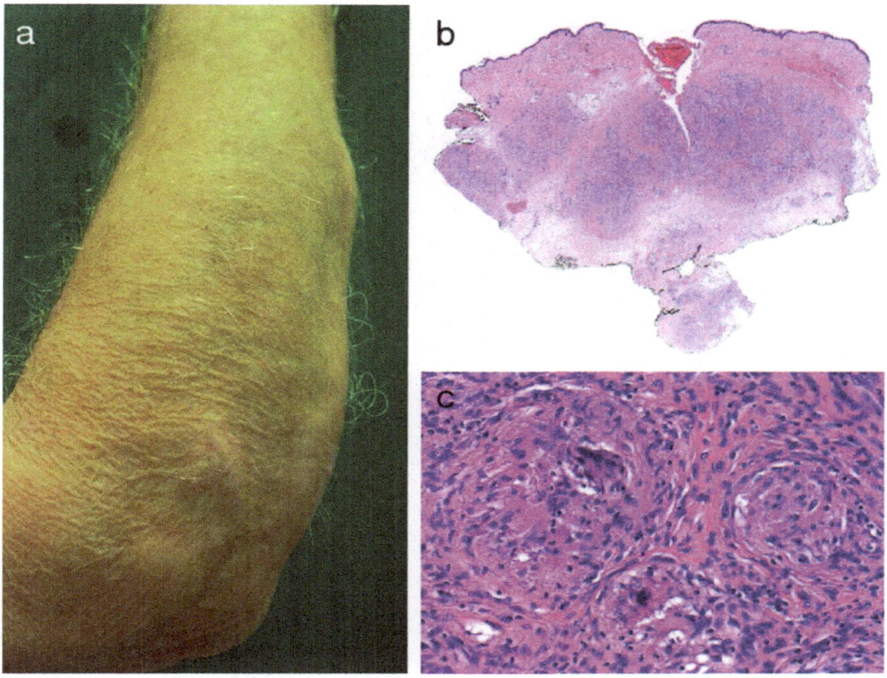

Subcutaneous nodules covered by normal-looking skin on the right forearm (a). Histology confirmed the presence of subcutaneous nodular infiltrates (×4, haematoxylin and eosin) (b), showing the typical features of sarcoid granuloma (×200, haematoxylin and eosin) (c). [Dalle Vedove C, Colato C, Girolomoni G. Subcutaneous sarcoidosis: report of two cases and review of the literature. Clinical Rheumatology. 2011 Aug;30(8):1123–8.] *Caption adapted from original*

- Lupus pernio is a specific complex of skin findings that involves the bridge of the nose, the area beneath the eyes, and the cheeks. This is more common in African Americans and it predicts a progression to chronic disease.

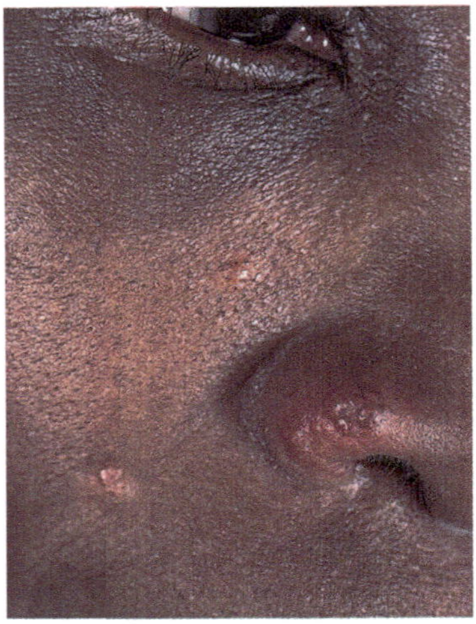

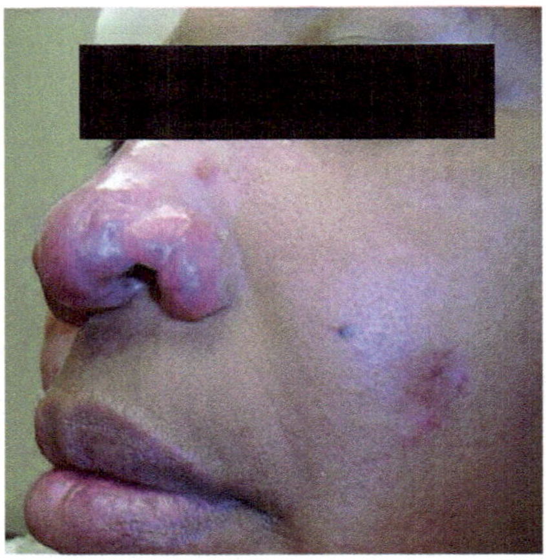

Lupus pernio in an African American female, left face [Jackson-Richards D. Sarcoidosis. In: Jackson-Richards D, Pandya AG, editors. Dermatology Atlas for Skin of Color [Internet]. Berlin, Heidelberg: Springer Berlin Heidelberg; 2014 [cited 2016 Mar 24]. p. 141–5. Available from: http://link.springer.com/10.1007/978-3-642-54446-0_26] *Caption from original*

- Eyes. Anterior uveitis is the most common ophthalmologic manifestation of sarcoidosis. Patients can note tearing, pain, and sometimes changes in visual acuity. In the U.S., only about 10–20 % of sarcoid patients will have eye involvement, but it is more common in African Americans. In Japan, greater than 70% may have eye involvement.

- Liver. Liver involvement can be found in about 50% of patients, but only 10–15 % have elevated liver function tests and clinically significant liver disease.
- Bone Marrow. Bone marrow involvement is often noted by the presence of lymphopenia and anemia. There is infiltration of the bone marrow with granulomas and also sequestration of blood cells in lymphoid tissue (splenomegaly).
- Renal. Seen in less than 5 % of patients. Direct granulomatous infiltration may cause nephritis. Most of the renal complications are secondary to hypercalcemia and hypercalciuria.
- Neurologic. Seen in about 5–10 % of patients. Sarcoidosis can affect any part of the central or peripheral nervous system. Neurosarcoid can cause cranial nerve abnormalities, seizures, and cognitive changes. Involvement of the optic nerve can cause an optic neuritis that is difficult to distinguish from multiple sclerosis.

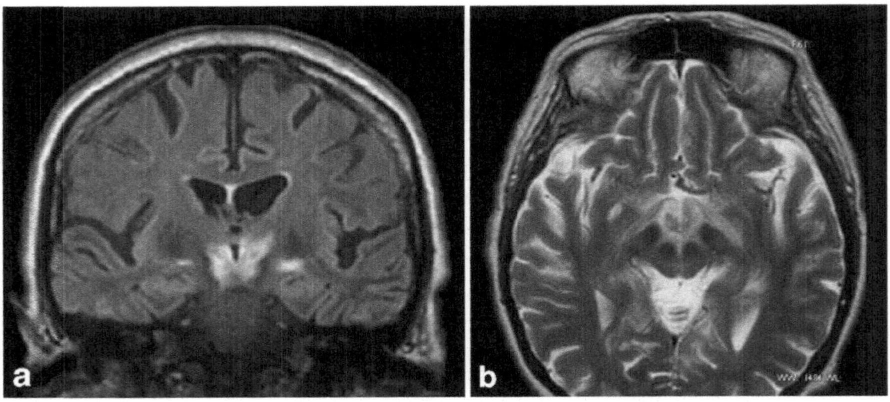

Presumed intracranial sarcoidosis. a The coronal FLAIR and b axial T2-weighted MRI scan show a hyperintense lesion involving the optic chiasm and hypothalamus with posterior extension along both optic tracts which appear hyperintense. [Jäger HR. Loss of vision: imaging the visual pathways. European Radiology. 2005 Mar;15(3):501–10.] *Caption from original*

- Cardiac. Cardiac manifestations are seen in about 2–5 % of patients in the U.S. and Europe, but in up to 25 % of patients in Japan. The most common cardiac manifestations are cardiomyopathy and CHF from diffuse myocardial infiltration, and conduction system abnormalities due to granulomatous infiltration of conduction tissue.
- Bone/joint/muscle. The patient can present with bone cysts that cause myalgias and arthralgias.

Primary Differential Considerations

- When patients present with signs and symptoms such as those that suggest pulmonary sarcoidosis, other diagnoses warranting early consideration include:
  - infection, especially with fungi and tuberculosis.
  - reactions to minerals and metals such as beryllium and aluminum.
  - Wegener granulomatosis.

History and Physical Exam

Findings That Confirm Diagnosis

- There are no pathognomonic historical or physical findings of sarcoidosis.
- Lung exam is often normal. Wheezing is present only when there is endobronchial involvement that causes airway obstruction.
- The diagnosis is confirmed only when typical noncaseating granulomas are found on biopsy of an involved organ in the presence of the usual clinical and radiographic findings and the exclusion of other causes. It is important to remember that there are causes of noncaseating granulomas other than sarcoidosis.
- The identification of classic Löfgren's Syndrome can usually confirm the diagnosis without a need for biopsy.

Factors That Suggest Diagnosis

- The diagnosis can be suggested by the presence of typical symptoms and bilateral hilar adenopathy on the CXR.
- Typical CXR findings can be found in asymptomatic patients who are having a CXR for other reasons.

Factors That Exclude Diagnosis

- The confirmation of an alternative diagnosis that can explain the patient's symptoms and findings can essentially exclude the diagnosis.

Ancillary Studies

Laboratory

- All patients being evaluated for sarcoidosis should have a complete laboratory evaluation that includes a CBC with differential, complete metabolic panel, liver function tests, and a urinalysis. These may not be helpful in diagnosing sarcoidosis, but may lead to a consideration of an alternative diagnosis.
- Testing for HIV should be considered.
- Patients should also have testing for tuberculosis with either a TB skin test, or an interferon gamma release assay.
- Angiotensin converting enzyme (ACE) levels are elevated in about three-quarters of patients with acute, untreated sarcoidosis, but this test is neither sensitive nor specific for the diagnosis of sarcoidosis, with about a 10 % false positive rate. Many diseases can cause a small elevation (about 10% above upper limit of normal) in the ACE level (such as diabetes), while fewer disease are associated with an ACE level that is greater than 1.5 times the upper limit of normal. These include: sarcoidosis, leprosy, Gaucher's disease, hyperthyroidism, miliary tuberculosis.
- Common laboratory abnormalities found in patients with sarcoidosis include:
  - Anemia, usually secondary to anemia of chronic disease (AOCD).
  - Leukopenia, seen in 5–10 % of patients.
  - Hypercalcemia/hypercalciuria are seen in about 10% of patients, and are more common in Caucasians. Sarcoid granulomas can produce 1,25-dihydroxyvitamin D, which leads to increased intestinal absorption of calcium with resultant hypercalcemia and hypercalciuria.
  - While sarcoid granulomas can produce 1,25-dihydroxyvitamin D, nearly all patients with sarcoidosis will have a deficiency of 25-hydroxyvitamin D. The pathologic basis of this has not been elucidated.
  - Elevated alkaline phosphatase (suggests liver involvement).

Imaging

- Imaging is necessary in the evaluation and diagnosis of sarcoidosis.
- The classic finding on plain chest x-ray is bilateral hilar adenopathy. The lung parenchyma may be normal (especially in early disease), or may show diffuse reticular or ground glass opacities.
- The chest x-ray findings have been classified into stages. These stages are only a reflection of the anatomic extent of pulmonary disease, and may not correspond to symptoms and disease activity. They may, however, offer some prognostic information.

- Stage I. Bilateral hilar adenopathy (with or without right paratracheal lymph node enlargement) with no parenchymal changes in the lung. Up to half of all patients will have this as their initial finding of sarcoidosis. Up to 75 % of patients with Stage 1 disease on presentation will have spontaneous regression of adenopathy within 1–3 years. Fewer than 10% will develop chronic enlargement.

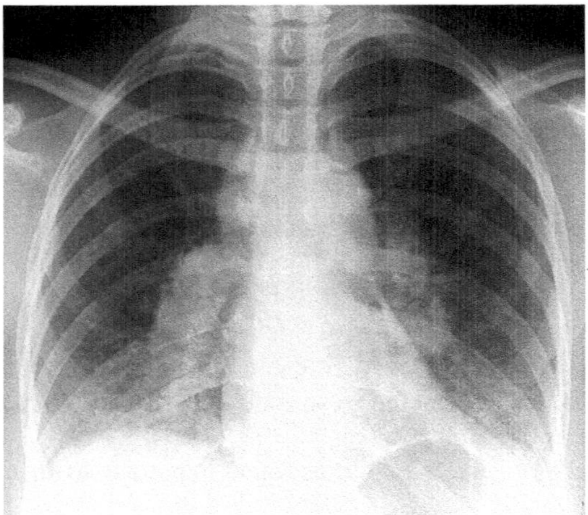

Chest radiograph of a patient with stage I sarcoidosis. [Tanoue L, Elias J. Sarcoidosis. In: Crapo J, editor. Bone's atlas of pulmonary medicine. 3rd ed. Philadelphia: Current Medicine; 2005. ISBN: 1-57340-211-7; 2005-01-14] *Caption adapted from original*

- Stage II. Bilateral hilar adenopathy with associated parenchymal changes, usually reticular opacities (upper lobes predominantly). These changes are found in about 25 % of patients at diagnosis. About two-thirds of patients with stage II findings on CXR at diagnosis will have spontaneous regression, and one-third will go on to have chronic changes. Patients with stage II disease at diagnosis are generally symptomatic.

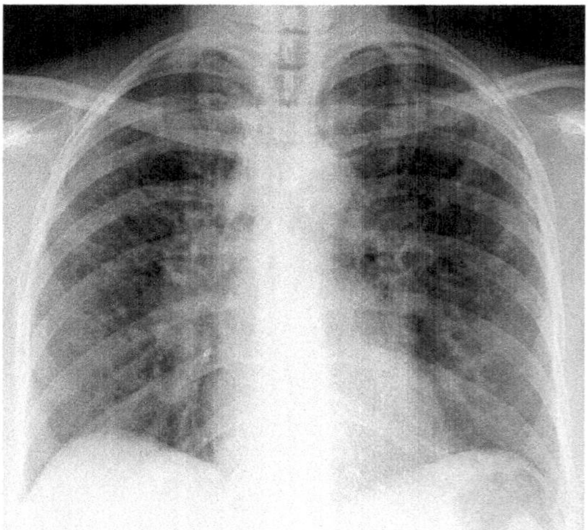

Stage II sarcoidosis. [Tanoue L, Elias J. Sarcoidosis. In: Crapo J, editor. Bone's atlas of pulmonary medicine. 3rd ed. Philadelphia: Current Medicine; 2005. ISBN: 1-57340-211-7; 2005-01-14] *Caption adapted from original*

- Stage III. Marked reticular opacities (again upper lungs >> lower lungs) with regression of hilar nodes.

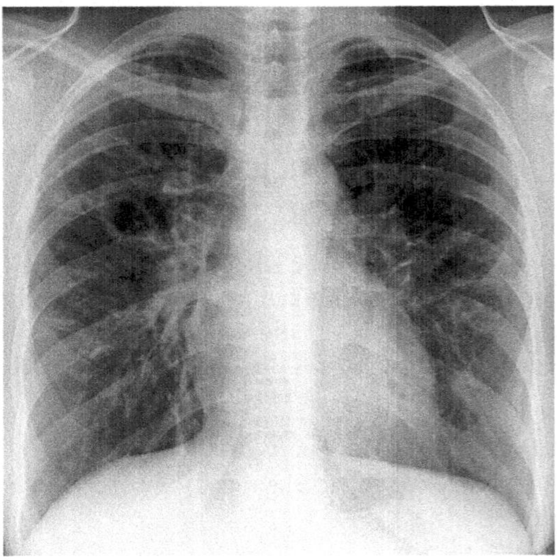

Stage III sarcoidosis. [Tanoue L, Elias J. Sarcoidosis. In: Crapo J, editor. Bone's atlas of pulmonary medicine. 3rd ed. Philadelphia: Current Medicine; 2005. ISBN: 1-57340-211-7; 2005-01-4] *Caption adapted from original*

- Stage IV. Reticular opacities with evidence of volume loss (upper lungs). Consolidated masses of granulomas causing traction bronchiectasis may be seen. Lung tissue calcification, cavitation, and cyst formation may be seen.

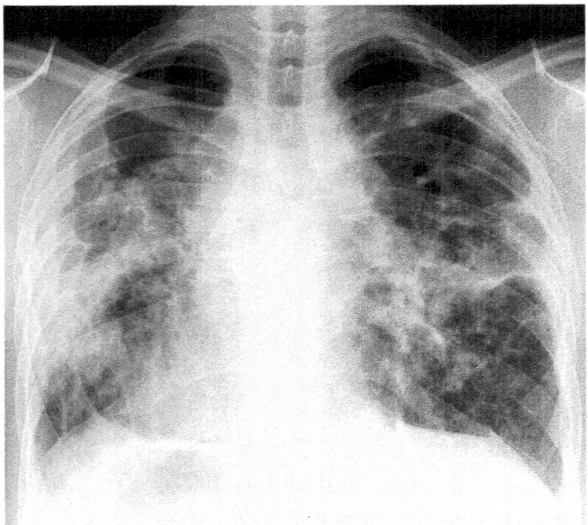

Stage IV sarcoidosis. With extensive fibrosis. [Tanoue L, Elias J. Sarcoidosis. In: Crapo J, editor. Bone's atlas of pulmonary medicine. 3rd ed. Philadelphia: Current Medicine; 2005. ISBN: 1-57340-211-7; 2005-01-4] *Caption adapted from original*

- Other radiologic studies (such as high resolution CT scan [HRCT], PET scanning, gallium scanning), are not necessary in the evaluation of suspected sarcoidosis, but may be obtained for other reasons. They may be helpful in evaluating for alternative diagnoses, and for further supporting the diagnosis of sarcoidosis.
  - HRCT may be performed for the evaluation of dyspnea and cough in a patient with an unremarkable CXR. Many patients will have a HRCT, as it is standard of care in the evaluation of suspected interstitial lung disease. Findings on HRCT in that situation may lead to earlier consideration of the diagnosis. Findings on HRCT that are highly suggestive of sarcoidosis include:
    - Hilar and mediastinal adenopathy
    - Beading or intermittent thickening of the bronchovascular bundles

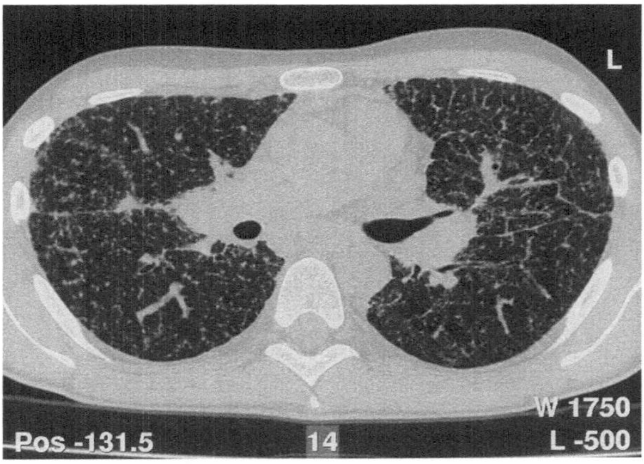

HRCT with the classical perilymphatic distribution of nodules in a patient with sarcoidosis. Note the occurrence of small nodules along subpleural surface and fissures, along interlobular septa and the peribronchovascular bundles giving these structures a "beaded" appearance. This is thought to be pathognomic for sarcoidosis. [Veltkamp M, Grutters JC. The Pulmonary Manifestations of Sarcoidosis. In: Judson MA, editor. Pulmonary Sarcoidosis [Internet]. New York, NY: Springer New York; 2014 [cited 2015 Jun 17]. p. 19–39. Available from: http://link.springer.com/10.1007/978-1-4614-8927-6_2] *Caption from original*

- The use of gallium scanning for the diagnosis of sarcoidosis is currently of only historic interest, as the sensitivity and specificity are low. Gallium scanning may be useful in the unlikely event that there are no easily amenable areas for biopsy. The presence of a panda sign (increased uptake in the parotid and lacrimal glands), and/or a lambda sign (increased activity in the right paratracheal and left hilar lymph nodes), is considered very suggestive of sarcoidosis.

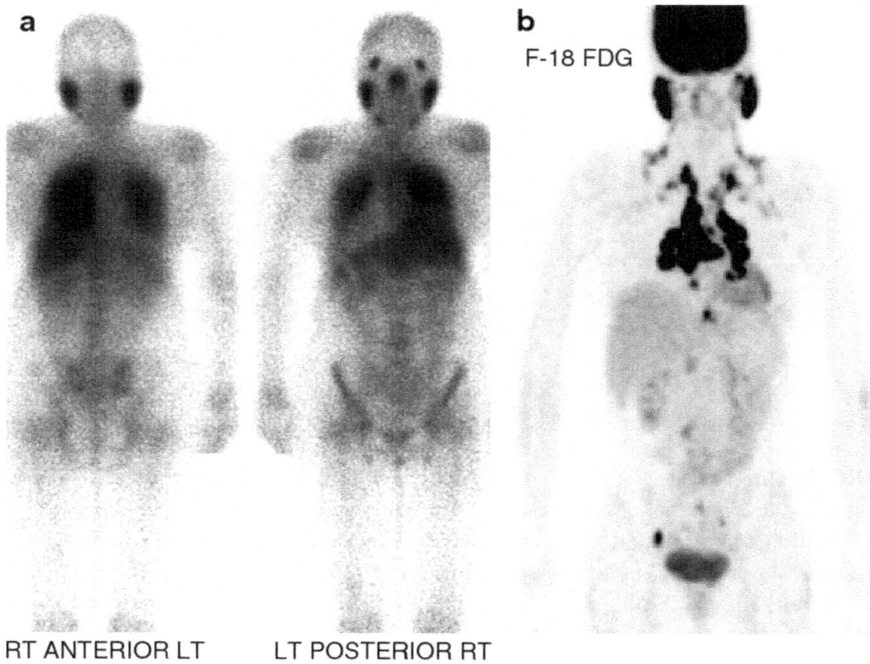

(a) Gallium-67 images for a patient with sarcoidosis illustrating diffuse lung uptake in addition to uptake in salivary glands, lacrimal glands, and inguinal lymph nodes. (b) 18 F-FDG image of a 35-year-old female with proven sarcoidosis. The study shows uptake in the areas of active inflammation in mediastinum, pulmonary hilus, salivary glands, cervical, supraclavicular, axillary, para-aortic, iliac, and inguinal lymph nodes. [Elgazzar AH. Respiratory System. Synopsis of Pathophysiology in Nuclear Medicine [Internet]. Cham: Springer International Publishing; 2014 [cited 2015 Aug 26]. p. 253–72. Available from: http://link.springer.com/10.1007/978-3-319-03458-4_11] *Caption from original*

- Cardiac MRI may be useful in the diagnosis of cardiac sarcoid.

Other

- All patients should have an ECG to screen for conduction abnormalities
- Pulmonary Function Testing. PFT's are not helpful in the diagnosis of sarcoidosis, but they are used to assess the severity of respiratory disease and to monitor the course of the disease. Most patients with early (stage I or II) disease will have normal PFT's. As symptoms worsen patients will usually demonstrate a restrictive pattern on PFT's with a reduced diffusing capacity for

carbon monoxide. If the patient has significant and lumen-narrowing endobronchial lesions, an obstructive pattern may be present on PFT's.

- Biopsies. The majority of patients with suspected sarcoidosis will need to have a biopsy to confirm the diagnosis. In general, biopsies should be obtained from the most accessible of the sites that are affected. This can include skin lesions (except for erythema nodosum), conjunctival lesions, and palpable lymph nodes, among others.
  - Patients who may not need a biopsy include asymptomatic patients with stage I disease on CXR, as the majority of these patients will have spontaneous resolution without progression, and those with classic Löfgren's syndrome.
- Fiber optic bronchoscopy (FOB). Flexible, fiber optic bronchoscopy can be a useful, minimally invasive procedure for the diagnosis of sarcoidosis. During FOB, Bronchoalveolar lavage (BAL), endobronchial biopsy, or transbronchial biopsy can be performed.
  - BAL via flexible bronchoscopy can be a useful and minimally invasive method to help diagnose sarcoidosis. BAL fluid can be evaluated for numbers of CD 4 and 8 cells. Sarcoid is usually associated with a reduced number of CD8 cells, with a ratio of CD4 to CD8 cells greater than 3.5–4:1. BAL is also useful to help exclude malignancy or infections as alternative diagnoses.
  - Endobronchial and transbronchial biopsies have a high yield for the diagnosis of sarcoidosis.

Special Populations

Age

- Sarcoidosis is unusual in children.
- It is, however, well described in patients less than 4 years of age, who most often present with skin, joint, and eye involvement without "typical" pulmonary disease.
- U.S. demographics indicate that southeastern and south central states contain more than 65% of reported cases (Virginia, North and South Carolina, and Arkansas)
- Sarcoidosis is most commonly diagnosed in young to middle-aged adults.

Co-morbidities

- The presence of HIV can make the diagnosis more challenging, as these patients may present atypically, and they are at risk for atypical presentations of many of the alternative diagnoses that need to be considered.
- All the diseases that can present with dyspnea and cough (such as asthma, COPD, CHF, other interstitial lung diseases) can make the diagnosis and management of sarcoidosis more challenging if they exist concurrently.
- However, many of the patients diagnosed with sarcoidosis are young adults and have few if any co-morbid conditions.

Pitfalls in Diagnosis

Critical Steps Not to Miss

- Consideration of the diagnosis is the first critical step.
- Consideration of all alternative diagnoses.
- Recognizing that a gold-standard diagnostic test does not exist, and that the diagnosis generally requires three elements: 1) consistent clinical and radiographic abnormalities; 2) detection of noncaseating granulomas on biopsy; and 3) the exclusion of alternative diagnoses.

Mimics

- As per the differential diagnosis section, many diseases can present with either symptoms consistent with sarcoid (dyspnea, cough, fever, fatigue), granulomas, or hilar adenopathy.

Time-Dependent Interventions

- Sarcoidosis is generally not an acute disease. Löfgren's syndrome (fever, erythema nodosum, arthralgias, and bilateral hilar adenopathy) may present acutely, but often will resolve spontaneously with no specific treatment.
- Symptoms that may indicate involvement of some extra-pulmonary organ systems, especially cardiac, central nervous system, or renal involvement, may require urgent diagnosis and treatment.

Overall Principles of Treatment

- When the diagnosis of sarcoidosis is considered likely, a thorough search should be undertaken to find the presence and extent of involvement of other organ systems.
- All patients should have a complete history that includes an occupational and hobby history.
- All patients should have a thorough skin examination.
- All patients should have an ophthalmologic examination to assess for ocular involvement.
- All patients should have an ECG to screen for conduction abnormalities.
- Laboratory testing as detailed above should be performed.
- Treatment is based upon symptoms. If the patient is asymptomatic and only has CXR findings, it is appropriate to just monitor for the development of symptoms.
- It also is appropriate to monitor patients with only mild symptoms, as about 50 % of cases will resolve spontaneously within 2–5 years.
- If there is mild-to-moderate skin or ocular involvement, it is reasonable to attempt a trial of topical treatment with topical steroids. This treatment should be guided and monitored by an experienced dermatologist/ophthalmologist.
- Systemic glucocorticoids (prednisone, methylprednisolone) are the treatment of choice if systemic treatment is warranted.
- Patients on long-term glucocorticoids, or with intolerable side effects from glucocorticoids, may be candidates for steroid-sparing therapy.
  - Hydroxychloroquine and minocycline may be useful for patients with predominant skin involvement.
  - Cytotoxic therapy may be necessary for patients with significant extrapulmonary sarcoidosis. Methotrexate is the cytotoxic agent with the most clinical experience. It is effective in managing symptoms in up to 65–70 % of those with extrapulmonary sarcoidosis. Other agents include, azathioprine, chlorambucil, and cyclophosphamide.
  - Infliximab, a monoclonal antibody against tumor necrosis factor, has recently been shown to improve lung function in those with chronic sarcoidosis already on glucocorticoids and cytotoxic agents. This agent is a potent immune suppressor, and has been associated with an increased risk for infections, especially reactivation tuberculosis.

Disease Course

- Fifty percent of cases will resolve within 2–5 years.
- About 20 % will go on to develop chronic sarcoidosis.

- The disease is generally non-life-threatening, but organ-threatening disease can occur, especially when there is ocular, cardiac, neurologic, and renal disease.
- Death due to sarcoidosis occurs in less than 5 % of cases, and mostly occurs due to progressive lung, cardiac, neurologic, or renal disease.
- The following factors have been found to be markers for progressive disease:
    - Fibrosis on CXR
    - Lupus pernio
    - Bone cysts
    - Cardiac or neurologic disease
    - Renal calculi due to hypercalciuria
    - Disease requiring systemic glucocorticoid treatment within the first six months of diagnosis

Related Evidence

Papers of particular interest have been highlighted as:
** Of key importance

Review

Hamzeh N, Steckman DA, Sauer WH, Judson MA. Pathophysiology and clinical management of cardiac sarcoidosis. Nat Rev Cardiol. 2015 May;12(5):278-88. https://doi.org/10.1038/nrcardio.2015.22. PMID: 25707386. http://www.ncbi.nlm.nih.gov/pubmed/25707386 **

Jamilloux Y, Kodjikian L, Broussolle C, Sève P. Sarcoidosis and uveitis. Autoimmun Rev. 2014 Aug;13(8):840-9. https://doi.org/10.1016/j.autrev.2014.04.001. PMID: 24704868. http://www.ncbi.nlm.nih.gov/pubmed/24704868

Amin EN, Closser DR, Crouser ED. Current best practice in the management of pulmonary and systemic sarcoidosis. Ther Adv Respir Dis. 2014 Jul 17;8(4):111-132. PMID: 25034021. http://www.ncbi.nlm.nih.gov/pubmed/25034021 **

Baughman RP, Lower EE. Medical therapy of sarcoidosis. Semin Respir Crit Care Med. 2014 Jun;35(3):391-406. https://doi.org/10.1055/s-0034-1376401. PMID: 25007090. http://www.ncbi.nlm.nih.gov/pubmed/25007090 **

Valeyre D, Bernaudin JF, Uzunhan Y, Kambouchner M, Brillet PY, Soussan M, Nunes H. Clinical presentation of sarcoidosis and diagnostic work-up. Semin Respir Crit Care Med. 2014 Jun;35(3):336-51. https://doi.org/10.1055/s-0034-1381229. PMID: 25007086. http://www.ncbi.nlm.nih.gov/pubmed/25007086 **

Heinle R, Chang C. Diagnostic criteria for sarcoidosis. Autoimmun Rev. 2014 Apr-May;13(4-5):383-7. https://doi.org/10.1016/j.autrev.2014.01.035. PMID: 24424172. http://www.ncbi.nlm.nih.gov/pubmed/24424172 **

Spagnolo P, Sverzellati N, Wells AU, Hansell DM. Imaging aspects of the diagnosis of sarcoidosis. Eur Radiol. 2014 Apr;24(4):807-16. https://doi.org/10.1007/s00330-013-3088-3. PMID: 24399491. http://www.ncbi.nlm.nih.gov/pubmed/24399491 **

Valeyre D, Prasse A, Nunes H, Uzunhan Y, Brillet PY, Müller-Quernheim J. Sarcoidosis. Lancet. 2014 Mar 29;383(9923):1155-67. https://doi.org/10.1016/S0140-6736(13)60680-7. PMID: 24090799. http://www.ncbi.nlm.nih.gov/pubmed/24090799 **

Judson MA. Advances in the diagnosis and treatment of sarcoidosis. F1000Prime Rep. 2014 Oct 1;6:89. https://doi.org/10.12703/P6-89. eCollection 2014. PMID: 25374667. http://www.ncbi.nlm.nih.gov/pubmed/25374667 **

Israel-Biet D, Valeyre D. Diagnosis of pulmonary sarcoidosis. Curr Opin Pulm Med. 2013 Sep;19(5):510-5. https://doi.org/10.1097/MCP.0b013e3283645950. PMID: 23880701. http://www.ncbi.nlm.nih.gov/pubmed/23880701 **

Müller-Quernheim J, Prasse A, Zissel G. Pathogenesis of sarcoidosis. Presse Med. 2012 Jun;41(6 Pt 2):e275-87. https://doi.org/10.1016/j.lpm.2012.03.018. PMID: 22595775. http://www.ncbi.nlm.nih.gov/pubmed/22595775 **

Use PubMed Clinical Queries to find the most recent evidence. Use this search strategy:

"Sarcoidosis"[Mesh] OR "Sarcoidosis"

Chapter 67
Sepsis

Charles V. Pollack, Jr., Melissa Platt, Richard M. Cantor, and Jaime Friel Blanck

Name and Synonyms

Sepsis; Severe Sepsis; Septic Shock; Systemic Inflammatory Response Syndrome (SIRS)

Incidence/Epidemiology

- Tenth leading cause of death in the United States.
- 750,000 patients will be hospitalized annually for sepsis in the United States.
    - Males have a higher incidence of sepsis than females.
- Two percent of all hospitalized patients in developed countries suffer from sepsis.
- More than 50 % of severe sepsis patients will require intensive care.
- Mortality rate of septic shock is nearly 50 %.

C. V. Pollack, Jr. (✉)
Department of Emergency Medicine, Thomas Jefferson University, Philadelphia, PA, USA

M. Platt
Department of Emergency Medicine, University of Louisville, Louisville, KY, USA

R. M. Cantor
Department of Emergency Medicine and Pediatrics, State University of New York Upstate Medical University, Syracuse, NY, USA

J. F. Blanck
Welch Medical Library, Johns Hopkins University, Baltimore, MD, USA

C. V. Pollack, Jr. (ed.), *Differential Diagnosis of Cardiopulmonary Disease*,
https://doi.org/10.1007/978-3-319-63895-9_67

- In developing countries sepsis is more common in younger people.
  - Gram negative and atypical pathogens are usually the cause (e.g., malaria)
- Improvement in treatments has decreased the fatality rate, but due to the increase of incidence the number of deaths has increased.
- Most cases of septic shock are hospital-acquired Gram-negative bacilli or Gram-positive cocci.
  - Immunocompromised and chronic illness are risk factors for sepsis.
- Candida or other fungi are rare causes of sepsis.

Differential Diagnosis

- Trauma
- Pancreatitis
- Adrenal insufficiency
- Toxic Shock Syndrome
- Cardiogenic shock
- Hemorrhage
- DIC-Disseminated Intravascular Coagulation
- Heatstroke
- MI
- Myocardial rupture
- Shock

Pathophysiology and Etiology

- Sepsis is a complex, multimediated state that is generally considered to be inflammatory in response to infection. Mediators of inflammation generally cause peripheral vasodilation which, if not reversed, causes blood pressure to drop ("septic shock") and tissues to be hypoperfused.
  - This can be identified by an increase in serum lactate.
  - If severe, this can result in multi-organ system failure.

Mediator	Potential role in intra-abdominal sepsis or injury	Reference(s)
CRP	A serum marker of sepsis that increases in concentration in plasma following abdominal surgery	[20-22]
Haptoglobulin	Elevated expression in blood leukocytes following severe blunt trauma	[23]
IL-1ra	Elevated in plasma following trauma; elevated expression in blood leukocytes following severe blunt trauma	[23,24]
IL-6	Potent inflammatory mediator and marker of sepsis; elevated levels correlate with length of hospital stay, complications, and mortality among patients with intra-abdominal sepsis; elevated levels in peritoneal fluid in a porcine model of intra-abdominal sepsis; elevated plasma/serum levels following abdominal surgery; elevated plasma levels following severe trauma associate with injury severity, development of organ dysfunction, and poor outcomes, including mortality	[21-23,25-28,44-50]
IL-8	Potent neutrophil chemoattractant; elevated expression in blood leukocytes following severe blunt trauma	[23,29]
IL-10	Elevated serum levels during intra-abdominal sepsis; blocks pro-inflammatory cytokine release; elevated after abdominal surgery	[30-32]
IL-15	Elevated levels in serum correlate with organ dysfunction and poor patient prognosis	[33]
IL-17	Potent pro-inflammatory mediator; promotes neutrophil recruitment to the peritoneal cavity and enhanced bacterial clearance in a mouse model of intra-abdominal sepsis; elevated plasma levels in select patients following severe trauma	[28,34,35]
IL-22	Elevated serum levels during intra-abdominal sepsis	[30]
IL-33	Mediates neutrophil recruitment to peritoneum; promotes bacterial clearance and reduces mortality in a mouse model of intra-abdominal sepsis	[36]
MCP-1 (CCL2)	Potent monocyte chemoattractant; serum levels elevated in a rat model of intra-abdominal sepsis; elevated expression in blood leukocytes following severe blunt trauma	[23,37]
M-CSF	Elevated in plasma following trauma	[24]
MIF	Present early in sepsis and remains elevated for a prolonged time period; significantly higher levels in non-survivors of sepsis compared to survivors; MIF neutralization reduces mortality in a mouse model of intra-abdominal sepsis	[38,39]
PDGF	Elevated in plasma following trauma	[24]
Procalcitonin	Marker of infectious complications following abdominal surgery and negatively associated with survival; elevated after abdominal surgery	[32,40]
TNF-α	Serum levels elevated in a rat model of intra-abdominal sepsis	[37]
tPA	Enhances bacterial clearance, reduces cellular influx, increases plasma and peritoneal IL-12 and IL-10 levels, and reduces lung and liver damage in a mouse model of intra-abdominal sepsis	[16]
TRAIL	Promotes inflammatory cell recruitment to the peritoneum, enhances bacterial clearance, and reduces mortality in a mouse model of intra-abdominal sepsis; modulates apoptosis	[41,42]

CCL2, Chemokine (C-C motif) ligand 2; CRP, C-reactive protein; IL-1ra, Interleukin-1 receptor antagonist; IL-6, Interleukin-6; IL-8, Interleukin-8; IL-10, Interleukin-10; IL-15, Interleukin-15; IL-17, Interleukin-17; IL-22, Interleukin-22; IL-33, Interleukin-33; MCP-1, Monocyte chemoattractant protein-1; M-CSF, Macrophage colony-stimulating factor; MIF, Macrophage migration inhibitory factor; PDGF, Platelet-derived growth factor; TNF-α, Tumor necrosis factor-alpha; tPA, Tissue plasminogen activator; TRAIL, Tumor necrosis factor-related apoptosis-inducing ligand.

Inflammatory mediators associated with intra-abdominal sepsis or injury, including abdominal surgery, among studies of animals or humans [From article: Efficacy and safety of active negative pressure peritoneal therapy for reducing the systemic inflammatory response after damage control laparotomy (the Intra-peritoneal Vacuum Trial): study protocol for a randomized controlled trial. Trials. 2013;14(1):141. https://doi.org/10.1186/1745-6215-14-141, at http://link.springer.com/article/10.1186%2F1745-6215-14-141; by Derek J Roberts, Craig N Jenne, Chad G Ball, Corina Tiruta, Caroline Léger, Zhengwen Xiao, Peter D Faris, Paul B McBeth, Christopher J Doig, Christine R Skinner, Stacy G Ruddell, Paul Kubes, Andrew W Kirkpatrick, © Roberts et al.; licensee BioMed Central Ltd. 2013; licensed under Creative Commons Attribution License BY 2.0 http://www.creativecommons.org/licenses/by/2.0] *Caption from original; See http://link.springer.com/10.1186/1745-6215-14-141 for references*

- Sepsis can result from any infectious etiology, bacterial, viral, or fungal. Nonbacterial causes are more common in immunocompromised patients.

Presentation

Typical/"Classic"

- Fever, dyspnea, altered mental status, nausea and vomiting, cough, SOA, abdominal pain, diarrhea and dysuria.
  - **SIRS**-4 criteria, **Sepsis = infection with ≥ 2 SIRS criteria**
    - Temperature > 38°C or < 36°C
    - HR > 90 bpm
    - RR > 20/min or $PaCO_2$ < 32 mm Hg
    - WBC > 12,000/mm^3, or > 10 % band forms

Stage	Clinical symptoms	Value
SIRS (≥2 symptoms)	Temperature	<36 °C or >38 °C
	Heart rate	>90 beats/minute
	Respiratory rate	>20 breaths/minute or $PaCO_2$<32 mmHg
	White blood cell count	>12,000 cells/mm^3 or < than 4,000 cells/mm^3
Sepsis	SIRS with proven infection	
Severe sepsis	Sepsis with organ dysfunction hypoperfusion and/or hypotension	
Septic shock	Severe sepsis, hypoperfusion and/or hypotension despite adequate fluid resuscitation	

Systemic Inflammatory Response Syndrome (SIRS) and sepsis stages [Loonen AJM, Wolffs PFG, Bruggeman CA, van den Brule AJC. Developments for improved diagnosis of bacterial bloodstream infections. European Journal of Clinical Microbiology & Infectious Diseases. 2014 Oct;33(10):1687–702.] *Caption from original*

- **Severe Sepsis** is indicated if the patient presents with an additional sign or symptom, such as those in the following list, that indicates an organ may be failing:
  - Decrease urine output
  - Confusion
  - Difficulty breathing
  - Decreased platelet count
- **Septic Shock:** The patient must present signs and symptoms of severe shock and decreased blood pressure that is not responding to fluid replacement treatments.

Atypical

- Older patients, immunocompromised patients, and patients on beta blockers may present without overt signs of shock. Younger patients with normal physiologic reserve may maintain normal vital signs and mentation for a relatively long period of time before suddenly manifesting shock.

Primary Differential Considerations

- Consider the following alternative diagnoses:
  - ARDS
  - Cardiogenic shock
  - DKA
  - Myocardial rupture
  - Toxic shock syndrome

History and Physical Exam

- **History and risk factors:**
  - Immunosuppressive states
  - Underlying terminal illnesses
  - Recent chemotherapy
  - Malignancy
  - Splenectomy
  - HIV
  - Diabetes
  - Nursing home
  - Source of infections: abdominal exam, rectal exam, chest exam, any rashes, decubitus ulcers, indwelling catheters, CNS infections.

Findings That Confirm Diagnosis

- Dyspnea
- Fever
- Nausea/vomiting
- Blood Pressure <90 mmHg, mean arterial pressure <70 mmHg, decrease in SBP>40 mmHg.
- Poor organ perfusion with early sign of flushed skin or later signs with cool skin due to redirection of blood flow to organs.
- Tachycardia >90 bpm
- Confusion/depressed consciousness-may be caused by encephalopathy
- Components of the "SIRS" (Systemic Inflammatory Response Syndrome) score are helpful in establishing the diagnosis of sepsis. A calculator and guidance for interpreting a SIRS score can be found at http://www.mdcalc.com/sirs-sepsis-and-septic-shock-criteria/.

Factors That Suggest Diagnosis

- Hyperthermia/hypothermia
- Tachypnea
- Tachycardia
- Prolonged capillary refill time

Factors That Exclude Diagnosis

- Negative blood cultures

Ancillary Studies

Laboratory

- CBC
- Lactate: Elevated lactate can be a manifestation of organ hypoperfusion.
- Blood cultures prior to antibiotics
- Platelet count
- Hematocrit
- Electrolytes
- BUN
- Creatinine
- Bilirubin
- Ca, Mg, pH
- C-reactive protein
- Cortisol level
- INR/prothrombin time/partial thromboplastin time
- LFT's
- Urine analysis and culture
- Pro calcitonin

Screening tests	Prothrombin time
	APTT
	Platelets
	Fibrinogen INR
Confirmatory tests	Soluble fibrin monomer complex
	Fibrinogen degradation products
	D-dimer
	Prothrombin fragments 1 and 2
	Antithrombin III

Screening and coagulopathy tests in the diagnosis of consumption coagulopathy (DIC) [Gullo A, Celestre CM, Paratore AL, Silvestri L, van Saene HK. Sepsis and Organ(s) Dysfunction. In: Gullo A, editor. Anaesthesia, Pharmacology, Intensive Care and Emergency APICE [Internet]. Milano: Springer Milan; 2014 [cited 2015 Aug 31]. p. 157–91. Available from: http://link.springer.com/10.1007/978-88-470-5516-2_14] *Caption from original*

Imaging

- Chest X-ray
- Soft tissue plain films
- Imaging to locate source of infections
  - CT of abdomen and pelvis
  - Ultrasound for gallbladder, etc.

Other

- Lumbar puncture
- Central Venous pressure measurement
- SvO_2 measurement

Special Populations

Age

Pediatric

- Reports of pediatric sepsis are increasing nationwide, accounting for nearly 8 percent of patients treated in Pediatric ICUs.
- Primary sources of sepsis are primary bacteremia and respiratory infection.
- Organisms to consider are:
  - Staphylococcus aureus, including MRSA
  - S pneumonia
  - S pyogenes
  - Group B streptococcus in neonates
  - Coagulase negative Staphylococcus in children with indwelling catheters
- Viral infections may mimic bacterial sepsis, particularly respiratory pathogens.
- It is not unusual to have co-infections with viral etiologies and bacterial superinfection.
- Hallmarks of treatment remain early recognition, culture acquisition, volume replacement, and the administration of broad spectrum antibiotics.
- When treating children for sepsis, check labs frequently, as it is important to avoid hyponatremia and hypoglycemia.
- Dexamethasone should be given early for streptococcal bacterial meningitis.

Neonate

- Septic shock often manifests with:
  - Hypoglycemia
  - Seizures
  - Disseminated intravascular coagulation (DIC)
  - Cardiovascular collapse and death if untreated

Antibiotic class	Oral bioavailability	Protein binding	CNS penetration	Metabolism	Excretion	$t_{½}$
Aminoglycosides						
Gentamicin	Poorly absorbed	<25 %	Extracellular fluids and vascularized tissues; poor CSF penetration	None	Renal	<1 week PGA: 5–14 h; ≥1 week PGA: 3–5 h[a]
Aminopenicillins						
Ampicillin	50 %	10 %	Penetrates most tissues; poor CSF penetration	Hepatic (10 %)	Renal (25–40 %)	2–7 days PNA: 4 h; 8–14 days PNA: 2.8 h; 15–30 days PNA: 1–1.8 h
Cephalosporins						
Cefotaxime	Not administered orally	30–50 %	Penetrates most tissues; adequate CSF penetration when meninges are inflamed	Hepatic	Renal (60 %)	BW ≤1.5 kg: 4.6 h BW >1.5 kg: 3.4 h
Glycopeptides						
Vancomycin	Poorly absorbed	30 %	Penetrates most tissues; erratic CSF penetration	None	Renal; minimal biliary	4–11 h (dependent upon renal maturation)

Comparative pharmacokinetic data are derived from DiCenzo et al., Yoshioka et al., Rodvold et al. [132–134]

[a] For neonates <1 week PGA, the $t_{½}$ of aminoglycoside agents is inversely associated with BW

BW birthweight, *CNS* central nervous system, *CSF* cerebrospinal fluid, *PGA* post-gestational age, *PNA* postnatal age, $t_{½}$ elimination half-life

Comparative pharmacokinetics, bioavailability, protein binding, central nervous system penetration, metabolism, and excretion of antibiotics used in the empiric treatment of neonatal sepsis [Stockmann C, Spigarelli MG, Campbell SC, Constance JE, Courter JD, Thorell EA, Olson J, Sherwin CMT. Considerations in the Pharmacologic Treatment and Prevention of Neonatal Sepsis. Pediatric Drugs. 2014 Feb;16(1):67–81.] *Caption from original*; *See http://link.springer.com/10.1007/s40272-013-0057-x for references*

Antifungal class	Oral bioavailability	Protein binding	CNS penetration	Metabolism	Excretion	$t_{½}$
Polyenes						
Amphotericin B	Poorly absorbed[a]	90 %[a]	Poor CSF penetration (<5 % of plasma concentration)[a]	Minimal hepatic[a]	Renal[a]	50 h
Liposomal amphotericin B	Poorly absorbed[a]	Unknown	Poor CSF penetration (<1 % of plasma concentration)[a]	Unknown	Unknown	100–153 h[a]
Cytosine analogs						
5-Fluorocytosine	80 %[a]	3–4 %[a]	Good CSF penetration (74 % of plasma concentration)[a]	Minimal hepatic[a]	Renal (90 %); feces (10 %)	3–6 h
Azoles						
Fluconazole	>90 %[a]	11–12 %[a]	Good CSF penetration (75 % of plasma concentration)[a]	Minimal[a]	Renal[a]	Pre-term: 74 h; 1 week PNA: 53 h; 2 weeks PNA: 47 h
Echinocandins						
Caspofungin	Poorly absorbed	97 %[a]	Poor CSF penetration (0 % of plasma concentration)[a]	Hepatic[a]	Renal (42 %); feces (35 %)	40 h
Micafungin	Poorly absorbed	>99 %	Poor CSF penetration (0 % of plasma concentration)[a]	Hepatic	Feces (71 %)	7 h

Comparative pharmacokinetic data are derived from Baley et al., Walsh et al., Smith et al., Wurthwein et al., Piper et al., Wade et al., and Doby et al. [69, 72, 74, 135–138]

CNS central nervous system, *CSF* cerebrospinal fluid, *PNA* postnatal age, $t_{½}$ elimination half-life

[a] Data obtained from adults (applicability to neonates is unclear)

Comparative pharmacokinetics, bioavailability, protein binding, central nervous system penetration, metabolism, and excretion of antifungals used in the empiric treatment of neonatal sepsis [Stockmann C, Spigarelli MG, Campbell SC, Constance JE, Courter JD, Thorell EA, Olson J, Sherwin CMT. Considerations in the Pharmacologic Treatment and Prevention of Neonatal Sepsis. Pediatric Drugs. 2014 Feb;16(1):67–81.] *Caption from original; See http://link.springer.com/10.1007/s40272-013-0057-x for references*

Co-morbidities

- Cancer
- Chronic-obstructive pulmonary Disease
- Immunosuppressed
- Congestive Heart Failure (CHF)
- Diabetes
- HIV/AIDS
- Renal Disease

Pitfalls in Diagnosis

Critical Steps Not to Miss

- Misdiagnosing septic arthritis
- In elderly and nursing home patients, watch for bedsores, UTI's, etc.
- Always consider the risk of sepsis in immunocompromised patients (diabetes, HIV, cancer on chemotherapy, etc.)
- Serum lactate should be done early and blood cultures prior to antibiotics. Placement of central line and broad spectrum of tests to identify source or infection.

Mimics

- Inflammatory colitis
- Hypovolemia
- Medication effects
- Adrenal insufficiency
- Acute myocardial infarction
- Acute pulmonary embolus

Time-Dependent Interventions

- Airway and breathing stabilization are a priority. Utilize supplemental oxygen with pulse oximetry. Intubation may be required.
- Assess perfusion. Utilize aggressive fluid resuscitation for hypotension (excluding patients with heart failure).
- Central line.
- Saline boluses until CVP > 8 cm H_2O
- Initiate pressors—Norepinephrine or dopamine.
- Administer antibiotics early, based on most likely organism.
- Additional therapies (conflicting evidence) include inotropic therapy or red blood cell transfusions

Sepsis resuscitation bundle—(to be started immediately and completed within 6 h)
• Serum lactate measured
• Blood cultures obtained prior to antibiotic administration
• Broad-spectrum antibiotics administered within 3 h for ED admissions and 1 h for non-ED ICU admissions
• In the event of hypotension and/or lactate >4 mmol/L:
– Deliver a minimum of 20 ml/kg of crystalloid (or colloid equivalent)
– Apply vasopressors for hypotension not responding to initial fluid resuscitation to maintain mean arterial pressure (MAP) ≥65 mmHg
• In the event of persistent arterial hypotension despite volume resuscitation (septic shock) and/or initial lactate >4 mmol/L (36 mg/dl):
– Achieve central venous pressure (CVP) of ≥8 mmHg
– Achieve central venous oxygen saturation ($ScvO_2$) of ≥70%[a]
Sepsis management bundle—(to be started immediately and completed within 24 h)
• Low-dose steroids administered for septic shock in accordance with a standardized ICU policy
• Glucose control maintained ≥lower limit of normal, but <150 mg/dl (8.3 mmol/L)
• For mechanically ventilated patients inspiratory plateau pressures maintained <30 cmH_2O

[a]Achieving a mixed venous oxygen saturation of 65% is an acceptable alternative

Sepsis Bundles: The goal is to perform all indicated tasks 100% of the time within the first 6 h (Sepsis Resuscitation Bundle) or first 24 h (Sepsis Management Bundle) of the diagnosis of severe sepsis [Kreiner LA, Moore LJ. Early Management of Sepsis, Severe Sepsis, and Septic Shock in the Surgical Patient. In: Moore LJ, Turner KL, Todd SR, editors. Common Problems in Acute Care Surgery [Internet].

New York, NY: Springer New York; 2013 [cited 2015 Aug 31]. p. 73–91. Available from: http://link.springer.com/10.1007/978-1-4614-6123-4_6] *Caption from original*

Overall Principles of Treatment

- The primary goal of managing sepsis is to address inflammation by restoring perfusion and treating the infection.
- Early goal-directed therapy (EGDT) targets to be measured:
  - Mean arterial pressure (MAP) $\geq$65 mmHg
  - Urine output $\geq$0.5 mL/kg/hr
  - Predictors of fluid responsiveness
  - Central venous oxyhemoglobin saturation ($Scv0_2$) $\geq$65 percent
  - Lactate clearance should be followed
- Protocol-directed therapies assist in management of septic patients.
- Early antimicrobial therapy is important and should be targeted at the likely primary site. Broad-spectrum coverage with at least two agents is usually indicated.
- Additional therapies:
  - Glucocorticoids: pathogenesis of sepsis involves host inflammatory response.
  - Nutrition: nutritional support improves nutritional outcomes.
  - Intensive insulin therapy: hyperglycemia and insulin resistance.
  - External cooling: controlling fever.
  - Investigational therapies: cytokine and toxin inactivation.

Prevention and Treatment Summary

Author (year)	Subject #	Method	Outcome
Primary Prevention			
Murugan (2012)	1,836	Prospective cohort	Statin use in patients with pneumonia not associated with reduction in acute kidney injury
Rothberg (2012)	121,254	Retrospective review	Modest reduction in non-ICU pneumonia mortality
Novack (2012)	17,802	Placebo controlled	No reduction in sepsis incidence. Modest reduction in pneumonia incidence
Nseir (2012)	342	Retrospective review	Mortality reduction in patients with bacteremia Statin use more than 12 weeks prior to bacteremia increased benefit
Leung (2012)	2,139	Retrospective cohort	Statin use not associated with improved survival in patients with bloodstream infection
Yende (2011)	1,895	Multicenter inception	No reduction in severe sepsis or 90-cohort day mortality
O'Neal (2011)	575	Prospective cohort	Reduction in risk of developing severe sepsis and acute lung injury
Al Harbi (2011)	763	Nested cohort	Reduction in severe sepsis related hospital mortality
Williams (2011)	2,642	Prospective cohort	No reduction in infection related 30-day mortality
Goodin (2011)	568	Retrospective cohort	No reduction of vasopressor duration, ICU length or stay, or hospital mortality
Secondary Prevention			
Kruger (2011)	150	Placebo-controlled	Continuation of statin in patients with infection did not reduce risk of developing sepsis
Novack (2009)	83	Placebo-controlled	Patients with infection randomized to statin therapy had reduced TNF-α and IL-6 levels
Treatment			
Patel (2011)	100	Placebo controlled	Atorvastatin reduced risk of sepsis progression
Dessap (2011)	76	Retrospective cohort	Continuation of statin in patients with severe sepsis and septic shock was not associated with reduction in severity of organ failure or mortality

Recent clinical reports on the prevention and treatment of sepsis [Mermis JD, Simpson SQ. HMG-CoA Reductase Inhibitors for Prevention and Treatment of Severe Sepsis. Current Infectious Disease Reports. 2012 Oct;14(5):484–92.] *Caption from original*

Severe Sepsis and Septic Shock Protocols

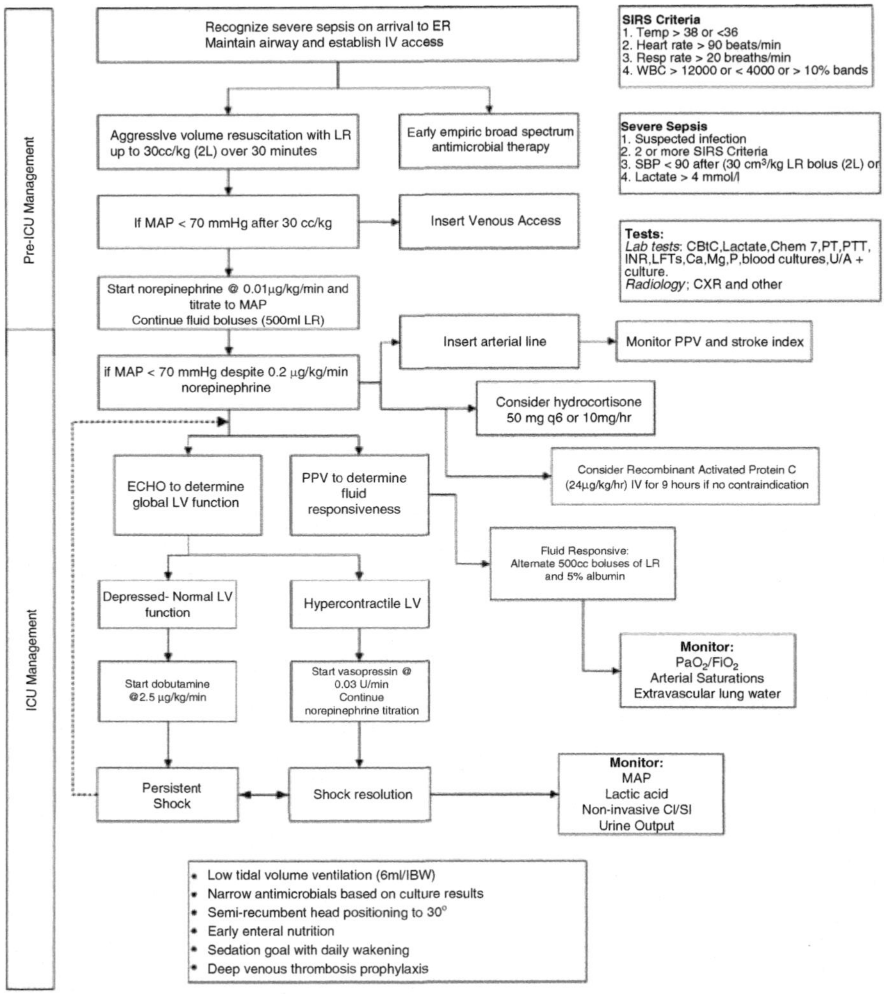

Sepsis Management Protocol. [Marik PE. Sepsis. Handbook of Evidence-Based Critical Care [Internet]. New York, NY: Springer New York; 2010 [cited 2015 Aug 31]. p. 95–116. Available from: http://link.springer.com/10.1007/978-1-4419-5923-2_10] *Caption from original*

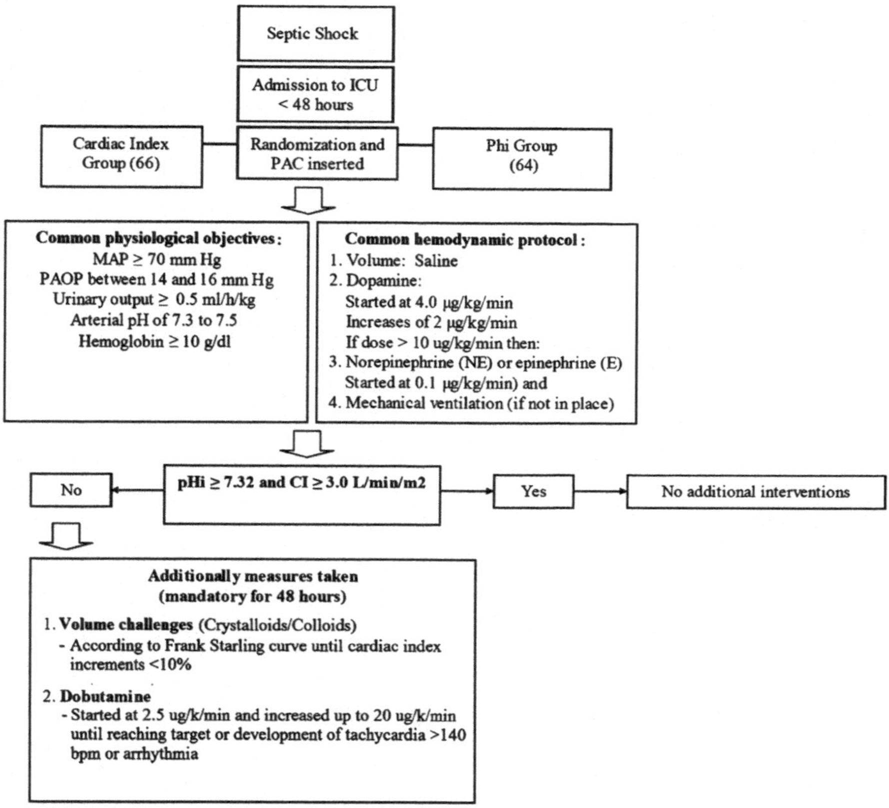

Septic-shock resuscitation protocol. [From article: Gastric tonometry versus cardiac index as resuscitation goals in septic shock: a multicenter, randomized, controlled trial. Critical Care. 2009;13(2):R44. https://doi.org/10.1186/cc7767, at http://link.springer.com/article/10.1186%2Fcc7767; by Fernando Palizas, Arnaldo Dubin, Tomas Regueira, Alejandro Bruhn, Elias Knobel, Silvio Lazzeri, Natalio Baredes, Glenn Hernández, © Palizas et al.; licensee BioMed Central Ltd. 2009; licensed under Creative Commons Attribution License BY 2.0 http://creativecommons.org/licenses/by/2.0] *Caption from original*

Disease Course

- Sepsis is a high-risk syndrome that is sometimes fatal even with aggressive treatment. Current literature suggests that early recognition and early, aggressive, goal-directed treatment are associated with better outcomes.

Related Evidence

Papers of particular interest have been highlighted as:
*** Of key importance*

Practice Guideline

Brady MT, Polin RA. Prevention and management of infants with suspected or proven neonatal sepsis. Pediatrics. 2013 Jul;132(1):166-8. https://doi.org/10.1542/peds.2013-1310. Epub 2013 Jun 10. PubMed PMID: 23753101. http://www.ncbi.nlm.nih.gov/pubmed/23753101 **

Dellinger RP, Levy MM, Rhodes A, Annane D, Gerlach H, Opal SM, Sevransky JE, Sprung CL, Douglas IS, Jaeschke R, Osborn TM, Nunnally ME, Townsend SR, Reinhart K, Kleinpell RM, Angus DC, Deutschman CS, Machado FR, Rubenfeld GD, Webb S, Beale RJ, Vincent JL, Moreno R; Surviving Sepsis Campaign Guidelines Committee including The Pediatric Subgroup. Surviving Sepsis Campaign: international guidelines for management of severe sepsis and septic shock, 2012. Intensive Care Med. 2013 Feb;39(2):165-228. https://doi.org/10.1007/s00134-012-2769-8. Epub 2013 Jan 30. PubMed PMID: 23361625. http://www.ncbi.nlm.nih.gov/pubmed/23361625 **

Dellinger RP, Levy MM, Rhodes A, Annane D, Gerlach H, Opal SM, Sevransky JE, Sprung CL, Douglas IS, Jaeschke R, Osborn TM, Nunnally ME, Townsend SR, Reinhart K, Kleinpell RM, Angus DC, Deutschman CS, Machado FR, Rubenfeld GD, Webb SA, Beale RJ, Vincent JL, Moreno R; Surviving Sepsis Campaign Guidelines Committee including the Pediatric Subgroup. Surviving sepsis campaign: international guidelines for management of severe sepsis and septic shock: 2012. Crit Care Med. 2013 Feb;41(2):580-637. https://doi.org/10.1097/CCM.0b013e31827e83af. PubMed PMID: 23353941. http://www.ncbi.nlm.nih.gov/pubmed/23353941 **

Brierley J, Carcillo JA, Choong K, Cornell T, Decaen A, Deymann A, Doctor A, Davis A, Duff J, Dugas MA, Duncan A, Evans B, Feldman J, Felmet K, Fisher G, Frankel L, Jeffries H, Greenwald B, Gutierrez J, Hall M, Han YY, Hanson J, Hazelzet J, Hernan L, Kiff J, Kissoon N, Kon A, Irazuzta J, Lin J, Lorts A, Mariscalco M, Mehta R, Nadel S, Nguyen T, Nicholson C, Peters M, Okhuysen-Cawley R, Poulton T, Relves M, Rodriguez A, Rozenfeld R, Schnitzler E, Shanley T, Kache S, Skippen P, Torres A, von Dessauer B, Weingarten J, Yeh T, Zaritsky A, Stojadinovic B, Zimmerman J, Zuckerberg A. Clinical practice parameters for hemodynamic support of pediatric and neonatal septic shock: 2007 update from the American College of Critical Care Medicine. Crit Care Med. 2009 Feb;37(2):666-88. https://doi.org/10.1097/CCM.0b013e31819323c6. Erratum in: Crit Care Med. 2009 Apr;37(4):1536. Skache, Sara [corrected to Kache, Saraswati]; Irazusta, Jose [corrected to Irazuzta, Jose]. PubMed PMID: 19325359; PubMed Central PMCID: PMC4447433. http://www.ncbi.nlm.nih.gov/pubmed/19325359

Meta-Analysis

Zhang L, Zhu G, Han L, Fu P. Early goal-directed therapy in the management of severe sepsis or septic shock in adults: a meta-analysis of randomized controlled trials. BMC Med. 2015 Apr 3;13:71. https://doi.org/10.1186/s12916-015-0312-9. PubMed PMID: 25885654; PubMed Central PMCID: PMC4393610. http://www.ncbi.nlm.nih.gov/pubmed/25885654

Bakhuizen SE, de Haan TR, Teune MJ, van Wassenaer-Leemhuis AG, van der Heyden JL, van der Ham DP, Mol BW. Meta-analysis shows that infants who have suffered neonatal sepsis face an increased risk of mortality and severe complications. Acta Paediatr. 2014 Dec;103(12):1211-8. https://doi.org/10.1111/apa.12764. Epub 2014 Sep 7. Review. PubMed PMID: 25073543. http://www.ncbi.nlm.nih.gov/pubmed/25073543

Review

Seymour CW, Rosengart MR. Septic Shock: Advances in Diagnosis and Treatment. JAMA. 2015 Aug 18;314(7):708-17. https://doi.org/10.1001/jama.2015.7885. Review. PubMed PMID: 26284722. http://www.ncbi.nlm.nih.gov/pubmed/26284722 **

Plunkett A, Tong J. Sepsis in children. BMJ. 2015 Jun 9;350:h3017. https://doi.org/10.1136/bmj.h3017. Review. Erratum in: BMJ. 2015;350:h3704. PubMed PMID: 26060188. http://www.ncbi.nlm.nih.gov/pubmed/26060188

Green JM. Essentials of sepsis management. Surg Clin North Am. 2015 Apr;95(2):355-65. https://doi.org/10.1016/j.suc.2014.10.006. Epub 2014 Dec 4. Review. PubMed PMID: 25814111. http://www.ncbi.nlm.nih.gov/pubmed/25814111 **

Cawcutt KA, Peters SG. Severe sepsis and septic shock: clinical overview and update on management. Mayo Clin Proc. 2014 Nov;89(11):1572-8. https://doi.org/10.1016/j.mayocp.2014.07.009. Epub 2014 Nov 3. Review. PubMed PMID: 25444488. http://www.ncbi.nlm.nih.gov/pubmed/25444488 **

de Montmollin E, Annane D. Year in review 2013: Critical Care--sepsis. Crit Care. 2014 Oct 15;18(5):578. https://doi.org/10.1186/s13054-014-0578-x. Review. PubMed PMID: 25673430; PubMed Central PMCID: PMC4331148. http://www.ncbi.nlm.nih.gov/pubmed/25673430

Yende S, Iwashyna TJ, Angus DC. Interplay between sepsis and chronic health. Trends Mol Med. 2014 Apr;20(4):234-8. https://doi.org/10.1016/j.molmed.2014.02.005. Epub 2014 Mar 14. Review. PubMed PMID: 24636941; PubMed Central PMCID: PMC4016696. http://www.ncbi.nlm.nih.gov/pubmed/24636941

Bloos F, Reinhart K. Rapid diagnosis of sepsis. Virulence. 2014 Jan 1;5(1):154-60. https://doi.org/10.4161/viru.27393. Epub 2013 Dec 11. Review. PubMed PMID:

24335467; PubMed Central PMCID: PMC3916369. http://www.ncbi.nlm.nih.gov/pubmed/24335467

Mayr FB, Yende S, Angus DC. Epidemiology of severe sepsis. Virulence. 2014 Jan 1;5(1):4-11. https://doi.org/10.4161/viru.27372. Epub 2013 Dec 11. Review. PubMed PMID: 24335434; PubMed Central PMCID: PMC3916382. http://www.ncbi.nlm.nih.gov/pubmed/24335434 **

Schorr CA, Zanotti S, Dellinger RP. Severe sepsis and septic shock: management and performance improvement. Virulence. 2014 Jan 1;5(1):190-9. https://doi.org/10.4161/viru.27409. Epub 2013 Dec 11. Review. PubMed PMID: 24335487; PubMed Central PMCID: PMC3916373. http://www.ncbi.nlm.nih.gov/pubmed/24335487

Angus DC, van der Poll T. Severe sepsis and septic shock. N Engl J Med. 2013 Aug 29;369(9):840-51. https://doi.org/10.1056/NEJMra1208623. Review. Erratum in: N Engl J Med. 2013 Nov 21;369(21):2069. PubMed PMID: 23984731. http://www.ncbi.nlm.nih.gov/pubmed/23984731

Coelho FR, Martins JO. Diagnostic methods in sepsis: the need of speed. Rev Assoc Med Bras. 2012 Jul-Aug;58(4):498-504. Review. PubMed PMID: 22930032. http://www.ncbi.nlm.nih.gov/pubmed/22930032

Martin GS. Sepsis, severe sepsis and septic shock: changes in incidence, pathogens and outcomes. Expert Rev Anti Infect Ther. 2012 Jun;10(6):701-6. https://doi.org/10.1586/eri.12.50. Review. PubMed PMID: 22734959; PubMed Central PMCID: PMC3488423. http://www.ncbi.nlm.nih.gov/pubmed/22734959

Soong J, Soni N. Sepsis: recognition and treatment. Clin Med. 2012 Jun;12(3):276-80. Review. PubMed PMID: 22783783. http://www.ncbi.nlm.nih.gov/pubmed/22783783 **

Lever A, Mackenzie I. Sepsis: definition, epidemiology, and diagnosis. BMJ. 2007 Oct 27;335(7625):879-83. Review. PubMed PMID: 17962288; PubMed Central PMCID: PMC2043413. http://www.ncbi.nlm.nih.gov/pubmed

Use PubMed Clinical Queries to find the most recent evidence. Use this search strategy:

("Shock, Septic"[Mesh] OR "Systemic Inflammatory Response Syndrome"[Mesh] OR "Sepsis"[Mesh] OR "sepsis" OR "septic shock" OR "SIRS" OR "Systemic inflammatory response syndrome")

Chapter 68
Tachyarrhythmias

Charles V. Pollack, Jr., Richard M. Cantor, and Jaime Friel Blanck

Name and Synonyms

Tachyarrhythmias

Incidence/Epidemiology

- "Tachyarrhythmias" include several distinct syndromes of varying incidence and epidemiology.
- A tachycardia (fast heart rate) is defined as a ventricular rate of 100 beats per minute or more, and may be regular or irregular in rhythm.
- The diagnoses addressed in this discussion include:
  - Sinus tachycardia, which is not a primary tachycardia (i.e., it is not caused by an abnormality of the cardiac conducting system).
  - Multifocal atrial tachycardia (MAT), which is most often seen in patients with lung disease such as COPD.
  - Atrial fibrillation (AFib), the most common arrhythmia, in which the atria do not beat in a coordinated fashion, and which may present with a "controlled" (less than 100 bpm) or "rapid" (greater than 100) ventricular rate.

C. V. Pollack, Jr. (✉)
Department of Emergency Medicine, Thomas Jefferson University, Philadelphia, PA, USA

R. M. Cantor
Department of Emergency Medicine and Pediatrics, State University of New York Upstate Medical University, Syracuse, NY, USA

J. F. Blanck
Welch Medical Library, Johns Hopkins University, Baltimore, MD, USA

C. V. Pollack, Jr. (ed.), *Differential Diagnosis of Cardiopulmonary Disease*,
https://doi.org/10.1007/978-3-319-63895-9_68

An American who lives until age 75 without atrial fibrillation has a one-in-four chance of developing AFib during the rest of his or her life.
- Atrial flutter (AFlutt), a less stable rhythm than AFib, where the atria beat regularly, but not every beat is transmitted to the ventricles.
- Paroxy mal supraventricular tachycardia (PSVT), which may be seen more often in younger patients than AFib or AFlutt.
- Wolff-Parkinson-White syndrome, in which an alternate transmission route for the electrical impulses through the heart is present.
- Ventricular tachycardia (VT), the most lethal of the tachyarrhythmias, is usually the result of myocardial ischemia.

- There are much rarer types of tachyarrhythmias that are beyond the scope of this review.

Differential Diagnosis

- Tachycardia is a straightforward diagnosis, confirmed with an ECG or even a manual pulse check. The important diagnostic inquiries related to tachycardia are centered on the actual rhythm (e.g., supraventricular vs ventricular) and underlying etiology of the rapid heart rate. Diagnostic considerations include but are not limited to:
  - Acute myocardial infarction
  - Acute heart failure
  - Pulmonary embolism
  - Sepsis
  - Myocarditis
  - Hypoxemia
  - Hypovolemia
  - Anemia
  - Hyperthyroidism
  - Poisoning or withdrawal syndrome

Pathophysiology and Etiology

- Tachyarrhythmias may be primary (i.e., the result of a defective cardiac electrical conduction system or cardiac injury) or secondary (e.g., tachycardia as a result of withdrawal syndromes, thyroid storm, or sepsis).
- Tachyarrhythmias may be associated with chest pain and dyspnea because they derive from a primary ischemic etiology such as acute myocardial ischemia, or they may cause ischemic pain because the rate does not allow sufficient time for perfusion of stressed myocardium.

- Sinus tachycardia is a normal physiologic response to stress, such as fever, anemia, exercise, anxiety, or hypotension. The patient's normal QRS morphology is present.

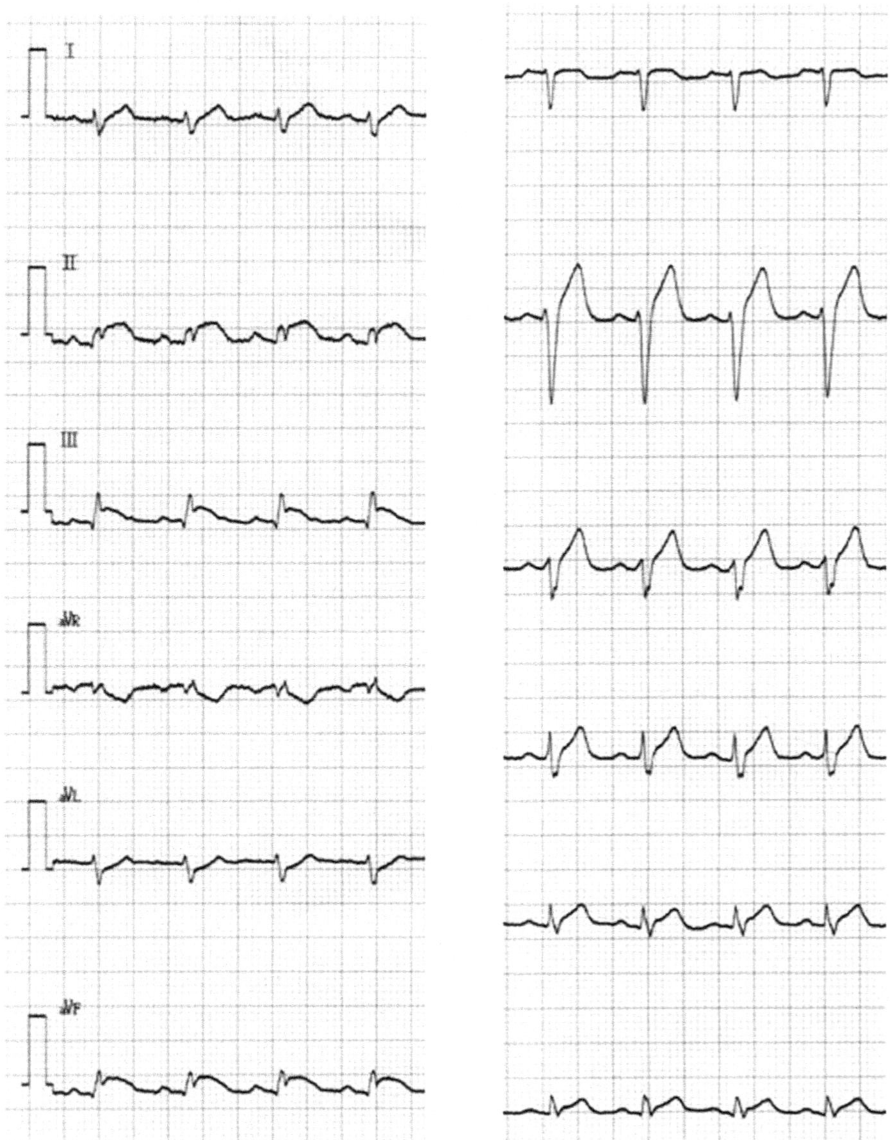

Electrocardiogram on admission showing sinus tachycardia with significant ST elevation in leads II, III, aVF, and V2–V4 [Okai I, Inoue K, Maruyama M, Maruyama S, Komatsu K, Nishizawa H, Okazaki S, Fujiwara Y, Sumiyoshi M, Daida H. Transbrachial intra-aortic balloon pumping for a patient with fulminant myocarditis. Heart Vessels. 2012 Nov 1;27(6):639–42.] *Caption from original*

Medical conditions	Physiological	Drugs, substances
Hyperthyroidism	Exercise	Caffeine
Cushing's disease	Emotion	Alcohol
Pheochromocytoma	Pain	Tobacco
Anemia	Fever	Catecholamines
Infection	Pregnancy	Vasodilators
Dehydration	Volume depletion	Atropinic substances
Cardiomyopathy		Theophylline
Panic attack		Illicit drugs: cocaine
Pericarditis		Decongestants
Aortic or mitral regurgitation		Sympathomimetics
Myocardial infarction		Thyroid hormones
Postural hypotension		

Explainable causes of sinus tachycardia that should be ruled out before making the diagnosis of inappropriate sinus tachycardia. [Peyrol M, Lévy S. Clinical presentation of inappropriate sinus tachycardia and differential diagnosis. J Interv Card Electrophysiol. 2016 Jun 1;46(1):33–41.] *Caption from original*

- Multifocal atrial tachycardia is caused by multiple sites of competing atrial electrical activity. The atrial rate by definition exceeds 100 bpm, and there are multiple morphologically identifiable p-waves. Conduction to the ventricles is 1:1, but the P-P intervals are variable. It is characterized by an irregular atrial rate greater than 100 beats per minute (bpm).

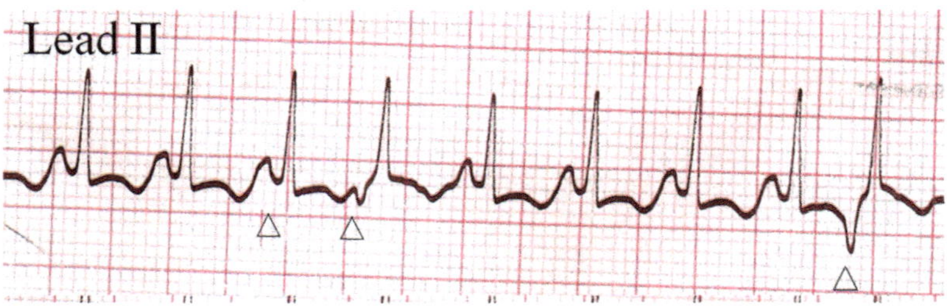

Three different morphologies of P-wave complexes (arrowheads) suggesting multifocal atrial tachycardia [Shabanian R, Kiani A, Rad EM, Eslamiyeh H. Lown-Ganong-Levine Syndrome in a 3-Month-Old Infant with Isolated Left Ventricular Noncompaction. Pediatr Cardiol. 2010 Feb 1;31(2):274–6.] *Caption from original*

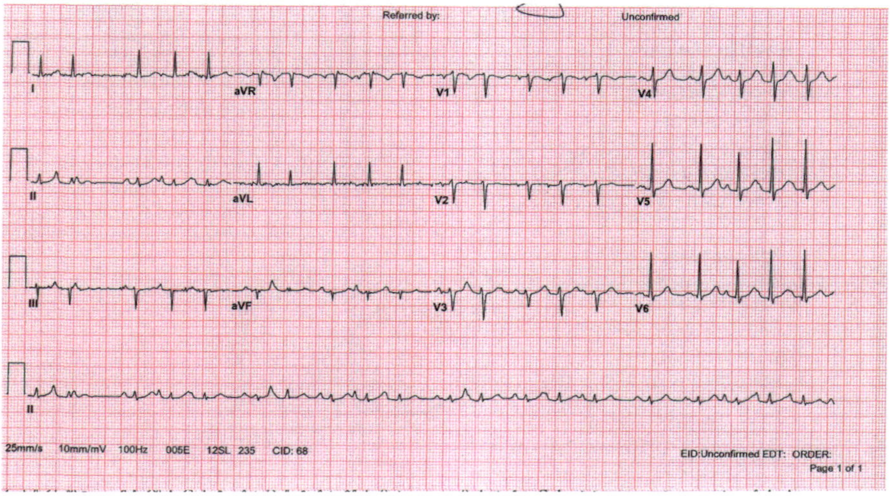

Multifocal atrial tachycardia (MAT). The diagnosis is made by three or more ectopic (i.e., not all sinus) P-waves. The heart rate (approximately 100–140 bpm) may be variable due to the site of ectopy or non-conduction of certain P-waves. MAT is commonly observed in patients with chronic obstructive pulmonary disease. [Chung EH, Martin DT. Management of Postoperative Arrhythmias. In: O'Donnell JM, Nácul FE, editors. Surgical Intensive Care Medicine [Internet]. Springer US; 2010 [cited 2017 May 24]. p. 209–27. Available from: http://link.springer.com/chapter/10.1007/978-0-387-77893-8_21] *Caption from original*

- Atrial fibrillation may be isolated, paroxysmal, or persistent. The first two are often prompted by an episode of emotional stress, hormonal stress, trauma, surgery, or intoxication. Persistent AFib usually is a manifestation of structural heart disease or chronic lung disease. It is manifest on the ECG and by manual pulse check as an "irregularly irregular" rhythm, reflecting uncoordinated, chaotic atrial activity that does not send the ventricles a clear and regular signal to contract. The ECG typically shows an erratic electrical baseline between QRS complexes.

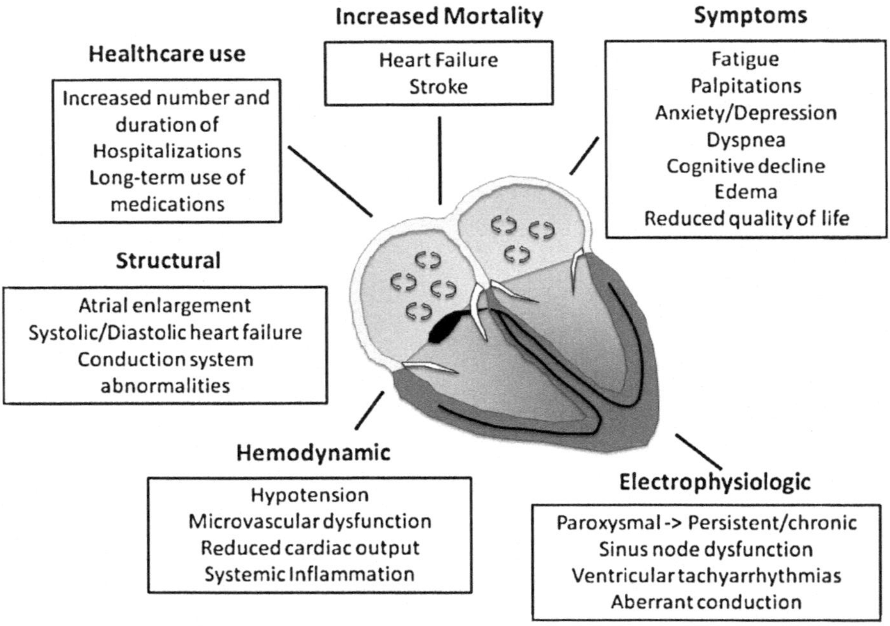

Broad consequences of atrial fibrillation. [Bunch TJ, Gersh BJ. Rhythm Control Strategies and the Role of Antiarrhythmic Drugs in the Management of Atrial Fibrillation: Focus on Clinical Outcomes. J GEN INTERN MED. 2011 May 1;26(5):531–7.] *Caption from original*

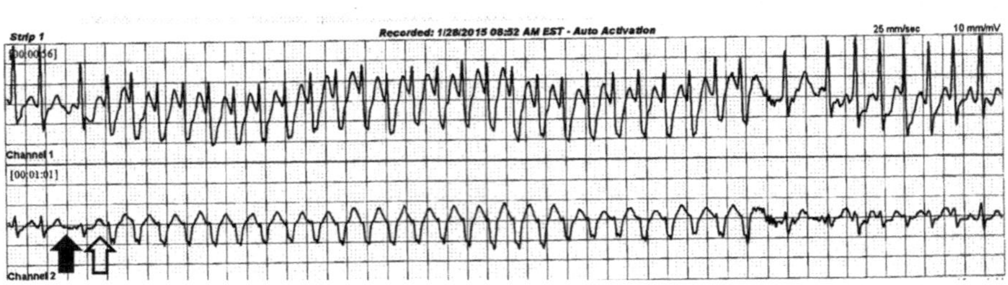

Ambulatory event monitor tracing showing long-short initiation of aberrant ventricular conduction during atrial fibrillation. The preceding long R-to-R interval is indicated by the *black-filled arrow* and the short R-to-R interval is indicated by the *unfilled arrow* [Winchester DE, Kaufmann MR, McKillop MS, Miles WM. Pitfalls in the Acute Management of Atrial Fibrillation. In: Peacock WF, Clark CL, editors. Short Stay Management of Atrial Fibrillation [Internet]. Springer International Publishing; 2016 [cited 2017 Jun 2]. p. 145–73. (Contemporary Cardiology). Available from: http://link.springer.com/chapter/10.1007/978-3-319-31386-3_14] *Caption from original*

- Atrial flutter is usually transient and is characterized by a regular atrial rate between 250 and 350 bpm, with a regular ventricular response to every third (3:1 conduction) or fourth (4:1 conduction) atrial beat. The ECG will typically show "sawtooth" p-waves in the inferior leads.

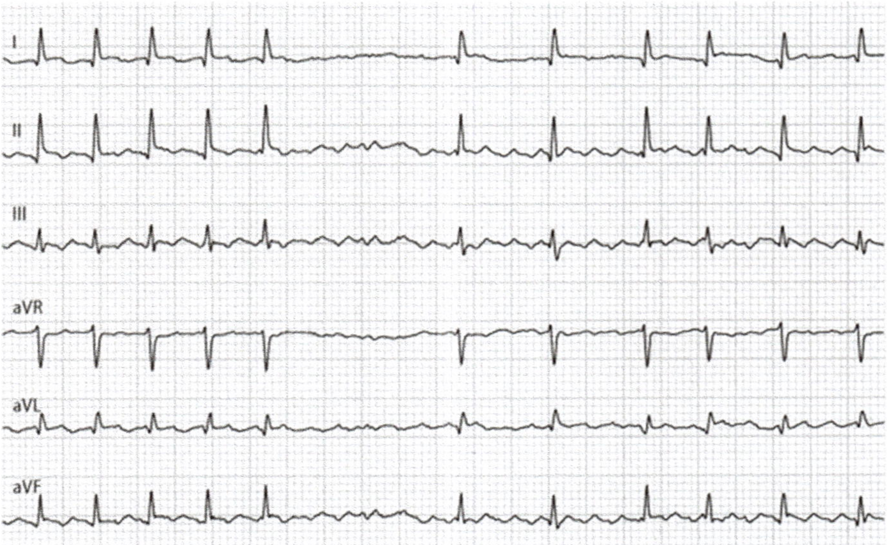

Six-lead ECG immediately after admission revealing the typical signs of atrial flutter [Haas NA, Wegendt C, Schäffler R, Kirchner G, Welisch E, Kind K, Blanz U, Kececioglu D. ECMO for cardiac rescue in a neonate with accidental amiodarone overdose. Clin Res Cardiol. 2008 Dec 1;97(12):878–81.] *Caption from original*

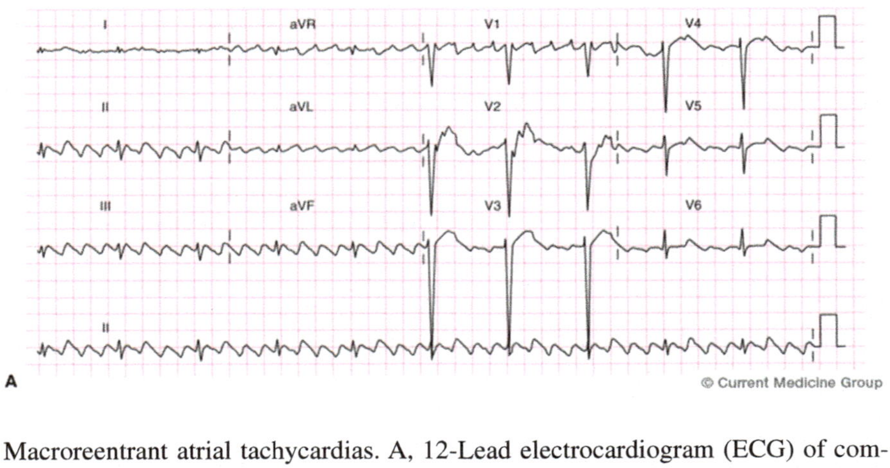

Macroreentrant atrial tachycardias. A, 12-Lead electrocardiogram (ECG) of common counterclockwise atrial flutter. Note the typical sawtooth P-waves in leads II, III, and aVF. [Epstein L, Stevenson W, Steven D, Seiler J, Roberts-Thomson K, See

V. Chapter 7 Arrhythmias. In: Libby P, editor. Essential atlas of cardiovascular disease. 4th ed. Philadelphia: Current Medicine Group; 2009.] *Caption adapted from original*

- PSVT is caused by functional differences in conduction and refractoriness in the AV node, or by the existence of an "accessory" or "bypass" tract involving the SA and AV nodes. The atrial rate is typically 120–180 bpm and conduction to the ventricles is usually 1:1 with a normal QRS morphology.

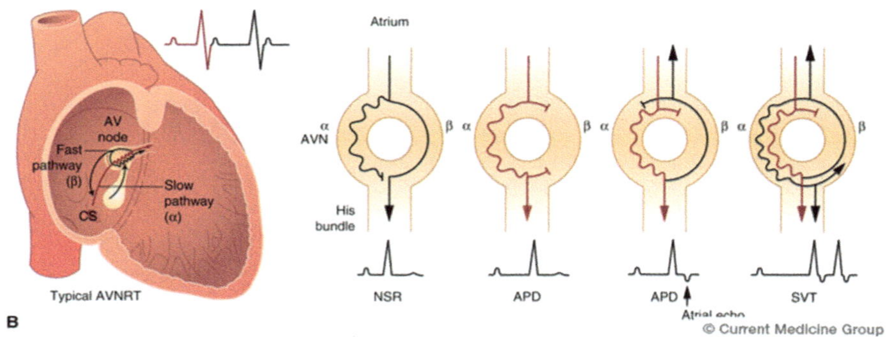

The mechanism of the common form of AVNRT. A lobe of the AV node extends inferiorly along the tricuspid annulus, anterior to the coronary sinus os, which functions as a slowly conducting pathway. During AVNRT-conduction occurs from inferior to superior through the slow pathway, then through the compact portion of the AV node to the His bundle and retrograde through this superior portion of the AV node to the atrium. The path from the compact AV node back down to the slow pathway may involve musculature around the coronary sinus, within the atrium, or may be largely confined to the AV node. Initiation of AV nodal reentry is shown in schematics on the right in which α is the slow AV nodal pathway and β is the fast pathway. During normal sinus rhythm (NSR), an impulse from the atrium enters the AV node and travels down both the slow and fast pathways with the impulse from the fast pathway reaching the His bundle first and activating the ventricles with a short PR interval. Collision of fast pathway and slow pathway impulses in the distal portion of the AV node prevents reentry. An atrial premature depolarization (APD) that blocks in the fast pathway (β) allows conduction of the impulse down the slow pathway to the ventricles, thus a longer PR interval. If this impulse blocks in the distal fast pathway, no reentry occurs. However, an APD can produce an atrial echo beat if the fast pathway has recovered allowing the impulse to continue retrogradely in the fast pathway back to the atrium. If the slow pathway has recovered to allow conduction, the impulse may continue circulating as supraventricular tachycardia (SVT). [Epstein L, Stevenson W, Steven D, Seiler J, Roberts-Thomson K, See V. Chapter 7 Arrhythmias. In: Libby P, editor. Essential atlas of cardiovascular disease. 4th ed. Philadelphia: Current Medicine Group; 2009.] *Caption adapted from original*

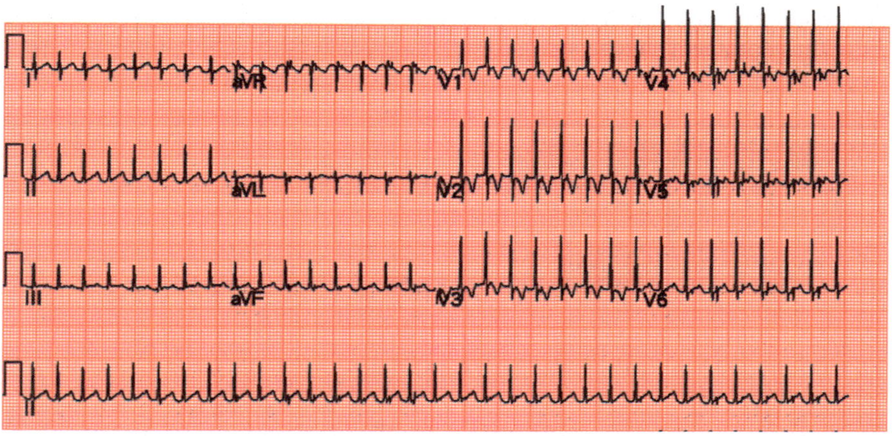

Electrocardiogram. Initial ECG with paroxysmal supraventricular tachycardia [From article: A male infant had subdural effusion and paroxysmal supraventricular tachycardia during the febrile episode of Kawasaki disease: a case report and literature review. BMC Pediatr. 2016 Dec 1;16(1):71. https://doi.org/10.1186/s12887-016-0606-x at https://link.springer.com/article/10.1186/s12887-016-0606-x by Chia-Pei Chou, I-Chun Lin, Kuang-Che Kuo, © Chou et al. 2016; licensee BioMed Central Ltd.; licensed under Creative Commons Attribution 4.0 International License http://creativecommons.org/licenses/by/4.0/] *Caption from original*

- WPW is a specific type of tachycardia that results from firing along an accessory electrical conduction tract. It is also called "pre-excitation syndrome" and often shows a particular upsloping of the QRS complex ("delta wave"). It can be associated with congenital cardiac anomalies such as Ebstein's anomaly. The QRS complex in WPW is often wide and the p-wave appears normal.

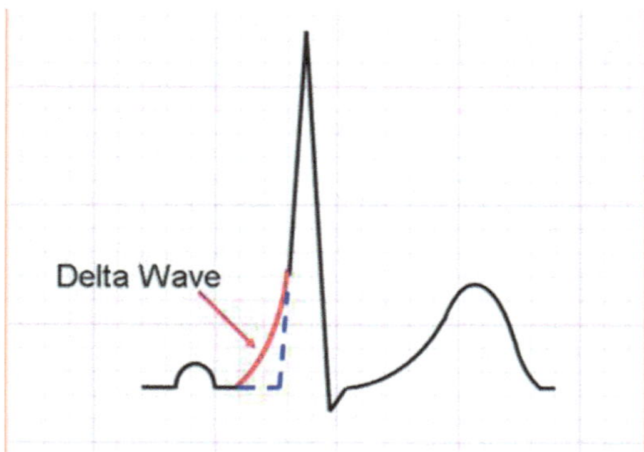

Delta wave, seen in WPW syndrome [Gnanaprakasam R, David S. Acute Cardiac Arrhythmias. In: David SS, editor. Clinical Pathways in Emergency Medicine

[Internet]. Springer India; 2016 [cited 2017 May 24]. p. 101–15. Available from: http://link.springer.com/chapter/10.1007/978-81-322-2710-6_8] *Caption from original*

Morphologic features of Ebstein anomaly	% of patients	Reference(s)
1. Adhesion of the posterior and septal leaflets to the underlying myocardium with displacement of the hinge point of the septal leaflet into the ventricular cavity, and atrialization of the right ventricle. [a]	100 %	[10]
[By echocardiography, exaggerated displacement of the septal leaflet into the ventricular cavity in the apical four-chamber view.]		
2. Dilatation of the tricuspid valve annulus[a]	100 %	[9]
3. Redundancy ± fenestrations of the anterior tricuspid valve leaflet [a]	100 %	[9]
4. Right ventricular dilatation	66 %	[7]
Associated echocardiographic abnormalities		
1. Varying degrees of tricuspid regurgitation	100 %	[11]
2. Atrial communication (patent foramen ovale or atrial septal defect)	50 % 89 %	[9, 11, 40••]
3. Ventricular septal defect	2 %	[40••]
4. Tricuspid stenosis		
5. Right ventricular outflow tract obstruction (functional or anatomic pulmonary atresia)	6 %	[40••]
6. Mitral valve prolapse	13 %	[9]
7. Bicuspid aortic valve	5 %	[9]
8. Left ventricular abnormalities (noncompaction, systolic and diastolic dysfunction)		
9. Partially anomalous pulmonary venous drainage	2 %	[40••]
Associated electrocardiographic abnormalities		
1. Right bundle branch block	58 % 68 %	[9, 11]
2. First degree heart block	31 %	[9]
3. Pre-excitation	18 % 44 %	[9, 11, 40••]
4. Nonspecific intraventricular conduction delay/block	15 %	[9]

[a] Required for diagnosis.

Morphologic features of Ebstein anomaly and associated abnormalities. References available at https://link.springer.com/article/10.1007/s11936-014-0338-x [Arya P, Beroukhim R. Ebstein Anomaly: Assessment, Management, and Timing of Intervention. Curr Treat Options Cardio Med. 2014 Oct 1;16(10):338.] *Caption adapted from original*

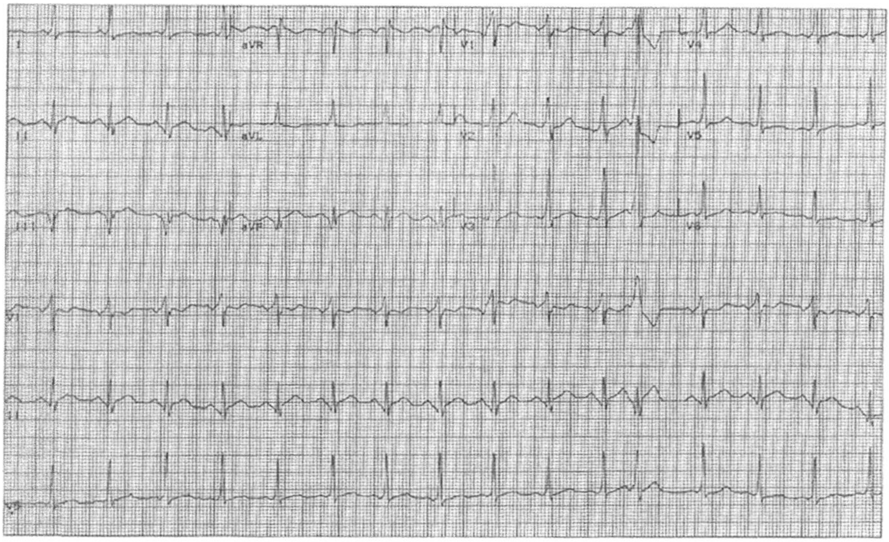

An electrocardiogram (ECG) from a 34-year-old asymptomatic aircrew member showing typical features of the Wolff-Parkinson-White (WPW) syndrome—ie, a short P-R interval and delta waves in multiple leads. [Ferry D, Anholm J, Blomqvist GC, Levine B, Lane L, Buckey J, Wachholz C. Chapter. In: Crawford C, editor. Heart Disease In Presence of Disorders of Other Organ Systems. 1st ed. Philadelphia: Current Medicine; 1996 (Braunwald E, editor. Atlas of heart diseases; vol. 6.)] *Caption adapted from original*

- Ventricular tachycardia is a potentially lethal tachyarrhythmia that is usually associated with structural heart disease, including ischemia. Occasionally it is seen in patients with intoxications, with metabolic derangements, with long QT syndrome, and, rarely, without identifiable precipitant. VT that persists more than 30 seconds is called sustained VT. Because it is driven by a ventricular pacemaker, the QRS complex is wide. VT may or may not generate a palpable pulse.

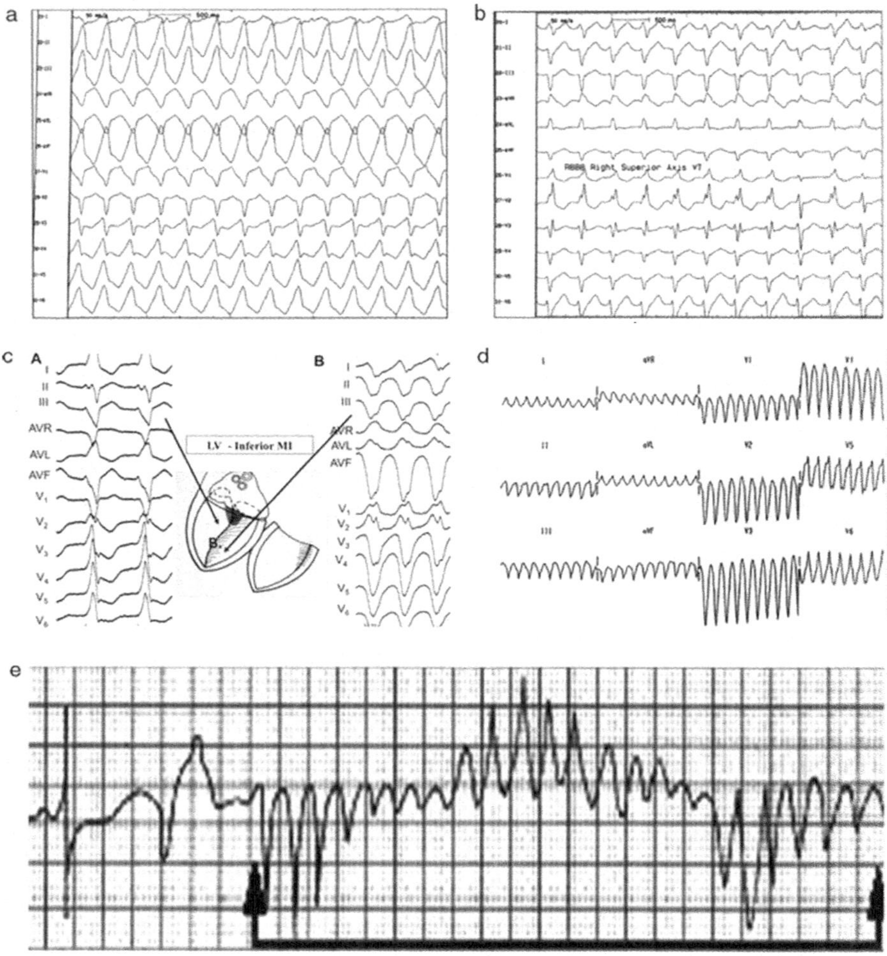

ECG types of VT and most common causes are shown with characteristic ECG features of selected VTs. LBBB indicates left bundle branch block; RBBB, right bundle branch block; L, left; and R, right. (a) Sustained monomorphic ventricular tachycardia with LBBB and inferior axis suggesting origin from RVOT. This tachycardia is idiopathic in origin. (b) Sustained monomorphic ventricular tachycardia with RBBB and right superior axis, suggesting origin in the left ventricular septum. This type of tachycardia is commonly idiopathic in origin. (c) Two different ventricular tachycardias originating in the left ventricle long after an inferior wall myocardial infarct. This type of VT is related to scars that form after myocardial infarct. (d) Fast ventricular tachycardia with LBBB and left superior axis. Morphology and rate are suggestive of bundle branch reentry ventricular tachycardia. This type of VT is related to nonischemic cardiomyopathy. (e) Polymorphic ventricular tachycardia. This type of tachycardia is frequently related to electrolyte abnormalities, ischemia, or drug toxicity. [Kocovic D. Ablation for Ventricular Tachycardia. In: Yan G-X, Kowey PR, editors. Management of Cardiac Arrhythmias [Internet]. Humana Press; 2011 [cited 2017 May 24]. p. 257–82. (Contemporary Cardiology). Available from: http://link.springer.com/chapter/10.1007/978-1-60761-161-5_12] *Caption from original*

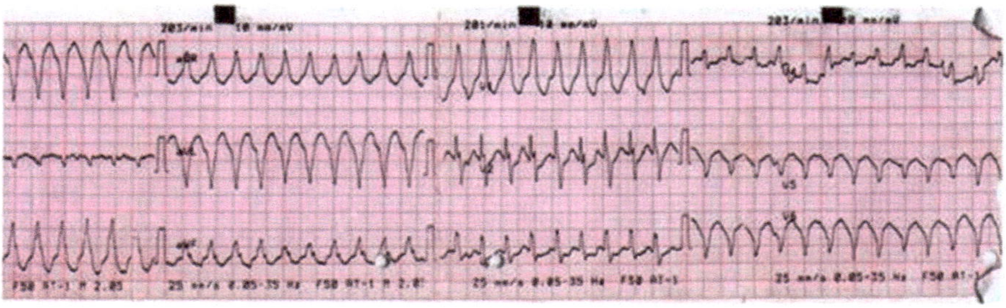

Electrocardiogram showing monomorphic ventricular tachycardia. [From article: Ventricular tachycardia – an atypical initial presentation of sarcoidosis: a case report. J Med Case Reports. 2013 Dec 1;7(1):196. https://doi.org/10.1186/1752-1947-7-196 at https://link.springer.com/article/10.1186/1752-1947-7-196 by Meera Ekka, Sanjeev Sinha, Raghunandan Purushothaman, Nitish Naik, Rajiv Narang, Lavleen Singh, © Ekka et al. 2013; licensee BioMed Central Ltd.; licensed under Creative Commons Attribution License BY 2.0 http://creativecommons.org/licenses/by/2.0] *Caption from original*

Presentation

Typical/"Classic"

- Patients with tachyarrhythmias typically present with:
  - Palpitations
  - Chest pain
  - Dizziness
  - Weakness

Atypical

- Patients with tachyarrhythmias, especially atrial fibrillation, may be largely asymptomatic.
- Sometimes the cardinal symptoms of underlying illness (e.g. sepsis, hyperthyroidism, withdrawal syndrome) may overwhelm the patient's perception of tachycardia

Primary Differential Considerations

- Patients with tachyarrhythmias should be evaluated for type of rhythm abnormality and for underlying cause. Among the important early considerations are:
  - Acute myocardial ischemia/infarction
  - Pulmonary embolism
  - Sepsis
  - Shock
  - Ventricular tachycardia
  - Sustained supraventricular tachycardia

History and Physical Exam

Findings That Confirm Diagnosis

- The ECG confirms the type of arrhythmia and may give clues of myocardial ischemia if present. The clinician should assess the patient's hemodynamic stability while the ECG is being performed. On first review of the ECG, focus on identifying the rhythm and on whether the QRS is narrow or wide.

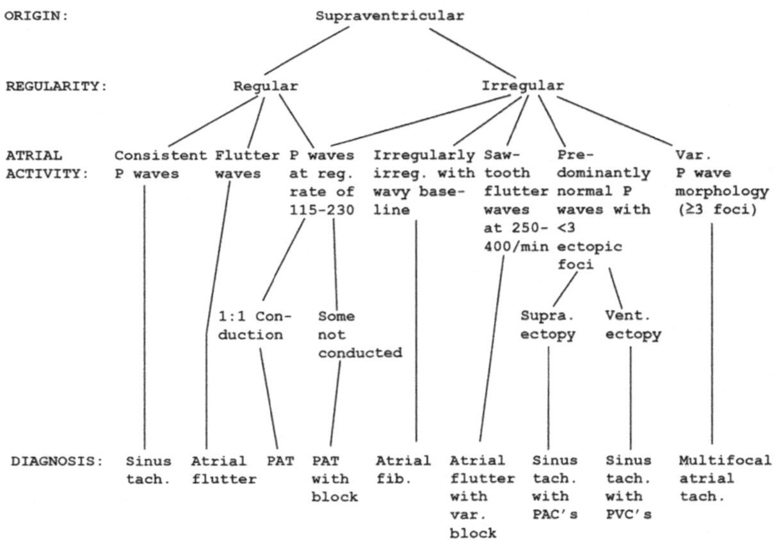

Flow sheet for supraventricular tachycardia [Petty BG. Arrhythmias. In: Basic Electrocardiography [Internet]. Springer New York; 2016 [cited 2017 May 24]. p. 101–35. Available from: http://link.springer.com/chapter/10.1007/978-1-4939-2413-4_7] *Caption from original*

Factors That Suggest Diagnosis

- Tachypalpitations, weakness, with or without chest pain or shortness of breath.
- ECG should be obtained immediately and will guide the diagnostic process.

Factors That Exclude Diagnosis

- A heart rate (on ECG, monitor, or manual pulse count) of < 100 bpm excludes tachyarrhythmia. A patient with suggestive symptoms, however, should be maintained on a monitor, because the abnormal rhythm may be paroxysmal.

Ancillary Studies

Laboratory

- It is helpful to send routine laboratory studies such as basic chemistries, a complete blood count, and cardiac biomarkers to evaluate for other causes for the patient's symptoms.
- Specialized studies should be ordered as pertinent to the presentation, such as thyroid studies, blood cultures, etc.
- If the patient is taking digoxin or theophylline, check drug levels.

Electrocardiography

- The ECG should be obtained and interpreted promptly.
  - Look first for signs of acute ischemia (in particular, ST-segment elevation).
  - Then look to see if QRS rhythm is regular or irregular.
  - Then evaluate the width of the QRS complex: narrow (normal conduction) or wide (abnormal conduction from above, or ventricular origin).

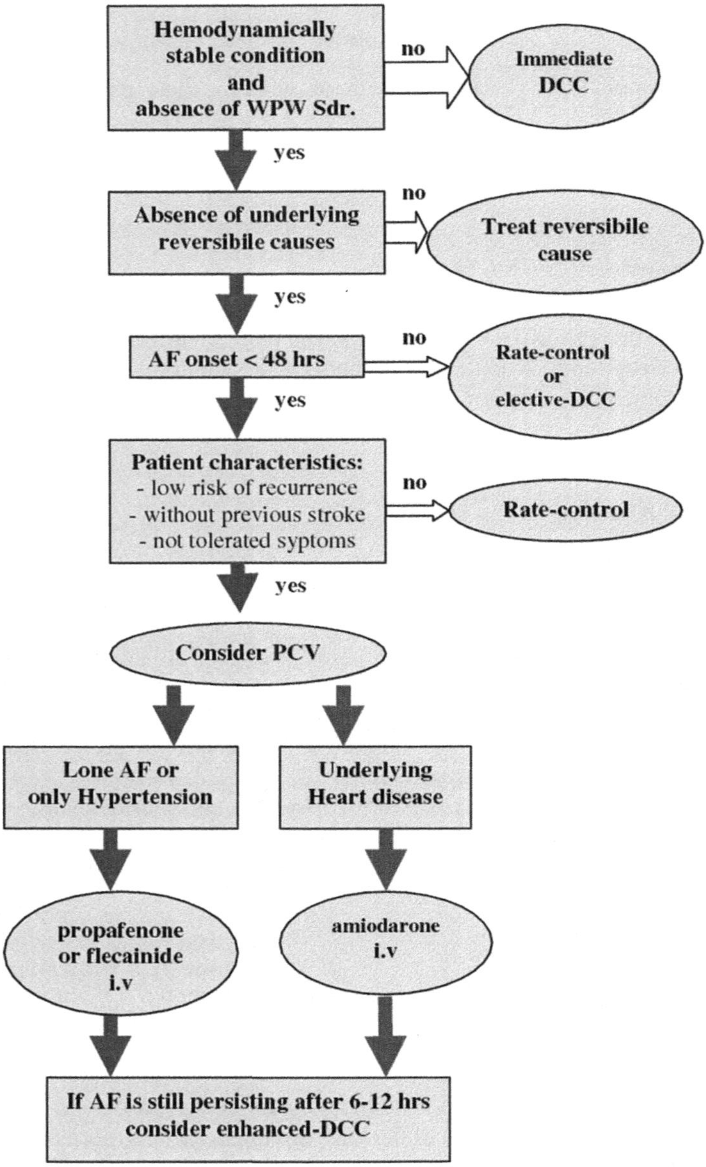

Key findings of common arrhythmias [Winchester DE, Kaufmann MR, McKillop MS, Miles WM. Pitfalls in the Acute Management of Atrial Fibrillation. In: Peacock WF, Clark CL, editors. Short Stay Management of Atrial Fibrillation [Internet]. Springer International Publishing; 2016 [cited 2017 May 24]. p. 145–73. (Contemporary Cardiology). Available from: http://link.springer.com/chapter/10.1007/978-3-319-31386-3_14] *Caption from original*

Imaging

- The chest x-ray may be helpful in the evaluation of tachyarrhthmias. Other imaging is typically not needed except in specific diagnostic evaluations for underlying problems, such as CT pulmonary angiogram for suspected pulmonary embolism.

Special Populations

Age

- Atrial fibrillation, atrial flutter, MAT, and VT are more likely to occur in older patients.
- PSVT and sinus tachycardia can occur at any age.
- Tachycardia is common in the pediatric age group; etiologies are often benign.
- Parental diagnosis is often accomplished by observing the neck veins or sensing a bounding pulse while holding the child.
- SVT is the most common symptomatic dysrhythmia of infancy and childhood.
- Symptoms of SVT in infancy range from minor to cardiogenic shock.
- In infants, lethargy, feeding problems, or irritability may be manifested.
- In newborns or infants with SVT, the heart rate is often > 220 bpm.

Co-morbidities

- The most important co-morbidities are underlying cardiopulmonary disease, including coronary artery disease, heart failure, structural heart abnormalities, and COPD.

Pitfalls in Diagnosis

Critical Steps Not to Miss

- It is imperative that all patients be monitored in an ongoing fashion for hemodynamic stability.
- Recognition of ventricular arrhythmia is critical, as VT is an unstable and potentially lethal rhythm.

- Patients with supraventricular arrhythmia (AFib, AFlut, PSVT) often present in relatively stable condition but may not tolerate the ongoing high myocardial oxygen demand for long, so early stabilization and rate control are warranted.

Mimics

- Palpitations can be caused by anxiety, but sometimes this is not a clear diagnosis, and a prompt ECG should still be obtained.

Time-Dependent Interventions

- The most important intervention is to stabilize patients with hemodynamic instability.
- Recognition of potentially lethal arrhythmias is important.
- Identification and management of underlying illness are important steps and may be life-saving (e.g., PE, sepsis).
- Rate control should be established as soon as possible in order to spare the myocardium ongoing high oxygen consumption that may lead to ischemia.

Overall Principles of Treatment

- Treatment approach is specific to the tachyarrhythmia diagnosis and/or underlying disease. Treatment may be very complex, but first-line actions typically are as follows:
  - Sinus tachycardia: identify and treat underlying cause.
  - MAT: focus on treating underlying pulmonary disease.
  - AFib: consider rate control with diltiazem (if hemodynamically stable) or with cardioversion (if unstable)

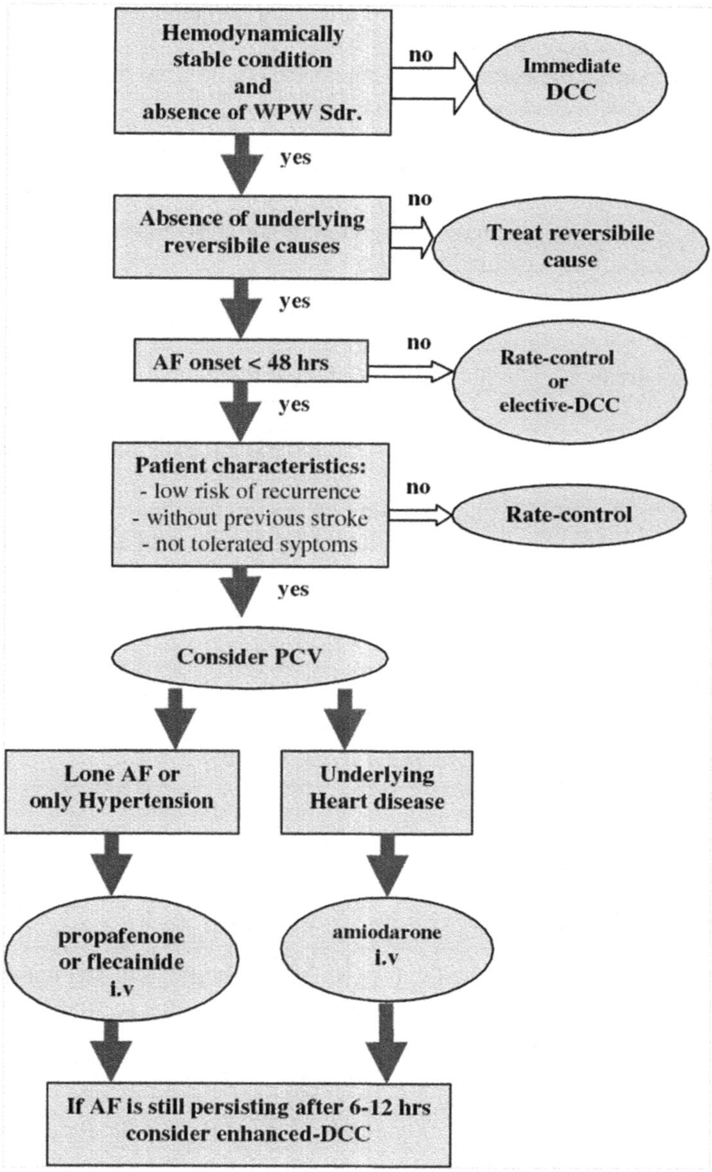

Proposed approach to the management of patients with recent-onset AF. Stratify thromboembolic risk and initiate appropriate prophylaxis in all patients. When elective DCC is considered in patients with AF >48 h or after a failed attempt at cardioversion, OAC treatment is required for at least 3 weeks before and 4 weeks after cardioversion [Tampieri A, Rusconi AM, Lenzi T. Cardioversion in atrial fibrillation. Focus on recent-onset atrial fibrillation. Intern Emerg Med. 2012 Oct 1;7(3):241–50.] *Caption from original*

  - AFlutt: consider rate control with diltiazem (if hemodynamically stable) or with cardioversion (if unstable).
  - PSVT: consider rate control with adenosine or diltiazem (if hemodynamically stable) or with cardioversion (if unstable).
  - WPW: if narrow complex QRS, can use adenosine or diltiazem; if wide-complex, treat as VT and avoid these drugs.
  - VT: synchronized cardioversion.
- Patients should be evaluated for any underlying or acute issues that, if treated, can help improve the cardiac function.

Disease Course

- Prognosis is dependent on the specific type of arrhythmia and underlying co-morbidities.
- The mortality of VT is highest within this group of diagnoses.
- Patients with AFib should be evaluated for chronic oral anticoagulation once stabilized.

Related Evidence

Papers of particular interest have been highlighted as:
*** Of key importance*

Practice Guideline

Page RL, Joglar JA, Caldwell MA, Calkins H, Conti JB, Deal BJ, Estes NA 3rd, Field ME, Goldberger ZD, Hammill SC, Indik JH, Lindsay BD, Olshansky B, Russo AM, Shen WK, Tracy CM, Al-Khatib SM; Evidence Review Committee Chair‡. 2015 ACC/AHA/HRS Guideline for the Management of Adult Patients With Supraventricular Tachycardia: A Report of the American College of Cardiology/American Heart Association Task Force on Clinical Practice Guidelines and the Heart Rhythm Society. Circulation. 2016 Apr 5;133(14):e506-74.https://doi.org/10.1161/CIR.0000000000000311. Erratum in: Circulation. 2016 Sep 13;134(11):e234-5. PubMed PMID: 26399663. https://www.ncbi.nlm.nih.gov/pubmed/26399663 **

Page RL, Joglar JA, Caldwell MA, Calkins H, Conti JB, Deal BJ, Estes NA 3rd, Field ME, Goldberger ZD, Hammill SC, Indik JH, Lindsay BD, Olshansky B, Russo AM, Shen WK, Tracy CM, Al-Khatib SM; Evidence Review Committee Chair‡. 2015 ACC/AHA/HRS Guideline for the Management of Adult Patients

With Supraventricular Tachycardia: Executive Summary: A Report of the American College of Cardiology/American Heart Association Task Force on Clinical Practice Guidelines and the Heart Rhythm Society. Circulation. 2016 Apr 5;133(14):e471-505. https://doi.org/10.1161/CIR.0000000000000310. Erratum in: Circulation. 2016 Sep 13;134(11):e232-3. PubMed PMID: 26399662. https://www.ncbi.nlm.nih.gov/pubmed/?term=26399662 **

Lane DA, Aguinaga L, Blomström-Lundqvist C, Boriani G, Dan GA, Hills MT, Hylek EM, LaHaye SA, Lip GY, Lobban T, Mandrola J, McCabe PJ, Pedersen SS, Pisters R, Stewart S, Wood K, Potpara TS, Gorenek B, Conti JB, Keegan R, Power S, Hendriks J, Ritter P, Calkins H, Violi F, Hurwitz J. Cardiac tachyarrhythmias and patient values and preferences for their management: the European Heart Rhythm Association (EHRA) consensus document endorsed by the Heart Rhythm Society (HRS), Asia Pacific Heart Rhythm Society (APHRS), and Sociedad Latinoamericana de Estimulación Cardíaca y Electrofisiología (SOLEACE). Europace. 2015 Dec;17(12):1747-69. https://doi.org/10.1093/europace/euv233. Review. PubMed PMID: 26108807. https://www.ncbi.nlm.nih.gov/pubmed/26108807

Macle L, Cairns JA, Andrade JG, Mitchell LB, Nattel S, Verma A; CCS Atrial Fibrillation Guidelines Committee. The 2014 Atrial Fibrillation Guidelines Companion: A Practical Approach to the Use of the Canadian Cardiovascular Society Guidelines. Can J Cardiol. 2015 Oct;31(10):1207-18. https://doi.org/10.1016/j.cjca.2015.06.005. PubMed PMID: 26429352. https://www.ncbi.nlm.nih.gov/pubmed/26429352 **

January CT, Wann LS, Alpert JS, Calkins H, Cigarroa JE, Cleveland JC Jr, Conti JB, Ellinor PT, Ezekowitz MD, Field ME, Murray KT, Sacco RL, Stevenson WG, Tchou PJ, Tracy CM, Yancy CW; ACC/AHA Task Force Members. 2014 AHA/ACC/HRS guideline for the management of patients with atrial fibrillation: a report of the American College of Cardiology/American Heart Association Task Force on practice guidelines and the Heart Rhythm Society. Circulation. 2014 Dec 2;130(23):e199-267. https://doi.org/10.1161/CIR.0000000000000041. Erratum in: Circulation. 2014 Dec 2;130(23):e272-4. PubMed PMID: 24682347; PubMed Central PMCID: PMC4676081. https://www.ncbi.nlm.nih.gov/pubmed/24682347 **

Whinnett ZI, Sohaib SM, Davies DW. Diagnosis and management of supraventricular tachycardia. BMJ. 2012 Dec 11;345:e7769. https://doi.org/10.1136/bmj.e7769. Review. PubMed PMID: 23233691. https://www.ncbi.nlm.nih.gov/pubmed/26701216

Estes NA 3rd, Halperin JL, Calkins H, Ezekowitz MD, Gitman P, Go AS, McNamara RL, Messer JV, Ritchie JL, Romeo SJ, Waldo AL, Wyse DG, Bonow RO, DeLong E, Goff DC Jr, Grady K, Green LA, Hiniker A, Linderbaum JA, Masoudi FA, Piña IL, Pressler S, Radford MJ, Rumsfeld JS; American College of Cardiology.; American Heart Association Task Force on Performance Measures.; Physician Consortium for Performance Improvement. ACC/AHA/Physician Consortium 2008 Clinical Performance Measures for Adults with Nonvalvular Atrial Fibrillation or Atrial Flutter: a report of the American College of Cardiology/

American Heart Association Task Force on Performance Measures and the Physician Consortium for Performance Improvement (Writing Committee to Develop Clinical Performance Measures for Atrial Fibrillation) Developed in Collaboration with the Heart Rhythm Society. J Am Coll Cardiol. 2008 Feb 26;51(8):865-84. https://doi.org/10.1016/j.jacc.2008.01.006. Erratum in: J Am Coll Cardiol. 2012 Aug 7;60(6):568. PubMed PMID: 18294574. https://www.ncbi.nlm.nih.gov/pubmed/18294574 **

Review

Bun SS, Latcu DG, Marchlinski F, Saoudi N. Atrial flutter: more than just one of a kind. Eur Heart J. 2015 Sep 14;36(35):2356-63. https://doi.org/10.1093/eurheartj/ehv118. Review. PubMed PMID: 25838435. https://www.ncbi.nlm.nih.gov/pubmed/25838435

de Riva M, Watanabe M, Zeppenfeld K. Twelve-lead ECG of ventricular tachycardia in structural heart disease. Circ Arrhythm Electrophysiol. 2015 Aug;8(4):951-62. https://doi.org/10.1161/CIRCEP.115.002847. Review. PubMed PMID: 26286304. https://www.ncbi.nlm.nih.gov/pubmed/26286304

Buttà C, Tuttolomondo A, Giarrusso L, Pinto A. Electrocardiographic diagnosis of atrial tachycardia: classification, P-wave morphology, and differential diagnosis with other supraventricular tachycardias. Ann Noninvasive Electrocardiol. 2015 Jul;20(4):314-27. https://doi.org/10.1111/anec.12246. Review. PubMed PMID: 25530184. https://www.ncbi.nlm.nih.gov/pubmed/25530184

Katritsis DG, Josephson ME. Differential diagnosis of regular, narrow-QRS tachycardias. Heart Rhythm. 2015 Jul;12(7):1667-76. https://doi.org/10.1016/j.hrthm.2015.03.046. Review. Erratum in: Heart Rhythm. 2016 Feb;13(2):629. PubMed PMID: 25828600. https://www.ncbi.nlm.nih.gov/pubmed/25828600

Nijjer SS, Sohaib SM, Whinnett ZI, Lefroy DC. Diagnosis of supraventricular tachycardias. Br J Hosp Med (Lond). 2014 Feb;75(2):C22-5. Review. PubMed PMID: 24521831. https://www.ncbi.nlm.nih.gov/pubmed/24521831

Buttà C, Tuttolomondo A, Di Raimondo D, Milio G, Miceli S, Attanzio MT, Giarrusso L, Licata G, Pinto A. Supraventricular tachycardias: proposal of a diagnostic algorithm for the narrow complex tachycardias. J Cardiol. 2013 Apr;61(4):247-55. https://doi.org/10.1016/j.jjcc.2012.11.008. Review. PubMed PMID: 23473762. https://www.ncbi.nlm.nih.gov/pubmed/23473762

Boateng S. Tachycardia. Dis Mon. 2013 Mar;59(3):74-82. https://doi.org/10.1016/j.disamonth.2012.12.003. Review. PubMed PMID: 23410668. https://www.ncbi.nlm.nih.gov/pubmed/23410668 **

Chen J. Atrial fibrillation and atrial flutter: medical management. Clin Geriatr Med. 2012 Nov;28(4):635-47. https://doi.org/10.1016/j.cger.2012.08.002. Review. PubMed PMID: 23101574. https://www.ncbi.nlm.nih.gov/pubmed/23101574

Link MS. Clinical practice. Evaluation and initial treatment of supraventricular tachycardia. N Engl J Med. 2012 Oct 11;367(15):1438-48. https://doi.

org/10.1056/NEJMcp1111259. Review. PubMed PMID: 23050527. https://www.ncbi.nlm.nih.gov/pubmed/?term=23050527 **

Mottram AR, Svenson JE. Rhythm disturbances. Emerg Med Clin North Am. 2011 Nov;29(4):729-46, vi. https://doi.org/10.1016/j.emc.2011.08.007. Review. PubMed PMID: 22040704. https://www.ncbi.nlm.nih.gov/pubmed/22040704

González-Torrecilla E, Arenal A, Atienza F, Datino T, Atea LF, Calvo D, Pachón M, Miracle A, Fernández-Avilés F. EGC diagnosis of paroxysmal supraventricular tachycardias in patients without preexcitation. Ann Noninvasive Electrocardiol. 2011 Jan;16(1):85-95. https://doi.org/10.1111/j.1542-474X.2010.00399.x. Review. PubMed PMID: 21251139. https://www.ncbi.nlm.nih.gov/pubmed/21251139

Medi C, Kalman JM, Freedman SB. Supraventricular tachycardia. Med J Aust. 2009 Mar 2;190(5):255-60. Review. PubMed PMID: 19296791. https://www.ncbi.nlm.nih.gov/pubmed/19296791

Jacobson C. Narrow QRS complex tachycardias. AACN Adv Crit Care. 2007 Jul-Sep;18(3):264-74. PubMed PMID: 18019517. https://www.ncbi.nlm.nih.gov/pubmed/18019517 **

Clinical Trial

Fromm C, Suau SJ, Cohen V, Likourezos A, Jellinek-Cohen S, Rose J, Marshall J. Diltiazem vs. Metoprolol in the Management of Atrial Fibrillation or Flutter with Rapid Ventricular Rate in the Emergency Department. J Emerg Med. 2015 Aug;49(2):175-82. https://doi.org/10.1016/j.jemermed.2015.01.014. PubMed PMID: 25913166. https://www.ncbi.nlm.nih.gov/pubmed/25913166

Siu CW, Lau CP, Lee WL, Lam KF, Tse HF. Intravenous diltiazem is superior to intravenous amiodarone or digoxin for achieving ventricular rate control in patients with acute uncomplicated atrial fibrillation. Crit Care Med. 2009 Jul;37(7):2174-9; quiz 2180. https://doi.org/10.1097/CCM.0b013e3181a02f56. PubMed PMID: 19487941. https://www.ncbi.nlm.nih.gov/pubmed/19487941

Use PubMed Clinical Queries to find the most recent evidence. Use this search strategy: "Tachycardia"[Mesh] OR "tachycardia" OR "tachycardias" OR "tachyarrhythmia" OR "tachyarrythmias"

Chapter 69
Tetralogy of Fallot

Richard M. Cantor, Charles V. Pollack, Jr., and Jaime Friel Blanck

Name and Synonyms

Tetralogy of Fallot (TOF): A constellation of four anatomic cardiac anomalies.

R. M. Cantor
Department of Emergency Medicine and Pediatrics, State University of New York Upstate Medical University, Syracuse, NY, USA

C. V. Pollack, Jr. (✉)
Department of Emergency Medicine, Thomas Jefferson University, Philadelphia, PA, USA

J. F. Blanck
Welch Medical Library, Johns Hopkins University, Baltimore, MD, USA

C. V. Pollack, Jr. (ed.), *Differential Diagnosis of Cardiopulmonary Disease*,
https://doi.org/10.1007/978-3-319-63895-9_69

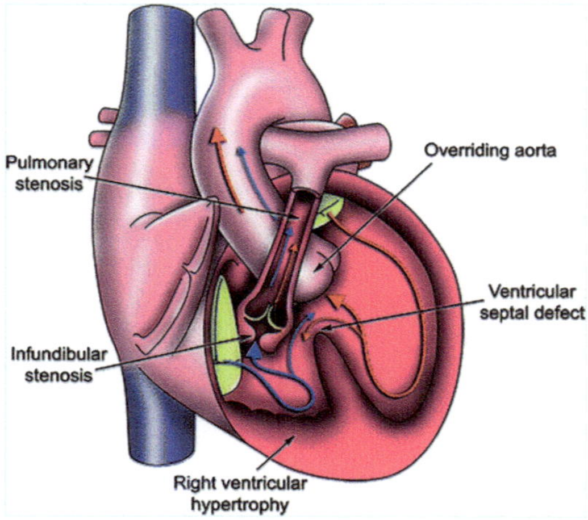

Schematic drawing of tetralogy of Fallot [Sridharan S, Price G, Tann O, Hughes M, Muthurangu V, Taylor AM. Tetralogy of Fallot. Cardiovascular MRI in Congenital Heart Disease [Internet]. Berlin, Heidelberg: Springer Berlin Heidelberg; 2010 [cited 2015 Sep 1]. p. 74–7. Available from: http://link.springer.com/10.1007/978-3-540-69837-1_31] *Caption from original*

Incidence/Epidemiology

- Tetralogy of Fallot is seen in 4 per 10,000 live births.
- It accounts for 7–10 % of reported cases of congenital heart disease.
- Repair is usually necessary within the first year of life.

Differential Diagnosis

- Should be considered in the differential diagnosis of cyanotic congenital heart disease, often represented by the "5 T's":
  - Truncus Arteriosus
  - Transposition of the Great Arteries
  - Tricuspid Atresia
  - Tetralogy of Fallot
  - Total Anomalous Pulmonary Venous Return

Pathophysiology and Etiology

- In patients with TOF, the degree of compromise is directly dependent on the severity of the right ventricular outflow obstruction. In most cases, the size of the VSD is generous enough to permit bidirectional blood flow. If left-sided pressures are high enough, the shunting will be "left-to-right," and the patient will be acyanotic. In the converse situation, shunting away from the pulmonary bed will present with cyanosis.
- In the most severe obstructive scenarios, episodes of profound cyanosis may occur (so-called "tet spells" or "hypercyanotic" spells). The etiology of these episodes is unclear.

Presentation

Typical/"Classic"

- As previously mentioned, in situations with severe right-sided outflow obstruction, infants will present with severe cyanosis. This most often occurs during the newborn period.
- In situations where pulmonary and systemic blood flows are equivocal, the infant will often present with a murmur, prompting further investigation.

Atypical

- In cases of minimal right-sided outflow obstruction, shunting across the large VSD will promote the development of congestive heart failure from pulmonary overperfusion.

Primary Differential Considerations

- The other components of the 5 T's (see above) are the most important differential diagnoses to consider.

History and Physical Exam

- Most infants will present with cyanosis in the first few days of life.
- In others, the diagnosis will often be difficult, since most patients with TOF will appear comfortable and in no distress.
- The development of a hypercyanotic (tet) spell will be heralded by the development of cyanosis, hyperpnea, and marked agitation.
- A prominent right ventricular impulse may be palpable.
- The murmur in TOF is secondary to right ventricular outflow obstruction (not from the VSD). As obstruction increases, the murmur will often diminish in intensity, as blood will preferentially be shunted across the VSD.

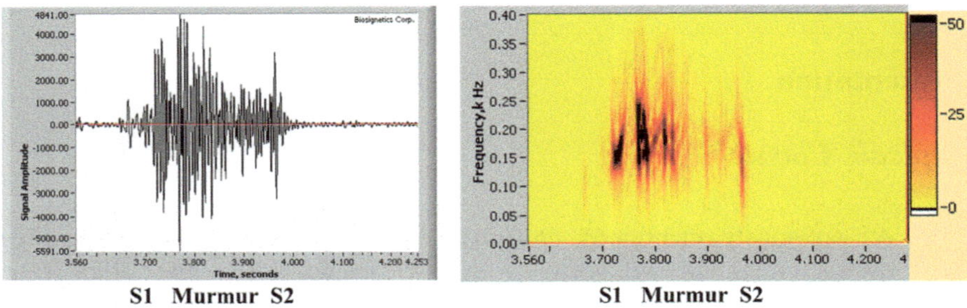

A) B)

(A, B). Abnormal heart sound of Severe Tetralogy of Fallot (acyanotic). A) PCG (single heart beat). B) HES (single heart beat). [From article: Heart energy signature spectrogram for cardiovascular diagnosis. BioMed Eng OnLine. 2007 May 4;6(1):1–22. DOI: 10.1186/1475-925X-6-16, at http://link.springer.com/article/10.1186/1475-925X-6-16; by Vladimir Kudriavtsev, Vladimir Polyshchuk, Douglas L Roy, © Kudriavtsev et al; licensee BioMed Central Ltd. 2007; licensed under Creative Commons Attribution License BY 2.0 http://creativecommons.org/licenses/by/2.0] *Caption from original*

http://www.easyauscultation.com/cases?coursecaseorder=5&courseid=29
Tetralogy of Fallot murmur. [Congenital Abnormalities: Tetralogy of Fallot; Easy Auscultation; www.easyauscultation.com; copyright 2015, MedEdu LLC]

Findings That Confirm Diagnosis

- Echocardiography is the gold standard for establishing the diagnosis of TOF.

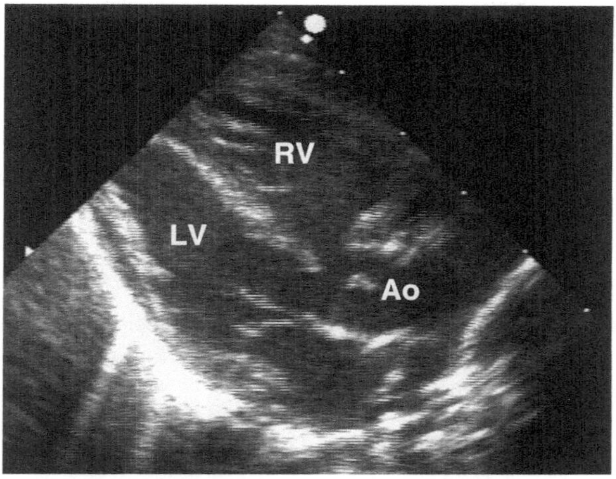

Tetralogy of Fallot. Both subxiphoid and parasternal long- and short-axis images demonstrate the most important aspects of tetralogy of Fallot. A,Parasternal long-axis view demonstrating the large anterior malalignment ventricular septal defect (VSD) with aortic overriding of the crest of the ventricular septum. Ao—aorta; LV—left ventricle; RV—right ventricle. [Hornberger L, Schwartz M. Chapter 2. In: Lee RT, Braunwald E, editors. Atlas of Cardiac Imaging. Atlas of Heart Diseases, Volume 01, Philadelphia: Current Medicine; 1998. ISBN: 0-443-07567-0] *Caption adapted from original*

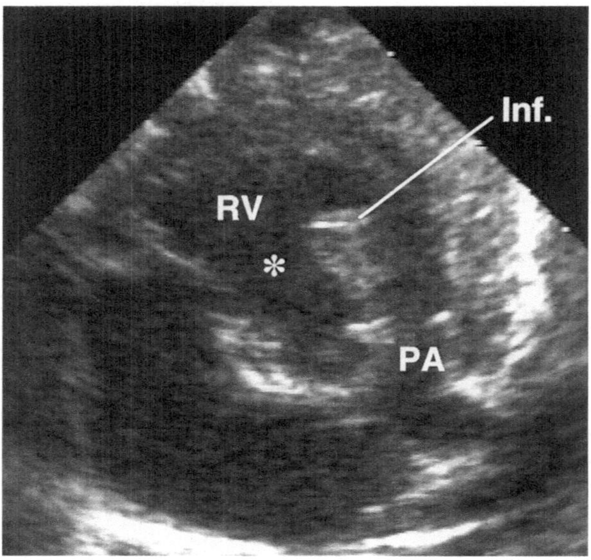

B, Parasternal short-axis view of the right ventricular outflow tract (RVOT) demonstrating anterior malalignment of infundibular septum (Inf). The large subaortic, malalignment VSD can be seen (asterisk). Other lesions to be excluded in tetralogy of Fallot include additional VSDs, branch pulmonary artery (PA) stenoses, mitral valve abnormalities, and coronary abnormalities, particularly the left anterior descending from the right coronary artery (which crosses over the RVOT) or a single right coronary artery. A prominent conal branch from the right coronary that partially crosses the infundibulum is common in tetralogy of Fallot. RV—right ventricle. [Hornberger L, Schwartz M. Chapter 2. In: Lee RT, Braunwald E, editors. Atlas of Cardiac Imaging. Atlas of Heart Diseases, Volume 01, Philadelphia: Current Medicine; 1998. ISBN: 0-443-07567-0] *Caption adapted from original*

- In more typical scenarios, the presence of cyanosis unresponsive to supplemental oxygen, combined with typical X-ray findings (boot-shaped heart), will point to the diagnosis.

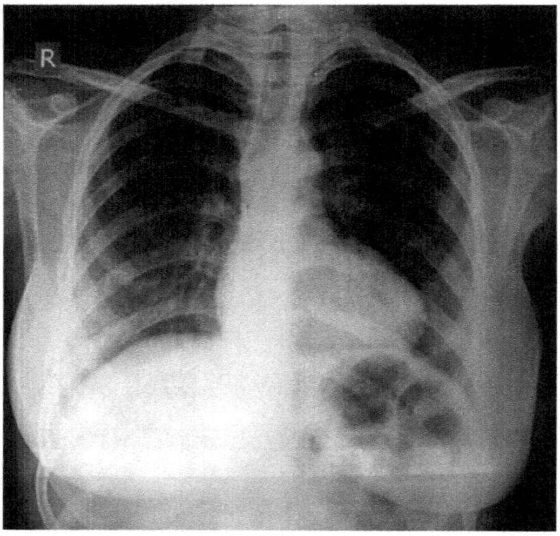

Boot-shaped heart, concave main pulmonary artery segment, and decreased pulmonary vasculature in a tetralogy of Fallot patient [Sadeghpour A, Alizadehasl A, Mahdavi M. Tetralogy of Fallot. In: Sadeghpour A, Kyavar M, Alizadehasl A, editors. Comprehensive Approach to Adult Congenital Heart Disease [Internet]. London: Springer London; 2014 [cited 2015 Sep 1]. p. 237–44. Available from: http://link.springer.com/10.1007/978-1-4471-6383-1_28] *Caption from original*

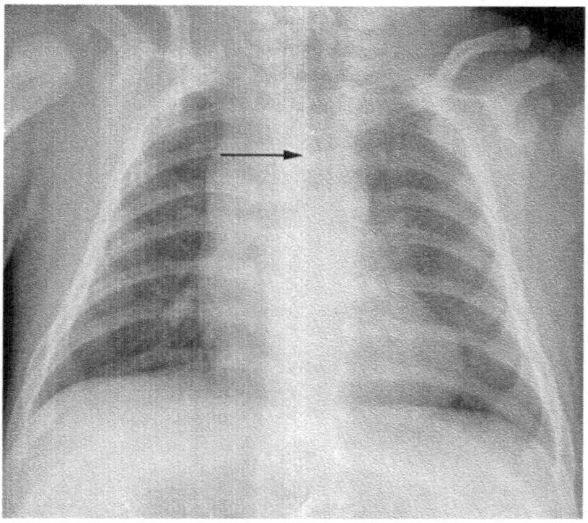

Tetralogy of Fallot. The "boot-shaped" heart is a result of upward tilting of the apex and attenuation of the main pulmonary artery segment. Note the leftward deviation of the trachea (black arrow) indicative of a right aortic arch, which is a common association. [Golding IF, Yoo S, Hamilton R. Cardiology. In: Laxer R, Ford-Jones EL, Friedman J, Gerstle T, editors. The Hospital for Sick Children: atlas of pediatrics. Philadelphia: Current Medicine; 2005. ISBN: 1-57340-188-9] *Caption adapted from original*

- CT scanning may also be helpful.

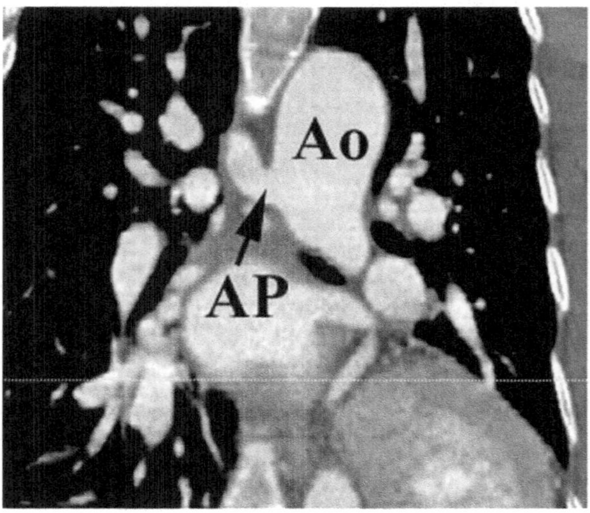

Unrepaired tetralogy of Fallot and pulmonary atresia: CT angiography. Electron beam angiogram of a cyanotic adult with unrepaired tetralogy of Fallot with pulmonary atresia and multiple aortopulmonary (AP) collaterals. A, Coronal slice demonstrating large AP collateral emerging rightward from the descending thoracic aorta (Ao). [Aboulhosn J. Chapter 11. In: Budoff MJ, Achenbach S, Narula J, Braunwald E, editors. Atlas of cardiovascular computed tomography. Philadelphia: Current Medicine; 2007] *Caption adapted from original*

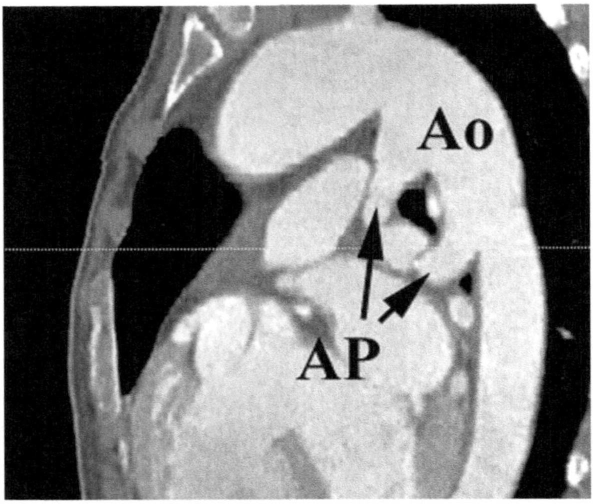

B, Sagittal slice demonstrating two AP collaterals emerging anteriorly from the descending thoracic aorta (Ao). Delineating the origin, course, and patency of these AP collaterals is challenging and time consuming but imperative to the management of these patients. Depending on anatomic findings patients may be candidates for complete surgical repair, unifocalization, or transcatheter interventions. [Aboulhosn J. Chapter 11. In: Budoff MJ, Achenbach S, Narula J, Braunwald E, editors. Atlas of cardiovascular computed tomography. Philadelphia: Current Medicine; 2007] *Caption adapted from original*

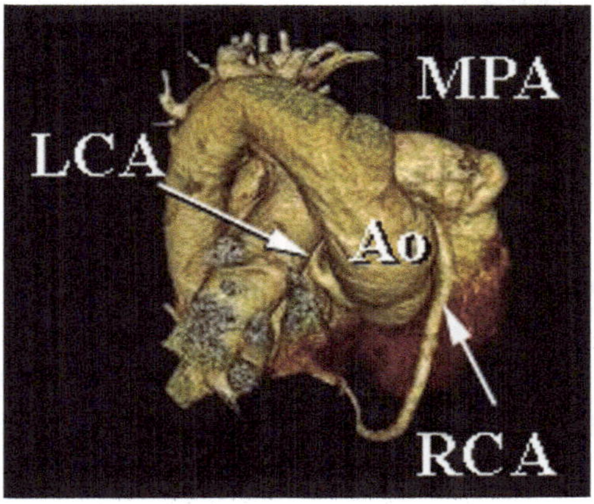

Repaired tetralogy of Fallot: CT angiography. Sixteenslice CT angiography with threedimensional volume rendering of a 21-year-old woman with repaired tetralogy of Fallot. A, Right anterior oblique and cranial projection, the right coronary artery (RCA) emerges from the anterior and left facing cusp and courses between the aortic root (Ao) and main pulmonary artery (MPA). The left coronary artery (LCA) emerges from the posterior facing cusp and courses leftward behind the Ao and below the MPA. [Aboulhosn J. Chapter 11. In: Budoff MJ, Achenbach S, Narula J, Braunwald E, editors. Atlas of cardiovascular computed tomography. Philadelphia: Current Medicine; 2007] *Caption adapted from original*

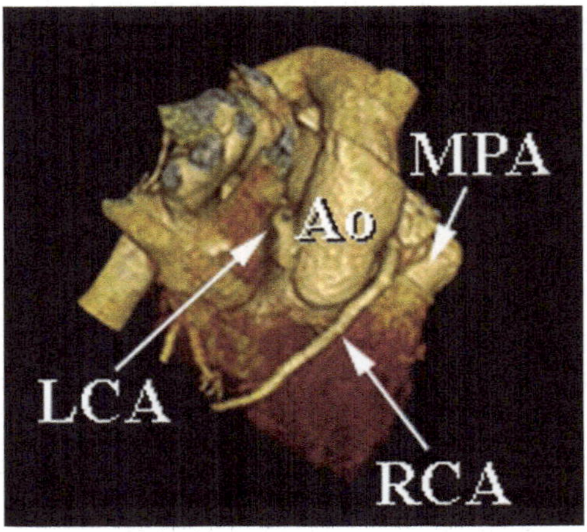

B, Right anterior oblique caudal projection. [Aboulhosn J. Chapter 11. In: Budoff MJ, Achenbach S, Narula J, Braunwald E, editors. Atlas of cardiovascular computed tomography. Philadelphia: Current Medicine; 2007] *Caption adapted from original*

Factors That Suggest Diagnosis

- A history of repeated cyanotic episodes, which may resolve spontaneously, should alert the clinician to the possibility of TOF.

Factors that Exclude Diagnosis

- The absence of cyanosis essentially rules out TOF except during periods of normal intracardiac shunting (the "pink" tet).

Ancillary Studies

Laboratory

- Basic laboratory tests are rarely indicated.
- As mentioned, arterial blood gas measurements will demonstrate low values for both partial pressures of oxygen and oxygen saturation.

Electrocardiography

- The ECG in TOF will show right ventricular hypertrophy. There will also be right axis deviation, along with varying degrees of R and T wave disruption.

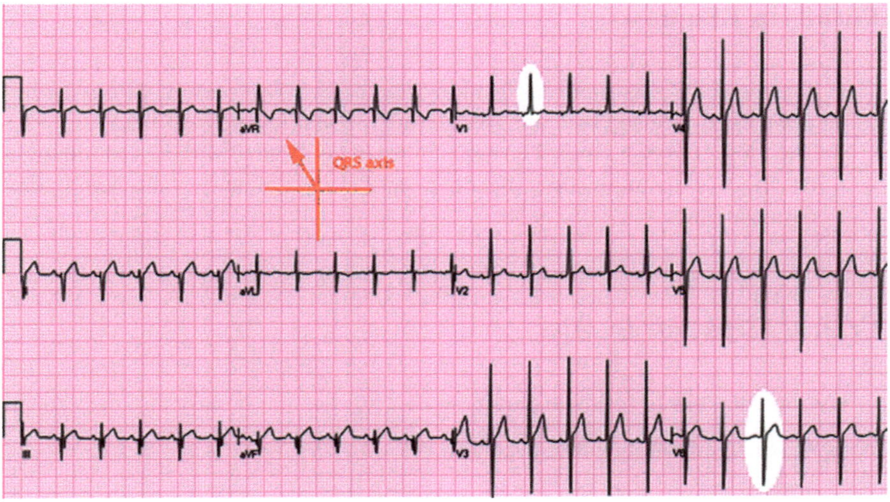

ECG in tetralogy of Fallot. Right ventricular hypertrophy is the dominant feature of ECG in patients with tetralogy of Fallot. RVH may manifest itself in different ways such as tall R in V1 and deep S in V6, rsR′, pure R-wave or qR pattern of QRS complex in right chest leads. In this ECG, RVH is manifested as a pure R in V1, deep S in V6, and right axis deviation [Luxenberg DM, Torchen L. Tetralogy of Fallot. In: Abdulla R, editor. Heart Diseases in Children [Internet]. Boston, MA: Springer US; 2011 [cited 2015 Sep 1]. p. 167–76. Available from: http://link.springer.com/10.1007/978-1-4419-7994-0_13] *Caption from original*

Cardiac Enzymes

- Not indicated,

Special Populations

Age

- The vast majority of patients will present in the neonatal period or early infancy.

Co-morbidities

- About 15–20 % of patients with TOF will present with other syndromes, including Trisomy 21, DiGeorge Syndrome, and velocardiofacial syndrome.

Pitfalls in Diagnosis

- The majority of cyanotic congenital heart defects will present within the first few days of life and be diagnosed during the first few days of life.
- The most common clinical error made when confronted with a cyanotic infant or child is distinguishing between cardiac, pulmonary, and hemoglobin derangements.

Critical Steps Not To Miss

- Clinical paths to follow include:
  - Recognition of central cyanosis.
  - Provision of hyperoxia.
    - If no clinical response is seen, consider cardiac etiologies.
    - If there is measured improvement in oxygenation, pulmonary causes are most likely.

Mimics

- Other causes of cyanosis.

Time-Dependent Interventions

- Immediate consultation with a Pediatric Cardiologist is recommended.
  - Focus is on diagnosis, not treatment, so this is limited.

Overall Principles of Treatment

- Provision of supplemental oxygen.
- In cases of hypercyanotic spells:
  - Placement in the knee-chest position.
  - Sedation with morphine (0.1 mg/kg/dose).
  - Administration of 10–20 cc/kg of normal saline.
  - Immediate consultation with a pediatric cardiologist.

Disease Course

- Short term is excellent after neonatal surgical repair; greater than 90% survival 25 years after neonatal repair.

Related Evidence

Papers of particular interest have been highlighted as:
*** Of key importance*

Review

Chai PJ, Jacobs JP, Quintessenza JA. Modern surgical management of patients with tetralogy of Fallot. Cardiol Young. 2013 Dec;23(6):905-9. doi: 10.1017/S1047951113001716. PubMed PMID: 24401265. http://www.ncbi.nlm.nih.gov/pubmed/24401265 **

Villafañe J, Feinstein JA, Jenkins KJ, Vincent RN, Walsh EP, Dubin AM, Geva T, Towbin JA, Cohen MS, Fraser C, Dearani J, Rosenthal D, Kaufman B, Graham TP Jr; Adult Congenital and Pediatric Cardiology Section, American College of Cardiology. Hot topics in tetralogy of Fallot. J Am Coll Cardiol. 2013 Dec 10;62(23):2155-66. doi: 10.1016/j.jacc.2013.07.100. Epub 2013 Sep 27. PubMed PMID: 24076489. http://www.ncbi.nlm.nih.gov/pubmed/24076489 **

Anderson RH, Spicer DE, Giroud JM, Mohun TJ. Tetralogy of Fallot: nosological, morphological, and morphogenetic considerations. Cardiol Young. 2013 Dec;23(6):858-66. doi: 10.1017/S1047951113001686. Review. PubMed PMID: 24401259. http://www.ncbi.nlm.nih.gov/pubmed/24401259 **

Monaco M, Williams I. Tetralogy of Fallot: fetal diagnosis to surgical correction. Minerva Pediatr. 2012 Oct;64(5):461-70. Review. PubMed PMID: 22992529. http://www.ncbi.nlm.nih.gov/pubmed/22992529 **

Sharkey AM, Sharma A. Tetralogy of Fallot: anatomic variants and their impact on surgical management. Semin Cardiothorac Vasc Anesth. 2012 Jun;16(2):88-96. doi: 10.1177/1089253211434566. Epub 2012 Jan 24. Review. PubMed PMID: 22275348. http://www.ncbi.nlm.nih.gov/pubmed/?term=22275348

Hughes D, Siegel MJ. MRI of complex cyanotic congenital heart disease: pre-and post surgical considerations. Int J Cardiovasc Imaging. 2010 Dec;26(Suppl 2):333-43. doi: 10.1007/s10554-010-9732-y. Epub 2010 Nov 3. Review. PubMed PMID: 21046255. http://www.ncbi.nlm.nih.gov/pubmed/21046255 **

Duro RP, Moura C, Leite-Moreira A. Anatomophysiologic basis of tetralogy of Fallot and its clinical implications. Rev Port Cardiol. 2010 Apr;29(4):591-630. Review. English, Portuguese. PubMed PMID: 20734579. http://www.ncbi.nlm.nih.gov/pubmed/20734579

Apitz C, Webb GD, Redington AN. Tetralogy of Fallot. Lancet. 2009 Oct 24;374(9699):1462-71. doi: 10.1016/S0140-6736(09)60657-7. Epub 2009 Aug 14. Review. PubMed PMID: 19683809. http://www.ncbi.nlm.nih.gov/pubmed/19683809 **

Bailliard F, Anderson RH. Tetralogy of Fallot. Orphanet J Rare Dis. 2009 Jan 13;4:2. doi: 10.1186/1750-1172-4-2. Review. PubMed PMID: 19144126; PubMed Central PMCID: PMC2651859. http://www.ncbi.nlm.nih.gov/pubmed/19144126 **

Rao PS. Diagnosis and management of cyanotic congenital heart disease: part I. Indian J Pediatr. 2009 Jan;76(1):57-70. doi: 10.1007/s12098-009-0030-4. Epub 2009 Apr 18. Review. PubMed PMID: 19391004. http://www.ncbi.nlm.nih.gov/pubmed/19391004

Anderson RH, Weinberg PM. The clinical anatomy of tetralogy of fallot. Cardiol Young. 2005 Feb;15 Suppl 1:38-47. Review. PubMed PMID: 15934690. http://www.ncbi.nlm.nih.gov/pubmed/15934690

Gutierrez FR, Siegel MJ, Fallah JH, Poustchi-Amin M. Magnetic resonance imaging of cyanotic and noncyanotic congenital heart disease. Magn Reson Imaging Clin N Am. 2002 May;10(2):209-35. Review. PubMed PMID: 12424944. http://www.ncbi.nlm.nih.gov/pubmed/12424944

Waldman JD, Wernly JA. Cyanotic congenital heart disease with decreased pulmonary blood flow in children. Pediatr Clin North Am. 1999 Apr;46(2):385-404. Review. PubMed PMID: 10218082. http://www.ncbi.nlm.nih.gov/pubmed/10218082 **

Comparative Study

Bernardes RJ, Marchiori E, Bernardes PM, Monzo Gonzaga MB, Simões LC. A comparison of magnetic resonance angiography with conventional angiography in the diagnosis of tetralogy of Fallot. Cardiol Young. 2006 Jun;16(3):281-8. PubMed PMID: 16725068. http://www.ncbi.nlm.nih.gov/pubmed/16725068

Gatzoulis MA, Soukias N, Ho SY, Josen M, Anderson RH. Echocardiographic and morphological correlations in tetralogy of Fallot. Eur Heart J. 1999 Feb;20(3):221-31. PubMed PMID: 10082155. http://www.ncbi.nlm.nih.gov/pubmed/10082155

Use PubMed Clinical Queries to find the most recent evidence. Use this search strategy: "Tetralogy of Fallot"[Mesh] OR "tetralogy of fallot"

Chapter 70
Thoracic Aortic Dissection

Charles V. Pollack, Jr., Richard M. Cantor, and Victoria G. Riese

Name and Synonyms

Thoracic Aortic Dissection (TAD)

- Occasionally referred to as "aortic syndrome" or "aortic disaster"

Incidence/Epidemiology

- TAD is the admitting diagnosis in 1 per 10,000 hospital admissions. Because TAD may be a rapidly fatal disease and autopsies are performed in very few deaths in the US, the true incidence remains unknown but likely is higher. A 2004 autopsy study found evidence of TAD in 1–3% of cadavers.
- TAD occurs more commonly in men than in women, roughly mirroring the prevalence of hypertension. It is more common in blacks than whites and more common in whites than in Asians.
- Peak age for TAD is 50–65 years. It may occur earlier in patients with Marfan's syndrome, in patients undergoing aortic and mitral valve replacements, in patients undergoing percutaneous coronary intervention, in patients with syphilis, and in those who abuse cocaine.

C. V. Pollack, Jr. (✉)
Department of Emergency Medicine, Thomas Jefferson University, Philadelphia, PA, USA

R. M. Cantor
Department of Emergency Medicine and Pediatrics, State University of New York Upstate Medical University, Syracuse, NY, USA

V. G. Riese
Librarian Consultant, Eldersberg, MD, USA

C. V. Pollack, Jr. (ed.), *Differential Diagnosis of Cardiopulmonary Disease*,
https://doi.org/10.1007/978-3-319-63895-9_70

- The dissection typically occurs either along the right lateral wall of the ascending aorta, where the shear stress of blood flow is highest, or in the ascending aorta just below the ligamentum arteriosum.

Differential Diagnosis

- Because the primary clinical manifestation of TAD is chest pain, the differential is broad. The other life-threatening etiologies of chest pain syndrome—acute myocardial infarction and pulmonary embolism—may present similarly, but because TAD is more often associated with back pain, the differential for this diagnosis may be broader.

Pathophysiology and Etiology

- The pathophysiology of TAD stems from the development of a split in the media of the aortic wall. The innermost layer of the aortic wall, the intima, is torn or interrupted, and blood dissects into the next layer (media) and with the aortic flow pressure behind it, may progress forward, creating a "false lumen." The outermost layer of the aortic wall, the adventitia, prevents the free flow of misdirected blood into the thoracic cavity. The split is usually a circumferential tear that leaves an "intimal flap," but also might result from an aortic ulcer.

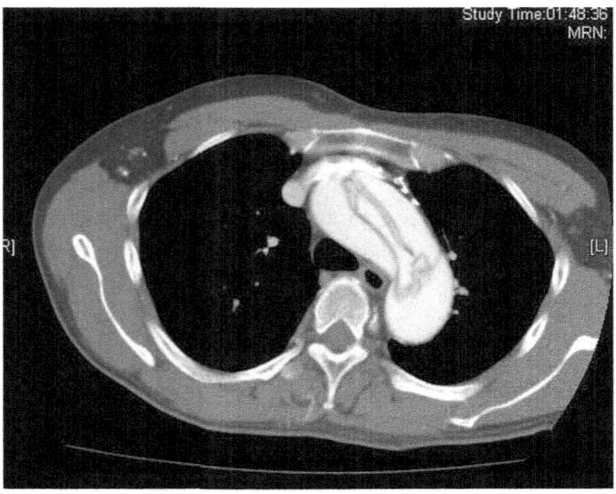

Intimal flap seen in the aortic arc. [Niino T, Unosawa S, Shimura K. Stanford type A aortic dissection with intimal intussusception. Gen Thorac Cardiovasc Surg. 2012 Sep;60(9):578-80. https://doi.org/10.1007/s11748-012-0051-1, 2012-09-04] *Caption adapted from original*

- This tearing down the middle of the aortic wall causes pain that is characteristically (but not universally) described by the patient as "ripping." As the false lumen develops and extends, driven by the hydrostatic pressure of continued pulsatile blood flow, it may prevent blood flow through the remaining true lumen into aortic branches that perfuse vital organs, including the heart itself, brain, lung, and kidneys (see Presentation).
- Several problems may predispose the thoracic aorta to dissection. The most important, by far, is hypertension. Problems with the aortic valve (aortic stenosis, bicuspid valve) and the aorta itself (coarctation) are associated with TAD. In addition, several connective tissue diseases are known to increase the risk of TAD, including Marfan's syndrome and Ehlers-Danlos syndrome.

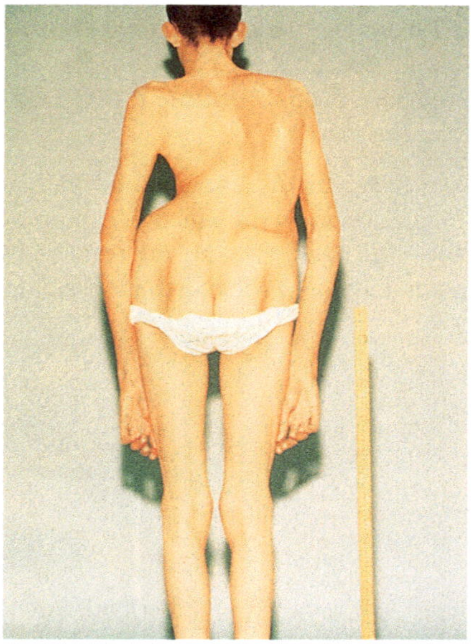

Marfan's syndrome. [Radio S, Godfrey M, Baxter T. Diseases of the aorta. In: McManus B, Braunwald E, editors. Atlas of cardiovascular pathology for the clinician. Philadelphia: Current Medicine; 2000. Chapter 17. ISBN: 1-57340-160-9; 2002-01-21]

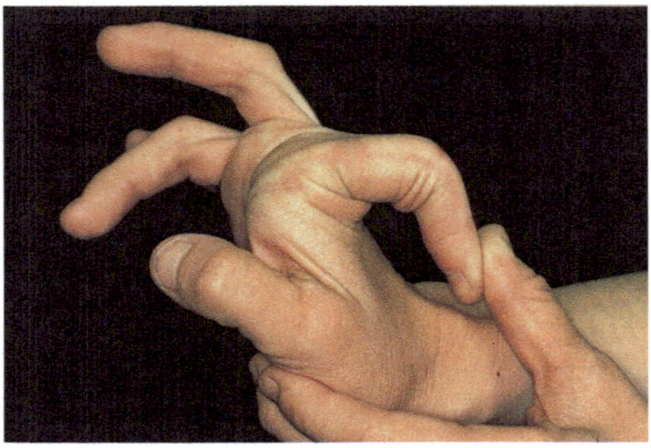

Joint hypermobility in Ehlers-Danlos syndrome. [Maricic M, Ko M. Diseases of bone and connective tissue. In Hunder G, editor. Atlas of rheumatology. 4th ed. Philadelphia: Current Medicine; 2005. Chapter 6. ISBN: 1-57340-210-9; 2002-03-07] *Caption adapted from original*

- Hypertension, connective tissue diseases, and the aging process itself may result in cystic medial necrosis, in which degenerative changes occur in the middle layer of the aortic wall. Elastin, collagen, and smooth muscle all start to break down, potentially predisposing to the development of TAD.

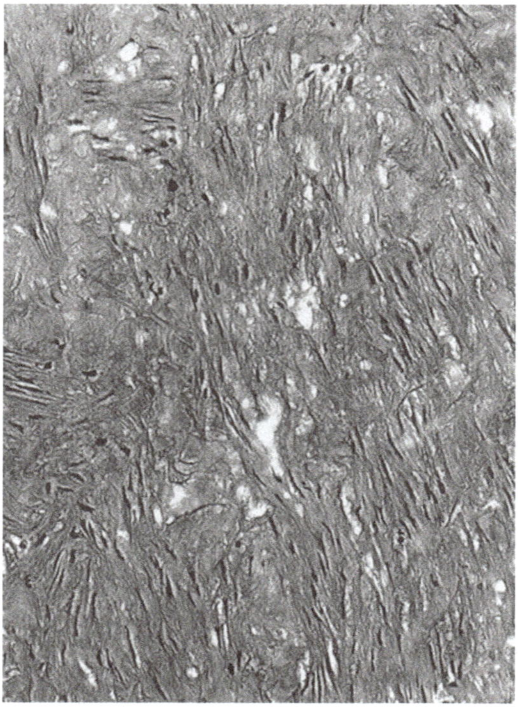

Cystic medial necrosis. [Elefteriades JA. Thoracic aortic aneurysm: reading the enemy's playbook. World J Surg. 2008 Mar;32(3):366-74. https://doi.org/10.1007/s00268-007-9398-3, 2008-02-20]

- Other diagnoses associated with TAD are:
  - Congenital
    - Polycystic kidney disease

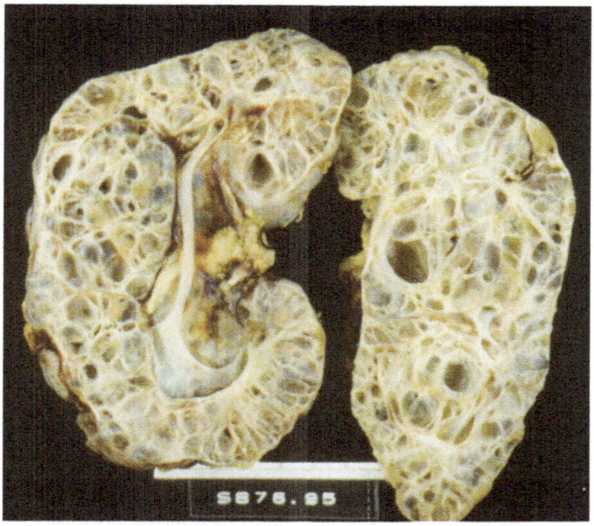

Evidence of cysts in autosomal recessive polycystic kidney disease. [Marks S, Geary DF. Nephrology. In: Laxer R, Ford-Jones EL, Friedman J, Gerstle T, editors. The Hospital for Sick Children: atlas of pediatrics. Philadelphia: Current Medicine; 2005. Chapter 17. ISBN: 1-57340-188-9, 2006-01-20] *Caption adapted from original*

- Turner syndrome

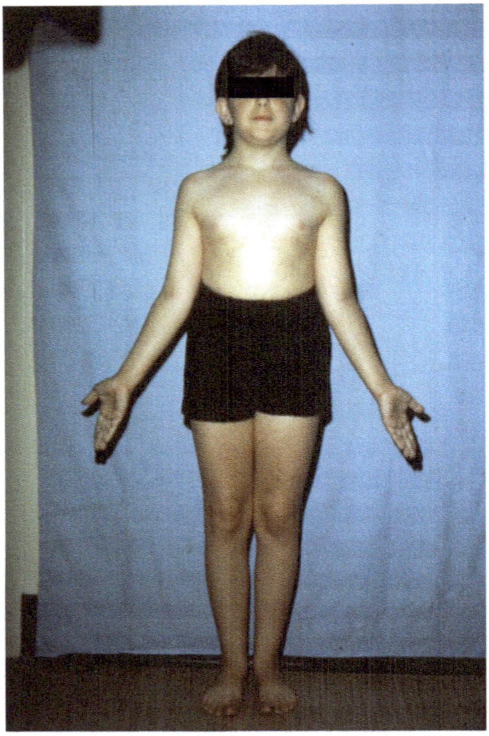

Turner syndrome. [Teebi A, Kennedy S, Chitayat D, Teshima I, Unger S, Babul-Hirji R, Shuman C, Weksberg R. Clinical genetics. In: Laxer R, Ford-Jones EL, Friedman J, Gerstle T, editors. The Hospital for Sick Children: atlas of pediatrics. Philadelphia: Current Medicine; 2005. Chapter 1. ISBN: 1-57340-188-9, 2006-01-20] *Caption adapted from original*

- Noonan syndrome

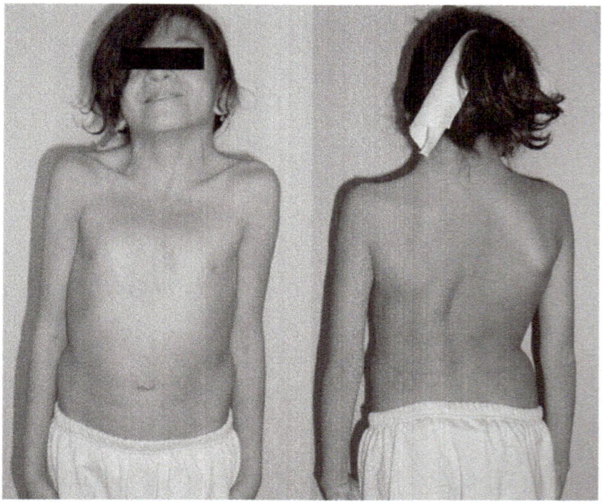

Noonan syndrome. Webbed neck and double structural curve with rib deformity evident. [From article: Rare causes of scoliosis and spine deformity: experience and particular features. Scoliosis. 2007 Oct;2(1):15. https://doi.org/10.1186/1748-7161-2-15, at http://link.springer.com/article/10.1186/1748-7161-2-15; by Konstantinos C Soultanis, Alexandros H Payatakes, Vasilios T Chouliaras, Georgios C Mandellos, Nikolaos E Pyrovolou, Fani M Pliarchopoulou, Panayotis N Soucacos, © Soultanis et al; licensee BioMed Central Ltd. 2007; licensed under Creative Commons Attribution License http://creativecommons.org/licenses/by/2.0] *Caption adapted from original*

- Osteogenesis imperfecta

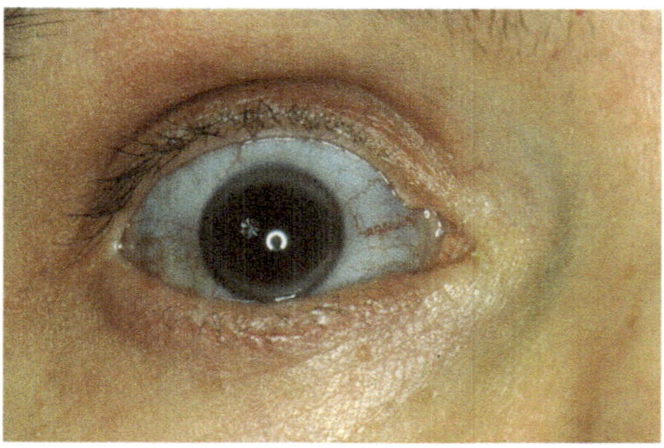

Blue sclera characteristic of osteogenesis imperfecta. [Teebi A, Kennedy S, Chitayat D, Teshima I, Unger S, Babul-Hirji R, Shuman C, Weksberg R. Clinical genetics. In: Laxer R, Ford-Jones EL, Friedman J, Gerstle T, editors. The Hospital for Sick Children: atlas of pediatrics. Philadelphia: Current Medicine; 2005. Chapter 1. ISBN: 1-57340-188-9, 2006-01-20]

  - Familial aortic dissections
- Infectious:
  - syphilis

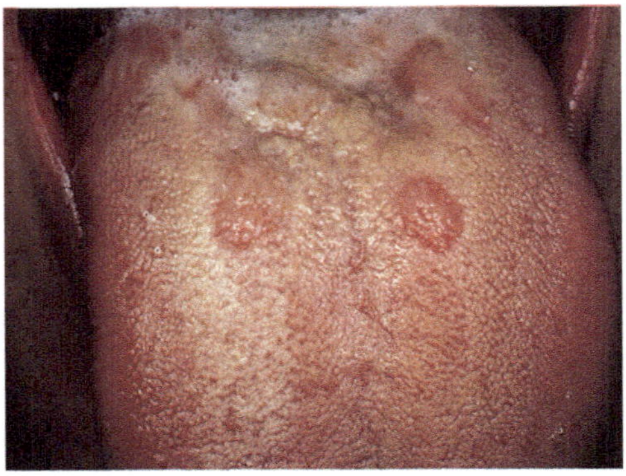

Papular lesions on the tongue in secondary syphilis. [Fiumara N. Primary and secondary syphilis. In: Rein M, editor. Sexually transmitted diseases. Philadelphia: Current Medicine; 1996. Chapter 9. (Mandell G, editor. Atlas of infectious diseases; vol. 5). ISBN: 0-443077-20-7, 2002-01-23] *Caption from original*

- Trauma:
  - Sudden deceleration injury
- Toxicologic:
  - Cocaine use
- Iatrogenic:
  - Catheter- or surgery-related aortic injury, especially near the aortic valve

Presentation

Typical/"Classic"

- Chest pain that is often described as "ripping" or "tearing" in nature is the classic presenting symptom in TAD. Less classically, but probably more commonly, the pain is described simply as "sharp." This pain may be felt in the front and/or back of the chest; when the latter, it is classically localized between the scapulae. The pain is usually noted to move with the extension of the dissection. Patients can often identify the exact time the pain started. Other symptoms may result from occlusion of branch arteries and compression of adjacent tissues and therefore are variable. Patients are usually hypertensive at presentation, although shock may also occur. Related signs and symptoms include:

- Syncope or stroke, when the dissection occludes the carotid arteries
  - Hemiplegia or hemianesthesia may result if just one carotid root is obstructed
- Dyspnea and a clinical picture of heart failure, when the dissection disrupts the aortic root, preventing valve closure and resulting in acute aortic regurgitation

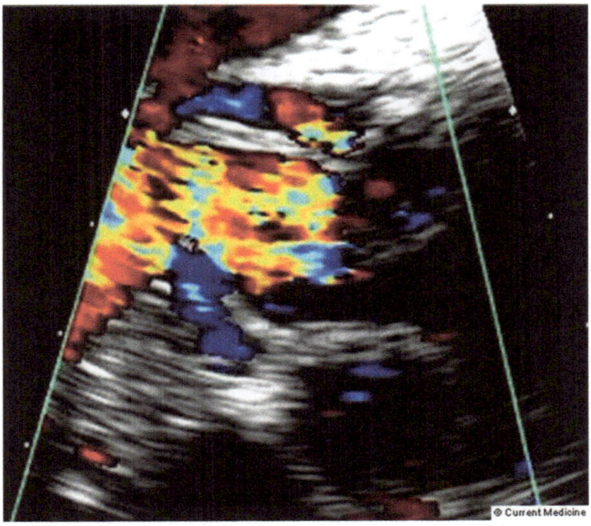

Severe aortic regurgitation from Stanford type A dissection. [Michelena H, Mankad S, Enriquez-Sarano M. Echocardiography in valvular heart disease: aortic valve disease. In: Solomon SD, Braunwald E, editors. Atlas of echocardiography. 2nd ed. Philadelphia: Current Medicine; 2008. Chapter 9. ISBN: 1-57340-217-6, 2008-10-22] *Caption from original*

- Classic signs of aortic regurgitation include a wide pulse pressure, bounding pulses, and a diastolic murmur heard best over the right sternal border.

http://www.easyauscultation.com/cases?coursecaseorder=1&courseid=27
Diastolic murmur. [Aortic Regurgitation – Mild; Easy Auscultation; www.easyauscultation.com; copyright 2015, MedEdu LLC]

- Hypotension, when the dissection spills false lumen blood into the pericardial sac, resulting in pericardial effusion and tamponade

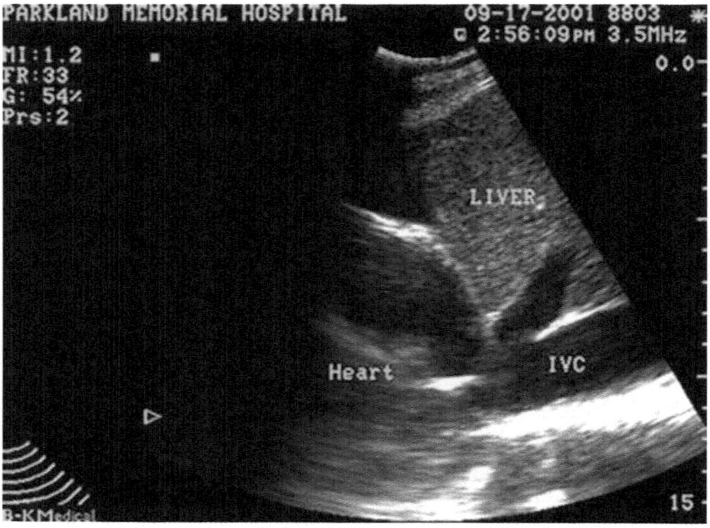

Ultrasound of acute pericardial effusion causing cardiac tamponade. [Tchorz KM. Ultrasound-guided drainage procedures for the intensivist. In: Frankel HL, deBoisblanc BP, editors. Bedside procedures for the intensivist. New York: Springer; 2010. p. 113-37. Book https://doi.org/10.1007/978-0-387-79830-1; Chapter: 6; Chapter https://doi.org/10.1007/978-0-387-79830-1_6, 2010-01-01] *Caption adapted from original*

    - Check for jugular venous distension and muffled heart sounds.

- Abdominal pain, from obstruction of mesenteric arteries
- Paraplegia, from obstruction of aortic branches perfusing the spinal cord (such as the great artery of Adamkiewicz)
- Hoarseness, difficulty swallowing, or dyspnea (perhaps with stridor) from pressure on the larynx, trachea, and esophagus caused by the expanding aortic hematoma

http://www.easyauscultation.com/cases.aspx?coursecaseorder=13&courseid=202 Stridor. [Stridor; Easy Auscultation; www.easyauscultation.com; copyright 2015, MedEdu LLC]

- Horner's syndrome, from compression of the superior cervical ganglia caused by the expanding aortic hematoma

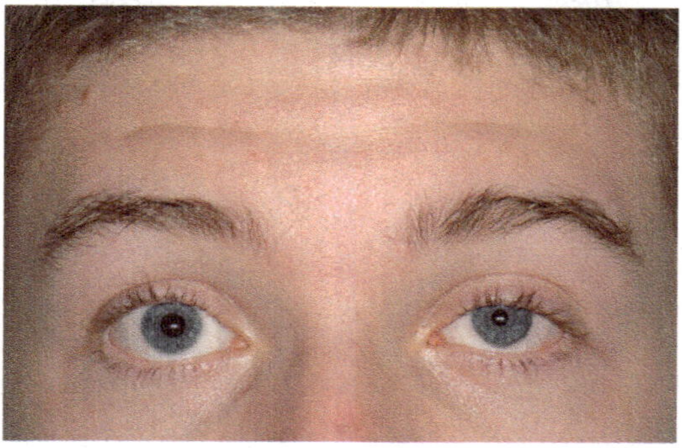

Left ptosis and miosis of Horner's syndrome. [Mutalib M, Vandervelde C, Varghese A, Sallomi DF, Silva P, Hickman CJM, Howlett DC. Horner's syndrome secondary to asymptomatic pneumothorax in an adolescent. Eur J Pediatr. 2007 May;166(5):507–8. https://doi.org/10.1007/s00431-006-0271-4, 2007-03-19] *Caption adapted from original*

- Horner's syndrome manifests as ipsilateral ptosis, miosis, and anhydrosis.

- Physical findings in TAD are highly variable because the location of the dissection and the direction (antegrade or retrograde) in which it extends will determine side branch involvement. If the dissection involves the aortic arch, there may be a difference in the blood pressure measured in each arm. A difference of 20 mm Hg is significant and suggestive of the diagnosis in the right clinical setting.

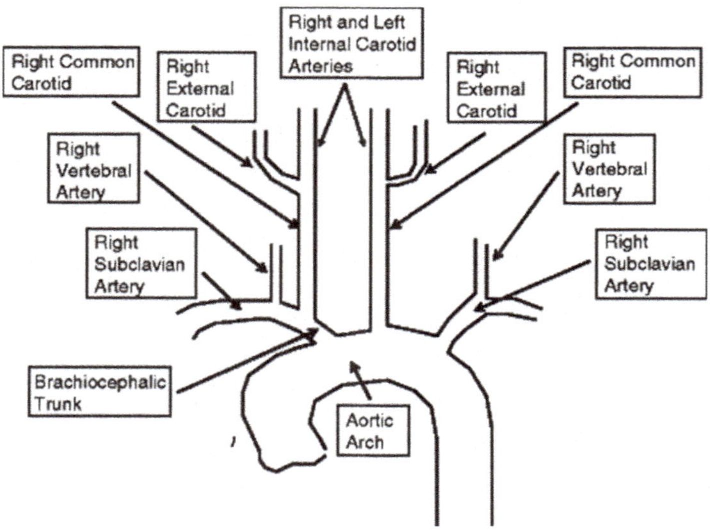

Anatomy of the aortic arch. [Pelberg RA, Mazur W. Vascular CT angiography manual. London: Springer; 2011. Chapter 5, Carotid and upper extremity CT angiography; p. 47-90. Book https://doi.org/10.1007/978-1-84996-260-5; Chapter https://doi.org/10.1007/978-1-84996-260-5_5, 2010-01-01]

Atypical

- The most vexing atypical presentation of TAD is a painless presentation. This may occur in elderly people who present with syncope or stroke only. In other cases, the TAD symptoms may simply be overwhelmed by other symptoms or findings, such as stroke, shock, or myocardial infarction (if the dissection extends to the ostium of a coronary artery and causes ST-segment elevation).

Primary Differential Considerations

- Primary differential considerations include pain mimics to TAD and other significant diagnoses (such as stroke) that distract the examiner. The most concerning pain mimics that may share other symptoms associated with TAD include myocardial infarction, pulmonary embolus, aortic aneurysm, and aortic regurgitation without dissection.

History and Physical Exam

Findings That Confirm Diagnosis

- Because there are so many mimics and related multisystem complications of TAD, the diagnosis cannot be confirmed without a definitive imaging study of the thoracic aorta.

Factors That Suggest Diagnosis

- Immediate onset of sharp, ripping, or tearing pain in the presence of ST-segment elevation, syncope, stroke, dyspnea, or weakness should raise suspicion for TAD and prompt consideration of an emergent diagnostic imaging study.
- Suggestive pain with a known diagnosis (or suggestive physiognomy) of Marfan's syndrome, Ehlers-Danlos syndrome, or syphilis should raise suspicion for TAD and prompt consideration of an emergent diagnostic imaging study.

- Suggestive pain and a difference in blood pressure readings between the two arms or between the arms and the legs should raise suspicion for TAD and prompt consideration of an urgent or emergent diagnostic imaging study.
- Any of the related symptoms or findings above *in the absence of suggestive pain in elderly patients* <u>*with*</u> *a history of hypertension* should raise suspicion for TAD and prompt consideration of an urgent or emergent diagnostic imaging study.

Factors That Exclude Diagnosis

- A normal imaging study (via CT scan, MRI, or transesophageal echocardiogram) of the thoracic aorta excludes the diagnosis of TAD.

Ancillary Studies

Laboratory

- Lab tests should include CBC; serum electrolyte, blood urea nitrogen (BUN), and creatinine levels; and coagulation studies. Generally, cardiac biomarker measurements are indicated because of the differential consideration of ACS and the possibility of a retrograde dissection that occludes a coronary artery and causes myocardial ischemia.
- If TAD is the presumed or confirmed diagnosis and surgical intervention is anticipated, a type and cross-match specimen should be sent.

Electrocardiography

- The ECG in most patients with TAD either is normal or shows only nonspecific ST-T changes. Because many patients with TAD have a longstanding history of hypertension, the ECG may show evidence of left ventricular hypertrophy with strain.
- A small minority of patients with TAD will have evidence of STEMI (usually inferior) due to occlusion of the right coronary artery as a complication of TAD.

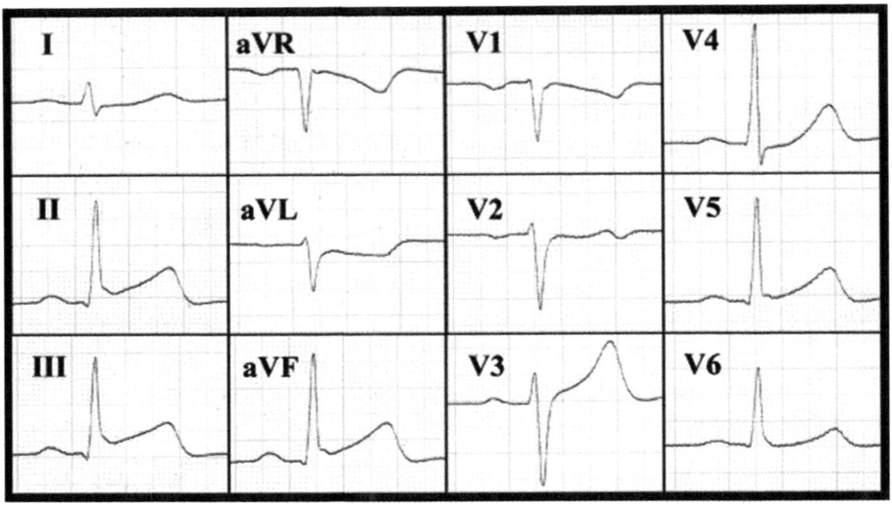

Twelve-lead ECG demonstrating inferiorly located STEMI with ST-segment elevation in the inferior leads (II, III, aVF) and ST-segment depression in leads I and aVL. [From article: Cardiovascular magnetic resonance of myocardial infarction after blunt chest trauma: a heartbreaking soccer-shot. J Cardiovasc Magn Reson. 2009 Oct;11(1):39. https://doi.org/10.1186/1532-429X-11-39, at http://link.springer.com/article/10.1186/1532-429X-11-39/fulltext.html; by Hannibal Baccouche, Torsten Beck, Martin Maunz, Peter Fogarassy, Martin Beyer, © Baccouche et al; licensee BioMed Central Ltd. 2009; licensed under Creative Commons Attribution License BY 2.0 http://creativecommons.org/licenses/by/2.0] *Caption adapted from original*

- An even smaller cohort will have ECG changes suggesting pericardial tamponade, such as low voltage or electrical alternans.

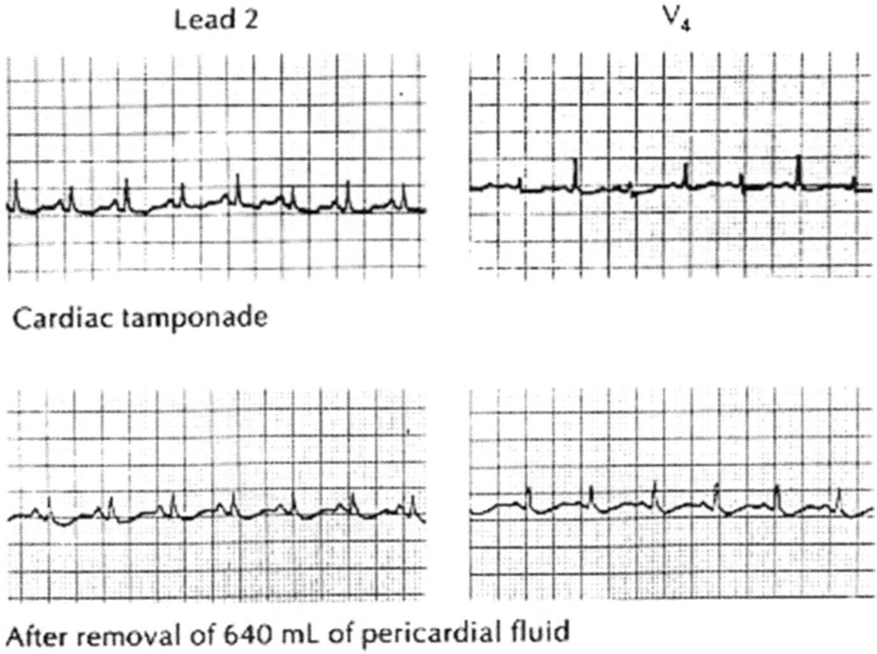

Electrical alternans of the QRS complex in a patient with cardiac tamponade. [Fowler N, Abelmann W. Chapter 13. In: Lee RT, Braunwald E, editors. Atlas of cardiac imaging. Philadelphia: Current Medicine; 1998. ISBN: 0-443-07567-0] *Caption from original*

Imaging

- Imaging studies are used definitively to confirm or refute the diagnosis of TAD.
- The plain chest radiograph (CXR) may suggest TAD but cannot be used to confirm or refute the diagnosis.
    - The most important finding on CXR is a widened mediastinum, which is seen in more than half the patients with TAD. Often these films are recorded with patients in the supine position because of their clinical status; this makes the mediastinum appear wider than on an erect film even in the absence of TAD.

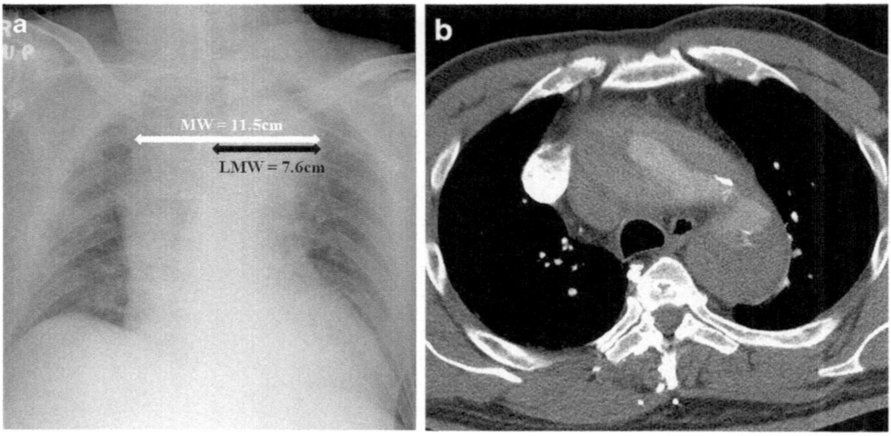

Acute type A aortic dissection in a 46-year-old man. A) AP chest radiograph showing marked widening of the mediastinum with MW and LMW measuring 11.5 and 7.6 cm, respectively. B) Corresponding selected image of CT aortogram confirms type A aortic dissection. [From article: Diagnostic accuracy of mediastinal width measurement on posteroanterior and anteroposterior chest radiographs in the depiction of acute nontraumatic thoracic aortic dissection. Emerg Radiol. 2012 Aug;19(4):309–15. https://doi.org/10.1007/s10140-012-1034-3, at http://link.springer.com/article/10.1007/s10140-012-1034-3/fulltext.html; by Vincent Lai, Wai Kan Tsang, Wan Chi Chan, Tsz Wai Yeung, © The Author(s) 2012; licensed under Creative Commons Attribution License http://creativecommons.org/licenses/by/2.0] *Caption from original*

  - Other findings suggestive of TAD that may appear on CXR include pleural effusion, inward displacement of aortic intimal calcifications, and a double aortic shadow.
  - The CXR is normal in more than 10% of cases of TAD.

- The choice of which definitive imaging study to use in suspected TAD is based on both the efficiency/availability of the test and the clinical stability of the patient. In the past, the diagnosis was made by invasive imaging (aortography). Less invasive modalities (CT, MRI, TEE) are more commonly used today. Of these, CT is the quickest and for the hemodynamically unstable or tenuous patient, is probably the safest approach. It does require iodinated contrast. CT has the additional benefit of potentially identifying another etiology of the patient's pain (such as pulmonary embolism). All three of these modalities allow classification of the TAD (Stanford or DeBakey models; See Overall Principles of Treatment), which directs the choice of medical vs surgical treatment.

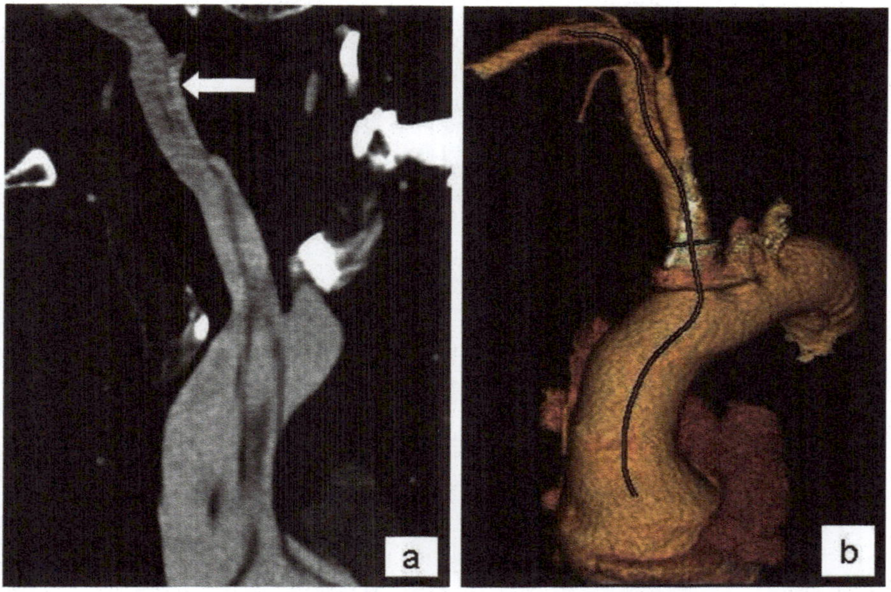

A, Contrast-enhanced CT scan showing the intimal flap due to dissection from the aortic root to the ascending aorta, innominate artery and subclavian artery. B, Enhanced reconstructed CT scan image showing the path of dissection. [From article: Postoperative peri-axillary seroma following axillary artery cannulation for surgical treatment of acute type A aortic dissection. J Cardiothorac Surg. 2010 May;5(1):43. https://doi.org/10.1186/1749-8090-5-43, at http://link.springer.com/article/10.1186/1749-8090-5-43; by Efstratios E Apostolakis, Nikolaos G Baikoussis, Konstantinos Katsanos, Menelaos Karanikolas, © Apostolakis et al; licensee BioMed Central Ltd.; licensed under Creative Commons Attribution License BY 2.0 http://creativecommons.org/licenses/by/2.0] *Caption adapted from original*

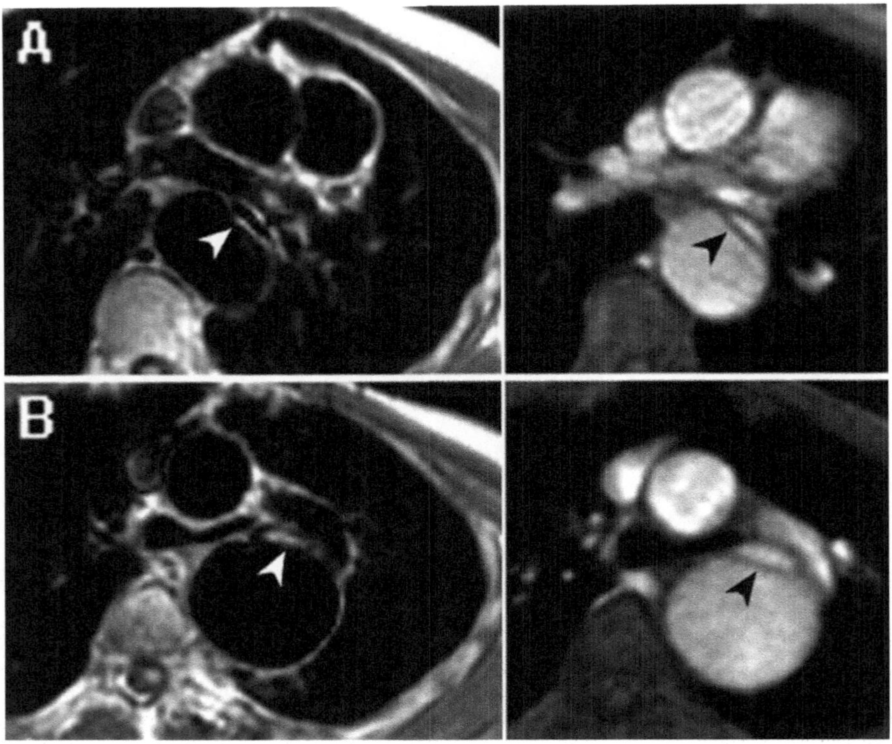
A
B

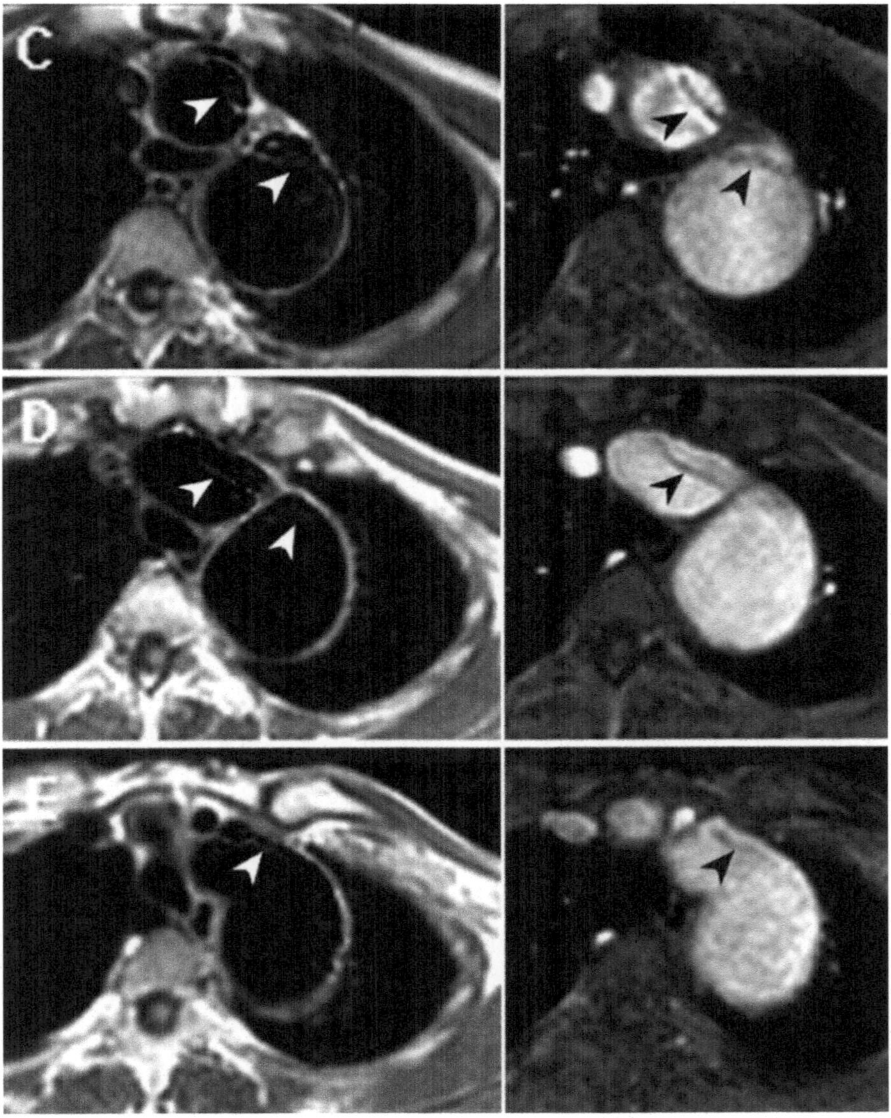

Type A aortic dissection in Marfan syndrome: the intimal flap (arrowhead) and the two channels are visible on sequential black blood (left) and bright blood cine-MRI (right) images. [Kastler B. MRI of cardiovascular malformations. Berlin Heidelberg: Springer; 2011. Chapter 6, Other aortic malformations; p. 147–75. https://doi.org/10.1007/978-3-540-30702-0] *Caption from original*

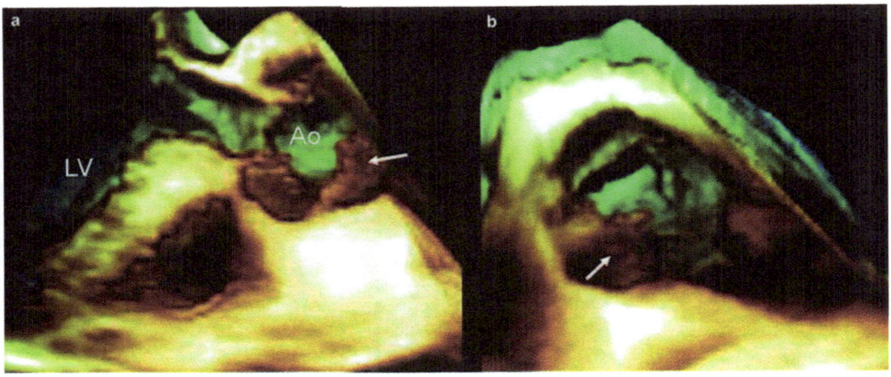

(a) RT 3D TEE image showing the dissection of the aortic wall (arrow) in longitudinal view and (b) from the aortic perspective. Ao aorta; LV left ventricle. [Faletra FF, de Castro S, Pandian NG, Kronzon I, Nesser H-J, Ho SY. The Aortic Valve and the Aorta. Atlas of Real Time 3D Transesophageal Echocardiography [Internet]. London: Springer London; 2010 [cited 2016 May 27]. p. 47–62. Available from: http://link.springer.com/10.1007/978-1-84996-083-0_4] *Caption from original*

Special Populations

Age

- TAD most commonly occurs between 50 and 65 years of age. Older patients may have less perception of the pain and more often present with stroke or syncope.
- Within the pediatric population, TAD is associated with Marfan syndrome, Turner syndrome, Ehler-Danlos syndrome, and homocystinuria.

Co-morbidities

- The most important comorbidities in TAD are hypertension and connective tissue disease.

Pitfalls in Diagnosis

Critical Steps Not to Miss

- Attributing chest pain to another, potentially less serious etiology may result in loss of valuable treatment time for TAD.
- Focusing on the sequelae of TAD—such as syncope, stroke, weakness, or dyspnea—without considering TAD as the source, may result in loss of valuable treatment time for TAD and further complications from ongoing extension of the false lumen.

Mimics

- The entire constellation of diagnoses that underlies chest pain syndrome can mimic the pain and overall presentation of TAD.

Time-Dependent Interventions

- Control of blood pressure and heart rate (the "pulse-pressure product" that creates shear stress on the aortic wall and may extend the dissection) is critical in stabilizing patients with TAD. Both alpha- and beta-adrenergic blockade is required, as reducing blood pressure alone with a potent agent such as nitroprusside will result in a reflex tachycardia that may be just as harmful as continued hypertension in promoting extension of the dissection.
- Adequate pain control (with attention to iatrogenic hypotension) is also important for reducing shear stress.

Overall Principles of Treatment

- Stabilization of the patient with control of blood pressure, pulse rate, and pain is critical. The patient may require resuscitation, intubation, and intensive support.
- Definitive treatment approaches for TAD are driven by the anatomic location of the dissection. There are two classification systems for TAD: DeBakey and Stanford. The Stanford system is simpler and more widely used: type A involves the ascending aorta, and type B does not involve the ascending aorta. In the DeBakey classification, there is involvement of the ascending aorta in types I and II but not in type III. Surgical management ordinarily is

indicated for type A (DeBakey I and II) lesions, whereas type B (DeBakey III) dissections may be managed medically or with (percutaneous) endovascular repair.

Steps in the Early Medical Management of a Patient Presenting With Suspected Acute Aortic Dissection
1. Immediate monitoring and stabilization of vital signs
2. Quick assessment: directed history, physical examination, chest radiograph, ECG, lab work
3. Reduce dP/dT with intravenous β-blockers: propranolol, labetalol, metoprolol, or esmolol
4. Treat hypertension to reduce dP/dT: intravenous nitroprusside (use in the presence of a β-blocker, because alone it may increase dP/dT); goal is to reduce systolic blood pressure to 100–120 mm Hg or the lowest level possible while still maintaining cerebral and vital organ perfusion
5. If β-blockers are absolutely contraindicated, consider using intravenous calcium channel blockers or enalaprilat
6. Pain control with morphine as needed
7. Select and proceed promptly to a diagnostic study
8. Decide on medical vs surgical therapy (and determine surgical candidacy as well)

Steps in the early medical management of a patient presenting with suspected aortic dissection. [Creager M. Vascular disease. In Libby P, editor. Essential atlas of cardiovascular disease. Philadelphia: Current Medicine; 2009. Chapter 4. ISBN: 978-1-57340-309-2, 2009-05-21] *Caption adapted from original*

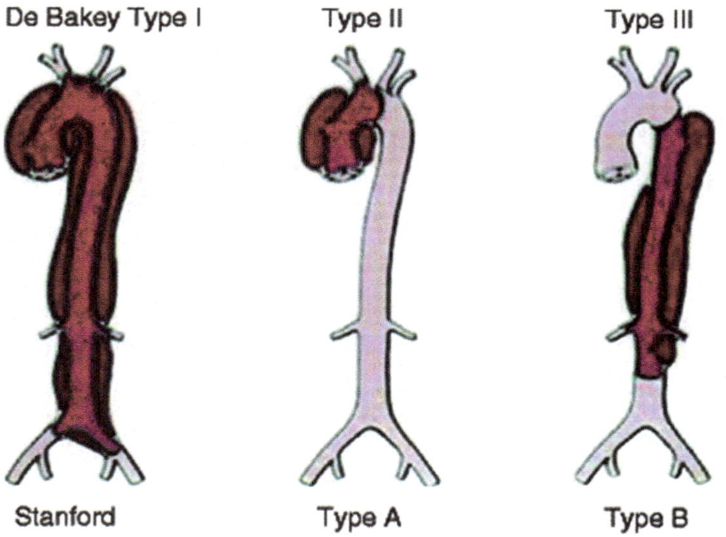

Acuity:

Acute	<2 weeks after onset
Subacute:	2–8 weeks after onset
Chronic:	>8 weeks after onset

Anatomic location:

Ascending aorta:	Stanford Type A, DeBakey Type II
Ascending and descending aorta:	Stanford Type A, DeBakey Type I
Descending aorta:	Stanford Type B, DeBakey Type III

Pathophysiology:

Class 1: Classical aortic dissection with initimal flap between true and false lumen
Class 2: Aortic intramural he matoma without identifiable intimal flap
Class 3: Intimal tear without hematoma (limited dissection)
Class 4: Atherosclerothic plaque rupture with aortic penetrating ulcer
Class 5: Iatrogenic or traumatic aortic dissection
(intra-aortic catherterization, high-speed deceleration injury, blunt chest trauma)

Classification of thoracic aortic dissection. [Akin I, Rehders TC, Kische S, Ince H, Nienaber CA. Endovascular treatment of thoracic aorta. In: Lanzer P, editor. Catheter-based cardiovascular interventions. Berlin Heidelberg: Springer; 2013. p. 957-70. Book https://doi.org/10.1007/978-3-642-27676-7; Chapter https://doi.org/10.1007/978-3-642-27676-7_59, 2013-01-01] *Caption from original*

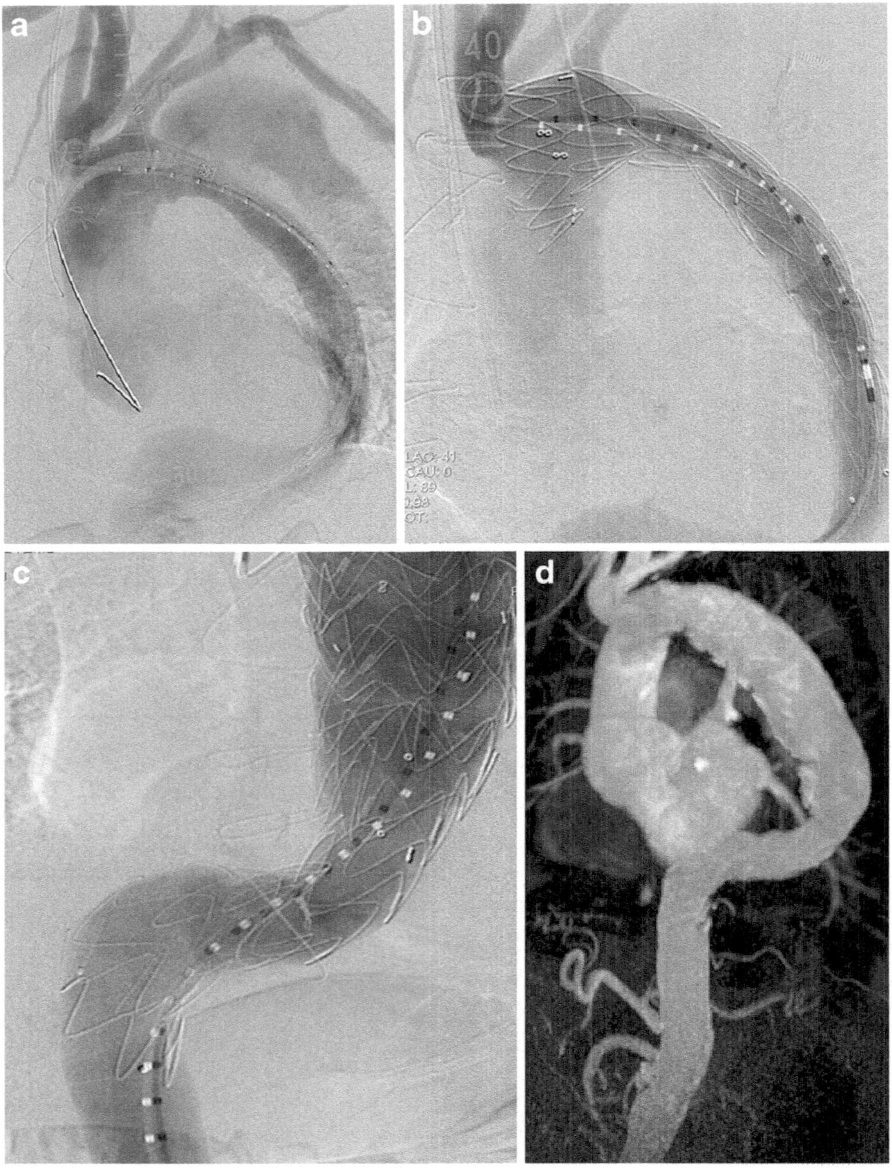

Thoracic endovascular aortic repair (TEVAR) of a type B aortic dissection extending from the arch to the abdominal aorta. (A) Pre- and (B, C) post-implantation angiograms showing two stent-grafts placed from the arch, covering the left subclavian artery (LSA), to the distal descending aorta in order to treat different entry tears and the true lumen compression. (D) MRA at 1 year from the implantation: the true lumen is well expanded at the proximal and middle descending aorta, while a smaller diameter is observed at the distal part of the vessel. [Midulla M, Moreno R, Baali A, Chau M, Negre-Salvayre A, Nicoud F, Pruvo JP, Haulon S, Rousseau H. Haemodynamic imaging of thoracic stent-grafts by computational fluid dynamics (CFD): presentation of a patient-specific method combining magnetic resonance imaging and numerical simulations. Eur Radiol. 2012 Oct;22(10):2094–102. https://doi.org/10.1007/s00330-012-2465-7, 2012-08-30] *Caption adapted from original*

Disease Course

- TAD carries a high mortality rate. Type A dissections have a 30% mortality even with surgical treatment, and twice that with medical treatment. Thrombotic complications of dissection carry their own risks of morbidity and mortality.

Related Evidence

Papers of particular interest have been highlighted as:
*** Of key importance*

Practice Guideline

Grabenwöger M, Alfonso F, Bachet J, Bonser R, Czerny M, Eggebrecht H, Evangelista A, Fattori R, Jakob H, Lönn L, Nienaber CA, Rocchi G, Rousseau H, Thompson M, Weigang E, Erbel R; European Association for Cardio-Thoracic Surgery (EACTS); European Society of Cardiology (ESC); European Association of Percutaneous Cardiovascular Interventions (EAPCI). Thoracic Endovascular Aortic Repair (TEVAR) for the treatment of aortic diseases: a position statement from the European Association for Cardio-Thoracic Surgery (EACTS) and the European Society of Cardiology (ESC), in collaboration with the European Association of Percutaneous Cardiovascular Interventions (EAPCI). Eur J Cardiothorac Surg. 2012 Jul;42(1):17–24. https://doi.org/10.1093/ejcts/ezs107. PMID: 22561652. http://www.ncbi.nlm.nih.gov/pubmed/2561652 **

Review

Wong SC, Cheung M, Zacharin M. Aortic dilatation and dissection in Turner syndrome: what we know, what we are unclear about and what we should do in clinical practice? Int J Adolesc Med Health. 2014;26(4):469–88. https://doi.org/10.1515/ijamh-2013-0336. PMID: 24887949. http://www.ncbi.nlm.nih.gov/pubmed/24887949

Paterick TE, Humphries JA, Ammar KA, Jan MF, Loberg R, Bush M, Khandheria BK, Tajik AJ. Aortopathies: etiologies, genetics, differential diagnosis, prognosis and management. Am J Med. 2013 Aug;126(8):670–8. https://doi.org/10.1016/j.amjmed.2013.01.029. PMID: 2380058. http://www.ncbi.nlm.nih.gov/pubmed/2380058 **

Kölbel T, Diener H, Larena-Avellaneda A, Debus S. Advanced endovascular techniques for thoracic and abdominal aortic dissections. J Cardiovasc Surg (Torino). 2013 Feb;54(1 Suppl 1):81–90. PMID: 23443592. http://www.ncbi.nlm.nih.gov/pubmed/23443592

Upadhye S, Schiff K. Acute aortic dissection in the emergency department: diagnostic challenges and evidence-based management. Emerg Med Clin North Am. 2012 May;30(2):307–27, viii. https://doi.org/10.1016/j.emc.2011.12.001. PMID: 22487109. http://www.ncbi.nlm.nih.gov/pubmed/22487109

Choi JC, LeMaire SA. Thoracic aortic dissection: genes, molecules, and the knife. Tex Heart Inst J. 2012;39(6):838-9. PMID: 23304027. http://www.ncbi.nlm.nih.gov/pubmed/23304027

Grubb KJ, Kron IL. Sex and gender in thoracic aortic aneurysms and dissection. Semin Thorac Cardiovasc Surg. 2011 Summer;23(2):124–5. https://doi.org/10.1053/j.semtcvs.2011.08.009. PMID: 22041041. http://www.ncbi.nlm.nih.gov/pubmed/22041041

Booher AM, Eagle KA. Diagnosis and management issues in thoracic aortic aneurysm. Am Heart J. 2011 Jul;162(1):38–46.e1. https://doi.org/10.1016/j.ahj.2011.04.010. PMID: 21742088 http://www.ncbi.nlm.nih.gov/pubmed/21742088

LeMaire SA, Russell L. Epidemiology of thoracic aortic dissection. Nat Rev Cardiol. 2011 Feb;8(2):103–13. https://doi.org/10.1038/nrcardio.2010.187. PMID: 21173794. http://www.ncbi.nlm.nih.gov/pubmed/21173794 **

Review. Thrumurthy SG, Karthikesalingam A, Patterson BO, Holt PJ, Hinchliffe RJ, Loftus IM, Thompson MM. A systematic review of mid-term outcomes of thoracic endovascular repair (TEVAR) of chronic type B aortic dissection. Eur J Vasc Endovasc Surg. 2011 Nov;42(5):632–47. https://doi.org/10.1016/j.ejvs.2011.08.009. Erratum in: Eur J Vasc Endovasc Surg. 2012 May;43(5):619. PMID: 21880515. http://www.ncbi.nlm.nih.gov/pubmed/21880515

Thrumurthy SG, Karthikesalingam A, Patterson BO, Holt PJ, Thompson MM. The diagnosis and management of aortic dissection. BMJ. 2011 Jan 11;344:d8290. https://doi.org/10.1136/bmj.d8290. PMID: 22236596. http://www.ncbi.nlm.nih.gov/pubmed/22236596 **

Hiratzka LF, Bakris GL, Beckman JA, Bersin RM, Carr VF, Casey DE Jr, Eagle KA, Hermann LK, Isselbacher EM, Kazerooni EA, Kouchoukos NT, Lytle BW, Milewicz DM, Reich DL, Sen S, Shinn JA, Svensson LG, Williams DM; American College of Cardiology Foundation/American Heart Association Task Force on Practice Guidelines; American Association for Thoracic surgery; American College of Radiology; American Stroke Association; Society of Cardiovascular Anesthesiologists; Society for Cardiovascular Angiography and Interventions; Society of Interventional Radiology; Society of Thoracic Surgeons; Society for Vascular Medicine. 2010 ACCF/AHA/AATS/ACR/ASA/SCA/SCAI/SIR/STS/SVM Guidelines for the diagnosis and management of patients with thoracic aortic disease: Executive summary: A report of the American College of Cardiology Foundation/American Heart Association Task Force on Practice Guidelines, American Association for Thoracic Surgery, American College of Radiology, American Stroke Association, Society of Cardiovascular Anesthesiologists, Society for Cardiovascular Angiography and Interventions, Society of Interventional Radiology, Society of Thoracic Surgeons, and Society for Vascular Medicine. Anesth Analg. 2010 Aug;111(2):279-315. https://doi.org/10.1213/ANE.0b013e3181dd869b. PMID: 20664093. http://www.ncbi.nlm.nih.gov/pubmed/20664093 **

Subramanian S, Roselli EE. Thoracic aortic dissection: long-term results of endovascular and open repair. Semin Vasc Surg. 2009 Jun;22(2):61–8. https://doi.org/10.1053/j.semvascsurg.2009.04.006. PMID: 19573743. http://www.ncbi.nlm.nih.gov/pubmed/19573743

Ramanath VS, Oh JK, Sundt TM 3rd, Eagle KA. Acute aortic syndromes and thoracic aortic aneurysm. Mayo Clin Proc. 2009 May;84(5):465–81. https://doi.org/10.1016/S0025-6196(11)60566-1. PMID: 19411444. http://www.ncbi.nlm.nih.gov/pubmed/19411444

Lin PH, Huynh TT, Kougias P, Huh J, LeMaire SA, Coselli JS. Descending thoracic aortic dissection: evaluation and management in the era of endovascular technology. Vasc Endovascular Surg. 2009 Feb-Mar;43(1):5–24. https://doi.org/10.1177/1538574408318475. PMID: 18583304. http://www.ncbi.nlm.nih.gov/pubmed/18583304

Golledge J, Eagle KA. Acute aortic dissection. Lancet. 2008 Jul 5;372(9632):55–66. https://doi.org/10.1016/S0140-6736(08)60994-0. PMID: 18603160. http://www.ncbi.nlm.nih.gov/pubmed/18603160

Shiga T, Wajima Z, Apfel CC, Inoue T, Ohe Y. Diagnostic accuracy of transesophageal echocardiography, helical computed tomography, and magnetic resonance imaging for suspected thoracic aortic dissection: systematic review and meta-analysis. Arch Intern Med. 2006 Jul 10;166(13):1350–6. PMID: 16831999. http://www.ncbi.nlm.nih.gov/pubmed/16831999

Hagan PG, Nienaber CA, Isselbacher EM, Bruckman D, Karavite DJ, Russman PL, Evangelista A, Fattori R, Suzuki T, Oh JK, Moore AG, Malouf JF, Pape LA, Gaca C, Sechtem U, Lenferink S, Deutsch HJ, Diedrichs H, Marcos y Robles J, Llovet A, Gilon D, Das SK, Armstrong WF, Deeb GM, Eagle KA. JAMA. 2000 Feb 16;283(7):897–903. The International Registry of Acute Aortic Dissection

(IRAD): new insights into an old disease. PMID: 10685714. http://www.ncbi.nlm.nih.gov/pubmed/10685714

Cohort Study

Pacini D, Di Marco L, Fortuna D, Belotti LM, Gabbieri D, Zussa C, Pigini F, Contini A, Barattoni MC, De Palma R, Di Bartolomeo R. Acute aortic dissection: epidemiology and outcomes. Int J Cardiol. 2013 Sep 10;167(6):2806-12. https://doi.org/10.1016/j.ijcard.2012.07.008. PMID: 22882963. http://www.ncbi.nlm.nih.gov/pubmed/22882963 **

Zipfel B, Czerny M, Funovics M, Coppi G, Ferro C, Rousseau H, Berti S, Tealdi DG, Riambau V, Mangialardi N, Sassi C; RESTORE Investigators. Endovascular treatment of patients with types A and B thoracic aortic dissection using Relay thoracic stent-grafts: results from the RESTORE Patient Registry. J Endovasc Ther. 2011 Apr;18(2):131–43. https://doi.org/10.1583/10-3233MR.1. PMID: 21521051. http://www.ncbi.nlm.nih.gov/pubmed/21521051

Comparative Study

Olsson C, Granath F, Ståhle E. Family history, comorbidity and risk of thoracic aortic disease: a population-based case-control study. Heart. 2013 Jul;99(14):1030–3. https://doi.org/10.1136/heartjnl-2013-303654. PMID: 23624484. http://www.ncbi.nlm.nih.gov/pubmed/23624484

Liao M, Zou S, Weng J, Hou L, Yang L, Zhao Z, Bao J, Jing Z. A microRNA profile comparison between thoracic aortic dissection and normal thoracic aorta indicates the potential role of microRNAs in contributing to thoracic aortic dissection pathogenesis. J Vasc Surg. 2011 May;53(5):1341-1349.e3. https://doi.org/10.1016/j.jvs.2010.11.113. PMID: 21334170. http://www.ncbi.nlm.nih.gov/pubmed/21334170

Case Study

Arnaoutakis GJ, Schneider EB, Arnaoutakis DJ, Black JH 3rd, Lum YW, Perler BA, Freischlag JA, Abularrage CJ. Influence of gender on outcomes after thoracic endovascular aneurysm repair. J Vasc Surg. 2013 Jul 26. doi:pii: S0741-5214(13)01242-1. https://doi.org/10.1016/j.jvs.2013.06.058. PMID: 23896176. http://www.ncbi.nlm.nih.gov/pubmed/23896176

Wanamaker KM, Amadi CC, Mueller JS, Moraca RJ. Incidence of aortic arch anomalies in patients with thoracic aortic dissections. J Card Surg. 2013 Mar;28(2):151-4. https://doi.org/10.1111/jocs.12072. PMID: 23488580. http://www.ncbi.nlm.nih.gov/pubmed/23488580

Lai V, Tsang WK, Chan WC, Yeung TW. Diagnostic accuracy of mediastinal width measurement on posteroanterior and anteroposterior chest radiographs in the depiction of acute nontraumatic thoracic aortic dissection. Emerg Radiol. 2012 Aug;19(4):309–15. https://doi.org/10.1007/s10140-012-1034-3. PMID: 22415593. http://www.ncbi.nlm.nih.gov/pubmed/22415593

General

Bhat SR, Garmel GM. Image diagnosis: thoracic aortic dissection and thoracic aortic aneurysm. Perm J. 2011 Spring; 15(2):88–9. PMID: 21841932. http://www.ncbi.nlm.nih.gov/pubmed/21841932

Culp WC Jr, Beyer EA. Three-dimensional transesophageal echocardiographic imaging of a thoracic aortic dissection. J Cardiovasc Med (Hagerstown). 2008 Aug;9(8):862–3. https://doi.org/10.2459/JCM.0b013e3282fa407a. PMID:18607258. http://www.ncbi.nlm.nih.gov/pubmed/18607258

PubMed Clinical Queries can provide the most recent evidence. Use this search strategy: ((“Aortic Aneurysm, Thoracic”[Mesh]) AND (“Aneurysm, Dissecting”[Mesh])) OR “thoracic aortic dissection”

Chapter 71
Total Anomalous Pulmonary Venous Connection

Richard M. Cantor, Charles V. Pollack, Jr., and Jaime Friel Blanck

Name and Synonyms

Total anomalous pulmonary venous connection (TAPVC) is also commonly referred to as Total Anomalous Pulmonary Venous Return (TAPVR).

The basic anomaly involves a failure of all four pulmonary arteries to normally connect to the left atrium.

Electronic supplementary material The online version of this chapter (https://doi.org/10.1007/978-3-319-63895-9_71) contains supplementary material, which is available to authorized users.

R. M. Cantor
Department of Emergency Medicine and Pediatrics, State University of New York Upstate Medical University, Syracuse, NY, USA

C. V. Pollack, Jr. (✉)
Department of Emergency Medicine, Thomas Jefferson University, Philadelphia, PA, USA

J. F. Blanck
Welch Medical Library, Johns Hopkins University, Baltimore, MD, USA

C. V. Pollack, Jr. (ed.), *Differential Diagnosis of Cardiopulmonary Disease*,
https://doi.org/10.1007/978-3-319-63895-9_71

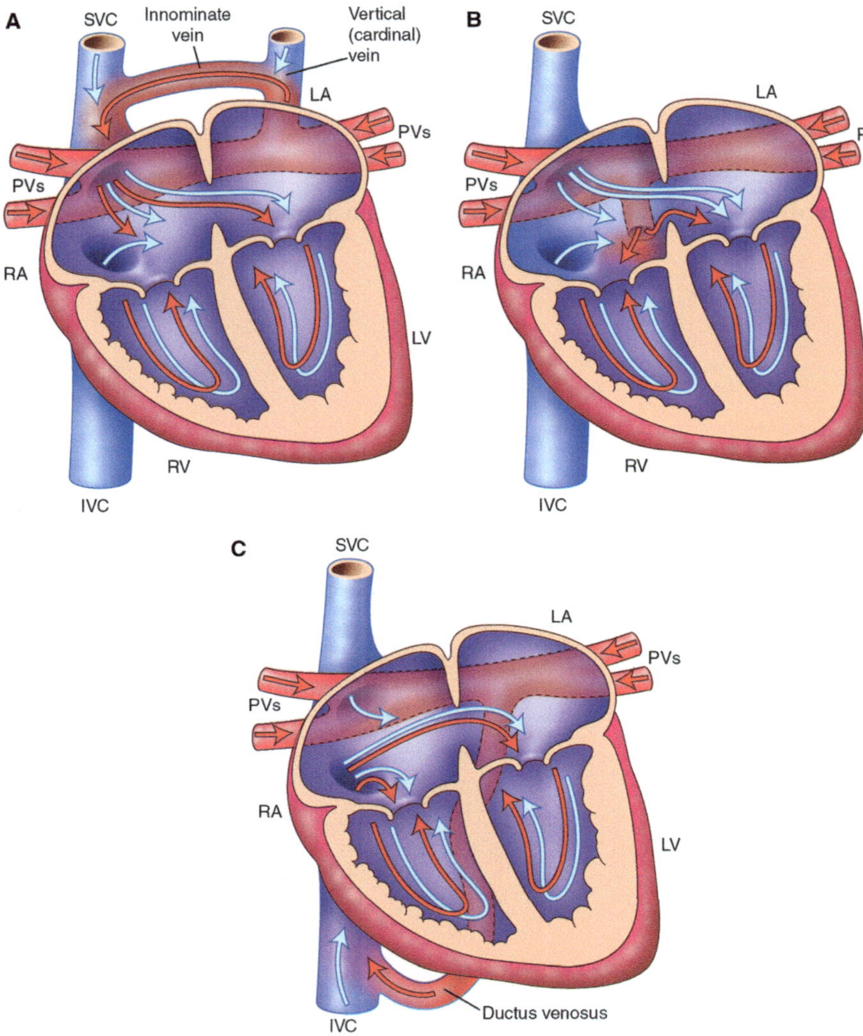

Graphic representation of total anomalous pulmonary venous return. Panel a, supracardiac drainage. In this lesion the path of pulmonary venous drainage is from a vertical vein to the innominate vein into the right atrium (RA). In most defects an associated atrial septal defect is present. Panel b, cardiac drainage. In this pathology, the pulmonary veins (PVs) typically empty into the coronary sinus, draining into the RA. Panel c, infracardiac drainage. In this setting, PVs drain through the ductus venosus to the RA. Frequently this anomaly is associated with pulmonary venous obstruction. IVC inferior vena cava, LA left atrium, LV left ventricle, RV right ventricle, SVC superior vena cava [Miller-Hance WC, Gottlieb EA, Motta P. Anesthesia for Cardiac Surgery in Neonates. In: Lerman J, editor. Neonatal

Anesthesia [Internet]. New York, NY: Springer New York; 2015 [cited 2015 Aug 31]. p. 291–357. Available from: http://link.springer.com/10.1007/978-1-4419-6041-2_12] *Caption from original*

Incidence/Epidemiology

- Within the population of infants with congenital heart disease, TAPVR accounts for approximately 1 percent of newborns.
- It is the fifth-most common cause of cyanotic heart disease.

Differential Diagnosis

- Should be considered in the differential diagnosis of cyanotic congenital heart disease, often represented by the "5 T's":
  - Truncus Arteriosus
  - Transposition of the Great Arteries
  - Tricuspid Atresia
  - Tetralogy of Fallot
  - Total Anomalous Pulmonary Venous Return

Pathophysiology and Etiology

- There are four variants of this defect:
  - Supracardiac (nearly 50 %): All blood returns form the pulmonary bed to the right atrium.

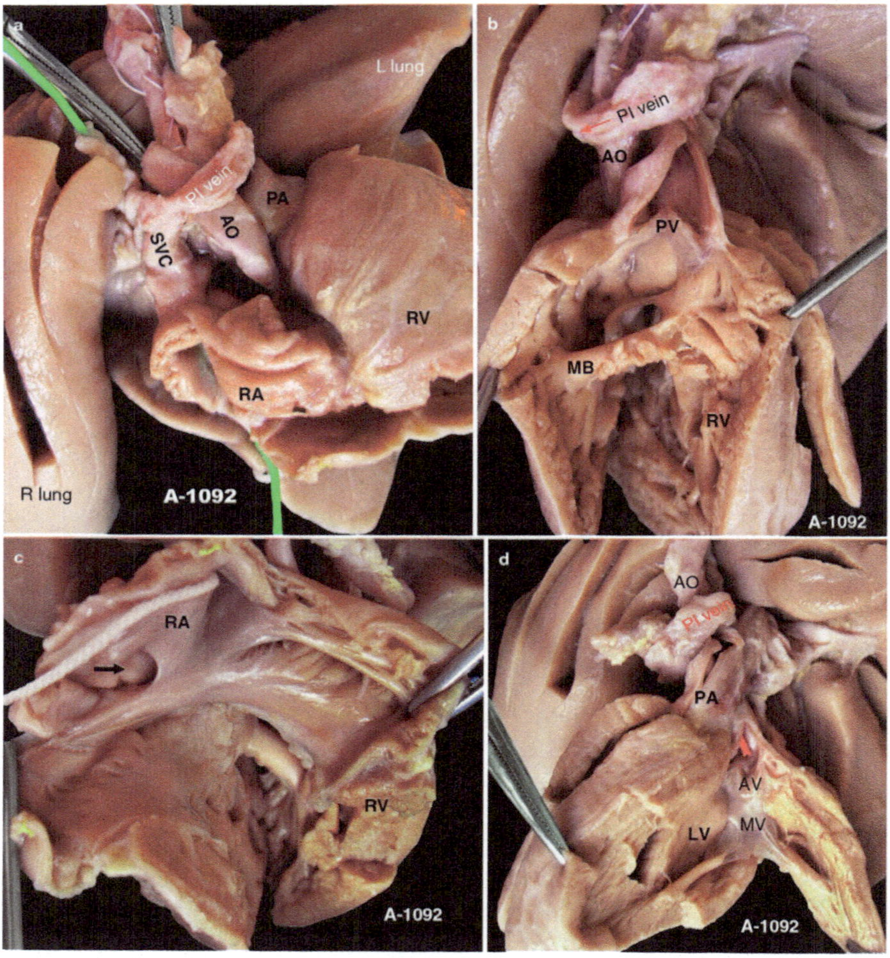
a
L lung
PI vein
PA
AO
SVC
RV
RA
R lung
A-1092
b
PI vein
AO
PV
MB
RV
A-1092
c
RA
RV
A-1092
d
AO
PI vein
PA
AV
LV
MV
A-1092

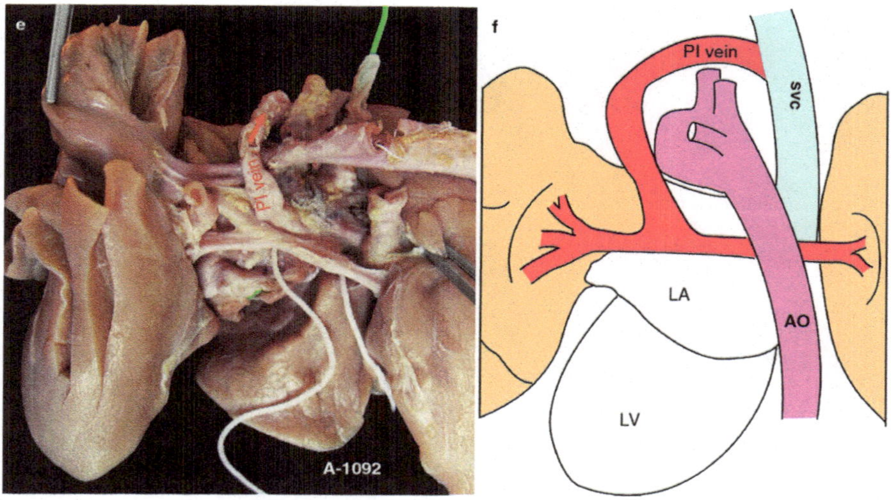

(**a**) Total anomalous pulmonary venous drainage, supracardiac type. Front view of the heart shows RA and RV cut open. At the root of the great vessels, the pulmonary vein is connected to anonymous veins and then to the SVC in front of the ascending aorta. The green probe is placed in the SVC. PI vein means that blood from the pulmonary vein flows through the anonymous vein. Ao aorta, RA right atrium, RV right ventricle, PA pulmonary artery, L lung left lung, R lung right lung. (**b**) View from the left to observe the pulmonary vein. PI vein: The pulmonary vein common trunk is connected to the anonymous vein in front of the aorta. This is the normal great artery relationship. The RV has a coarse moderator band. MB moderate band, PV pulmonary valve, RV right ventricle, AO ascending aorta. (**c**) View from right atrium and right ventricle. The arrow indicates the foramen ovale, RA right atrium, RV right ventricle. (**d**) View from left ventricle outlet tract. The left heart is normal. Red probe is in the aorta (Ao). The pulmonary vein (PI vein) originates from the left and right lungs, then passes by the aorta and returns to the SVC. LV left ventricle, MV mitral valve, PA main pulmonary vein, AV aortic valve. (**e**) Dorsal view of the heart and lung. The left and right pulmonary veins converge, then go forward and return to the SVC. The red arrow indicates the pulmonary artery blood flow. (**f**) Schematic diagram (dorsal view). PI vein means that blood from the pulmonary vein flows through the anonymous vein. LA left atrium, LV left ventricle, AO ascending aorta, SVC superior vena cava and PI vein[Zhu X. Anomalous Pulmonary Venous Drainage. In: Zhu X, editor. Surgical Atlas of Cardiac Anatomy [Internet]. Dordrecht: Springer Netherlands; 2015 [cited 2015 Aug 31]. p. 215–24. Available from: http://link.springer.com/10.1007/978-94-017-9409-1_14] *Caption from original*

- Cardiac (20 %): Pulmonary venous return connects to the coronary sinus.

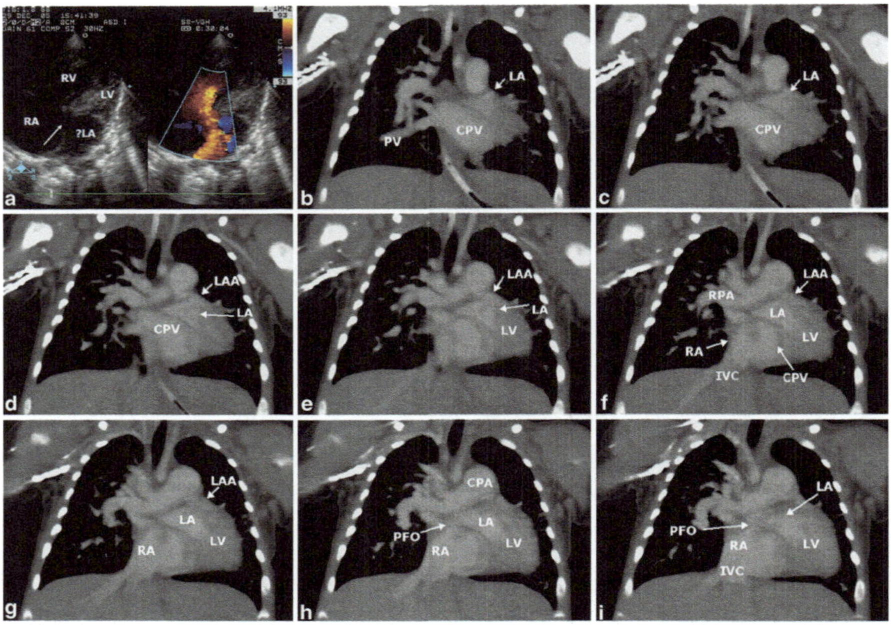

A 26-day-old boy with cardiac type total anomalous pulmonary venous return (TAPVR) who presented to our hospital for evaluation of progressive dyspnoea. aEchocardiography shows a large septal defect (long arrow) between the right atrium and suspected left atrium. The initial impression was a primum-type atrial septal defect. The paediatric cardiologist also noted the unusually early heart failure and dilated right atrium and right ventricle. MDCT was undertaken for further evaluation. b–i Sequential coronal MIP images from posterior to anterior clearly demonstrate cardiac type TAPVR. The pulmonary veins drain into a large common pulmonary vein and then into the right atrium. The common pulmonary vein and left atrium are separated by a septum. The patent foramen ovale, which is necessary for survival, is also visualized (h, i). After discussion, the paediatric cardiologist believed the misdiagnosis was probably related to the limited spatial resolution of echocardiography. Even on retrospective review, the anatomical detail shown by echocardiography was not as clear as identified on MDCT (?LAechocardiography-proposed LA, but is actually a common pulmonary vein; CPA central pulmonary artery; CPV common pulmonary vein; IVC inferior vena cava; LA left atrium;LAA left atrial appendage; LV left ventricle; PFO patent foramen ovale; PV pulmonary vein; RA right atrium; RPA right pulmonary artery; RV right ventricle) [Lee T, Tsai I-C, Fu Y-C, Jan S-L, Wang C-C, Chang Y, Chen M-C. Using multidetector-row CT in neonates with complex congenital heart disease to replace diagnostic cardiac catheterization for anatomical investigation: initial experiences in technical and clinical feasibility. Pediatric Radiology. 2006 Nov 10;36(12):1273–82.] *Caption adapted from original*

- Infracardiac (30 %): Pulmonary blood return connects to parts of the portal system.
- Mixed (10 %): Return at multilevels.

- Regardless of the anatomic derangement, there is admixing of oxygenated blood with deoxygenated blood, resulting in varying degrees of cyanosis.
- Eventually, right-sided cardiac enlargement will develop in response to volume overload on a chronic basis.

Presentation

Typical/"Classic"

- Presentations vary, depending on the degree of pulmonary venous obstruction.
- Severely obstructed infants present in the early hours after birth, with cyanosis and poor perfusion. Many of these newborns are difficult to diagnose, since premature lung disease is often considered at first.
- In infants with no or mild obstruction, presentations mimic clinical situations encountered in any patient with large volume left-to-right shunts (such as a VSD or ASD). Findings may include poor weight gain, tachycardia, and tachypnea. Oxygen saturations vary, from normal to slightly diminished.

Atypical

- As mentioned, mild cases may not present for months, until right-sided volume overload dominates.
- Older patients may present with TAPVR.

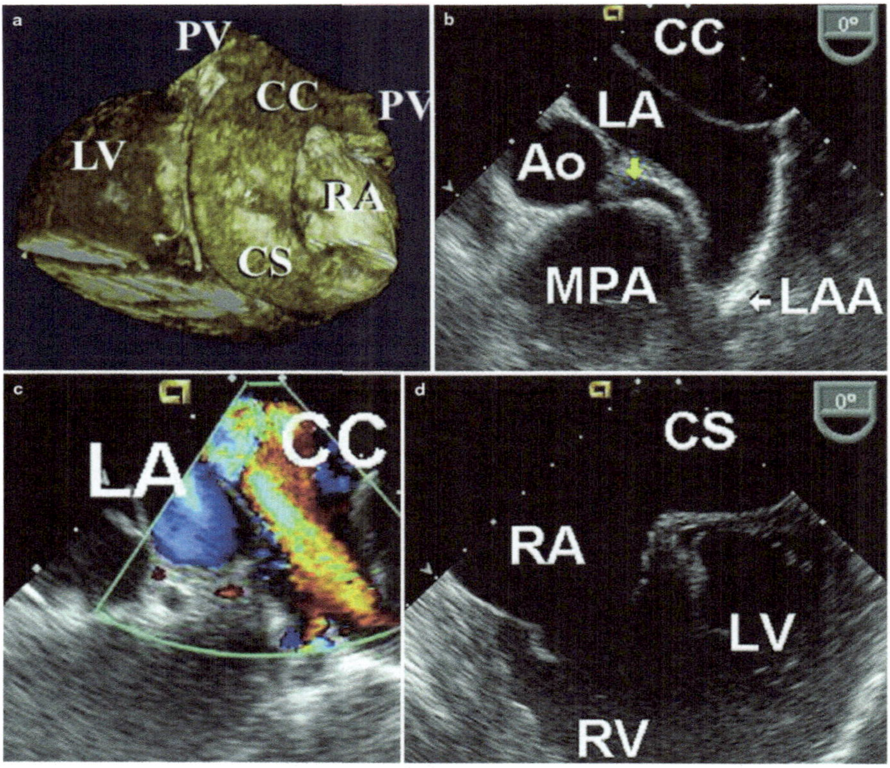

(a) Three-dimensional reconstruction of ECG gated CT angiogram in a 27-year-old cyanotic patient with uncorrected total anomalous pulmonary venous return. Two pulmonary veins (PV) connect to a posterior confluence chamber (CC) that courses inferiorly behind the left atrium (LA) into a dilated coronary sinus (CS) that in turn connects to the right atrium (RA). (b) TEE in the same patient, in the mid esophageal aortic valve short axis view with leftward probe position. Note the posterior CC closely apposing but not connected to the LA. The left main coronary artery (yellow arrow) is seen emerging from the aortic root (Ao) and coursing anterior to the left atrial appendage (LAA) and posterior to a dilated main pulmonary artery (MPA). (c) Color flow Doppler imaging demonstrating low velocity flow towards the transducer from the left sided pulmonary veins to the CC. Note the absence of flow between the CC and LA. (d) Mid esophageal four chamber view with the transducer in a more inferior position at the level of entry of the dilated CS into an enlarged RA. The right ventricle (RV) is also dilated, in comparison to the left ventricle (LV) [Aboulhosn JA, Child JS. Transesophageal Echocardiography in Adults with Congenital Heart Disease. In: Wong PC, Miller-Hance WC, editors. Transesophageal Echocardiography for Congenital Heart Disease [Internet]. London: Springer London; 2014 [cited 2015 Aug 31]. p. 455–73. Available from: http://link.springer.com/10.1007/978-1-84800-064-3_18] *Caption from original*

Primary Differential Considerations

- The other components of the 5 T's (see above) are the most important differential diagnoses to consider.

History and Physical Exam

- Assuming an uneventful neonatal course (i.e., no serious obstruction), these infants will demonstrate the signs and symptoms of progressive heart failure, including, but not limited to, poor weight gain, diaphoresis while feeding, and signs of respiratory distress.
- Heart sounds vary widely. Hepatomegaly will eventually develop.

Findings That Confirm Diagnosis

- Echocardiography remains the gold standard.

The video represents a representative sweep in an infant with total anomalous pulmonary venous connection to the left innominate vein. The exam is initiated at the midesophageal four chamber view. From this window, modified views at the level of the mid esophagus display the right upper and lower pulmonary veins (RUPV, RLPV) and left pulmonary veins (LPVs) are seen returning to a large horizontal confluence. A large vertical vein (VV) arises from the left side of the confluence and travels anteriorly and superiorly, coursing over the left pulmonary artery (LPA) to insert into the left innominate vein (Inn V). The length of the vertical vein is best seen in a sagittal plane, with the midesophageal ascending aortic and upper esophageal aortic arch short axis views, and leftward rotation of the probe. There is no obstruction at any point to pulmonary venous return. A catheter placed in the left internal jugular vein is seen in the vertical vein by two-dimensional imaging. On this video, prominent electrocautery and Doppler mirror image artifacts are seen (MPG 38454 kb) [Tacy TA. Systemic and Pulmonary Venous Anomalies. In: Wong PC, Miller-Hance WC, editors. Transesophageal Echocardiography for Congenital Heart Disease [Internet]. London: Springer London; 2014 [cited 2015 Aug 31]. p. 145–69. Available from: http://link.springer.com/10.1007/978-1-84800-064-3_6] *Caption from original*

- TAPVR should be considered in any infant who presents with cyanosis associated with pulmonary over-circulation.

Factors That Suggest Diagnosis

- TAPVR remains a difficult diagnosis.
- Since eventual echocardiography is often considered in the workup of neonatal cyanosis or CHF, the diagnosis will reveal itself.

Factors That Exclude Diagnosis

- A normal echocardiogram rules out TAPVR diagnosis.

Ancillary Studies

Laboratory

- Laboratory results will demonstrate hypoxia, acidosis, and hypercarbia in severe cases (nonspecific findings).

Electrocardiography

- ECG findings, unfortunately, are nonspecific and cannot be utilized in making the diagnosis of TAPVR.

Cardiac Enzymes

- Not indicated.

Special Populations

Age

- As discussed, most cases are diagnosed in the first few days of life.

Co-morbidities

- TAPVR is associated with asplenia or polysplenia.

Pitfalls in Diagnosis

- Cyanotic variant:
  - Pediatric cardiology consultation is emergently warranted.
- Acyanotic variety:
  - Adherence to strict algorhythmic workups of neonatal CHF or respiratory distress will eventually uncover the lesion.

Critical Steps Not to Miss

- Provision of supplemental oxygen
- Early ventilator support
- Immediate PICU or Pediatric Cardiology consultation

Mimics

- Any congenital cardiac lesion causing cyanosis and/or CHF.

Time-Dependent Interventions

- All interventions are emergent.

Overall Principles of Treatment

- Surgical repair of TAPVR is required; catheter-based treatments have not been shown to be effective. The timing of surgery varies by case.

Disease Course

- Surgical correction is almost always indicated – the earlier the better.

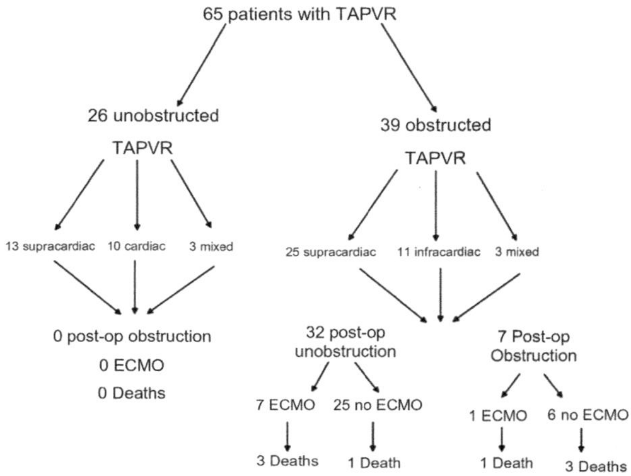

Surgical outcome. The flow chart summarizes the outcome of the cohort presenting for surgical repair of total anomalous pulmonary venous return (TAPVR) at Children's Hospital of Wisconsin from 1991 to 2007 [Frommelt PC, Sheridan DC, Deatsman S, Yan K, Simpson P, Frommelt MA, Litwin SB, Tweddell JS. Unobstructive Total Anomalous Pulmonary Venous Return: Impact of Early Elective Repair on the Need for Prolonged Mechanical Ventilatory Support. Pediatric Cardiology. 2010 Nov;31(8):1191–7.] *Caption from original*

- Long-term outcomes are dramatically improved after full correction (less than 5 %).

Related Evidence

Papers of particular interest have been highlighted as:
*** Of key importance*

Review

Spentzouris G, Zandian A, Cesmebasi A, Kinsella CR, Muhleman M, Mirzayan N, Shirak M, Tubbs RS, Shaffer K, Loukas M. The clinical anatomy of the inferior vena cava: a review of common congenital anomalies and considerations for clinicians. Clin Anat. 2014 Nov;27(8):1234-43. https://doi.org/10.1002/ca.22445. Epub 2014 Jul 17. Review. PubMed PMID: 25042045. http://www.ncbi.nlm.nih.gov/pubmed/25042045

Yoshimura N, Fukahara K, Yamashita A, Doki Y, Takeuchi K, Higuma T, Senda K, Toge M, Matsuo T, Nagura S, Aoki M, Sakata K, Obi H. Current topics in surgery for isolated total anomalous pulmonary venous connection. Surg Today. 2014 Dec;44(12):2221-6. https://doi.org/10.1007/s00595-014-0877-5. Epub 2014 Mar 16. Review. PubMed PMID: 24633930. http://www.ncbi.nlm.nih.gov/pubmed/24633930 **

Ciçek S, Arslan AH, Ugurlucan M, Yildiz Y, Ay S. Scimitar syndrome: the curved Turkish sabre. Semin Thorac Cardiovasc Surg Pediatr Card Surg Annu. 2014;17(1):56-61. https://doi.org/10.1053/j.pcsu.2014.01.003. Review. PubMed PMID: 24725718. http://www.ncbi.nlm.nih.gov/pubmed/24725718 **

Odenthal C, Sarikwal A. Anomalous unilateral single pulmonary vein versus scimitar syndrome: Comparison of two paediatric cases and a review of the literature. J Med Imaging Radiat Oncol. 2012 Jun;56(3):247-54. https://doi.org/10.1111/j.1754-9485.2012.02385.x. Epub 2012 May 14. Review. PubMed PMID: 22697320. http://www.ncbi.nlm.nih.gov/pubmed/22697320 **

Korkmaz AA, Yildiz CE, Onan B, Guden M, Cetin G, Babaoglu K. Scimitar syndrome: a complex form of anomalous pulmonary venous return. J Card Surg. 2011 Sep;26(5):529-34. https://doi.org/10.1111/j.1540-8191.2011.01309.x. Epub 2011 Aug 31. Review. PubMed PMID: 21883462. http://www.ncbi.nlm.nih.gov/pubmed/21883462 **

van der Bom T, Zomer AC, Zwinderman AH, Meijboom FJ, Bouma BJ, Mulder BJ. The changing epidemiology of congenital heart disease. Nat Rev Cardiol. 2011 Jan;8(1):50-60. https://doi.org/10.1038/nrcardio.2010.166. Epub 2010 Nov 2. Review. PubMed PMID: 21045784. http://www.ncbi.nlm.nih.gov/pubmed/21045784

Midyat L, Demir E, Aşkin M, Gülen F, Ulger Z, Tanaç R, Bayraktaroğlu S. Eponym. Scimitar syndrome. Eur J Pediatr. 2010 Oct;169(10):1171-7. https://doi.org/10.1007/s00431-010-1152-4. Epub 2010 Mar 12. Review. PubMed PMID: 20225123. http://www.ncbi.nlm.nih.gov/pubmed/20225123 **

Dillman JR, Yarram SG, Hernandez RJ. Imaging of pulmonary venous developmental anomalies. AJR Am J Roentgenol. 2009 May;192(5):1272-85. https://doi.org/10.2214/AJR.08.1526. Review. PubMed PMID: 19380552. http://www.ncbi.nlm.nih.gov/pubmed/19380552 **

Ferguson EC, Krishnamurthy R, Oldham SA. Classic imaging signs of congenital cardiovascular abnormalities. Radiographics. 2007 Sep-Oct;27(5):1323-34. Review. PubMed PMID: 17848694. http://www.ncbi.nlm.nih.gov/pubmed/17848694 **

Chowdhury UK, Malhotra A, Kothari SS, Reddy SK, Mishra AK, Pradeep KK, Venugopal P. A suggested new surgical classification for mixed totally anomalous pulmonary venous connection. Cardiol Young. 2007 Aug;17(4):342-53. Epub 2007 Jun 25. Review. PubMed PMID: 17588283. http://www.ncbi.nlm.nih.gDov/pubmed/17588283

Stein P. Total anomalous pulmonary venous connection. AORN J. 2007 Mar;85(3):509-20; quiz 521-4. Review. PubMed PMID: 17352891. http://www.ncbi.nlm.nih.gov/pubmed/17352891

Gudjonsson U, Brown JW. Scimitar syndrome. Semin Thorac Cardiovasc Surg Pediatr Card Surg Annu. 2006:56-62. Review. PubMed PMID: 16638549 http://www.ncbi.nlm.nih.gov/pubmed/16638549 **

Kanter KR. Surgical repair of total anomalous pulmonary venous connection. Semin Thorac Cardiovasc Surg Pediatr Card Surg Annu. 2006:40-4. Review. PubMed PMID: 16638546. http://www.ncbi.nlm.nih.gov/pubmed/16638546 **

Johnson BA, Ades A. Delivery room and early postnatal management of neonates who have prenatally diagnosed congenital heart disease. Clin Perinatol. 2005 Dec;32(4):921-46, ix. Review. PubMed PMID: 16325670. http://www.ncbi.nlm.nih.gov/pubmed/16325670

Lodge AJ, Rychik J, Nicolson SC, Ittenbach RF, Spray TL, Gaynor JW. Improving outcomes in functional single ventricle and total anomalous pulmonary venous connection. Ann Thorac Surg. 2004 Nov;78(5):1688-95. Review. PubMed PMID: 15511457. http://www.ncbi.nlm.nih.gov/pubmed/15511457

Comparative Study

Dusenbery SM, Geva T, Seale A, Valente AM, Zhou J, Sena L, Geggel RL. Outcome predictors and implications for management of scimitar syndrome. Am Heart J. 2013 May;165(5):770-7. https://doi.org/10.1016/j.ahj.2013.01.016. Epub 2013 Feb 22. PubMed PMID: 23622914. http://www.ncbi.nlm.nih.gov/pubmed/23622914

Use PubMed Clinical Queries to find the most recent evidence. Use this search strategy:

"Scimitar Syndrome"[Majr] OR "pulmonary venous return anomaly"[tiab] OR "TAPVR"[tiab] OR "anomalous pulmonary venous return"[tiab] OR "anomalous pulmonary venous connection"[tiab] OR "scimitar syndrome"[tiab] OR "scimitar anomaly"[tiab]

Chapter 72
Tracheal Tumors

Christopher J. Rees, Charles V. Pollack, Jr., and Jaime Friel Blanck

Name and Synonyms

Tracheal Tumors

Incidence/Epidemiology

- Tracheal tumors are very rare. They account for only 2 % of all tumors of the respiratory tract.
- Tracheal tumors account for less than one-half of one percent of all malignant tumors.
- Tumors found in the tracheae are more commonly seen from direct extension of primary lung cancer.
- Metastatic lesions in the trachea arising from non-pulmonary cancers are rare.
- Tracheal tumors have an estimated annual incidence of 0.1/100,000 people per year.
- Tracheal tumors are exceptionally rare in children. Most tracheal tumors in children are benign.
- The majority of tracheal tumors in adults are malignant (80–90 %).

C. J. Rees
Emergency Department, Pennsylvania Hospital, Philadelphia, PA, USA

C. V. Pollack, Jr. (✉)
Department of Emergency Medicine, Thomas Jefferson University, Philadelphia, PA, USA

J. F. Blanck
Welch Medical Library, Johns Hopkins University, Baltimore, MD, USA

C. V. Pollack, Jr. (ed.), *Differential Diagnosis of Cardiopulmonary Disease*,
https://doi.org/10.1007/978-3-319-63895-9_72

- Squamous cell carcinoma (SCC) accounts for up to two-thirds of all tracheal malignancies.
    - SCC is more common in older adults (>60), has a significant male predominance, and is almost always associated with cigarette smoking (90 %).
- Adenoid cystic carcinoma (ACC/cylindroma) accounts for 10–15 % of all tracheal malignancies.
    - ACC is more common in younger age groups (40 and up), and has equal distribution between genders.

Differential Diagnosis

- Tracheal tumors are frequently misdiagnosed as adult-onset asthma. Pulmonary function tests (PFTs) in both may show a similar obstruction pattern. The diagnosis of tracheal tumor should be considered in any patient diagnosed with adult-onset asthma who doesn't respond or worsens despite usual treatment with steroids and bronchodilators.
- The most common symptoms of tracheal tumors are cough and dyspnea, so the differential can be very broad, and includes all the causes of cough and dyspnea such as asthma, chronic bronchitis, chronic obstructive pulmonary disease (COPD), pneumonitis, interstitial lung disease (ILD), congestive heart failure (CHF).
- Tracheal tumors can also be initially misdiagnosed as invasive thyroid cancers.

Pathophysiology and Etiology

- Tumors of the trachea can be primary (arising from tracheal tissue), secondary (metastatic from other tissues), or from direct invasion from tumors arising in other contiguous structures.
- The majority (about 80 %) of primary tracheal tumors in adults are malignant.
- Malignant tumors of the trachea include the following cell types.
    - Squamous Cell Carcinoma (SCC). Squamous cell carcinomas account for up to two-thirds of all malignant tracheal tumors. They are pathologically identical to SCC of the lung. They are predominately related to cigarette smoking. There is a male predominance, and most cases occur in those over age 60.

    - SCC are rapid-growing tumors. About half are not amenable to surgical removal when diagnosed.
  - Adenoid Cystic Carcinoma (ACC) has also been called cylindroma. These account for about 10–15 % of malignant tracheal tumors. They arise from bronchial/salivary glandular tissue. These occur about a decade earlier than SCC (in 40's and up), are not associated with cigarette smoking, and occur equally in men and women.
    - ACC grow more slowly than SCC and are usually more amenable to surgical removal.
  - Others. Mucoepidermoid carcinoma, non-small cell bronchogenic cancer, sarcomas, and carcinoid tumors can occur primarily in the trachea, but all are very rare.
- Benign tumors of the trachea also occur. These include chondromas, hemangiomas, hamartomas, neurogenic tumors, granular cell tumors, and squamous papillomas.
  - Chondromas are the most common (but still very rare) non-malignant tracheal tumors. They arise from the tracheal rings. These do have metastatic potential.
  - Papillomas. These are usually associated with infection from human papilloma virus (HPV) types 6 and 11. They commonly arise in areas of prior tracheal injury (tracheotomy sites). They have a tendency to extend down into the lungs, instead of out into the tracheal lumen, making them difficult to diagnose until they are large. Malignant transformation is possible.

Presentation

Typical/"Classic"

- As noted above, tracheal tumors are very uncommon, so there is no "classic" presentation.
- The two most common symptoms of tracheal tumors are cough and dyspnea.
- Other symptoms that can be seen include wheezing, stridor (when the mass is large and nearly obstructing), hoarseness (when the recurrent laryngeal nerve is involved), hemoptysis (more common with SCC) and dysphagia (from external compression of the esophagus).
- As these symptoms are non-specific and frequently seen with much more common diagnoses (asthma, chronic bronchitis, COPD, CHF, etc.), the diagnosis of a tracheal tumor may not have even been considered in the initial differential diagnosis.

- It is important to consider the diagnosis in a patient diagnosed with adult-onset asthma, especially when they are not responding appropriately to usual treatment.
- These tumors are usually large at diagnosis. They don't usually cause symptoms until the tracheal lumen is narrowed by at least 75 %.

Atypical

- As tracheal tumors are uncommon, all presentations could be considered atypical.
- Many patients will have the diagnosis considered only when an imaging study performed for other reasons shows a tracheal mass.

Primary Differential Considerations

- Patients with tracheal tumors may present with symptoms suggestive of other diagnostic considerations, including but not limited to:
  - Tuberculosis and other infectious masses
  - Inflammation
  - Scar tissue

History and Physical Exam

Findings That Confirm Diagnosis

- There are no historical or physical examination findings that can confirm the diagnosis.
- The diagnosis is generally confirmed by imaging or direct visualization by bronchoscopy.

Factors That Suggest Diagnosis

- It is important to consider the diagnosis in a patient diagnosed with adult-onset asthma.
- The diagnosis should also be considered in a patient with a significant smoking history and with cough and dyspnea.
- Inspiratory stridor that worsens with recumbency can be a clue to an obstructing lesion of the trachea.

Factors That Exclude Diagnosis

- There are no historical or physical examination findings that can exclude the diagnosis.
- The diagnosis can only be excluded by a normal bronchoscopic examination.

Ancillary Studies

Laboratory

- Laboratory studies are not helpful in the diagnosis of tracheal tumors.

Imaging

- Plain chest x-ray (PA and lateral) will show an abnormality in only about 25 % of cases.
- Computed tomography (CT) of the chest and trachea is the imaging study of choice for the diagnosis of tracheal tumors. Appearance on CT may be able to help distinguish benign from malignant lesions.

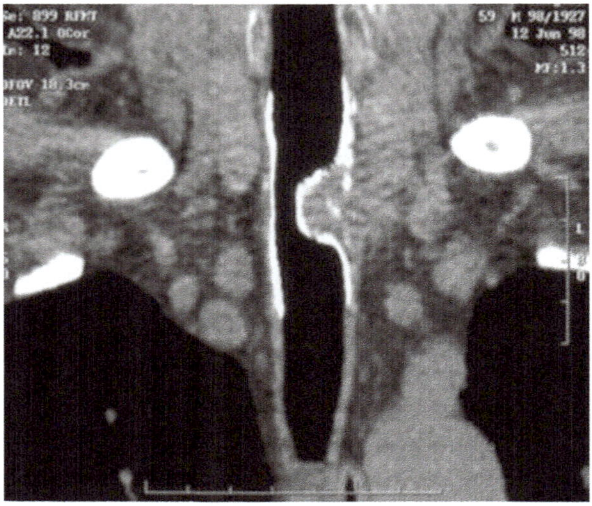

A 59-year-old man with upper tracheal squamous cell carcinoma. [Ferretti GR, Kocier M, Calaque O, Arbib F, Righini C, Coulomb M, Pison C. Follow-up after stent insertion in the tracheobronchial tree: role of helical computed tomography in comparison with fiberoptic bronchoscopy. Eur Radiol. 2003 Feb 7;13(5):1172–8.] *Caption adapted from original.*

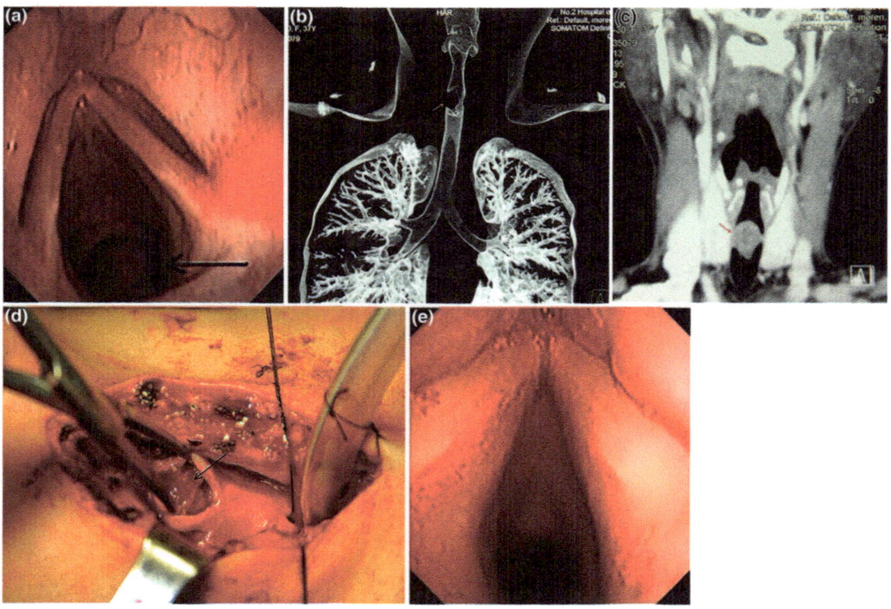

a Female, 37 years old, with tracheal adenocystic carcinoma which is located beneath the annular cartilage under tracheobronchoscope (the black arrow). b 3-D CT scan frontal image reconstruction shows there is a tracheal tumor presenting an irregular filling defect inside the trachea cavity (the red arrow). c 3-D CT scan image reconstruction shows the tracheal tumor is a nodular round tumor protruding inside the tracheal cavity with an even density and a smooth border. Its narrow base is connected to the tracheal wall. There is no increase in the thickness of the tracheal wall (the red arrow). d After the first tracheal rings were incised, there is a tumor protruding into the tracheal cavity from the tracheal wall on the right, and there is no increase in the thickness of the wall (the black arrow). e Electronic fiberoptic bronchoscopy shows that the tracheal wall is smooth and there is no stenosis of the first tracheal rings after postoperative radiotherapy [Li Y, Peng A, Yang X, Xiao Z, Wu W, Wang Q. Clinical manifestation and management of primary malignant tumors of the cervical trachea. European Archives of Oto-Rhino-Laryngology. 2014 Feb;271(2):225–35.] *Caption from original.*

- Bronchoscopy (either flexible or rigid) is currently considered the gold standard test for the diagnosis and evaluation of tracheal tumors. Not only can the tumor be directly visualized, tissue biopsy can be done to allow for pathologic examination and cell typing.

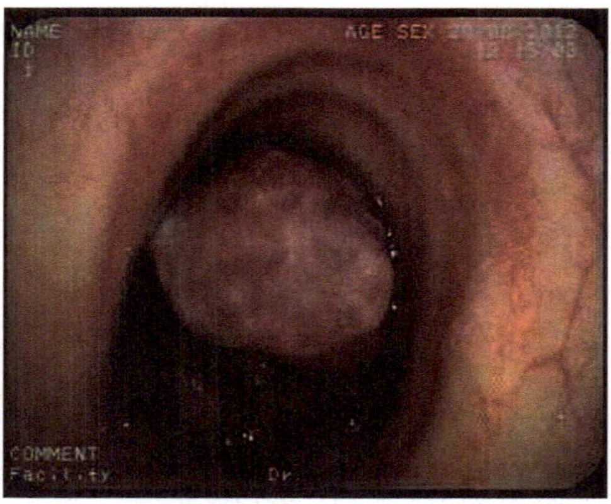

Bronchoscopy showing broad based pedunculated intraluminal tracheal mass which markedly narrow the lumen [Sukumaran R, Nair RA, Jacob PM, Koshy SM, Mathew AP. Extramedullary Plasmacytoma of the Trachea. Head and Neck Pathology. 2014 Jun;8(2):220–4.] *Caption from original.*

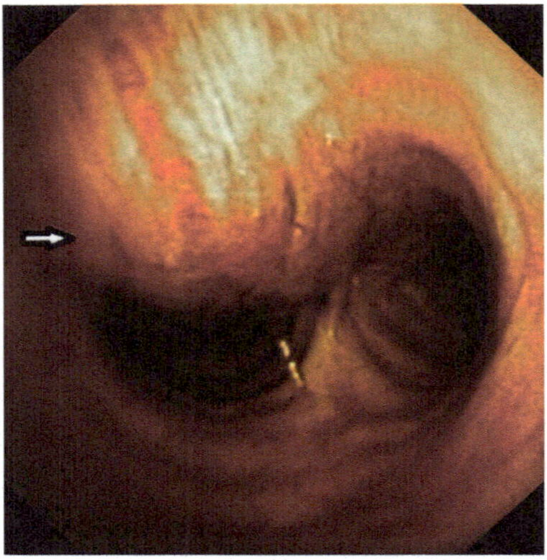

Fiberoptic bronchoscopy showed a submucosal tracheal tumor (arrow). [From article: About a submucosal tracheal tumor. World Journal of Surgical Oncology. 2013;11(1):229. https://doi.org/10.1186/1477-7819-11-229, at http://link.springer.com/article/10.1186/1477-7819-11-229; by Mounia Serraj, Marouane Lakranbi, Jamal Ghalimi, Yassine Ouadnouni, Siham Tizniti, Mohamed Smahi, © Serraj et al.; licensee BioMed Central Ltd. 2013; licensed under Creative Commons Attribution License BY 2.0 http://creativecommons.org/licenses/by/2.0] *Caption from original.*

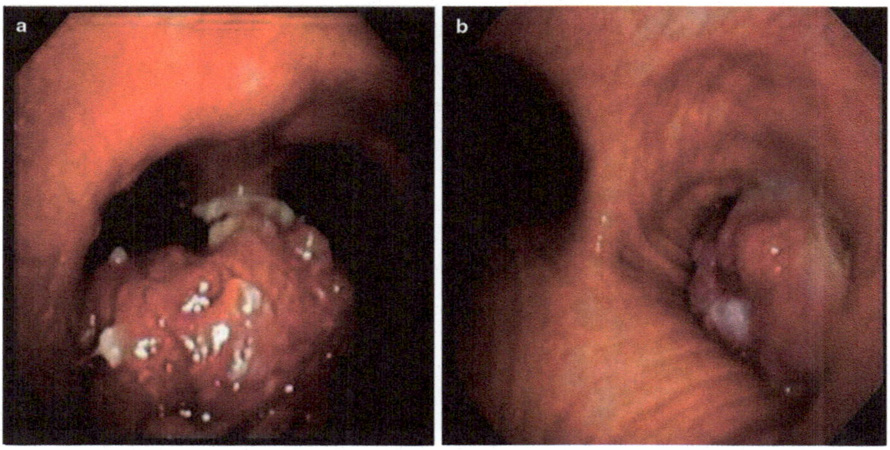

(a) Tracheal tumor obstructing left mainstem bronchus. (b) Right upper lobe tumor obstructing the right mainstem bronchus [Gorden JA. Rigid Bronchoscopy. In: Ernst A, Herth FJ, editors. Principles and Practice of Interventional Pulmonology [Internet]. New York, NY: Springer New York; 2013 [cited 2015 Dec 4]. p. 285–95. Available from: http://link.springer.com/10.1007/978-1-4614-4292-9_27] *Caption adapted from original.*

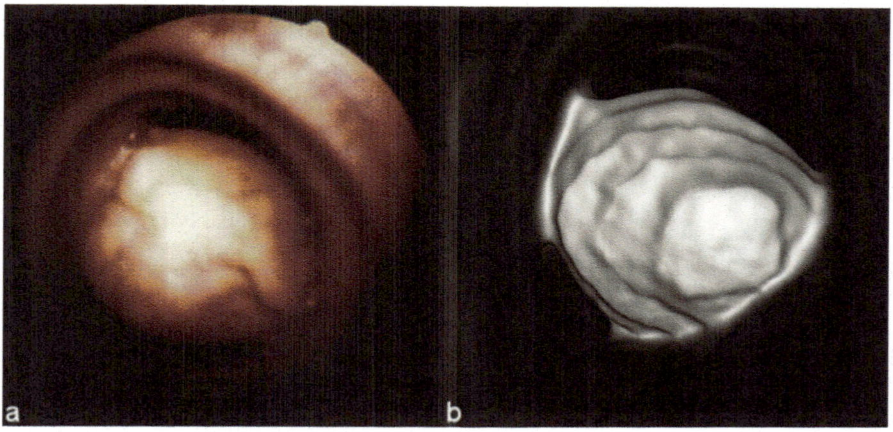

Intraluminal tracheal tumor causing severe airway obstruction. [From article: Tumoral and non-tumoral trachea stenoses: evaluation with three-dimensional CT and virtual bronchoscopy. Journal of Cardiothoracic Surgery. 2007;2(1):18. https://doi.org/10.1186/1749-8090-2-18, at http://link.springer.com/article/10.1186/1749-8090-2-18; by Efstratios N Koletsis, Christine Kalogeropoulou, Eleni Prodromaki, George C Kagadis, Konstantinos Katsanos, Konstantinos Spiropoulos, Theodore Petsas, George C Nikiforidis, Dimitris Dougenis, © Koletsis et al; licensee BioMed Central Ltd. 2007; licensed under Creative Commons Attribution License BY 2.0 http://creativecommons.org/licenses/by/2.0] *Caption adapted from original.*

- Positron emission tomography (PET/CT). This is often done to help "stage" the disease and to help make treatment decisions.

Special Populations

Age

- Tracheal tumors are very rare in children. When found they are almost universally benign. They can include papillomas, hemangiomas, and granular cell tumors.

Co-morbidities

- A large majority of the patients with SCC of the trachea are smokers, so they often have co-morbidities (COPD, coronary disease, CHF) that can make the diagnosis more difficult. Many of these patients will have the diagnosis considered when an imaging study performed for other reasons shows a tracheal mass.

Pitfalls in Diagnosis

Critical Steps Not to Miss

- It is critical to consider the diagnosis in any patient diagnosed with adult-onset asthma.
- Patients diagnosed with adult-onset asthma should probably have a chest CT as part of their evaluation to exclude competing diagnoses.
- It is important to remember that "all that wheezes is not asthma."

Mimics

- Adult-onset asthma is the most significant mimic of tracheal tumors.
- Chronic bronchitis can also mimic tracheal mass lesions.

Time-Dependent Interventions

- In patients who present with respiratory distress, it is helpful to start humidified oxygen and avoid the recumbent position. It may be helpful to also use heliox (a mixture of helium and oxygen) to aid with ventilation. Some patients may benefit from tracheal stents or bronchoscopic laser ablation as bridges to surgery or for palliation of symptoms.

Overall Principles of Treatment

- The primary treatment for tracheal tumors is surgical resection.
  - Resectability is decided based upon the physical characteristics of the tumor (such as how much of the trachea is involved, how large the tumor is, and whether there is evidence of spread/metastases.
  - SCC's are usually rapidly growing tumors that metastasize early in their course. Only about one-half of SCC's are amenable to surgical removal when diagnosed.
- As these are rare tumors, there are few clinical trials to help guide treatment; most treatments are guided by expert opinion.
- Because they are so uncommon, there is no validated staging system for any of these tumors.

- Radiation therapy (RT) is often used after surgical resection, especially if the surgical margins were positive, or if the tumor could only be incompletely resected.
- Chemotherapy is often used (usually combined with RT) in unresectable tumors, but there are no good clinical trials documenting benefit.

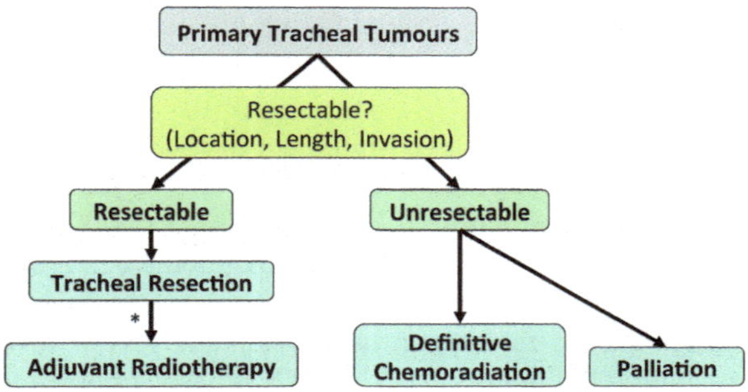

Management algorithm for primary tracheal tumors. [Sudarshan M, Alamri H, Al-Mahroos M. Lung and Airway Disorders. In: Madani A, Ferri L, Seely A, editors. Pocket Manual of General Thoracic Surgery [Internet]. Cham: Springer International Publishing; 2015 [cited 2015 Dec 4]. p. 35–83. Available from: http://link.springer.com/10.1007/978-3-319-17497-6_3] *Caption adapted from original.*

- Bronchoscopy with laser ablation may be helpful in alleviating symptoms in tumors not amenable to resection, and to control symptoms prior to surgery.
- Non-malignant tumors are also usually treated primarily surgically. Papillomas may respond to bronchoscopic laser ablation, but the treatment may need to be repeated several times. Some papillomas may respond to intralesional injection of cidofovir.

Disease Course

- The five-year survival rate for resectable SCC is about 39 %.
- The five-year survival rate for unresectable SCC is 7 %.
- The five-year survival rate for ACC is about 50 %.
- Benign tumors of the trachea that can be surgically repaired should not recur.
- The only non-malignant tumor associated with long-term complications is the papilloma associated with HPV. It may require numerous endoscopic-guided procedures and treatments and can lead to an increased incidence of tracheal stenosis and tracheomalacia from recurrent "injury" to the trachea. It is important to start treatment only for symptomatic lesions to avoid all unnecessary tracheal injury.

Related Evidence

Papers of particular interest have been highlighted as:
*** Of key importance*

Review

Sherani K, Vakil A, Dodhia C, Fein A. Malignant tracheal tumors: a review of current diagnostic and management strategies. Curr Opin Pulm Med. 2015 Jul;21(4):322-6. https://doi.org/10.1097/MCP.0000000000000181. PubMed PMID: 25978628. http://www.ncbi.nlm.nih.gov/pubmed/25978628 **

Jindal A, Bal A, Agarwal R. Inflammatory myofibroblastic tumor of the trachea in the pediatric age group: case report and systematic review of the literature. J Bronchology Interv Pulmonol. 2015 Jan;22(1):58-65. https://doi.org/10.1097/LBR.0000000000000105. Review. PubMed PMID: 25590486. http://www.ncbi.nlm.nih.gov/pubmed/25590486

El Marjany M, Arsalane A, Sifat H, Andaloussi K, Oukabli M, Hadadi K, Kabiri el H, Mansouri H. Primary adenoid cystic carcinoma of the trachea: a report of two cases and literature review. Pan Afr Med J. 2014 Sep 15;19:32. https://doi.org/10.11604/pamj.2014.19.32.4878. eCollection 2014. Review. PubMed PMID: 25667694; PubMed Central PMCID: PMC4314152. http://www.ncbi.nlm.nih.gov/pubmed/25667694

Jamjoom L, Obusez EC, Kirsch J, Gildea T, Mohammed TL. Computed tomography correlation of airway disease with bronchoscopy–part II: tracheal neoplasms. Curr Probl Diagn Radiol. 2014 Sep-Oct;43(5):278-84. https://doi.org/10.1067/j.cpradiol.2014.02.005. Review. PubMed PMID: 25088220. http://www.ncbi.nlm.nih.gov/pubmed/25088220 **

Junker K. Pathology of tracheal tumors. Thorac Surg Clin. 2014 Feb;24(1):7-11. https://doi.org/10.1016/j.thorsurg.2013.09.008. Review. PubMed PMID: 24295655. http://www.ncbi.nlm.nih.gov/pubmed/24295655 **

Wu CC, Shepard JA. Tracheal and airway neoplasms. Semin Roentgenol. 2013 Oct;48(4):354-64. https://doi.org/10.1053/j.ro.2013.03.018. Review. PubMed PMID: 24034267. http://www.ncbi.nlm.nih.gov/pubmed/24034267

Honings J, Gaissert HA, van der Heijden HF, Verhagen AF, Kaanders JH, Marres HA. Clinical aspects and treatment of primary tracheal malignancies. Acta Otolaryngol.2010Jul;130(7):763-72.https://doi.org/10.3109/00016480903403005. Review. PubMed PMID: 20569185. http://www.ncbi.nlm.nih.gov/pubmed/20569185 **

Gaissert HA, Honings J, Gokhale M. Treatment of tracheal tumors. Semin Thorac Cardiovasc Surg. 2009 Fall;21(3):290-5. https://doi.org/10.1053/j.semtcvs.2009.06.001. Review. PubMed PMID: 19942130. http://www.ncbi.nlm.nih.gov/pubmed/19942130 **

Ferretti GR, Bithigoffer C, Righini CA, Arbib F, Lantuejoul S, Jankowski A. Imaging of tumors of the trachea and central bronchi. Radiol Clin North Am. 2009 Mar;47(2):227-41. https://doi.org/10.1016/j.rcl.2008.11.010. Review. PubMed PMID: 19249453. http://www.ncbi.nlm.nih.gov/pubmed/19249453

Gaissert HA, Mark EJ. Tracheobronchial gland tumors. Cancer Control. 2006 Oct;13(4):286-94. Review. PubMed PMID: 17075566. http://www.ncbi.nlm.nih.gov/pubmed/17075566 **

Macchiarini P. Primary tracheal tumours. Lancet Oncol. 2006 Jan;7(1):83-91. Review. PubMed PMID: 16389188. http://www.ncbi.nlm.nih.gov/pubmed/16389188

Cohort Study

Urdaneta AI, Yu JB, Wilson LD. Population based cancer registry analysis of primary tracheal carcinoma. Am J Clin Oncol. 2011 Feb;34(1):32-7. https://doi.org/10.1097/COC.0b013e3181cae8ab. PubMed PMID: 20087156. http://www.ncbi.nlm.nih.gov/pubmed/20087156 **

Case Study

Romão RL, de Barros F, Maksoud Filho JG, Gonçalves ME, Cardoso S, Tannuri AC, Tannuri U. Malignant tumor of the trachea in children: diagnostic pitfalls and surgical management. J Pediatr Surg. 2009 Nov;44(11):e1-4. https://doi.org/10.1016/j.jpedsurg.2009.07.045. PubMed PMID: 19944203. http://www.ncbi.nlm.nih.gov/pubmed/19944203

General

Chen F, Huang M, Xu Y, Li T, Xie K, Zhang L, Cheng D, Liu L, Che G, Hou M, Wang J, Luo Z, Lu Y. Primary tracheal adenoid cystic carcinoma: adjuvant treatment outcome. Int J Clin Oncol. 2015 Aug;20(4):686-92. https://doi.org/10.1007/s10147-014-0771-6. Epub 2014 Nov 21. PubMed PMID: 25412605. http://www.ncbi.nlm.nih.gov/pubmed/25412605

Li W, Hua W, Yan FG, Shen HH, Xu H. Adenoid cystic carcinoma of trachea: a case report and review of literature. Chin Med J (Engl). 2012 Jun;125(12):2238-9. Review. PubMed PMID: 22884161. http://www.ncbi.nlm.nih.gov/pubmed/22365629

Gaissert HA, Grillo HC, Shadmehr MB, Wright CD, Gokhale M, Wain JC, Mathisen DJ. Uncommon primary tracheal tumors. Ann Thorac Surg. 2006 Jul;82(1):268-

72; discussion 272-3. PubMed PMID: 16798228. http://www.ncbi.nlm.nih.gov/pubmed/16798228

Use PubMed Clinical Queries to find the most recent evidence. Use this search strategy: "Tracheal Neoplasms"[Mesh] OR "tracheal tumor" OR "tracheal tumors"

Chapter 73
Tracheomalacia

Christopher J. Rees, Charles V. Pollack, Jr., and Jaime Friel Blanck

Name and Synonyms

Tracheomalacia/Tracheobronchomalacia

Incidence/Epidemiology

- The incidence and prevalence are unknown.
- Acquired tracheomalacia (TM) seems to be more common in men over the age of 40.
- The estimated incidence of primary TM in children is one in 2,100 births.

Differential Diagnosis

- The predominant symptoms and signs of TM in adults are dyspnea and cough, so the differential includes all diseases associated these complaints.

C. J. Rees
Emergency Department, Pennsylvania Hospital, Philadelphia, PA, USA

C. V. Pollack, Jr. (✉)
Department of Emergency Medicine, Thomas Jefferson University, Philadelphia, PA, USA

J. F. Blanck
Welch Medical Library, Johns Hopkins University, Baltimore, MD, USA

C. V. Pollack, Jr. (ed.), *Differential Diagnosis of Cardiopulmonary Disease*,
https://doi.org/10.1007/978-3-319-63895-9_73

- This includes asthma, chronic obstructive pulmonary disease (COPD), congestive heart failure (CHF), cigarette smoking, chronic aspiration, gastroesophageal reflux disease (GERD), interstitial lung disease (ILD), and others.

Pathophysiology and Etiology

- Tracheomalacia (TM) is the term used to describe tracheal weakness. This weakness can be focal/segmental (confined to small lengths of the trachea) or diffuse (involving long portions of the trachea.) When the weakness extends into one or both mainstem bronchi, the term tracheobronchomalacia (TBM) is often used. The disorders are similar and share symptoms, pathophysiology, and treatment, so the following discussion will relate to both, and will be referred to as TM.
- The physiologic result of the tracheal cartilage and surrounding connective tissue weakening is exaggerated luminal narrowing during expiration, and excessive widening during inspiration.
- The trachea can completely collapse during periods of increased expiratory flow, such as coughing and crying (in infants and children).
- The severity appears to be related to the length of the involved segment and the degree of narrowing.
  - TM is generally classified as primary or acquired. Acquired TM is much more common in adults.
    - Congenital TM usually presents in childhood.
      - TM in children more commonly involves the distal third of the trachea and is associated a congenital abnormality.
      - These congenital abnormalities include:
        - Cardiovascular abnormalities (vascular rings, anomalous innominate artery)
        - Developmental delay
        - Severe GERD
        - Tracheoesophageal fistula
        - Esophageal atresia
      - Idiopathic giant trachea is a type of congenital TM that presents in adulthood. It is due to atrophy of the longitudinal elastic fibers and thinning of the muscularis mucosa of the trachea. There is diffuse tracheomegaly. When the process extends into the central bronchi, it is called, Mounier-Kuhn Syndrome. These are exceedingly rare conditions.

  - Acquired TM. Acquired TM is more common in adults. There are many causes.
    - Prolonged endotracheal intubation and tracheostomy can lead to tracheal cartilage destruction and usually segmental tracheomalacia.
    - Other causes of direct tracheal injury that can lead to cartilage destruction include direct chest trauma and surgery such as lung transplantation.
    - Chronic compression from extrinsic masses can also lead to cartilage destruction. This can result from vascular compression from aortic aneurysms, vascular rings, malignancies, goiter, and other mediastinal mass lesions.
    - Recurrent cartilaginous inflammation from relapsing polychondritis can cause cartilage injury and destruction leading to tracheomalacia.
    - Recurrent tracheobronchial infections (especially associated with cystic fibrosis and COPD) can lead to tracheomalacia.
    - Prolonged exposure to known airway irritants (tobacco smoke, chronic GERD with aspiration) can also be associated with tracheomalacia.
- Appearance of the trachea: Some patients have predominantly posterior tracheal wall weakness and this results in a crescent-shaped trachea. Other patients have lateral wall tracheal weakness, resulting in a fissure-shaped trachea.
- Distribution: Segmental vs. diffuse distribution of weakness. This classification is important for guiding treatment.

Presentation

Typical/"Classic"

- The predominant symptoms and signs of TM in adults are dyspnea, cough, and sputum retention.
- The disease tends to be slowly progressive and goes through a prolonged asymptomatic period.
- As the disease progresses and symptoms develop, they may only be noticed first during periods of physiologic stress such as infections and while undergoing general anesthesia.
- Dyspnea tends to be less associated with exertion and more with maneuvers that force expiration, such as coughing, valsalva, and a recumbent position.

- Coughing can occur in severe paroxysms and be associated with expiratory wheezing or stridor. The wheezing with asthma and COPD tends to be inspiratory or both inspiratory and expiratory, and the presence of purely expiratory wheezing may be a subtle clue to the diagnosis.
- The symptoms and signs of TM are very nonspecific and can be seen with multiple other diseases, such as asthma, COPD, and CHF.
- Infants with TM are often noted to have expiratory stridor (sometimes called laryngeal crow) within the first few weeks of life. The stridor tends to be worsened and exacerbated by crying, supine position, and feeding.
- Infants may also be noted to have feeding difficulties, e.g., coughing and choking while feeding.

https://www.youtube.com/watch?v=X7xgW5-AFUw
Audio of infant with tracheomalacia.

https://www.youtube.com/watch?v=DFqL3bFQpTE&list=PLRr91eakaLBZvq7dUGWiXlhLRME0SDr3Y
Audio of stridor associated with laryngomalacia, tracheomalacia, and bronchomalacia.

Atypical

- As noted above, the symptoms and signs of TM can be very nonspecific.
- Initial symptoms may be thought to be caused by many other conditions.
- Patients may be noted to have recurrent pulmonary infections due to the inability to clear their sputum.
- When TM develops in the presence of other conditions, the symptoms of dyspnea and cough may seem to be worse than what would be predicted by the severity of the underlying condition.
- Some patients may present with cough syncope.

Primary Differential Considerations

- Patients with tracheomalacia may present with signs and symptoms of other diagnostic considerations, including but not limited to:
  - Laryngomalacia
  - Laryngeal cysts
  - Vocal cord paralysis

History and Physical Exam

Findings That Confirm Diagnosis

- There are no historical or physical examination findings that can confirm the diagnosis.
- The diagnosis can only be confirmed by appropriate findings (airway collapse upon forced expiration) on bronchoscopy.

Factors That Suggest Diagnosis

- The diagnosis can be suspected when a patient presents with a chronic cough or dyspnea that can be related historically or on exam to forced expiratory maneuvers such as coughing and valsalva.
- Predominantly expiratory wheezing should suggest the diagnosis.
- Early symptoms may only be noted during periods of physiologic stress, such as infections, and while undergoing general anesthesia.

Factors That Exclude Diagnosis

- There are no historical or physical examination findings that can completely exclude the diagnosis.

Ancillary Studies

Laboratory

- Laboratory studies are generally not helpful in the diagnosis of TM.

Imaging

- Chest x-ray. Plain chest x-ray is generally not helpful in the diagnosis of TM. The CXR may help if TM is caused by compression from other processes (goiter, mass, aneurysm, etc.).

- Chest CT. Chest CT can be helpful in the diagnosis and evaluation of TM. Ultrafast, multidetector CT performed both normally, and then under forced expiration or cough can document airway collapse. Airway collapse can even be quantified and used to help guide treatment decisions. Chest CT can also help diagnose the cause of acquired TM.

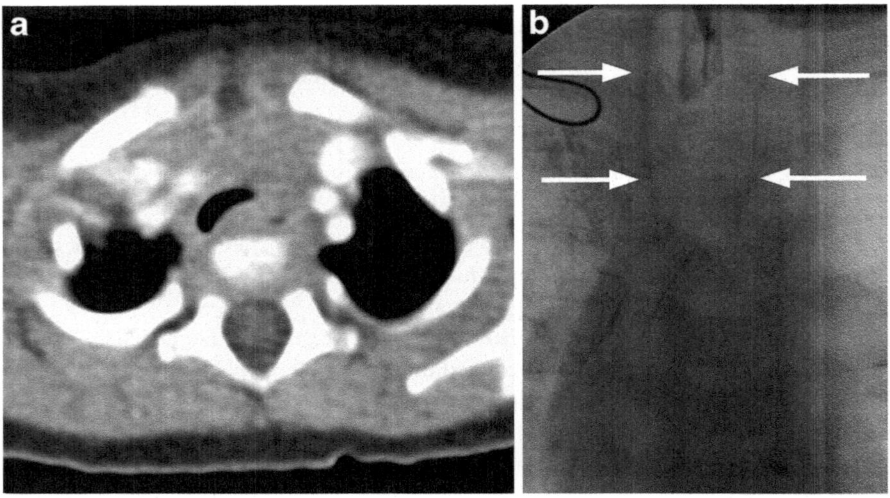

a. Axial CT shows anteroposterior narrowing of the upper trachea suggesting tracheomalacia (W 412, L 55). b. Massive tracheal dilatation is seen at bronchography with only 5 cmH2O CPAP (arrows) [McHugh K, Afaq A, Broderick N, Gabra HO, Roebuck DJ, Elliott MJ. Tracheomegaly: a complication of fetal endoscopic tracheal occlusion in the treatment of congenital diaphragmatic hernia. Pediatric Radiology. 2010 May;40(5):674–80.] *Caption from original.*

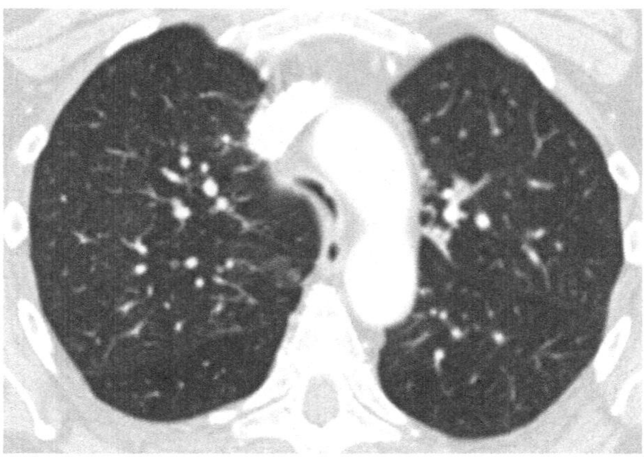

CT scan of the chest of a 57-year-old man with severe tracheomalacia demonstrating the “frown sign” [Maldonado F, Tomassetti S, Ryu JH. Orphan Tracheopathies.

In: Cottin V, Cordier J-F, Richeldi L, editors. Orphan Lung Diseases [Internet]. London: Springer London; 2015 [cited 2015 Dec 4]. p. 73–89. Available from: http://link.springer.com/10.1007/978-1-4471-2401-6_6] *Caption from original.*

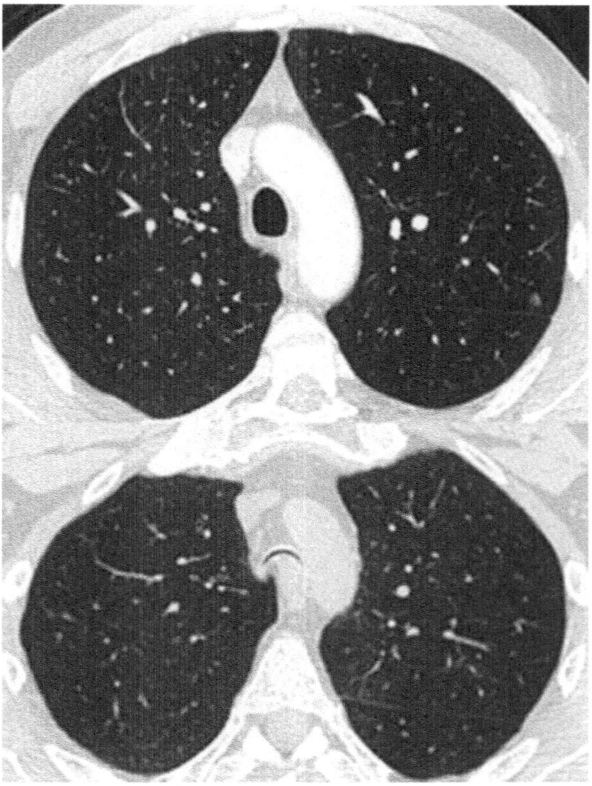

Tracheomalacia. The tracheal lumen has a normal appearance on the inspiratory transverse CT scan (top). This lumen collapses on the expiratory transverse scan (bottom). The posterior tracheal wall bows anteriorly tremendously reducing the airway lumen. [Grenier PA. Airway Disease. In: Baert AL, editor. Encyclopedia of Diagnostic Imaging [Internet]. Berlin, Heidelberg: Springer Berlin Heidelberg; 2008 [cited 2015 Dec 4]. p. 57–60. Available from: http://www.springerlink.com/index/10.1007/978-3-540-35280-8_85] *Caption from original.*

Other

- Bronchoscopy. Currently, the diagnostic gold standard for the diagnosis of TM is direct visualization of dynamic airway collapse during bronchoscopy. Bronchoscopy allows the direct visualization and measurement for grading the severity of TM. Mild TM is defined as luminal narrowing of less than 50 % during expiration. Moderate TM is defined as narrowing of 25–50 %, and severe TM is diagnosed if the anterior and posterior tracheal walls touch during expiration.

https://www.youtube.com/watch?v=rNADYJySIl4
Video of focal tracheomalacia.

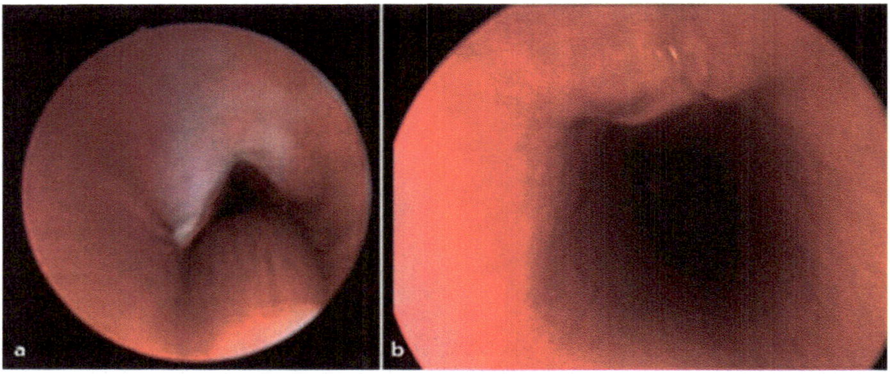

Tracheomalacia. Severe tracheomalacia (a) and after aortopexy (b) [Masciopinto F, Gentili A, Bianchini A, Baroncini S. Airway Endoscopy. In: Lima M, editor. Pediatric Thoracic Surgery [Internet]. Milano: Springer Milan; 2013 [cited 2015 Dec 4]. p. 181–91. Available from: http://link.springer.com/10.1007/978-88-470-5202-4_15] *Caption from original.*

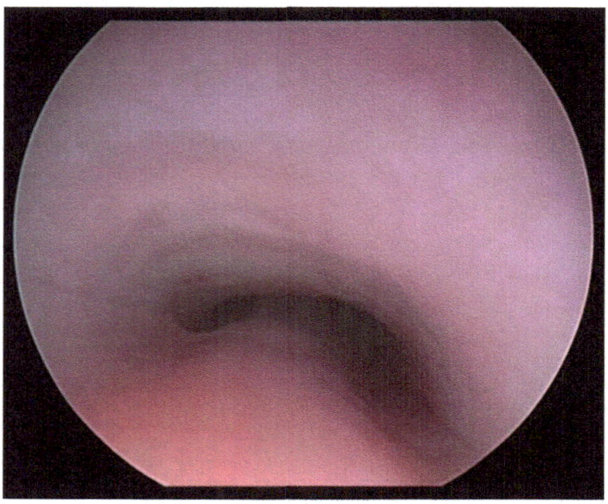

Primary tracheomalacia with soft, collapsible cartilaginous support proximal to the carina [Berg EE, McClay J. Tracheobronchomalacia. In: Lioy J, Sobol SE, editors. Disorders of the Neonatal Airway [Internet]. New York, NY: Springer New York;

2015 [cited 2015 Dec 4]. p. 87–95. Available from: http://link.springer.com/10.1007/978-1-4939-1610-8_11] *Caption from original.*

- Pulmonary Function Tests (PFTs). PFTs can help support a diagnosis of TM, but they cannot make or confirm the diagnosis. PFTs will often show reduction in the expiratory flow rate on a flow volume curve and the expiratory curve will have a "notched" appearance.

Special Populations

Age

- Acquired TM is more common in adults over age 40.
- Congenital TM is more common in children.
- TM in children more commonly involves the distal third of the trachea and is associated a congenital abnormality.
    - These congenital abnormalities include:
        - Cardiovascular abnormalities (vascular rings, anomalous innominate artery)
        - Developmental delay
        - Severe GERD
        - Tracheoesophageal fistula
        - Esophageal atresia
- TM in infants generally disappears spontaneously by the age 0f 18–24 months.
- Infants with TM are often noted to have expiratory stridor (sometimes called laryngeal crow) within the first few weeks of life. The stridor tends to be worsened and exacerbated by crying, supine position, and feeding.
- Infants may also be noted to have feeding difficulties with coughing and choking with feeding.
- Treatment in children is more guided by the pattern (focal or diffuse) of disease.
- Infants and children with mild-to-moderate symptoms can often be managed with conservative measures until the disease spontaneously remits. Conservative treatment includes:
    - Humidified air
    - Chest physiotherapy
    - Slow feedings
    - Meticulous control of secretions
    - Appropriate treatment of infections
- Surgery may be indicated for infants/children with severe disease who do not respond to conservative treatments.
- Infants with reflex apnea should be managed surgically.

Co-morbidities

- Patients with tracheomalacia will frequently have other medical issues that can complicate and worsen TM.
- TM can occur in patients with long-standing asthma and COPD.
- Gastroesophageal reflux disease (GERD) can both cause and worsen TM. Aggressively treating (when present) may prevent worsening.

Pitfalls in Diagnosis

Critical Steps Not to Miss

- Consideration of the diagnosis is the first critical step.
- TM can coexist with other cardio-pulmonary and laryngeal diseases, so it is important to consider even if a competing/alternative diagnosis has been confirmed.
- TM should be considered if the patients' cough and dyspnea seem out of proportion to the severity of the current diagnosis.

Mimics

- Asthma and COPD can both mimic TM.
- Severe GERD can also cause similar symptoms to TM.

Time-Dependent Interventions

- TM is generally a slowly progressive disease, and as such there are usually no immediately time-sensitive interventions.
- Patients with TM who are admitted to the hospital with another acute illness may benefit from the use of continuous positive airway pressure (CPAP). This can help maintain an open airway and secretion mobilization.

Overall Principles of Treatment

- Treatment is guided by the symptoms and graded severity of TM.
- There is no indication for treatment of asymptomatic patients.

- All patients with suspected TM should have both bronchoscopy and CT chest to help gauge severity and guide therapy.
- The underlying cause of TM should be sought and treated.
- The treatment of contributing, comorbid diseases (COPD, asthma, GERD, CHF) should be maximized.
- If patients remain symptomatic after treatment of all contributing factors, primary therapy for TM should be considered.
- Prior to starting primary therapy, patients should have functional respiratory testing with PFTs, six-minute walk test, and a quality-of-life assessment. This assessment will be used to guide and assess the success of therapy.
- In general, primary therapy for TM can involve stenting and primary surgical repair.
- Many experienced centers will start with stenting and assess response to guide long-term treatment.
    - If patients are not surgical candidates, but they improve with stent insertion, they may be managed with long-term silicone stents. Stents tend to be most helpful in focal, proximal disease.

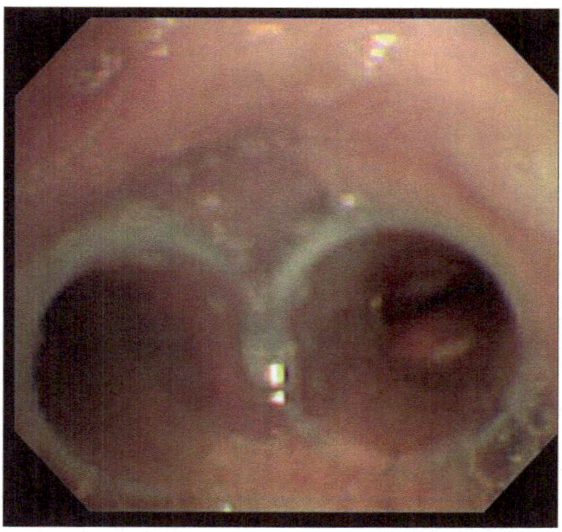

Silicone Y-stent inserted in a patient with tracheomalacia [Anantham D. Management Principles of Nonmalignant Airway Obstruction. In: Ernst A, Herth FJ, editors. Principles and Practice of Interventional Pulmonology [Internet]. New York, NY: Springer New York; 2013 [cited 2015 Dec 4]. p. 269–83. Available from: http://link.springer.com/10.1007/978-1-4614-4292-9_26] *Caption from original.*

- Patients who are surgical candidates and improve with stenting should be offered definitive surgical repair. Definitive surgical repair generally involves tracheobronchoplasty (the application of a mesh to the posterior tracheal wall, which increases the rigidity of the wall).

    - Patients who do not improve with stenting should have the stent removed and be managed with positive airway pressure when needed.
- Future treatments:
    - There is ongoing research on biogenic stents and tracheal replacement.

Disease Course

- In infants, TM usually resolves spontaneously by 18 – 24 months of age
- TM is a slowly progressive disease in adults.
- Almost all patients will worsen over time.
- There have been no reports of spontaneous remission or improvement in adults.

Related Evidence

Papers of particular interest have been highlighted as:
*** Of key importance*

Review

de Trey LA, Dudley J, Ismail-Koch H, Durward A, Bellsham-Revell H, Blaney S, Hore I, Austin CB, Morrison GA. Treatment of severe tracheobronchomalacia: Ten-year experience. Int J Pediatr Otorhinolaryngol. 2016 Apr;83:57-62. doi: 10.1016/j.ijporl.2016.01.022. Epub 2016 Jan 27. PubMed PMID: 26968054. http://www.ncbi.nlm.nih.gov/pubmed/26968054

Krustins E. Mounier-Kuhn syndrome: a systematic analysis of 128 cases published within last 25 years. Clin Respir J. 2016 Jan;10(1):3-10. doi: 10.1111/crj.12192. Epub 2014 Aug 26. Review. PubMed PMID: 25130790. http://www.ncbi.nlm.nih.gov/pubmed/25130790 **

Snijders D, Barbato A. An Update on Diagnosis of Tracheomalacia in Children. Eur J Pediatr Surg. 2015 Aug;25(4):333-5. doi: 10.1055/s-0035-1559816. Epub 2015 Aug 15. PubMed PMID: 26276910. http://www.ncbi.nlm.nih.gov/pubmed/26276910

Payandeh J, McGillivray B, McCauley G, Wilcox P, Swiston JR, Lehman A. A Clinical Classification Scheme for Tracheobronchomegaly (Mounier-Kuhn Syndrome). Lung. 2015 Oct;193(5):815-22. doi: 10.1007/s00408-015-9757-z. Epub 2015 Jul 19. PubMed PMID: 26189148. http://www.ncbi.nlm.nih.gov/pubmed/26189148 **

Hysinger EB, Panitch HB. Paediatric Tracheomalacia. Paediatr Respir Rev. 2016 Jan;17:9-15. doi: 10.1016/j.prrv.2015.03.002. Epub 2015 Mar 17. Review. PubMed PMID: 25962857. http://www.ncbi.nlm.nih.gov/pubmed/25962857

Acar T, Bayraktaroglu S, Ceylan N, Savas R. Computed tomography findings of tracheobronchial system diseases: a pictorial essay. Jpn J Radiol. 2015 Feb;33(2):51-8. doi: 10.1007/s11604-014-0380-3. Epub 2014 Dec 11. Review. PubMed PMID: 25504056. http://www.ncbi.nlm.nih.gov/pubmed/25504056 **

Lawrence DA, Branson B, Oliva I, Rubinowitz A. The wonderful world of the windpipe: a review of central airway anatomy and pathology. Can Assoc Radiol J. 2015 Feb;66(1):30-43. doi: 10.1016/j.carj.2014.08.003. Review. PubMed PMID: 25623009. http://www.ncbi.nlm.nih.gov/pubmed/25623009

Kugler C, Stanzel F. Tracheomalacia. Thorac Surg Clin. 2014 Feb;24(1):51-8. doi: 10.1016/j.thorsurg.2013.09.003. Review. PubMed PMID: 24295659. http://www.ncbi.nlm.nih.gov/pubmed/24295659 **

Krustins E, Kravale Z, Buls A. Mounier-Kuhn syndrome or congenital tracheobronchomegaly: a literature review. Respir Med. 2013 Dec;107(12):1822-8. doi: 10.1016/j.rmed.2013.08.042. Epub 2013 Sep 6. Review. PubMed PMID: 24070565. http://www.ncbi.nlm.nih.gov/pubmed/24070565 **

Murgu S, Colt H. Tracheobronchomalacia and excessive dynamic airway collapse. Clin Chest Med. 2013 Sep;34(3):527-55. doi: 10.1016/j.ccm.2013.05.003. Epub 2013 Jun 27. Review. PubMed PMID: 23993822. http://www.ncbi.nlm.nih.gov/pubmed/23993822 **

Choo EM, Seaman JC, Musani AI. Tracheomalacia/Tracheobronchomalacia and hyperdynamic airway collapse. Immunol Allergy Clin North Am. 2013 Feb;33(1):23-34. doi: 10.1016/j.iac.2012.10.005. Epub 2012 Nov 27. Review. PubMed PMID: 23337062. http://www.ncbi.nlm.nih.gov/pubmed/23337062 **

Damle SS, Mitchell JD. Surgery for tracheobronchomalacia. Semin Cardiothorac Vasc Anesth. 2012 Dec;16(4):203-8. doi: 10.1177/1089253212464276. Epub 2012 Oct 29. Review. PubMed PMID: 23108414. http://www.ncbi.nlm.nih.gov/pubmed/23108414 **

Tan JZ, Ditchfield M, Freezer N. Tracheobronchomalacia in children: review of diagnosis and definition. Pediatr Radiol. 2012 Aug;42(8):906-15; quiz 1027-8. doi: 10.1007/s00247-012-2367-5. Epub 2012 Mar 18. Review. Erratum in: Pediatr Radiol. 2012 Dec;42(12):1536. PubMed PMID: 22426568. http://www.ncbi.nlm.nih.gov/pubmed/22426568

Ridge CA, O'donnell CR, Lee EY, Majid A, Boiselle PM. Tracheobronchomalacia: current concepts and controversies. J Thorac Imaging. 2011 Nov;26(4):278-89. doi: 10.1097/RTI.0b013e3182203342. Review. PubMed PMID: 22009081. http://www.ncbi.nlm.nih.gov/pubmed/22009081 **

Murgu SD, Colt HG. Tracheobronchomalacia and excessive dynamic airway collapse. Respirology. 2006 Jul;11(4):388-406. Review. PubMed PMID: 16771908. http://www.ncbi.nlm.nih.gov/pubmed/23993822 **

General

van der Zee DC, Straver M. Thoracoscopic aortopexy for tracheomalacia. World J Surg. 2015 Jan;39(1):158-64. doi: 10.1007/s00268-014-2798-2. PubMed PMID: 25231705. http://www.ncbi.nlm.nih.gov/pubmed/25231705

Use PubMed Clinical Queries to find the most recent evidence. Use this search strategy: "Tracheomalacia"[Mesh] OR "tracheomalacia" OR "tracheomalacias" OR "tracheobronchomalacia"

Chapter 74
Tuberculosis

Charles V. Pollack, Jr. and Victoria G. Riese

Name and Synonyms

Tuberculosis, TB

Incidence/Epidemiology

- Tuberculosis is a multisystem disease with many varied presentations, all of which evolve from infection with the atypical pathogen *Mycobacterium tuberculosis*, an acid-fast bacterium that is endemic in some parts of the world, especially underdeveloped regions where living conditions and access to health care are poor.
- Chest pain due to tuberculosis tends to be pleuritic in nature, and may result from lung infection and/or pleural or pericardial involvement.
- In the United States, the current incidence of TB is 3–4/100,000 persons, with the highest incidence in states with the most immigrants—California, Texas, Florida, and New York. The prevalence of HIV disease in those states also may be a contributing factor.
- Globally, the highest incidence of TB is found in India, China, South Africa, Indonesia, and Pakistan.

C. V. Pollack, Jr. (✉)
Department of Emergency Medicine, Thomas Jefferson University,
Philadelphia, PA, USA

V. G. Riese
Librarian Consultant, Eldersberg, MD, USA

C. V. Pollack, Jr. (ed.), *Differential Diagnosis of Cardiopulmonary Disease*,
https://doi.org/10.1007/978-3-319-63895-9_74

Differential Diagnosis

- The differential considerations for chest pain due to TB are primarily other pleuritic pain processes, such as pulmonary embolism, pericarditis, pneumonia, pneumothorax, and pleurisy.
- As in all chest pain presentations, immediate life threats such as acute coronary syndrome and aortic dissection should always be considered.
- Acute chest syndrome in sickle cell disease is a differential consideration in at-risk patients.

Pathophysiology and Etiology

- The clinical manifestations of TB result from a variable combination of actual infection and the host's inflammatory response to the infection.
- Chest pain syndrome in patients with TB typically arises from actual pneumonia or from involvement of the pleura or pericardium.
- There may also be chest wall pain from coughing.

Presentation

Typical/"Classic"

- The classic presentation of pulmonary or extrapulmonary thoracic TB that causes chest pain is marked by most or all of the following:
  - Cough
  - Weight loss/anorexia
  - Fever
  - Night sweats
  - Hemoptysis
  - Fatigue
  - Lymphadenopathy
- TB is a more likely presentation in patients with such symptoms if they have risk factors for exposure, such as:
  - Recent travel to an endemic area
  - Recent imprisonment, homelessness, or living in a shelter
  - HIV infection

- Prior TB exposure or infection
- Known positive prior PPD (purified protein derivative) test

Atypical

- TB may affect multiple organ systems, including the spine and other bones, the gastrointestinal and genitourinary (GU) tracts, and the meninges. These types of tuberculous infections are less likely to present with chest pain.

Primary Differential Considerations

Pulmonary TB has protean manifestations. In patients with a history concerning for TB exposure, other diagnoses must still be considered, including:

- Necrotizing bacterial pneumonia
- Fungal pneumonia
- Lung abscess
- Lung cancer
- Bronchiectasis

History and Physical Exam

Findings That Confirm Diagnosis

- History and physical examination cannot confirm the presence of tuberculosis.

Factors That Suggest Diagnosis

- A history of fever, chills, weight loss, and hemoptysis is suggestive of TB in the patient with chest pain.
- Findings of consolidation on pulmonary exam—such as egophony and percussion dullness, especially in the upper lung fields—are suggestive of TB in the patient with chest pain.

http://www.easyauscultation.com/egophony
Egophony. [Egophony Page; Easy Auscultation; www.easyauscultation.com; copyright 2015, MedEdu LLC]

- Evidence of malnutrition or chronic illness on physical exam should raise suspicion for TB in the patient with chest pain.

Factors That Exclude Diagnosis

- There are no history or physical findings that conclusively exclude TB in the patient with chest pain.

Ancillary Studies

Laboratory

- Confirmation of TB infection is provided by the finding of acid-fast bacilli (AFB) on smear and/or culture of a bodily fluid, such as sputum

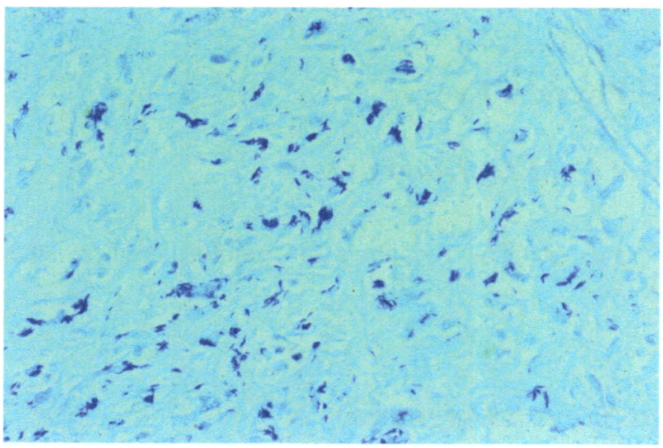

Granulomatous area with acid-fast bacilli in a lung biopsy specimen. Lung biopsy specimen showing a granulomatous area with numerous acid-fast bacilli. Diagnostic fiberoptic bronchoscopy with transbronchial biopsy and bronchial washings is an effective way to obtain diagnostic materials when sputum examination is unrevealing, in the early diagnosis of miliary disease, and in lower lobe tuberculosis when the number of bacilli may be small. (Kinyoun stain.) [Maslow M. Tuberculosis and nontuberculosis mycobacterial infections of the lungs. In: Simberkoff MS, editor. Pleuropulmonary and bronchial infections. Philadelphia: Current Medicine; 1996.

283 p. (Mandell GL, editor. Atlas of infectious diseases; vol. 6). ISBN: 0-443-07740-1] *Caption from original*

- An HIV test should be obtained in patients with TB and unknown HIV status.
- Basic laboratory tests are of limited clinical value in assessing the patient with chest pain for TB, but they may be appropriate in the evaluation of potential differential considerations.
- Patients suspected of having pulmonary TB should undergo urinalysis; sterile pyuria is a common manifestation of GU TB.

Imaging

- Chest radiography and CT may strongly suggest pulmonary TB.

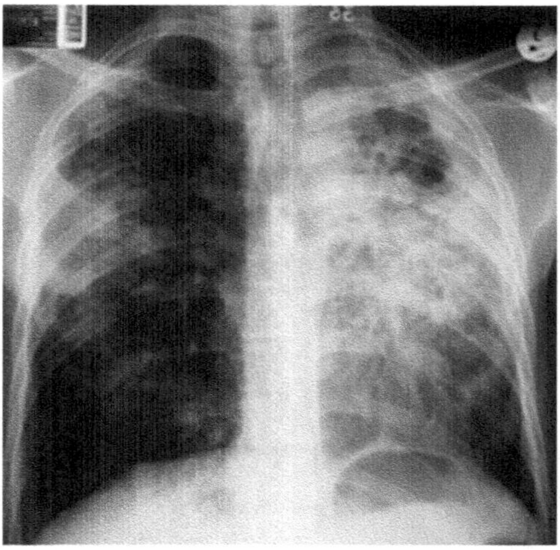

Multidrug-resistant tuberculosis (MDR TB). Chest radiograph of a black African man aged 31 years with a CD4 count of 79 cells/mm3 showing bilateral patchy confluent consolidation with cavitatory changes in the left upper lobe. Left apical pleural thickening and features of volume loss suggest previous TB. Tubular lucencies in the left upper lobe suggest underlying bronchiectasis. [Lalloo UG, Ambaram A, Vawda F. Pulmonary complications. In: Mildvan D, editor. International atlas of AIDS. 4th ed. Philadelphia: Current Medicine; 2008. 366 p. ISBN: 1-57340-270-2] *Caption adapted from original*

- The classic findings on x-ray are apical infiltrate(s), often with a cavitary lesion.

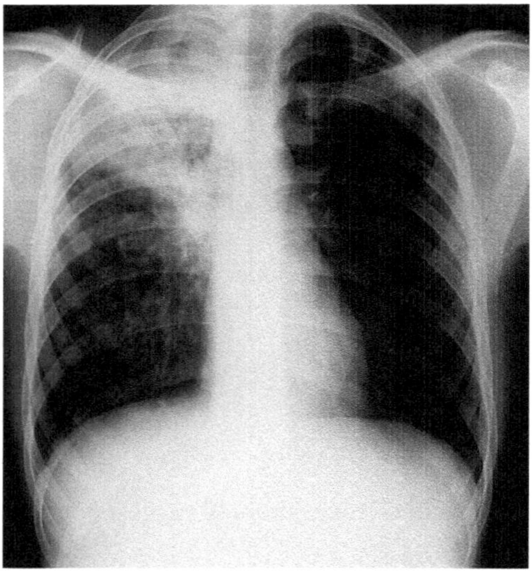

Pulmonary tuberculosis (TB) presenting as a right upper lobe infiltrate. [Jacobs R. Tuberculosis. In: Wilfert CM, editor. Pediatric infectious diseases. Philadelphia: Current Medicine; 1999. 283 p. (Mandell GL, editor. Atlas of infectious diseases; vol. 11). ISBN: 0-443-06526-8] *Caption adapted from original*

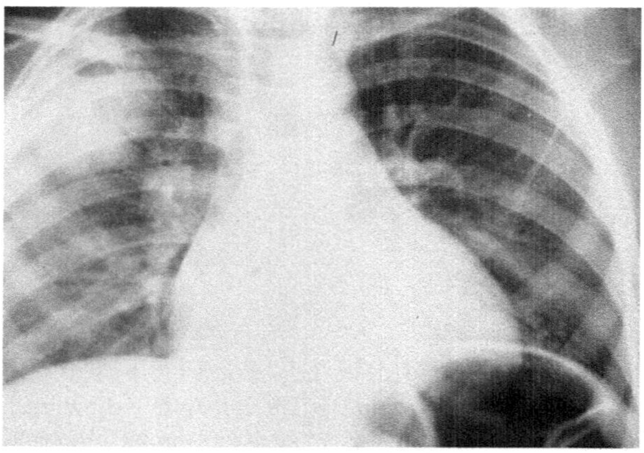

Pulmonary tuberculosis (TB) presenting as a lung abscess. [Jacobs R. Tuberculosis. In: Wilfert CM, editor. Pediatric infectious diseases. Philadelphia: Current Medicine; 1999. 283 p. (Mandell GL, editor. Atlas of infectious diseases; vol. 11). ISBN: 0-443-06526-8] *Caption adapted from original*

- A normal chest radiograph *does not* exclude TB, but casts doubt on the diagnosis if chest pain features prominently in the patient's presentation.

Special Populations

Age and Gender

- TB occurs in all age, ethnic, and socioeconomic groups. It occurs in both males and females.
- Pulmonary TB often has poorer outcomes at the extremes of age.
- In the United States, foreign-born patients with TB most often are Hispanic or Asian.

Comorbidities

- Comorbidities associated with pulmonary TB include but are not limited to:
  - HIV

TB—Tuberculosis

Transmission
1 of 3 TB cases in HIV patients is recently acquired
Immunity is not conferred by previous exposure to TB organisms
Lack of cavitary disease with HIV may render patients less contagious
Spread of TB facilitated by grouping HIV patients together in health care facilities, homeless shelters, and prisons
Clinical manifestations
Positive purified protein derivative with early stages of HIV only
Usual symptoms (fever, sweats, cough, and weight loss) are usually more exaggerated
Rapid progression from exposure to active disease (from loss of cell-mediated immunity)
Higher rate (40%–89%) of extrapulmonary manifestations
Lymphadenitis with fistula formation and abscesses
Radiographic features
Nonapical distribution
Infiltrates in any lung zone
Cavitation rare late in the disease
Intrathoracic adenopathy in 1 of 3 cases
Miliary infiltrates and pleural effusions
Normal chest radiograph in early stages of pulmonary

Tuberculosis and HIV. All patients with tuberculosis should be screened for HIV, and conversely, all HIV positive patients should have a purified protein derivative (PPD) skin test. The sensitivity of the test is inversely proportional to the degree of immunosuppression. Anergy is common, so a negative PPD should be interpreted with caution. Prophylactic regimens should be continued for 9 months. Tuberculosis should be considered in any HIV-positive patient with unexplained fevers, cough, infiltrate, adenopathy, meningitis, brain abscess, pericarditis, pleural effusion, or an abscess anywhere in the body. The diagnosis is difficult because the symptoms are nonspecific, the PPD is often negative despite active disease, atypical radiographs are the rule, and extrapulmonary manifestations are common (American Thoracic Society: Targeted tuberculin testing and treatment of latent tuberculosis infection. MMWR Recomm Rep. 2000; 49(RR-6):1 -43.) [Bates JH, Huitt GA. Infections. In: Crapo JD, editor. Bone's atlas of pulmonary medicine. 3rd ed. Philadelphia: Current Medicine; 2005. 338 p. ISBN: 1-57340-211-7] *Caption from original*

- Other immunocompromise
- Cancer
- COPD and chronic respiratory failure
- Chronic hepatic disease
- Alcoholism
- Neurologic disease

Pitfalls in Diagnosis

Critical Steps Not to Miss

- Early consideration of the diagnosis of TB in the patient with chest pain is essential in order to protect other people—family members as well as health-care providers—from possible exposure to the disease.

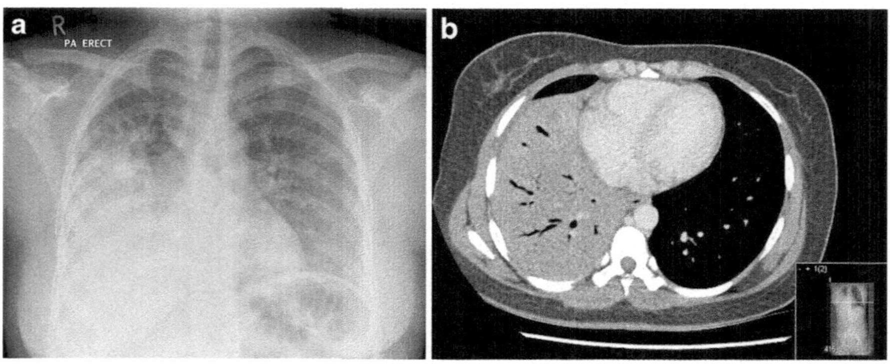

Case example: a 39-year-old Zambian woman presented with a 4-day history of pleuritic chest pain, cough and breathlessness, and a 6-week history of weight loss and night sweats. She was initially treated with amoxicillin and clavulanic acid, which resulted in symptomatic improvement. Tests on admission demonstrated

HIV-1 infection, with a CD4 count of 192 cells/μL. a Chest radiograph demonstrates right-sided middle and lower zone consolidation. b CT image of the thorax demonstrates nodular shadowing in both upper lobes, with dense consolidation of the right middle and lower lobes. Sputum microscopy was 3+ positive for acid-fast bacilli and culture confirmed Mycobacterium tuberculosis. This emphasizes the importance of testing for HIV and mycobacterial disease in patients with community-acquired pneumonia [Brown J, Lipman M. Community-acquired pneumonia in HIV-infected individuals. Curr Infect Dis Rep [Internet]. 2014 Mar [cited 2015 May 29];16(3)397. Available from: http://link.springer.com/10.1007/s11908-014-0397-x] *Caption from original*

- Accessible, pertinent body fluids (especially sputum in patients with chest pain) should be sent for AFB smear and culture as soon as possible.

Mimics

- The entire constellation of diagnoses underlying pleuritic chest pain, especially those often accompanied by dyspnea and/or fever, can mimic the pain and overall presentation of TB.
- Pericarditis may mimic pleuritic chest pain from TB in presentation. Listen for a pericardial friction rub.

Time-Dependent Interventions

- Anti-infective therapy, usually with empiric antibiotic therapy initially, should be initiated when the diagnosis of pneumonia is strongly considered or confirmed. Consult your local antibiogram for guidance in choosing a specific agent.
- Choice of antimicrobial also is driven by the classification of the pneumonia (community-acquired vs hospital-acquired vs ventilator-associated pneumonia).

Overall Principles of Treatment

- Respiratory isolation should be implemented immediately upon serious consideration of the presence of TB.
- There are several drugs used to treat TB, often in combination. Resistance patterns evolve; therefore, treatment is guided by microbiologic studies.

Categories	Patients	Treatment
Category I	New smear-positive pulmonary TB, smear-negative pulmonary TB with parenchymal involvement, seriously ill pulmonary TB, extrapulmonary TB, severe concomitant HIV disease	2HRZE + 4HR
Category II	Previously treated sputum/smear-positive pulmonary TB relapse, treatment after interruption, treatment failure	2HRZES/1HRZE + 5HRE
Category III	New smear-negative pulmonary TB, less severe form of extrapulmonary TB	2HRZE + 4HR
Category IV	Chronic and MDR-TB	Specially designed/individualized regimens

The number before the letters refers to the number of months of treatment

H isoniazid, *R* rifampicin, *Z* pyrazinamide, *E* ethambutol, *S* streptomycin

Categories of tuberculosis and their treatment regimens as recommended by WHO (Toman K [2004] Toman's tuberculosis case detection, monitoring, treatment, 2nd edn. WHO, Geneva) [Rajasekaran S, Khandelwal G. Drug therapy in spinal tuberculosis. Eur Spine J. 2013 Jun;22(S4):587–93.] *Caption from original*

- Chest pain associated with TB usually improves quickly as the infection resolves. Nonsteroidal anti-inflammatory drugs or narcotics may be given to patients with persistent or severe pain.

Disease Course

- The course of TB is determined by multiple factors, most important of which are:
  - The overall health and immune status of the individual host
  - The number of organ systems involved
  - The extent of infection prior to initiation of treatment
  - Age (older patients have poorer prognoses)
  - Patient adherence to the treatment regimen

Related Evidence

Papers of particular interest have been highlighted as:
*** Of key importance*

Practice Guideline

Abubakar I, Griffiths C, Ormerod P; Guideline Development Group. Diagnosis of active and latent tuberculosis: summary of NICE guidance. BMJ. 2012 Oct 17;345:e6828. https://doi.org/10.1136/bmj.e6828. PMID: 23077351. http://www.ncbi.nlm.nih.gov/pubmed/23077351 **

Meta-Analysis

Bauer M, Leavens A, Schwartzman K. A systematic review and meta-analysis of the impact of tuberculosis on health-related quality of life. Qual Life Res. 2013 Oct;22(8):2213-35. https://doi.org/10.1007/s11136-012-0329-x. PMID: 23232952. http://www.ncbi.nlm.nih.gov/pubmed/23232952

Review

Matteelli A, Roggi A, Carvalho AC. Extensively drug-resistant tuberculosis: epidemiology and management. Clin Epidemiol. 2014 Apr 1;6:111-8. https://doi.org/10.2147/CLEP.S35839. PMID: 2472972. http://www.ncbi.nlm.nih.gov/pubmed/24729727

Cruz-Knight W, Blake-Gumbs L. Tuberculosis: an overview. Prim Care. 2013 Sep;40(3):743-56. https://doi.org/10.1016/j.pop.2013.06.003. PMID: 23958367. http://www.ncbi.nlm.nih.gov/pubmed/23958367 **

Wong EB, Cohen KA, Bishai WR. Rising to the challenge: new therapies for tuberculosis. Trends Microbiol. 2013 Sep;21(9):493-501. https://doi.org/10.1016/j.tim.2013.05.002. PMID: 23764389. http://www.ncbi.nlm.nih.gov/pubmed/23764389 **

Lawn SD. Diagnosis of pulmonary tuberculosis. Curr Opin Pulm Med. 2013 May;19(3):280-8. https://doi.org/10.1097/MCP.0b013e32835f1b70. PMID: 23528956. http://www.ncbi.nlm.nih.gov/pubmed/23528956 **

Zar HJ, Udwadia ZF. Advances in tuberculosis 2011-2012. Thorax. 2013 Mar;68(3):283-7. https://doi.org/10.1136/thoraxjnl-2012-203127. PMID: 23321600. http://www.ncbi.nlm.nih.gov/pubmed/23321600 **

Zumla A, Raviglione M, Hafner R, von Reyn CF. Tuberculosis. N Engl J Med. 2013 Feb 21;368(8):745-55. https://doi.org/10.1056/NEJMra1200894. PMID: 23425167. http://www.ncbi.nlm.nih.gov/pubmed/23425167 **

Dheda K, Ruhwald M, Theron G, Peter J, Yam WC. Point-of-care diagnosis of tuberculosis: past, present and future. Respirology. 2013 Feb;18(2):217-32. https://doi.org/10.1111/resp.12022. PMID: 23190246. http://www.ncbi.nlm.nih.gov/pubmed/23190246 **

Philips JA, Ernst JD. Tuberculosis pathogenesis and immunity. Annu Rev Pathol. 2012;7:353-84. https://doi.org/10.1146/annurev-pathol-011811-132458. .PMID: 22054143. http://www.ncbi.nlm.nih.gov/pubmed/22054143

Lawn SD, Zumla AI. Tuberculosis. Lancet. 2011 Jul 2;378(9785):57-72. https://doi.org/10.1016/S0140-6736(10)62173-3. PMID: 21420161. http://www.ncbi.nlm.nih.gov/pubmed/21420161 **

Fair E, Hopewell PC, Pai M. International Standards for Tuberculosis Care: revisiting the cornerstones of tuberculosis care and control. Expert Rev Anti Infect Ther. 2007 Feb;5(1):61-5. PMID: 17266454. http://www.ncbi.nlm.nih.gov/pubmed/17266454

Use PubMed Clinical Queries to find the most recent evidence. Use this search strategy:

"Tuberculosis"[Mesh] OR "Tuberculosis"

Printed by Printforce, the Netherlands